4th edition

physiology

The National Medical Series for Independent Study

4th edition
physiology

John Bullock, M.S., Ph.D.
Adjunct Associate Professor of Physiology
Department of Pharmacology and Physiology
New Jersey Medical School
University of Medicine and Dentistry of New Jersey
Newark, New Jersey

Joseph Boyle, III, M.D.
Retired
Department of Pharmacology and Physiology
University of Medicine and Dentistry of New Jersey
Newark, New Jersey

Michael B. Wang, Ph.D.
Professor of Physiology
Department of Physiology
Temple University Health Sciences Center
Philadelphia, Pennsylvania

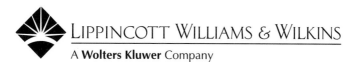

LIPPINCOTT WILLIAMS & WILKINS
A **Wolters Kluwer** Company
Philadelphia · Baltimore · New York · London
Buenos Aires · Hong Kong · Sydney · Tokyo

Editor: Elizabeth A. Nieginski
Editorial Director: Julie P. Scardiglia
Development Editors: Virginia Barishek, Martha Cushman, Emilie Linkins
Editorial Assistants: Veronica McBride, Estelle Elliott , Joan Coper
Marketing Manager: Kelley Ray
Illustrators: Pat MacAllen, Chris Wikoff, Tina Pavlatos
Managing Editor: Darrin Kiessling

351 West Camden Street
Baltimore, Maryland 21201-2436 USA

530 Walnut Street
Philadelphia, Pennsylvania 19106 USA

Printed in the United States of America

The publishers have made every effort to trace the copyright holders for borrowed material. If they have inadvertently overlooked any, they will be pleased to make the necessary arrangements at the first opportunity.

We'd like to hear from you! If you have comments or suggestions regarding this Lippincott Williams & Wilkins title, please contact us at the appropriate customer service number listed below, or send correspondence to **book_comments@lww.com.** If possible, please remember to include your mailing address, phone number, and a reference to the book title and author in your message. To purchase additional copies of this book call our customer service department at **(800) 638-3030** or fax orders to **(301) 824-7390.** International customers should call **(301) 714-2324.**

02 03
2 3 4 5 6 7 8 9 10

Contents

Preface

Since its first publication in 1984, NMS Physiology has garnered considerable response from medical students around the world. Based on these written and oral commentaries, the authors have revised the text to conform better to the needs of students preparing for course examinations and standardized medical or other health science examinations. Accordingly, this new edition of NMS Physiology contains a well-defined fund of knowledge the authors consider essential for medical practitioners. Although this book does not focus specifically on pathology, it does provide an insight into the pathophysiologic aspects of disease by comparing normal processes in the body with the abnormal.

The outline format has allowed the authors to emphasize the relative importance of the facts presented and to provide students with a source of fundamental information about physiology. Such a core guide to the discipline should prove especially valuable now that medical students are expected to assume more and more responsibility for their own learning.

John Bullock
Joseph Boyle, III
Michael B. Wang

Acknowledgments

We collectively wish to express our thanks to Virginia Barishek, Martha Cushman, and, especially, Emilie Linkins for their personal support, perseverance, understanding, and editorial expertise over the course of the development of this edition of NMS Physiology. We also recognize the special contribution of Pat MacAllen as medical illustrator.

GENERAL PHYSIOLOGY

Michael B. Wang

Chapter 1

Membrane and Cellular Physiology

I. **HOMEOSTASIS.** The compositions of the extracellular fluid (ECF) and the intracellular fluid (ICF) differ from each other (Table 1-1; see also Chapter 22) and are maintained in a steady-state condition, distinct from equilibrium by a variety of regulatory processes called **homeostatic mechanisms.**

A. **Extracellular fluid (ECF)** consists of the blood plasma and interstitial fluid. The composition of the ECF is maintained by the cardiovascular, pulmonary, renal, gastrointestinal (GI), endocrine, and nervous systems acting in a coordinated fashion.

B. **Intracellular fluid (ICF).** The composition of the ICF is maintained by the cell membrane, which mediates the transport of material between the ICF and ECF by diffusion, osmosis, active transport, and vesicular transport.

II. **CELL MEMBRANE.** All animal cells are enveloped by a cell membrane composed of **lipids** and **proteins.**

A. The **lipids** form the basic structure of the membrane.

1. The lipid molecules (primarily phospholipids, cholesterol, and glycolipids) are **amphipathic;** in other words, they have a hydrophilic polar region at one end of the molecule and a hydrophobic hydrocarbon tail at the other end (Figure 1-1).

2. The lipid molecules arrange themselves into **bilayers** when they are placed in an aqueous solution (see Figure 1-1).
   a. The hydrophilic ends of the lipid molecules line up facing the ICF and ECF.
   b. The hydrophobic tails of the molecules face each other in the interior of the bilayer.

B. The **proteins** assist the membrane in carrying out a large variety of physiologic processes (see Figure 1-1).

1. According to the **fluid mosaic model** of membrane structure, membrane proteins are embedded in the lipid bilayer.

2. Some proteins (called **integral** or **intrinsic proteins**) bind to the hydrophobic center of the lipid bilayer.
   a. **Transmembrane proteins** are integral proteins that **span the entire bilayer.** Transmembrane proteins serve as:
   (1) **Channels,** through which small, water-soluble substances can diffuse
   (2) **Carriers,** which transport materials across the bilayer
   (3) **Pumps,** which actively transport ions across the bilayer

TABLE 1-1. Major Ions Within the Intracellular and Extracellular Fluids

Ion	Intracellular Concentration		Extracellular Concentration	
	(mOsm/L)	(mEq/L)	(mOsm/L)	(mEq/L)
Na^+	15	15	1–12	1–12
K^+	135	135	4	4
Ca^{2+}	10^{-4}	2×10^{-4}	1.5	3
Mg^{2+}	20	40	1	2
Cl^-	4	4	106	106
HCO_3^-	10	10	24	24
Unchanged particles	5	0	10	0
Other anions	131	136	12	19

The osmolarity of the intracellular fluid (ICF) is the same as that of the extracellular fluid (ECF). Also, the milliequivalents of cations and anions are equal in the ICF as well as in the ECF.

 (4) **Receptors,** which, when activated, initiate intracellular processes
 b. Integral proteins that are **present on only one side of the membrane** serve primarily as **enzymes** that activate or inactivate various metabolic processes.
 3. Other proteins **(peripheral or extrinsic proteins)** bind to the hydrophilic polar heads of the lipids or the integral proteins.
 a. Peripheral proteins that bind to the **intracellular surface** of the membrane contribute to the **cytoskeleton.**
 b. Peripheral proteins that bind to the **extracellular surface** of the membrane contribute to the **glycocalyx** (i.e., a structure composed of glycolipids and glycoprotein that covers cell membranes).

III. **TRANSPORT ACROSS CELL MEMBRANES.** Substances move through cell membranes by **diffusion, osmosis, active transport,** and **vesicular transport.**

A. Diffusion

 1. Simple diffusion is a passive process by which particles in solution flow down a concen-

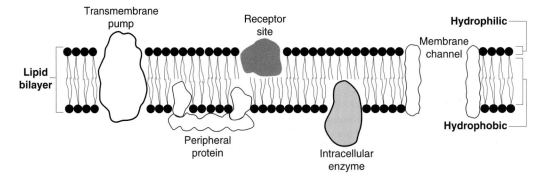

FIGURE 1-1. Some of the functions performed by proteins within the lipid bilayer of cell membranes.

tration (chemical) gradient (i.e., particles move from areas of high concentration to areas of low concentration).

  a. Process. No external source of energy (or driving force) is required to move particles by diffusion. Simple diffusion occurs because the heat content of the solution keeps the solvent and solute particles of the solution in constant motion.

  (1) Although each particle moves in an unpredictable (random) fashion, it is more likely that a particle will move from an area of high concentration to an area of low concentration (i.e., down the gradient).

  (2) Net movement ceases when the concentration of the particles is equal everywhere within the solution **(diffusional equilibrium).**

  (3) Although random movement of the particles continues after diffusional equilibrium is achieved, the concentration of the particles throughout the solution remains the same.

  b. Rate. Fick's law of diffusion describes the rate at which a material diffuses through a membrane as a function of its concentration gradient. It has two forms:

  (1)

$$\text{Flux} = - \frac{D \cdot A}{X} (C_{in} - C_{out})$$

  where D = diffusion coefficient (cm^2/sec) [see III A 1 c]; A = area of the membrane (cm^2); x = diffusion distance, or thickness of the membrane (cm); and C_{in} and C_{out} = concentrations of the material on the inside and outside of the membrane, respectively (mmol/L or mmol/1000 cm^3). The negative sign indicates that the material is moving down its concentration gradient.

  (2) Fick's law can also be expressed as:

$$\text{Flux} = - P \cdot A \cdot (C_{in} - C_{out})$$

  where P is the permeability coefficient (cm/sec) and is equal to D/x.

  c. Permeability. The **permeability coefficient** (and the **diffusion coefficient**) depend on the solute and the membrane through which diffusion occurs.

  (1) Lipid-soluble particles diffuse through the lipid bilayer of the cell membrane. Thus, their permeability is proportional to their lipid solubility.

  (2) Water-soluble particles diffuse through the aqueous channels formed by transmembrane proteins. Thus, their permeability is proportional to their molecular size, shape, and charge, as well as the number of channels through which they can diffuse.

2. Facilitated diffusion is a carrier-mediated process that enables particles that are too large to flow through membrane channels by simple diffusion to pass through the membrane. For example, facilitated diffusion is used to transport glucose into red blood cells (RBCs) and into muscle and adipose tissue when insulin is present.

  a. Process. No external source of energy (or driving force) is required to move particles by facilitated diffusion.

  (1) The carrier protein undergoes repetitive spontaneous conformational changes during which the binding site for the substance is alternately exposed to the ICF and ECF (Figure 1-2A).

  (2) The substance is more likely to bind to the carrier where it is more highly concentrated and dissociate from the carrier where it is less highly concentrated. (Therefore, it flows down its concentration gradient.)

  b. Rate. Unlike simple diffusion, the rate of facilitated diffusion rises as the concentration gradient increases until all of the binding sites are filled. At this point, the rate of diffusion can no longer rise with increasing particle concentration. This is called **saturation,** or **Michaelis-Menten, kinetics** (Figure 1-2B).

B. **Osmosis** is the passive flow of water across a selectively permeable membrane down an osmotic pressure gradient (Figure 1-3).

  1. The **osmotic pressure gradient** is created by the presence of different concentrations of solutes in the solutions on either side of the membrane.

A

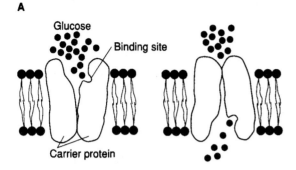

B

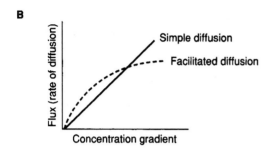

FIGURE 1-2. (*A*) The transmembrane carrier protein responsible for the facilitated diffusion of glucose undergoes a conformational change when glucose binds to it. The conformational change allows glucose to diffuse across the membrane down its concentration gradient. (*B*) In facilitated diffusion, the diffusion rate reaches a maximum when all the binding sites on the carrier protein are filled.

a. Osmotic pressure is a **colligative property** of solutions, which means that it is related to the number of particles dissolved in the solution, not their size, shape, molecular weight, or charge. Thus, the osmotic concentration difference (ΔC) of a substance reflects the difference in particle concentrations, not molar concentrations. For example, a 1 mmol/L glucose solution has an osmotic concentration of 1 mOsm/L, but a 1 mmol/L sodium chloride solution, which forms two particles when dissolved in water, has an osmotic concentration of 2 mOsm/L.

b. **Calculating osmotic pressure**

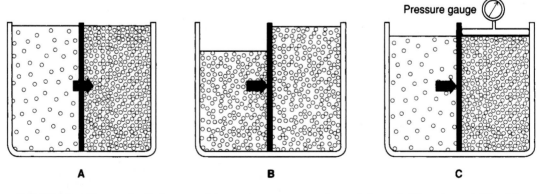

FIGURE 1-3. When a selectively permeable membrane separates two solutions of different osmolalities (*A*), water flows from the solution with the lower osmotic pressure (concentration) to the solution with the higher osmotic pressure (concentration). (*B*) Water flows into the chamber until the pressure (i.e., hydrostatic and osmotic) difference between the two chambers is zero. (*C*) The application of pressure to the chamber that contains the higher solute concentration prevents the flow of water. The amount of pressure that must be applied to prevent the flow of water is a measure of the osmotic pressure between the two chambers.

(1) The osmotic pressure difference across a membrane can be calculated using the **van't Hoff equation:**

$$\pi = \Delta C \cdot R \cdot T$$

where Π = osmotic pressure (mm Hg), ΔC = difference in the concentration of particles between the two solutions (mOsm/L), R = natural gas constant (62 mm Hg $\cdot$ L/mmol $\cdot$ °K), and T = absolute temperature (°K).

(2) The osmotic pressure produced by a concentration difference can also be determined experimentally (see Figure 1-3).

2. Flow. The flow of water caused by osmotic pressure differences can be calculated using the **osmotic flow equation:**

$$\text{Flow} = L \cdot A \cdot (\pi_1 \, 2 \, \pi_2)$$

where L = hydraulic conductivity of the membrane (L/sec/cm^2/mm Hg), A = area of the membrane (cm^2), and π_1 and π_2 = osmotic pressures on either side of the membrane (mm Hg).

a. If the particles in the solution are permeable to the membrane, the osmotic pressure difference created by the concentration difference is less than predicted by the van't Hoff equation. The reduction in osmotic pressure may be determined from the **reflection coefficient,** which is a measure of the relative membrane permeabilities of the solute and solvent.

(1) If the particle is totally impermeable to the membrane (i.e., it is totally reflected from the membrane), it has a reflection coefficient of 1.

(2) If the particle is as permeable to the membrane as the solvent (i.e., it is not at all reflected from the membrane), it has a reflection coefficient of 0.

(3) The actual reflection coefficient can be calculated using the expression:

$$\sigma = 1 - \frac{P_{solute}}{P_{water}}$$

where σ is the reflection coefficient and P_{solute} and P_{water} are the membrane permeabilities of the solute and solvent, respectively.

b. The osmotic flow equation can be used to calculate the osmotic flow of water if it is modified to include the reflection coefficient:

$$\text{Flow} = \sigma \cdot L \cdot A \cdot (\pi_1 \, 2 \, \pi_2)$$

3. Clinical importance

a. Cells. Changes in plasma osmolarity cause cells to shrink or swell.

(1) Calculating cell volume change. The final volume of the cell subjected to a change in extracellular osmolality can be calculated using the expression:

$$\pi_i \cdot V_i = \pi_f \cdot V_f$$

where i and f refer to the initial and final osmolalities and volumes of the cell.

(a) For example, if an RBC with an initial volume of 100 μm^3 and a normal osmolality of 285 mOsm/L is placed in a solution with an osmolality of 325 mOsm/L, its final volume (V_f) is:

$$285 \cdot 100 = 325 \cdot V_f$$
$$V_f = 88 \, \mu m^3$$

(b) The volume of water leaving the RBC is so small compared to the volume of the extracellular solution that the osmolarity of the extracellular solution is assumed to remain constant.

(2) The ability of a particle to cause a steady-state change in cell volume is referred to as its **tonicity.** Osmotic pressure differences can only cause a steady-state change in cellular volume if the particles creating the osmotic pressure difference are impermeable to the membranes.

    (a) An extracellular solution that causes water to flow into the cell is called **hypotonic.**

    (b) An extracellular solution that causes water to flow out of the cell is called **hypertonic.**

    (c) A solution that causes no change in intracellular volume is called **isotonic.**

    (d) Na^+ is the major somatically active constituent of extracellular fluid. Therefore changes in plasma Na^+ concentration result in an osmotic flow of water between the extracellular and intracellular compartments. (Chapter 22, Section III). The increase in extracellular urea concentration caused by renal failure does not cause water to flow out of cells because urea is permeable to the cell membrane. (The extracellular fluid is hyperosmotic but not hypertonic).

        On the other hand, the rise in glucose concentration produced by diabetes does cause water to flow out of cells because the lack of insulin decreases the permeability of the cell membranes to glucose (the extracellular fluid is both hyperosmotic and hypertonic).

b. Capillaries. Almost all particles dissolved in blood plasma, except proteins, easily cross the capillary and thus do not cause water to flow between capillary and the interstitial fluid. Plasma proteins have an osmolar concentration of approximately 1.2 mOsm/L, thus creating an osmotic pressure of approximately 23 mm Hg.

    (1) The osmotic pressure produced by the plasma proteins, called the **colloid oncotic pressure,** draws water into the capillaries from the interstitial fluid and is counteracted by the hydrostatic pressure of the blood produced by the heart. The movement of water through the capillary walls as a result of hydrostatic or osmotic pressure differences is called **bulk flow** (see also Chapter 12 I C 5 b).

    (2) Whether water flows into or out of the capillaries depends on whether the colloid osmotic pressure is greater or less than the hydrostatic pressure of the blood. When water flows into or out of capillaries, it carries dissolved particles with it. This is known as **solvent drag.**

C. Active transport

1. Primary active transport processes directly use the energy obtained from the hydrolysis of adenosine triphosphate (ATP) to transport material against an energy (e.g., concentration, electrical) gradient.

    a. The most common of these active transport systems is the **sodium–potassium (Na–K) pump (Na–K–ATPase),** which uses the membrane-bound ATPase as a carrier molecule (Figure 1–4).

        (1) Function. The Na–K pump is responsible for maintaining the high K^+ and low Na^+ concentrations in the ICF.

        (2) Pump cycle. Each cycle of the pump uses 1 molecule of ATP to remove 3 Na^+ ions from the intracellular fluid and transport 2 K^+ ions into the intracellular fluid.

        (3) Inhibition of the pump

            (a) Digitalis, a drug used in the treatment of heart failure, produces its therapeutic effect by binding to the extracellular face of the α subunit and interfering with the dephosphorylation step of the transport process.

            (b) The pump requires binding by Na^+, K^+, and ATP for its operation. Therefore, if the concentration of any of these substances is too low, the pump does not function.

    b. Other primary active transport systems that directly rely on the hydrolysis of ATP to transport ions across membranes are:

        (1) The **calcium (Ca^{2+}) pump** on the sarcoplasmic reticulum (SR) of muscle cells, which maintains the intracellular ionic Ca^{2+} concentration below 0.1 μmol/L

        (2) The **potassium–hydrogen (K–H) pump** of the gastric mucosa cells, which affects the secretion of H^+ into the stomach during the digestive process

2. Secondary active transport processes use the energy stored in the Na^+ concentration gradient to transport material against an energy gradient (Figure 1-5).

    a. Function. The transport of many ions and nutrients against their electrochemical en-

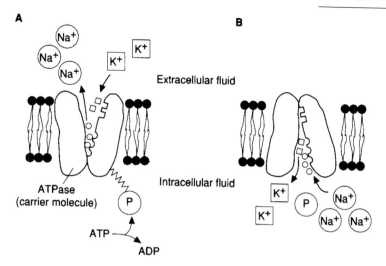

FIGURE 1-4. (*A*) The energy contained in the high-energy phosphate bond produces a conformational change in the carrier, during which three ions of Na^+ are transported out of the cell. A second conformational change occurs after two K^+ ions bind to the carrier on the outside of the cell, (*B*) transporting K^+ into the cell and causing the phosphate (P) to dissociate from the carrier.

ergy gradients is accomplished by Na^+-dependent secondary active transport. For example:

(1) Glucose and amino acids are reabsorbed from the proximal tubule and absorbed from the intestinal lumen by Na^+-dependent secondary active transport mechanisms.

(2) Calcium is removed from the cytoplasm of muscle cells such as the ventricular muscle of the heart by a Na^+-dependent secondary active transporter called the Na^+–Ca^{2+} exchanger. The Na-Ca exchanger uses the energy contained in 3 Na^+ ions to transport 1 ca^{2+} ion out of the cell. This mechanism [along with the SR Ca^{2+} pump described in III C 1 b (1)] causes muscle relaxation.

FIGURE 1-5. Glucose is transported through the membrane by secondary active transport (i.e., active transport that uses an indirect energy source). (*A*) As indicated by the length of the arrows, the affinity of the carrier for glucose is increased in the presence of Na^+. The glucose and Na^+ pass through the membrane together. (*B*) Once inside the cell, the Na^+ dissociates from the carrier, reducing the carrier's affinity for glucose and causing the glucose to dissociate from the carrier.

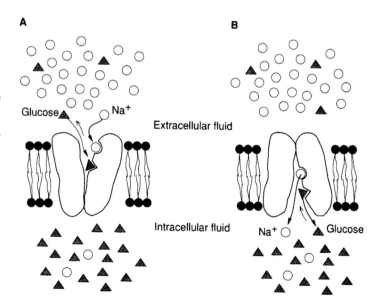

(3) H$^+$ produced by cellular metabolism is pumped out of cells by a Na$^+$-dependent secondary active transporter. This mechanism is important for maintaining normal intracellular pH in all cells, and it is necessary for the reabsorption of bicarbonate in the proximal tubule of the kidney.

b. Electrochemical gradient. The energy stored in the Na$^+$ electrochemical gradient is the sum of the membrane potential, E_M (the electrical energy driving Na$^+$ into the cell) and the equilibrium (Nernst) potential, E_{ion}, (the electrical energy equivalent of the energy in the concentration gradient).

(1) the energy in the electrochemical gradient for Na$^+$ is -140 mV.

$$(E_M - E_{Na}) = -80 \text{ mV} - +60 \text{ mV} = -140 \text{ mV}$$

(2) the energy in the electrochemical gradient for Ca^{2+} is -209 mV.

$$(E_M - E_{Ca}) = -80 \text{ mV} - +127 \text{ mV} = -207 \text{ mV}$$

(3) Therefore 3 Na$^+$ ions have enough energy ($3 \cdot -140$ mV $= -420$ mV) to transport 2 mEq (1 ion) of Ca^{2+} ($2 \cdot -207$ mV $= 414$ mV) out of the cell.

c. Glucose transport. The energy contained in the Na$^+$ electrochemical gradient is used to transport glucose into the epithelial cells lining the small intestine and the nephron (see figure 1-5).

(1) When Na$^+$ binds to the carrier molecule, the carrier molecule increases its affinity for glucose.

(2) Glucose binds to the carrier.

(3) The carrier undergoes a conformation change in which both Na$^+$ and glucose are transported into the cell.

D. **Vesicular transport.** Many substances are transported across the cell membrane by **endocytosis** and **exocytosis.**

1. In **endocytosis,** extracellular material is trapped within vesicles that are formed by the invagination of the cell membrane.

a. The endocytotic vesicle pinches off from the cell membranes and fuses with another intracellular vesicle (e.g., an endosome or lysosome), from which the ingested material is released into the ICF.

b. In receptor-mediated endocytosis, the material to be transported first binds to a receptor, and then the receptor–substance complex is ingested by endocytosis. Iron and cholesterol are two important substances transported into cells by receptor-mediated endocytosis.

2. In **exocytosis,** intracellular material is trapped within vesicles.

a. The vesicles fuse with the cell membrane and release their contents to the ECF.

b. Hormones, digestive enzymes, and synaptic transmitters (see Chapter 3 II B 3) are examples of materials transported out of the cell by exocytosis.

Case

A 72-year-old woman with congestive heart failure presents in the emergency department complaining of nausea and heart palpitations. She is receiving treatment with furosemide, a diuretic, to prevent edema, and digoxin, a cardiac glycoside, to increase cardiac performance. To counteract her recent weight gain, she has been taking extra doses of furosemide for several days. The treating physician suspects digitalis intoxication and prescribes oral potassium.

1. *What effect does digitalis have on cellular function?*

DISCUSSION

Digitalis, an extract of the foxglove plant, is the original cardiac glycoside. It has been used in the treatment of heart failure since 1785. Its physiologic effects are produced by its ability to inhibit the sodium–potassium (Na–K) pump. (see III C 1 a (4)) Digitalis depolarizes cell membranes directly by inhibiting the electrogenic Na–K pump and indirectly by allowing the concentration gradient of Na^+ and K^+ to decrease.

    2. *What physiologic effect does digitalis have on the heart? What conditions does it cause?*

DISCUSSION

In the heart, the reduced activity of the Na–K pump causes accumulation of Na^+ within the cytoplasm. The increase in intracellular Na^+ decreases the electrochemical gradient of Na^+, thus reducing the activity of the Na–Ca^2 (see III C 2) exchanger. The decrease in the activity of the Na–Ca^2 exchanger leads to an increase in intracellular Ca^{2+}, which causes an increase in contractile performance by the heart muscle.

    Digitalis leads to heart palpitations as a result of membrane depolarization and the subsequent increased automaticity. In addition, digitalis produces arrhythmias by shortening the duration of the ventricular action potential and depolarizing the membrane. Digitalis can also cause bradycardia or complete heart block because of its vagolytic activity. Nausea results from the direct effect of the drug on the vomiting center within the area postrema of the medulla.

    3. *Why does the physician prescribe potassium to treat digitalis intoxication?*

DISCUSSION

Adequate extracellular K^+ is necessary for proper functioning of the Na–K pump. Increasing extracellular K^+ is often effective in eliminating the signs of digitalis intoxication, particularly if the patient is hypokalemic. In this case, serum K^+ is likely to be low because furosemide increases the renal excretion of K^+.

Chapter 2

Membrane Potentials

I. **INTRODUCTION.** All cells have membrane potentials.

A. **Definition.** A membrane potential (E_m) is the electrical energy difference between the inside and outside of the cell. It is measured in millivolts (mV).

B. **Origin.** The membrane potential is produced by the **separation of charge.** Charge separation can occur in either an equilibrium or a steady-state condition.

II. **EQUILIBRIUM POTENTIALS**

A. **Equilibrium (Nernst) potential.** The equilibrium potential is **the membrane potential that prevents an ion from flowing down its concentration gradient.**

1. The equilibrium potential is **calculated using the Nernst equation:**

$$E_{ion} = - \frac{R \cdot T}{Z \cdot F} \cdot \ln \frac{C_{in}}{C_{out}}$$

E_{ion} = the electrical potential (mV)

R = the natural gas constant (8.2 joules/mol K)

T = the absolute temperature (°k)

Z = the valence of the ion

F = the Faraday constant (96,500 coulombs/mol)

C_{in} = the concentration of the ion inside the cell (mmol/L)

C_{out} = the concentration of the ion outside the cell (mmol/L)

2. The Nernst equation can be **simplified** by substituting for the constants (R, T, and F) and converting to common logarithms, yielding:

$$E_{ion} = - \frac{61}{Z} \cdot \log \frac{C_{in}}{C_{out}}$$

The valence (z) is usually omitted from the equation because it is +1 for both Na^+ and K^+. However, if the Nernst potential for Ca^{2+} is calculated, −61 must be divided by +2; similarly, if the Nernst potential for chloride (Cl^-) is calculated, −61 must be divided by −1. Table 2-1 gives the Nernst potentials for several important electrolytes.

3. **When the membrane potential equals** the **equilibrium potential** for an ion, the **net flux** of that ion across the membrane **is zero.**

4. The equilibrium potential for an ion is the energy (in volts) contained in the concentration gradient.

B. **Donnan Equilibrium.** When a membrane separating two solutions is permeable to several, but not all, of the ions, a Donnan equilibrium is established.

1. The membrane potential (E_M) balances the concentration gradient for each of the ions permeable to the membrane (i.e. $E_M = E_{ion}$).

TABLE 2-1. Nernst Potential for Ions Commonly Found in Nerve and Muscle Cells

Ion	Concentration (mmol/L)		Nernst Potential (mV)
	Intracellular	Extracellular	
Na^+	15	142	+ 60
K^+	135	4	− 92
Ca^{2+}	10^{-4}	1.5	+ 127
H^+	10^{-4}	40×10^{-6}	− 24
Cl^-	4	106	− 87
HCO_3^-	10	24	− 23

2. A cell in Donnan equilibrium is **not in osmotic equilibrium.** There are more particles inside the cell because of the presence of intracellular proteins (i.e., nondiffusible anions). The osmotic gradient causes water to flow into the cell.
   a. Normal cells are prevented from reaching a Donnan equilibrium by the action of the Na-K pump, which maintains an intracellular Na^+ concentration low enough to keep the inside and outside of the cell in osmotic equilibrium.
   b. In brain ischemia, for example, decreased activity of the Na-K pump allows the Na^+ concentration to rise. The increase in intracellular osmolarity causes water to flow into the cell, producing neuronal swelling and damage.

3. A Donnan equilibrium exists between the plasma and interstitial fluids because the capillary membranes are not permeable to the plasma proteins.
   a. The plasma has a higher osmolarity than the interstitial fluid
   b. The flow of water from the interstitial fluid to the plasma fluid is prevented by the capillary hydrostatic pressure.

III. STEADY-STATE MEMBRANE POTENTIALS

A. **Definition. The membrane potential in normal cells is called a steady state potential because the Na^+-K^+ pump prevents the intracellular and extracellular concentration of Na+ and K+ from reaching equilibrium.**

B. **The steady state potential is called the resting membrane potential.**

C. The **magnitude of the resting membrane potential** is determined by the concentration gradients and the conductances (or permeabilities) of the ions that are able to diffuse across the membrane.

D. **Calculating the resting membrane potential.** The resting membrane potential is calculated using the **transference (chord conductance) or Goldman equation.**

1. Transference equation

$$E_M = T_K \cdot E_K + T_{Na} \cdot E_{Na} + T_{ion} \cdot E_{ion} + \ldots + E_{pump}$$

   a. Definition of terms
      (1) E_{ion} = **Equilibrium (Nernst) potential** and represents the **energy in the concentration gradient** for each of the ions permeable to the membrane.
      (2) T_{ion} = **transference** and represents the **relative conductance (g)** of each of the ions permeable to the membrane. For example

$$T_K = \frac{g_K}{g_K + g_{Na}} \text{ and } T_{Na} = \frac{g_{Na}}{g_K + g_{Na}}$$

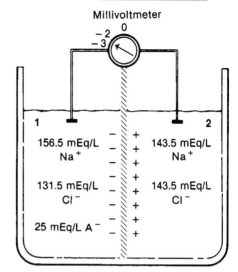

FIGURE 2-1. An established Donnan equilibrium. Compared with chamber 2, chamber 1 is negatively charged and has a larger solute concentration, a greater cation concentration (Na^+), and a smaller concentration of diffusible anions (Cl^-). Because the nondiffusible anion (A^-) is in chamber 1, the membrane potential is negative on the left side of the membrane and can be calculated by finding the Nernst potential for either of the diffusible ions. There are more particles in chamber 1 (because of the presence of the nondiffusible anion); therefore, the solutions are not in osmotic equilibrium.

      (3) E_{pump} = **the membrane potential produced by the Na–K pump.** Because **the Na–K pump is electrogenic** (i.e., it pumps three Na^+ ions out of the cell while pumping two K^+ ions into the cell), it makes the cell slightly negative. However, in most cells except cardiac cells, the magnitude of the **pump potential is so small that it can be ignored.**

   b. Example. In the steady state, g_K is approximately nine times g_{Na+} Therefore,

$$T_K = \frac{9}{9 + 1} = 0.9 \text{ and } T_{Na} = \frac{1}{9 + 1} = 0.1$$

$$E_M = 0.9 \cdot -92 \text{ mV} + 0.1 \cdot +60 \text{ mV} = 76.8 \text{ mV}$$

2. Goldman equation. The Goldman equation is derived from the laws of diffusion rather than Ohm's law, and therefore uses permeability (P) rather than conductance (g) as a measure of the ease with which an ion passes through the membrane

$$E_M + -61 \cdot \log \frac{K^+\text{in} + a \cdot Na^+ \text{ in}}{K^+ \text{ out} + a \cdot Na^+ \text{ out}}$$

   a. Definition of terms
      (1) K^+ and Na^+_{in} represent the intracellular concentrations of K^+ and Na^+.
      (2) K^+_{out} and Na^+_{out} represent the extracellular concentrations of K^+ and Na^+.
      (3) α represents the relative permeabilities (P) or K^+ and Na^+.

$$\alpha = \frac{P_{NA}}{P_K}$$

     Although permeability and conductance are both measures of how easily an ion passes through a membrane, they are not identical. In the resting state the ratio of P_{Na} to P_K is 1/40 while the ratio of g_{Na} to g_K is 1/9.
   b. Example

$$E_M = -61 \times \log \frac{135 \text{ mM} + \dfrac{1}{40} \times 15 \text{ nM}}{4 \text{ mM} + \dfrac{1}{40} \times 152 \text{ mM}} = -76.5 \text{ mV}$$

E. The magnitude of the resting membrane potential is determined primarily by the concentration of extracellular K^+ because the resting membrane is much more permeable to K^+ than it is to Na^+.

1. **Increases in extracellular K^+,** which make the equilibrium potential for K^+ more positive, cause the membrane potential to **depolarize** (i.e., become more positive).

2. **Decreases in extracellular K^+,** which make the equilibrium potential for K^+ more negative, cause the membrane potential to **hyperpolarize** (i.e., become more negative).

IV. ACTION POTENTIALS

A. **Definition.** The action potential is a transient change in the membrane potential that conveys information within excitable cells and the nervous system.

B. **Origin.** Electrically excitable cells (e.g., nerve and muscle cells β-cells) generate action potentials when they are stimulated by a change in membrane potential (i.e., by the flow of current into and out of the cell).

C. **Recording action potentials**

1. **Intracellular recordings** of action potentials are made by inserting glass microelectrodes that have tip diameters of less than 0.5 μm through the cell membrane. The small tips prevent damage to the cell.
   a. **Nerve cells**
      (1) Figure 2-2A shows the recording made as a microelectrode is inserted into a nerve cell at rest. The electrical potential is 0 mV when the microelectrode is outside the cell and drops to −80 mV as soon as the microelectrode passes through the membrane and enters the intracellular fluid (ICF). Note that this is the **resting membrane potential.**
      (2) When the cell is stimulated, the microelectrode records the changes in membrane potential (i.e., the **action potential**).
   b. **Other cell types**
      (1) Figure 2-2B illustrates an action potential recorded from a **cardiac ventricular muscle cell** (Chapter 10 II C).
      (2) Figure 2-2C illustrates an action potential recorded from a **stomach smooth muscle cell** (see Chapter 41 II C).

2. **Extracellular recordings** usually are made with metal electrodes that are placed on or near the nerve or muscle.
   a. Because these electrodes are outside the cell, they can record only changes in membrane potential (i.e., action potentials but not resting potentials). They cannot record the exact magnitude or time-course of the action potentials.
   b. Extracellular recordings are useful in clinical situations when the electrical activity of excitable tissues must be monitored. For example, electroencephalograms (EEGs) are used to aid in the diagnosis of brain disease; electrocardiograms (EKGs) are used to detect damage to the heart; and electromyograms (EMGs), which are recordings from skeletal muscle, are used to aid in the diagnosis of neuropathies and myopathies.

D. **Phases.** The phases of action potentials produced by various cell types differ slightly, but in all action potentials, the change in membrane potential is caused by the flow of current through ion-specific channels that open or close in response to changes in membrane potential. The phases of the **nerve cell** action potential are discussed here. Detailed information about the cardiac and gastric action potentials is found in Chapters 10 and 41, respectively.

1. **Threshold.** Excitable cells undergo rapid depolarization if the membrane potential is reduced to a critical level (i.e., the threshold potential).

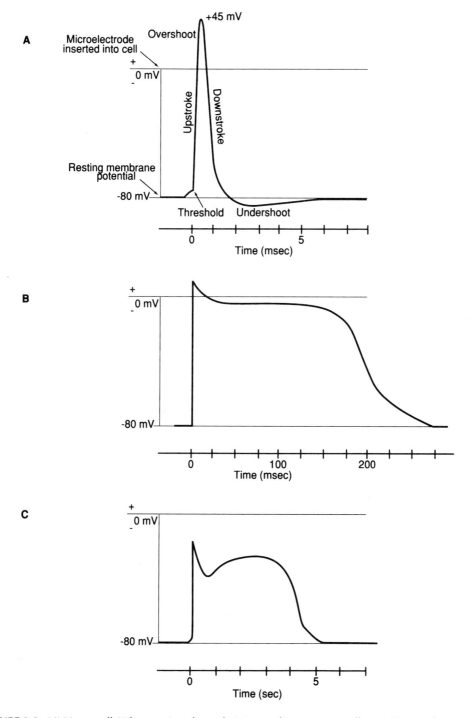

FIGURE 2-2. (*A*) Nerve cell. When a microelectrode is inserted into a nerve cell, a resting membrane potential of −80 mV is recorded. Stimulation produces an action potential, which is also recorded. Note that during upstroke, depolarization takes place as the conductance for sodium (G_{Na}) increases, and that during downstroke, repolarization occurs as the conductance for potassium (G_K) increases, allowing K⁺ to flow out of the cell. (*B*) Cardiac ventricular muscle cell. As in the nerve cell, depolarization and repolarization take place as G_{Na}, and G_K, respectively, increase; however, an increased conductance for calcium (G_{Ca}^{2+}) maintains the plateau phase that occurs during the cardiac action potential. (*C*) Gastric antrum smooth muscle cell. In these cells, the flow of Ca^{2+} into the cell causes the upstroke phase and maintains the plateau phase. As in the nerve and cardiac cells, an increased G_K and the flow of K⁺ out of the cell cause the downstroke.

  a. Once the threshold potential is reached, the remainder of the depolarization is spontaneous.

  b. The action potential is an **all-or-none response** to a stimulus; that is, if the stimulus is strong enough to reach threshold, the changes in membrane potential that characterize the action potential are always the same.

2. Upstroke. The rapid depolarization of the membrane after threshold is reached is the **depolarization phase,** or upstroke, of the action potential. **The upstroke is produced by the flow of Na⁺ into the cell.**

3. Overshoot. The portion of the action potential during which the membrane is positive is the overshoot. The peak of the action potential is the overshoot potential.

4. Downstroke. The rapid return of the membrane toward its resting potential is the **repolarization phase,** or downstroke, of the action potential. **The downstroke is produced by the flow of K⁺ out of the cell.**

5. Undershoot. The membrane potential becomes more negative than its resting value at the end of the action potential. This is the **hyperpolarization phase,** also known as after-hyperpolarization potential (AHP) or undershoot, of the action potential.

E. **Activation of the action potential**

  1. Ion-specific channels. The all-or-none characteristic of the action potential is based on the behavior of the regulatory gates that cover the ion-specific channels present in electrically excitable cells. In nerve cells, there are two voltage-gated channels: one specific for Na⁺ ions and the other specific for K⁺ ions.

  a. General composition. The ion-specific channels are transmembrane integral proteins that form aqueous pores through the membrane (Figure 2-3). They are composed of several thousand amino acids. Each channel contains:

   (1) Selectivity filters, which give the channel its ion-selective characteristics

   (2) Gating particles, which open and close the channels

  b. Regulation of the Na⁺ channel. The Na⁺ channel has **two gating particles** (an **m gate** and an **h gate**).

   (1) The **m gate** covers the **extracellular side** of the Na⁺ channel, and the **h gate** covers the **intracellular side** of the Na⁺ channel.

   (2) **Both** the m and the h gates **must be open for Na+ to flow through the Na⁺ channel.**

    (a) When the **m gate** is **open,** the channel is said to be **activated.**

    (b) When the **h gate** is **closed,** the channel is said to be **inactivated.**

  c. Regulation of the K⁺ channel. The K⁺ channel has one gating particle, the **n gate.**

   (1) The **n gate** covers the **extracellular side** of the K⁺ channel.

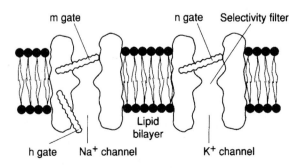

Extracellular space

m gate   n gate   Selectivity filter

Lipid bilayer

h gate   Na⁺ channel   K⁺ channel

Intracellular space

FIGURE 2-3. The gates that cover the Na⁺ and K⁺ channels. The negative resting potential tends to keep the m and n gates closed and the h gate opened.

(2) The n gate must be open for K$^+$ to flow through the K$^+$ channel.
  (a) When the **n gate** is **open,** the K$^+$ channel is **activated.**
  (b) The K$^+$ channel **does not have an inactivation gate.**
  d. **Recording channel activity.** The opening and closing of the channels can be recorded with **patch electrodes,** which are small (1–5 μm) glass capillary tubes with smooth edges that are attached to the membrane by applying suction to the electrode. One or more channels are typically contained in the patch of membrane covered by the patch electrode (Figure 2-4).

2. **Voltage and time dependency.** Changes in the membrane potential cause the opening and closing of the gates in a time-dependent fashion. This phenomenon is called the **voltage and time dependency of the gating particles.**
  a. The **voltage- and time-dependent nature** of the gating particles produces an action potential when the nerve membrane is depolarized to threshold.
    (1) When the membrane is at rest (−70 to −90 mV), almost all of the channels are closed (see Figure 2-3).
      (a) The Na$^+$ channel is closed by the m gate. However, the h gate is in the open

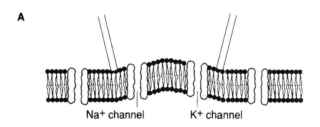

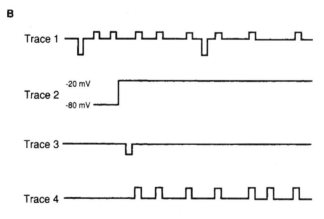

FIGURE 2-4. (*A*) The patch electrode is sealed tightly against the membrane by applying a partial vacuum to the electrode. (*B*) The currents passing through the Na$^+$ and K$^+$ channels underneath the patch electrode are illustrated in trace 1. The channels open rapidly, remain open for approximately 1 millisecond, and then close rapidly. The inward flow of Na$^+$ is shown as a downward current. It is larger than the current generated by the outward flow of K$^+$ because the driving force on Na$^+$ ($E_m - E_{Na}$ = −70 + −60, or −130 mV) is larger than the driving force on K$^+$ ($E_m - E_K$ = −70 − −90, or +20 mV). Because the K$^+$ channels open more often at the resting membrane potential, the resting K$^+$ conductance is greater than the resting Na$^+$ conductance. By alternately blocking the K$^+$ and Na$^+$ channels, the response of each channel to membrane depolarization can be studied in isolation. When the membrane potential is changed to −20 mV (trace 2), the Na$^+$ channel opens only once (trace 3) because the h gate inactivates the channel. The K$^+$ channel opens after the Na$^+$ channel (trace 4) closes. The K$^+$ channel is able to open repetitively because it does not have an h gate and, therefore, it is not inactivated.

position. In this condition, the Na^+ channel is described as being closed but available for excitation.

    (b) The K^+ channel is closed by the n gate.

    (c) Although almost all of the channels are closed, there are approximately 10 times as many open K^+ channels as open Na^+ channels; therefore, the membrane potential is close to E_K.

  (2) When the membrane is depolarized to threshold (approximately −65 to −60 mV), a **positive feedback** (regenerative) **process** produces the all-or-none upstroke of the action potential. That is, the response of the membrane to the stimulus (the opening of the m gates) causes an effect (membrane depolarization) that produces an even greater response (Figure 2-5).

  (3) The downstroke follows the upstroke as part of the all-or-none response.

    (a) Depolarization of the membrane causes the inactivation of the Na^+ channels, and the flow of Na^+ into the cell stops.

    (b) Depolarization of the membrane activates the K^+ channels, and K^+ flows out of the cell, causing the membrane to repolarize.

  (4) The undershoot also occurs as part of the all-or-none response.

    (a) The n gates close slowly as the membrane repolarizes; therefore, the K^+ conductance (G_K) is higher at the end of the action potential than during the resting state. The high G_K causes the membrane to hyperpolarize (i.e., become more negative than the resting membrane potential).

    (b) Eventually, the n gates close and the membrane potential returns to its resting level.

b. The **time-dependent nature** of the gating particles is essential for the production of the all-or-none action potential.

  (1) If the h gates closed as rapidly as the m gates opened (i.e., if the Na^+ channel was inactivated and activated at the same time), Na^+ could not flow into the cell.

  (2) Similarly, if the n gates opened as fast as the m gates opened (i.e., if Na^+ and K^+ activation occurred at the same time), the upstroke could not occur.

c. The **refractory period** (i.e., interval during which it is more difficult to elicit an action potential) is produced by the behavior of the voltage and time-dependent gating particles (Figure 2-6). There are two refractory periods.

  (1) **Absolute refractory period.** During this interval, another action potential cannot be elicited, regardless of the strength of the stimulus.

    (a) The absolute refractory period begins at the start of the upstroke and extends into the downstroke.

      (i) During the upstroke, a second action potential cannot occur because the m gates are opening as fast as possible (see Figure 2-6A).

      (ii) During the early portion of the downstroke, an action potential cannot occur because the Na^+ channels are inactivated by the h gates (see Figure 2-6B).

    (b) The absolute refractory period ends when the number of inactivated Na^+ channels is reduced by repolarization and another action potential can be initiated. The Na^+ channels are once again available for excitation when the h gates open during the downstroke.

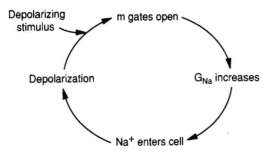

FIGURE 2-5. When the cell is depolarized to threshold, Na^+ channels open, causing an increase in the conductance for Na^+ (G_{Na}). This allows Na^+ to enter the cell, causing further depolarization. The positive feedback system represented by this cycle is responsible for the upstroke of the action potential.

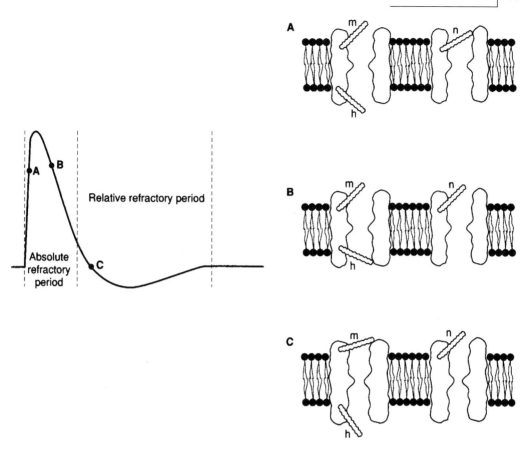

FIGURE 2-6. Diagram illustrating how the position of the Na$^+$ and K$^+$ gates changes during the action potential. (*A*) Both the m and h gates are opened during the upstroke of the action potential, allowing Na$^+$ to flow into the cell. (*B*) The closing of the h gates (inactivation) stops the flow of Na$^+$ into the cell. The opening of the n gates allows K$^+$ to flow out of the cell and initiates downstroke. (*C*) During the undershoot, the n gates are open, the m gates are closed, and the h gates are open. The high K$^+$ conductance causes the cell to hyperpolarize.

    (2) Relative refractory period. During this interval, a second action potential can be elicited if the stimulus is sufficient. The stimulus must be greater than normal because some Na$^+$ channels are still inactivated and more K$^+$ channels than normal are still open (see Figure 2-6C).

      (a) The relative refractory period begins when the absolute refractory period ends.

      (b) The action potential elicited during the relative refractory period has a lower upstroke velocity and a lower overshoot potential than does the normal action potential.

        (i) These changes result from the increased number of inactivated Na$^+$ channels and activated K$^+$ channels that exist during the relative refractory period compared with the resting state.

        (ii) The changes do not violate the all-or-none principle of the action potential but demand that the principle be revised. If a stimulus is sufficient to bring the membrane to threshold, the strength of the stimulus does not affect the magnitude and time-course of the action potential.

   d. Changes in extracellular K$^+$ and Ca^{2+} concentrations affect the **excitability** of neurons.

(1) Increasing the extracellular K^+ concentration depolarizes the membrane, causing inactivation of the Na^+ channels. With fewer Na^+ channels available for activation, a greater stimulus is necessary for production of an action potential.

(2) Decreasing the extracellular K^+ concentration hyperpolarizes the membrane. Because the membrane potential is more negative, a greater stimulus is necessary for depolarization of the membrane to threshold.

(3) Decreasing the extracellular Ca^{2+} concentration allows activation of Na^+ channels at more negative potentials. Therefore, production of an action potential requires a smaller stimulus. The increased excitability of nerve and muscle produced by lowering of the extracellular Ca^{2+} concentration is called **tetany.**

F. **Conduction of the action potential** occurs along the axon.

1. **Propagation.** The action potential generated at one location on the axon acts as a stimulus for the production of an action potential on the adjacent region of the axon (Figure 2-7). The magnitude of the action potential does not change as it is conducted along the axon because new action potentials are being generated constantly. This is different from the spread of an electrotonic potential (see III G), which diminishes in size along the axon.

2. The speed of propagation depends on the **type of fiber.** Propagation is faster in myelinated fibers than in unmyelinated fibers.
   a. In **myelinated fibers,** action potentials are generated only at the nodes of Ranvier, the region of the axonal cell membrane exposed to the extracellular fluid (ECF).
      (1) The nodes occur every 100–500 μm. In general, the internodal distance increases as the diameter of the axon increases. The membrane area between the nodes is covered by an insulating sheath of myelin formed from Schwann cell membranes.
      (2) Because the action potential appears to jump from node to node, this type of propagation is called **saltatory** ("jumping" or "dancing") **propagation.**
   b. In **unmyelinated fibers,** new action potentials must be generated at each contiguous patch of membrane.

3. The speed of propagation is proportional to the **fiber diameter.**
   a. In **myelinated fibers,** the speed of propagation is approximately six times the fiber diameter. The diameter of myelinated fibers ranges from 1–20 μm; therefore, propagation velocities vary from **6–120 m/sec.**
   b. In **unmyelinated fibers,** the speed of propagation is proportional to the square root of the diameter. The largest unmyelinated fibers are approximately 1 μm in diameter; their action potentials propagate at a velocity of approximately **1 m/sec.**

G. **Electrotonic potentials** are passive changes in membrane potential that do not propagate.

1. **Types**
   a. A **local (subthreshold) response** is produced on an excitable membrane when a stim-

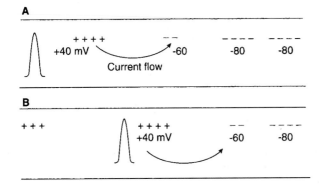

FIGURE 2-7. (A) The intracellular positive potential (+40 mV) produced during the overshoot of the action potential causes current to flow toward the negative, resting portion of the axon. The flow of current acts as a stimulus that depolarizes the axon toward threshold. (B) When threshold is achieved, an action potential is elicited, and the entire process is repeated, causing propagation of the action potential along the axon.

ulus does not open enough m gates to elicit an action potential. Because of the small number of open m gates, the amount of Na^+ entering the cell is insufficient to initiate a positive feedback cycle.

b. A **receptor potential,** which is produced by a sensory stimulus on a receptor (see Chapter 5 II C 2–3), **and a synaptic potential,** which is produced by neurotransmitters on a postsynaptic membrane [see Chapter 3 II C 2 b (2)], are not propagated because these membranes do not have the voltage- and time-dependent channels responsible for the production of action potentials.

2. **Cable properties of the membrane.** The membrane changes produced by graded, non-propagated responses spread passively, or electrotonically, along the membrane. Cable properties of the membrane determine the time-course and voltage changes of an electrotonic potential.

a. The **time constant** is the time required for the change in membrane potential to reach approximately 63% of its final magnitude (Figure 2-8A).

b. The **space constant** is the distance at which the change in membrane potential is reduced to approximately 37% of its original magnitude (Figure 2-8B).

c. The cable properties of a neuron play an important role in determining the ability of a stimulus to elicit an action potential and the propagation velocity of action potentials. Graded, nonpropagating responses (e.g., synaptic and receptor potentials) must spread passively from the patch of membrane where they are produced to a patch of membrane that is able to produce an action potential.

(1) If the graded response is produced too far from the action potential–producing portion of the membrane (e.g., at the end of a long dendrite), it decays too much to be able to depolarize the action potential–generating portion of the membrane to threshold.

(2) If the membrane resistance is reduced (e.g., by an inhibitory synaptic transmitter), the space constant is reduced, and the ability of an excitatory response to spread passively to the action potential–generating region of the membrane is reduced.

(3) If the time constant is increased, it takes longer for the action potential produced at one point along the axon to depolarize its adjacent region to threshold, and the propagation velocity slows.

(a) In demyelinating diseases such as multiple sclerosis, the loss of myelin increases the membrane capacitance, which increases the time constant.

(b) The increase in the time constant causes action potential propagation to fail, producing the sensory and motor deficits characteristic of multiple sclerosis (e.g., paresis, diplopia, paresthesia).

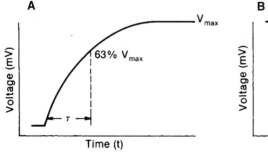
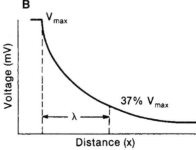

FIGURE 2-8. (*A*) When a stimulus is applied to a nerve membrane, the membrane depolarizes exponentially. When t = τ (the time constant), $V_t = 0.63 \cdot V_{max}$. (*B*) The magnitude of depolarization decreases as the distance from the stimulus increases. When the distance from the stimulus equals λ (the space constant), $V_x = 0.37 \cdot V_{max}$.

Case

Prior to his final examination in physiology, a 22-year-old medical student reports dyspnea, dizziness, a tingling sensation in the fingers, and muscle spasms in the hands and feet. Laboratory tests reveal an abnormally low arterial $PaCO_2$ and a low serum ionized calcium level.

> **1.** *What caused low arterial $PaCO_2$ and low serum ionized calcium concentration.*

DISCUSSION

The student hyperventilated because he was nervous about his upcoming physiology examination. The increased ventilation, decreased his arterial CO_2 tension (Cross reference to respiratory section). The decreased, arterial $PaCO_2$ increased his plasma pH which, in turn, caused serum Ca^{2+} to bind to the plasma proteins. The binding of serum Ca^{2+} to plasma protein decreased the concentration of ionized Ca^{2+} in the plasma.

> **2.** *How does the low plasma calcium concentration produce paresthesias and muscle spasms?*

DISCUSSION

Decreasing ionized Ca^{2+} concentration increases membrane excitability leading to spontaneous activity of motor and sensory nerves and skeletal muscle. The increased motor neuron and skeletal muscle activity produces muscle spasms. The sensory nerve activity is responsible for the paresthesias. Membrane excitability is increased because the voltage sensitivity of activation gates on the sodium channels is increased in a low Ca^{2+} environment. The increased sensitivity (decreased threshold) makes it easier to excite cardiac cells and therefore leads to automaticity and arrhythmias.

> **3.** *How does the low arterial PCO_2 produce dizziness?*

DISCUSSION

Cerebral arterial resistance is controlled by arterial PCO_2 causes cerebral arterial resistance to increase decreasing cerebral blood flow. The decrease in blood flow to the brain produces dizziness and could leak to syncope (fainting caused by decreased blood flow to the brain).

Chapter 3

Synaptic Transmission

I. **INTRODUCTION.** This chapter describes synaptic transmission in the peripheral and central nervous systems (PNS and CNS).

A. **Synaptic transmission** is the process by which nerve cells communicate among themselves and with muscles and glands.

B. The **synapse** is the anatomic site where this communication occurs.

C. Most synaptic transmission is carried out by a chemical called a **neurotransmitter.** However, in some instances, synaptic transmission may be **electrical** and occur through **gap junctions.**

D. The neurotransmitter is released from a **neuron (presynaptic cell)** and diffuses to its **target (postsynaptic cell),** where it produces a **postsynaptic response.** The postsynaptic response may be **excitatory** or **inhibitory.**

1. **Excitation** causes an action potential (if the target cell is another neuron), contraction (if the target cell is a muscle), or secretion (if the target cell is a gland).

2. **Inhibition** reduces or blocks the activity of the postsynaptic cell.

II. **NEUROMUSCULAR TRANSMISSION** is synaptic transmission between an alpha motoneuron and a skeletal muscle fiber that occurs at the neuromuscular junction.

A. **Physiologic anatomy.** Figure 3-1 illustrates the anatomic structure of the neuromuscular junction.

1. **Light microscopic appearance** (see Figure 3-1A)
   a. The **alpha motoneuron branches** as it approaches the muscle, sending axon terminals to several skeletal muscle fibers.
      (1) The number of skeletal muscle fibers innervated by an alpha motoneuron depends on the type of muscle fiber involved.
         (a) Alpha motoneurons innervating large muscles used primarily for strength or postural control innervate hundreds to thousands of skeletal muscle fibers.
         (b) Alpha motoneurons innervating muscles used for precision movements innervate just a few skeletal muscle fibers.
      (2) Each skeletal muscle fiber receives only one axon terminal.
   b. The **axon terminal** lies in a groove called the **synaptic trough,** which is formed by an invagination of the skeletal muscle fiber.
   c. Synaptic transmission occurs at the **end-plate region** (i.e., the postsynaptic membranes) of the skeletal muscle fiber.

2. **Electron microscopic appearance.** Figure 3-1B illustrates the details of the presynaptic and postsynaptic (end-plate) membranes.
   a. **Synaptic vesicles** (approximately 50 nm in diameter) containing the neurotransmitter **acetylcholine (ACh)** are located in the presynaptic nerve terminal. They are concentrated around specialized presynaptic membrane structures called the **active zones.**
   b. The **synaptic cleft** (approximately 60 nm wide) is filled with an amorphous network of connective tissue called the basal lamina, in which the enzyme **acetyl-**

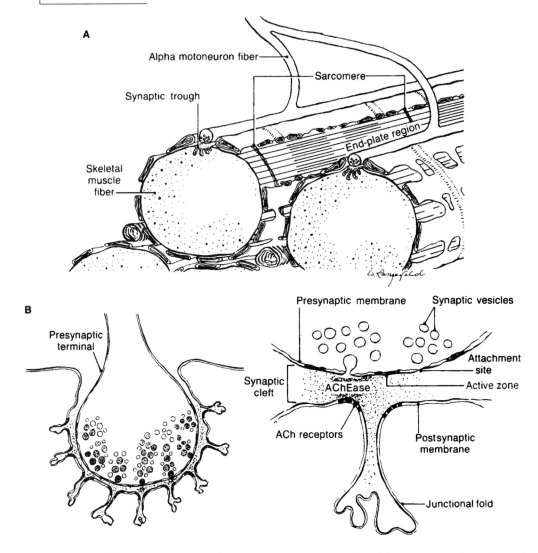

FIGURE 3-1. (*A*) Light microscopic view of a neuromuscular junction. The alpha motoneuron branches as it reaches the muscle, and each branch forms a synapse with a single muscle fiber at the end-plate region of the muscle. The axon terminal lies in the synaptic trough. Junctional folds increase the surface area of the postsynaptic membrane. (*B*) Electron microscopic view showing the synaptic vesicles within the presynaptic terminal, the acetylcholinesterase (AChEase) within the synaptic cleft, and the postsynaptic receptor sites. ACh = acetylcholine.

cholinesterase (AChEase) is bound. AChEase degrades ACh after it has produced its effect on the postsynaptic membrane of the skeletal muscle fiber.

c. The **postsynaptic membrane** contains numerous **junctional folds,** which are membrane invaginations located opposite the active zones. The receptor sites for ACh are found on the postsynaptic membranes near the junctional folds.

B. Synthesis, storage, and release of ACh

1. **Synthesis.** ACh is synthesized in the presynaptic nerve terminal from **choline** and **acetyl coenzyme A (acetyl-CoA)** by **choline acetyltransferase (CAT).**

2. **Storage.** Newly synthesized ACh is pumped into synaptic vesicles by a secondary active transport system.

    a. H$^+$ is accumulated within the vesicle by an H$^+$–ATPase active transport system. The energy contained within the H$^+$ electrochemical gradient is used to pump ACh into the vesicle.

    b. Approximately 5000–10,000 molecules of ACh are stored within each vesicle.

3. Release. Secretion of ACh occurs by **exocytosis** (Figure 3-2).

    a. The vesicle fuses with the presynaptic membrane, exposing its contents to the extracellular fluid (ECF).

    b. ACh diffuses out of the vesicle into the synaptic cleft, and the vesicle merges with the presynaptic membrane.

C. | Events in synaptic transmission

1. Neurotransmitter release is triggered by the **depolarization** of the presynaptic nerve terminal. Depolarization occurs when an action potential propagates into the nerve terminal.

    a. Depolarization of the nerve terminal by the action potential causes voltage-dependent Ca^{2+} channels (which are located in the active zones) to open, allowing Ca^{2+} to enter the cell down its electrochemical gradient.

    b. The increase in intracellular Ca^{2+} concentration causes synaptic vesicles to dock with and fuse with an attachment site on the presynaptic membrane.

        (1) The fusion of synaptic vesicles with the presynaptic terminal involves three proteins (SNAREs).

            (a) Synaptobrevin, a vesicular-associated membrane protein

            (b) Syntaxin, a presynaptic membrane protein

            (c) A fusion–protein complex, which functions as an ATPase

        (2) Activation of the fusion–protein complex causes synaptobrevin and syntaxin to form a membrane channel through which the transmitter diffuses from the vesicle to the extracellular space.

        (3) Tetanus and botulinum toxins, which hydrolyze the SNAREs, block synaptic release.

2. Postsynaptic response. When ACh binds to the postsynaptic receptor, it causes a depolarization of the postsynaptic membrane called the **end-plate potential (EPP).**

    a. The ACh receptor

        (1) ACh receptors in the end-plate region of skeletal muscle are called **nicotinic** (as opposed to muscarinic) receptors, because they are stimulated by nicotine (as well as ACh) and inhibited by curare.

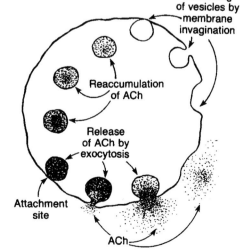

FIGURE 3-2. The life cycle of a synaptic vesicle. After binding to its attachment site, the vesicle releases its transmitter, acetylcholine (ACh), via exocytosis and then merges with the membrane. Later, a new vesicle is formed from invaginations of the presynaptic membrane. These vesicles are filled with transmitter and can be reused.

    (2) The ACh receptor (Figure 3-3) is a transmembrane protein consisting of five sub-
units that form an aqueous channel within the lipid bilayer.

        (a) Two of the subunits, called α subunits, contain binding sites for ACh.

        (b) When the two α subunits are occupied by ACh, the proteins undergo a con-
formational change that opens a gate within the channel.

        (c) The channel is equally permeable to Na^+ and K^+. Unlike the Na^+ and K^+
channels found on electrically excitable membranes (which are activated by
changes in membrane voltage), the ACh-activated channel is **opened by the
binding of the neurotransmitter to the receptor,** not by membrane depolarization. Therefore, it is a **chemically activated channel.**

b. Depolarization

    (1) Opening the channel causes the cell to depolarize.

        (a) When the channel is opened, Na^+ enters and K^+ leaves the cell down their
respective electrochemical gradients.

        (b) The magnitude of the Na^+ current (I_{Na}) is greater than the K^+ current (I_K). Be-
cause the electrochemical gradient for Na^+ is greater than that for K^+ (and the
conductances for Na^+ and K^+ are equal), the amount of Na^+ entering the cell
exceeds the amount of K^+ leaving the cell, and the cell depolarizes.

    (2) The EPP is a **graded response,** not an all-or-none response. The magnitude of de-
polarization is proportional to the number of open ACh channels.

        (a) If a **single ACh channel** is opened (as occurs when two ACh molecules bind
to it—one to each α unit), the membrane depolarizes by only a few micro-
volts (μV).

        (b) If a **single vesicle** releases its contents of 5000–10,000 ACh molecules (i.e., a
quantum of ACh), the membrane depolarizes by approximately 1 mV. The
depolarization is called a miniature end-plate potential (MEPP).

        (c) The **100–300 vesicles** that release their contents when an action potential in-
vades the presynaptic nerve terminal produce a depolarization of approximately 50 mV. This depolarization is the **EPP.**

    (3) The **reversal potential** is the **maximum depolarization** that can occur on the end-
plate membrane.

        (a) The reversal potential is the potential at which no net current flows through
the channel (i.e., when the Na^+ and K^+ currents are equal and opposite to
each other).

        (b) These currents are equal and opposite to each other when the membrane po-
tential is -16 mV. [This can be verified by substituting the appropriate values
of E_{Na} ($+58$ mV) and E_K (-92 mV) into the transference equation (see Chapter
2 III B 1).] Recall that the membrane potential calculated with the transference equation is the membrane potential at which inward and outward currents are equal and opposite.

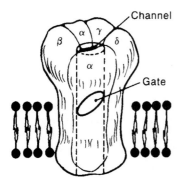

FIGURE 3-3. Acetylcholine (ACh) receptor. The receptor contains
five subunits, two of which (the α subunits) contain binding sites for
ACh. When both subunits are occupied, the channel's gate opens,
allowing Na^+ and K^+ to pass through the membrane. (Adapted with
permission from Anholdt R, Lindstrom J, Montal M: In *Enzymes of
Biological Membranes.* Edited by Martonosi A. New York, Plenum
Press, 1985, pp 335–401.)

    (c) The reversal potential is analogous to the equilibrium potential because it is the potential at which there is no net current through the channel.

        (i) At the reversal potential, no net current flows because the inward (in this case, Na^+) currents and the outward (in this case, K^+) currents are equal and opposite.

        (ii) At the equilibrium potential, however, no net current flows because the driving force for the ion down its electrical gradient is equal and opposite to the driving force for the ion down its concentration gradient.

3. The **EPP initiates an action potential on the muscle fiber membrane.**

  a. There are no electrically excitable Na^+ and K^+ channels on the end-plate region; however, Na^+ and K^+ channels are located on the muscle membrane contiguous to the end-plate.

  b. The EPP depolarizes the contiguous membrane regions to threshold, and an action potential is generated.

  c. The action potential is propagated along the muscle membrane and is responsible for initiating a muscle contraction (see Chapter 4 II B).

4. ACh is degraded rapidly.

  a. After binding to the ACh receptor, the ACh dissociates from the receptor and is hydrolyzed by the AChEase in the synaptic cleft.

  b. Degradation of ACh is necessary to prevent it from causing multiple muscle contractions.

  c. **Enzymatic destruction** is a unique method for inactivating the transmitter and occurs only at ACh synapses. Inactivation of the transmitter at all other synapses occurs when the transmitter diffuses out of the synaptic region or is actively transported back into the nerve terminal.

III. AUTONOMIC SYNAPTIC TRANSMISSION

A. **Organization of the autonomic nervous system (ANS)** [Figure 3-4]

  1. The ANS is divided into the **parasympathetic** and **sympathetic** systems, each of which has a **preganglionic neuron** in the **CNS** and a **postganglionic neuron** in the **PNS.**

  2. Synaptic transmission within the PNS involves several neurotransmitters (e.g., ACh, norepinephrine) and a variety of postsynaptic responses (e.g., inhibitory, excitatory), which are summarized in Table 3-1.

B. **Modes of transmission**

  1. Ganglionic transmission within the sympathetic and parasympathetic divisions of the ANS. Transmission is essentially the same as at the neuromuscular junction. ACh is released from the preganglionic (presynaptic) fiber, diffuses across the synaptic cleft, and binds to receptors on the postganglionic (postsynaptic) fiber, causing it to depolarize by opening channels that are equally permeable to K^+ and Na^+. Differences between neuromuscular transmission and ganglionic transmission include the following:

  a. Unlike the presynaptic fibers of neuromuscular transmission, a single preganglionic fiber does not release enough neurotransmitter to depolarize the postganglionic fiber to threshold. The postganglionic fiber can discharge an action potential only when there is a **summation** of the postsynaptic responses (see IV B 2).

  b. Although the ACh receptors at the synapses of the pre- and postganglionic fibers are nicotinic receptors, they are not identical to those on the skeletal muscle end-plate, because the pharmacologic agents needed to block the two receptors are different. The extreme toxicity of high concentrations of nicotine (it causes vomiting, diarrhea, diaphoresis, and high blood pressure) is primarily due to its action on the ANS.

    (1) Hexamethonium blocks ganglionic transmission.

    (2) Curare blocks neuromuscular transmission.

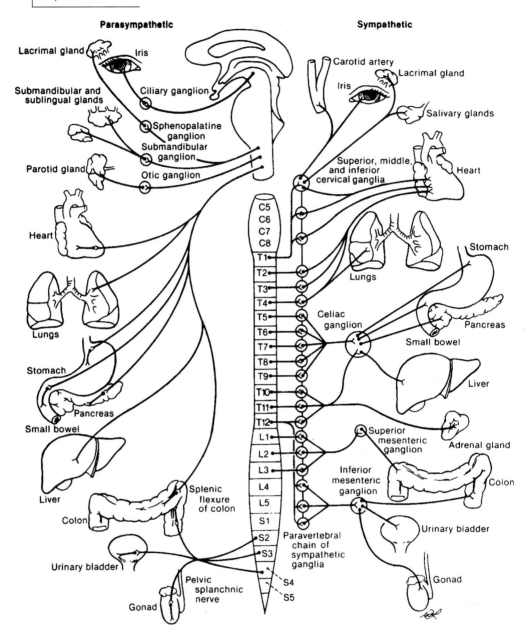

FIGURE 3-4. The autonomic nervous system (ANS). The parasympathetic division (*left*) arises from cranial nerve (CN) III, CN VII, CN IX, and CN X and from spinal cord segments S2 to S4. The sympathetic division (*right*) arises from spinal cord segments T1 to L3. (Reprinted with permission from NMS *Neuroanatomy.* Malvern, PA, Harwal Publishing, 1988, p 88.)

2. **Postganglionic (parasympathetic) transmission. ACh** is the neurotransmitter released from most **parasympathetic postganglionic** fibers. The postganglionic receptors are **muscarinic** (i.e., they respond to muscarine but not to nicotine). Muscarinic receptors are blocked by atropine. ACh can have either an excitatory or inhibitory effect, depending on the postsynaptic receptor that is activated.
   a. **Excitatory effects** of the parasympathetic fibers are produced on a variety of **smooth**

muscles (e.g., those within the stomach, intestine, bladder, and bronchi) and on **glands.** ACh can produce its excitatory effect by a variety of mechanisms.

  (1) ACh can bind to receptors that cause the membrane to depolarize, much in the **same way** ACh receptors effect the **depolarization of the skeletal muscle end-plate** (see Table 3-1).

  (2) ACh can bind to receptors that **increase Ca^{2+} conductance.** The increase in Ca^{2+} conductance does not produce a major effect on membrane potential. However, the Ca^{2+} entering the cell through the channels opened by ACh can be used to initiated contraction in smooth muscles (see Chapter 4 IV B 2 b).

  (3) ACh can bind to receptors that activate the membrane-bound protein **guanosine triphosphate (GTP) binding protein,** or **G protein.** When the G protein is activated, it initiates a series of membrane and intracellular events that lead to muscle contraction (Figure 3-5; see also Chapter 4 II B).

b. Inhibitory effects of parasympathetic fibers are produced on the **heart.**

  (1) ACh acts primarily on the pacemaker regions of the sinoatrial (SA) node to decrease the heart rate and the atrioventricular (AV) node to slow conduction of the action potential from the atria to the ventricles (see Chapter 10 III A 1).

  (2) When ACh binds to a receptor on the SA node, it slows the rate of pacemaker activity by two mechanisms:

  (a) Hyperpolarization. ACh causes a K^+ channel to open. K^+ flows out of the cell (down its electrochemical gradient) and the cell hyperpolarizes. The hyperpolarization acts to decrease the rate of pacemaker activity and to slow the conduction of the action potential through the AV node.

TABLE 3-1. Neurotransmitters Within the Peripheral Nervous System (PNS)

Transmitter	Receptor	Presynaptic Neuron	Postsynaptic Cell	Response
ACh	Nicotinic	Alpha motoneuron	Skeletal muscle fiber	Contraction
	Muscarinic	Postganglionic parasympathetic	Secretory cells	Secretion
			SA and AV nodes	Slow pacemaker activity and conduction
			Smooth muscle of GI tract	Relaxation of sphincters; contraction of other muscle
Norepinephrine, epinephrine	α	Postganglionic sympathetic	Smooth muscle of GI tract	Contraction of sphincters; relaxation of other muscle
			Vascular smooth muscle	Contraction
	β		Ventricular muscle	Contraction
			Bronchial and vascular smooth muscle	Relaxation
			Adipose tissue	Fatty acid mobilization

The table lists some of the most important actions of ACh and the catecholamines (e.g., norepinephrine and epinephrine) within the PNS. Although muscarinic, α, and β receptors all have several subtypes, these have not been listed in the table. ACh = acetylcholine; AV = atrioventricular; GI = gastrointestinal; SA = sinoatrial.

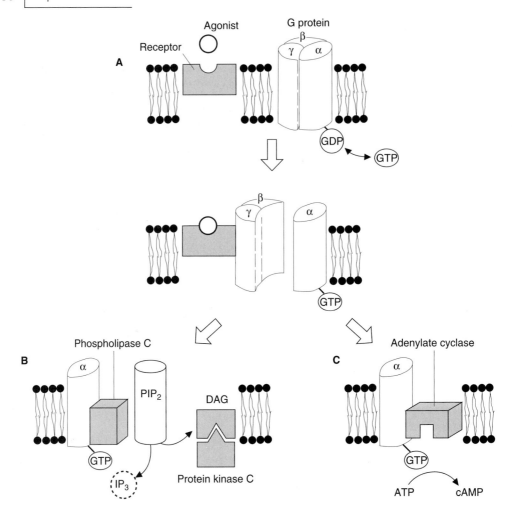

FIGURE 3-5. (*A*) When a neurotransmitter or other agonist binds to a receptor that is linked to a G protein–mediated second messenger system, the receptor diffuses within the membrane until it encounters a G protein complex. When the activated receptor binds to the G protein, it induces the G protein to exchange the guanosine diphosphate (GDP) molecule that is bound to the α subunit for a guanosine triphosphate (GTP) molecule. The presence of GTP causes the α subunit to separate from the G protein. The α subunit diffuses within the membrane until it encounters the enzyme that initiates the second messenger response. The G protein is inactivated when GTP is converted to GDP. (*B*) If the agonist binds to a muscarinic of α_1 receptor, the α subunit of the G protein activates phospholipase C, a membrane-bound lipase. The phospholipase C, in turn, hydrolyzes phosphatidylinositol diphosphate (PIP_2) into inositol triphosphate (IP_3) and diacylglycerol (DAG). IP_3 enters the cytoplasm, where it liberates Ca^{2+} from internal stores. The increase in intracellular Ca^{2+} leads to muscle contraction. DAG remains in the membrane and activates protein kinase C, a cytoplasmic enzyme that activates a series of cytoplasmic proteins by phosphorylating them. (*C*) If the agonist binds to a β receptor, the α subunit of the G protein activates adenylate cyclase. The adenylate cyclase catalyzes the conversion of adenosine triphosphate (ATP) to cyclic adenosine 3′,5′-monophosphate (cAMP). cAMP activates protein kinase A, which catalyzes the phosphorylation of cellular proteins.

      (b) Direct inhibition. ACh acts directly to inhibit the pacemaker channel, slowing the rate of spontaneous depolarization.

    3. Postganglionic (sympathetic) transmission. Norepinephrine is the neurotransmitter released from most **sympathetic postganglionic** fibers. Norepinephrine can have an excitatory or inhibitory effect, depending on the type and location of the receptor activated.

  a. Norepinephrine receptors are either β or α receptors.

    (1) β-Adrenergic receptors. When norepinephrine binds to the β receptors, it activates a G protein similar to that activated by ACh (see Figure 3-5). However, in this case, the activated G protein activates a different membrane-bound protein: **adenylate cyclase.**

      (a) Adenylate cyclase stimulates the formation of **cyclic adenosine 3′,5′-monophosphate (cAMP)** from adenosine triphosphate (ATP). The G protein that stimulates the formation of cAMP is called the G_s protein.

      (b) cAMP activates the cytoplasmic enzyme **protein kinase A** (or **cAMP-dependent protein kinase**), which, in turn, produces a variety of physiologic responses by phosphorylating the amino acids serine and threonine on an assortment of intracellular proteins.

        (i) **Heart.** The **phosphorylation of the Ca^{2+} channels** in cardiac ventricular muscle cells by **protein kinase A** increases the amount of Ca^{2+} entering the cell with each action potential, thus, **increasing the force of contraction** (see Chapter 4 III B 2 a).

            The **phosphorylation of phospholamban** [a protein located on the sarcoplasmic reticulum (SR)] by **protein kinase A** enhances the activity of the sarcoplasmic reticular Ca^{2+} pump. Although phospholamban is normally inhibitory to the sarcoplasmic reticular Ca^{2+} pump, the inhibition is removed when phosphorylation occurs. The increased activity of the sarcoplasmic reticular Ca^{2+} pump removes Ca^{2+} from the cytoplasm of the cardiac ventricular muscle cells, **reducing the duration of the contraction.**

            The **phosphorylation of membrane channel proteins** increases the rate of pacemaker depolarization and shortens the duration of the action potential by activating the K^+ channels responsible for phase 3 repolarization (see Chapter 10 II C 4), thus **increasing the heart rate.**

        (ii) **Lungs.** In bronchiole smooth muscle cells, the **phosphorylation of phospholamban** (and the resulting increase in sarcoplasmic reticular Ca^{2+} pump activity) **relaxes the bronchiole smooth muscle.**

    (2) α-Adrenergic receptors

      (a) When norepinephrine binds to the **$α_2$ receptor** (a subtype of the α-adrenergic receptors), it activates a G protein that inhibits adenylate cyclase, thus reducing the amount of cAMP in the cell. The G protein that inhibits the formation of cAMP is called the **G_i protein.**

      (b) When norepinephrine binds to the **$α_1$ receptor** (another subtype of the α-adrenergic receptors), it activates a G protein that, similar to its action at the muscarinic receptor, results in the formation of inositol triphosphate (IP_3) and diacylglycerol (DAG). Activation of the $α_1$ receptor by sympathetic nerve activity causes constriction of vascular smooth muscle.

  b. Adrenergic receptors can be distinguished by the types of drugs that activate and inhibit them.

    (1) α-Adrenergic receptors are **activated** preferentially **by epinephrine** and are **blocked by phenoxybenzamine.**

    (2) β-Adrenergic receptors are **activated** preferentially **by isoproterenol** and are **blocked by propranolol.**

  c. **Inactivation of norepinephrine** occurs by active transport into the nerve terminal and diffusion out of the synaptic cleft. In contrast to ACh, enzymatic degradation is not an important mechanism for inactivating norepinephrine.

C. The **enteric nervous system** is an independent component of the ANS. Composed of the ganglia found within the wall of the gastrointestinal (GI) tract, it is responsible for coordinating the activity of GI smooth muscle and gastric secretions.

  1. The enteric nervous system **receives synaptic input from the sympathetic and parasympathetic postganglionic fibers.**

  2. **Known active neurotransmitters** used by the enteric nervous system include serotonin, the enkephalins and endorphins, somatostatin, vasoactive intestinal peptides (VIPs), the purines ATP and adenosine, and nitric oxide. However, many active neurotransmitters have not yet been identified.

   a. Nitric oxide is a gas that is synthesized from the amino acid L-arginine by **nitric oxide synthetase.**
      (1) Nitric oxide synthetase activates guanylate cyclase, which stimulates the formation of cyclic guanosine monophosphate (cGMP) from GTP.
      (2) Nitric oxide is **unique** among neurotransmitters because, unlike other neurotransmitters, which are stored in and released from synaptic vesicles, nitric oxide is **synthesized as needed** and **diffused from the cytoplasm of the postsynaptic cell.**
   b. In the **GI system,** nitric oxide is found within the myenteric plexus and acts (along with the VIPs) as the **major relaxer of smooth muscle contraction.**

IV. CENTRAL NERVOUS SYSTEM (CNS) SYNAPTIC TRANSMISSION. An enormous variety of synaptic mechanisms occur within the CNS.

A. Electrical synaptic transmission. In a few locations (e.g., within the retina and olfactory bulb), synaptic transmission is accomplished by the **passive electrotonic spread of current between two cells.**

   1. Specialized junctions called **gap junctions** allow the spread of current between two cells.
      a. Only 2 nm separate the pre- and postsynaptic membranes at the site of gap junctions.
      b. Gap junctions are formed by **membrane bridges** that are constructed from integral membrane proteins called **connexin.**
         (1) An **aqueous channel** is formed in the membrane by six molecules of connexin (Figure 3-6A).
         (2) The channel in one cell merges with a channel in the membrane of another cell to form the gap junction (Figure 3-6B), enabling small molecules and ions to pass from one cell to the other, thus establishing **cytoplasmic continuity.**
            (a) When an action potential propagating along the membrane in one cell reaches the gap junction, an electrical current flows passively through the gap from one cell to another.

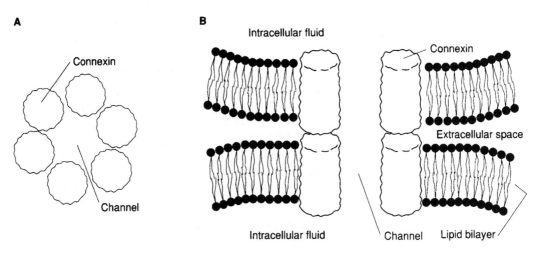

FIGURE 3-6. A gap junction. (*A*) *Top view,* Showing the six connexin molecules and the channel they form. The hexagonal unit is called a connexin. (*B*) *Side view,* Showing how the connexin proteins from two cells align at the gap junction to form a channel that permits the passage of water-soluble molecules and electrical currents from cell to cell. The extracellular space between the two lipid bilayers measures approximately 2 nm; the channel itself is approximately 1.5 nm wide.

    (b) Electrical current can pass through the gap in both directions, allowing either cell to serve as the pre- or postsynaptic cell.

2. Although gap junctions are not common in CNS synaptic transmission, they play an important role in coordinating **muscle contraction in the heart and viscera.** Gap junctions rapidly transmit an action potential that is generated in one cell to all of the other cells within the organ, permitting the entire tissue to act as a **syncytium** and contract in a co-ordinated fashion.

B. **Chemical synaptic transmission**

1. Most synapses within the CNS use chemical neurotransmitters.
   a. The synaptic transmitter is synthesized in the nerve terminal, stored in vesicles, and released by exocytosis when an action potential invades the nerve terminal.
   b. After being released from the presynaptic terminal, the transmitter diffuses across the synaptic cleft, binds to a postsynaptic receptor, and causes the opening of channels through which ions can flow. Both **excitatory** and **inhibitory receptors** exist on the postsynaptic cell.
      (1) **Excitatory neurotransmitters** produce a depolarization of the postsynaptic membrane called the **excitatory postsynaptic potential (EPSP).** The most common excitatory neurotransmitter within the CNS is **glutamate.**
      (2) **Inhibitory neurotransmitters** produce a hyperpolarization of the postsynaptic membrane called the **inhibitory postsynaptic potential (IPSP).** The most common inhibitory neurotransmitters within the CNS are **glycine** and **γ- aminobutyric acid (GABA).**
   c. The transmitter is inactivated in one of three ways.
      (1) It diffuses out of the synaptic cleft.
      (2) It is actively transported into the presynaptic terminal.
      (3) It is enzymatically degraded (if the transmitter is ACh).

2. **Summation.** The postsynaptic effects of the thousands of excitatory and inhibitory synapses that converge on a single neuron within the CNS (Figure 3-7) are integrated by

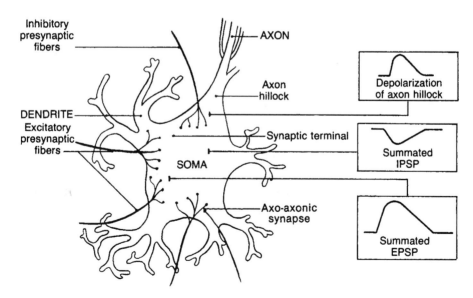

FIGURE 3-7. Inhibitory and excitatory synapses are formed on an alpha motoneuron. (Although synaptic junctions cover most of the soma and proximal dendrites, only a few are shown here.) When the amplitude of the summated excitatory postsynaptic potentials (EPSPs) exceeds the amplitude of the summated inhibitory postsynaptic potentials (IPSPs), the axon hillock is depolarized to the threshold and an action potential is generated.

the process of summation. Because the presynaptic terminals are only a few micrometers in diameter (and therefore can only release a few synaptic vesicles at a time), summation is required.

   a. Summation occurs because the duration of the postsynaptic effect is relatively long, and additional neurotransmitters can be released by the axon terminals before the effect of the first synaptic event has dissipated. Although the synaptic channel is open for only a few milliseconds, the membrane capacitance causes the postsynaptic response to decay more slowly.

     (1) Temporal summation occurs if another action potential invades the nerve terminal before the first postsynaptic potential has disappeared. The second postsynaptic potential adds to the first, producing a larger response.

     (2) Spatial summation occurs if several nerve terminals fire at approximately the same time.

   b. The summated potentials produced by the excitatory and inhibitory neurotransmitters spread passively to the **axon hillock,** where the action potential is generated.

     (1) The threshold for producing an action potential at the axon hillock is approximately −65 mV.

     (2) If the summates EPSPs are large enough to depolarize the axon hillock to threshold, an action potential is generated.

     (3) The summated IPSPs can prevent the axon hillock from being depolarized to threshold by hyperpolarizing the cell.

3. Presynaptic inhibition. The amount of neurotransmitter released from an axon terminal can be reduced by presynaptic inhibition.

   a. GABA, which is released from a neuron synapsing on the presynaptic nerve terminal, produces presynaptic inhibition. The synapse between the GABA-containing neuron and the presynaptic nerve terminal is called an **axo-axonic synapse.**

   b. GABA reduces the amount of neurotransmitter released from the nerve terminal by reducing the amount of Ca^{2+} entering the presynaptic nerve terminal during synaptic transmission. The mechanism by which the amount of Ca^{2+} is reduced depends on the type of GABA receptor present on the presynaptic nerve terminal.

     (1) When GABA binds to a receptor called the **$GABA_A$ receptor,** it opens Cl^- channels (Figure 3-8).

       (a) The opened Cl^- channels allow the negative Cl^- ion to flow into the cell.

       (b) When an action potential invades the presynaptic nerve terminal, the size of the action potential is reduced because of the increased Cl^- conductance.

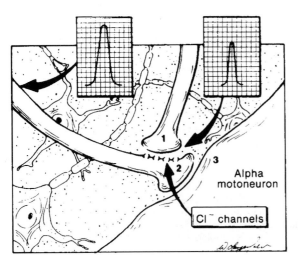

Alpha motoneuron

Cl^- channels

FIGURE 3-8. One way the axo-axonic synapse facilitates presynaptic inhibition. Neuron 1 releases γ-aminobutyric acid (GABA), which binds to a $GABA_A$ receptor on neuron 2, causing Cl^- channels to open. The increased Cl^- conductance reduces the amplitude of the action potential as it approaches the nerve terminal. Because the action potential is smaller, less Ca^{2+} enters the nerve terminal, less transmitter is released from the nerve terminal, and the magnitude of the excitatory postsynaptic potential (EPSP) produced on the postsynaptic membrane of neuron 3 is reduced.

      (c) Because the size of the action potential is smaller, less Ca^{2+} enters the nerve terminal, and the amount of neurotransmitter released is diminished.

   (2) When GABA binds to a receptor called a **$GABA_B$ receptor,** it activates a G protein. The G protein aids in reducing the amount of neurotransmitter that is released by acting in one of two ways.

      (a) The G protein may open a K^+ channel that reduces the size of the action potential invading the nerve terminal by hyperpolarizing the presynaptic nerve terminal.

      (b) Alternatively, the G protein may directly block the opening of Ca^{2+} channels that normally occurs when an action potential invades the nerve terminal.

  c. In presynaptic inhibition, the excitability of the postsynaptic cell is not diminished, whereas an IPSP reduces the effectiveness of all excitatory input to a cell. Presynaptic inhibition allows a particular excitatory input to be inhibited without affecting the ability of other excitatory synapses to fire the cell.

Chapter 4

Muscle Contraction

I. INTRODUCTION

A. Muscle fibers are divided into **two types** based on their appearance in light micrographs.

   1. **Striated muscle,** which includes **skeletal** and **cardiac** muscle, is characterized by alternating light and dark bands.

   2. **Smooth muscle** has no distinguishing surface features.

B. Although all muscles function in a similar way, several important differences exist. In the following discussion, the structural and contractile properties of skeletal muscle are noted first, and the major differences between cardiac and smooth muscle are then discussed (Table 4-1).

TABLE 4-1. Comparison of Muscle Types

Muscle Type	Role of Ca^{2+}	Source of Ca^{2+}	Mechanism of Ca^{2+} Mobilization	Regulation of Force
Skeletal	Initiates contraction by binding to troponin	Intracellular from SR. Enough Ca^{2+} is released to activate all muscle protein	Depolarization of T-tubule	Summation, recruitment, and preload are varied to vary force
Cardiac	Initiates contraction by binding to troponin	Intracellular from SR. Extracellular through DHP receptor (L type) Ca^{2+} channels. Amount of Ca^{2+} released can be varied to vary contractile force	Ca^{2+}-induced Ca^{2+} release	Contractility and preload are varied to vary force; variations in contractility affect speed of contraction
Smooth	Activates calmodulin, which in turn activates MLCK	Intracellular from SR. Extracellular through voltage- and receptor-activated Ca^{2+} channels	IP_3 increases release of Ca^{2+}; protein kinase A increases uptake of Ca^{2+} by SR	Recruitment, summation, preload, and contractility are varied to force. Formation of latch-bridges reduces speed of contractility

DHP = dihydropyridine; IP_3 = inositol triphosphate; MLCK = myosin light-chain kinase; SR = sarcoplasmic reticulum.

II. SKELETAL MUSCLE contraction maintains posture and produces movement.

A. Structure. Skeletal muscle is composed of multinucleated skeletal muscle fibers (Figure 4-1). The fibers vary from approximately 10–100 μm in diameter and may be several centimeters in length.

1. **Fascicles.** The skeletal muscle fibers are grouped into fascicles of approximately 20 fibers by the **perimysium,** a connective tissue sheath that is continuous with the connective tissue surrounding the entire muscle.

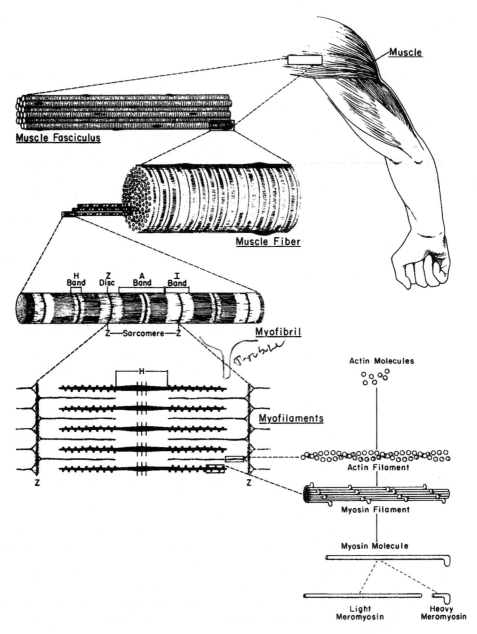

FIGURE 4-1. Skeletal muscle and its components as observed by light and electron microscopy. (Adapted from Fawcett DW: *Bloom and Fawcett's Textbook of Histology,* 11th ed. Philadelphia, WB Saunders, 1986, p 282.)

a. The perimysium is continuous with the **endomysium** surrounding each muscle fiber.

b. The endomysium is continuous with the **sarcolemma,** a sheath that contains glyco-protein and closely envelops the true cell membrane of the muscle fiber.

c. The tight connection between the cell membranes and the surrounding connective tissue structures enables the force developed by the muscle fibers to be transmitted effectively to the tendons.

2. **Myofibrils.** The individual skeletal muscle fibers are divided into myofibrils by a tubular network called the **sarcoplasmic reticulum (SR).**

   a. The myofibrils are approximately 1 to 2 μm in diameter and extend from one end of the muscle fiber to the other.

   b. The myofibrils are divided into functional units, or **sarcomeres,** by a transverse sheet of α-actinin protein called the **Z line.**

   c. The Z lines of neighboring myofibrils are aligned with each other so that in histologic slides, a Z line spans the entire width of the fiber.

3. **Filaments.** The myofibrils contain both **thick and thin filaments** composed of contractile proteins.

   a. **Thick filaments,** which are composed of approximately 300 **myosin** molecules, are approximately 11 nm in diameter and 1.6 μm in length.

      (1) A portion of the myosin molecule, called the **cross-bridge,** which extends out of the thick filament, is the **force-generating component of muscle.**

      (2) The center of the thick filament contains two important proteins, **myomesin** and **creatine phosphokinase.**

   b. **Thin filaments,** which contain the proteins **actin, tropomyosin,** and **troponin,** are approximately 5 nm in diameter and 1 μm in length.

   c. **Organization of filaments.** The thick filaments, which are interspersed between the thin filaments, are held in place by **myomesin** and **titin.**

      (1) **Myomesin** is part of the thick filament.

      (2) **Titin attaches to the Z line** at one end of the sarcomere **and** to myomesin in the center of the sarcomere.

         (a) **Titin,** the largest known protein, is approximately 1 μm long, contains almost **27,000 amino acids** and has a molecular weight of over 3 million.

         (b) An **elastic protein** that stretches when the muscle stretches and shortens when the muscle contracts, titin is responsible for the **passive tone** in skeletal muscle [parallel elastic component (PEC)].

      (3) The **overlap** between thick and thin filaments varies with sarcomere length and determines how much force skeletal muscle develops when it is stimulated (see II C).

4. **Tubules.** Two tubular networks are present in skeletal muscle fibers.

   a. The **transverse (T) tubule** is formed as an invagination of the surface of the muscle membrane. In mammalian skeletal muscle, the T tubules are located at the junction of the A and I bands. (In frog muscle, the T tubules are at the Z line.)

   b. An action potential spreading over the surface of the muscle membrane is propagated into the network of T tubules, which forms specialized contacts with the **SR,** the internal tubular structure that runs between the myofibrils.

      (1) The SR has a **high concentration of Ca^{2+},** which is used to initiate muscle contraction when the muscle is stimulated.

      (2) The ends of the SR expand to form **terminal cisternae (TC),** which make contact with the T tubule. Small projections, or **foot processes,** span the 20 nm separating the two tubular membranes (Figure 4-2).

         (a) The SR membrane contains a protein called the **ryanodine receptor** that contains the foot process and a Ca^{2+}-release channel.

         (b) The T tubule membrane contains a **voltage-sensitive dihydropyridine (DHP) receptor** that opens the ryanodine Ca^{2+}-release channel on the SR membrane.

B. **Excitation–contraction (EC) coupling** is the process by which an action potential initiates the contractile process. EC coupling involves **four steps:** the propagation of the action poten-

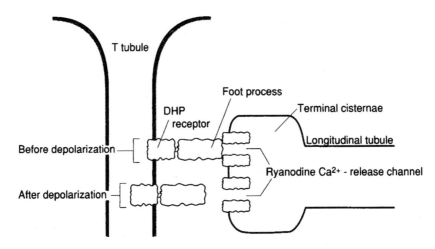

FIGURE 4-2. The dihydropyridine (*DHP*) receptor on the T tubule functions as a voltage sensor in skeletal muscle. When the T tubule is depolarized, the voltage sensor pulls the foot process away from the ryanodine Ca^{2+}-release channel in the sarcoplasmic reticulum (SR) membrane. The release of Ca^{2+} from the SR initiates muscle contraction. In cardiac muscle, the DHP receptor is associated with a Ca^{2+} channel. When Ca^{2+} enters the cell through the DHP Ca^{2+} channel, it opens the ryanodine Ca^{2+}-release channel in the SR. In smooth muscle, another receptor, called the inositol triphosphate (IP_3) receptor, is linked to the Ca^{2+}-release channel.

tial into the T tubule and release of Ca^{2+} from the TC, the activation of the muscle proteins by Ca^{2+}, the generation of tension by the muscle proteins, and the relaxation of the muscle.

1. **Release of Ca^{2+} from the TC.** Depolarization of the T tubule causes the ryanodine Ca^{2+} channels to open, which leads to the release of Ca^{2+}. Ca^{2+} flows out of the TC and into the cytoplasm.

2. **Activation of muscle proteins.** For a muscle to contract, the thick and thin filaments must interact. When the cell is at rest, this interaction is inhibited; the influx of Ca^{2+} removes the inhibition.
   a. Ca^{2+} binds to **troponin,** one of two regulatory proteins located on the thin filament (Figure 4-3A).
   b. The troponin undergoes a conformational change that alters the position of the **tropomyosin,** the other regulatory protein located on the thin filament.
   c. The movement of tropomyosin (deeper into the groove of the thin filament) exposes the myosin binding sites on the actin, allowing the myosin cross-bridge on the thick filament to bind to actin on the thin filament (Figure 4-3B). A rise in Ca^{2+} concentration, from 0.1 to 10 μmol/L, is sufficient to activate all of the muscle protein within the skeletal muscle fiber.

3. **Generation of tension.** The activated muscle proteins undergo **repetitive cross-bridge cycling** during which the muscle uses the energy obtained from the hydrolysis of ATP to shorten and generate tension. The cross-bridge cycle can be divided into four steps.
   a. The **first step** is the binding of the cross-bridge to actin, as described in II B 2 c (see Figure 4-3B). Binding occurs spontaneously after Ca^{2+} binds to troponin.
   b. The **second step** is the bending of the cross-bridge (Figure 4-3C), which pushes the thin filament over the thick filament, generating tension (see II C).
      (1) The energy used to bend the cross-bridge is generated when ATPase splits the ATP molecule into **adenosine diphosphate (ADP)** and **inorganic phosphate (P_i).**
      (2) Both the ATP molecule and the ATPase required for its hydrolysis are located on the cross-bridge; however, ATPase is activated only when myosin binds to actin. Therefore, hydrolysis occurs only during the cross-bridge cycle.

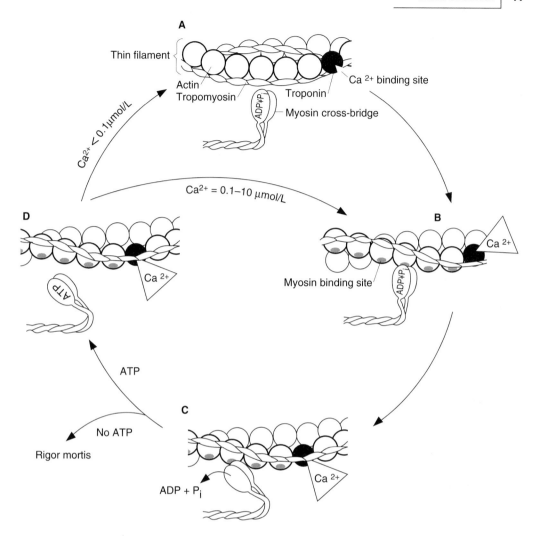

FIGURE 4-3. (*A*) Resting position. (*B*) When Ca^{2+} binds to troponin, the troponin undergoes a conformational change, pulling the tropomyosin away from the myosin binding site and allowing the cross-bridge cycle to begin. During this step of the cycle, the myosin binds to actin. (*C*) In the second step, the cross-bridge bends and the thin filament slides over the thick filament. During this step, the products of hydrolysis [i.e., adenosine diphosphate (*ADP*) and inorganic phosphate (*P_i*)] are released from the cross-bridge. (*D*) In the third step, a new molecule of adenosine triphosphate (*ATP*) binds to the cross-bridge and the cross-bridge detaches from the thin filament. The cross-bridge then stands up, and a new cycle begins if the intracellular Ca^{2+} concentration is sufficient to maintain troponin in its active state. Otherwise, the muscle relaxes.

    c. The **third step** is the detachment of the cross-bridge from the thin filament. This occurs after the cross-bridge has bent (Figure 4-3D).
        (1) For detachment to occur, ADP and P_i must be removed from the cross-bridge and replaced with a new molecule of ATP. If no ATP is available, the thick and thin filaments cannot be separated (i.e., rigor mortis occurs).
        (2) As soon as myosin separates (or, perhaps, while it is separating) from actin, the initial steps of ATP hydrolysis occur, producing myosin · ADP · P_i, a high-energy ATP intermediate. Complete dissociation of the phosphate from the ADP does not occur until after myosin has bound to actin and completed its bending cycle.

    d. In the **fourth step,** the cross-bridge returns to its original upright position. Once there, it can participate in another cycle. Cycling continues as long as Ca²⁺ is bound to troponin.

   4. Relaxation of muscle occurs when the Ca²⁺ is removed from the cytoplasm by Ca pumps (Ca–ATPase) located on the SR membrane. When the intracellular Ca²⁺ concentration falls below 0.1 μmol/L, troponin returns to its original conformational state, tropomyosin inhibition of myosin–actin interaction is restored, and cross-bridge cycling stops.

C. **Shortening and force development** is produced by the sliding of thin filaments over thick filaments. The contractile properties of muscle can be studied in two types of mechanical conditions: **isometric** and **isotonic contractions.**

   1. Mechanical basis. The thin filaments are drawn to the center of the sarcomere by the repetitive cycling of the cross-bridge (Figure 4-4).
     a. Each time an attached cross-bridge bends, it generates a force that pulls the Z line toward the center of the sarcomere.
     b. The force developed by the bending of the cross-bridge is transmitted through the thin filament to the Z line and then through the sarcolemma and tendinous insertions of the muscle to the bones.
     c. In Figure 4-5, the thick and thin filaments are represented by the **contractile component,** and the tendons and other compliant structures of the muscle are represented by the **series elastic component (SEC).**

   2. An **isometric contraction** occurs when the ends of the muscle (or bones) do not move

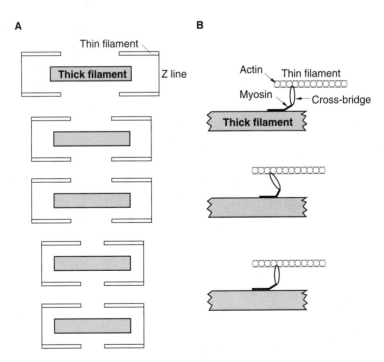

FIGURE 4-4. Shortening of the sarcomere. (*A*) Repetitive cycling of cross-bridges causes the thin filament to slide over the thick filament, dragging the Z lines toward the center of the sarcomere and causing the muscle to shorten. (*B*) During the cross-bridge cycle, the myosin head binds to actin and pulls the thin filament toward the center of the sarcomere, advancing the Z line 7–10 nm. The myosin then detaches, unbends, and reattaches to another actin molecule on the thin filament, and a second cross-bridge cycle begins.

Relaxed

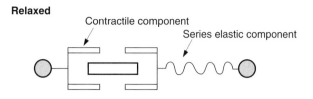

Contracted

FIGURE 4-5. The contractile properties of a muscle can be explained using a mechanical analog consisting of a force-generating contractile component in series with an elastic element.

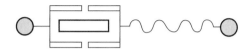

during the contraction; therefore, the length of the muscle remains constant, but the **tension changes.**

a. The intracellular Ca^{2+} concentration and the force developed during an isometric muscle **twitch** are illustrated in Figure 4-6.

  (1) Contraction begins when the Ca^{2+} released from the SR binds to troponin.

  (2) The muscle relaxes after the Ca^{2+} is resequestered into the SR by the Ca–ATPase pump on the SR.

  (3) The duration of the twitch is longer than the duration of the **Ca^{2+} transient** (i.e., the period during which the intracellular Ca^{2+} concentration is above resting values and the cross-bridges are cycling) because the cross-bridges remain attached to actin for a period of time after the Ca^{2+} is removed from the sarcoplasm.

b. Increasing the force of an isometric contraction. The motor control system increases the force of an isometric contraction by either:

  (1) Increasing the number of active alpha motoneurons. When an alpha motoneuron fires, all the muscle fibers that it innervates contract; therefore, recruitment of additional alpha motoneurons increases the number of active muscle fibers (and, consequently, the force of the contraction).

  (2) Increasing the frequency of alpha motoneuron firings (Figure 4-7)

    (a) The duration of the Ca^{2+} transient and, hence, the force of the isometric contraction, can be increased by increasing the frequency of alpha motoneuron firings because more Ca^{2+} is released from the SR each time the muscle is stimulated.

      (i) Summation. If the frequency increase is moderate, individual twitches "accumulate," increasing the force of contraction.

      (ii) Tetanus. If the frequency of stimulation is rapid, individual twitches become one continuous contraction (i.e., a maximal force is generated). The

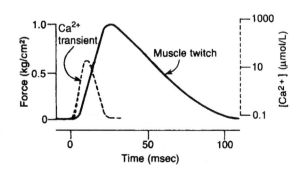

FIGURE 4-6. When intracellular Ca^{2+} concentration (*right ordinate*) increases to greater than 0.1 μmol/L, cross-bridge cycling causes an increase in muscle force (*left ordinate*). The resulting force development is the muscle twitch.

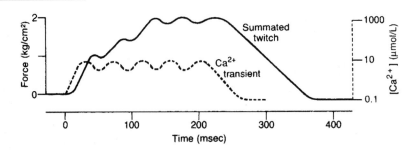

FIGURE 4-7. When the duration of the Ca^{2+} transient is increased by repetitive firing of the muscle, force development increases because there is sufficient time for the series elastic component (SEC) to be stretched completely.

frequency required to produce a maximal force is called a tetanic frequency, and the resulting contraction is called tetanus.
- **(b)** The force generated by the cross-bridge can only be transmitted to the bones if the SEC is stretched.
  - **(i)** Each time the cross-bridge bends, the Z line moves approximately 7.5–10 nm, and the SEC is stretched by the same amount. (Although the sarcomere is shortening, the contraction is still considered isometric because the total length of the muscle does not change.)
  - **(ii)** The total shortening of the sarcomere (and the accompanying lengthening of the SEC) depends on the number of cross-bridge cycles that occur during the Ca^{2+} transient. The more the SEC is stretched, the more force is transmitted.
- **c. Length–tension relationships.** The force of an isometric contraction can be altered by altering the initial length of the muscle fiber. Figure 4-8 illustrates this relationship, which is called the length–tension relationship.
  - **(1)** The **overlap** between the thick and thin filaments determines the number of cross-bridges that bind to actin when the muscle is stimulated.
    - **(a)** At an initial sarcomere length of 2.2 μm, each cross-bridge can bind to an actin molecule on the thin filament. A maximum force is generated.
    - **(b)** If the muscle is stretched to a sarcomere length of 3.5 μm, there is no overlap between the thick and thin filaments. Therefore, no force develops when the muscle is stimulated.

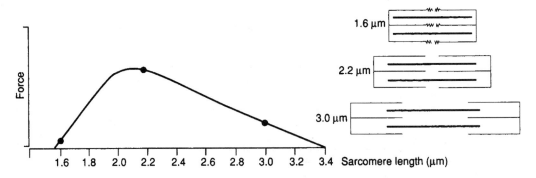

FIGURE 4-8. The length-tension relationship results from the overlap between thick and thin filaments. At a sarcomere length of 2.2 μm, overlap is optimal and force development is maximal. At lengths greater than 2.2 μm, force decreases because cross-bridge overlap is lessened. At lengths less than 2.2 μm, force is diminished because the thin filaments meet at the center of the sarcomere, causing an increased resistance to shortening.

    (c) If the sarcomere shortens to lengths below 2.0 μm, the thin filaments from opposite sides of the sarcomere interfere with each other, and the force of contraction decreases.

    (d) If the sarcomere shortens to 1.5 μm, the Z lines abut the thick filaments and no force can be generated.

  (2) Preload. Force must be applied to the skeletal muscle fiber to stretch it beyond 2.0 μm. The force is used to overcome elastic elements called **PECs,** one of which is the protein **titin,** which connects the thick filaments to the Z line. The force required to stretch the muscle to lengths beyond 2.0 μm is called the preload. The term preload is also used to indicate the length of the sarcomere or muscle before contraction.

    (a) The elastic portion of titin in cardiac muscle contains fewer amino acids than in skeletal muscle and is therefore stiffer.

    (b) Because cardiac muscle is stiffer than skeletal muscle, more force must be applied to stretch cardiac muscle.

  (3) Varying the preload is not an important method of varying the contractile force of skeletal muscle. Often, the muscle length is determined by the particular motor task being performed. However, if muscle length is not constrained by the motor activity, more force can be obtained by holding the muscle at its optimal length (i.e., where the sarcomere length is 2.2 μm).

3. An **isotonic contraction** occurs when the muscle shortens. Therefore, the tension remains constant, but the **length changes.**

  a. The development of force and the change in muscle length that occurs during an isotonic contraction is illustrated in Figure 4-9.

    (1) The initial portion of the contraction is isometric, because the muscle only begins to shorten when the force developed by the muscle equals the load on the muscle. The weight that a muscle lifts during an isotonic contraction is called the **afterload.**

    (2) Constants

      (a) Force. While the muscle is shortening, the force remains equal to the after-

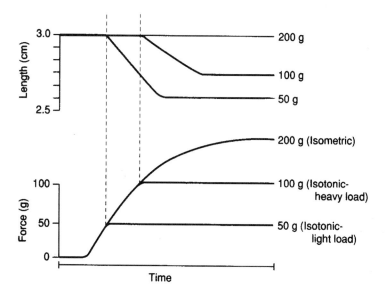

FIGURE 4-9. During an isotonic contraction, sufficient force must be generated for the muscle to shorten against the afterload on the muscle. Once sufficient force is developed, the muscle shortens at a constant velocity. Increasing the afterload increases the amount of force that must be developed before shortening can begin and decreases the velocity and extent of shortening.

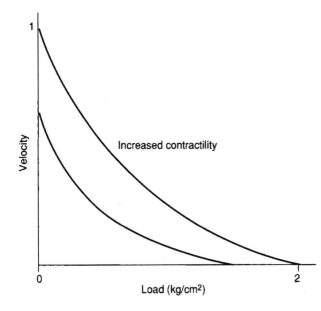

FIGURE 4-10. The load-velocity relationship illustrates that velocity of shortening increases when the afterload on the muscle decreases. Velocity is zero when the afterload equals or exceeds the maximum force that the muscle is capable of generating (F_{max}). Maximum velocity of shortening (V_{max}) is achieved when the afterload is zero. In cardiac muscle, the intrinsic force-generating capability of the muscle (i.e., the muscle's contractility) can be increased by increasing the amount of Ca^{2+} that is released from the sarcoplasmic reticulum (SR). When contractility is increased, both F_{max} and V_{max} increase.

load. The contraction is called isotonic because the force remains constant during the contraction.

    (b) The **velocity** of shortening remains constant.

  b. The **characteristics** of the contraction vary with the **magnitude of the afterload.** Increasing the afterload has the following effects.

    (1) The **duration of the isometric portion** of the contraction **increases,** because the SEC must stretch more to transmit the force required to lift the greater afterload.

    (2) The **velocity of shortening decreases** as the afterload increases.

      (a) Velocity decreases because each cross-bridge cycle takes longer.

      (b) The relationship between afterload and velocity is called the **load–velocity relationship** (Figure 4-10). The load–velocity relationship is an important char-

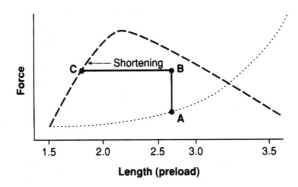

FIGURE 4-11. The relationship between force and length during an isotonic contraction (*solid line*). The sometric length-tension relationship (*dashed line*) indicates the maximum force the muscle can develop at any preload. The passive length-tension relationship (*dotted line*) indicates the amount of force required to stretch the resting muscle. When the muscle is stimulated (*point A*), it develops force but does not begin to shorten until its force equals the afterload (*point B*). At this point, the muscle shortens isotonically (i.e., its force remains equal to the afterload). As the muscle shortens to lengths below 2.2 μm, its ability to develop force (based on the isometric length-tension relationship) decreases. Eventually, depending on the afterload, the maximum force the muscle can develop equals the afterload and additional shortening cannot occur (*point C*).

acteristic of muscle because it indicates that the greatest velocity of shortening is generated when the afterload on the muscle is zero. The peak velocity of shortening is an indication of the cross-bridge cycling speed.

(3) The **amount of shortening decreases** as the afterload increases (Figure 4-11).

    (a) As the muscle shortens below a sarcomere length of 2.2 μm, its ability to generate force decreases.

    (b) At some length, the maximal force the muscle can develop becomes slightly less than the afterload and shortening stops.

    (c) The greater the afterload, the longer the muscle when shortening stops.

III. CARDIAC MUSCLE allows the heart to contract and propel blood through the circulatory system.

A. **Composition.** Although cardiac muscle fibers are striated, their structure differs somewhat from that of skeletal muscle.

  1. Cardiac muscle fibers have a **single nucleus** and are smaller than skeletal muscles. Each fiber is approximately 15–20 μm wide, approximately 100 μm long, and only approximately 5 μm thick.

  2. The T tubule is larger in cardiac muscle than in skeletal muscle and is located at the Z line rather than at the junction of the A and I bands. The SR makes contact with the T tubule and the cell membrane.

B. **EC coupling** of cardiac muscle differs in significant ways from that of skeletal muscle.

  1. Ca^{2+}**-induced Ca^{2+} release.** Ca^{2+} release from the SR is triggered by Ca^{2+}, not by membrane depolarization. The Ca^{2+} responsible for Ca^{2+}-induced Ca^{2+} release enters the sarcoplasm during the plateau phase of the cardiac action potential.

    a. The T tubule DHP receptor in cardiac muscle, unlike the DHP receptor in skeletal muscle, contains a Ca^{2+} channel through which Ca^{2+} enters the cell during the action potential.

    b. The SR ryanodine receptor containing the Ca^{2+}-release channel is opened by the influx of Ca^{2+} from the T tubule. In contrast, the skeletal muscle Ca^{2+}-release channel is opened by a voltage-induced conformational change of the DHP receptor (see Figure 4-2).

  2. The amount of Ca^{2+} released from the SR is under physiologic control.

    a. The amount of Ca^{2+} entering the cell during the plateau phase of the cardiac action potential may be increased by norepinephrine and epinephrine. Increasing the amount of Ca^{2+} entering the cell increases the amount of Ca^{2+} released from the SR by Ca^{2+}-induced Ca^{2+} release.

    b. The amount of Ca^{2+} within the SR can be increased by catecholamine stimulation. When the Ca^{2+} concentration within the SR increases, the amount of Ca^{2+} released by Ca^{2+}-induced Ca^{2+} release increases.

    c. The amount of intracellular Ca^{2+} is regulated by the **Na–Ca exchanger,** an antiport mechanism driven by the Na^+ gradient that transports one Ca^{2+} molecule out of the cell for every three Na^+ molecules that enter [see Chapter 1 III C 2 a (2)].

      (1) **Reduced intracellular Ca^{2+}**

        (a) **During the plateau phase** of the cardiac action potential, the driving force for Na^+ is reduced. Because the exchange rate is proportional to the Na^+ concentration gradient, the amount of Ca^{2+} leaving the cell is also reduced.

        (b) **Cardiac glycosides. Ouabain** and other cardiac glycosides can also affect Na^+–Ca^{2+} exchange. These drugs inhibit the Na–K pump, causing Na^+ to accumulate in the cell. The increase in intracellular Na^+ reduces the driving force for Na^+ and thus decreases the ability of the Na–Ca exchanger to remove Ca^{2+}.

      (2) **Increased intracellular Ca^{2+}.** Under certain circumstances, the driving force for Ca^{2+} entry may exceed the driving force for Na^+ entry. Under these conditions,

Ca^{2+} is pumped into the cell by the Na–Ca exchanger and Na$^+$ is pumped out of the cell.

C. **Shortening and force development** of cardiac muscle differs from that in skeletal muscle because of the duration of the action potential and the ability of cardiac muscle to regulate the amount of Ca^{2+} entering the cell.

1. The action potential and the period of time that Ca^{2+} remains in the cytoplasm (the Ca^{2+} transient) are nearly equal in duration; thus, **summation and tetanus are not possible.** This is not a physiologic disadvantage for the heart, which must relax after each beat so blood can enter it.

2. The sarcomere length in a cardiac muscle before contraction (the preload) depends on how much blood has entered the heart. Because this amount is under physiologic control, it is an important regulator of the force of cardiac muscle contraction.

3. The force of contraction can vary at a given sarcomere length if the amount of Ca^{2+} entering the cell is changed. This also is under physiologic control and, thus, is an important regulator of cardiac muscle contractile force.

IV. **SMOOTH MUSCLE** plays a major role in the physiologic regulation of the airways, blood vessels, and gastrointestinal (GI) tract.

A. **Composition.** The structure of smooth muscle differs from that of striated muscle.

1. **Fibers.** Smooth muscle is composed of **elongated** (10–500 μm long), **thin** (5–10 μm wide) muscle fibers that contain a single nucleus.

2. **Filaments**
   a. **Organization. Sarcomeres are absent** in smooth muscle; instead, the thick and thin filaments are **dispersed throughout the cell.**
      (1) The thin filaments are attached to **dense bodies.** Some of the dense bodies are anchored to the cell membrane, but most float within the cytoplasm.
      (2) The dense bodies are composed of **α-actinin,** the same protein found in the Z lines.
   b. **Proteins.** The thick filaments contain myosin, and the thin filaments contain actin and tropomyosin; however, the thin filaments **lack troponin** in smooth muscle.

3. **T tubules are absent** and unnecessary in smooth muscle because the cells are small enough for a stimulus present on the cell surface to activate the contractile machinery effectively. Instead, smooth muscle fibers contain **caveolae,** small invaginations of the surface membrane that increase the smooth muscle surface area and may (like T tubules) function to couple membrane potential changes to the SR.

B. **EC coupling** in smooth muscle is fundamentally different from that in striated muscle. In smooth muscle, cross-bridge cycling is regulated by **Ca^{2+}-induced phosphorylation of myosin** (Figure 4-12).

1. The myosin cross-bridges contain **four light chains,** two associated with each one of the head portions of the myosin molecule.

2. Myosin cannot bind to actin unless one of these light chains (called **LC$_{20}$** because it has a molecular weight of 20 kD) is phosphorylated.
   a. Phosphorylation of LC$_{20}$ is catalyzed by the enzyme **myosin light-chain kinase (MLCK).** MLCK is activated by **calmodulin,** which in turn is activated by Ca^{2+}.
   b. Ca^{2+} can enter the cells in a variety of ways.
      (1) **Stimulation by a neurotransmitter.** When smooth muscle is stimulated by a neurotransmitter, a receptor-activated Ca^{2+} channel may open, allowing Ca^{2+} to enter the cell.
      (2) **Voltage-operated Ca^{2+} channels.** Ca^{2+} may also enter the cell through voltage-operated Ca^{2+} channels that open during the smooth muscle action potential.

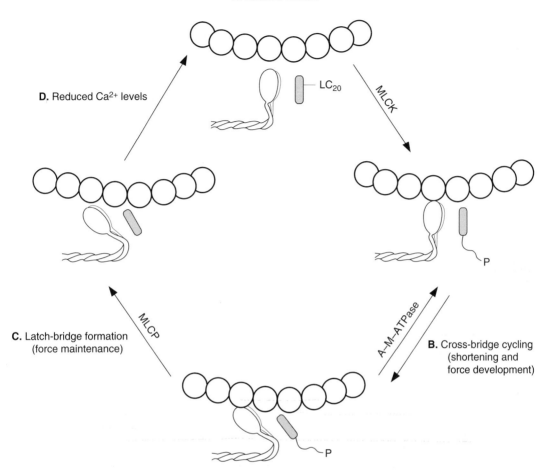

A. Relaxed muscle

D. Reduced Ca^{2+} levels

MLCK

LC$_{20}$

C. Latch-bridge formation
(force maintenance)

MLCP

A–M–ATPase

B. Cross-bridge cycling
(shortening and
force development)

P

P

FIGURE 4-12. Activated smooth muscle can exist in a phosphorylated and an unphosphorylated (latch) state. (A) Relaxed muscle. When myosin light-chain kinase (*MLCK*) catalyzes the phosphorylation (*P*) of light chain 20 (*LC$_{20}$*), rapid cross-bridge cycling ensues, enabling the muscle to develop force and shorten. (*B*) Each time the cross-bridge cycles, a molecule of adenosine triphosphate (*ATP*) is used. Actin—myosin—ATPase (*A—M—ATPase*) catalyzes the hydrolysis of ATP. (*C*) When the LC$_{20}$ is dephosphorylated by myosin light-chain phosphatase (*MLCP*), a latch-bridge forms. In the latch-bridge state, cross-bridge cycling slows, enabling the muscle to maintain force with minimal energy consumption. (*D*) When the cytoplasmic Ca^{2+} concentration falls to resting levels, the latch-bridges dissociate and the muscle relaxes.

     (3) Release from SR. Ca^{2+} may be released from the SR. The Ca^{2+}-release channel on smooth muscle SR is activated by inositol triphosphate (IP$_3$). This channel is called the **IP$_3$ receptor** to distinguish it from the ryanodine receptor found in striated muscle.

   3. The light chains are **dephosphorylated by** the enzyme **myosin light-chain phosphatase (MLCP).**

C. **Shortening and force development** in smooth muscle differs from that in striated muscle.

   1. The **speed of shortening** (i.e., the rate of cross-bridge cycling) is dependent on the phosphorylation of the myosin light chain. When the light chains are dephosphorylated by MLCP, the speed of shortening decreases.

2. **Latch-bridges.** These **dephosphorylated** cross-bridges **remain attached to actin in latch-bridges** and provide smooth muscle with the ability to maintain tone with little energy consumption. Because the latch-bridges do not cycle, or cycle very slowly, they do not use much ATP.

Case

A 45-year-old man undergoing a routine hernia operation, and he is anesthetized with isoflurane. During the surgery he develops sudden tachycardia, metabolic acidosis, and a rapid increase in body temperature. Dantrolene, a ryanodine receptor antagonist is administered to relieve malignant hyperthermia.

> **1.** *What are the consequences of malignant hyperthermia?*

DISCUSSION

Malignant hyperthermia, which is caused by a genetic defect in the ryanodine receptor, results in excessive release of calcium from the sarcoplasmic reticulum (SR) when patients are given gaseous anesthetics such as halothane and isoflurane, as well as the muscle relaxant succinylcholine. The excess calcium causes continuous muscle activity with massive heat production. The body, unable to dissipate the heat, undergoes a rapid rise in temperature.

> **2.** *How does dantrolene relieve the signs of malignant hyperthermia?*

DISCUSSION

Dantrolene blocks the ryanodine receptor, preventing the release of calcium from the SR. The recognition of the signs of malignant hyperthermia by physicians and the use of dantrolene to prevent a rise in body temperature has dramatically reduced the number of deaths from this condition, which is one of the most common causes of mortality resulting from anesthesia.

> **3.** *What is the function of the ryanodine receptor in muscle contraction?*

DISCUSSION

Ryanodine is the calcium release channel on the SR of skeletal and cardiac muscle. In skeletal muscle, the ryanodine receptor is opened by depolarization of the T tubule (voltage-induced calcium release). In cardiac muscle, the ryanodine receptor is opened by calcium entering the cell through L-type calcium channels during the ventricular muscle action potential. In smooth muscle, the calcium release channel is open by inositol triphosphate (IP_3) and is called the IP_3 channel.

STUDY QUESTIONS

1. According to Fick's law of diffusion, particle flux will decrease if there is an increase in which of the following?

(A) A particle's concentration difference across the membrane
(B) The thickness of the membrane
(C) The area of the membrane
(D) The temperature of the solution
(E) The diameter of the particle

2. When activated by β-adrenergic receptors, the G protein

(A) activates phospholipase C
(B) activates adenylate cyclase
(C) activates protein kinase C
(D) converts guanosine diphosphate (GDP) to guanosine triphosphate (GTP)
(E) stimulates the release of Ca^{2+} from the sarcoplasmic reticulum (SR)

3. Significantly decreasing the extracellular concentration of K^+ would do which of the following?

(A) Increase the transport of Na^+ out of the cell by the Na^+-K^+ pump
(B) Decrease the negativity of the membrane potential
(C) Increase the conductance of the membrane to K^+ (G_K)
(D) Increase the driving force on Na^+
(E) Decrease the negativity of the equilibrium potential for K^+

4. Assuming that the extracellular concentration of Na^+ is 10 times the intracellular concentration, the equilibrium potential for Na^+ would be the same as the equilibrium potential for Ca^{2+} if the extracellular concentration of Ca^{2+} was

(A) 2 times the intracellular concentration of Ca^{2+}
(B) 10 times the intracellular concentration of Ca^{2+}
(C) 20 times the intracellular concentration of Ca^{2+}
(D) 100 times the intracellular concentration of Ca^{2+}
(E) the same as the intracellular concentration of Ca^{2+}

5. Which of the following is true about the synaptic channels on the endplate of skeletal muscle?

(A) They are highly selective for Na^+.
(B) They are opened when the cell membrane depolarizes.
(C) They are activated by acetylcholine (ACh).
(D) They are inhibited by atropine.
(E) They are responsible for the relative refractory period.

6. Increasing the afterload on a skeletal muscle fiber

(A) increases the velocity of shortening
(B) decreases the force produced by the muscle during shortening
(C) decreases the interval between excitation and shortening
(D) increases the amount of shortening
(E) none of the above

7. Which one of the following statements regarding a Donnan equilibrium is true?

(A) The concentration of permeable anions is higher in the solution with the impermeable proteins.
(B) The concentration of particles is greater in the solution that contains no impermeable proteins.
(C) The membrane potential is more negative on the side with the impermeable proteins.
(D) There is a net flux of cations into the solution that contains no impermeable proteins.

8. The equilibrium potentials for K^+ and Na^+ are -90 mV and $+60$ mV, respectively. If the conductance for K^+ (G_K) is 4 times the conductance for Na^+ (G_{Na}), what is the resting membrane potential?

(A) -50 mV
(B) -60 mV
(C) -70 mV
(D) -80 mV
(E) -90 mV

9. In a nerve axon, which phase of the action potential is caused by the inactivation of the Na^+ channels?

(A) Upstroke
(B) Absolute refractory period
(C) Downstroke
(D) Undershoot
(E) Relative refractory period

10. The velocity of propagation along an axon will increase if there is a decrease in which of the following?

(A) Membrane resistance (r_m)
(B) Membrane capacitance (c_m)
(C) Axon diameter
(D) Refractory period
(E) Axon excitability

11. Release of synaptic transmitter by exocytosis would be blocked most effectively by preventing the

(A) propagation of the action potential into the nerve terminal membrane
(B) depolarization of the nerve terminal membrane
(C) flow of Na^+ into the nerve terminal membrane
(D) flow of K^+ out of the nerve terminal membrane
(E) flow of Ca^{2+} into the nerve terminal membrane

12. In smooth muscle, Ca^{2+} is released from the sarcoplasmic reticulum (SR) by which of the following?

(A) Diacylglycerol (DAG)
(B) The guanosine triphosphate (GTP) binding protein (G protein)
(C) Phospholipase C
(D) Inositol triphosphate (IP_3)
(E) Adenylate cyclase

13. The production of cyclic guanosine monophosphate (cGMP) is associated with the postsynaptic effect of

(A) acetylcholine (ACh)
(B) epinephrine
(C) γ-aminobutyric acid (GABA)
(D) glutamate
(E) nitric oxide

14. A red blood cell is placed in a saline (NaCl) solution, and the cell's volume increases to 1.5 times its original volume. This finding indicates that the Na^+ concentration in the saline solution is approximately

(A) 50 mEq/L
(B) 75 mEq/L
(C) 100 mEq/L
(D) 200 mEq/L
(E) 600 mEq/L

15. Which one of the following proteins is important for skeletal muscle contraction but not for smooth muscle contraction?

(A) Actin
(B) Myosin
(C) Troponin
(D) Myosin—adenosine triphosphatase (ATPase)
(E) Ca^{2+}-ATPase

16. The osmotic flow of water across a membrane will decrease if there is a decrease in

(A) the permeability of the membrane to the particles in solution
(B) the particle's concentration difference across the membrane
(C) both A and B
(D) neither

17. Depolarization of the T tubule is directly linked to the opening of Ca^{2+} channels on the sarcoplasmic reticulum (SR) of

(A) skeletal muscle
(B) cardiac muscle
(C) both A and B
(D) neither

18. Alteration in preload alters the force of contractions in which of the following muscle type or types?

(A) Cardiac muscle
(B) Skeletal muscle
(C) Smooth and cardiac muscle
(D) Smooth and skeletal muscle
(E) Smooth, cardiac, and skeletal muscle

19. All of the following transport processes display saturation (Michaelis-Menten) kinetics EXCEPT

(A) Na^+-coupled active transport
(B) primary active transport
(C) facilitated diffusion
(D) simple diffusion
(E) Na^+-Ca^{2+} exchanger

ANSWERS AND EXPLANATIONS

1. The answer is B [Chapter 1 III A 1 b]. According to Fick's law of diffusion, particle flux is inversely proportional to the thickness of the membrane and directly proportional to the area of the membrane, the concentration difference across the membrane, and the diffusion coefficient. The diffusion coefficient depends on the physical properties of the particle and the membrane through which it is diffusing. In general, the larger the diameter of the particle, the slower the rate of diffusion. Increasing temperature will increase the rate of diffusion.

2. The answer is B [Chapter 3 III B 3 a (1); Figure 3-5]. When norepinephrine binds to a β-adrenergic receptor, it activates a G protein [i.e., a guanosine triphosphate (GTP) binding protein], which, in turn, activates adenylate cyclase. Adenylate cyclase catalyzes the formation of cyclic adenosine 3',5'-monophosphate (cAMP), which activates a variety of kinases. One of these kinases (protein kinase A) phosphorylates phospholamban, which reduces the inhibition of the sarcoplasmic reticular Ca^{2+} pump, increasing resequestration of Ca^{2+} from the cytoplasm.

3. The answer is D [Chapter 1 III C 1; Chapter 2 II A; III D 1]. Decreasing the extracellular K^+ concentration increases the equilibrium potential for K^+ (i.e., makes it more negative) and causes the membrane to hyperpolarize. Hyperpolarization increases the driving force on Na^+. The conductance of K^+ (G_K) will decrease when the cell hyperpolarizes because some of the K^+ activation gates close, and because there are fewer ions to carry current through the K^+ channels that remain open. The activity of the Na^+-K^+ pump decreases if the fall in K^+ is significant enough, because there is not enough K^+ to occupy all of the binding sites on the pump.

4. The answer is D [Chapter 2 II A]. The equilibrium potential (E_{ion}) is calculated using the Nernst equation [$E_{ion} = -61 \cdot \log (C_{in}/C_{out})$], where C is the concentration of the ion. Because Ca^{2+} has a valence of 2, the log of the Ca^{2+} ratio would have to be twice the log of the Na^+ ratio to produce the same equilibrium potential. Since the log of 1/10 (the Na^+ ratio)

= −1, a log of −2 would require a ratio of 1/100. Thus, the extracellular Ca^{2+} concentration would have to be 100 times the intracellular concentration of Ca^{2+}.

5. The answer is C [Chapter 3 II C 2; III B 2]. Acetylcholine (ACh) is released from the alpha motoneuron nerve terminal and activates the synaptic channels on the skeletal muscle endplate. These channels, unlike the channels that produce the action potential, are not affected by changes in the membrane potential. The ACh receptor is inhibited by curare; atropine blocks ACh receptors activated by postganglionic parasympathetic neurons. The channel opened by the ACh receptor is equally permeable to Na^+ and K^+.

6. The answer is E [Chapter 4 II C 3 b]. The afterload is the weight that a muscle lifts during an isotonic contraction. When the afterload on an isotonically contracting skeletal muscle is increased, the velocity of shortening slows, the amount of force produced by the muscle increases (because force must equal load for the muscle to shorten), the interval between excitation and shortening increases (because it takes longer for the muscle to build up enough force to lift the load), and the amount of shortening decreases.

7. The answer is C [Chapter 2 II B; Figure 2-1]. A Donnan equilibrium occurs when two solutions are separated by a membrane that is impermeable to one of the charged particles in solution. In biologic solutions, the impermeable particle is a negatively charged protein. The solution containing the protein will have a higher concentration of particles (and thus a greater osmotic pressure), a higher concentration of permeable cations, and a negative charge (compared to the solution without the proteins). Because the solutions are in equilibrium (i.e., the concentration differences between the permeable ions are balanced by the membrane potential differences), no net flux of particles occurs.

8. The answer is B [Chapter 2 III D]. The resting potential can be calculated using the transference equation ($E_m = E_K \cdot T_K + E_{Na} \cdot T_{Na}$). Since the conductance for K^+ (G_K) is 4 times the conductance for Na^+ (G_{Na}), T_K (the transference for K^+) is 0.8 and T_{Na} is 0.2. Substituting the appropriate values in the transference equation ($-90 \cdot 0.8 + 60 \cdot 0.2$) yields a membrane potential of -60 mV.

9. The answer is B [Chapter 2 IV D, E 2 c; Figure 2-6]. The absolute refractory period is caused by the inactivation of Na^+ channels that occurs during the depolarization phase of the action potential. During this time, another action potential cannot be elicited because the closing of the h gates prevents Na^+ from entering the cell. The absolute refractory period ends when some of the h gates open during the downstroke. At this point, another action potential can be elicited but its threshold is above normal because some of the Na^+ channels are still inactivated and the conductance of the membrane to K^+ (G_K) is higher than at rest. This period of time is referred to as the relative refractory period. Although inactivation of the Na^+ channels contributes to the downstroke, the downstroke is caused primarily by K^+ channel activation. Na^+ channel inactivation that occurs during the upstroke opposes depolarization. Almost all Na^+ channel activation occurs before the undershoot phase.

10. The answer is B [Chapter 2 III G 2; Figure 2-8]. Propagation occurs because the current entering the axon during one action potential acts as a stimulus for the production of another action potential further along the axon. The velocity of propagation is proportional to the cable properties of the axon that modulate the passive flow of charge along the axon. The lower the membrane capacitance (c_m), the smaller the charge needed to depolarize the membrane to threshold and thus the greater the velocity of propagation. Decreasing the membrane resistance (r_m) causes charge to leak out of the cell, slowing propagation. Decreasing the axon diameter increases the axoplasmic resistance (r_a), decreasing the amount of charge that flows along the axon. Decreasing axon excitability makes it more difficult to elicit an action potential and, therefore, slows conduction velocity. The refractory period may affect the frequency of action potential firing, but not the propagation velocity.

11. The answer is E [Chapter 3 II B 3, C 1]. Preventing the flow of Ca^{2+} into the cell would prevent the release of transmitter, because Ca^{2+} initiates the intracellular events leading to the docking of the vesicle to its binding site on the active zone. Although Ca^{2+} normally enters the cell through voltage-operated channels that are opened by the depolarization of the nerve terminal that occurs as the action potential propagates along the nerve axon, release of transmitter will not occur if Ca^{2+} does not enter the nerve terminal. The flow of Na^+ into the nerve terminal would depolarize the membrane and open Ca^{2+} channels, leading to Ca^{2+} entry and exocytosis. However, Na^+ entry does not directly stimulate exocytosis. K^+ does not affect the nerve terminal membrane.

12. The answer is D [Figure 3-5; Chapter 4 IV B 2 b]. In smooth muscle, Ca^{2+} is released from the sarcoplasmic reticulum (SR) by an inositol triphosphate (IP_3)-activated channel. In striated muscle, Ca^{2+} is released from the SR through a ryanodine receptor that is activated by depolarization in skeletal muscle and by Ca^{2+} in cardiac muscle. Diacylglycerol (DAG), the guanosine triphosphate (GTP) binding protein (the G protein), and phospholipase C all play a role in excitation-contraction (EC) coupling but do not directly cause the release of Ca^{2+} into the cytoplasm. Adenylate cyclase catalyzes the conversion of adenosine triphosphate (ATP) to cyclic adenosine $3',5'$-monophosphate (cAMP). cAMP activates protein kinase A, which phosphorylates phospholamban, leading to an increase in Ca^{2+} sequestration by the sarcoplasmic reticular Ca^{2+} pump.

13. The answer is E [Chapter 3 III C 2 a]. Nitric oxide acts as a paracrine agent and as a neurotransmitter. It stimulates the action of guanylate cyclase which, in turn, promotes the formation of cyclic guanosine monophosphate (cGMP). The physiologic effects of nitric oxide are produced by cGMP-dependent kinases that phosphorylate a variety of intracellular proteins. In the gastrointestinal (GI) system, nitric oxide facilitates smooth muscle relaxation, and in the cardiovascular system, it relaxes blood vessels.

14. The answer is C [Chapter 1 III B 3 a (1)]. The steady-state volume of a cell placed in a solution containing an osmotic concentration different from the cell's can be found using the equation: $\pi_i \cdot V_i = \pi_f \cdot V_f$. The normal tonicity of red blood cells is approximately 285 mOsm/L. In this problem, a red blood cell is placed in a solution of unknown osmolality and swells to 1.5 times its original volume. Solving the equation for the osmolality of the extracellular fluid (π_f) yields 285/1.5, or 190 mOsm. A saline solution of this osmolality will have a Na^+ concentration of 95 mEq/L.

15. The answer is C [Chapter 4 II B 2; IV B]. In skeletal muscle, contraction is initiated when Ca^{2+} binds to troponin. Smooth muscle contraction is initiated by the phosphorylation of the myosin light-chain proteins. Both smooth and skeletal muscle rely on actin, myosin, and myosin-adenosine triphosphatase (ATPase) for cross-bridge cycling and on Ca^{2+}-ATPase for Ca^{2+} resequestration.

16. The answer is B [Chapter 1 III B 1]. Decreasing the membrane's permeability to the particle will increase the particle's effective osmolality and thus increase the osmotic flow of water. The osmotic flow of water is proportional to the osmotic pressure difference across a membrane, which is, in turn, proportional to the concentration difference across the membrane. However, the osmotic pressure actually produced depends on the particle's permeability to the membrane. The smaller the particle's permeability (or the greater its reflection coefficient), the greater the osmotic pressure produced for a given concentration difference.

17. The answer is A [Chapter 4 II B 1; III B 1]. Release of Ca^{2+} from the sarcoplasmic reticu-

lum (SR) in both skeletal and cardiac muscle is activated by T tubule depolarization. However, in skeletal muscle, the Ca^{2+}-release channel in the SR is opened directly by the depolarization of the T tubule membrane. In cardiac muscle, Ca^{2+} is released from the SR by a Ca^{2+}-induced Ca^{2+} release process. The Ca^{2+} used in this process enters the cell through a voltage-activated Ca^{2+} channel [the dihydropyridine (DHP) receptor Ca^{2+} channel] associated with the T tubule membrane.

18. The answer is E [Chapter 4 II C 2 c (2); III C 2; Table 4-1]. Smooth, cardiac, and skeletal muscles all are able to influence the force of contraction by varying the initial length (preload) of their sarcomeres.

19. The answer is D. [Chapter 1 III A 1 b, 2 b]. Saturation, or Michaelis-Menten, kinetics occurs in all carrier-mediated transport processes because in these transport processes, the flux is proportional to the concentration of substrate-carrier complexes that are formed. Saturation (i.e., maximum flux) occurs when all of the carrier proteins are occupied. There is a limit to the number of particles that can pass through membrane channels by simple diffusion so, theoretically, saturation can also be achieved via this process. However, under physiologic conditions, simple diffusion obeys Fick's law, which indicates that flux increases linearly with increases in the concentration difference across a membrane.

NEUROPHYSIOLOGY

Michael B. Wang

Chapter 5

Cutaneous, Olfactory, and Gustatory Sensation

I. INTRODUCTION

A. **Sensory receptors transform (transduce) stimulus energy** into a local change in membrane potential called a **receptor (generator) potential.**

1. The **receptor potential** serves as a **stimulus for the generation of an action potential** or for the **release of neurotransmitter** by the sensory receptor.

2. In either case, information about the stimulus is **transmitted to the central nervous system (CNS),** where it is used to elicit a reflex response, alter behavior, or produce a conscious sensation.

B. This chapter first considers the general mechanisms used by the nervous system to encode sensory information, and then describes receptors that are stimulated by direct contact with the stimulus (i.e., those in the skin, nose, and tongue). Chapter 6 describes receptors that are stimulated by energy transmitted from a distance (i.e., those in the ear and eye).

II. GENERAL SENSORY MECHANISMS

A. **Receptor classification.** Receptors can be classified in four ways.

1. **Source of the stimulus**
   a. **Exteroceptors** such as the eye, ear, taste, and cutaneous receptors receive stimuli from outside the body.
   b. **Enteroreceptors** such as the chemoreceptors that measure blood gases, the baroreceptors that measure blood pressure, and the proprioceptors that measure the position of the limbs or the force of muscle contraction receive stimuli from within the body.

2. **Type of stimulus energy**
   a. **Mechanoreceptors** detect skin deformation and sounds.
   b. **Thermoreceptors** detect environmental temperatures.
   c. **Photoreceptors** detect light.
   d. **Chemoreceptors** detect substances that produce the sensations of smell and taste.

3. **Type of sensation** (e.g., touch, heat, cold, pain, light, sound, taste, and smell receptors)

4. **Rate of adaptation** (see also II C 3)
   a. **Slowly adapting (tonic, static) receptors** fire action potentials continuously during stimulus application.
   b. **Rapidly adapting (phasic, dynamic) receptors** fire action potentials at a decreasing rate during stimulus application.

B. **Sensory neuron classification**

1. Sensory neurons are classified on the basis of axon diameter or propagation velocity (Table 5-1). The information provided by the larger, more rapidly conducting fibers is more precise than that provided by the smaller, more slowly conducting fibers.
   a. **Roman numerals** are used to classify axons according to **size.**
   b. The **letters A** and **C** are used to classify axons according to **propagation velocity.**

2. Examples of sensorimotor neurons and their classifications are given in Table 5-2.

C. **Energy transduction**

1. **Adequate (appropriate) stimulus.** Each receptor is specialized to receive a particular type of stimulus.
   a. Although each receptor is exquisitely sensitive to its adequate stimulus, receptors can respond to other forms of energy if the intensity is high enough.
   b. For example, the retina can detect the presence of a single photon of light. However, a mechanical stimulus (e.g., rubbing the eyes) can produce a sensation of light.

2. **Conversion of stimulus energy.** A **transducer region** and a **spike generation region** are contained within most receptor membranes (Figure 5-1). In some receptors (e.g., those in the eye or the ear) the transducer and spike generation functions are served by separate cells.
   a. The **transducer region** is responsible for converting the stimulus energy into an electrical signal [i.e., the receptor (generator) potential]. The mechanism used by the

TABLE 5-1. Classification of Sensory Neurons

Classification Diameter	Classification Velocity	Fiber Type	Axon Diameter	Propagation Velocity
I	Aα	Myelinated	12–20 μm	80–120 m/sec
II	Aβ	Myelinated	6–12 μm	35–75 m/sec
III	Aδ	Myelinated	1–6 μm	5–30 m/sec
IV	C	Unmyelinated	< 1 μm	0.5–2 m/sec

TABLE 5-2. Examples of Sensorimotor Neuron Classification

Classification		Efferent Nerve	Afferent Cutaneous Nerve	Afferent Muscle Nerve
I	Aα	Motoneurons to skeletal muscle	. . .	Ia: All intrafusal (nuclear chain and nuclear bag) fibers
				Ib: Golgi tendon organs
II	Aβ	. . .	Mechanoreceptors	Nuclear chain fibers
III	Aδ, Aγ	Motoneurons to intrafusal muscle fibers	Nociceptors, thermoreceptors	. . .
IV	C	. . .	Nociceptors, thermoreceptors	. . .

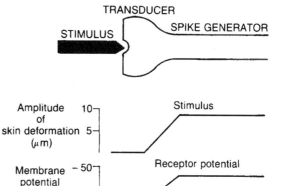

FIGURE 5-1. When a stimulus is applied to a sensory nerve ending, a receptor potential results. For example, in mechanoreceptors, the stimulus produces the receptor potential by deforming the nerve terminal. The deformation opens channels that are permeable to Na⁺ and K⁺, causing the membrane to depolarize. Note that the receptor potential follows the time-course of the mechanical stimulus. The magnitude of the receptor potential and the frequency of the action potential are proportional to the magnitude of the stimulus.

transducer region to produce the receptor potential varies depending on the type of receptor.

   b. The **spike generator region** of the receptor is responsible for converting the receptor potential into a train of action potentials.

      (1) The receptor potential spreads passively from the transducer region to the spike generator region. If the spike generator is depolarized to threshold, an action potential is generated.

      (2) At the end of one action potential, the receptor potential causes the spike generator membrane to depolarize toward threshold.

         (a) If threshold is reached again, another action potential is generated.

         (b) Figure 5-1 illustrates the repetitive discharge of action potentials by the receptor axon in response to a receptor potential.

3. Adaptation causes the receptor's response to decrease, despite the continued presence of a stimulus.

   a. Functions

      (1) Sensory adaptation functions primarily to **encode information about the rate of stimulus application.**

         (a) In **rapidly adapting receptors,** the discharge rate increases as the rate of stimulus application increases.

            (i) When a stimulus is applied too slowly, adaptation of the spike generator occurs before an action potential can be generated.

            (ii) When a stimulus is applied rapidly enough, excitation exceeds adaptation, and a steady discharge of action potentials occurs.

         (b) In **slowly adapting receptors,** the discharge continues at a steady rate as long as the stimulus is applied.

      (2) In some cases, sensory adaptation is used to **decrease the amount of information reaching the brain.** Brain stem mechanisms responsible for consciousness and attention are capable of keeping the information flow to the brain within tolerable limits, however, so sensory adaptation is not often required for this purpose.

   b. Mechanisms. Sensory adaptation takes place via two major mechanisms.

      (1) In one, the **transducer mechanism fails to maintain a receptor potential** despite continued stimulus application.

      (2) In the other, the **spike generator fails to sustain a train of action potentials.** Although a receptor potential is present, the excitability of the spike generator membrane is diminished. An increase in the membrane conductance to K^+ or the activity of the electrogenic Na^+–K^+ pump, or the inactivation of Na^+ channels may be responsible for the decreased excitability of the membrane.

4. **Encoding.** The **intensity, location,** and **quality of a stimulus** are encoded by the sensory system.
   a. **Stimulus intensity** is encoded by the **firing frequency** of a sensory neuron and by the **number of sensory neurons** activated. The firing frequency is proportional to the magnitude of the receptor potential.
      (1) **As the intensity of a stimulus increases, the magnitude of the receptor potential increases** (Figure 5-2). This relationship is expressed by the **Steven's power law function**

      $$V = k \cdot [I - I_0]^n$$

   or by the **Weber-Fechner law**

   $$V = k \cdot \log \frac{I}{I_0}$$

      where V = the magnitude of the receptor potential, k = a constant, I = the intensity of the stimulus, I0 = the threshold, and n = a constant.
      (2) The perception of stimulus strength is also related to the intensity of the stimulus by the Weber-Fechner and Stevens equations (see Figure 5-2). This concept substantiates the idea that the strength of a stimulus is encoded by the firing frequency of a sensory neuron.
   b. **Stimulus location** is encoded primarily by the location of the sensory projection in the cerebral cortex. This mechanism of encoding, called topographic representation, is used by the visual and somatosensory systems to localize the point of stimulus application.

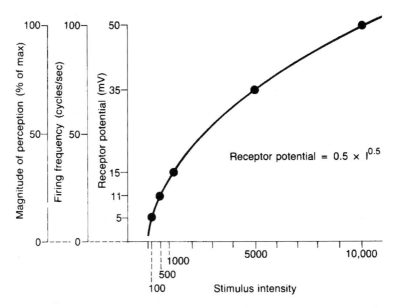

FIGURE 5-2. The proportionality between the receptor potential and the stimulus can be expressed as a power function. This same relationship can be used to describe the proportionality between the stimulus magnitude and firing frequency, and between the magnitude of the stimulus and its perceived intensity. *I* = intensity.

(1) Receptive field. Each sensory neuron receives information from a particular sensory area called its receptive field. The smaller the receptive field, the more precise the encoding of stimulus localization.

    (a) For example, the receptive fields of the fovea are the smallest within the eye.

    (b) Similarly, the receptive fields within the fingertips are much smaller than those on the hands and back, where it is difficult to locate the point of a mechanical stimulus precisely.

(2) Lateral inhibition. Stimulus localization can be made more precise by lateral inhibition (Figure 5-3).

    (a) Two stimuli are applied to the skin, and the sensory task is to indicate whether one or two stimuli are present. The closest that two stimuli can be to each other and still be distinguished as separate stimuli is called the **two-point threshold.**

    (b) Without lateral inhibition (see Figure 5-3A), the two stimuli are recognized as separate only if they are applied in receptive fields that are separated from each other by a nonstimulated receptive field.

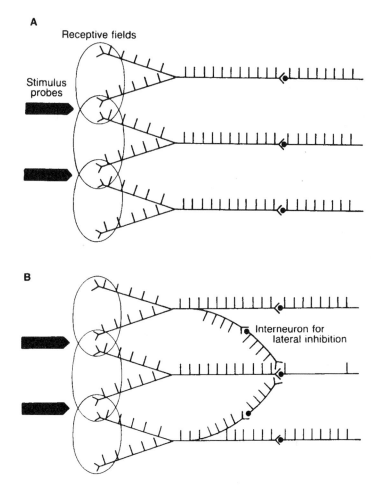

FIGURE 5-3. In order for two distinct stimuli to be perceived, they must stimulate receptive fields separated by an unstimulated receptive field. (*A*) Without lateral inhibition, the stimuli produce equal amounts of discharge in all three neurons. (*B*) With lateral inhibition, the neuron with the receptive field in the center is presynaptically inhibited by collaterals from the neurons with receptive fields located laterally. As a result, the receptive field in the center does not fire, and two stimuli are perceived.

(c) Lateral inhibition (see Figure 5-3B) can decrease the two-point threshold by reducing the discharge of the neuron innervating the receptive field in the center, thus making it apparent to the CNS that two stimuli are present.

c. **Stimulus quality** is encoded by a variety of mechanisms.

   (1) The simplest mechanism uses a **labeled line,** in which the stimulus is encoded by the particular neural pathway that is stimulated.

      (a) The basic sensory modalities are encoded in this way. Thus, the sensation of touch is elicited whether the receptors on the skin are excited by mechanical deformation or by electrical stimulation. Similarly, light sensation always is evoked no matter how the retina is activated, and sound sensation always results from stimulation of the cochlea.

      (b) The same type of sensation results no matter where along the sensory pathway the stimulus is applied. For example, stimulating electrodes placed on the visual cortex evoke the sensation of light, and seizures within the olfactory cortex produce sensations of smell.

   (2) A more complex mechanism of coding uses the **pattern of activity** within the neural pathway that is carrying information to the brain.

      (a) In **temporal pattern coding,** the same neuron can carry two different types of sensory information depending on its pattern of activity. For example, cutaneous cold receptors indicate temperatures below and above 30°C by firing with or without bursts, respectively.

      (b) In **spatial pattern coding,** the activity of several neurons is required to elicit a sensation. For example, three neurons may be required to encode different taste sensations. A sour taste may result if all three neurons are activated, whereas a salty taste may result if only two neurons fire.

   (3) The most sophisticated mechanism of sensory coding uses **feature detectors.** These are neurons within the brain that integrate information from a variety of sensory fibers and fire to indicate the presence of a complex stimulus.

      (a) For example, the location of an object in space can be encoded by cortical cells receiving information from a single eye. However, special feature detectors receiving information from both eyes are required to specify the depth of an object in space.

      (b) Similarly, the location of a sound in space requires integration of information from both ears by feature detectors within the brain stem.

III. **CUTANEOUS SENSATION.** The skin contains receptors that are adapted to encode information about touch, pain, and temperature. Approximately 1 million sensory nerve fibers innervate the skin. Most of these are unmyelinated nerve fibers that are responsible for crude somatosensory mechanical sensation. Although far fewer in number, the large myelinated (group II) sensory fibers encode the important sensory qualities of touch, vibration, and pressure. The sensations of temperature and pain are encoded by small myelinated (Aδ) fibers and unmyelinated (C) fibers.

A. **Mechanoreceptors.** Precise information about mechanical stimulation from the hairless (glabrous) region of the skin is provided by four receptors (Table 5-3).

   1. The **pacinian corpuscle** is a very rapidly adapting receptor with a large receptive field that is used to encode **vibratory sensation.**

      a. **Description.** The receptor is located on the end of a group II myelinated fiber, which is inserted into an onion-like lamellar capsule that is approximately 1 mm in diameter (see Table 5-3).

      b. **Conversion of stimulus energy**

         (1) When a mechanical stimulus deforms the outer lamellae of the capsule, the **deformation** is **transmitted through the capsule to the nerve terminal.**

            (a) The deformation of the nerve terminal increases the membrane permeability to Na^+ and K^+, producing a depolarizing receptor potential.

TABLE 5-3. Cutaneous Mechanoreceptors

	Receptor	Receptive Field Size	Speed of Adaptation	Encoded Sensation
	Pacinian corpuscle	Large	Very rapid	Vibration
	Meissner's corpuscle	Small	Rapid	Speed of stimulus application
	Merkel's disk	Small	Slow	Location of stimulus
	Ruffini's corpuscle	Large	Slow	Magnitude and duration of stimulus

       (b) The size of the receptor potential increases in proportion to the magnitude of the deformation. However, because the pacinian corpuscle is a very rapidly adapting receptor, only a few action potentials are generated, regardless of stimulus intensity.

    (2) A **vibratory stimulus** produces a **steady discharge** of the pacinian corpuscle. Each time the stimulus is removed and reapplied, the pacinian corpuscle discharges another action potential.

  c. Adaptation. The deformation of the nerve terminal is not maintained during continuous stimulus application, resulting in adaptation.

    (1) Only rapid deformations are transmitted effectively to the core of the capsule.

    (2) If the stimulus is applied slowly or is left in place, the inner lamellae become rearranged so that they no longer deform the nerve terminal. This is an example of adaptation caused by failure to maintain the receptor potential.

  d. Encoding. The frequency of discharge by the pacinian corpuscle equals the frequency of a vibratory stimulus in the range of 50–500 Hz (cycles/sec).

    (1) This is about the same range of frequencies identifiable by humans, indicating that the **frequency of firing is encoding the frequency,** not the intensity, of vibration.

    (2) **Intensity** is encoded by the number of action potentials generated by each deformation (limited to two or three) and the number of pacinian corpuscles responding to the vibration.

2. Meissner's corpuscle is a rapidly adapting receptor with a small receptive field that is used to encode the **rate of stimulus application.**

  a. Description. The receptor is located at the end of a single group II afferent fiber that is inserted into a small capsule (see Table 5-3).

  b. Receptive field. Meissner's corpuscle can be stimulated only by **deformation of the small region of the skin lying just above the receptor;** therefore, it has a **small receptive field.**

    c. Adaptation. Meissner's corpuscle **rapidly adapts to a maintained or slowly applied stimulus** (Figure 5-4).

      (1) Because the frequency of action potentials is proportional to the magnitude of the receptor potential, a slowly applied stimulus produces a lower frequency of nerve discharge than a rapidly applied stimulus.

      (2) Thus, the CNS uses the frequency of firing in a neuron innervating a Meissner's corpuscle to detect the speed of stimulus application.

        (a) Rapid deformation of the skin occurs when the skin is jabbed quickly with a probe or when the fingers move over a rough object.

        (b) The ability to detect the rate of skin deformation when the skin is moved over an object is especially important to individuals using braille.

3. Merkel's disk is a slowly adapting receptor with a small receptive field that is used to encode the **location of a stimulus.**

    a. Description. Merkel's disk is unique because the transducer is not on the nerve terminal but on the epithelial cells that make up the disk. The epithelial sensory cells form synaptic connections with branches of a single group II afferent fiber (see Table 5-3).

    b. Receptive field. The disk is about 0.25 mm in diameter and can be stimulated only if the stimulus is applied directly to the disk. The small receptive field of the Merkel's disk makes it an ideal receptor to encode information about the location of the stimulus.

4. Ruffini's corpuscle is a slowly adapting receptor with a large receptive field that is used to encode the **magnitude of a stimulus.**

    a. Description. The receptor is located on the terminal of a group II axon that is covered by a liquid-filled collagen capsule. Collagen strands within the capsule make contact with the nerve fiber and the overlying skin (see Table 5-3).

    b. Receptive field. Any deformation or stretch of the skin causes the nerve terminal to depolarize and generate action potentials.

B. **Thermoreceptors.** Temperature sensation is encoded by thermoreceptors located on the free endings of small myelinated ($A\delta$) and unmyelinated (C) fibers. Separate receptors with discrete receptive fields exist for encoding warm and cold sensations.

    1. Warm fibers are active when the skin temperature is between 30°C and 43°C (Figure 5-5A).

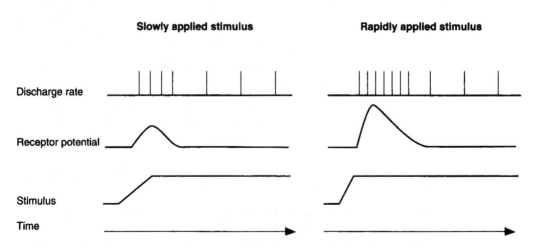

FIGURE 5-4. Meissner's corpuscle encodes the rate of stimulus application. If the stimulus is applied fairly slowly, adaptation occurs during the application of the stimulus and the magnitude of the receptor potential is reduced. If the stimulus is applied very rapidly, little adaptation occurs during the application of the stimulus and a large receptor potential is produced.

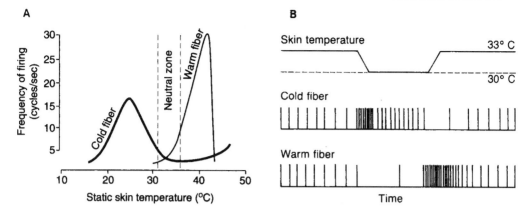

FIGURE 5-5. (A) Graph illustrating the tonic level of firing in both warm and cold fibers as a function of temperature. At temperatures within the neutral (comfort) zone, complete perceptual adaptation occurs (i.e., awareness of temperature disappears). (B) Spike trains illustrating the dynamic response of warm and cold fibers to a change in temperature. When the temperature decreases, cold fibers increase their rate of firing and then adapt to the firing rate indicated by the graph. Similarly, when the temperature increases, warm fibers phasically increase their firing rate before adapting to the rate indicated by the graph.

    a. The steady-state firing rate of warm fibers reaches a peak at temperatures of approximately 42°C.

    b. Warm fibers transiently increase their firing rate when skin temperatures increase, and decrease their firing rate when skin temperatures decrease (Figure 5-5B). Because the thermoreceptors respond transiently to the direction of a temperature change, the sensation produced by a small change in temperature depends on the current skin temperature. For example, a stimulus of 35°C feels warm if the skin is at 30°C, and cool if the skin is at 40°C.

  2. Cold fibers are active when the skin temperature is between 15°C and 38°C (see Figure 5-5A).

    a. The steady-state firing rate of cold fibers reaches a peak at temperatures between 23°C and 28°C. Paradoxically, temperatures between approximately 45°C and 49°C stimulate cold fibers as well as pain fibers, producing a mixed sensation of cold and pain.

    b. Cold fibers transiently increase their firing rate when skin temperatures decrease, and transiently decrease their firing rate when skin temperatures increase (see Figure 5-5B).

C. **Nociceptors.** Pain sensation is different from other sensations because its purpose is not to inform the brain about the quality of a stimulus, but rather to indicate that the stimulus is physically damaging. Although unpleasant, pain is a useful sensation if it leads to removal of the damaging stimulus. Much more information is required about the physiologic and psychologic mechanisms of pain before its elimination becomes a routine part of medical practice.

  1. Peripheral mechanisms

    a. The **receptors for pain,** which are called nociceptors to indicate that they respond to noxious stimuli, are on the free nerve endings of small myelinated (Aδ) and unmyelinated (C) fibers.

      (1) Nociceptors are **specific for painful stimuli,** responding to damaging or potentially damaging mechanical, chemical, and thermal stimuli. Cutaneous receptors that respond to nonpainful levels of these stimuli do not elicit pain sensations no matter how intense the stimulus.

      (2) Although the **adequate stimulus** for nociceptors is not known, it is assumed that a chemical such as histamine or bradykinin is released from cells damaged by the pain stimulus and that the chemical substance activates the nociceptors.

    b. Two types of pain sensation result from the application of a strong, noxious stimulus to the skin.

       (1) Fast (initial) pain is a discrete, well-localized, pinprick sensation that results from activating the nociceptors on the Aδ fibers.

       (2) Slow (delayed) pain is a poorly localized, dull, burning sensation that results from activating the nociceptors on the C fibers.

   c. Different **pathways** are used to reach the centers of consciousness in the brain.

      (1) Somatic sensation

         (a) Fast pain. Action potentials that are propagated by the fast pain fibers travel faster, and thus reach the brain before those conducted by the slow pain fibers. The sensory fibers for fast pain have small receptive fields, travel to the cortex through the spinothalamic tract, and are topographically represented on the cortex—all factors that account for the ability of these fibers to encode the location of the stimulus producing the fast pain.

         (b) Slow pain. This pain sensation, which has a more diffuse pathway, travels to the brain through the spinoreticulothalamic system. Collaterals of this system pass through the reticular formation to activate fiber tracts that produce the emotional perceptions accompanying pain sensations. These pathways account for the intense unpleasantness associated with slow pain.

      (2) Visceral sensation. Referred pain (i.e., pain originating in visceral organs that is referred to sites on the skin) most likely occurs because the visceral and somatic pain fibers share a common pathway to the brain.

         (a) Because the **skin is topographically mapped and the viscera are not,** the pain is identified as originating on the skin and not within the viscera.

         (b) Because of this anatomic relationship, **diagnosis of visceral disease can be made based on the location of the referred pain.** For example, ischemic heart pain is referred to the chest and the inside of the arm.

      (3) Projected pain. Referred pain should not be confused with projected pain, which occurs as a result of directly stimulating fibers within a pain pathway.

         (a) Because a **labeled-line mechanism** is used to encode the location of the pain, stimulation anywhere along the pathway will result in the same perception. For example, striking the elbow causes pain to be projected to the hand.

         (b) Amputees often have sensations that appear to come from the severed limb. This is known as **phantom limb sensation** and presumably results from activation of the sensory pathway either at the site of amputation or within the CNS. Occasionally, the phantom sensation is one of pain, but with no obvious source of stimulation, it is difficult to eliminate the pain.

  d. Reflexes

      (1) Fast pain evokes a **withdrawal reflex** (see Chapter 7 III A) and a **sympathetic response,** including an increase in blood pressure and a mobilization of body energy supplies.

      (2) Slow pain produces nausea, profuse sweating, a lowering of blood pressure, and a generalized reduction in skeletal muscle tone. (Pain sensations originating in the muscles, blood vessels, and viscera produce similar reflexes.)

2. The **central mechanisms** of pain sensation are not well known.

  a. Generally, it is assumed that pain sensation is conveyed to the CNS through the **anterolateral quadrant.**

  b. Chronic pain (i.e., a sensation of pain that endures long after the stimulus is removed and the injury is healed) is an extremely debilitating condition that is difficult to treat. Treatment is based on attempts to remove the pain area within the brain by surgery or to reduce the activity of the pain pathways by activating inhibitory pathways projecting to the pain areas. However, surgical section of the cord through the anterolateral quadrant is not very successful in relieving chronic pain.

      (1) Failure to relieve pain with this procedure may result from the existence of **parallel pain pathways** outside the anterolateral tracts.

      (2) Alternatively, chronic pain may result from the spontaneous activity of pain centers within the CNS.

(a) Reverberating circuits that develop because of continuous pain input may fail to stop firing when the input is removed.

(b) Denervation supersensitivity (i.e., increased sensitivity to circulating neurotransmitters that occurs when the normal synaptic input is removed from a neuron) may develop in pain centers subsequent to the removal of pain fiber input.

IV. OLFACTORY SENSATION.

Olfactory stimuli are detected by specialized receptors located on the free nerve endings of the olfactory nerve (cranial nerve I) fibers.

A. **Olfactory (nasal) mucosa.** The olfactory receptors are located within the olfactory mucosa, which is distinguished from the surrounding respiratory mucosa by the presence of tubular **Bowman's glands,** the **absence of** the **rhythmic ciliary beating** that characterizes the respiratory mucosa, and a distinctive **yellow-brown pigment.** A mucous layer covers the entire epithelium.

1. **Innervation.** The olfactory mucosa is innervated by the olfactory nerve (cranial nerve I) and some branches of the trigeminal nerve (cranial nerve V). The irritative character of some odorants results from stimulation of the free nerve endings of the trigeminal nerve.

2. **Histologic structure. Three cell types** comprise the olfactory mucosa (Figure 5-6).
   a. The **receptor cells** are **bipolar neurons.**
      (1) Their **dendrites** terminate in a knob. Cilia project from the knob into the mucous layer of the olfactory mucosa.
      (2) Their **axons** form the olfactory nerve.
   b. The **supporting cells** have a columnar shape. Microvilli extend from the surface of these cells into the mucous layer covering the nasal mucosa.
   c. The **basal cells** are **stem cells** from which new receptor cells are formed. There is a continuous replacement of receptor cells by mitosis of basal cells.

3. **Location.** The olfactory mucosa is located on the **superior nasal concha,** adjacent to the nasal septum. Because of its superior position in the nasal cavity, the olfactory mucosa is not directly exposed to the flow of inspired air entering the nose. Odorant molecules come in contact with the olfactory mucosa by **sniffing** (i.e., by short, forceful inspirations). Sniffing produces turbulence in the airflow and thereby transports molecules to the receptor cells.

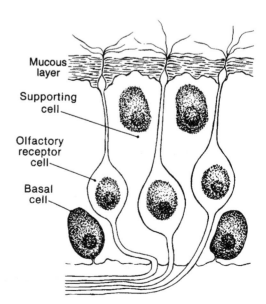

Mucous layer

Supporting cell

Olfactory receptor cell

Basal cell

FIGURE 5-6. The olfactory mucosa. Olfactory receptor cells are situated among supporting cells. The cilia lie within the mucous layer that covers the epithelium. New receptors are generated from basal cells. Bowman's glands, which contribute to mucus secretion, are not shown.

B. **Stimuli. Odorant molecules** must dissolve in the mucous layer lining the nose before they can come in contact with the olfactory receptors. To be effective, an odorant molecule must be:

1. **Volatile,** because the olfactory receptors respond to chemicals transported by the air into the nose

2. **Water-soluble** (to some degree), to penetrate the watery mucous layer lining the nasal epithelium to reach the receptor cell membrane

3. **Lipid-soluble** (to some degree), to penetrate the cell membranes of the olfactory receptor cells to stimulate those cells

C. **Receptors**

1. **Sensitivity.** The olfactory receptors are extremely sensitive. For many odorants, the sensitivity is so high that interaction of a few molecules with receptors is sufficient to produce excitation.

   a. **Number of odorants.** The olfactory system can discriminate among a vast number of odorants. In some instances, the olfactory system can discriminate dextro- and levorotatory forms as well as *cis-* and *trans-* conformations of a molecule.

   b. **Concentration.** The olfactory system has limited ability to discriminate differences in odorant concentration in ambient air.

   c. **Adaptation.** Olfactory sensation adapts very rapidly with continued exposure to an odorant.

2. **Receptor potential.** The adsorption of odorant molecules to the plasma membrane of the cilia of the receptor cells generates a depolarizing receptor potential in the receptor cell.

   a. When an odorant molecule stimulates a receptor, it activates a **G protein,** which, in turn, **activates adenylate cyclase.** Adenylate cyclase catalyzes the formation of **cyclic adenosine 3′5′-monophosphate (cAMP),** which **directly opens Ca^{2+} channels.** The Ca^{2+} **activates Cl^- channels. Cl^- flows out of the cell,** causing the membrane to depolarize and generate a train of action potentials.

   b. A specific olfactory receptor does not respond to a particular compound or category of compounds. Instead, an individual receptor responds to many odors. Furthermore, no two receptor cells have identical responses to a series of stimuli. **Sensory perception,** therefore, **is based on the pattern of receptors activated by the stimulus.**

   c. The electrical response recorded from the olfactory mucosa in response to an olfactory stimulus is called an **electro-olfactogram (EOG).** The amplitude of the EOG increases when the intensity of the stimulus increases.

V. **GUSTATORY SENSATION.** Gustatory (taste) stimuli are detected by taste receptors within the tongue, mouth, and pharynx. Taste must be distinguished from flavor, which includes the olfactory, tactile, and thermal attributes of food in addition to taste.

A. **Stimuli. Sapid (taste-producing) substances** must dissolve in the saliva before they can stimulate the taste receptors. There are **four basic types** of taste sensations; all taste sensations are assumed to result from various combinations of these four primary types (Figure 5-7A).

1. A **sweet sensation** is produced by various classes of organic molecules, including sugars, glycols, and aldehydes. The **tip of the tongue** is the area most sensitive to sweet stimuli.

2. A **bitter sensation** is produced by alkaloids such as quinine and caffeine. Many alkaloids are harmful when swallowed. The **back of the tongue** is the area most sensitive to bitter stimuli.

3. A **salty sensation** is produced by the anions of ionizable salts. The **front half of each side of the tongue** is the area most sensitive to salty stimuli.

4. A **sour sensation** is produced by acids; this sensation relates, to some degree, to the pH of stimulus solutions. The **posterior half of each side of the tongue** is the area most sensitive to sour stimuli.

B. **Receptors.** Taste cells are located within **taste buds,** which, in turn, are located within **papillae.**

A

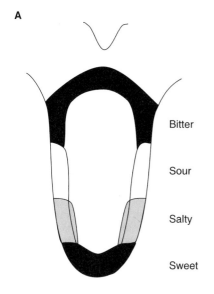

Bitter

Sour

Salty

Sweet

B

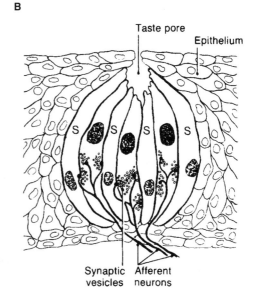

C

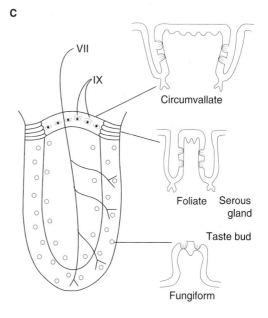

FIGURE 5-7. (*A*) View of the dorsal lingual surface, showing the distribution of the four primary taste sensations. (*B*) Structure of a taste bud. Taste receptor cells contain synaptic vesicles and receive afferent nerve terminals. Supporting cells (*S*) are not innervated. (*C*) Distribution of the gustatory papillae. Innervation by the cranial nerves (*roman numerals*) is also indicated. (*A* and *C* redrawn and modified from Kandel EK, Schwartz JH, Jessell TM: *Principles of Neural Science,* 3rd ed. New York, Elsevier, 1991, p. 519.)

1. **Taste buds**
   a. **Distribution.** Taste buds are located on the tongue papillae, hard and soft palate, epiglottis, and in the pharynx.
   b. **Structure.** Each taste bud is a cluster of 40–60 taste cells and numerous supporting and basal cells (Figure 5-7B).
      (1) **Taste pore.** Each taste bud contains a taste pore that allows substances to reach the interior of the taste bud. The taste receptors are located on **microvilli,** which project from the taste cells into the taste pores.

(2) **Taste cells.** These modified epithelial cells communicate with gustatory nerve endings by synaptic transmission.

    (a) **Innervation** (Figure 5-7C). Taste cells are innervated by branches of the facial, glossopharyngeal, and vagus nerves (cranial nerves VII, IX, and X, respectively). The tactile and temperature receptors of the mouth, tongue, and pharynx are innervated by the trigeminal nerve (cranial nerve V).

        (i) The taste buds in the **anterior two-thirds** of the tongue are innervated by lingual branches of the **facial nerve;** the lingual nerve, which branches from the chorda tympani, is part of the facial nerve. The cell bodies are located in the geniculate ganglion, and the nerve terminals end in the **nucleus solitarius** of the medulla.

        (ii) The taste buds in the **posterior third** of the tongue are innervated by the **glossopharyngeal nerve.** The cell bodies lie in the superior and inferior ganglia of this nerve. The fibers relating to taste sensation terminate in the nucleus solitarius.

        (iii) Taste receptors in the **pharyngeal aspect** of the tongue and on the hard palate, soft palate, and epiglottis are innervated by fibers of the **vagus nerve.** The cell bodies are located in the superior and inferior ganglia of the vagus nerve and terminate in the nucleus solitarius.

    (b) **Regeneration.** Each taste cell has a life cycle of only a few days.

        (i) The degenerating taste cell is replaced by a cell that arises from the basal epithelial cells.

        (ii) Contact with the afferent neuron is required to maintain the taste cell cycle. Nerve transection causes the taste cells to atrophy.

2. **Papillae.** There are four types of papillae. Three contain taste buds, and one contains mechanical receptors.

    a. **Gustatory papillae** (see Figure 5-7C)

      (1) **Fungiform papillae** are located in the anterior two-thirds of the tongue. There are 8–10 taste buds on each papilla.

      (2) **Circumvallate papillae** are arranged in a V-shaped row of 7–12 on the posterior part of the tongue. Each papilla has approximately 200 taste buds. These taste buds are located on the sides of these large structures.

      (3) **Foliate papillae,** located on the lateral border of the tongue anterior to the circumvallate papillae, have numerous taste buds.

    b. **Mechanical papillae. Filiform papillae** are not gustatory structures. However, they may play a role in breaking up food particles.

C. **Transduction.** Taste receptors respond to taste stimuli in a variety of ways.

1. **Sweet-tasting substances** depolarize taste cells by:

    a. **Opening Na^+-selective channels.** These channels are blocked by amiloride and are similar to Na^+ channels found in renal and other epithelial cells.

    b. **Activating adenylate cyclase.** The cAMP produced by adenylate cyclase leads to the closing of K^+-selective channels.

2. **Bitter-tasting substances** stimulate the production of inositol triphosphate (IP_3) by taste cells. IP_3 increases intracellular Ca^{2+} levels, which leads to the release of synaptic transmitter and the activation of the gustatory nerve fiber.

3. **Salty-tasting substances** depolarize taste cells by activating an amiloride-sensitive Na^+ channel. No specific Na^+ receptor has been identified.

4. **Sour-tasting substances** (e.g., citric acid) depolarize taste cells directly by raising the intracellular H^+ ion concentration, which blocks K^+ channels.

D. **Encoding.** Each nerve fiber in the gustatory nerves responds to more than one taste stimulus. However, each fiber responds best to one of the four primary taste qualities. Therefore, the coding of a gustatory sensation is not a simple, labeled-line, chemical sensory system; instead, it **depends on the pattern of nerve fibers** activated by a particular stimulus.

Chapter 6

Vision and Audition

I. VISION

A. **Introduction.** A mental image of the external world is created by the visual system.

   1. An **image is formed on the retina** by the refractive surfaces of the eye.

   2. The **light energy is transduced into an electrical signal** by the rods and the cones.

   3. The **information needed to create the mental image is encoded** by the neurons within the retina. It is used by the **visual cortex** to create the visual perception described as "seeing."

B. **Image formation**

   1. **Principles of image formation. Convex (converging) lenses** form real images of illuminated objects (Figure 6-1).

     a. **Converging power.** The converging power of a lens is a measure of how well the lens bends light rays passing through it. Converging power is measured in **diopters.**

       (1) **Focal point.** When parallel rays of light pass through a lens, they converge at the focal point.

       (2) **Focal distance.** The distance from the lens to the focal point is called the focal distance.

       (3) **Measurement.** The converging power of the lens in **diopters** is equal to the reciprocal of the focal length when the focal length is measured in meters:

$$P = \frac{1}{f}$$

       where P = the converging power in diopters (D) and f = the focal distance in meters (m).

     b. **Image formation by the eye.** The eye forms an image of an object on its retina by the process of **accommodation**—adjusting the refractive power of its lens (Figure 6-2).

       (1) **Relaxed eye.** Normally, the image of a distant object [6 m (20 ft) from the eye] is focused on the retina without accommodation. In this case, the rays of light are practically parallel to each other, and therefore, the image is formed at the focal point.

       (2) **Accommodated eye.** When objects are moved closer to the eye, the lens must accommodate (increase its power of refraction, decrease its focal length) to keep the image in focus. The **power of accommodation** is the difference between the power of the eye before and after accommodation.

       (3) **Lens formula.** The relationship between the object distance, the image distance and the focal distance is given by the lens formula:

$$P = P\frac{1}{o} + \frac{1}{i} = \frac{1}{f}$$

       where o, i, and f are the object, image, and focal distances, respectively (in meters) and P is the power of the lens (in diopters).

   2. **Eye structures.** The **cornea** and **lens** provide the converging power of the eye.

     a. The **cornea** is the **avascular, transparent outer surface** of the eye.

       (1) **Refractive power.** The cornea is responsible for approximately two-thirds of the refractive power of the eye, and its refractive power **cannot be altered physiologically.**

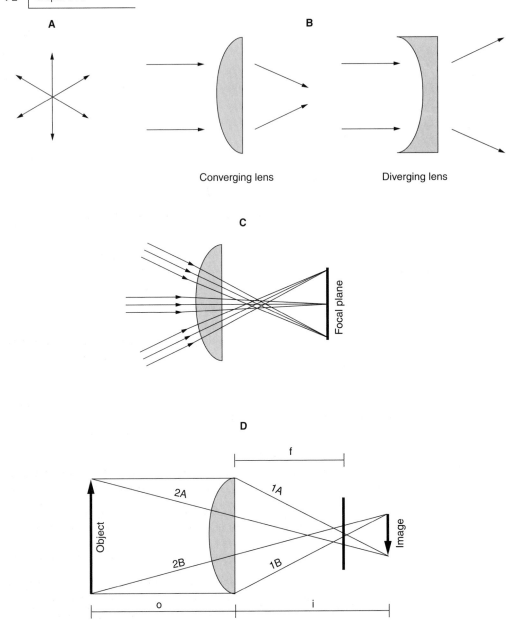

FIGURE 6-1. Fundamental optical principles. (*A*) Although light rays travel in all directions from a source of light, only those passing through the lens are used to form an image. (*B*) Converging lenses focus all rays of light coming from a point on an object onto a single image point. Diverging lenses cannot form an image. (*C*) If the rays of light are parallel to each other when they enter a converging lens, they will converge at the focal point. (*D*) If the rays of light are diverging from each other when they enter the lens, the image will be formed behind the focal plane. The relationship between the object distance (o), focal distance (f), and image distance (i) is given by the lens formula.

    (2) Transparency. The absence of blood vessels in the cornea allows light to pass through unhindered. Because it has no blood vessels, the cornea must receive O_2 and nutrients via diffusion through the **aqueous humor.**

        (a) The aqueous humor is continuously secreted into the eye from the capillaries of the ciliary body in the posterior chamber, passes through the pupil into the

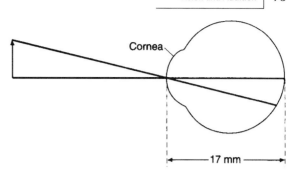

FIGURE 6-2. Reduced eye model. The converging power of the unaccommodated lens (approximately 20 D) and the cornea (approximately 40 D) are combined into a single refractive surface having a converging power of 58.8 D and a focal distance of 17 mm. The axial length of the reduced eye is 17 mm, so images of distant objects (i.e., objects > 20 ft away) are formed on the retina.

anterior chamber, and returns to the circulation through the trabecular mesh located where the iris and cornea meet.

    (b) Increased formation of aqueous humor or blockage of outflow can cause intraocular pressure to rise above its normal value of 10–20 mm Hg. Increased intraocular pressure is called **glaucoma** and can lead to blindness if not treated.

  b. The **lens,** like the cornea, is avascular and transparent.

    (1) Refractive power. Unlike the cornea, the **refractive power** of the lens is **under physiologic control** (see I B 3).

    (2) Transparency. As an individual ages, the lens develops opacities called **cataracts.** Normal vision can be restored by surgically removing the opaque lens and replacing it with a plastic lens.

3. Image focusing

  a. Accommodation reflex. Objects closer than 6 m (20 ft) can be focused on the retina by the accommodation reflex, which has three components.

    (1) Bulging of the lens. Contraction of the ciliary muscle releases tension on the zonular fibers. The elastic capsule surrounding the lens retracts, increasing the convexity (and thus the power) of the lens.

    (2) Pupillary constriction. By reducing the area through which light can enter the eye, **spherical aberration** is reduced. Reducing spherical aberration increases the **depth of focus** (i.e., the degree to which the image can form in front of or behind the retina and still appear to be in focus). **Squinting** also increases the depth of focus.

    (3) Convergence. The gaze of the two eyes shifts toward the center of the head to keep both eyes focused on the object.

  b. The **near point** and **far point define the range of distances over which a clear image can be formed** by the eye.

    (1) The **near point** is the nearest point at which an object can be seen clearly. A typical young adult can increase his or her converging power 12 D from a basic value of 58.8 D. Therefore, at a maximum lens power of 70.8 D, the near point is approximately 8.3 cm from the eye.

    (2) The **far point** is the distance from the eye that an object must be placed so that it can be seen clearly without accommodation. For a normal person, this is 6 m.

    (3) Presbyopia is the loss of accommodative power that occurs with age. As an individual ages, the near point increases, making it difficult to see objects placed close to the eye. Reading glasses are converging lenses that compensate for the loss of accommodation.

  c. Refractive errors, in which distant objects cannot be seen clearly, are caused by variations in the converging power of the cornea, lens, or both.

    (1) Myopia (nearsightedness) results when the focal distance of the eye is less than the axial distance. In this case, the **focal point is in front of the retina;** thus, distant objects are not focused on the retina.

      (a) The object can be seen clearly if it is moved closer to the eye so that the image forms on the retina (i.e., behind the focal point). In severe myopia, the far point may be only 10–15 cm from the eye.

(i) Because the **far point** is close to the eye in myopia, objects must be brought near to the eye to be seen clearly (hence the term "nearsightedness").

(ii) Myopes have **near points** very close to the eye. Thus, they are able to do fine work without magnifying glasses.

(b) A **diverging lens** can be placed in front of a myopic eye, reducing its converging power. When wearing such a lens, the myope can see distant objects clearly.

(2) **Hyperopia (farsightedness)** results when the focal distance of the eye is greater than the axial distance. In this case, the **focal point is behind the retina;** thus, distant objects are not focused on the retina.

(a) A distant object can be seen clearly if the hyperope increases his or her converging power by accommodating. If the degree of hyperopia is minimal, the person is usually unaware of the refractive error. However, if a large amount of **accommodation** is required to focus distant objects, the constant contraction of the ciliary muscle causes **eye strain.**

(b) Because some degree of accommodation is used to see distant objects, less is available for near vision. Thus, the near point in hyperopes is farther from the retina than normal. That is, objects must be placed farther from the eyes to be seen clearly (hence the term "farsightedness").

(c) A **converging lens** can be placed in front of a hyperopic eye to increase its converging power. When wearing a converging lens, a hyperope can see distant objects clearly without accommodation.

(3) **Astigmatism** results from an **uneven cornea.** Normally, the cornea has a spherical surface; in astigmatism, it has more of an egg-shaped surface. As a result, the power of the lens is different in different axes.

(a) **Images** formed with an astigmatic lens **are distorted.** For example, a point is seen as a line, and a line appears to have a halo on either side of it.

(b) **Cylindrical lenses** can be worn by an astigmatic individual. These lenses increase converging power in only one axis, allowing the lens system to behave as a spherical surface.

C. **Energy transduction.** The **rods** and **cones** (Figure 6-3) are the photoreceptors of the eye.

1. **Morphology.** Both cell types have similar parts.
   a. An **inner segment containing the nucleus, abundant mitochondria,** and **synaptic vesicles**
   b. An **outer segment containing membranous disks**
      (1) The membranous disks are **continuously formed at the base of the outer segment and migrate toward the apex,** where they are sloughed off.
      (2) The membranous disks **contain a visual pigment,** called **rhodopsin,** which absorbs light rays.
         (a) **Rhodopsin** consists of a protein called **opsin** and a light-absorbing analogue of vitamin A (retinol) called **11-*cis* retinal** (Figure 6-4A).
         (b) The amino acid composition of opsin determines the wavelength of light absorbed by the photopigment.
            (i) **Rods** contain a **single type of opsin.** The gene encoding for rod opsin is located on chromosome 3.
            (ii) **Cones** contain **three types of opsins (blue, green, or red,** depending on the portion of the visual spectrum they absorb best). The genes for the red and green pigments are located on the X chromosome; red–green color blindness is sex-linked. The gene for the blue pigment is located on chromosome 7.

2. **Phototransduction.** When light is absorbed by rhodopsin, a photoisomerization occurs in which the 11-*cis* retinal is isomerized to all-*trans* retinal.
   a. **Activation of rhodopsin.** Following the formation of all-*trans* retinal by light, rhodopsin undergoes a series of spontaneous transformations leading to the formation of **metarhodopsin II,** the active form of rhodopsin.

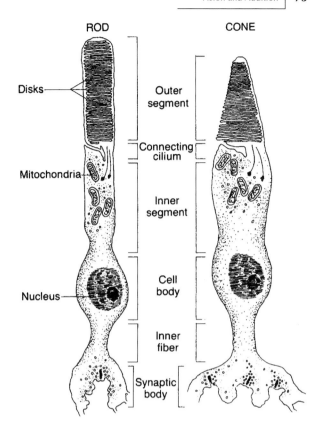

FIGURE 6-3. Morphology of rod and cone receptor cells. Cones, which are responsible for color perception and high visual acuity, are found in the fovea. Rods, which are responsible for night vision, are located in the peripheral retina.

ROD   CONE

Disks

Outer segment

Connecting cilium

Mitochondria

Inner segment

Nucleus

Cell body

Inner fiber

Synaptic body

   b. The **visual cycle.** Metarhodopsin II ultimately splits into opsin and all-*trans* retinal. Some of the isolated all-*trans* retinal is converted to all-*trans* retinol (vitamin A). An isomerase in the pigment epithelium reconverts the all-*trans* forms of retinal and retinol to the 11-*cis* form. After reattachment of the 11-*cis* retinal to opsin, it is once again available to capture a photon of light.

   c. **Excitation of photoreceptors.** Metarhodopsin II activates a G protein, which, in turn, activates a phosphodiesterase that hydrolyzes cyclic guanosine monophosphate (cGMP). The reduction in cGMP concentration leads to the closing of Na^+ channels and the hyperpolarization of the cell (Figure 6-4B).

3. Electrophysiology

   a. Rods and cones are **depolarized** in the **dark.** Their resting membrane potential is approximately -40 mV.

      (1) The low resting membrane potential results from the **high Na^+ conductance of the outer segment** (see Figure 6-4A).

         (a) Na^+ flows into the cell through Na^+ channels in the outer segment and is transported out of the inner segment by Na^+–K^+ pumps.

            (i) **Na^+ channels** are **maintained in the open state** by **cGMP,** which is synthesized from guanosine triphosphate (GTP) by guanylate cyclase. When cGMP binds to the Na^+ channel, the channel opens. That is, in this case, cGMP acts by activating the channel directly, not by activating a protein kinase.

            (ii) The numerous mitochondria in the inner segment provide the large quantities of adenosine triphosphate (ATP) required to maintain the high Na^+–K^+ pump activity.

      (2) **Neurotransmitter** is released from the photoreceptors as long as the cells are depolarized.

A. Membrane depolarized

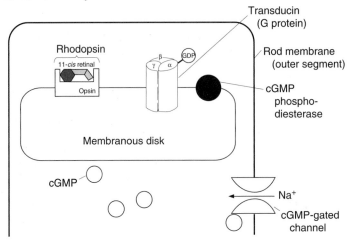

B. Membrane hyperpolarized

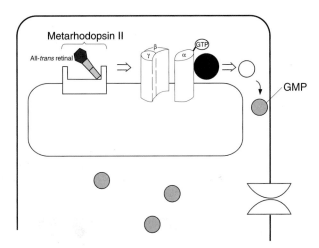

FIGURE 6-4. (*A*) In the dark, Na$^+$ channels are kept open by cyclic guanosine monophosphate (cGMP) and the membrane is depolarized. (*B*) When rhodopsin absorbs light, the 11-*cis* retinal is converted to its more stable isomer, all-*trans* retinal. The photoisomerization of 11-*cis* retinal to all-*trans* retinal produces metarhodopsin II, the active form of rhodopsin. Metarhodopsin II activates transducin, a G protein located within the outer segment disk membrane. The activated transducin activates a cGMP phosphodiesterase that hydrolyzes cGMP, forming guanosine monophosphate (GMP). As the concentration of cGMP falls, cGMP dissociates from the Na$^+$ channels, causing them to close. The reduced Na$^+$ conductance causes the receptor to hyperpolarize. GDP = guanosine diphosphate; GTP = guanosine triphosphate.

  b. Photoreceptors are **polarized** by **light.** Hydrolysis of cGMP (see I C 2 c) leads to the closing of the Na$^+$ channels and **hyperpolarization,** which causes synaptic release to decrease or stop.

 4. Functions. The rods and cones perform different sensory functions.
  a. The **rods,** which are **more sensitive to light** than cones, are responsible for **night vision.**
   (1) Rods can **absorb more light** than cones.

      (a) Rods contain more rhodopsin in their outer segments.

      (b) Rods can detect light entering the eye from any direction, whereas cones respond only to light directly along their axis.

    (2) Rods **produce a greater response for each photon of light absorbed.**

    (3) Rods **remain polarized for a longer time** than cones. Therefore, the response produced by several photons of light can be added together to create a larger response in rods than in cones.

  b. The **cones,** which have **three different photopigments,** are responsible for **daylight, high acuity,** and **color vision.**

    (1) Cones can **respond to light over a large range of intensities** (e.g., from that produced by a light bulb to that produced by sunlight on a snow-covered field).

    (2) Cones achieve **high visual acuity** because they are **concentrated in the center of the retina** (where the clearest images are formed), they **do not respond to scattered light,** and their **response to light is brisk.** That is, the same properties that reduce the cones' sensitivity to light enhance their ability to produce an image of high quality.

    (3) **Color vision** is achieved by combining the information contained in cones, which absorb light in the red, green, or blue range of the visual spectrum (see I E 5 a,b).

D. **Encoding of the visual stimulus.** Cells in the **retina** perform this function.

  1. Morphology of the retina (Figure 6-5). The retina is a thin sheet of cells consisting of

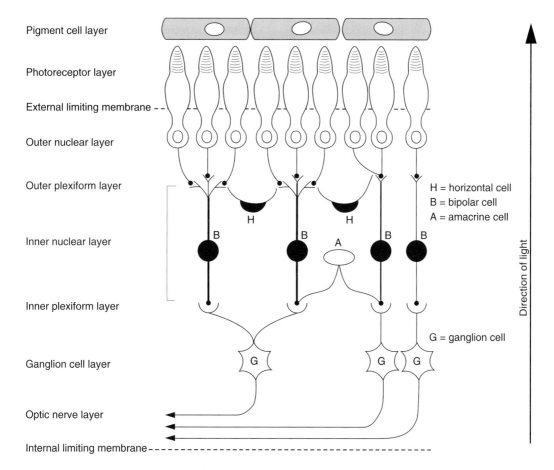

FIGURE 6-5. Organization of the retina. Photoreceptors converge on bipolar cells, which converge on ganglion cells. All of the receptors that convey information to a ganglion cell are part of that ganglion cell's receptive field.

three cellular and two synaptic layers. Light has to pass through all of the retinal layers before it reaches the photoreceptors.

a. The **pigment epithelium** is a single sheet of melanin-containing epithelial cells.

    (1) Functions

        (a) Light absorption. Most of the light reaching the back of the eye is absorbed by the pigment epithelium so that light scattering does not degrade visual acuity.

        (b) Phagocytosis. The membranous disks and other debris sloughed from the photoreceptors is phagocytosed by the cells of the pigment epithelium.

        (c) Vitamin A (retinol) storage. The pigment epithelium serves as a repository for vitamin A, which is needed for the synthesis of rhodopsin.

    (2) Clinical significance. Retinal detachment (i.e., detachment of the rest of the retina from the pigment epithelium) can lead to **blindness.** However, reattachment can be accomplished by laser surgery.

b. Cellular layers

    (1) Outer nuclear layer (ONL). The **nuclei of the photoreceptors** form the ONL.

    (2) Inner nuclear layer (INL). The **nuclei of the retinal neurons (i.e., bipolar, horizontal, and amacrine cells)** form the INL.

    (3) Ganglion cell layer. The **third cellular layer** of the retina is the ganglion cell layer, where **axons** of the ganglion cells **form the optic nerve.**

c. Synaptic layers

    (1) Outer plexiform layer (OPL). Synaptic connections between the photoreceptors and the horizontal and bipolar cells occur within the OPL.

    (2) Inner plexiform layer (IPL). Synapses between the bipolar and ganglion cells, as well as the amacrine and ganglion cells, occur in the IPL.

2. Receptive fields. Each ganglion cell collects information from a group of receptors called its receptive field (Figure 6-6).

a. Circular region. The cells within the receptive field of each ganglion cell are contained within a circular region of the retina. In the fovea (where visual acuity is greatest), the receptive field may be only 10 μm in diameter. Near the periphery of the retina, receptive fields are much larger (up to 1 mm in diameter).

    (1) The cones in the center of the receptive field (the **field center**) convey information **directly** to the ganglion cell by synapsing with **bipolar cells.**

    (2) The cones at the periphery of the receptive field (the **field surround**) reach the ganglion cell **indirectly** through **horizontal cells.**

b. Receptive field properties

    (1) The receptive fields of ganglion cells are organized into **center-surround antagonistic regions** (Figure 6-6A).

    (2) The properties of the center-surround receptive fields result from the synaptic organization of the retina.

        (a) Illuminating the center of an on-center receptive field increases ganglion cell firing, and illuminating the center of an off-center receptive field decreases ganglion cell firing.

            (i) In an on-center receptive field, glutamate released by cones depolarizes bipolar cells by **opening cation selective channels** (Figure 6-6B).

            (ii) In an off-center receptive field, glutamate released by cones hyperpolarizes bipolar cells through a G protein–mediated second messenger system that either **opens K+-selective ion channels** or **closes Na+-selective ion channels** (Figure 6-6C).

        (b) Illuminating the surround of an on-center receptive field decreases ganglion cell firing, and illuminating the surround of an off-center receptive field increases ganglion cell firing (Figure 6-6D). The cones within the surround of a receptive field stimulate horizontal cells.

            (i) The horizontal cells synapse with the axons of cones within the center of the receptive fields and release **γ-aminobutyric acid (GABA).**

            (ii) GABA **produces both its inhibitory effect** (on on-center bipolar cells)

and its excitatory effect (on off-center bipolar cells) **by depolarizing cone axons,** thus decreasing the amount of transmitter they release (i.e., GABA returns cones to the membrane potential they were at before being activated by light).

(c) Illuminating both the **center and surround of an on-center or an off-center receptive field has little or no effect on ganglion cell firing** (Figure 6-6E).

3. **Visual pathways.** Visual information is relayed from the ganglion cell to the cortex by cells within the **lateral geniculate nucleus.**

   a. **Optic tract.** The axons of the ganglion cells are rearranged at the **optic chiasm.** Axons from the right half of each retina project to the **right lateral geniculate,** and axons from the left half of each retina pass to the **left lateral geniculate.** This means that fibers of the **temporal** retina on each side pass through the chiasm without crossing, while fibers of the **nasal** half of each retina decussate at the chiasm.

   b. **Lateral geniculate nucleus.** The input from each eye remains segregated in the lateral geniculate; uncrossed fibers go to layers 2, 3, and 5, and crossed fibers go to layers 1, 4, and 6. Neurons in the lateral geniculate also retain the on-center, off-surround (or the off-center, on-surround) organization of the ganglion cells.

E. **Visual perception.** The receptive field organization of the retina and cortex are used to encode information about intensity, contrast, form, and color and depth of the visual image.

1. **Intensity.** Light intensity is encoded by the firing rate of ganglion cells.

   a. **At very low light levels, only rods are active.** Rods are not organized into center-surround receptive fields, Therefore, every rod that is stimulated by light contributes to the overall response.

   b. **At high light levels, only cones are involved** in the stimulation of ganglion cells. The overall response is attenuated by the receptors in the surround of the receptive field.

2. **Contrast.** Contrast is encoded when one ganglion cell is stimulated and its neighbor is inhibited.

   a. Neighboring cells respond in opposite ways at the border between light and dark areas of the image (Figure 6-7).

      (1) In the lighted portions of the border between light and dark, the center of the receptive field is illuminated, while its surround is not. Therefore, the on-center ganglion cell activity is increased.

      (2) In the darkened portions, the surround of the receptive field is illuminated, while its center is not. Therefore, the on-center ganglion cell activity is decreased.

   b. When both the center and surround of the receptive field are totally in the illuminated or darkened portions of the image, no change in ganglion cell activity occurs.

3. **Form.** Information about form is decoded by cells within the primary visual cortex (area 17) that are referred to as **simple cells.**

   a. Simple cells have **center-surround receptive fields.** Unlike the circular receptive fields of ganglion cells, simple cell receptive fields are **rectangularly organized.**

   b. Ganglion cells from each area of the retina project, via the lateral geniculate nucleus, to a group of cortical cells organized into **columns.** Each column contains simple cells oriented in a particular direction.

      (1) The orientation of the simple cells in a small (approximately 50 μm wide) columnar region of the cortex is the same.

      (2) Adjacent columns have orientations that are approximately 10° apart; therefore, lines of any angle at any point on the retina are decoded by a specific column of cells in the cortex.

4. **Depth.** Information about depth is provided by cells within extrastriate regions of the visual cortex (areas 18 and 19). The cells responsible for depth perception are organized into **hypercolumns.**

   a. **Ocular-dominant cells** are **binocular** (i.e., they receive input from both eyes). The binocular ocular-dominant cells in the hypercolumns fuse the images.

A. Center-surround organization

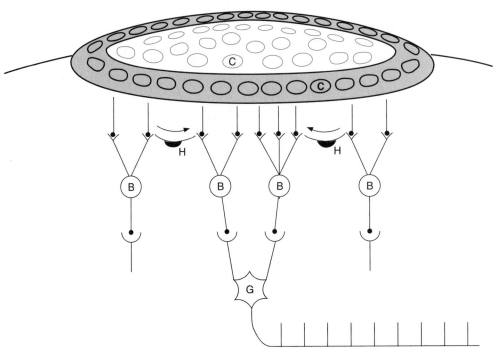

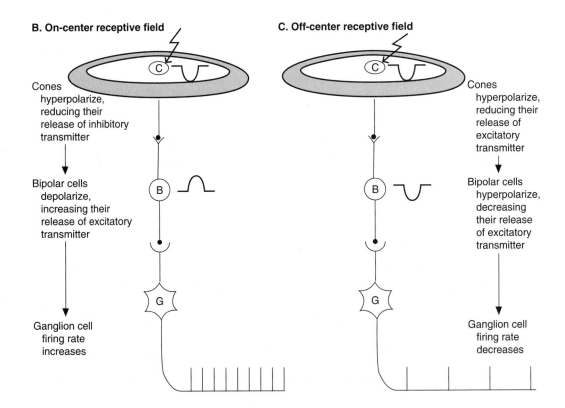

B. On-center receptive field

Cones
hyperpolarize,
reducing their
release of inhibitory
transmitter

↓

Bipolar cells
depolarize,
increasing their
release of excitatory
transmitter

↓

Ganglion cell
firing rate
increases

C. Off-center receptive field

Cones
hyperpolarize,
reducing their
release of
excitatory
transmitter

↓

Bipolar cells
hyperpolarize,
decreasing
their release
of excitatory
transmitter

↓

Ganglion cell
firing rate
decreases

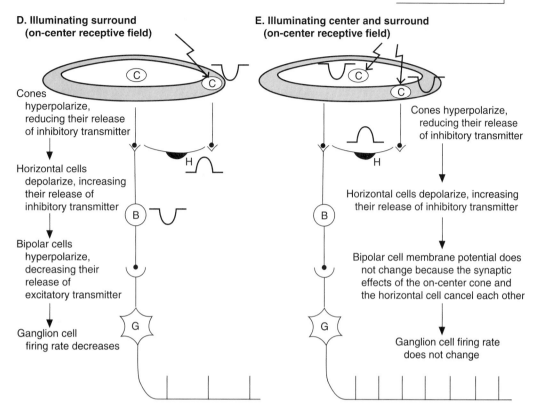

FIGURE 6-6. (*A*) Center-surround organization of a ganglion cell. Those cones that converge on a ganglion cell (*unshaded circles*) are part of the field center. Those cones that affect ganglion cells via horizontal cells (*shaded circles*) are part of the field surround. The ganglion cell fires at a constant rate, even when the retina is not exposed to light. (*B,C*) On- and off-center receptive fields occupy overlapping regions of the retina so that light striking any region of the retina will cause on-center cones to increase their firing rate and off-center cones to decrease their firing rate. The intensity of the light stimulus is signaled by the difference in firing rate between on- and off-center receptive fields. (*D*) Illuminating cones in the field surround of an on-center receptive field decrease the ganglion cell firing rate. (*E*) When light strikes the center and surround of an on-center receptive field, it produces opposite effects on the cones. The cones in the center of the field are hyperpolarized by light. At the same time, the horizontal cells that were activated by light striking the cones in the surround depolarize the cones in the center of the field. As a result, there is no change in transmitter release by the cones, no change in bipolar cell membrane potential, and no change in the ganglion cell firing rate. B = bipolar cell; C = cone; G = ganglion cell; H = horizontal cell.

    b. The amount of disparity between the images perceived by each eye is used to assign depth to the image. **Depth perception** (i.e., **stereopsis**) is possible because each eye perceives a slightly different image.

5. Color. The cells responsible for color perception are organized into **oblong regions** called **blobs.** The blobs are located **within the hypercolumn** of cells that decode form and depth.

    a. Ganglion cells relaying information about color to the lateral geniculate nucleus respond oppositely to red and green light; therefore, they are called **color-opponent cells.**

    b. Cortical cells interpret the information received from the lateral geniculate to assign color to each region of the image formed on the retina. For example, if green center and red center cortical cells are equally excited, the color assigned that region of the cortex is yellow.

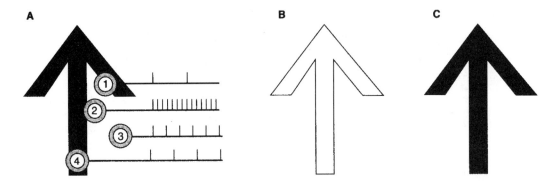

FIGURE 6-7. (*A*) Receptive fields of four ganglion cells are represented on an area of the retina covered by an image of a black arrow. When the center of an on-center receptive field is covered by a dimmer portion of the image than its surround (receptive field 1), the ganglion cell decreases its firing rate. When the center of an on-center receptive field is covered by a brighter portion of the image than its surround (receptive field 2), the ganglion cell increases its firing rate. If both the center and surround are illuminated equally (receptive fields 3 and 4), the ganglion cell's firing rate does not change. The ganglion cell associated with receptive field 3 has a slightly higher firing rate because it is in the light. (*B*) Because only the ganglion cells on the border of the arrow display a change in activity, only the outline of the arrow is transmitted to the cortex. (*C*) The brain creates the correct image of the arrow by assuming that the level of illumination does not change within or outside the borders of the arrow.

     c. Color blindness results from the absence of the gene that codes for either the red, green, or blue opsin.
        (1) Red–green color blindness results from the inability to synthesize either red or green pigment. This genetic defect is sex-linked. Approximately 9% of the male population has some sort of red or green color deficit.
        (2) Blue color blindness is very rare.

II.   AUDITION.
The detection of distant sounds may serve to warn of impending danger or to localize friends. But most importantly, audition allows social communication.

A. **Structure of the ear.** Sound waves must travel through the **three divisions** of the ear, the **external, middle,** and **inner ear** (Figure 6-8), before reaching the auditory receptor cells within the organ of Corti.
    1. The **external ear** consists of the **pinna** (auricle) and the **external auditory canal.**
      a. Pinna. By transforming the sound field, the convoluted pinna **helps identify sound sources.**
        (1) In **lower animals,** the cartilaginous pinna can be moved by muscular action in the direction of a sound source to collect sound waves for the receptor organ.
        (2) In **humans,** these muscles have little action, but the shape of the pinna aids in discerning the source of a sound (e.g., in front of versus behind the head).
      b. The **external auditory canal** extends from the pinna to the tympanic membrane of the middle ear. Its outer portion is cartilaginous and its inner portion is osseous.
    2. The **middle ear (tympanic cavity)** is an **air-filled** cavity within the temporal bone that contains the **tympanic membrane (eardrum)** and three small bones called the **auditory ossicles (ossicular chain).**
      a. Tympanic membrane. Sound stimuli that pass through the pinna and external auditory canal strike the tympanic membrane, causing it to vibrate.
      b. Auditory ossicles. The vibrating tympanic membrane causes the middle ear bones to vibrate.

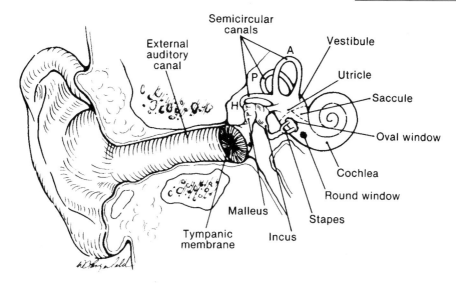

FIGURE 6-8. Major anatomic components of the human ear. The bony labyrinth consists of the saclike otolith organs (i.e., the saccule and utricle) and three semicircular canals: the horizontal (H), anterior (A), and posterior (P) canals.

      (1) The **malleus** resembles a **mallet.** The manubrium (handle) of the malleus is connected to the inner surface of the tympanic membrane (see Figure 6-8).

      (2) The **incus,** which resembles an **anvil,** articulates with the head of the malleus (see Figure 6-8).

      (3) The **stapes** looks like a **stirrup.** The head of the stapes articulates with the incus, and the oval footplate contacts the membrane of the oval window of the cochlea (see Figure 6-8).

  3. The **inner ear** is a **fluid-filled** cavity within the temporal bone that contains the **vestibular** and **auditory receptor apparatuses.**

    a. The **vestibular receptors** are contained within the **saccule, utricle,** and **semicircular canals** and are described in Chapter 7.

    b. The **auditory receptors** are contained within the **cochlea.**

      (1) Cochlear organization. The cochlea is a spiral tube which, in humans, has two and one-half turns (see Figure 6-8).

        (a) Two membranes divide the cochlea into **three compartments** (Figure 6-9).

          (i) **Reissner's membrane** separates the **scala vestibuli** from the **scala media.**

          (ii) The **basilar membrane** separates the **scala tympani** from the **scala media.**

        (b) Helicotrema. Reissner's membrane and the basilar membrane meet near the apex of the cochlea, allowing the scala tympani and scala vestibuli to join. The junction between the two scalae is called the helicotrema.

        (c) Fluid composition

          (i) **Perilymph,** the fluid within the **scala tympani** and **scala vestibuli,** is similar to extracellular fluid (ECF) in that it is high in Na^+ and low in K^+.

          (ii) **Endolymph,** the fluid within the **scala media,** is more like **intracellular fluid (ICF)** in that it is high in K^+ and low in Na^+. Endolymph is secreted by the stria vascularis, which covers the lateral wall of the scala media.

        (d) The vibrating middle ear bones cause the fluid within the cochlea to vibrate. The vibrating fluid ultimately stimulates the auditory receptors (i.e., the hair cells in the organ of Corti).

          (i) The footplate of the stapes contacts the cochlea at the **oval window,** which is the membrane-covered opening of the **scala vestibuli.**

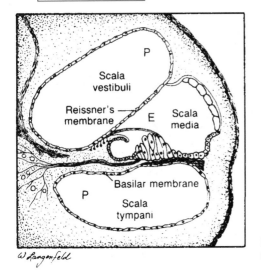

FIGURE 6-9. The components of the cochlea shown in cross-section. P = perilymph; E = endolymph.

     (ii) When the sound pressure wave impinges on the oval window, the **round window** (i.e., the membrane-covered opening of the **scala tympani**) bulges outward.

     (iii) As the sound energy passes from the scala vestibuli to the scala tympani, it causes the basilar membrane to vibrate, stimulating the organ of Corti.

  (2) The **organ of Corti,** which is situated on top of the basilar membrane, contains **hair (auditory receptor) cells.**

    (a) **Two groups of hair cells** lie on the basilar membrane (Figure 6-10).

      (i) The **inner layer** is a **single row** of hair cells. The inner hair cells are responsible for **fine auditory discrimination.** Over 90% of the auditory nerve fibers innervate these cells.

      (ii) The **outer layer** consists of **three rows** of hair cells. The outer hair cells are responsible for **detecting the presence of sound.** They receive approximately 10% of the auditory nerve fibers.

    (b) The hair cells contain **stereocilia,** which protrude into the overlying **tectorial membrane.**

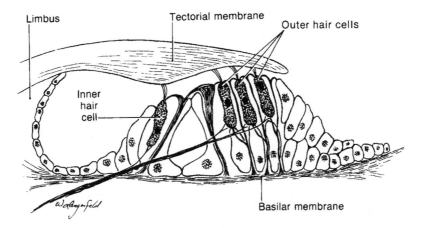

FIGURE 6-10. The organ of Corti, showing the connection between the tectorial membrane and the cilia of the hair cells.

B. **Stimuli. Sound waves** are produced by vibrating objects, which cause alternating phases of compression and rarefaction in the medium surrounding the object. The compressions and rarefactions spread out as a sound wave.

1. **Speed of sound**
   a. In **air,** sound travels at a rate of approximately **330 m/sec** (1100 ft/sec, 700 miles/hr).
   b. In **water,** sound travels much faster, at a rate of approximately **1500 m/sec.**

2. **Frequency** and **amplitude** characterize sound waves (Figure 6-11).
   a. The **frequency of sound** is measured in **hertz (Hz).**
      (1) The **range of human hearing** is approximately 20–20,000 Hz.
      (2) The **range of the average speaking voice** is approximately 2000–5000 Hz.
   b. The **amplitude (intensity) of sound** is measured using a logarithmic scale. The unit of intensity is the **decibel (dB).**
      (1) Decibels are measured using the formula:

$$dB = 20 \cdot \log \frac{P_{sound}}{P_{SPL}}$$

      where dB = the number of decibels, P_{sound} = the pressure of the sound stimulus, and P_{SPL} = the sound pressure level (SPL) at the threshold for human hearing.
      (a) Thus, sound intensities are measured on a ratio scale using a subjective intensity (i.e., the threshold), rather than an arbitrary intensity, as a base.
      (b) The actual SPL intensity is 0.0002 dynes/cm^2.
      (2) The formula can be used to calculate the decibels above threshold for any sound for which the amplitude is known. Sound pressures above 140 dB (10^7 times threshold) are painful and damaging to the auditory receptors.
      (a) The sound pressures used during normal conversation are approximately 1000 times as great as threshold, or 60 dB.
      (b) An airplane produces a sound pressure of approximately 100,000 times that of threshold, or 100 dB.

C. **Conduction of stimulus energy.** The sound stimulus must be amplified if it is to be effectively transferred from the air-filled middle ear to the fluid-filled cochlea.

1. **Impedance mismatching.** Effective transfer of sound energy from an air to a fluid medium is difficult because most of the sound is reflected as a result of the different mechanical (i.e., elastic, resistive, and inertial) properties of the two media.

2. **Impedance matching.** The **middle ear** functions as an impedance matching device, primarily by amplifying the sound pressure.

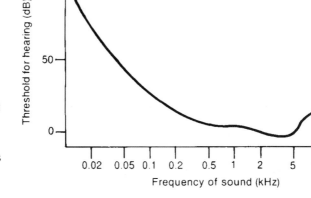

FIGURE 6-11. The minimum audibility curve traces the threshold for hearing at different frequencies in the human hearing range. Maximum sensitivity occurs at about 4 kHz. The actual threshold at this frequency is 0.0002 dynes/cm^2 (or 0 dB).

a. Amplification of sound pressure

(1) Mechanisms. Together, the following effects increase the sound pressure 22-fold (i.e., by 27 dB).

(a) Most amplification occurs because the area of the tympanic membrane (55 mm²) is approximately 17 times greater than the **stapes–oval window surface area.** The size difference means that the force produced by the sound is concentrated over a smaller area, thus amplifying the pressure.

(b) A small additional amount of amplification is obtained by the mechanical advantage that results from the leverage of the **auditory ossicles.**

(2) The ability of the middle ear to amplify some sounds better than others accounts for the shape of the **minimum audibility curve** (see Figure 6-11).

(a) Amplification is greatest for sounds between 2000 and 5000 Hz, the frequencies used for speech.

(b) Sounds below 20 Hz or above 20,000 Hz are not amplified at all.

b. Reduction of sound pressure. The **middle ear muscles** reduce sound pressure amplitude by affecting the mobility and transmission properties of the auditory ossicles, thereby reducing the pressure of sounds reaching the inner ear.

(1) Description. There are **two middle ear muscles.**

(a) The **tensor tympani** is an elongated muscle that inserts on the manubrium of the malleus and is innervated by the **trigeminal nerve** (cranial nerve V).

(b) The **stapedius** is a small muscle that inserts on the neck of the stapes and is innervated by the **facial nerve** (cranial nerve VII).

(2) Significance. These muscles **contract reflexively in response to intense sounds.** Although the middle ear muscles may act to prevent receptors from being damaged by high-intensity sounds, contraction occurs too long after the stimulus to provide much protection. Muscle contraction also occurs just **prior to vocalization and chewing,** which suggests that the middle ear muscles may act to reduce the intensity of the sounds produced by these activities.

D. Conversion of stimulus energy. Auditory transduction occurs in the organ of Corti.

1. Movement of the organ of Corti

a. The in-and-out motion of the oval window produced by the pressure wave is converted into an up-and-down motion of the basilar membrane.

(1) Sound waves entering the inner ear from the oval window spread along the scala vestibuli as a traveling wave.

(2) Most of the sound energy is transferred directly from the scala vestibuli to the scala tympani. Very little of the sound wave ever reaches the helicotrema at the apex of the cochlea.

(3) As the sound energy passes from the scala vestibuli to the scala tympani, it causes the basilar membrane to vibrate.

b. The up-and-down motion of the basilar membrane causes the organ of Corti to vibrate up and down, which, in turn, causes the stereocilia to bend back and forth (Figure 6-12).

(1) The **attachment of the stereocilia to the tectorial membrane** makes it possible for the up-and-down movement of the organ of Corti to be translated into the back-and-forth movement of the stereocilia.

(a) The **bottoms of the hair cells** are anchored to the **basilar membrane,** and the **stereocilia** are connected to the overlying **tectorial membrane.**

(b) Because the **tectorial and basilar membranes** are attached at different points on the limbus (Figure 6-12A), they slide past each other as they vibrate up and down, causing the stereocilia on the hair cells to bend back and forth.

(i) When the organ of Corti moves **up,** the **stereocilia bend away** from the limbus (Figure 6-12B).

(ii) When the organ of Corti moves **down,** the **stereocilia bend toward** the limbus (Figure 6-12C).

(2) Polarization of the stereocilia

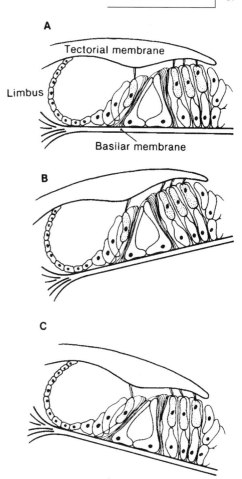

FIGURE 6-12. Up-and-down movement of the basilar and tectorial membrane causes the stereocilia extending from the hair cells to bend back and forth. (*A*) The tectorial and basilar membranes are attached to the limbus at different points. (*B*) When the membranes rotate upward, the tectorial membrane slides forward relative to the basilar membrane, bending the stereocilia away from the limbus. (*C*) When the membranes rotate downward, the stereocilia bend toward the limbus.

  (a) When the organ of Corti moves **upward,** the stereocilia bend **away** from the limbus and they **depolarize.**

  (b) When the organ of Corti moves **downward,** the stereocilia bend **toward** the limbus and they **hyperpolarize.**

 2. Receptor potential. The hair cells are depolarized by the movement of K$^+$ into the cell.

  a. The electrochemical gradient for K$^+$ on the apical surface of the hair cells (where the stereocilia are located; see Figure 6-9) favors the movement of K$^+$ into the cell.

   (1) The **endolymph** contains a high concentration of K$^+$ (135 mEq/L) and is **electrically positive** in comparison to the perilymph.

   (2) Hair cells, like all other cells, contain a high concentration of K$^+$ and are **electrically negative** in comparison to the perilymph. The high intracellular K$^+$ concentration is maintained by Na$^+$–K$^+$ pumps on the basal surface of the hair cell (i.e., the surface that faces the perilymph of the scala tympani).

   (3) Because the endolymph is electrically positive and the hair cell is electrically negative, a **very large potential difference** (in excess of -100 mV) exists across the hair cell membrane.

   (4) The large negative potential and lack of a K$^+$ concentration difference between the inside and outside of the hair cell create a **driving force, pushing K$^+$ into the cell.**

  b. The **gating of the K$^+$ channels** is controlled by the bending of the stereocilia.

   (1) When the **stereocilia bend away** from the limbus, they cause **K$^+$ channels** to **open.** K$^+$ then flows into the cell and the **hair cell depolarizes.**

       (2) When the **stereocilia bend toward** the limbus, they cause **K$^+$ channels** to **close** and the **hair cell hyperpolarizes.**

   c. Release of synaptic transmitter

       (1) When the hair cell depolarizes, a Ca^{2+} channel opens, allowing **Ca^{2+}** to enter the cell. Ca^{2+} initiates the release of a synaptic transmitter, which stimulates the auditory nerve fiber.

       (2) The cell bodies of the auditory nerve fibers are located within the **spiral ganglion.** Their axons join those from the vestibular apparatus to form the **vestibulocochlear nerve (cranial nerve VIII).**

E. Encoding

1. Frequency

   a. Place principle of frequency determination. The frequency of sound that activates a particular hair cell depends on the location of the hair cell along the basilar membrane. The basilar membrane is narrowest and stiffest at the base of the cochlea (near the oval and round windows) and widest and most compliant at the apex of the cochlea (near the helicotrema).

       (1) The energy contained in high-frequency sounds passes through the organ of Corti near the base of the cochlea.

       (2) In contrast, the energy in low-frequency sounds passes through the organ of Corti near the apex of the cochlea.

   b. Encoding of frequency. The auditory nerve fiber activated by a particular sound frequency is similarly dependent on the location of the hair cell it innervates.

       (1) There are about 30,000 nerve fibers in each auditory nerve.

       (2) For low-frequency sounds, the auditory nerve fibers can fire at the same frequency as the sound wave. This mechanism of sensory encoding is called the **volley principle of frequency discrimination.**

       (3) The sound frequency producing the greatest response in an auditory nerve fiber is called the **characteristic frequency** of that nerve fiber.

2. Intensity. The frequency of firing in an auditory nerve fiber increases as the intensity of the sound wave increases. In addition, a larger portion of the basilar membrane is vibrated as the sound intensity increases so that more auditory nerve fibers are activated. Thus, sound intensity is encoded by the frequency of auditory nerve discharge and by the number of auditory nerve fibers that are active.

3. Inhibitory innervation. The hair cells receive a very prominent efferent innervation from the superior olivary nucleus via the olivocochlear bundle. Although such a large pathway probably plays an important role in auditory transduction, its purpose has not been deciphered.

4. Auditory pathways and cortex

   a. Tonotopic organization. Generally, any neuron of the auditory pathway can be tested with tones of different frequencies to determine a characteristic frequency for that cell. Neurons responding best to low-frequency tones are located at one end of a nucleus, while neurons responding best to high-frequency tones are represented at the opposite end of the nucleus. This orderly arrangement of frequency sensitivity, termed tonotopic organization, resembles the retinotopic organization of the visual system and the somatotopic organization of the somatosensory system. The tonotopic map reflects the methodical arrangement of frequency sensitivity along the length of the basilar membrane from base to apex. Tonotopic organization is prominent in the cochlear nuclei but becomes less precise in more rostral structures of the auditory pathway.

   b. Feature detection. Higher auditory centers respond to particular features of sound stimuli. For example, cortical neurons may respond specifically to a shift from high- to low-frequency notes, which is why lesions of the auditory cortex may not impair the ability to discriminate frequency. Instead, lesions of the auditory cortex cause a loss of ability to recognize a patterned sequence of sounds. In addition, the ability to identify the position of a sound source is impaired.

c. **Localization of sound in space.** Detection of the position of a sound source depends on the ability of the central nervous system (CNS) to compare intensity differences and phase differences. A sound source located behind the head, closer to one ear than the other, produces a slightly more intense sound in the near ear than in the remote ear. Sound absorption by the tissues of the head attenuates sound intensity in the remote ear. In addition, at low frequencies there may be phase differences in the sound waves striking the two ears. These minute phase and intensity differences between the two ears are detected and discriminated by the auditory system. The extensive decussation and complex circuitry of the auditory pathway provide the CNS with the information necessary to identify a sound source.

F. **Hearing impairments**

1. **Tinnitus.** This ringing sensation in the ears is caused by irritative stimulation of either the inner ear or the vestibulocochlear nerve.

2. **Deafness.** Two classes of deafness are distinguished based on the location of the abnormality or lesion.
   a. **Conduction deafness** is caused by interference with the transmission of sound to the sensory mechanism of the inner ear. Conduction deafness represents a defect of the external or middle ear.
   b. **Nerve deafness** results from defects of either the inner ear or the vestibulocochlear nerve. Deafness due to a lesion in the CNS structures generally is not found clinically because of the redundancy and bilateral nature of the central auditory pathways.

Chapter 7

Motor Control System

I. COMPONENTS OF THE MOTOR CONTROL SYSTEM (Figure 7-1).

A. **Cerebral cortex.** The cerebral cortex is responsible for generating the idea for voluntary movements and issuing the motor commands for their execution.

B. **Subcortical centers** are responsible for modulating and coordinating the motor commands so that tasks are properly carried out.

1. The **basal ganglia** provide the motor patterns necessary to maintain the postural support required for motor commands to be carried out properly. → *cerebrocerebellum*

2. The **cerebellum** receives information from the motor cortex about the nature of the intended movement and from the spinal cord about how well it is being performed. This information is used to adjust the motor command so that the intended movement is executed smoothly. → *spino-cerebellum*

3. The **brain stem** is the major relay station for all motor commands except those requiring the greatest precision, which are transferred directly from the cortex to the spinal cord. In addition, the brain stem is responsible for maintaining normal body posture during motor activities.

C. **Spinal cord.** The spinal cord contains the final common pathways through which a movement is executed. By selecting the proper motoneurons for a particular task and by reflex-

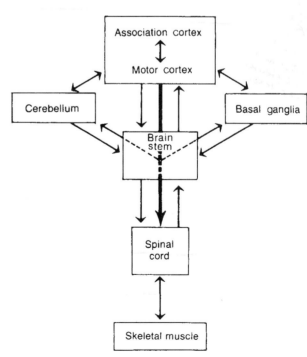

FIGURE 7-1. Diagram illustrating the extensive interconnections between the components of the motor control system. Note that all of the descending pathways except for the pyramidal tract (*thick arrow*) communicate with the spinal cord through the brain stem.

ively adjusting the amount of motoneuron activity, the spinal cord contributes to the proper performance of a motor task.

D. **Receptors** provide sensory feedback to the central nervous system (CNS) that can be used to adjust the motor commands during a movement.

    1. **Proprioceptive information** (i.e., **unconscious information** about the position of the limbs in space and the tension produced by the contracting skeletal muscles) is provided by the **muscle, joint, and skin receptors.**

    2. **Conscious information** about the position of the body and limbs in space is provided primarily by the **visual** and **cutaneous sensory organs.**

II. **MOTOR UNITS.** The motor unit is the functional module used by the motor control system to carry out a movement.

A. **Components.** A motor unit consists of a **motoneuron** and **all the muscle fibers it innervates.**

    1. **Alpha motoneurons** are the final common pathway over which the motor control system coordinates the activity of skeletal muscle fibers.

       a. **Function.** If an alpha motoneuron is stimulated, skeletal muscle fibers contract. If the alpha motoneuron is not stimulated, the skeletal muscle fibers relax. Therefore, each component of the motor control system produces its effect on movement by altering the amount of excitation or inhibition impinging on the alpha motoneurons within the CNS.

       b. **Organization.** The alpha motoneurons are organized into **motoneuron pools.** Gamma motoneurons are randomly interspersed among alpha motoneurons within the pool, and some overlap among neurons from separate motoneuron pools takes place.

          (1) Motoneurons innervating distal muscle are located more laterally within the ventral horn than motoneurons innervating proximal muscles.

          (2) Motoneurons innervating extensor muscles are located more dorsally within the ventral horn than motoneurons innervating flexor muscles.

          (3) Usually, the motoneurons leave the spinal cord in several contiguous ventral roots and then combine into a single motor nerve containing the alpha and gamma motoneurons as well as the Ia, Ib, and II afferent fibers from the muscle [see III B 1 a (2)].

    2. **Muscle fibers.** All of the muscle fibers in a motor unit are of the same physiologic type and are categorized according to their **histochemical** and **contractile characteristics.**

       a. **Fast-twitch fatigable fibers** contract quickly, fatigue easily, and have the following characteristics.

          (1) **Rapid contractile speeds** result from the high myosin–adenosine triphosphatase (ATPase) activity of the cross-bridges and the rapid sequestering of Ca^{2+} by the sarcoplasmic reticulum (SR).

          (2) **Rapid fatigue** occurs because fast-twitch fatigable fibers have few mitochondria and, thus, cannot make use of oxidative metabolism. They rely on glycolysis for their adenosine triphosphate (ATP) supply and fatigue when their glucose stores are depleted.

          (3) **Sparse capillary supply.** Because fast-twitch fatigable fibers do not make use of oxidative metabolism, the growth of surrounding capillaries is limited.

          (4) **Large size.** Although fast-twitch fatigable fibers cannot sustain activity for long periods of time, they can generate large contractile forces. Their large size is not a disadvantage from a diffusional point of view because they do not make use of oxidative metabolism.

       b. **Slow-twitch fibers** contract slowly, are virtually untiring, and have the following characteristics.

(1) Slow contractile speeds result from the low myosin–ATPase activity of the cross-bridges and the slow sequestering of Ca^{2+} by the SR. The long contraction times make summation and tetanus possible at low frequencies of stimulation.

(2) Great resistance to fatigue is a consequence of the ability of slow-twitch fibers to use oxidative metabolism as a primary source of ATP. The low myosin–ATPase activity and slow sequestering of Ca^{2+} by slow-twitch fibers reduce the amount of ATP they require.

(3) Rich capillary supply. O_2 needed by slow-twitch fibers during oxidative metabolism encourages the growth of surrounding capillaries.

(4) Small size. Although slow-twitch fibers cannot produce a large amount of force, they can sustain force for a long time. Their small size allows O_2 to diffuse into the center of the fiber and waste products to diffuse out of the fiber.

   c. Fast fatigue-resistant fibers have characteristics of both fast-twitch fatigable and slow-twitch muscle fibers.

B. Characteristics

1. The motor units within a muscle vary in size from a few muscle fibers to several thousand muscle fibers. Muscles that perform precise movements (e.g., the extraocular muscles or those responsible for finger movements) have smaller motor units than those responsible for large body movements and for maintaining posture.

2. Whenever an alpha motoneuron fires, all of the muscle fibers in its motor unit are activated.

3. The muscle fibers belonging to a single motor unit are dispersed throughout the muscle so that the force they produce is distributed evenly.

C. Recruitment. The orderly recruitment of motor units during a contraction enhances the ability of the motor control system to carry out its task. During the performance of a motor task, the small motor units, because they are more excitable, are recruited before the large ones. This **size principle of motor unit selection** has significant physiologic advantages.

1. **Simplification of motor command structure.** Because of the size principle, the motor cortex does not need to specify the particular motoneuron to be recruited during a movement. Therefore, the number of cortical neurons that are involved in generating a movement is reduced.

   a. Force. To perform a precision movement requiring small amounts of force, it is advantageous to use small motor units. When more force is required, larger motor units must be activated.

      (1) When a small amount of force must be applied, the motor cortex provides a minimal amount of input to the motoneuron pool, activating only the smallest motor units.

      (2) If more force is required, the motor cortex increases its input to the motoneuron pool, and larger motor units are recruited.

   b. Endurance. To perform a task requiring endurance, the smaller, fatigue-resistant motor units must be recruited. When power is required, the larger motor units must be recruited.

      (1) When an endurance movement must be performed, the motor cortex provides a minimal input to the spinal cord, and the smallest, most fatigue-resistant motor units are recruited.

      (2) When the amount of force being generated by the muscle is not sufficient to execute the movement, the motor cortex increases its input and recruits more motor units. In all cases, the most fatigue-resistant fibers are recruited first without requiring that the motor cortex determine which motoneuron to activate.

2. **Development of fatigue resistance.** The relationship between fatigue resistance and muscle fiber size is a consequence of the size principle. A muscle fiber's fatigability can be altered by its activity. Small motor units are recruited first. Thus, they are involved in all movements and, consequently, develop fatigue resistance.

III. **SPINAL CORD REFLEXES** enhance the ability of the motor control system to produce a coordinated movement. A reflex is an automatic response to a stimulus carried out by a relatively simple neuronal network consisting of a receptor, an afferent pathway, and an effector organ. Spinal cord reflexes are categorized according to the receptor from which they originate.

A. **Cutaneous reflexes.** The most important of the cutaneous reflexes is the **withdrawal (flexor, pain) reflex,** which effects the removal of a body part from a painful stimulus.

1. **Receptors** for the withdrawal reflex are the **nociceptors** located on the free nerve endings of Aδ and C fibers.

2. **Effector organs** of the withdrawal reflex are the **skeletal muscles** that cause withdrawal of the limb. Although they are called flexors, these muscles are **flexors in the physiologic, not anatomic, sense.** For example, the muscles that cause the fingers to open to drop a hot coal, although anatomically referred to as extensors, are considered flexors, because they are involved in the withdrawal reflex.

3. **Polysynaptic (multisynaptic) pathway.** Limb withdrawal is produced by a polysynaptic pathway that begins with the stimulation of a cutaneous pain afferent and ends with the firing of the alpha motoneuron that excites flexor muscles.
   a. **Excitation of flexor muscles.** On entering the spinal cord, the pain fibers synapse on many **interneurons.** Some of these convey information to the CNS. Other interneurons contribute to reflex pathways that coordinate the withdrawal of the limb.
      (1) **Afterdischarge** refers to the continuation of reflex withdrawal even after the sensory receptor has stopped firing. Afterdischarge is produced by **reverberating circuits** (i.e., a branch from the axon of one interneuron in the reflex pathway feeds back onto previously excited neurons, reexciting them and prolonging alpha motoneuron firing).
      (2) **Local sign** refers to the ability of the reflex to confine the withdrawal to the portion of the body affected by the noxious stimulus. For example, if an individual accidentally touches a hot stove, it is likely that he or she will jerk only the hand away from the stove.
      (3) **Irradiation** refers to the activation of a large number of muscles when the noxious stimulus is strong enough. For example, if an individual picks up a hot coal, not only will the fingers open to drop it, but the entire arm will withdraw and the individual may even leap away from the fire.
      (4) **Crossed extensor reflex** refers to interneurons that form pathways crossing the spinal cord to innervate the extensor motoneurons on the contralateral side. In the lower limbs, the crossed extensor reflex allows one limb to support the body while the other is raised off the ground.
   b. **Inhibition of the antagonist to the flexor muscle** is produced by a polysynaptic pathway that begins with the stimulation of a cutaneous pain afferent and ends with the inhibition of the alpha motoneuron that innervates the antagonistic muscles. This type of neuronal organization, in which the reflex pathway activating one group of alpha motoneurons also inhibits its antagonistic motoneuron, is quite common within the spinal cord and is called **reciprocal innervation.** By inhibiting the motoneurons that innervate muscles antagonistic to those withdrawing the limb, reciprocal innervation **ensures that the flexion movement is not impeded by contraction of the extensors.**
   c. **Integration of the withdrawal reflex** occurs on the alpha motoneuron, the final common pathway through which all the afferent fibers act. If the excitatory pathways dominate, the alpha motoneuron discharges a train of action potentials; if the inhibitory pathways dominate, the neuron does not fire.
   d. **Characteristics of the withdrawal reflex**
      (1) **Long latency.** The withdrawal reflex has a relatively long latency because the afferent pathway uses small, slowly conducting fibers and involves many synapses.
      (2) **Response outlasts stimulus.** The afterdischarge that results from the parallel path-

ways and reverberating circuits causes the response to outlast the stimulus, keeping the affected limb away from the painful stimulus while the brain determines where to place it next.

(3) **Patterned response.** The crossed extensor reflex produces a patterned response in which the affected limb flexes while the contralateral limb extends.

B. Muscle reflexes. Two important reflexes originate in the muscles: the stretch reflex and the lengthening reaction.

1. The **stretch reflex** causes the reflex contraction of a muscle that is stretched. For example, when the patellar tendon is tapped by a reflex hammer, it stretches the quadriceps muscle. The stretched muscle contracts reflexively, elevating the leg (i.e., the **knee jerk reflex** takes place).

   a. **Receptor.** The receptor for the stretch reflex is the **muscle spindle.** The number of spindles in each muscle depends on the task performed by the muscle. Muscles involved in precision movements contain many more spindles than muscles used to maintain posture. For example, hand muscles have approximately 80 spindles, which is 20% of the number of spindles contained in back muscles weighing 100 times as much. This complex, spindle-shaped, encapsulated receptor contains muscle fibers that have both sensory and motor innervation (Figure 7-2).

   (1) **Intrafusal muscle fibers.** The muscle fibers within the spindle are called **intrafusal muscle fibers,** in contrast to **extrafusal muscle fibers,** which are responsible for generating tension.

   (a) There are **two major types** of intrafusal muscle fibers.

   (i) The **nuclear bag fibers** are 30 μm in diameter and 7 mm in length. Their **nuclei** appear to be **gathered in the center of the cell** as if in a bag. Approximately **2–5** nuclear bag fibers exist in a typical spindle.

   (ii) The **nuclear chain fibers** are 15 μm in diameter and 4 mm in length. Their **nuclei** are **lined up** in a **single file** in the center of the fiber. Approximately **6–10** nuclear chain fibers exist in each spindle.

   (b) The connective tissue surrounding the intrafusal fibers is continuous with that of the extrafusal fibers. As a result, when the extrafusal fiber contracts, the intrafusal fiber is shortened, and when the extrafusal fiber stretches the intrafusal fiber is lengthened. Thus, the **muscle spindle** is **in parallel** with the **extrafusal muscle fibers.**

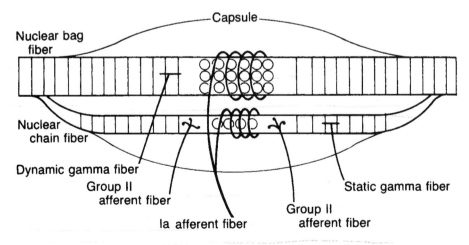

FIGURE 7-2. Diagram of an intrafusal muscle fiber, showing its nuclear bag and nuclear chain fibers. The afferent innervation (Ia and II fibers) and efferent innervation (gamma dynamic and gamma static fibers) of the intrafusal muscle fiber also are illustrated.

    (2) Afferent sensory neurons
        (a) There are **two types** of sensory neurons that emerge from the muscle spindle.
            (i) A **single large fiber,** called a **group Ia fiber (primary ending),** sends branches to **every intrafusal fiber** within the muscle spindle.
            (ii) **Several smaller neurons,** called **group II fibers (secondary endings),** innervate the **nuclear chain fibers.**
        (b) The **primary endings surround the center** of the intrafusal muscle fiber, and the **secondary endings terminate on either side** of the primary endings.
    (3) Efferent fibers. The efferent fibers to the muscle spindle are called **gamma fibers** because their axons belong to the Aγ group of fibers. Gamma efferent fibers **control the sensitivity of the receptors to stretch** [see III B 1 d (2)].
        (a) There are **two types** of gamma fibers.
            (i) **Dynamic gamma fibers** primarily **innervate nuclear bag fibers** and **increase the sensitivity of the Ia afferent fiber to stretch.** That is, the Ia afferent firing rate for a given velocity of stretch is increased by the discharge of the dynamic gamma fibers.
            (ii) **Static gamma fibers** primarily **innervate nuclear chain fibers** and **increase the tonic activity** in the Ia afferent fibers at any given muscle length.
        (b) Some nuclear bag fibers have characteristics similar to those of nuclear chain fibers. These fibers, called static nuclear bag fibers, are innervated by the static gamma fibers.
  b. Effector organs. Both **extensor** and flexor muscles exhibit stretch reflexes, which are elicited routinely during neurologic examinations to test for damage to either the spinal cord or the sensory or motor neurons.
  c. Monosynaptic pathway. The Ia fiber enters the spinal cord through the dorsal root and sends branches to every alpha motoneuron that goes to the muscle from which the Ia originated.
    (1) Monosynaptic pathway. Because of its monosynaptic pathway, the stretch reflex **does not exhibit afterdischarge or radiation.**
    (2) Reciprocal innervation. Like the withdrawal reflex, the stretch reflex is characterized by reciprocal innervation. When a stretch reflex is elicited, the muscle antagonistic to the stretched muscle is inhibited, allowing the agonistic muscle to contract without interference.
    (3) Integration. Like the withdrawal reflex, the **alpha motoneuron** is the final common pathway, serving as both and **integrating center and efferent pathway.**
    (4) Characteristics of the stretch reflex. The rapidly conducting afferent fiber of the stretch reflex allows for a **short latency.**
  d. Role. The stretch reflex is used by the motor control system to aid in the performance of a movement. During activity generated by the motor command center, the Ia fibers from the muscle spindle inform the motor control system about the changes in muscle length and provide the alpha motoneuron with a source of excitatory input in addition to that coming from higher centers.
    (1) Ia afferent discharge increases when the muscle stretches and decreases when the muscle contracts (Figure 7-3).
        (a) In parallel. Because the extrafusal and intrafusal muscle fibers are in parallel, stretching the extrafusal muscle fibers stretches the intrafusal muscle fibers as well.
        (b) Central region. Most of the stretch occurs in the central, more compliant region of the intrafusal fiber, which lacks sarcomeres.
        (c) Deformation. Stretching the central region deforms the primary endings of the Ia afferents, opening ion channels that cause the membrane to depolarize and generate a train of **action potentials.** The action potentials **discharge phasically** at a frequency proportional to the **velocity of stretch** and then adapt to **discharge statically** at a frequency proportional to the **amount of stretch.**
            (i) The central region of the **nuclear bag fiber** stretches rapidly when the muscle is rapidly stretched and then returns to its initial length. Thus, the

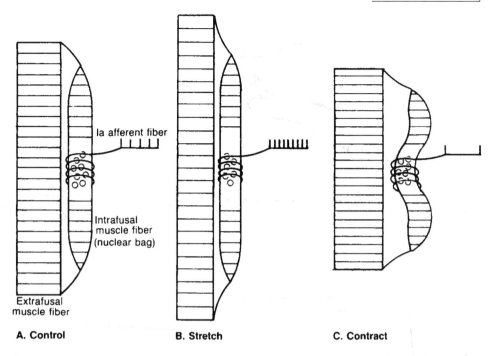

FIGURE 7-3. (*A*) Ia afferent fiber. (*B*) The firing rate of the Ia afferent fiber increases when the extrafusal muscle fiber is stretched because the intrafusal muscle fiber also is stretched. Most of the stretch occurs at the center region of the intrafusal muscle fiber. (*C*) Contraction of the extrafusal muscle fiber compresses the central region of the intrafusal fiber, reducing the deformation of the Ia fiber terminal and reducing the firing rate of the Ia fiber.

Ia listed in TLE as ∆L only, not rate

nuclear bag fiber produces a **phasic discharge** of the Ia afferents that is proportional to the rate of stretch.

(ii) The central region of the **nuclear chain fiber** stretches as the muscle stretches and then maintains its length. Thus, the nuclear chain fiber produces a **static discharge** that is proportional to actual muscle length.

(2) **Gamma efferent discharge.** The decreased rate of Ia afferent discharge that occurs during muscle contraction, called **unloading,** is functionally disadvantageous because the CNS stops receiving information about the rate and extent of muscle shortening. Unloading can be prevented by the activity of the gamma efferent motoneurons (Figure 7-4). The gamma motoneurons cause the sarcomeres of the intrafusal muscle fibers to shorten as the extrafusal muscle fiber shortens. As a result, the central region of the intrafusal muscle fiber remains stretched during muscle contraction, and unloading does not occur.

  (a) When the **dynamic gamma motoneurons** are fired, only the **nuclear bag fibers shorten.** Because the nuclear bag fibers are responsible for the phasic (i.e., velocity-sensitive) portion of the Ia afferent response to stretch, stimulation of the dynamic gamma fibers increases phasic activity without affecting the static activity.

  (b) When the **static gamma motoneurons** are fired, only the **nuclear chain fibers shorten.** Because the nuclear chain fibers are responsible for the static (i.e., length-sensitive) component of the Ia afferent response to stretch, stimulation of the static gamma fibers increases static activity without affecting phasic activity.

(3) **Coactivation of alpha and gamma motoneurons**

  (a) During a **normal movement** (e.g., **lifting a weight**), the motor control system

Ia → ∆L and ∆V of contraction

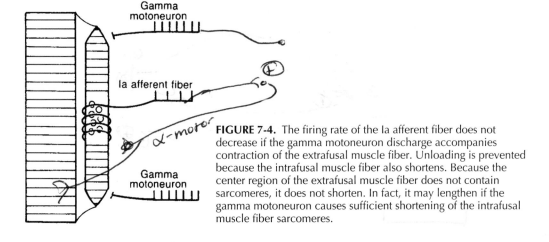

Gamma
motoneuron

la afferent fiber

α-motor

Gamma
motoneuron

FIGURE 7-4. The firing rate of the Ia afferent fiber does not decrease if the gamma motoneuron discharge accompanies contraction of the extrafusal muscle fiber. Unloading is prevented because the intrafusal muscle fiber also shortens. Because the center region of the extrafusal muscle fiber does not contain sarcomeres, it does not shorten. In fact, it may lengthen if the gamma motoneuron causes sufficient shortening of the intrafusal muscle fiber sarcomeres.

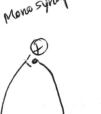

Mono synaptic

α-motor

Ia

coactivates both the alpha and gamma motoneurons, diminishing the amount of unloading that occurs during muscle contraction and allowing the CNS to determine if its motor commands are being carried out.

   (i) As the extrafusal muscle fiber shortens, the intrafusal muscle fiber sarcomeres also shorten.

   (ii) If the two muscle fibers shorten at the same rate, then the central region of the intrafusal fiber is neither compressed nor lengthened, keeping Ia activity at a constant level.

   (iii) The constant level of Ia input to the CNS during a movement indicates that the motor command is being carried out.

(b) If the **weight to be lifted is underestimated** by the CNS, the motor command system does not activate a sufficient number of alpha motoneurons to lift the weight and the extrafusal muscle fibers do not shorten.

   (i) The intrafusal muscle fibers do shorten, however, and because the tendon ends of the muscle cannot move, the central portion of the intrafusal fiber lengthens.

   (ii) Stretching the central region of the fiber causes Ia activity to increase, indicating that the motor command is not being carried out. The CNS uses this information to readjust its command to the spinal cord.

   (iii) Even before the CNS responds to the information provided by the Ia fibers, the Ia activity is used at the spinal cord level to adjust the alpha motoneuron activity to meet the unexpectedly high load. Because the Ia fiber synapses on the alpha motoneuron, its activity increases the excitability of the alpha motoneuron, leading to an increase in the frequency of action potential generation and an increase in muscle force development.

(4) Gamma loop. Theoretically, the CNS is capable of initiating movements directly by stimulating only the gamma motoneurons, using a pathway called the gamma loop (Figure 7-5).

(a) Increasing gamma motoneuron activity causes the intrafusal muscle fiber sarcomeres to shorten, which, in turn, leads to stretching of the central portion of the intrafusal fiber and activation of the Ia fiber. Firing the Ia fibers causes alpha motoneuron activity to increase, which results in an increased amount and force of skeletal muscle activity.

(b) Although the gamma loop can elicit movement on its own, it normally does not do so. However, because of coactivation, the gamma loop is activated during all movements and thus contributes to the excitability and firing rate of the alpha motoneurons.

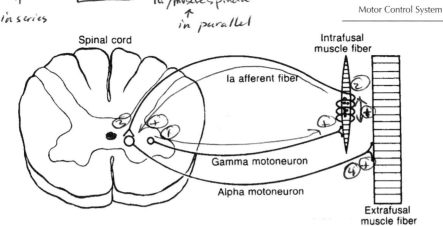

Handwritten annotations above figure:
— GTO —
↑
in series

Muscle
Ia /muscle spindle
↑
in parallel

— GTO —

FIGURE 7-5. The gamma loop increases the firing of the alpha motoneuron during muscle contraction. The loop begins with the gamma motoneuron, which discharges to cause intrafusal muscle fiber contraction. This leads to an increase in Ia afferent fiber activity, which, in turn, causes increased alpha motoneuron discharge via a monosynaptic reflex.

2. The **lengthening reaction** causes inhibition of the alpha motoneurons that innervate muscles that are under tension, allowing them to lengthen.
   a. **Receptor.** The receptors for the lengthening reaction are the **Golgi tendon organs.** These small (0.5–1 mm long), encapsulated receptors are located in the tendons, between the muscles and tendon insertions.
      (1) The Golgi tendon organs have neither muscle fibers nor an efferent innervation.
      (2) The Golgi tendon organs are stretched whenever the muscle contracts and, thus, in contrast to the muscle spindle, are **in series** with the extrafusal muscle fibers.
   b. **Effector organs.** Both **extensor** and **flexor muscles** exhibit the lengthening reaction.
   c. **Disynaptic pathway.** The afferent fiber innervating the Golgi tendon organ is a **group Ib fiber.** It enters the dorsal root and forms a disynaptic pathway, which ends on the alpha motoneurons that send axons to the muscle from which the Ib fiber originated.
      (1) The disynaptic pathway of the Golgi tendon organ is **inhibitory to the alpha motoneuron.** The Ib fiber, like all sensory fibers, releases an excitatory transmitter. To produce inhibition, an **inhibitory interneuron** must be activated.
      (2) The lengthening reaction displays reciprocal innervation but lacks afterdischarge and irradiation.
   d. **Role**
      (1) Historically, the lengthening reaction has been described as a **protective reflex** in which a strong and potentially damaging muscle force reflexively inhibits the muscle, causing the muscle to lengthen instead of trying to maintain the force and risking damage.
      (2) Although the lengthening reaction is a protective reflex, it is now clear that the reflex plays a more important role in **regulating tension during normal muscle activity.** The lengthening reaction is described as **autogenic inhibition,** which indicates that the force generated when the muscle contracts is the stimulus for its own relaxation.

Handwritten annotations in left margin:
Disynaptic
↑GTO
inhibitory IN ⊖(+)
α-motor ⊖

IV. **BRAIN STEM.** The brain stem contains the medulla, pons, midbrain, and parts of the diencephalon. Neuronal circuits within these areas control many physiologic functions (e.g., blood pressure, respiration, body temperature, sleep, wakefulness). In addition, the **reticular formation** and **vestibular nuclei** are **important components of the motor control system.**

A. The **reticular formation** plays an important role in coordinating normal movements.

1. The **motor control centers** within the reticular formation are a relay station for all descending motor commands, except those traveling directly to the spinal cord through the medullary pyramids (e.g., fine movements performed by the distal muscles of the fingers and hands).
   a. The motor control centers **receive and modify the motor commands to the proximal and axial muscles** of the body.
   b. These centers are **responsible for maintaining normal postural tone.**
      (1) Neurons within the pontine reticular formation send axons to the spinal cord in the medial reticulospinal tract and are **excitatory to the alpha and gamma motoneurons that innervate the extensor antigravity muscles.**
      (2) These neurons are prevented from firing too rapidly by **inhibitory input** derived from the cerebral and cerebellar components of the motor control system.
         (a) The amount of inhibition is increased to reduce postural tone and is decreased to enhance postural tone.
         (b) The withdrawal of inhibition, called **release of inhibition,** frequently is used to increase neuronal activity within the CNS.

2. **Lesions**
   a. **Lesions within the motor control centers** of the reticular formation produce the syndrome of **spinal shock.**
      (1) The **initial result** of removing the spinal cord from the control of the brain stem is the **complete loss of reflex activity,** which can last for days in cats and for months in humans.
      (2) **When reflexes return,** they no longer are under the influence of the brain stem and, therefore, **do not follow their normal patterns.** For example, the local sign that characterizes the withdrawal reflex disappears. Instead, even a light touch on the foot can cause activation of all the flexor muscles in the body.
      (3) **Ultimately,** the **excitability of the motoneurons becomes excessive,** causing particular groups of muscles to contract continuously.
   b. **Lesions within the cerebrum** that interfere with inhibitory input to the motor control centers within the reticular formation cause **spasticity.** When discussing the effects of the brain stem on antigravity muscles, the terms spasticity and **rigidity** are used interchangeably. Clinically, however, spasticity and rigidity are not alike. Spasticity refers to the condition in which the stretch reflexes of the antigravity muscles are increased as a result of increased activity of the alpha or gamma motoneurons. Rigidity refers to the condition seen in Parkinson's disease [see V C 4 a (1)], in which there is increased activity in all of the muscles at a joint.
      (1) Without the inhibitory input from the higher centers, the pontine reticular formation fires uncontrollably, subjecting both the alpha and gamma antigravity motoneurons to intense excitation.
         (a) **Excessive firing of the alpha motoneurons** causes the antigravity muscles (i.e., the leg extensors and the arm flexors) to contract continuously.
         (b) **Firing of the gamma motoneurons** activates the gamma loop, increasing discharge of the Ia afferent fibers and reflexively adding to the alpha motoneuron excitation produced by the reticulospinal tract. Because the gamma motoneurons are firing at higher than normal rates, the muscle spindles become more sensitive to stretch. Therefore, spasticity is increased further when the affected muscle is stretched.
      (2) Cutting the dorsal roots reduces the amount of Ia input to the spinal cord and reduces spasticity by eliminating the reflex excitation of the alpha motoneurons.
   c. **Severing the pathways between the cerebrum and cerebellum** and **the motor control centers** within the reticular formation causes **decorticate posturing** or **decerebrate rigidity.**
      (1) **Decorticate posturing** is produced by lesions that involve the internal capsule or rostral cerebral peduncle. It is characterized by flexion of the arms and extension and internal rotation of the legs.
      (2) **Decerebrate rigidity** occurs when the brain stem is severed above the pontine

reticular formation. It is characterized by an increased tone in all the antigravity muscles, resulting in **opisthotonos** (arching of the back and neck), extension and hyperpronation of the arms, and extension and internal rotation of the legs.

B. The **vestibular nuclei,** located within the brain stem and cerebellum, receive information from **vestibular receptors** via **vestibular nerve fibers** (cranial nerve VIII). **Vestibular system reflexes** maintain tone in antigravity muscles, coordinate the adjustments made by the limbs and trunk to maintain balance, and adjust the position of the eyes to maintain visual fixation when the position of the head changes.

1. **Vestibular receptors**
   a. **Location.** The vestibular organ is located within the temporal bone of the skull. The receptors are located within a system of fluid-filled, membrane-bound structures called the **labyrinth.** The labyrinth consists of **two otolith organs** (i.e., the **saccule** and **utricle**) and **three semicircular canals.**
   b. **Function**
      (1) The receptors within the **otolith organs** are responsible for detecting **linear acceleration** and the **static position of the head.**
      (2) The receptors within the **semicircular canals,** which are located in the expanded end of the each canal (i.e., the **ampulla**), are responsible for detecting **angular accelerations of the head.** Each canal is oriented in a different plane. Therefore a movement in any direction can be detected.
   c. **Receptor cells.** The receptor cells of the vestibular system, called **hair cells,** are **polarized** (Figure 7-6). A large cilium, called the **kinocilium,** is located at one end of the cell. When the stereocilia are bent toward the kinocilium, the cell depolarizes. When the stereocilia are bent away from the kinocilium, the cell hyperpolarizes.
      (1) **Otolith organs.** The hair cells of the utricle and saccule are located on a mass of tissue called the **macula.** The cilia are enmeshed in a gelatinous substance filled with small calcium carbonate crystals called **otoconia.** Because the **otoconia** are heavier than the fluid of the otolith organs, they **bend the cilia when the hair cells are moved from their vertical position.**
         (a) **Tilting.** The kinocilium of each hair cell is oriented in a different plane so that, regardless of the direction in which the head is moved, some of the hair cells are stimulated while others are inhibited.
         (b) **Linear acceleration** (i.e., the type of movement experienced when one jumps down stairs or pulls away from a traffic light in a car) also displaces otoconia and stimulates the otolith organs.

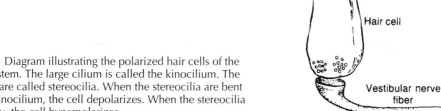

FIGURE 7-6. Diagram illustrating the polarized hair cells of the vestibular system. The large cilium is called the kinocilium. The smaller cilia are called stereocilia. When the stereocilia are bent toward the kinocilium, the cell depolarizes. When the stereocilia are bent away, the cell hyperpolarizes.

(2) Semicircular canals (Figure 7-7). The hair cells of the semicircular canals are located on the **crista,** a mass of tissue within the ampulla. The cilia are embedded in a gelatinous structure called the **cupula,** which completely fills the ampullar space.

(a) Movement of the cupula causes the cilia to bend.

  (i) When the head begins to move, the fluid within the semicircular canals lags behind and pushes the cupula backward, causing the cilia of the hair cells to bend. Depending on whether the stereocilia are pushed toward or away from the kinocilium, the hair cell depolarizes or hyperpolarizes.

  (ii) After 15–20 seconds of continuous movement at a constant velocity (e.g., the movement of a twirling dancer), the velocity of fluid movement catches up to that of the head, and the cupula returns to its resting position. The return of the cupula to the resting position causes the cilia to return to their upright position and the hair cell to return to its resting membrane potential. Thus, **the semicircular canals signal changes in motion (acceleration) but are insensitive to movements at a constant angular velocity.**

  (iii) When the head stops moving, the fluid within the semicircular canals continues to move, pushing the cupula forward, causing the cilia to bend in the opposite direction. Thus, if the original movement caused the hair cell to depolarize, the hair cell hyperpolarizes when the movement ceases.

(b) Side-to-side movements cause the cilia of the horizontal canal to bend (see Figure 7-7).

  (i) Movements to the right **(clockwise movements) stimulate** the hair cells in the **right horizontal canal** and **inhibit** those in the **left horizontal canal.**

  (ii) Movements to the left **(counterclockwise movements) stimulate** the hair cells in the **left horizontal canal** and **inhibit** those in the **right horizontal canal.**

(c) Because each of the three canals is oriented in a different plane, movement of the head in any direction generates a unique pattern of activity within the semicircular canals. This information is used by the CNS to interpret the speed and direction of head movement and to make the appropriate adjustments in posture and eye position.

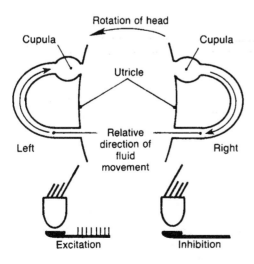

FIGURE 7-7. (*A*) The vestibular organ, which is located within the temporal bone, consists of three semicircular canals (horizontal, anterior vertical, and posterior vertical)and two otolith organs (utricle and saccule). The three semicircular canals are oriented at right angles to each other. (*B*) Activation of the left horizontal canal occurs when the head is rotated toward the left. The endolymph lags behind the bone, preventing the cupula from moving. As a result, the cupula displaces the stereocilia on the hair cells. The stereocilia on the hair cells in the left horizontal canal are bent toward the kinocilium, depolarizing the hair cell and stimulating the vestibular nerve fiber. At the same time, the stereocilia on the hair cells within the right horizontal canal are pushed away from the kinocilium, causing them to hyperpolarize. When the head stops rotating, the fluid continues to move, pushing the cupula in the opposite direction. This action causes the hair cells in the left horizontal canal to hyperpolarize and those in the right horizontal canal to depolarize.

2. Vestibular nuclei. The vestibular nuclei send their axons into the spinal cord through a number of **vestibulospinal tracts.**
  a. The **input from the vestibular nuclei is excitatory to antigravity alpha motoneurons.**
  b. The vestibular nuclei, like the motor control centers within the reticular formation, **receive inhibitory input from the cerebrum and cerebellum.** If the inhibitory input from the cerebrum and cerebellum is removed, the vestibular nuclei greatly increase their firing rate, leading to signs of spasticity similar to those observed after the inhibitory input to the reticular formation is severed.
    (1) The spasticity produced by the vestibular nuclei differs from that produced by the reticular formation in that the vestibular nuclei primarily affect the alpha motoneurons, rather than both alpha and gamma motoneurons. Spasticity caused by the vestibular nuclei is called **alpha rigidity** to distinguish it from spasticity caused by the reticular formation, which is called **gamma rigidity.**
    (2) Because gamma motoneurons are not involved in spasticity produced by the vestibular nuclei, alpha rigidity is not reduced greatly by cutting the dorsal roots and eliminating the Ia input.

3. Vestibular reflexes
  a. The **vestibulo-ocular reflex** maintains visual fixation during movements of the head. For example, if the head is rotated to the left, the eyes move slowly toward the right in order to keep an image on the fovea. When the eyes have rotated as far as they can, they are rapidly returned to the center of the socket. These movements of the eyes are called **nystagmus.**
    (1) The **slow movement** of the eyes to maintain visual fixation is **initiated by the receptors of the semicircular canals.** When the head rotates to the left, receptors in the left horizontal canal are stimulated. Their axons activate the reflex movement of the eyes towards the right.
    (2) After the body has been rotated and the movement ceases, the receptors within the right horizontal canal are stimulated. These receptors cause **postrotatory** nystagmus to occur. The postrotatory nystagmus rotates in a direction opposite to the original nystagmus. Postrotatory nystagmus continues until the cupula returns to its resting position.
  b. **Otolith reflexes.** The otolith organs initiate a reflex that prevents leg injuries when an individual walks down stairs or jumps from a platform. When making such a descent, the muscles in the leg begin to contract before the feet reach the ground to cushion the force of impact.
    (1) The otolith receptors responsible for this reflex are **stimulated by the linear acceleration of the head** that occurs during the descent.
    (2) Individuals lacking otolith reflexes are prone to leg injuries because of the large contact forces that occur during descent (e.g., stepping off a bus).

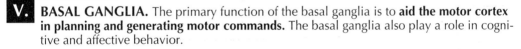

V. BASAL GANGLIA. The primary function of the basal ganglia is to **aid the motor cortex in planning and generating motor commands.** The basal ganglia also play a role in cognitive and affective behavior.

A. Basal nuclei

  1. The basal ganglia consist of five nuclei (Figure 7-8):
    a. Caudate nucleus
    b. Putamen
    c. Globus pallidus
    d. Subthalamic nucleus
    e. Substantia nigra

  2. Together, the **caudate nucleus** and **putamen** are considered the **striatum (neostriatum).**

B. Pathways. The basal ganglia form extensive interconnections with the cortex and the thalamus (Figure 7-9). Because the basal ganglia do not make any direct sensory or motor con-

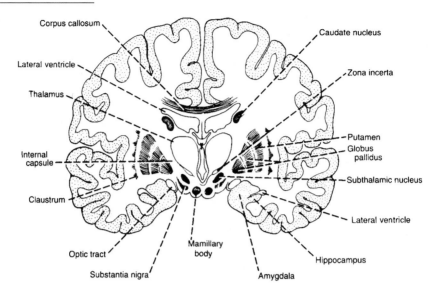

FIGURE 7-8. Coronal section through the midthalamus at the level of the mamillary bodies. The basal ganglia are prominent at this level and include the caudate nucleus, putamen, globus pallidus, subthalamic nucleus, and substantia nigra. (Reprinted from Fix JD: *BRS Neuroanatomy,* Malvern PA, Harwal Publishing, 1992, p 266.)

nections with the spinal cord, their contribution to the control of movement is made indirectly through the sensorimotor cortex.

1. **Primary feedback loop**
   a. **Afferent fibers** from all areas of the cortex **project to the striatum.**
      (1) The **putamen** receives information related to **motor control.**
      (2) The **caudate nucleus** receives information related to the **control of eye movement.** In addition, the caudate nucleus receives information from the cortex that is related to cognitive and affective behavior, rather than to motor control.
   b.The **striatum sends most of its output to the globus pallidus** and to **the reticular nucleus of the substantia nigra.**
   c. **Efferent fibers** from the striatum and the reticular nucleus of the substantia nigra **project to the thalamus. The information received by the thalamus is conveyed back to the cortex,** completing the feedback loop.

2. **Additional pathways**
   a. **Fibers from the pars compacta of the substantia nigra project to the putamen.** This pathway utilizes dopamine as a neurotransmitter and damage to it produces **parkinsonism.**
   b. **Fibers from the subthalamic nucleus project to the globus pallidus.** Because the subthalamic nucleus receives input from the motor cortex, lesions within the subthalamic nucleus lead to uncontrolled flinging movements of the limbs (i.e., **ballismus**).

C. **Lesions** in the basal ganglia produce characteristic deficits in motor behavior.

1. **Lesions in the globus pallidus** result in an inability of the trunk muscles to maintain postural support. The head bends forward so that the chin touches the chest, and the body bends at the waist.
   a. The motor deficits are not the result of muscular weakness or failure of voluntary control because individuals with these lesions can stand upright when requested to do so.
   b. Because the globus pallidus is the major outflow tract of the basal ganglia, it is possible that the motor deficits occur because the cortex is deprived of information it needs to automatically control the trunk muscles.

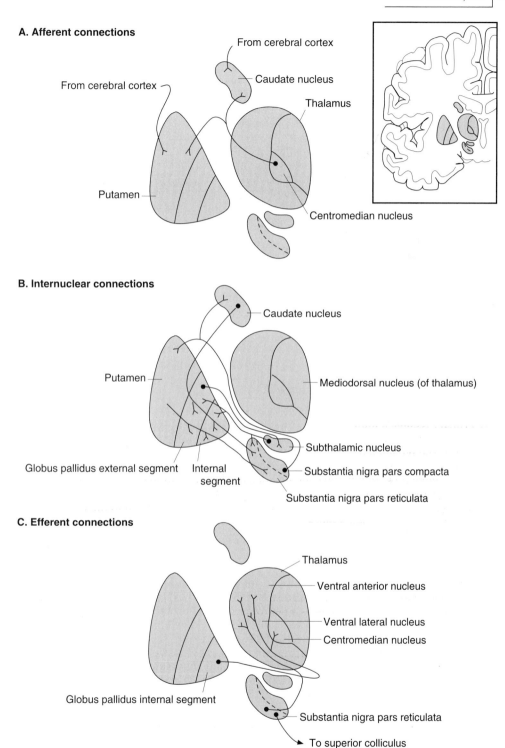

FIGURE 7-9. The basal ganglia form extensive connections with the cortex and thalamus. (*A*) The striatum (i.e., the caudate nucleus and putamen) receives afferent input from all areas of the cortex. (*B*) Extensive connections exist among the nuclei of the basal ganglia. (*C*) The thalamus receives efferent fibers from the basal ganglia. (Redrawn with permission from Kandel ER, Schwartz JH, Jessell TM: *Principles of Neural Science,* 3rd ed. New York, Elsevier, 1991, p 649.)

2. **Lesions in the subthalamic nucleus** cause spontaneous, wild, flinging movements of the limbs. This syndrome is called **hemiballismus.**
   a. The movements, which are **caused by a release of inhibition, appear on the side opposite the lesion.** The subthalamic nucleus inhibits the cortex indirectly.
      (1) Efferent fibers from the subthalamic nucleus release glutamate, which excites thalamic neurons.
      (2) The thalamic neurons use γ-aminobutyric acid (GABA) to inhibit the cortex.
      (3) Damage to the subthalamic nucleus reduces the excitation of inhibitory fibers in the thalamus and leads to excitation of the cortex.
   b. Because the movements of hemiballismus appear to be like those performed when an individual is thrown off balance, the subthalamic nucleus is believed to be involved with controlling the centers that issue the motor commands for **balance.**
      (1) Normally, the subthalamic nucleus responds to the need for initiating the balancing movement by momentarily withdrawing its inhibition from these centers.
      (2) When there is a lesion in the subthalamic nucleus, these centers no longer are under inhibitory control, and the movements are generated spontaneously.

3. **Lesions within the striatum** produce a variety of motor syndromes that are also related to a release of inhibition.
   a. **Huntington's chorea,** an inherited disorder, is characterized by continuous uncontrollable movements of the limbs that resemble the movements of hemiballism.
      (1) In Huntington's chorea, the **GABA-containing neurons** that originate **within the striatum** are **destroyed.** These GABA-ergic neurons normally inhibit neurons within the globus pallidus, which, in turn, inhibit neurons within the subthalamic nucleus.
      (2) When the striatal neurons are destroyed, the pallidal cells are released from inhibition and thus increase their inhibitory effect on the subthalamic nucleus.
      (3) Reduction in subthalamic nucleus activity may produce spontaneous movements resembling those observed when the subthalamic nucleus is destroyed.
   b. **Athetosis** is characterized by continuous, slow, irregular, twisting motions of the limbs, fingers, and hands.
   c. **Dystonia** is typified by twisting, tonic-type movements of the head and trunk.

4. **Lesions within the pars compacta of the substantia nigra** produce **Parkinson's disease.**
   a. **Characteristics.** Parkinson's disease is characterized by rigidity, hypokinesia (i.e., reduction in voluntary movement), and tremor.
      (1) The **rigidity** in Parkinson's disease involves all of the muscles at a joint and, thus, is different from spasticity that is associated with cortical lesions.
         (a) The rigidity of Parkinson's disease has been described as **lead-pipe rigidity** because the rigid limb, when moved, remains where it is placed.
         (b) The rigidity seen in Parkinson's disease also has been described as **cogwheel rigidity.** When an examiner tries to move the limb, the limb periodically gives way and then reestablishes its resistance to movement like cogs on a wheel.
      (2) The **hypokinesia** reduces the movement patterns normally associated with motor activity. For example, a Parkinson's disease patient may not swing his or her arms when walking, or display varied facial expressions during conversation.
         (a) The hypokinesia is **not related to a loss of muscle strength** or power, because normal movements occur under certain conditions.
         (b) The hypokinesia is **not caused by rigidity,** because hypokinesia may occur in the absence of rigidity.
      (3) The **tremor** in Parkinson's disease occurs at rest and usually disappears during voluntary activity. It occurs at a frequency of approximately 4–7 cycles/sec. (A normal physiologic tremor has a frequency of approximately 10 cycles/sec.)
   b. **Therapy.** Because the lesion of Parkinson's disease involves a pathway that uses dopamine as its neurotransmitter, some success has been achieved in treating the disease with L-dopa, a precursor of dopamine that can cross the blood–brain barrier. Dopamine inhibits the striatum sufficiently to reduce some of the clinical signs of the disease.

VI. **CEREBELLUM.** The cerebellum is intimately associated with control of the **timing, duration,** and **strength of a movement.** Its removal produces no deficits in emotional or intellectual function but causes profound disturbances in the ability to produce smooth, coordinated movements.

A. Lobes. Two transverse fissures divide the cerebellum into three lobes: the **anterior, posterior,** and **flocculonodular lobes** (Figure 7-10).

1. **Phylogenetic nomenclature.** These lobes developed at different times during evolution.
   a. The **flocculonodular lobe** evolved early in the evolution of vertebrates and is therefore called the **archicerebellum.**
   b. The **anterior lobe** evolved next and is called the **paleocerebellum.**
   c. The **posterior lobe** was the last to evolve and is called the **neocerebellum.**

2. **Functional nomenclature.** These lobes are also named according to the connections they make with other components of the motor control system.
   a. The **flocculonodular lobe** is functionally related to the vestibular apparatus. Therefore, it is also called the **vestibulocerebellum.**
   b. The **entire anterior lobe,** and those parts of the posterior lobe that receive information from the spinal cord, are called the **spinocerebellum.** The spinocerebellum occupies the medial portion of the cerebellar cortex.
   c. The **remainder of the posterior lobe** receives input from the cerebral cortex. Therefore, it is called the **cerebrocerebellum.** It occupies the more lateral regions of the cerebellar cortex.

B. Pathways. The organization of the synaptic connections within each lobe is the same.

1. **Layers.** The cerebellar cortex is divided into **three** layers (Figure 7-11).
   a. **Granule cell layer.** The **innermost layer** contains **10 billion granule cells,** as well as a smaller number of interneurons called **Golgi cells.**
   b. **Purkinje cell layer.** The **middle layer** contains **Purkinje cells.** The highly branched dendritic tree of the Purkinje cells extends vertically into the outer portion of the cortex, and the axon of the Purkinje fiber descends to the cerebellar nuclei (located in the granule cell layer).
   c. **Molecular layer.** The **outer layer** contains two types of **interneurons,** the **basket cells** and the **stellate cells.**

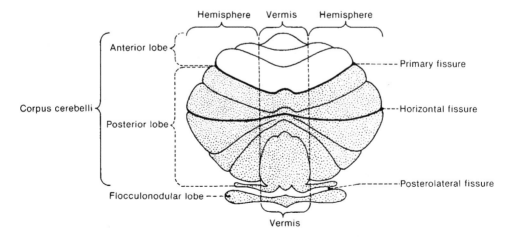

FIGURE 7-10. Diagrammatic dorsal view of the cerebellum, showing the anterior, posterior, and flocculonodular lobes. (Reprinted with permission from *NMS Neuroanatomy*. Malvern PA, Williams & Wilkins, 1988, p 189.)

Cerebellar cortex

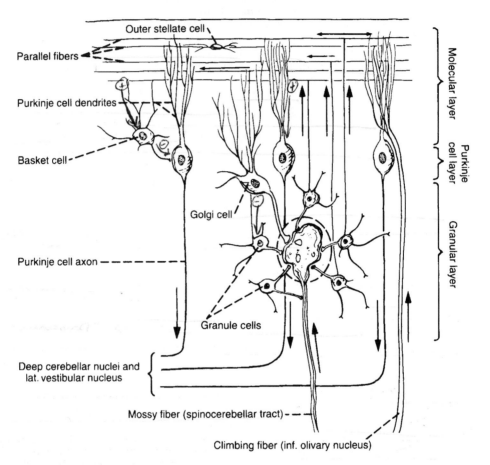

FIGURE 7-11. Schematic diagram of the three layers of the cerebellar cortex, showing the neuronal elements and their connections. The *circular broken line* contains a cerebellar glomerulus. Climbing and mossy fibers provide excitatory input. Purkinje cell axons provide the sole output from the cerebellar cortex, which is inhibitory. (Reprinted from Fix JD: *BRS Neuroanatomy,* Malvern PA, Harwal Publishing, 1992, p 198.)

　　　　(1) The axons of the granule cells project vertically into the molecular layer, where they form two branches (i.e., the **parallel fibers**), which extend parallel to the cortical surface.
　　　　(2) The parallel fibers synapse with the dendrites of the Purkinje cells in the outer layer.
　2. Afferent fibers
　　　a. Excitatory. The Purkinje cells receive **two types of excitatory input.**
　　　　(1) Mossy fibers arise from cells within all levels of the nervous system that send projections to the cerebellum.
　　　　　(a) Mossy fibers **excite granule cells** which, in turn, **excite Purkinje cells** via the parallel fiber axons. Each Purkinje fiber receives axons from approximately 20,000 granule cells.
　　　　　(b) The Purkinje cells lie along a narrow path several millimeters in length.
　　　　(2) Climbing fibers arise from cells within the inferior olivary nucleus. Each climbing fiber excites approximately ten Purkinje cells.
　　　b. Inhibitory

       (1) Basket cells inhibit Purkinje cells.
         (a) The basket cells, like Purkinje cells, are excited by parallel fibers.
         (b) The axons of the basket cells run perpendicular to the parallel fibers and act
            to inhibit the Purkinje cells on either side of the Purkinje cells activated by the
            parallel fibers. Thus, granule cell excitation produces a strip of excited Purk-
            inje cells surrounded by parallel strips of inhibited Purkinje cells.
       (2) Golgi cells inhibit granule cells.
         (a) The dendrites of the Golgi cells ascend vertically from the granule cell layer to
            the molecular layer, where they receive excitatory input from the parallel fibers.
         (b) The axons of the Golgi cell inhibit the granule cells. Thus, excitation of the
            granule cell is rapidly extinguished by a **negative feedback loop:** Granule cell
            axons (parallel fibers) excite Golgi cell dendrites, whose axons inhibit the
            granule cells.

3. Efferent fibers. The **Purkinje cell axons,** which are **inhibitory,** provide the only output
   from the cerebellum.
   a. Axons originating in the **cerebrocerebellum** and **spinocerebellum project to the deep
      cerebellar nuclei.**
   b. Axons originating in the vestibulocerebellum project to the **vestibular nuclei.** *(Brainstem)*

C. **Lesions** in the various lobes produce characteristic motor deficits.

   1. Lesions in the vestibulocerebellum cause deficits related to the loss of vestibular func-
      tion (e.g., loss of equilibrium, **ataxia**). Individuals with vestibulocerebellar lesions are
      unable to maintain their balance and tend to fall over when standing. When walking,
      these individuals tend to stagger and have a wide stance.   → *"Drunkeness"*

   2. Lesions in the spinocerebellum have **no obvious effects** in humans, probably because
      spinocerebellar functions can be assumed by the cerebrocerebellum. In cats, lesions in
      the anterior lobe increase the tone of the antigravity muscles. → *Project to Red Nucleus?*

   3. Lesions in the cerebrocerebellum cause **small motor deficits,** unless an extensive area
      of the cerebellar cortex is affected. **If the outflow pathways are damaged,** however, **the
      ability to produce smooth, coordinated movements is lost.**
     a. A major sign of cerebrocerebellar disease is **decomposition of movement.** Instead of
        acting in a coordinated way to produce a movement, the muscles act individually. For
        example, when reaching for an object, extension of the arm first takes place at the
        shoulder, followed by extension at the elbow, and finally by extension of the hand.
     b. Dysmetria (i.e., the inability to stop a movement at the appropriate time or to direct it
        in the appropriate direction) is another sign of cerebrocerebellar disease. Dysmetria
        results from the loss of the neuronal circuitry required to control the duration and
        strength of a movement.
     c. The **intention tremor** that results from cerebrocerebellar lesions also is related to the
        inability to time and sequence movements properly. The intention tremor is different
        from the resting (spontaneous) tremor of Parkinson's disease and appears to occur be-
        cause an entire movement cannot be directed by a single motor command. Instead,
        the movement is partially directed and then halted. Several other motor commands
        are required before the movement is completed.
     d. Adiadochokinesia is the inability to make rapidly alternating movements (e.g., turning
        the hands back and forth). This, too, appears related to the inability to time the dura-
        tion of a movement.

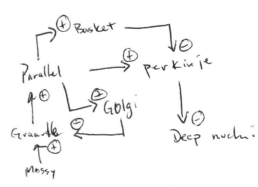

Chapter 8

Cortical Control of Movement and Consciousness

I. **CORTICAL CONTROL OF MOVEMENT.** The cerebral cortex contains the neuronal circuits responsible for the conception, planning, and generation of motor commands. **Two parallel** systems of **descending pathways** originate in the cerebral cortex: the **pyramidal** and **extrapyramidal systems.** Clinically, these systems are considered together because lesions within the cortex almost always involve both of them; however, these systems are functionally different.

A. Motor areas. The cerebral cortex contains three motor areas.

1. The **primary motor cortex** is located within the precentral gyrus and corresponds to Brodmann's area 4.
   a. **Organization**
      (1) The primary motor cortex is **organized somatotopically** (i.e., each area of the body is controlled by a specific area of the primary motor cortex). For example, the head is controlled by cells located laterally, and the feet are controlled by cells located on the medial surface of the cortex.
      (2) The **area of the cortex devoted to each part** of the body **is proportional to the amount of motor control that is exerted over that part.** Therefore, the hands and face have a much larger representation than the trunk and legs.
   b. **Role.** Neurons within the primary motor area are responsible for continuously **exciting spinal motoneurons** during the performance of a movement.
      (1) Although primary motor area neurons responsible for performing fine dextrous movements of the fingers may send axons to a group of motoneurons controlling a single muscle, most corticospinal tract neurons send axons to several synergistic motoneuron pools.
      (2) The firing frequency of the primary motor area neurons is proportional to the force that must be generated by the muscle to carry out its motor command.
      (3) The primary motor area neurons receive sensory input from the spinal cord. This information is used to modify ongoing motor commands.

2. The **supplementary motor cortex** is located on the lateral and medial surface of the cortex in Brodmann's area 6.
   a. **Organization.** The supplementary motor cortex is organized **somatotopically.** However, unlike the primary motor area, which controls muscles on the contralateral side of the body, the supplementary motor cortex controls muscles on both sides of the body.
   b. **Role.** Neurons within the supplementary motor area are responsible for **generating the plan for a movement;** therefore, they are activated before those of the primary motor area. **Lesions** within the supplementary motor area interfere with the coordination of complex motor tasks, particularly those requiring both limbs.

3. The **premotor motor cortex** is located on the lateral surface of the cortex (in Brodmann's area 6), just in front of the primary motor cortex.
   a. **Organization.** The premotor motor cortex is organized **somatotopically.**
   b. **Role.** The premotor motor cortex **coordinates the proximal and axial muscles** during a motor task.

B. Pathways. Two major descending pathways emerge from the motor areas.

1. **Corticospinal tract**
   a. **Organization.** The corticospinal tract originates in the motor cortex, crosses to the

contralateral side within the pyramids on the ventral medulla, and terminates within the spinal cord or the cranial nerves controlling facial muscles. Because its axons pass through the pyramids on their way to the spinal cord, the corticospinal tract is also referred to as the **pyramidal system.**

(1) **Axons.** The corticospinal tract contains approximately 1 million axons.

   (a) The cell bodies of these axons are in layer V of the cerebral cortex. A small number of the axons (approximately 30,000) **originate from** large pyramidal cells called **Betz cells.** The remainder come from **smaller pyramidal cells.**

   (b) Approximately half of the axons come from the primary motor cortex. A third come from the other motor areas, and the remainder come from the somatosensory cortex.

(2) **Collaterals** from the corticospinal tract travel to the basal ganglia and cerebellum, which use this information to modify and coordinate ongoing movements.

b. **Role.** The corticospinal tract is responsible for **controlling muscles that make precision movements** (e.g., the muscles that move the fingers and hands and the muscles that produce speech). **Lesions** within the pyramidal tract system produce only **minor deficits** in motor control. Most movements are not affected because they can be adequately controlled by cortical fibers descending in the extrapyramidal system (see I B 2).

(1) Muscle weakness or paralysis, particularly of the distal muscles responsible for fine, highly coordinated movements, occurs with pure pyramidal tract lesions.

(2) A number of cutaneous reflexes (e.g., the cremasteric reflex) are abolished or more difficult to elicit and a positive Babinski sign is produced when the plantar surface of the foot is stroked.

2. **Corticoreticular and corticovestibular tracts**

a. **Organization.** These pathways are referred to as the **nonpyramidal or extrapyramidal system,** because their influence over motoneurons is not exerted through axons that travel through the pyramids. In the past, the basal ganglia were also referred to as the extrapyramidal system; the two usages of this term should not be confused.

(1) Axons from cells within the nuclei of the pontine reticular formation (the primary nucleus reticularis pontis oralis and caudalis) and the lateral vestibular nucleus pass ipsilaterally to the spinal cord, where they excite motoneurons controlling antigravity muscles of the limbs.

(2) Motoneurons controlling motoneurons going to antigravity muscles of the neck and back muscles are excited by axons originating within the medial and inferior vestibular nuclei.

b. **Role.** The corticoreticular and corticovestibular tracts provide inhibitory input to contralateral nuclei within the pontine reticular formation and the vestibular system. They are responsible for **maintaining postural tone** and for **directing voluntary movement. Lesions** to the extrapyramidal system remove inhibition from the pontine reticular formation and lead to spasticity (see Chapter 7 IV A 2 b).

II. SLEEP AND CONSCIOUSNESS

A. **Diurnal (circadian) rhythms.** Many of the body's regulatory mechanisms vary in their activity during the day. For example, body temperature is approximately 1°C higher during the early evening than it is at dawn, and adrenocortical hormones are secreted at levels that are higher in the morning than they are at night. The cycle of these diurnal rhythms is roughly **24 hours.**

1. If an individual is isolated from the environmental stimuli that indicate the normal day–night periods, the cycle time lengthens, demonstrating that the circadian rhythms are not rigidly linked to the rotation of the earth but can be driven by an individual's internal biological clock.

2. It is necessary to understand normal variations in physiologic activities when evaluating

pathologic functions. For example, it would be misleading to compare temperatures obtained at different times of the day.

B. **Sleep–wake cycle.** The most obvious, and probably most important, diurnal rhythm is the sleep–wake cycle. When awake, an individual is able to perform all activities that are required for individual and species survival. When asleep, an individual is not aware of the environment and is unable to perform activities that require consciousness.

1. **Assessment of sleep states.** The presence of sleep can be assessed by **behavioral analysis** (e.g., an individual who does not move and does not respond when spoken to or touched is often asleep). A more accurate assessment of sleep can be obtained from an **electroencephalogram (EEG).**

   a. **Obtaining the EEG**
      (1) The EEG is obtained by placing electrodes on the scalp. The location of the electrodes and the amplification and paper speed of the polygraph used for recording the EEG are standardized.
      (2) The brain waves recorded by an EEG represent the summated activity of millions of cortical neurons. The inhibitory postsynaptic potentials (IPSPs), excitatory postsynaptic potentials (EPSPs), and the passive spread of electrical activity into the dendrites of these neurons, rather than their action potentials, form the basis for the EEG.

   b. **Variations in the EEG during sleep and wakefulness** (Figure 8-1). The two states of sleep—**slow-wave** and **fast-wave** sleep—have characteristic EEG patterns.
      (1) When an individual is **awake,** the electrical activity recorded from the brain is asynchronous and of low amplitude. This type of brain electrical recording is called a **beta wave.**
      (2) If an individual sits quietly for a while, the brain waves gradually become larger and highly synchronized. The **typical resting EEG pattern** has a frequency of 8–13 cycles/sec and is called an **alpha wave.** When the eyes open or when conscious mental activity is initiated, the EEG shifts from an alpha to a beta pattern (i.e., **alpha blocking** takes place).
      (3) As consciousness is reduced still further, an individual enters a state of sleep called **slow-wave sleep,** which progresses in an orderly way from **light to deep sleep.** Behaviorally, slow-wave sleep is characterized by a progressive reduction in consciousness and an increasing resistance to being awakened. Muscle tone is reduced, the heart and respiratory rates decrease, and, in general, body metabolism slows.
         (a) **Light sleep** is characterized by an EEG that shows high-amplitude waves of

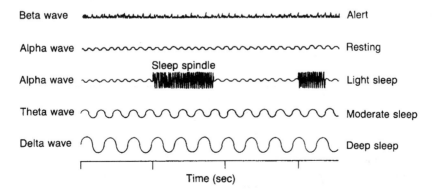

FIGURE 8-1. As an individual passes from wakefulness to deep sleep, the electroencephalogram (EEG) wave increases in amplitude and decreases in frequency. Sleep spindles indicate the presence of light sleep.

approximately 12–15 cycles/sec, called **sleep spindles,** which periodically interrupt the alpha rhythm.

    (b) Moderate sleep is characterized by an EEG that displays slower and larger waves called **theta waves.**

    (c) Deep sleep produces an EEG pattern with very slow (4–7 cycles/sec), large waves called **delta waves.**

(4) Fast-wave (desynchronized) sleep is characterized by the same high-frequency and low-amplitude EEG pattern that is seen in the waking state; however, the individual clearly is unresponsive to environmental stimuli and, thus, is asleep. For this reason, fast-wave sleep also is called **paradoxical sleep.**

    (a) Because this state of sleep is characterized by the presence of rapid eye movements, it also is called **rapid eye movement (REM) sleep.**

    (b) Because dreaming occurs during REM sleep, it is also called **dream sleep.**

    (c) Behaviorally, REM sleep is quite different from slow-wave sleep.

        (i) It is as difficult to arouse an individual from REM sleep as it is from deep sleep. However, when awakened from REM sleep, the individual is immediately alert and aware of the environment.

        (ii) The eyes are not the only organs that are active during REM sleep. The middle ear muscles are active, penile erection occurs, heart rate and respiration become irregular, and there are occasional twitches of the limb musculature. Because muscle tone is reduced tremendously during REM sleep, the frequency and intensity of muscle twitching do not produce injuries or awaken the individual.

2. The sleep cycle. There is an orderly progression of sleep stages and states during a typical sleep period (Figure 8-2).

    a. When an individual falls asleep, the light stage of slow-wave sleep is entered first. During the next hour or so, the individual passes into progressively deeper stages of sleep until deep sleep is reached. After approximately 15 minutes of deep sleep, the depth of sleep starts to decrease and continues to do so until the individual reenters the light stage of sleep (about 90 minutes after the start of the first sleep cycle). At this point, the individual passes from slow-wave sleep to REM sleep.

    b. This cycle repeats itself about five times during the night. However, as Figure 8-2 demonstrates, after the second cycle, the intervals between periods of REM sleep shorten and the duration of each period of REM sleep lengthens. As morning approaches, an individual spends less time in the deeper stages of slow-wave sleep and periodically awakens.

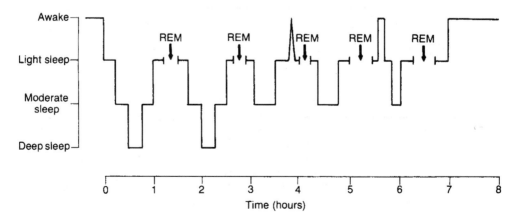

FIGURE 8-2. Diagram indicating the pattern of sleep during one sleep cycle. As the night progresses, the depth of slow-wave sleep decreases, and the duration and frequency of rapid eye movement (REM) sleep episodes increase. Note that occasional periods of wakefulness occur during the night.

   c. The sleep cycle shown in Figure 8–2 is typical of an adult. The cycle varies greatly with age.

      (1) During infancy, approximately 16 hours of every day are spent asleep. This figure drops to 10 hours during childhood and to 7 hours during adulthood. Elderly individuals spend less than 6 hours of each day sleeping.

      (2) It is interesting to note that prematurely born infants spend approximately 80% of their sleep time in REM sleep, whereas full-term infants spend only 50% of their sleep time in REM sleep. The total time spent in REM sleep is reduced to about 1.5–2 hours by puberty and remains unchanged thereafter.

      (3) During infancy and childhood, therefore, the reduction in sleep time from 16 hours to 10 hours occurs almost entirely by a reduction of the amount of time spent in REM sleep. In adulthood, the reduction in sleep time is caused by a reduction in the time spent in the deep stages of slow-wave sleep.

3. Physiologic basis for sleep. Areas throughout the entire brain participate in the sleep–wake cycle.

   a. The **waking state** is maintained by the **ascending reticular activating system (RAS),** a diffuse collection of neurons within the medulla, pons, midbrain, and diencephalon. Electrical stimulation anywhere within this area causes the EEG pattern to change abruptly from that of the sleep state to that of the waking state [i.e., a **cortical alerting (arousal) response** takes place].

   b. The **sleep state** does not result from the passive withdrawal of arousal. **Two sleep centers** exist in the brain stem; one is responsible for producing **slow-wave sleep,** and the other produces **REM sleep.**

4. Sleep disorders. As noted previously, there is a cycling between slow-wave sleep and REM sleep during a normal sleep period.

   a. In **narcolepsy,** REM sleep is entered directly from the waking state.

      (1) Individuals suffering from narcolepsy often report an intense feeling of sleepiness just prior to an attack, although sleep sometimes occurs without warning.

      (2) In some narcoleptics, the profound reduction in muscle tone characteristic of REM sleep can occur without loss of consciousness. During such an attack, called **cataplexy,** the individual suddenly becomes paralyzed, falls to the ground, and is unable to move.

      (3) Another symptom associated with narcolepsy is the presence of a dream-like state during wakefulness, which narcoleptics describe as a hallucination.

   b. Most of the other symptoms of sleep disorders are associated with slow-wave sleep. These include **sleepwalking (somnambulism), bed- wetting (nocturnal enuresis),** and **nightmares (pavor nocturnus),** all of which occur during stages of slow-wave sleep.

      (1) During a nightmare that occurs in slow-wave sleep, the individual wakes up screaming and appears terrified. However, no reason for the acute anxiety is recalled. These episodes are called night terrors.

      (2) By contrast, terrifying dreams that occur during REM sleep are graphically remembered.

5. Disturbances of consciousness

   a. Coma. A lesion blocking the connection between the ascending RAS and the thalamus produces a permanent state of sleep, or coma. In this situation, stimulation of sensory pathways can cause a momentary desynchronization of the EEG but does not produce any behavioral signs of arousal.

      (1) Coma is not simply a deep sleep state. It is characterized by a loss of consciousness from which **arousal cannot be elicited.**

      (2) O_2 **consumption by the brain is reduced** during coma. This is in marked contrast to normal sleep, in which there is no change in brain O_2 consumption from the waking state.

   b. Syncope (fainting). A transient pathologic loss of consciousness is called syncope. More persistent losses of consciousness (from which arousal can be obtained) are called stupor.

   c. Brain death occurs when the brain no longer can achieve consciousness. Because of the desire to obtain organs for transplant operations and the desire to remove heroic life-support systems, an objective standard for determining the presence of brain death has been developed.

     (1) Brain death is said to occur when a loss of consciousness is accompanied by a flat EEG (i.e., an EEG with no brain waves) and a loss of all brain stem regulatory systems (e.g., those systems that control respiration and blood pressure).

     (2) Moreover, these clinical signs must be due to traumatic or ischemic anoxia and not to hypothermia or metabolic poisons, from which later recovery is possible.

     (3) Finally, the criteria for brain death must be present for 6–12 hours.

PART II

STUDY QUESTIONS

1. Which one of the following stimuli normally activates a receptor that is located on the free nerve ending of a sensory neuron?

(A) Taste
(B) Gravity
(C) Light
(D) Sound
(E) Smell

2. Which one of the following statements about the optical properties of a myopic eye is correct?

(A) A converging lens can be used to correct the optical defect
(B) The image of a distant object is formed in front of the retina
(C) The power of accommodation for near vision is greater than normal
(D) The refractive power of the lens is less than normal
(E) The far point is greater than normal

3. If the refractive power of the unaccommodated eye of an emmetropic woman is 60 diopters (D), the axial length of her eye is closest to

(A) 14.5 mm
(B) 15.5 mm
(C) 16.5 mm
(D) 17.5 mm
(E) 18.5 mm

4. A sound stimulus of 20 decibels (dB) is

(A) 10 times threshold
(B) 20 times threshold
(C) 50 times threshold
(D) 100 times threshold
(E) 200 times threshold

5. Which one of the following statements best describes the muscle fibers that are recruited first during a normal movement?

(A) They have a very limited capillary supply
(B) They store large quantities of glycogen
(C) They have low myosin—adenosine triphosphatase (ATPase) activity
(D) They fatigue easily
(E) They rapidly sequester Ca^{2+} into their sarcoplasmic reticulum (SR)

6. Which one of the following sensory systems uses unmyelinated fibers to convey information to the central nervous system (CNS)?

(A) Proprioception
(B) Vision
(C) Vibration
(D) Temperature
(E) Pressure

7. Which of the following statements correctly describes the role played by transducin during the response of rods and cones to light?

(A) Transducin reduces membrane conductance by closing Na^+ channels
(B) Transducin stimulates synaptic transmitter release by opening Ca^{2+} channels
(C) Transducin initiates the photoreceptor response by converting 11-*cis* retinal to all-*trans* retinal
(D) Transducin enhances the action of rhodopsin by converting vitamin A to 11-*cis* retinal
(E) Transducin reduces the concentration of cyclic guanosine monophosphate (cGMP) by activating a phosphodiesterase enzyme

8. Which one of the following statements about pain sensation is correct?

(A) Painful sensations can be elicited by any sensory neuron if its firing frequency is high enough
(B) Painful sensations arising from a particular area of the skin occur only when pain fibers from that area of the skin are stimulated
(C) Cutting the anterolateral tract on both sides of the spinal cord will permanently eliminate painful sensations arising from skin regions innervated by sensory neurons located below the site of the lesion
(D) Pain fibers conduct impulses to the spinal cord and to skin regions surrounding the site of a painful stimulus

9. Which one of the following is more descriptive of rods than of cones?

(A) Not located within the fovea
(B) Provide information about the color of an object
(C) Recover their sensitivity more rapidly after exposure to bright light
(D) Responsible for the high visual acuity of the visual system
(E) Organized into on-center, off-surround receptor fields

10. Which of the following will occur in a girl who suddenly stops spinning after several seconds of spinning to the left?

(A) The hair cells in the right semicircular canal will depolarize
(B) Her eyes will move slowly to the right
(C) When asked to point to a target, the girl will point to the right of the target
(D) The cupula in the right semicircular canal will move away from the utricle
(E) The objects in the visual field will appear to be spinning to the right

11. Which of the following is most closely related to slow-wave sleep?

(A) Dreaming
(B) Atonia
(C) Bed-wetting
(D) High-frequency electroencephalogram (EEG) waves
(E) Irregular heart rates

12. Production of endolymph is the function of which component of the auditory system?

(A) Stria vascularis
(B) Scala media
(C) Auditory ossicles
(D) Oval window
(E) Basilar membrane

13. Which characteristic of a sensory stimulus is encoded better by phasic receptors than by tonic receptors?

(A) How strong the stimulus is
(B) The type of energy producing the stimulus
(C) How rapidly the stimulus is applied
(D) The duration of the stimulus
(E) Where the stimulus is located

14. Which of the following refractive problems most closely resembles presbyopia?

(A) Hyperopia
(B) Myopia
(C) Astigmatism
(D) Cataract
(E) Diplopia

15. Movement disorders related to the removal of inhibition are produced by lesions to all of the following components of the motor control system EXCEPT the

(A) striatum
(B) internal capsule
(C) substantia nigra
(D) medullary pyramids
(E) subthalamic nucleus

16. The flow of K^+ into the cell produces the receptor potential for which of the following sensory systems?

(A) Taste
(B) Olfaction
(C) Audition
(D) Touch
(E) Vision

17. Which one of the following statements best describes cold receptors?

(A) Cold receptors produce a sensation of warmth when their firing frequency is very low
(B) Sudden decreases in temperature always increase the firing frequency of cold receptors
(C) Cold receptors are tonic receptors that slowly increase their firing rate when the temperature is decreased
(D) Cold receptors do not fire at skin temperatures above body temperature
(E) Cold receptors produce a sensation of pain when their firing frequency is very high

18. Which one of the following receptors is responsible for monitoring the rate of muscle stretch?

(A) Nuclear bag intrafusal fibers
(B) Nuclear chain intrafusal fibers
(C) Golgi tendon organs
(D) Pacinian corpuscles
(E) Ruffini's corpuscles

ANSWERS AND EXPLANATIONS

1. The answer is E [Chapter 5 IV A 1]. Olfactory receptors are on the free nerve endings of the olfactory nerve (cranial nerve I). Gravity is detected by hair cells in the utricle and saccule, sound by hair cells in the organ of Corti, light by rods and cones, and taste by epithelia cells within the taste buds. Hair cells, rods and cones, and epithelial taste cells then communicate with afferent nerves via synaptic transmission.

2. The answer is B [Chapter 6 I B 3 c (1)]. A myopic eye is one in which the power of the unaccommodated lens is too high for the axial length of the eye, so that the image is formed in front of the retina. The refractive error can be corrected by a diverging lens that reduces the strength of the high converging power that characterizes a myope's eye. The far point is the point at which the image can be clearly seen by the unaccommodated eye (i.e., the image is located on the retina). Myopes must bring the object close to the eye to be seen (hence the term "nearsighted"); therefore, the myope's far point is closer than the far point of a person with normal vision.

3. The answer is C [Chapter 6 I B 3]. The focal point of an optical system (in meters) is the reciprocal of the refractive power of the system. Therefore, the focal point is 1/60 diopter (D), or 16.7 mm. An emmetropic eye forms a focused image of a distant object on the retina without accommodation. If the axial length is 16.5 mm, the image will be focused on the retina.

4. The answer is A [Chapter 6 II B 2 b (1)]. A decibel (dB) is a unit of sound intensity based on the formula:

$$dB = 20 \cdot \text{Log} \frac{I}{I_0}, \text{ where}$$

$$I = \text{stimulus intensity}$$
$$I_0 = \text{threshold stimulus}$$

According to this formula, a sound intensity of 20 dB is 10 times threshold:

$$20 = 20 \cdot \text{Log} \frac{10 \cdot I_0}{I_0}$$

5. The answer is C [Chapter 7 II A 2 b, c]. The first muscles to be recruited during a movement are the slow-twitch muscle fibers. Slow-twitch fibers are characterized by low myosin—adenosine triphosphatase (ATPase) activity associated with slow contractile speeds, slow sequestering of Ca^{2+} that facilitates summation, and high oxidative enzyme activity and a rich capillary supply that render them fatigue-resistant.

6. The answer is D [Chapter 5 III B]. The thermoreceptors are on the free nerve endings of unmyelinated C fibers and small myelinated ($A\delta$) sensory fibers. Proprioception (i.e., the sense of muscle tension and length) is conveyed by Ia and Ib afferent fibers, which innervate muscle spindles and Golgi tendon organs. Vibration is detected by Pacinian corpuscles and pressure is detected by Ruffini's corpuscles. Both are innervated by large, myelinated (group II) afferent neurons.

7. The answer is E [Chapter 6 I C; Figure 6-4]. Transducin is a G protein that, when activated by the photoisomerization of 11-*cis* retinal to all-*trans* retinal, activates a cyclic guanosine monophosphate (cGMP) phosphodiesterase. The hydrolysis of cGMP by the phosphodiesterase leads to the closing of Na^+ channels, the hyperpolarization of the membrane, and a reduction in the release of synaptic transmitter. Formation of 11-*cis* retinal from vitamin A requires two steps; the vitamin A must be isomerized to its 11-*cis* isomer by an isomerase enzyme and then the 11-*cis* retinol must be oxidized to the aldehyde, 11-*cis* retinal.

8. The answer is D [Chapter 5 III C]. Small myelinated and unmyelinated nociceptive fibers that convey information to the spinal cord have collateral branches that innervate blood vessels in the region of the pain stimulus. Antidromically conducted action potentials cause the release of bradykinins from the blood vessels, which stimulates the release of pain-producing substances (e.g., histamine) from neighboring cells. The pain-producing substances enlarge the area from which painful sensations arise and produce hyperalgesia (an increase in the sensitivity to painful stimuli). Only stimulation of pain fibers produces the sensation of pain. Other sensory neurons do not elicit a painful stimulus. Visceral pain can be referred to areas of the skin where there are no painful stimuli to activate the pain fibers in that region. Although cutting the anterolateral tract eliminates the acute pain and temperature sensations arising from areas below the lesion, chronic pain is not eliminated and occasionally worsens.

9. The answer is A [Chapter 6 I C 4]. Rods are not located within the fovea; only cones are present. The three types of cones (red, green, and blue) make color vision possible. Because cones are smaller than rods, have a greater sensitivity to light, and are organized into smaller center-surround receptor fields, they are capable of high visual acuity. After being exposed to bright light, cones recover their sensitivity about five times faster than rods.

10. The answer is A [Chapter 7 IV B 1 b; Figure 7-7]. When the head spins to the left, the vestibular nerve innervating the left horizontal semicircular canal will be stimulated. When the girl stops spinning, the endolymph within the horizontal semicircular canals will continue to move toward the left, pushing the cupula in both horizontal semicircular canals toward the left. In the right horizontal semicircular canal, the cupula moves toward the utricle and bends the stereocilia toward the kinocilium, causing the hair cell to depolarize. Depolarization of the hair cells stimulates the right vestibular nerve, which cause the eyes to move slowly toward the left. Stimulation of the right vestibular nerve also causes the girl to feel that she is spinning to the right or that the world is spinning to the left. As a result, when she reaches for a target, she points to the left of the target (toward the direction she senses the target is moving).

11. The answer is C [Chapter 8 II B 1 b (3), 4 b]. A variety of sleep disturbances, including bed-wetting, sleepwalking, and night terrors all occur during slow-wave sleep. Dreaming occurs most often during rapid eye movement (REM) sleep, which is also characterized by high-frequency electroencephalogram (EEG) waves, irregular heart rates and breathing patterns, and total inhibition of alpha motoneurons.

12. The answer is A [Chapter 6 II A 3 b (1) (c) (ii). The stria vascularis is a profusely perfused

layer of epithelial cells that is responsible for the production of endolymph. Endolymph resembles intracellular fluid (ICF) in that it contains a high concentration of K^+ and a low concentration of Na^+. It is secreted into the scala media, where it surrounds the cells of the organ of Corti. The scala media is bounded above by Reissner's membrane and below by the basilar membrane.

13. The answer is C [Chapter 5 II A 4, C 3 a (1)]. Phasic (rapidly adapting) receptors are better suited than tonic receptors to encode the rate of stimulus application. When stimulated, phasic receptors produce a high frequency discharge that declines rapidly after the stimulus reaches its peak amplitude. The rate of decline depends on the rate of stimulus application. If the stimulus reaches its peak rapidly, very little adaptation occurs during the stimulus application and the initial rate of firing is very high. However, if the stimulus rises slowly to its peak, adaption limits the maximum frequency that can be obtained. Therefore, the firing encodes the rate of stimulus application. Tonic receptors are required to encode stimulus strength. Both types of receptors can provide information about stimulus quality, location, and duration. Phasic receptors encode duration by firing when the stimulus is applied and when it is removed. Tonic receptors encode duration by firing for as long as the stimulus is applied.

14. The answer is A [Chapter 6 I B 3 b (3), c (2)]. Presbyopia is the loss of accommodative power that occurs as a person ages. Because accommodation cannot occur, the near point moves away from the eye and images must be held at some distance from the eye to be clearly seen. This is similar to the situation in hyperopia where the converging power is too weak for the axial length of the eye. Hyperopes must accommodate to see distant objects clearly and thus have less accommodation available for near vision. Thus hyperopes, like presbyopes, must hold objects at a distance to see them clearly (hence the term "farsighted").

15. The answer is D [Chapter 7 V C 2–4; Chapter 8 I B 1 b]. The medullary pyramids contain the axons of the corticospinal tract. These axons provide excitatory input directly to alpha motoneurons within the spinal cord or to interneurons that excite alpha motoneurons. Lesions to these axons, therefore, reduce excitability. The striatum, substantia nigra, and subthalamic nucleus are components of the basal ganglia, which normally inhibit motor activity. Lesions in these structures increase motor tone or spontaneous movements. The internal capsule contains axons of upper motor neurons that normally inhibit brain stem neurons that are, in turn, excitatory to antigravity muscles. When these axons are damaged, the brain stem neurons are released from inhibition, causing the antigravity muscles to become hyperexcitable.

16. The answers is C [Chapter 6 II D 2]. The stereocilia and apical surface of hair cells in the organ of Corti are surrounded by the endolymph that fills the scala media. Endolymph contains high levels of K^+. When the vibration of the basilar membrane causes the stereocilia to bend toward the kinocilium, K^+ channels open, allowing K^+ to enter the cell. The flow of K^+ into the cell causes the hair cell to depolarize. K^+ is forced into the cell by the large potential difference between the endolymph (which is made positive by the secretion of K^+ from the scala vestibuli) and the intracellular fluid (ICF) of the hair cell (which is negative because the basolateral potions of the hair cell are bathed in the Na^+-containing perilymph of the scala vestibuli.

17. The answer is B [Chapter 5 III B 2; Figure 5-5]. Specific cold receptors are located on the free nerve endings of small myelinated and unmyelinated neurons. These receptors are distinguished from warm receptors because they produce a phasic burst of action potentials whenever their temperature is decreased and reduce their firing rate when they are warmed. Their steady-state firing rate reaches a peak at skin temperatures of about 23°C–28°C and declines as the temperature is raised or lowered from this point. If the temperature is raised to about 45°C, the cold fibers start firing again. At the same time, pain fibers are activated, producing a burning cold sensation.

18. The answer is A [Chapter 7 III B 1 a (1) (a) (i); Figure 7-3]. The Ia afferent fibers innervating the intrafusal muscle fibers contained within muscle spindles convey proprioceptive information about muscle length to the central nervous system (CNS). When nuclear bag intrafusal fibers are stretched, the Ia afferents respond by generating a burst of action potentials with a frequency proportionate to the rate of muscle stretch. Stretching the nuclear chain fibers produces a steady discharge proportional to the amount of stretch. Golgi tendon organs respond to the force developed by muscles, pacinian corpuscles respond to vibratory stimuli, and Ruffini's corpuscles respond to pressure applied to the skin.

PART III

CARDIOVASCULAR PHYSIOLOGY

Joseph Boyle, III

Chapter 9

Hemodynamics

I. CARDIOVASCULAR SYSTEM

A. **Primary functions,** which are carried out by **convection** (i.e., the mass movement of fluid caused by a difference in pressure between two points)

1. Distribution of substrates and oxygen (O_2) to all body cells

2. Collection of waste products and carbon dioxide (CO_2) for excretion

B. **Secondary functions**

1. Control of blood flow to the skin and extremities to enhance or retard heat loss

2. Distribution of hormones

3. Delivery of antibodies, platelets, and leukocytes to aid body defense mechanisms

C. **Components**

1. **Heart,** the driving force for blood flow

2. **Arteries,** the distribution channels to the organs

3. **Microcirculation,** including the capillaries, which serves as the exchange region

4. **Veins,** the blood reservoirs that collect the blood to return it to the heart

II. THE HEART AS A PUMP. The heart is two pumps in series (i.e., the right and left sides) that are connected by the pulmonary and systemic circulations.

A. **Valves** (Figure 9-1). Each side of the heart is equipped with two valves that normally maintain one-way blood flow.

1. **Atrioventricular (AV) valves [tricuspid (right) and mitral (left)]** separate the atria from the ventricles. These valves open during **ventricular diastole** to allow blood to fill the ventricles and close during **ventricular systole** to prevent **regurgitation** of blood from the ventricles into the atria.

2. **Semilunar valves (aortic and pulmonary)** open to allow the ventricles to eject blood into the aorta or pulmonary artery during systole and close to prevent **regurgitation** of blood into the ventricles during diastole.

3. **Systemic versus pulmonary flow.** Both ventricles must pump the same volume of blood over any significant time period because of the series arrangement of the systemic and

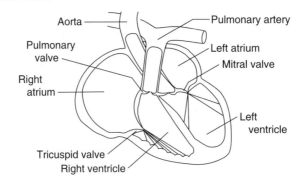

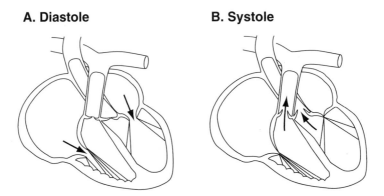

FIGURE 9-1. Heart valves. A schematic depiction of the heart valves during diastole (*A*) and systole (*B*). The direction of blood flow is indicated.

pulmonary circulations (Figure 9-2). The balanced output is achieved by an intrinsic property of cardiac muscle known as the **Frank-Starling mechanism** (see Chapter 11 III A).

B. **Ventricles**

1. The **right ventricle** pumps blood at low pressures through the pulmonary circulation.
   a. This ventricle ejects blood by the concurrent shortening of the free wall and bulging of the interventricular septum into the right ventricle **(bellows function).**
   b. The **normal cross-section** of the right ventricular chamber is **crescent-shaped.** If the right ventricle ejects blood against a high pressure for prolonged periods (e.g., secondary to pulmonary disease), it becomes more **cylindrical,** and thickening of the right ventricular free wall (ventricular hypertrophy) develops.

2. The **left ventricle,** which normally has a thicker wall than the right ventricle, pumps blood through the systemic circulation.
   a. This ventricle, which is cylindrical in shape, ejects blood primarily by reducing its cross-sectional area (a function of the square of the radius).
   b. The left ventricle works much harder than the right ventricle because of the higher pressures in the systemic circulation. Consequently, the left ventricle is more commonly affected by disease processes than the right ventricle.

C. **Cardiac output** (CO) equals the average stroke volume (SV) multiplied by the heart rate (HR):

$$CO = SV \cdot HR$$

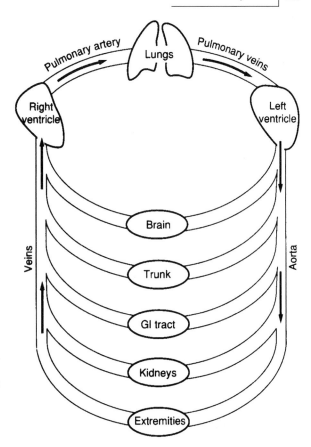

FIGURE 9-2. A schematic illustration of the organization of the cardiovascular system. Note that the right and left sides of the heart are connected in series, but the body organs receive blood through a parallel arrangement of vessels. GI = gastrointestinal.

1. **Normal cardiac output.** The stroke volume for each ventricle averages 70 ml, and a normal heart rate is approximately 70–75 beats/min. Therefore, the cardiac output at rest is approximately 5 L/min.
   a. Cardiac sympathetic efferent activity increases heart rate, whereas parasympathetic (vagal) efferent impulses decrease heart rate.
   b. The stroke volume varies with changes in the ventricular contractility, the arterial pressure, and the end-diastolic volume of the ventricle.

2. **Parallel distribution to the organs** (see Figure 9-2)
   a. The various systemic organs receive blood flow through parallel distribution channels.
   b. The parallel arrangement of vessels supplies the body organs with blood of the same arterial composition (e.g., same O_2 and CO_2 tensions, pH, glucose levels, and so on) and essentially the same arterial pressure.

III. **HEMODYNAMICS** is the study of the factors that determine blood flow and blood pressure in the body.

A. **Pressure,** a force per unit area (dynes/cm^2), is usually expressed in terms of the height of a column of fluid that the pressure will support. The common units of pressure are mm Hg and cm H_2O [1 mm Hg = 1.36 cm H_2O = 1330 dynes/cm^2].

1. **A pressure gradient (ΔP)** [i.e., a difference in the total energy or pressure between two points] is required to generate flow. Fluid always flows from an area of higher pressure

to one of lower pressure; in other words, water (or blood) always flows downhill (Figure 9-3).

2. The **total energy** at any point equals the sum of the potential energy and the kinetic energy.
   a. **Kinetic energy** is the momentum that blood gains because of its mass and velocity:

   $$\text{kinetic energy} = \frac{m \cdot v^2}{2}$$

   where m = mass and v = velocity.
   b. **Potential energy**
      (1) **Hydrostatic pressure (P_h)** results from a difference in vertical height in a fluid-filled system. Because of gravity, fluid has weight that generates force, which is proportional to its vertical height (e.g., the pressure at the bottom of a lake is higher than it is at the surface):

      $$P_h = \delta \cdot h \cdot g$$

      where δ = fluid density, h = height of the fluid column above or below a reference level, and g = gravitational constant.
      (a) In an upright person, assuming that the foot is 150 cm below the heart, the pressure in the vessels of the foot is 150 cm H_2O (110 mm Hg) higher than the pressure at the root of the aorta (Figure 9-4).
      (b) In a supine person, the hydrostatic effect is eliminated because the entire cardiovascular system is at essentially the same horizontal level. To measure blood pressure accurately, it is important to place the gauge or the sphygmomanometer cuff at the **zero reference (phlebostatic) level,** which is equivalent to the level of the right atrium.

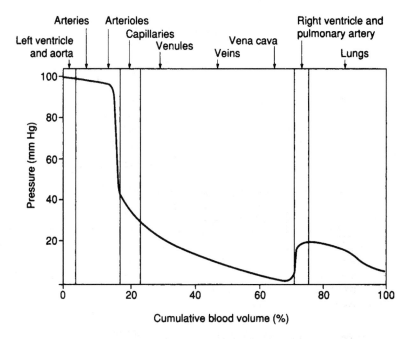

FIGURE 9-3. Mean (average) lateral pressure in various components of the cardiovascular system. Note the progressive decrease in pressure from the left ventricle through the systemic circulation until the blood enters the right ventricle. The right ventricle pumps the blood through the pulmonary circulation. The resistance of the large vessels is minimal. The greatest pressure drop occurs in the arterioles, which represent the highest resistance segment of the systemic circulation.

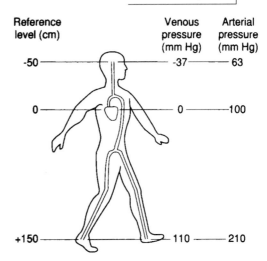

Reference level (cm)	Venous pressure (mm Hg)	Arterial pressure (mm Hg)
-50	-37	63
0	0	100
+150	110	210

FIGURE 9-4. Effects of a hydrostatic column of blood on arterial and venous pressures. The zero reference level is at the right atrium.

    (c) Both arteries and veins at any given horizontal level are affected by the same hydrostatic pressure of blood so that the pressure gradient between arteries and veins is not altered (see Figure 9-4). However, the hydrostatic pressure causes distention of dependent blood vessels, which alters flow by reducing the resistance. This distention is especially significant in compliant vascular beds such as the veins or the pulmonary vessels.

  (2) Lateral (static) pressure represents the pressure in the cardiovascular system that is usually measured with a gauge or transducer after eliminating the hydrostatic pressure effect. (It does not include kinetic energy.)

 c. Conversion of energy. Energy can be converted between potential and kinetic energy.

  (1) The difference in total pressure between any two points in a system represents the **pressure gradient** that generates flow. (Figure 9-5).

  (2) As the fluid flows through the pipe, as shown in Figure 9-5, there is progressive loss of energy along the pipe as a result of resistance (see III B 2 b). If there is no flow, then the fluid level (pressure) in all the columns equals the fluid level at the source.

  (3) The narrowed section of the pipe is a high-resistance segment. The greater resistance leads to a greater loss of total energy per unit length of pipe. Because velocity through this narrowed segment is very high, some of the total energy is converted into kinetic energy, which is recovered when the tube widens.

B. **Flow (Q)** is the mass movement of a volume of fluid per unit time. Usually expressed in ml/sec or L/min, it may be represented as the average velocity of movement (cm/sec) multiplied by the cross-sectional area of the tube (cm²).

 1. Continuity principle. In any system arranged in series, the flow through each vascular segment must be equal to the flow through every other, unless one segment becomes progressively distended. The limit for distention can be rapidly reached. The cross-sectional area of different vascular segments varies in the body. To keep the flow rate equal, the velocity of flow must vary inversely with the cross-sectional area for each vascular segment (Figure 9-6).

 2. Poiseuille's law for laminar flow is expressed as:

$$Q = \frac{\Delta P \cdot \pi \cdot r^4}{8 \cdot \eta \cdot L}$$

 where ΔP = pressure gradient, r = tube radius, η = fluid viscosity, and L = tube length.

 a. Flow, pressure gradient, and resistance. Poiseuille's law is valid for straight, rigid tubes that contain a fluid with constant flow rate and constant viscosity; therefore, it

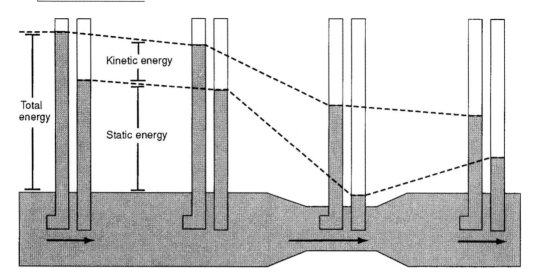

FIGURE 9-5. A system of pitot tubes demonstrating the variation in total energy (pressure), potential energy, and kinetic energy in relation to flow velocity. The *arrows* represent relative velocities in the different segments of the system. The narrowed section, a high-resistance segment, causes a large pressure drop as a result of the conversion of potential energy to kinetic energy. In addition, resistance (frictional) forces contribute to the drop in pressure. In the right segment, potential energy increases as the velocity of flow slows again.

does not strictly apply to the vascular system. Nevertheless, important principles relating flow, pressure gradient, and resistance remain applicable.

(1) If resistance (R) is defined as $\Delta P/Q$, then Poiseuille's law simplifies to a relationship analogous to Ohm's law: current (flow) = voltage (pressure gradient)/R. Therefore, blood flow equals the difference in pressure between two points in the vascular system divided by the resistance to flow: $Q = \Delta P/R$.

    (a) Elevating the arterial pressure usually leads to an increase in the pressure gradient.

    (b) An increase in the pressure gradient causes a rise in blood flow, whereas an increase in resistance causes a decrease in blood flow.

(2) **Measures of resistance**

    (a) **Total peripheral resistance (TPR)** is usually expressed as the ratio of the difference in pressure to the flow: TPR = $\Delta P/Q$ (in mm Hg/L/min).

    (b) The **peripheral resistance unit (PRU)** equals 1 mm Hg/ml/sec. The resistance of the normal systemic circulation is approximately 1 PRU, and the pulmonary vascular resistance is 0.1–0.2 PRU.

b. **Factors that affect resistance.** The major factors that determine the resistance to blood flow are the **radius of the vessels** and the **viscosity of the blood.** Although an increase in the length of blood vessels in the body would cause a proportional increase in resistance, the length is generally fixed.

(1) **Vessel radius.** Because the vessel radius is raised to the fourth power, any change in the vessel radius produces a marked change in the flow (e.g., for a constant pressure gradient, if the radius is reduced by a factor of 2, the flow is decreased by a factor of 16).

    (a) **Arteriolar radius.** Control of blood flow to organs or tissues is regulated primarily by altering the radius of the arterioles. Because the arterioles control the flow to various vascular beds, they are considered the **stopcocks** of the circulation. Arteriolar radius is controlled by altering the number of sympathetic impulses to the blood vessels, by various drugs or hormones, or by the

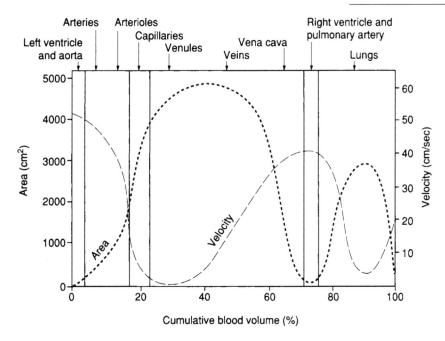

FIGURE 9-6. Relationships between velocity, cross-sectional area, and pressure in various segments of the cardiovascular system plotted as a function of the cumulative blood volume. Velocity of blood flow and area are inversely related.

release of various chemicals from the tissues (e.g., histamine, prostaglandin, CO_2, H^+).

- **(b) Distensibility.** Blood vessels in the body are not rigid but distensible; the diameter of the vessels varies as a function of the transmural pressure. Increasing arterial pressure not only increases the driving force but also decreases vascular resistance. Thus, blood flow in the body increases to a greater extent than would be predicted from the increased arterial pressure, per se.

(2) Viscosity is the internal friction to flow in a fluid. Blood, which contains cells and proteins, is a complex fluid, and its viscosity varies as a function of flow rate and vessel size.

- **(a)** Variation in the **hematocrit** is the major factor that changes the viscosity of blood. An increase in hematocrit tends to reduce flow rate because of increased viscosity.
- **(b)** The normal hematocrit for men is 40–45, whereas the normal value for premenopausal women is 35–40. The viscosity of blood with a hematocrit of 40 is approximately three times that of water.

IV. ARTERIAL BLOOD VOLUME AND PRESSURE

A. **Arterial blood volume,** the amount of blood within the arterial vessels, is **normally 10%–15% of the total blood volume.**

1. The **arterial blood volume is one determinant of arterial pressure,** because the blood in the arteries stretches the walls of the blood vessels, which then recoil, generating pressure (Figure 9-7). This recoil force is termed **elastance.**

   a. The **equilibrium (unstressed) volume** of the arterial tree is the volume of blood in the arteries when the transmural pressure is zero.

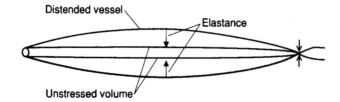

Distended vessel

Elastance

Unstressed volume

FIGURE 9-7. Diagram showing that the vascular system exhibits elastic properties similar to a balloon. The blood volume distends the vessel, which then recoils and generates a pressure.

    b. The **arterial elastance** represents the ratio of change in pressure to a change in volume.

        (1) **Elastance** is the **reciprocal of compliance** (i.e., distensibility).

        (2) The **slope** of the pressure–volume curves for the various age groups in Figure 9–8 represents the elastance.

  2. Acute changes. The arterial pressure varies constantly as a result of changes in the arterial blood volume, which depends on changes in heart rate, peripheral resistance, and stroke volume (Figure 9-9).

  3. Long-term changes in arterial pressure are caused by changes in the unstressed (resting) volume or the elastance of the arterial system (the arterial system enlarges and becomes more rigid with age).

B. **Arterial blood pressure**

  1. Factors that increase arterial pressure

    a. Increased heart rate

        (1) Increasing the heart rate raises pressure, because the time the blood has to leave the arterial tree is reduced (i.e., decreased duration of the cardiac cycle). In addition, the **cardiac output usually increases.**

        (2) After an increase in heart rate, the arterial pressure rises, increasing the driving pressure for flow, until the amount of blood exiting the arterial system equals the amount entering. At this time, the transfer of blood from the venous to the arterial system has raised the arterial pressure and lowered the venous pressure.

    b. Increased peripheral resistance raises the arterial volume by reducing the amount of blood that leaves the arterial system. The arterial pressure rises until the new pressure is sufficient to overcome the additional resistance to flow, and arterial outflow again equals inflow.

    c. Increased stroke volume raises the arterial pressure by increasing the cardiac output (flow rate). The arterial pressure rises until outflow equals inflow.

    d. Increased elastic constant. The elastic constant refers to stiffness of the arterial system, which progressively increases from birth until death (see Figure 9-8). Increased stiffness or elastance of the arterial system causes a rise in pressure for any increase in arterial volume.

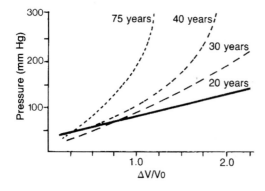

FIGURE 9-8. The average pressure–volume relationships of arterial systems in 20-, 30-, 40-, and 75-year-old individuals. Note the increasing elastance (decreased distensibility) that occurs with aging. ΔV = volume change, V_0 = unstressed arterial volume.

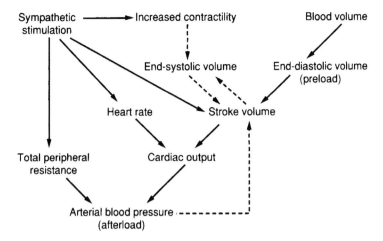

FIGURE 9-9. A flow diagram showing the relationships among factors that determine cardiac output and mean arterial pressure. Increases are indicated by *solid arrows;* decreases are indicated by *dashed arrows.*

2. **Factors that decrease arterial pressure**
   a. **Reductions in heart rate, peripheral resistance, stroke volume,** or **elastic constant** decrease arterial pressure.
   b. **Hemorrhage** and **blood pooling** reduce the arterial pressure by **decreasing the circulating blood volume. Gravity or marked vasodilation** by neural, chemical, or mechanical factors may lead to blood pooling in dependent portions of the body and decrease circulating blood volume.

3. **Arterial pressure** varies continuously because although the heart ejects blood into the arteries intermittently, the blood flows out through the capillaries continuously.
   a. **Terminology**
      (1) **Systolic pressure** is the highest pressure in the arterial system and occurs during ventricular ejection. The normal systemic arterial systolic pressure is approximately 120 mm Hg.
      (2) **Diastolic pressure** is the lowest pressure in the arterial system during any cardiac cycle and occurs just before the onset of ventricular ejection. The normal systemic arterial diastolic pressure is approximately 80 mm Hg.
   b. **Factors that affect pulse pressure.** Pulse pressure, the arithmetic difference between systolic and diastolic pressures, is normally 40 mm Hg. The **pulse pressure** depends on three factors: **arterial volume, stroke volume,** and the **arterial elastic constant.**

$$\Delta P = \frac{\Delta V}{V} \cdot \frac{1}{K_a}$$

where ΔV = arterial uptake volume (approximately equal to, but less than, the stroke volume), V = arterial volume [proportional to the mean arterial pressure (MAP)], and K_a = arterial elastic constant.
      (1) Figure 9-10 depicts the relationship among these factors, which is integral to properly interpreting changes in a patient's heart rate and blood pressure. The effects of age and increased stroke volume raise the pulse pressure, while increases in heart rate or TPR reduce this pressure.
      (2) **Mean arterial pressure (MAP)** equals TPR divided by cardiac output. MAP can also be expressed as:

$$MAP = \frac{PP}{3} + DP$$

where MAP = mean arterial pressure, PP = pulse pressure, and DP = diastolic pressure.

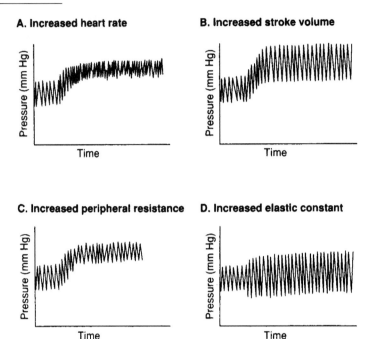

FIGURE 9-10. Factors that alter pulse pressure. (A) An increased heart rate but constant stroke volume increase cardiac output and mean arterial pressure (MAP). Because the elastic constant remains unchanged, the pulse pressure must decline to maintain equality. (B) An increased stroke volume at a constant heart rate also increases cardiac output and MAP, but pulse pressure increases. (C) An increased peripheral resistance transiently reduces capillary flow, and arterial volume and pressure increase. The result is a decrease in pulse pressure. (D) An increased elastic constant increases the pulse pressure, but the MAP remains normal.

Case 9

A 67-year-old man has a heart rate of 80 beats/min at rest and an arterial blood pressure of 135/90 mm Hg (mean = 105 mm Hg). Cardiac catheterization reveals a right atrial pressure of 0 mm Hg and a cardiac output of 4.5 L/min. During a cardiac stress test, the patient's heart rate is 120 beats/min with an arterial blood pressure of 170/100 mm Hg (mean = 125 mm Hg). Cardiac output now is 8.0 L/min, and the right atrial pressure is 5 mm Hg.

    1. *What causes the increased pulse pressure during exercise?*

DISCUSSION

The equation for Young's elastic modulus ($\Delta P = (\Delta V/V)/K_a$) can be used to analyze the different factors that control pulse pressure. The elastic modulus changes only over extended periods with aging, so that is not a factor. An increased arterial volume [V, proportional to mean arterial pressure (MAP)] would produce a decrease in pulse pressure. Therefore, the increased pulse pressure occurs primarily as the result of increased stroke volume.

    2. *How does the peripheral resistance change during exercise?*

DISCUSSION

The peripheral resistance equals the driving force for blood flow through the systemic circulation divided by the cardiac output. Aortic pressure minus right atrial pressure is the driving force. At rest, the peripheral resistance is 26.7 mm Hg/L/min (125—5/4.5), while during exercise, it decreases to 15 (120/8). The reduction in peripheral resistance during exercise occurs as a result of vasodilation in the skeletal muscles.

3. *Why does the MAP increase during exercise?*

DISCUSSION

The elevated arterial pressure during exercise is due to a higher cardiac output, which increases to a greater extent than peripheral resistance decreases.

Chapter 10

Electrical Events

I. INTRODUCTION

A. **Terminology.** The terms systole (contractile phase) and diastole (relaxation phase) usually refer to ventricular events but may be prefixed by "atrial" to refer to atrial contraction and relaxation, respectively.

B. **Rate.** The heart has an intrinsic contraction rate because it contains its own **pacemaker,** normally located in the **sinoatrial (SA) node.**

1. **Noradrenergic (sympathetic postganglionic) neurons** increase the pacemaker rate.

2. **Cholinergic (parasympathetic) neurons** decrease the pacemaker rate. The parasympathetic nerve to the heart is the **vagus nerve (cranial nerve X).**

C. **Myocardial syncytium.** The heart muscle (myocardium) is composed of separate cardiac muscle cells that are electrically connected with one another by gap junctions (see Chapter 3 IV A 1–2).

1. Depolarization of one cardiac cell is transmitted to adjacent cells via the gap junctions; thus, the myocardium is a functional syncytium (a mass of cytoplasm with numerous nuclei).

2. The heart actually functions as two syncytia (i.e., the atria and the ventricles).
   a. These two masses of muscle are separated by the fibrous atrioventricular (AV) valve ring, which insulates the electrical events of the atria from those of the ventricles.
   b. Normally, there is only one functional electrical connection between the atria and the ventricles—the AV node and its continuation, the bundle of His.

II. ELECTRICAL ACTIVITY

A. **Resting membrane potential** (see Chapter 2 III). The myocardial cells maintain a voltage difference across their cell membranes of 60–90 mV.

B. **Slow and fast fibers.** Myocardial cells are either slow or fast fibers, depending on the membrane potential and the shape and conduction velocity of the action potential (AP) [Figure 10-1].

1. **Slow fibers** are normally present only in the **SA and AV nodes.** The effects of hypoxia or certain drugs can convert fast fibers to slow fibers.
   a. **Resting membrane potential.** In slow fibers, this value is **60–70 mV.**
   b. **Action potential (AP).** In slow fibers, the inward movement of positive ions (Na^+ and Ca^{2+}) neutralizes the normally negative intracellular charge, producing an AP. During the AP, the membrane potential approaches zero and the cell is said to be depolarized.
      (1) **Slow channels.** Ions enter cells through "slow channels" in slow fibers.
         (a) These slow channels limit the rate of ion entry, slowing the rate of cell depolarization.
         (b) The upstroke of the AP requires approximately 100 msec in slow fibers, compared with 1 msec in fast fibers.
      (2) The **conduction velocity** is directly related to the resting membrane potential and

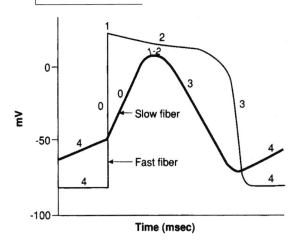

FIGURE 10-1. Action potentials (APs) from fast and slow cardiac fibers showing the different phases of the AP. Note the diastolic depolarization (phase 4) and the gradual phase 0 in the slow fiber.

the rate of membrane depolarization. The conduction velocity of slow fibers is only 0.02–0.10 m/sec.

(3) The **absolute refractory period** (see Chapter 2 IV E 2 c) lasts for the duration of the AP in all myocardial fibers.

(4) The **relative refractory period** may last for several seconds in slow fibers.

   (a) A stimulus applied during the relative refractory period must be stronger than normal to elicit an AP, which has a slower-than-normal conduction velocity.

   (b) A prolonged refractory period frequently interferes with the conduction of impulses within the AV node, preventing some or all of the atrial depolarizations from reaching the ventricles.

2. **Fast fibers** include the normal atrial and ventricular myocardial cells and the specialized conducting tissues of the heart.

   a. **Resting membrane potential.** In fast fibers, this is **80–90 mV.**

   b. **Action potentials (APs)** [Figure 10-2]

   (1) **Na$^+$ channels.** The AP of fast fibers exhibits an extremely rapid rate of rise be-

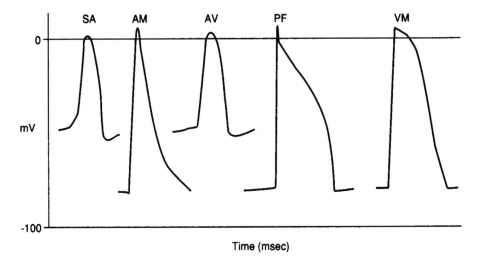

FIGURE 10-2. The form of the action potentials (APs) from various cardiac tissues. SA = sinoatrial node; AM = atrial muscle; AV = atrioventricular node; PF = Purkinje fiber; VM = ventricular muscle.

cause once the threshold potential is reached, the cell membrane becomes extremely permeable to Na^+. (See Chapter 2 III for a discussion of ionic events during an AP.)

   (a) The duration of the AP, which varies in fast fibers, is longest in Purkinje and bundle of His fibers (see Figure 10-2).

   (b) The long AP and absolute refractory period protect the heart somewhat against certain arrhythmias by limiting the maximal ventricular rate.

   (2) The **conduction velocities** of fast fibers vary from 0.3–1.0 m/sec in myocardial cells to approximately 4 m/sec in Purkinje fibers. The high conduction velocity ensures that the entire myocardium is depolarized almost instantaneously, which improves the effectiveness of myocardial contraction.

   (3) The **absolute refractory period** in fast fibers lasts until the repolarization has reached a membrane potential of 50–60 mV.

   (4) The **relative refractory period** ends when the resting membrane potential of 80–90 mV is reestablished.

C. **The cardiac AP** is the change in membrane potential that occurs after a myocyte is depolarized to the threshold potential (see Chapter 2 IV D 1 a). The cardiac AP has five phases (see Figure 10-1).

1. **Phase 0 (upstroke).** The resting membrane is relatively impermeable to Na^+, but once the threshold potential is reached, the Na^+ channels open and Na^+ rushes into the cell. This is a positive feedback (regenerative) system (see Chapter 2, Figure 2-5). The movement of Na^+ ions is a current-carrying process that results in the depolarization of the cell membrane (phase 0).

   a. This process is extremely rapid in fast fibers (see II B).

   b. In slow fibers, Ca^{2+} is the current-carrying ion; therefore, phase 0 coincides with an increase in the Ca^{2+} conductance.

2. **Phase 1.** The Na^+ conductance is rapidly reduced when the Na^+ channels close, but the membrane conductance for both Ca^{2+} and K^+ increases. The overall effect is a small amount of repolarization.

3. **Phase 2.** The plateau of the AP in fast fibers coincides with an increased membrane conductance for Ca^{2+}. The inward movement of Ca^{2+} and the decreased efflux of K^+ maintain the membrane potential near zero.

4. **Phase 3** is a rapid repolarization resulting from a reduction of the inward Na^+ and Ca^{2+} currents and a large increase in the outward K^+ current.

5. **Phase 4**

   a. **Nonpacemaker cells** (e.g., atrial and ventricular myocardium) exhibit a constant membrane potential during phase 4.

   b. In **pacemaker tissues** (e.g., SA and AV nodes and Purkinje fibers), a slow diastolic depolarization occurs, which indicates the presence of **automaticity** (i.e., ability of the heart to generate its own beat).

      (1) The diastolic depolarization **(pacemaker potential)** brings the membrane potential toward threshold. The cell whose membrane potential first reaches threshold is the pacemaker of the heart, and the depolarization then spreads to the remainder of the heart.

      (2) The **normal pacemaker** of the heart is the **SA node** because its cells usually have the steepest slope of phase 4. Elimination of SA nodal activity or an increased slope of phase 4 in other areas of the heart produces an **ectopic pacemaker.**

III. **CONDUCTION PATHWAYS** (Figure 10-3A&B)

A. **SA node.** The normal pacemaker of the heart, the SA node is located near the junction of the superior vena cava and the right atrium. The isolated SA node has a firing rate of

A

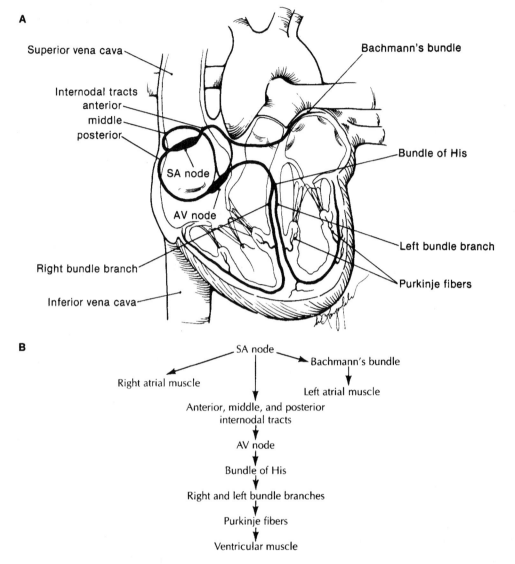

FIGURE 10-3. (*A*) The specialized conducting tissues of the heart. (*B*) Flow diagram summarizing the path of depolarization in the heart. SA = sinoatrial; AV = atrioventricular.

90–120 beats/min. This rate is higher in young individuals and declines with advancing age. The rate of the intrinsic firing rate of the SA node rises as a result of temperature increases and hyperthyroidism.

1. **Vagus nerve.** The right vagus nerve densely innervates the SA node and liberates **acetylcholine** from its nerve endings when stimulated.
   a. Vagal activity (vagal tone) slows the firing rate of the SA node from its intrinsic rate of 90–120 beats/min to the actual heart rate of approximately 70 beats/min.
   b. Strong vagal stimulation can completely eliminate SA node impulses **(sinus arrest),** leading to **asystole.** The heart will begin to beat again if an ectopic pacemaker takes over or if vagal escape occurs.
2. **Sympathetic nerves.** Stimulation of cardiac sympathetic nerves or the injection of sym-

pathomimetic drugs **increases heart rate** (i.e., has a **positive chronotropic effect**) and increases the automaticity of ectopic sites. Such nerve stimulation markedly **increases the force of contraction (positive inotropic effect).**

B. **Interatrial tract (Bachmann's bundle).** This band of specialized muscle fibers runs from the SA node to the left atrium. The interatrial tract causes almost simultaneous depolarization and contraction of both atria, because the conduction velocity through this tissue is very fast (Table 10-1).

C. **Internodal tracts.** The **anterior, middle,** and **posterior internodal tracts** connect the SA and AV nodes. The internodal tracts increase the likelihood that impulses from the SA node will reach the AV node and initiate ventricular depolarization, because the internodal tracts are more resistant than atrial muscle to the blockade of impulses.

D. **AV node.** The AV node is normally the **only path for excitation** from the atria to the ventricles. The AV node is located just beneath the endocardium on the right side of the interatrial septum near the tricuspid valve.

1. **AV nodal delay.** The conduction velocity through the AV node is extremely slow (see Table 10-1), so that ventricular depolarization is delayed for 100–150 msec after atrial depolarization. This delay provides time for atrial contraction to occur, which enhances ventricular filling, especially at fast heart rates.

2. **Stimulation.** The AV node is richly supplied by fibers from both the sympathetic and vagal nerves, which affect the conduction of impulses.
   a. **Sympathetic stimulation** shortens the duration of the AP and increases the conduction rate through the AV node. These effects enhance the transmission of impulses.
   b. **Parasympathetic (vagal) stimulation** slows the conduction velocity and prolongs the refractory periods, making it more likely that AV block will occur.

E. **Ventricular conduction.** The impulses conducted through the AV node are distributed to the ventricles by specialized fibers.

1. The **bundle of His,** the continuation of the AV node, is located beneath the endocardium on the right side of the interventricular septum. The bundle of His **splits into the right and left bundle branches.**

2. The **right** and **left bundle branches** proceed on each side of the interventricular septum to their respective ventricles (see Figure 10-3A).
   a. **Congenital or acquired lesions** may lead to blockage of the depolarization process in either bundle branch. The affected ventricle is eventually depolarized by the spread of impulses through the regular ventricular muscle fibers. This leads to delayed activation of the affected ventricle as a result of the slow depolarization of ventricular muscle fibers.

TABLE 10-1. Cardiac Conductive Properties

Tissue	Fiber Diameter (μm)	Resting Membrane Potential (mV)	Conduction Velocity (m/sec)
Sinoatrial node	. . .	40–50	0.05
Atrial muscle	8–10	70–80	0.3–0.5
Internodal tracts	15–20	80–90	1.0
Atrioventricular node	Variable	50	0.02–0.05
Purkinje fibers	70–80	70	2.0–4.0
Ventricular muscle	10–16	80	<1.0

b. A right or left bundle branch block produces characteristic electrocardiographic (EKG) changes (see V C 4).

3. Purkinje fibers arise from both bundle branches and radiate extensively just beneath the endocardium of both ventricles. These cells have the largest diameter of any fibers in the heart and possess the highest conduction velocity (see Table 10-1). The high conduction velocity ensures that both ventricles normally contract almost simultaneously, which increases the effectiveness of contraction.

F. | **Ventricular muscle.** Depolarization of this muscle occurs from the endocardial surface to the epicardium.

1. The first part of the ventricle to undergo depolarization is the interventricular septum, and the last area to be depolarized is the base of the left ventricle.

2. The conduction velocity of the AP through the ventricular myocardium is 0.3–0.4 m/sec.

IV. | **ELECTROCARDIOGRAPHY.** The technique of recording electrical activity from the heart originally was developed by Willem Einthoven, a Dutch physiologist. The acronym EKG (from *elektrokardiogramm*) is used here in deference to Dr. Einthoven, who received a Nobel prize for his work. The EKG provides a method of evaluating excitation events, arrhythmias, cardiac hypertrophy, myocardial damage, and the presence of ischemia or necrosis. The EKG does not provide information concerning the mechanical performance of the heart, and at times, standard EKG leads do not record even abnormal electrical activity.

A. | **Volume conduction.** Body tissues function as electrical conductors because they contain electrolytes. The heart is assumed to lie centrally within the thorax, and its electrical activity is conducted to the body surface through the body fluids.

1. Electrodes. Attaching electrodes to the body surface allows the voltage changes within the body to be recorded after adequate amplification of the signal. A **galvanometer** within the EKG machine (electrocardiograph) is used as a recording device. Galvanometers record potential (voltage) differences between two electrodes.

2. Surface potentials. EKGs are merely the recordings of voltage differences between two electrodes on the body surface as a function of time.

a. Zero potentials. During diastole, the cardiac cells are positively charged on the outside and negatively charged on the inside. Electrodes on the skin do not detect voltage differences because all parts of the heart are equally polarized. Thus, the recording shows no deflection from the **zero potential line** (Figure 10-4A).

b. Action potentials (APs)

(1) Depolarization of a portion of the heart causes a reversal of membrane potential in the area. The outside of these cells is now negatively charged with respect to ground. Thus, a potential difference exists between the depolarized cells and the neighboring, nonexcited cells (Figure 10-4B).

(a) Surface electrodes record this potential difference, and the direction of its deflection depends on the polarity of the electrodes.

(b) When the entire heart has been depolarized, all of the cells are negatively charged outside. Both electrodes again "see" the same potential, and the galvanometer reading returns to zero (Figure 10-4C).

(2) Repolarization. Assuming that repolarization proceeds in the same direction as depolarization, the galvanometer will be deflected in the opposite direction (Figure 10-4D&E) during the repolarization process.

(3) The resulting record of depolarization and repolarization is termed a **biphasic AP** because there are two opposite waves.

3. Equivalent dipole. The voltage differences among resting, depolarized, and repolarizing cells function as a battery. The sum of the various charges is termed an **equivalent dipole.**

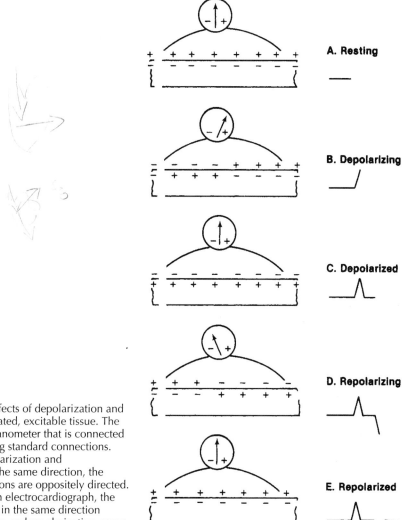

FIGURE 10-4. The effects of depolarization and repolarization on isolated, excitable tissue. The dial represents a galvanometer that is connected to the tissue bath using standard connections. Note that when depolarization and repolarization are in the same direction, the galvanometer deflections are oppositely directed. In the limb leads of an electrocardiograph, the QRS and T waves are in the same direction because depolarization and repolarization occur in opposite directions.

A. Resting

B. Depolarizing

C. Depolarized

D. Repolarizing

E. Repolarized

   a. The total charge depends on the mass of tissue involved as well as the magnitude of the membrane potentials.
   b. The cardiac dipole is a **vector quantity,** with both **magnitude** and **direction.** Vectors are represented as arrows, with the arrowhead indicating the direction, and the length of the arrow indicating the magnitude.
4. The magnitude of the voltage recorded at the body surface is a function of electrode position and the orientation and magnitude of the dipole. Figure 10-5 depicts these relationships, which are essential to understanding analysis of EKG recordings.
   a. By convention, a wave of depolarization approaching the positive electrode results in an upward deflection of the EKG tracing.
   b. A wave of depolarization proceeding parallel to an electrode axis (the line connecting two electrodes) produces the maximal deflection for that dipole.
   c. A depolarization wave perpendicular to the electrode axis produces no net deflection of the tracing (i.e., the positive and negative waves are equal).

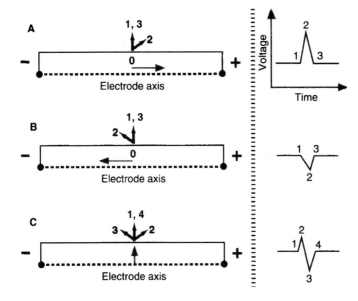

FIGURE 10-5. The deflection of a galvanometer needle using standard connections. (*A*) A wave of depolarization approaching a positive electrode causes an upward (positive) deflection. (*B*) A wave of depolarization approaching a negative electrode causes a downward deflection. (*C*) A wave of depolarization proceeding perpendicular to the electrode axis produces no net deflection.

B. The **standard 12-lead EKG** consists of three bipolar limb leads (I, II, and III), three augmented limb leads (aVR, aVL, and aVF), and six chest leads (V_1–V_6). Each lead shows the same cardiac events as the other leads, but from a different view. Additional leads are used in special circumstances.

1. **Einthoven's triangle.** In this conformation, the torso forms an equilateral triangle, with the right and left shoulders and the left leg as the apices. The right leg serves as a ground connector (Figure 10-6A). The extremities merely serve as conductors from the torso.

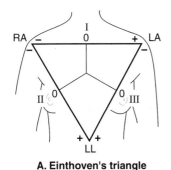

A. Einthoven's triangle

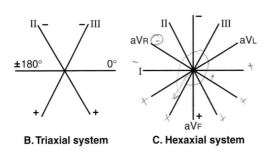

B. Triaxial system **C. Hexaxial system**

FIGURE 10-6. (*A*) Einthoven's triangle showing connections, bipolar limb leads, and lead polarity. The electrical zero occurs at the center of each of the bipolar leads. (*B*) The triaxial reference system in which leads I, II, and III are collapsed onto their respective zero points. (*C*) The hexaxial reference system, obtained by adding the augmented unipolar limb leads (aVR, aVL, aVF) to the triaxial system. RA = right arm; LA = left arm; LL = left leg.

a. **Zero potential lines.** If lines are drawn perpendicularly from the center of each side of an equilateral triangle, they will meet at the center of the triangle. These lines represent the zero potential lines for the three axes (see Figure 10-6A).
   b. **Bipolar limb leads.** Three leads are formed by measuring the potential differences between any two of the active limb electrodes [i.e., the **right arm (RA), left arm (LA), and left leg (LL)**]. These leads are selected by a switch on all standard EKG machines.
   (1) **Lead I** (mV) = LA − RA.
   (2) **Lead II** (mV) = LL − RA.
   (3) **Lead III** (mV) = LL − LA.

2. **Unipolar (V) leads.** If the three limb leads are connected to a common terminal, the combined voltage from the three leads theoretically will be zero. This common terminal can be attached to the negative pole of a galvanometer and a fourth, or exploring, electrode can be attached to the positive pole. If the common electrode is at zero volts, the exploring electrode will provide the actual or absolute voltage at the body surface. This arrangement of connections, which is termed a **unipolar electrode,** is used to record the **precordial** or **chest leads** from standardized sites. There are six precordial (V) leads in the standard EKG (Figure 10-7).

3. **Augmented unipolar (aV) leads.** Alternatively, the unipolar exploring electrode may be placed on the limbs to record cardiac potentials; however, the deflections are small. The size of the recordings is increased by eliminating the electrode of interest from the common terminal. The potentials recorded in this manner from the **RA, LA,** and **LL** are termed **aVR, aVL,** and **aVF,** respectively. The "a" refers to augmented, because the deflections are enlarged.

C. **Reference systems**

1. **Triaxial reference system.** This system involves moving the sides of Einthoven's triangle so that they intersect at the center of the triangle. Lead I then divides the system into an upper (negative) and a lower (positive) hemisphere (Figure 10-6B).

2. **Hexaxial reference system.** Superimposing the axes of the aV leads on the triaxial system provides a hexaxial reference system with axes every 30°. The aV lead axes bisect the angles of Einthoven's triangle (Figure 10-6C). In this system, leads I and aVF divide the system into quadrants with the **zero potential point** for all leads at the central intersection.

D. **EKGs** are the tracings of the surface cardiac potentials recorded against time. These records usually are made at a standard recording speed (25 mm/sec) and amplification (1 mV = 1

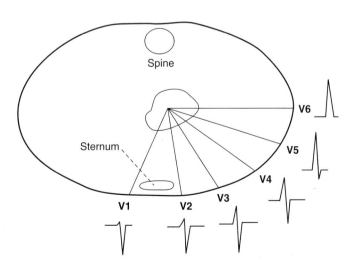

FIGURE 10-7. Standard placement sites for the precordial or chest electrodes of an electrocardiograph, showing typical complexes recorded from each site.

cm deflection). Using standard EKG paper, each small horizontal division represents 0.04 sec and each large division 0.2 sec. Each small vertical division represents 0.1 mV.

1. **EKG waves and intervals** (Figure 10-8)

   a. A **P wave** results from **atrial depolarization** and is normally positive (upright) in the standard limb leads and inverted in aVR.

   b. The **QRS complex** is caused by **ventricular depolarization,** and its duration is normally less than 0.08 sec.

      (1) **Terminology.** The **ventricular depolarization complex** is termed the **QRS complex** regardless of whether all three components are present.

         (a) A **Q wave** is a **negative wave before a positive wave.**

         (b) An **R wave** is a **positive wave.** If there are two positive waves, the second is designated **"R'"** and the smaller of the two is designated by **"r."** For example, an rSR' complex would consist of a small, initial R wave, an S wave, and a large, final R wave (see Figure 10-19B).

         (c) An **S wave** is a negative wave following an R wave. If no R wave is present, a **completely negative wave** is termed a **QS complex.**

      (2) Prolongation of the QRS complex indicates either an intraventricular conduction block or the presence of a ventricular pacemaker.

   c. The **T wave** is caused by **ventricular repolarization** and normally is in the same direction as the QRS complex, because ventricular repolarization follows a path opposite to depolarization.

   d. The **P-R interval,** which is measured from the onset of the P wave to the onset of the QRS complex, normally is between 0.12 and 0.21 sec, depending on heart rate. The P-R interval is a measure of the **AV conduction time,** including the delay through the AV node.

   e. The **R-R interval,** the time between successive QRS complexes, is the **cardiac cycle duration.** The heart rate equals 60 divided by the R-R interval in seconds.

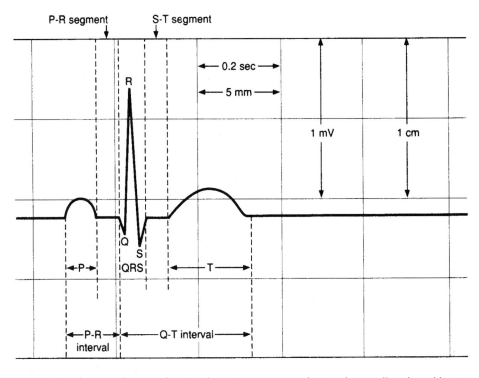

FIGURE 10-8. An electrocardiogram showing the various waves and intervals as well as the calibration times and voltages.

f. The **Q-T interval** is the time from the start of the QRS complex to the end of the T wave. Ischemia and any ventricular conduction defects prolong the Q-T interval.

2. The **mean electrical axis (MEA)** is the average vector produced by the P, QRS, and T waves in the EKG.
   a. **Derivation.** The MEA in the frontal plane can be derived using any two standard (i.e., bipolar) limb leads or any two augmented limb leads. The MEA in the horizontal plane is derived using the precordial leads.
   b. **Method of measurement.** Clinically, the frontal MEA of the QRS complex is determined algebraically by summing the heights of the Q, R, and S waves in each of two leads. The resultant sum represents the magnitude of the vector for the respective lead. The direction of the vector is toward either the positive or negative electrode depending on the value of the summation. Figure 10-9 summarizes this method of determining the MEA.
      (1) **Plotting lead vectors.** The vector from each lead is plotted on an appropriate scale using the Einthoven triangle or the triaxial or hexaxial reference systems.
      (2) **Plotting the MEA.** The tail of the vector for each lead is placed on the zero potential point of that lead, and the vector is drawn along the respective lead, with the head of the arrow pointing toward the correct pole (positive or negative). Perpendiculars are then drawn from the heads of the two vectors until they intersect.
      (3) **Drawing the mean vector.** The head of an arrow is drawn at the intersection of the two perpendiculars, and the tail is drawn to the center of the triangle or the zero potential point. The length of this arrow represents the magnitude of the MEA, and its direction (in degrees) represents the electrical axis in the frontal plane.
   c. **Electrical axis in the frontal plane** (Figure 10-10A)
      (1) A **normal axis** is present if the MEA lies between $-30°$ and $+120°$ when plotted on the hexaxial reference system (or 2 and 7 o'clock, respectively, if the hexaxial system is considered a clock face).
      (2) **Right axis deviation (RAD)** is present when the MEA lies between $+120°$ and $+180°$ (or 7 and 9 o'clock). Causes of RAD include **right ventricular hypertrophy** secondary to chronic lung disease or pulmonary valve stenosis as well as **delayed activation of the right ventricle** (as occurs in right bundle branch block). Figure 10-10B shows QRS complexes characteristic of RAD.
      (3) **Left axis deviation (LAD)** is present when the MEA lies between $-30°$ and $-90°$ (or 2 and 12 o'clock). Conditions such as **obesity, left ventricular hypertrophy,** or

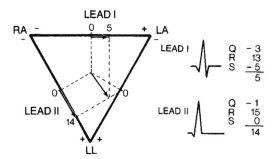

FIGURE 10-9. Mean electrical axis (MEA) determination by vector analysis. The Q and S waves (negative values) are added algebraically to the R waves (positive values) for each of two leads. The result gives the magnitude and the direction of the QRS vector (+ or −) in each lead. The QRS magnitude is plotted along the respective leads from the zero point toward the appropriate polarity. Perpendiculars to each axis are drawn through the arrowheads, and the intersection marks the head of the mean electrical vector. The MEA is drawn from the center of the triangle (electrical zero for the system) to the perpendiculars' intersection. The MEA (in degrees) and the magnitude are given by the direction and the length of the mean electrical vector. RA = right arm; LA = left arm; LL = left leg.

A

B

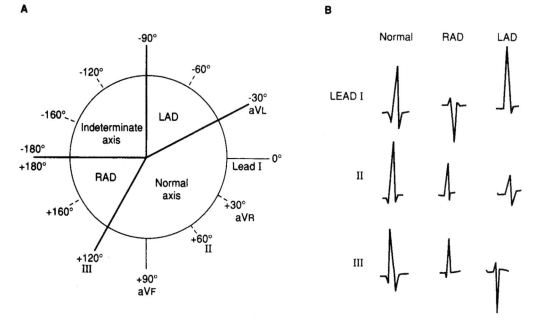

FIGURE 10-10. (A) Axis definitions in the frontal plane (using the hexaxial reference system). Lead I divides the frontal plane into upper (negative) and lower (positive) hemispheres and the aVF lead divides the frontal plane into quadrants. Note the degree designations and the division into various axis designations. (B) QRS configuration as seen in leads I, II, and III for a normal axis and right and left axis deviations. RAD = right axis deviation; LAD = left axis deviation.

left bundle branch block may lead to LAD. Figure 10-10B shows typical QRS complexes that occur with LAD.

(4) An **indeterminate axis** is present if the MEA lies between −90° and −180° (or 12 and 9 o'clock). Indeterminate axis may result from either **extreme RAD or extreme LAD.**

E. **Vector loops.** The instantaneous cardiac vector represents the electrical vector generated by the cardiac dipole during the depolarization process. This vector begins at the zero isopotential point and inscribes a loop as the tissues are depolarized. Three loops can be recorded during one cardiac cycle. The **P loop** is caused by atrial depolarization, the **QRS loop** is caused by ventricular depolarization, and the **T loop** results from ventricular repolarization (Figure 10-11). Atrial repolarization cannot be recorded with standard techniques because of the prolonged time course and the small voltages involved.

1. The **P loop** is small and is directed leftward and inferiorly, resulting in a positive P wave in the three bipolar limb leads.

2. The normal **QRS loop** is inscribed counterclockwise and is directed leftward, inferior and posterior.

   a. **Stages.** Ventricular depolarization is a continuous process, but it can be divided into stages for purposes of discussion (Figure 10-12A).

   (1) **Stage 1,** the initial phase of ventricular depolarization, involves the left endocardial surface of the interventricular septum. Depolarization spreads superiorly and to the right, resulting in a small vector directed toward the right shoulder. This initial vector produces small negative waves in leads I and II and small positive waves in the right precordial leads (Figure 10-12B).

   (2) **Stage 2** represents depolarization of the remainder of the interventricular septum and the subendocardial areas of both ventricles. The resultant vector is directed

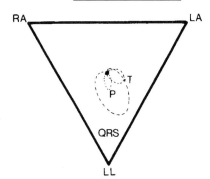

FIGURE 10-11. The vectorcardiographic loops P, QRS, and T, which can be recorded with appropriate equipment and electrode placement. RA = right arm; LA = left arm; LL = left leg.

inferiorly and produces large positive waves in leads II, III, and aVF (see Figure 10-12B).

(3) **Stage 3** depolarization involves the remainder of the right ventricle and a large portion of the left ventricle. Because the left ventricle normally has a larger muscle mass than the right, the stage 3 vector is directed toward the left. This vector produces R waves in lead I and causes a progressive increase in the R waves in the left precordial leads V_2–V_6.

(4) **Stage 4** represents the last portion of the ventricle to depolarize (i.e., the posterior base of the left ventricle). This vector is directed toward the left shoulder and produces small S waves in leads II, III, and aVF (see Figure 10-12B).

(5) **Stage 5** is the return of the cardiac potential to the zero potential point and the end of the depolarization process.

b. **Relationship between the QRS loop and QRS complex.** Depolarization of the cardiac tissue generates the vector loop.

(1) A **scalar EKG** records the depolarization process by plotting voltage as a function of time. Figure 10-12B depicts how the vector loop generates the QRS complex on the different leads.

(2) It is possible to reconstruct the vector loops from scalar EKGs (and vice versa) if basic electrical principles are understood.

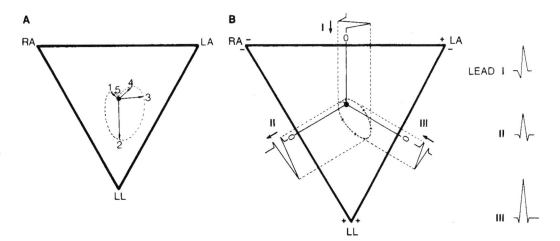

FIGURE 10-12. (A) Arbitrary stages of ventricular depolarization. (B) Reconstruction of the QRS complex from the QRS loop for the three bipolar limb leads. Arrows indicate the direction of the loop recording. RA = right arm; LA = left arm; LL = left leg.

3. The **T loop** represents the repolarization process, which is roughly opposite in direction to that of depolarization. This reversal of direction results in T waves that normally are in the same direction as the QRS complex.

V. CARDIAC RATE, RHYTHM, AND CONDUCTION DISTURBANCES

A. Cardiac rates

1. Normocardia, a normal heart rate, varies between 60 and 100 beats/min.

2. Tachycardia is a heart rate of more than 100 beats/min.

3. Bradycardia is a heart rate of less than 60 beats/min.

B. Cardiac rhythms

1. Sinus rhythm is present when the SA node is the pacemaker. Sinus rhythm can be assumed if each P wave is followed by a normal QRS complex, the P-R and Q-T intervals are normal, and the R-R interval is regular.

    a. Sinus arrhythmia (Figure 10-13) is characterized by a normal QRS complex, P-R interval, and Q-T interval, but the R-R interval (cardiac rate) varies in a set pattern.

        (1) Sinus arrhythmia is usually, but not always, synchronized with respiration. Usually, heart rate increases during inspiration (note the shorter cycles during inspiration in Figure 10-13) and slows during expiration as a result of variations in vagal tone that affect the SA node.

        (2) Sinus arrhythmia is common in children and in endurance athletes with slow heart rates.

    b. Sinus tachycardia is a normal response to exercise and also occurs with fever, hyperthyroidism, and as a reflex response to low arterial pressures (Figure 10-14).

    c. Sinus bradycardia may be abnormal, but is more commonly seen in highly trained endurance athletes (see Figure 10-14).

2. Atrial rhythms are generated when there is an ectopic atrial pacemaker.

    a. Atrial tachycardia is characterized by very regular rates ranging from 140–220 beats/min. Atrial tachycardia may be caused by overindulgence in caffeine, nicotine, or alcohol and may also occur during anxiety attacks.

    b. Paroxysmal atrial tachycardia (PAT) may result from discharge of a single ectopic site. Alternatively, a **reentry phenomenon,** which occurs when an AP reexcites an area of myocardium that had been depolarized previously, may lead to PAT.

    c. Premature atrial contractions (PACs, atrial extrasystoles) occur if an atrial ectopic site fires and becomes the pacemaker for one beat.

        (1) EKG appearance. A premature P wave is present, followed by a normal QRS complex and T wave. The premature P wave may have an aberrant configuration or an abnormal P-R interval because of the different path of atrial depolarization.

        (2) Diagnosis. Bedside diagnosis is usually possible because the premature beat dis-

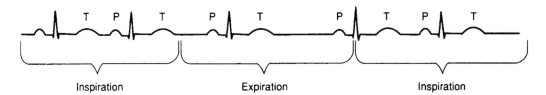

FIGURE 10-13. Sinus arrhythmia. The heart rate increases (i.e., the cycle length decreases) during inspiration. Note the differences in the T-P intervals during inspiration and expiration.

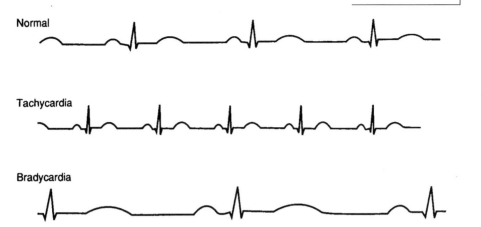

FIGURE 10-14. Electrocardiograms showing normal sinus rhythm, sinus tachycardia, and sinus bradycardia.

charges the SA node, which then repolarizes and fires after the normal interval; this results in a shift in cardiac rhythm (Figure 10-15A).

    (3) Significance. Atrial extrasystoles occur normally, and the patient may or may not be aware of an occasional irregularity in the cardiac rhythm.

  d. Atrial flutter (Figure 10-16A), which differs from atrial tachycardia only with regard to the atrial rate, occurs with atrial rates of 220–350 beats/min. The **AV node is unable to transmit all of the atrial impulses.** A physiologic AV block develops, and the ventricular rate is one-half, one-third, or one-fourth of the atrial rate. For example, changes in the AV block from 4:1 to 3:1 may cause rapid shifts in the ventricular rate.

    (1) Cause. Like atrial tachycardia, atrial flutter may result from either a single ectopic focus or a reentry phenomenon.

    (2) EKG appearance. The P waves have a saw-toothed appearance that is virtually diagnostic of atrial flutter.

  e. Atrial fibrillation (Figure 10-16B) is an irregular, rapid atrial rate. **Contraction of only small portions of the atrial musculature occurs at any one time because large por-**

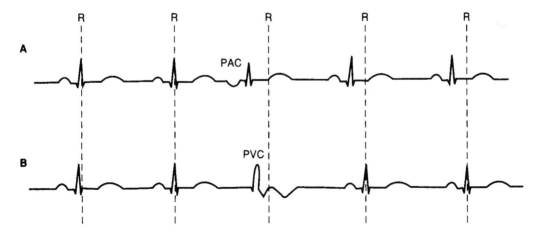

FIGURE 10-15. Effects of premature atrial (PAC) and ventricular (PVC) contractions on rhythm. The vertical lines represent the normal R-R interval. Note that the rhythm shifts with a PAC because the sinus node is reset, but the rhythm does not shift after a PVC because the following beat occurs after a compensatory pause.

A. Atrial flutter

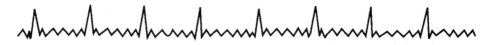

B. Atrial fibrillation

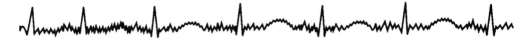

FIGURE 10-16. (*A*) Atrial flutter, which exhibits a characteristic saw-toothed appearance. (*B*) Atrial fibrillation, which shows very small baseline fluctuations on the electrocardiogram as small portions of the atria are depolarized in an uncoordinated manner.

> **tions of the atria are still in the refractory period.** The ventricular rate is completely (irregularly) irregular because only a fraction of the atrial impulses that reach the AV node are transmitted to the ventricles.
> (1) **EKG appearance.** The baseline of the EKG shows **small, irregular oscillations (F waves)** that result from the depolarization of small units of the atrial musculature. There are **no recognizable P waves,** and the **R-R interval is irregularly irregular.** The QRS and T waves are normal because the impulses that are transmitted through the AV node are conducted normally through the ventricles.
> (2) **Significance.** Atrial fibrillation represents an even higher rate of atrial activity than atrial flutter.
>   (a) Atrial fibrillation frequently is associated with **enlarged atria** secondary to AV valve disease. Reduction in cardiac output may occur as a result of the valve disease and the loss of an effective atrial contraction.
>   (b) Long-term atrial fibrillation is associated with **thrombi** in the atrial appendages. Atrial thrombi may be the source of pulmonary emboli (right atrium) or systemic emboli (left atrium).

3. **AV junctional (nodal) rhythms.** Pacemaker cells have been found in the AV node. The term "junctional rhythms" is used if there is an ectopic pacemaker located in the AV node.
   a. **Junctional premature beats**
      (1) **EKG appearance.** Junctional premature beats are characterized by an **inverted P wave** (as the result of retrograde transmission) and **normal QRS complexes.** They have been subdivided into **high or low** junctional beats depending on whether the P wave precedes or follows the onset of the QRS complex.
      (2) **Significance.** Junctional beats have the same significance as PACs. If the AV nodal tissues recover excitability, a retrograde impulse may return and cause a second ventricular depolarization (known as a **reciprocal beat**).
   b. **Transient or permanent junctional rhythms** may develop in otherwise healthy individuals if the SA node is suppressed. Permanent junctional rhythms may occur secondary to a large number of organic heart diseases.
   c. **Junctional tachycardias** are similar to atrial tachycardias and may be indistinguishable on EKG. They should be considered supraventricular tachycardias.

4. **Ventricular rhythms**
   a. **Premature ventricular contractions (PVCs)** can arise from any portion of the ventricular myocardium and occasionally occur in otherwise healthy individuals.
      (1) **Cause.** Frequent PVCs occur with many forms of heart disease, especially coronary artery disease (because ischemia increases the irritability of the myocardium).
      (2) **EKG appearance.** PVCs are characterized by a **prolonged** (> 0.1 sec), **bizarre**

QRS complex that does not have a preceding P wave. The T wave is usually oppositely directed from the QRS complex (Figure 10-15B).

(3) **Compensatory pause.** Retrograde transmission of depolarization to the atria usually does not occur with PVCs; thus, the atrial rate remains unaltered.

    (a) The atrial depolarization that follows a PVC usually arrives while the AV node is still refractory and, therefore, it is not conducted to the ventricles, creating a pause in the ventricular rhythm.

    (b) This pause is usually fully compensatory so that the R-R interval of the beat preceding the PVC and the PVC interval together equal two normal cycle lengths (see Figure 10-15B). **The beat following the PVC, which is stronger than normal because of the added stroke volume, is usually detectable by the patient.**

(4) **Interpolated beats.** If the sinus rhythm is slow, a PVC may occur without altering the normal R-R interval. The PVC is termed an interpolated beat.

b. **Ventricular tachycardias** result from a rapid, repetitive discharge from a ventricular site, usually as a result of a reentry phenomenon. Alterations in vagal tone (carotid sinus massage, Valsalva maneuver) do not affect ventricular tachycardias because the ventricles do not receive any efferent vagal innervation.

    (1) **Causes.** Ventricular tachycardias are almost always associated with **serious heart disease** or **drug toxicity.** These arrhythmias also occur when **catheters** (e.g., Swan-Ganz) stimulate the endocardial surface of the ventricles. A slight movement or withdrawal of the catheter may terminate the tachycardia.

    (2) **EKG appearance** (Figure 10-17). The EKG reveals **wide, bizarre QRS complexes** that occur at a rapid rate. The P waves are usually indistinguishable, although the SA node activity continues independently of the ventricles.

    (3) **Significance.** Sustained ventricular tachycardia can be a life-threatening arrhythmia if it degenerates into ventricular fibrillation.

        (a) Cardiac output is lower because ventricular filling time is less, causing a decrease in stroke volume.

        (b) Cardiac output may also be less because the effectiveness of ventricular contraction is reduced by **asynchrony** of the contractile process. During ventricular tachycardia, APs travel over the slowly conducting ventricular muscle, rather than the Purkinje fibers, causing prolonged depolarization. Asynchrony occurs.

c. **Ventricular fibrillation** results from rapid, irregular, ineffective contractions of small segments of the ventricular myocardium. The peripheral pulse is absent, and **cardiac**

A. Ventricular tachycardia

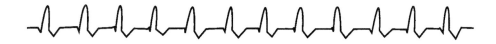

B. Ventricular fibrillation

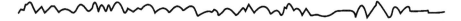

FIGURE 10-17. (*A*) Ventricular tachycardia, which is characterized by wide, bizarre QRS complexes that are caused by an ectopic ventricular pacemaker. (*B*) Ventricular fibrillation, like atrial fibrillation, results from uncoordinated depolarization of small segments of the myocardium.

output is zero. **To distinguish ventricular fibrillation from cardiac standstill,** the EKG must be used.

(1) EKG appearance (see Figure 10-16B). The EKG shows **undulating waves of varying frequency and amplitude.** Ventricular fibrillation is **often precipitated by** one or more **PVCs,** one of which falls on the **vulnerable interval** of the T wave (i.e., the interval near the peak of the T wave when the ventricle is partially repolarized). A PVC during the vulnerable interval produces fibrillation because the likelihood of reentry occurring is increased.

(2) Significance. Cardiopulmonary resuscitation must be started immediately to prevent tissue death and continued until cardioversion (defibrillation) can be performed.

C. **Conduction disturbances**

1. SA nodal block (sick sinus syndrome) consists of the disappearance of the P wave for several seconds while an ectopic pacemaker, usually in a junctional or ventricular site, drives the ventricles.

a. SA block results in a **bradycardia** and is seen especially in the elderly and in patients recovering from a coronary occlusion.

b. Various drugs and implanted pacemakers may be used to increase the heart rate to normal levels.

2. AV nodal block (Figure 10-18)

a. First-degree AV nodal block is a prolongation of the P-R interval beyond 0.21 sec due to slowed conduction through the AV node (see Figure 10-18A).

Normal

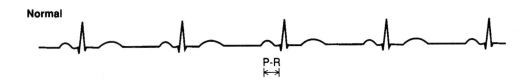

A. First-degree AV block

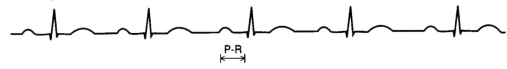

B. Second-degree AV block

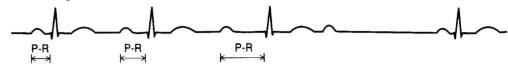

C. Third-degree AV block

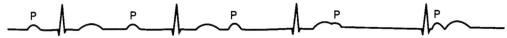

FIGURE 10-18. Various types of atrioventricular (AV) nodal block. (*A*) First-degree AV block. Note the prolonged P-R interval, which is diagnostic. (*B*) Second-degree AV block exhibits occasional dropped beats. Wenckebach block (Mobitz type I) is characterized as a series of progressively longer P-R intervals ending with a dropped beat. (*C*) Third-degree (complete) AV block represents a condition in which the atria and ventricles beat independently at their own rates.

(1) Causes. Increased vagal tone and many systemic diseases may lead to first-degree AV nodal block.

(2) Significance. This condition has no effect on the pumping ability of the ventricles but indicates that some conduction disturbance is present.

b. Second-degree AV nodal block occurs when the AV node fails to transmit all of the atrial impulses. It is usually associated with organic heart disease.

(1) Wenckebach block (Mobitz type I) is characterized by a progressive lengthening of the P-R interval in successive beats and finally a failure of one impulse to be transmitted (see Figure 10-18B).

(2) Periodic block (Mobitz type II) is characterized by an occasional failure of conduction that results in an atrial-to-ventricular rate of, for example, 6:5 or 8:7. The P-R interval is constant.

(3) Constant block represents a higher degree of block than the periodic type. The atrial-to-ventricular rate is a constant small-number ratio (e.g., 2:1 or 3:1).

c. Third-degree (complete) AV nodal block occurs when AV node conduction is completely interrupted, causing the atria and ventricles to beat at independent rates (see Figure 10-18C).

(1) Cause. As in second-degree AV nodal block, organic heart disease is often the cause.

(2) Significance. Third-degree AV nodal block may be associated with prolonged ventricular standstill until a ventricular focus begins firing. If prolonged, the cardiac arrest may result in cerebral ischemia, syncope, or death; the condition is termed **Stokes-Adams syndrome.**

3. Wolff-Parkinson-White syndrome, also termed **ventricular preexcitation** or **accelerated conduction,** results from an aberrant conduction pathway between the atria and the ventricles. The aberrant pathway eliminates or reduces the normal delay between atrial and ventricular activation.

a. EKG appearance (Figure 10-19A). The EKG shows a shortened P-R interval, usually less than 0.1 sec, and a widened QRS complex with a slurred initial upstroke (delta wave). The slurred upstroke is caused by the slow conduction through the ventricular muscle.

b. Significance. The **accessory bundle** (i.e., aberrant pathway) predisposes to paroxysmal tachycardias because of a reentry phenomenon. The atrial impulse is conducted to the ventricles through the AV node and returns to the atria via the accessory bundle. The circular depolarization pathway triggers the reentry mechanism. Surgical ablation of the accessory bundle is possible if it can be adequately localized.

4. Bundle branch block. Blockage of the right or left common bundles or the left anterior or posterior fascicles results in an abnormal sequence of ventricular excitation.

a. Right bundle branch block delays the activation of the right ventricle.

(1) Causes. Right bundle branch block may occur in otherwise healthy individuals as a transient or a permanent manifestation. It also occurs secondary to chronic pulmonary disease and may appear acutely as a consequence of pulmonary embolism.

(2) EKG appearance

(a) The **QRS duration** is prolonged beyond 0.12 sec, except in **incomplete right bundle branch block,** in which the QRS duration is only 0.08–0.10 sec.

(b) The sequence of excitation produces a typical QRS pattern in the right precordial leads, a wide S wave in lead I, and an RAD (Figure 10–19B).

b. Left bundle branch block

(1) Causes. Left bundle branch block is common in association with coronary artery disease or conditions leading to **left ventricular hypertrophy** (e.g., hypertension, aortic valve stenosis). It is **rare in the absence of organic heart disease.**

(2) EKG appearance. Left bundle branch block is best diagnosed using the left precordial leads (Figure 10-19C). The QRS duration is greater than 0.12 sec, and the initial and final QRS vectors are directed toward the left.

A. Wolff-Parkinson-White syndrome

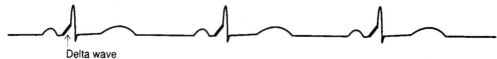

Delta wave

B. Right bundle branch block

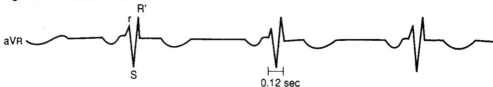

aVR

R'

r

S

0.12 sec

C. Left bundle branch block

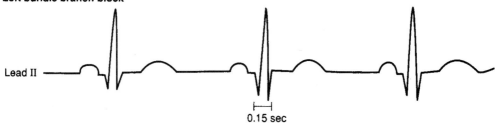

Lead II

0.15 sec

FIGURE 10-19. (*A*) The characteristic deformity of the QRS complex that results from an aberrant connection between the atria and ventricles, as seen in Wolff-Parkinson-White syndrome. (*B*) Right bundle branch block is caused by an interruption in the right bundle branch. The right ventricle is depolarized last, leading to a widening of the QRS complex. (*C*) Left bundle branch block causes late activation of the left ventricle and a widening of the QRS complex.

D. **Other sources of cardiac dysfunction**

1. **Narrowing** or **occlusion of coronary arteries** leads to the reduction or absence of blood flow to an area of the myocardium. The most common causes of coronary artery narrowing and occlusion are atherosclerotic plaque and arteriosclerotic coronary thrombosis, respectively. Reduction of coronary blood flow results in **myocardial ischemia** or **infarction.**
   a. **Myocardial ischemia**
      (1) **Symptoms.** The cardinal sign of coronary artery insufficiency is **angina** related either to exertion or emotional stress. The pain may be precordial or may radiate to the shoulder, arm, or jaw. The pain is typically described as a tight band or weight on the chest that results in a **strangling sensation;** the term **angina pectoris** is truly apt. This symptom typically lasts 1–10 minutes and is relieved by rest.
      (2) **EKG appearance.** The ischemic area of the myocardium has a reduced membrane potential compared with normal regions of the heart, which leads to a current flow from the normal regions to the ischemic area.
         (a) This current produces **ST-segment elevation** from leads overlying the ischemic area. **ST-segment depression** occurs in leads on the opposite side of the heart.
         (b) Ischemia alters the path of repolarization, usually resulting in **T-wave inversion.**
      (3) **Diagnosis. Patient history is the usual basis of diagnosis,** because the resting EKG may be within normal limits. **Twenty-four hour EKG (Holter) monitoring** may provide evidence of ischemic changes during anginal attacks. **Stress (exercise) testing with EKG monitoring** is used to precipitate ischemic episodes for diagnostic purposes.

   b. Myocardial infarction occurs when coronary blood flow ceases or is reduced below a critical level. The left ventricle is almost always the site of a myocardial infarction.

     (1) Symptoms are similar to those of coronary insufficiency, except that the pain is more intense, it generally lasts for more than 15–20 minutes, it may not be related to exertion or exercise, and it is not relieved by nitrates.

     (2) EKG appearance. The EKG undergoes a series of changes following a myocardial infarction. These changes must be recorded with daily EKG tracings for diagnostic purposes.

       (a) ST-segment and T-wave changes are present similar to those seen in ischemia.

       (b) Q waves occur in leads overlying the infarct if the infarcted area is transmural. Because there is no functioning myocardium under the electrode, the Q wave indicates that the electrode is "seeing" the luminal EKG pattern.

2. Ventricular hypertrophy occurs if the work of one or both ventricles is increased sufficiently (a common complication of pulmonary or systemic hypertension). In ventricular hypertrophy, the number of myocardial cells remains the same, but the diameter of the individual cells increases, raising the diffusion distance for O_2 and other metabolites. The increased diffusion distance may produce ischemia.

   a. EKG appearance

     (1) R wave. There is a direct correlation between the thickness of the ventricular wall and the height of the R wave in the overlying leads. The increased height is a reflection of the greater magnitude of the depolarization vector.

     (2) QRS duration is increased slightly because of the increased muscle mass that is present. The duration of the QRS complex is usually less than 0.12 sec, but occasionally it may exceed this value.

   b. Left ventricular hypertrophy

     (1) Axis. The MEA is shifted toward the left and superiorly. The transition zone of the precordial leads is also shifted to the left.

     (2) QRS configuration. Left ventricular hypertrophy is usually present if the R wave in V_5 or V_6 together with the S wave in V_1 are greater than 35 mm.

   c. Right ventricular hypertrophy

     (1) Axis. The MEA is usually vertical or greater than +110° in the frontal plane.

     (2) QRS configuration. Right precordial leads generally show tall R waves, rather than normal S waves. The QRS is usually prolonged, but less than 0.12 sec; the ST segment is depressed; and the T wave is inverted in the right precordial leads.

Case 10

A 47-year-old man develops chest pain and shortness of breath at 2:00 A.M. Previously diagnosed with coronary insufficiency, he has been using nitrate skin patches to relieve mild chest pain. He describes the present chest pain as crushing, and nitrates do not relieve the pain.

   1. *What is the most likely diagnosis?*

DISCUSSION

This patient has a classic history of coronary insufficiency. The history of prolonged, intense chest pain that is not relieved by nitrates is typical of a myocardial infarction.

In the emergency department, the man's blood pressure is 140/105 mm Hg, and his pulse rate is 114 beats/min. An electrocardiograph (EKG) reveals large Q waves in V3 and V4, ST-segment elevation, and T-wave inversion in the left precordial leads.

   2. *What do the Q waves in the precordial leads indicate?*

DISCUSSION

Q waves, which are generated by the wave of depolarization proceeding away from the electrode, are similar in appearance to recordings taken with the exploring electrode within the ventricular cavity. The presence of large Q waves indicates the absence of viable myocardium under the electrodes.

   3. *What does the T-wave inversion in the precordial leads indicate?*

DISCUSSION

T waves are normally upright in the precordial leads, because the direction of ventricular repolarization is usually opposite from depolarization. The T-wave inversion results from hypoxia of the myocardium, which alters the pathway of repolarization and prolongs the period of repolarization.

Chapter 11

Cardiodynamics

I. **GENERAL TERMINOLOGY. Cardiodynamics** is the study of the mechanical events associated with the contraction and relaxation of the heart. The **cardiac cycle** includes both electrical and mechanical events (e.g., myocardial cell shortening leading to pressure generation and volume changes).

II. **CARDIAC CYCLE**

A. **Sequence of events** (Figure 11-1). A complete understanding of the events of the cardiac cycle is essential for interpretation of the physical signs of cardiovascular disease that are elicited during physical examination. The electrocardiogram (EKG) records the electrical events that precede and initiate the corresponding mechanical events.

1. **Atrial contraction**
   a. **Electrical events.** The **P wave** initiates atrial contraction.
   b. **Function.** Atrial contraction forces more blood into the ventricles.
      (1) The effects of atrial contraction are especially important when the heart rate is rapid and the ventricular filling time is reduced.
      (2) The **ventricular end-diastolic pressure (VEDP),** the pressure of the blood in the ventricles at the termination of the atrial contraction, is normally less than 12 mm Hg in the left ventricle and 5 mm Hg in the right ventricle.
   c. **Clinical significance.** Atrial contraction generates the **a wave,** which is reflected back into the large veins. The a wave may be recorded from the jugular vein with appropriate transducers for diagnostic purposes.
      (1) The **right ventricular filling pressure** may be estimated from the level of blood in the jugular veins. In an upright position, the jugular veins are normally collapsed because right atrial pressure is less than 6–7 cm H_2O. In a supine position, the jugular veins fill with blood because they are at the same level as the heart.
      (2) Distended jugular veins indicate excessive pressures in the right atrium. **Depressed right ventricular function** (i.e., congestive heart failure) or **tricuspid valve** dysfunction usually cause these high pressures.
      (3) The **fourth heart sound (S_4),** which occurs during atrial contraction, is caused by the forcing of additional blood into a distended ventricle. S_4 is occasionally heard in individuals with congestive heart failure; in these patients, a triple sound called a **gallop rhythm** is audible.

2. **Ventricular contraction (systole)**
   a. **Terminology. Ventricular volume** (i.e., volume of blood in the ventricles) is difficult to measure clinically. However, **echocardiography** can be used to measure ventricular dimensions as well as ventricular wall and valve motion during the cardiac cycle.
      (1) The **ventricular end-diastolic volume (VEDV)** is the volume of blood in the ventricle just before the onset of ventricular contraction. The normal left VEDV is 120–140 ml.
      (2) The **ventricular end-systolic volume (VESV)** is the volume of blood remaining in the ventricle at the end of ejection. The normal left VESV is 40–70 ml.
      (3) The **stroke volume** is the volume of blood that is ejected with each beat. It is equal to the VEDV minus the VESV (e.g., 75–80 ml). The **ejection fraction** equals the stroke volume divided by the VEDV. Normally, the ejection fraction is 60%–70%, but it declines markedly with ventricular dysfunction.

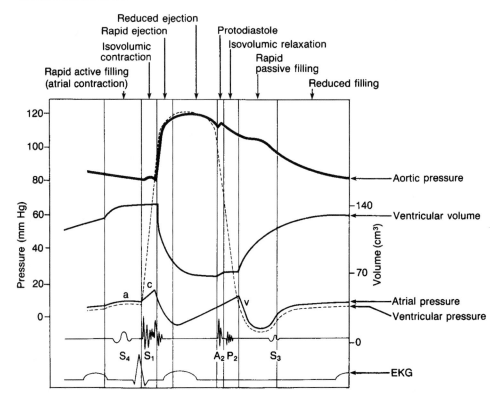

FIGURE 11-1. The events of the cardiac cycle. S_1, S_2 (A_2 and P_2), S_3, and S_4 are the heart sounds. The a wave (a) is caused by atrial contraction. The c wave (c) is caused by the atrioventricular (AV) valves ballooning back into the atria during isovolumic contraction. The peak of the v wave (v) results from the opening of the AV valves.

b. Stages

(1) Atrioventricular (AV) valve closure. Shortly after the QRS complex begins, the ventricles begin to contract, and the pressure in the ventricular cavities rises. The increasing ventricular pressure exceeds the atrial pressure, which causes the AV valves to close.

(a) The **first heart sound (S_1)** results primarily from closure of the AV valves.

(b) S_1, a low-frequency sound that occurs just after the onset of ventricular contraction, **signals the onset of ventricular systole** (see Figure 11-1).

(2) Isovolumic (isovolumetric) contraction. Closure of the AV valves seals off the ventricular chambers from the atria. The ventricular volume remains constant (isovolumic) until the ventricular pressure exceeds the arterial pressure.

(3) Ventricular ejection. When the ventricular pressure exceeds the arterial pressure, ventricular ejection begins (see Figure 11-1). Right ventricular ejection occurs before left ventricular ejection because the pressure in the pulmonary artery is low compared with that in the aorta.

(a) **Rapid ejection.** As soon as ventricular ejection begins, the arterial pressure starts to increase because the arterial volume rises. During the first third of systole, approximately two-thirds of the stroke volume is ejected (see the ventricular volume tracing, Figure 11-1).

(b) **Reduced ejection.** During the last two-thirds of systole, the rate of ejection declines, and the ventricles begin to relax. Both ventricular and arterial pressures begin to decrease as the rate of blood flow through the peripheral vessels exceeds the rate of blood flow from the ventricles.

(4) Semilunar valve closure. Closure of the semilunar (i.e., aortic and pulmonic) valves, which prevents the movement of blood back into the ventricles, produces the **second heart sound (S_2).** S_2, a relatively high-frequency sound, indicates the end of systole and the onset of ventricular diastole.

    (a) Normal splitting of S_2. Under normal conditions, the aortic and pulmonic valves do not close simultaneously. Normally, the aortic valve closes first, producing the aortic component of $S_2(A_2)$. Then the pulmonic valve closes, producing the P_2 component. During inspiration, the increased venous return causes prolongation of right ventricular ejection and an increased separation between A_2 and P_2. The aortic valve closes first because the ejection rate from the left ventricle is higher than that from the right ventricle.

    (b) Paradoxical splitting of S_2. Paradoxical splitting occurs if the splitting of S_2 decreases during inspiration, indicating that P_2 precedes A_2. Delayed aortic valve closure indicates a **disease process affecting the left ventricle** [e.g., left bundle branch block (delayed activation), myocardial depression leading to prolongation of systole, or prolonged ejection caused by aortic stenosis].

3. Ventricular relaxation (diastole)

  a. Isovolumic (isovolumetric) relaxation begins with the closure of the semilunar valves.

    (1) Ventricular pressure falls rapidly as the ventricles relax; isovolumic relaxation lasts only approximately 0.04 sec.

    (2) Isovolumic relaxation ends when the AV valves open, as indicated by the peak of the **v wave** on the atrial pressure tracing (see Figure 11-1).

  b. Rapid passive filling. During ventricular systole, venous return continues so that the atrial pressure is high when the AV valves first open.

    (1) The high atrial pressure causes a rapid, initial flow of blood into the ventricles (see Figure 11-1).

    (2) Once the AV valves open, the atria and ventricles are a common chamber, and the pressure in both cavities falls as ventricular relaxation continues.

    (3) The **third heart sound (S_3),** which occurs during the **rapid passive filling stage,** is not normally audible in adults but may be heard in children.

  c. Reduced filling and diastasis. Toward the end of diastole, the pressure in the atria and ventricles rises slowly as blood continues to return to the heart.

    (1) With very slow heart rates, ventricular filling virtually ceases because the ventricles reach their volume limit. This phase is termed **diastasis.**

    (2) When the heart rate increases, the length of the cardiac cycle obviously shortens. Diastasis and the reduced filling phase are most affected by shortening of the cycle.

    (a) Increases in heart rate of up to 140–150 beats/min do not cause a significant decrease in ventricular filling. At these levels, cardiac output rises in almost direct proportion to the increased heart rate.

    (b) Heart rates in excess of 180–200 beats/min result in decreased cardiac output, because the ventricular filling time is markedly reduced. The decreased ventricular filling time lowers the VEDV and, consequently, the stroke volume.

B. | **Aortic and pulmonary arterial pressures.** The pulsatile pressure changes in the aorta and pulmonary artery are termed **pressure pulses.**

  1. Systole. During the period of rapid ejection, the pressure in the aorta is slightly less than that in the ventricle. The peak arterial pressure is the arterial systolic pressure, which occurs at the end of the rapid ejection phase.

    a. The normal aortic systolic pressure is approximately 120 mm Hg, and the normal pulmonary artery systolic pressure is 15–18 mm Hg.

    b. The **incisura,** which is produced by the closure of the semilunar valves, indicates the end of ventricular systole. The incisura coincides with S_2.

  2. Diastole. The arterial pressure declines as blood continues to flow from the arteries, through the capillaries, and into the veins.

    a. The arterial diastolic pressure is the lowest arterial pressure during a cardiac cycle, and it occurs just before the onset of the next ventricular ejection, which is actually during systole.

b. The normal diastolic pressure in the aorta is approximately 80 mm Hg, and in the pulmonary artery, it is 8–10 mm Hg.

3. The **pulse pressure** is the difference between the systolic and the diastolic pressures (e.g., the normal aortic pulse pressure is 120–80, or 40 mm Hg). The **recorded blood pressure** is normally written as the arterial systolic pressure/diastolic pressure (e.g., 120/80 mm Hg).

C. **Valve lesions and murmurs.** The cardiac valves may be abnormal as a result of either congenital or acquired heart disease.

1. Abnormal cardiac valves lead to **abnormal blood flow and pressure gradients,** which in turn, produce signs of dysfunction that are **recognizable during physical examination.** Valve lesions affect the circulation by:
   a. Reducing cardiac output
   b. Imposing additional work on the heart by creating an extra pressure or volume load
   c. Producing the backup of blood

2. **Murmurs** are important physical signs of valve lesions.
   a. **Causes.** Murmurs are caused by turbulent blood flow or by changes in the direction of the blood flow. **Laminar (normal) flow** is streamlined and silent, whereas **turbulent flow** produces vibrations in the tissues that are heard as murmurs.
      (1) Turbulent blood flow occurs when the Reynold's number exceeds 2000.
      (2) The Reynold's number is a dimensionless value that is given by:

$$\frac{D \cdot \delta \cdot v}{\eta}$$

where D = vessel diameter, δ = blood density, v = velocity, and η = blood viscosity.
   b. **Timing.** Murmurs may be **systolic, diastolic,** or **continuous** throughout the cardiac cycle. They may also be more specifically classified (e.g., presystolic, pansystolic, early, or middiastolic). Timing of murmurs is associated with specific valve lesions.
   c. **Location and radiation of murmurs.** Murmurs are best heard on the chest wall closest to their origin and in the downstream direction of blood flow.

3. **Valvular stenosis** is a narrowing of the valve orifice that impedes the forward flow of blood.
   a. **Stenosis of the aortic or pulmonary valves** forces the left and right ventricles, respectively, to generate high pressures to eject blood through the narrowed orifice, a high-resistance segment of the vascular system.
      (1) **Diagnosis.** A ventricular systolic pressure that is much higher than the systolic pressure in the respective artery is pathognomonic of semilunar valve stenosis (Figure 11-2A).
         (a) **Cardiac catheterization** allows detection of the pressure gradient.
         (b) The murmur of semilunar valve stenosis is a systolic **ejection-type (crescendo–decrescendo or diamond-shaped) murmur.**
      (2) **Clinical significance.** Semilunar valve stenosis may lead to **ventricular hypertrophy** and eventually produce ventricular failure.
   b. **Stenosis of the AV (mitral or tricuspid) valves** impedes the filling of the ventricles so that a pressure gradient develops between the atria and the ventricles during diastole (Figure 11-2B). Atrial (and, consequently, venous) pressure tends to be high.
      (1) **Diagnosis.** AV valve stenosis produces diastolic murmurs that occur during atrial contraction (presystolic murmur) and the rapid passive filling stage (middiastolic murmur). These two murmurs are described as crescendo and decrescendo murmurs, respectively.
      (2) **Clinical significance**
         (a) Mitral valve stenosis may lead to pulmonary edema (because of the high pulmonary venous pressures), enlargement of the left atrium, or atrial fibrillation.
         (b) Tricuspid stenosis elevates systemic venous pressure leading to dependent edema. It may also produce giant **a waves** that are visible as pulsations in the distended jugular veins.

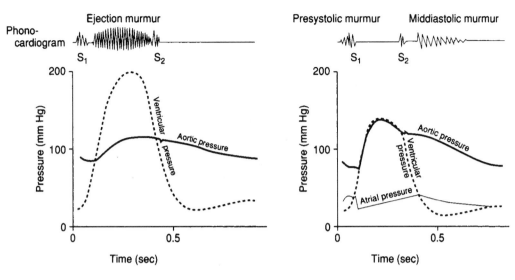

A. Semilunar valve stenosis

B. Atrioventricular valve stenosis

FIGURE 11-2. Valvular stenosis. (*A*) Semilunar (aortic or pulmonic) valve stenosis. The large pressure gradient between the ventricular and aortic pressures during ventricular ejection is pathognomonic. (*B*) Atrioventricular (AV; mitral or tricuspid) valve stenosis results in a sizable pressure gradient between the atria and the ventricles during diastole. Pressure builds in the veins behind the ventricle and may lead to edema. Presystolic and middiastolic murmurs are usually audible.

4. **Valvular insufficiency (regurgitation)** allows backward flow of blood from the ventricles to the atria or from the arteries to the ventricles.
    a. **Insufficiency of the semilunar valves** reduces the effective cardiac output because blood flows back into the ventricular cavities during diastole.
        (1) **Pandiastolic murmur.** Semilunar valve insufficiency results in a pandiastolic murmur that is relatively constant in intensity (Figure 11-3A).
        (2) **Arterial pressures.** The backward flow of blood causes a rapid fall in arterial pressure, producing **very low diastolic arterial pressures.** In addition, the backflow augments the next stroke volume, leading to **high systolic pressures.**
        (3) **Clinical significance.** Extremely large pulse pressures of more than 100 mm Hg are sometimes diagnostic of aortic insufficiency.
            (a) Large pulse pressures, called **Corrigan's (water-hammer) pulses,** are seen in patients with **aortic insufficiency.** The large pulse pressure, which may be transmitted to the capillaries, is **detectable in the nail beds.**
            (b) Semilunar valve insufficiency produces **marked ventricular dilation,** which eventually leads to **ventricular failure.**
    b. **Insufficiency of the AV valves** allows blood to flow from the ventricles to the atria during systole.
        (1) **Diagnosis.** The backflow of blood results in very high atrial pressures during systole (Figure 11-3B).
        (2) **Clinical significance.** Dilation of one or more heart chambers, which occurs to compensate for the regurgitant blood, may eventually lead to heart failure.

III. CARDIAC CONTRACTILE FORCE

A. **Frank-Starling effect. Starling's law of the heart** states that the energy produced by the heart when it contracts is a function of the end-diastolic length of its muscle fibers.

A. Semilunar valve insufficiency

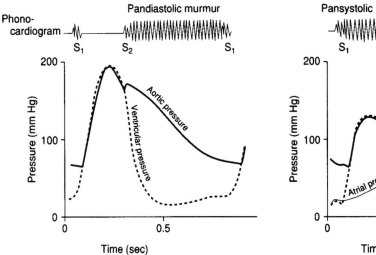

B. Atrioventricular valve insufficiency

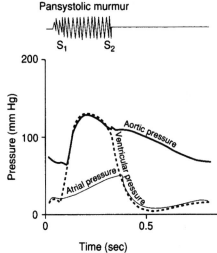

FIGURE 11-3. Valvular insufficiency (regurgitation), (*A*) Semilunar (aortic or pulmonic) valve insufficiency is caused by incomplete closure of the semilunar valves during diastole. The murmur is termed pandiastolic because it lasts throughout diastole, as the pressure gradient would lead one to predict. (*B*) AV (mitral or tricuspid) valve insufficiency causes a reflux of blood from the ventricles into the atria during systole. The regurgitant flow of blood creates a pansystolic murmur.

1. **Factors.** One of the major factors that controls the force of cardiac contraction is the **initial length** (i.e., the **preload**) of the muscle fibers.
   a. The **preload** depends on the volume of blood in the ventricles at the onset of contraction (i.e., the **VEDV**). The VEDV is considered to be proportional to either the VEDP or the central venous pressure (which are essentially equivalent).
   b. **Cross-bridges.** Increases in preload raise the number of available cross-bridges by changing the overlap of the actin and myosin filaments.
      (1) The strength of the cardiac contraction is proportional to the number of available cross-bridges.
      (2) An increase in preload (or venous pressure) produces a stronger contraction, allowing the heart to pump more blood per beat (Figures 11-4A and 11-5).
2. **Usefulness.** The Frank-Starling mechanism is extremely important in **balancing the output of the two sides of the heart** over extended periods.

B. **Contractility.** Changes in stroke volume also depend on the contractility of the ventricles.

1. **Increased contractility (positive inotropism)** is a greater contractile force at a constant preload or ventricular volume. Positive inotropism allows the ventricles to eject more blood from the same diastolic volume; consequently, the stroke volume increases.
   a. **Positive inotropic mechanisms**
      (1) **Activation of the β_1 receptors** (via **sympathetic nerve stimulation** or the **administration of β-adrenergic drugs**) increases the concentration of Ca^{2+} within the myocardial cells and results in a more rapid and forceful contraction. In addition, the Ca^{2+} is taken up more rapidly by the sarcoplasmic reticulum (SR), which shortens the duration of both the action potential and the contraction (Figure 11-4B).
      (2) **Digitalis** glycosides (e.g., **ouabain, digoxin**) also increase the force of cardiac contraction by raising the intracellular Ca^{2+} concentration. Digitalis, which was initially prepared from the plant *Digitalis purpurea,* has been used for centuries to treat heart failure.

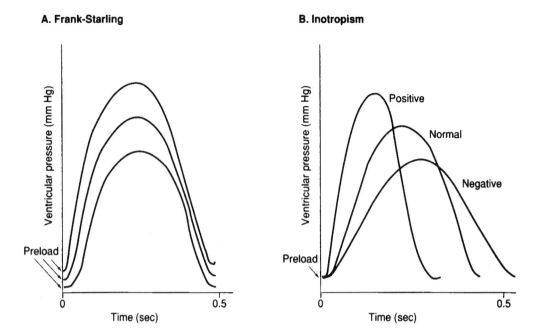

A. Frank-Starling

B. Inotropism

FIGURE 11-4. Effects of preload and contractility on ventricular pressure generated. (*A*) Increasing ventricular end-diastolic volume and pressure (i.e., the preload) increases the force of contraction by means of the Frank-Starling mechanism; the time required to generate peak pressure is unchanged. (*B*) Changes in contractility alter the peak force developed and the duration of the contractile process.

b. **Positive inotropic effects.** Figure 11-5, a family of ventricular function (Frank-Starling) curves, depicts ventricular performance as a function of preload. Positive inotropic effects produce a shift upward or toward the left [i.e., a greater stroke volume (more cardiac force) can be generated at a constant ventricular volume, or the same force can be generated from a smaller VEDV].

c. **Maximal velocity of shortening.** Positive inotropism also can be defined as an increase in the **maximal** velocity of shortening (V_{max}) when it is plotted as a function of afterload. For the ventricles, the afterload is the arterial pressure during the ejection

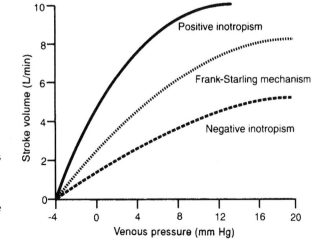

FIGURE 11-5. A family of Frank-Starling curves. Changes in stroke volume can be accomplished by alterations in the venous pressure (i.e., ventricular end-diastolic volume), causing movement along one of the curves (Frank-Starling mechanism) or by shifting from one curve to another. The latter mechanism indicates changes in ventricular contractility (inotropism).

phase (Figure 11-6). During any muscle contraction, the velocity of shortening and the force developed are inversely related.

(1) In Figure 11-6, the intercept of each line with the x-axis represents the load that prevents shortening of the muscle fibers. This condition is referred to as an **isometric** or **isovolumic contraction.**

(2) In Figure 11-4B, increased contractility allows the ventricle to generate a greater amount of force from the same preload (venous pressure or VEDV). This contrasts with the Frank-Starling mechanism, where an increase in the force of contraction is produced by an increase in fiber length or preload (see Figure 11-4A).

2. Decreased contractility (negative inotropism) represents a decrease in the force of contraction at any fiber length or ventricular volume.

a. Causes. This condition results from **hypoxia, acidosis, myocardial ischemia,** or **infarction.**

(1) The damaged or dead tissue leads to a decrease in stroke volume and a decline in cardiac output. The decreased pumping ability of the ventricle results in an increase in ventricular size as the venous pressure increases.

(2) The increased ventricular volume invokes the Frank-Starling mechanism, increasing the force of contraction and returning the stroke volume toward normal. However, as the ventricle dilates, it faces a double disadvantage because of the **Laplace effect.**

b. Law of Laplace. For a thick-walled structure such as the ventricle, the **law of Laplace** can be expressed as:

$$T = \frac{(P \cdot r)}{h}$$

where T = wall tension, P = pressure difference across the ventricular wall, r = radius of the ventricle, and h = ventricular wall thickness.

(1) Wall tension. Any hollow organ such as the ventricle generates pressure by increasing wall tension, which squeezes down on the contained volume.

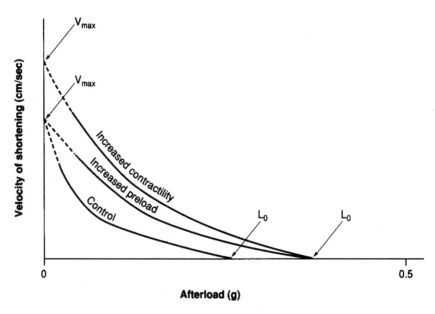

FIGURE 11-6. The velocity of shortening as a function of afterload. Changes in preload (i.e., venous pressure, ventricular end-diastolic pressure or volume) do not cause an increase in the maximal velocity of shortening (V_{max}). Sympathomimetic substances (e.g., epinephrine) increase contractility and result in an increased V_{max}. L_O = initial length of muscle.

(2) **Ventricular dilation** causes a thinning of the ventricular wall because a given ventricular muscle mass must enclose a larger volume of blood.

   (a) Because there are fewer myocytes per cross-sectional area of the ventricular wall, each myocyte must develop more force than was previously required to accomplish the same amount of work.

   (b) Eventually, the ability of the myofibrils to generate force is exceeded, and the amount of shortening or force generated is reduced. This represents a negative inotropic effect; less work is performed by the heart from any given VEDV.

(3) **Ventricular radius.** Because ventricular dilation is equivalent to an increased ventricular radius, the ventricle must generate a greater wall tension to maintain any given force generation or systolic pressure (i.e., a larger ventricle must work harder to generate the same stroke volume).

c. **Clinical significance**

   (1) **Diminished cardiac reserve.** Decreased contractility means that the ability of the heart to increase the stroke volume is limited; therefore, cardiac output is primarily maintained by **increasing the heart rate.** Patients' ability to increase cardiac output in response to stress is limited, causing them to tire easily. Eventually, the compensatory mechanisms fail, and cardiac output further declines.

   (2) **Edema.** In **severe ventricular failure,** VEDP is high. Increased VEDP raises venous pressure, which is reflected back to the capillaries and produces leakage of fluid into the tissues (edema).

      (a) In **left-sided heart failure,** fluid accumulates in the lungs, causing difficulty breathing (dyspnea) and the inability to breathe when lying down (orthopnea).

      (b) In **right-sided heart failure,** dependent edema occurs in the feet and ankles, because the high venous pressures are reflected into the systemic capillaries.

   (3) **Hypertrophy.** Any increase in the work of the heart causes the ventricular muscle to enlarge, like any other muscle that is exercised sufficiently.

      (a) The ventricles first dilate, producing thinning of the wall as noted previously; later the muscle hypertrophies. Myocytes have a limited ability to multiply; therefore, hypertrophy entails an increase in the diameter of the muscle fibers.

      (b) The increased muscle dimensions may cause ischemia because the diffusion distance between capillaries increases. The hypertrophy also may be harmful if the blood supply does not increase proportionately.

IV. **PRESSURE–VOLUME LOOPS.** It is possible to record changes in ventricular pressure and volume during a cardiac cycle. These records result in a **loop (Figure 11-7A),** which provides a great deal of information regarding the **function and integrity of the ventricles.**

A. **Afterload.** The afterload represents an impediment to the shortening of muscle fibers or to ejection in the heart.

1. The afterload for the ventricles is the **arterial pressure,** which normally increases progressively throughout most of the ejection phase.

2. The normal ventricle is able to maintain a relatively normal stroke volume in response to an increased afterload, but an increased afterload markedly reduces stroke volume in the failing ventricle (Figure 11-7B).

B. **Ventricular end-diastolic volume (VEDV).** The VEDV affects the stroke volume because of the Frank-Starling mechanism. The greater the VEDV, the stronger the contraction and the larger the stroke volume at any one level of contractility (Figure 11-7C).

1. The VEDV increases when the filling pressure in the atria or the central veins increases, because the higher pressure stretches the ventricular walls.

2. The VEDV also increases if the distensibility of the ventricles increases or if the heart rate slows, allowing more time for the blood to enter the ventricles during diastole.

A. Normal pressure–volume curve

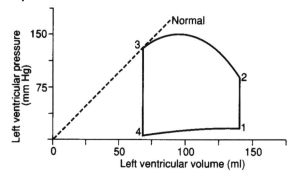

B. Effects of afterload

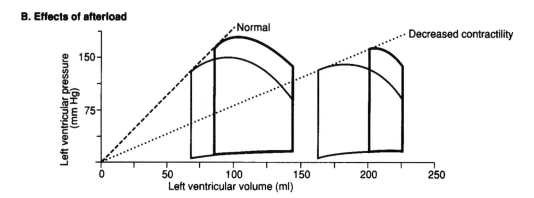

C. Increases in stroke volume

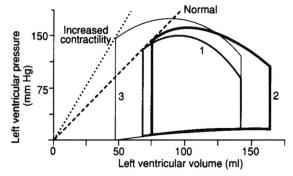

FIGURE 11-7. The effects of changes in afterload and ventricular end-diastolic volume (VEDV) on the ventricular pressure–volume loop. (*A*) Normal pressure–volume loop. Point 1 represents the beginning of isovolumic contraction (or the VEDV) point 2 marks the onset of ejection, point 3 is the beginning of isovolumic relaxation, and point 4 is the onset of ventricular filling [or the ventricular end-systolic volume (VESV)]. The stroke volume equals the VEDV minus the VESV. The *dashed line* represents the end-systolic pressure–volume relationship, which is determined by the level of contractility. (*B*) In the normal heart (curve 1) an increased afterload (*thick line*) reduces the stroke volume because the increased afterload abbreviates myocardial shortening. The VESV is greater than normal, indicating that the stroke volume has been slightly reduced. If the contractility of the heart decreases (curve 2), the VEDV increases as a Frank-Starling response to depressed ventricular function. The slope of the maximal pressure–volume relationship is reduced. An increased afterload markedly decreases stroke volume in a depressed ventricle. (*C*) Curve 1 is the control curve. An increase in VEDV (curve 2) results in an increased stroke volume (i.e., the Frank-Starling effect), but the maximal pressure–volume relationship is unchanged. The slight increase in VESV is caused by the increased aortic pressure (i.e., afterload) that results from the larger stroke volume. An increased contractility (curve 3) increases the stroke volume because of the greater myocardial force and shortening that occurs (i.e., the VESV is reduced).

C. **Cardiac work,** a reflection of the size of the pressure–volume loop (see Figure 11-7), is proportional to both the pressure generated by the ventricular contraction and the stroke volume. Because both ventricles pump the same average stroke volume, and because the systolic pressure of the right ventricle is approximately one-seventh that of the left ventricle, the work of the right ventricle is approximately one-seventh that of the left ventricle.

1. **Myocardial oxygen consumption.** The amount of oxygen (O_2) that is used by the heart depends on the amount of work performed. The coronary arterial–venous O_2 difference multiplied by the coronary blood flow equals the O_2 consumption by the heart (Fick's Law).

2. **Factors that affect cardiac work**
   a. **Hypertension.** The work of the ventricles is markedly greater in the presence of hypertension. Hypertension can occur in either the right or left side of the circulation.
      (1) **Pulmonary (right-sided) hypertension** almost invariably is caused by lung disease, whereas **systemic hypertension** most commonly is caused by an unknown mechanism and is termed **essential hypertension.**
      (2) Hypertension can also be caused by endocrine, renal, or congenital conditions.
   b. **Myocardial oxygen supply.** Normal cardiac function requires a continuous delivery of O_2 to the heart. Impaired O_2 delivery to the heart is almost always caused by the partial or complete obstruction of a coronary artery secondary to atherosclerosis.

D. **Positive inotropic mechanisms** cause the end-systolic pressure–volume relationships to shift toward the left (see Figure 11-7C). Positive inotropism allows the ventricles to achieve greater stroke volumes in the face of greater aortic pressures or afterloads. The resultant increased stroke volume is an important mechanism for increasing cardiac output during exercise.

Case 1

A 25-year-old woman complains of tiredness and shortness of breath of several months' duration. Until these symptoms appeared, she was in excellent health. Examination reveals significant findings that relate only to cardiac function. Percussion indicates an enlarged left ventricle. A pansystolic murmur that radiates toward the axilla is most audible near the apex of the heart.

    1. *What valve lesion could cause these findings?*

DISCUSSION

A pansystolic murmur begins with the first heart sound and extends beyond the second heart sound, and this indicates that the lesion involves an atrioventricular (AV) valve. The location and radiation of the murmur point to involvement of the mitral valve. This case is typical of the condition called prolapse of the mitral valve.

    2. *What is the cause of the shortness of breath?*

DISCUSSION

Mitral valve insufficiency causes a large increase in the pressure of the left atrium and pulmonary veins. The increased venous pressure may lead to pulmonary edema, which makes the lungs harder to distend and interferes with gas exchange.

Case 2

A 54-year-old patient undergoes cardiac catheterization to evaluate left ventricular function. Pressure–volume loops during a dobutamine stress test are constructed. The sloped

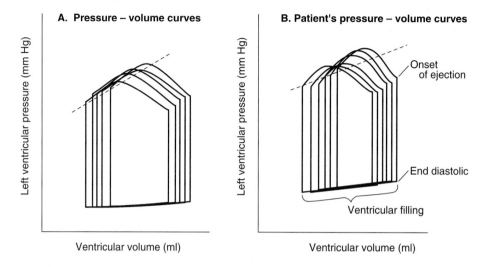

A. Pressure – volume curves

B. Patient's pressure – volume curves

Left ventricular pressure (mm Hg)

Ventricular volume (ml)

Onset of ejection

End diastolic

Ventricular filling

Patient #2

CASE 11-2 FIGURE. End-systolic pressure–volume relationships under normal conditions versus those in a particular patient.

straight lines in the pressure–volume curves in the figure indicate the end-systolic pressure–volume relationship for a normal individual (A) and for this patient (B).

> **1.** *What does the marked decrease in slope of the end-systolic pressure–volume relationship denote?*

DISCUSSION

The slope of the end-systolic pressure–volume relationship denotes the systolic elastance of the ventricle. This indicates how much force the ventricle can generate against an increased afterload. Decreased slope indicates a dysfunction of the ventricle, decreased contractility, which leads to an inappropriate increase in ventricular volume as a response to increased aortic pressure.

> **2.** *What phase of the cardiac cycle do the straight vertical lines on the pressure–volume loops represent?*

DISCUSSION

The vertical lines represent isovolumic contraction (right) and isovolumic relaxation (left) phases of the cardiac cycle. Isovolumic contraction is initiated when the mitral valve closes at the beginning of systole and ends when the aortic valve opens at the beginning of the rapid ejection phase of the cycle.

Chapter 12

The Vascular System

I. VESSELS

A. Arteries

1. **Elastic arteries** consist of the **aorta** and the **carotid, iliac,** and **axillary arteries.**
   a. **Distensibility.** The distensibility (compliance) of the elastic arteries allows them to accommodate the stroke volume of the heart with only a moderate increase in pressure.
   b. **Elastic recoil.** The vessels also generate elastic recoil during diastole. Elastic recoil creates potential energy (pressure), which maintains blood flow during the diastolic phase of the cardiac cycle.

2. **Muscular arteries** comprise most of the named arteries in the body. These arteries serve as the **distributing channels** to the organs. Their relatively large lumen minimizes the pressure drop that occurs as a result of resistance.

B. **Arterioles.** These vessels are the site of the major pressure drop in the cardiovascular system (see Chapter 9; Figure 9-3).

1. **Structure.** The arterioles contain a **thick layer of smooth muscle** and have a **relatively narrow lumen.**

2. **Functions**
   a. **Flow control.** Arterioles are the **stopcocks (valves) of the circulation.** The smooth muscle permits a fine control over the distribution of the cardiac output. This control depends on the activity of the sympathetic nerves; the arterial pressure; and the local concentration of metabolites, various hormones, and many other mediators (e.g., prostaglandins, thromboxanes, histamine).
   (1) **Autoregulation** is the ability of an organ or tissue to adjust its vascular resistance and maintain a relatively constant blood flow in the presence of changes in arterial pressure (Figure 12-1). Autoregulation is well developed in the kidneys, brain, heart, skeletal muscle, and mesentery.
   (a) The **metabolic theory** proposes that an increase in arterial blood pressure initially raises blood flow to a tissue or organ. This increased blood flow washes out vasodilator substances in the area. Vascular resistance increases, and blood flow returns to normal. Many vasodilator substances have been identified, including carbon dioxide (CO_2), H^+, nitric oxide (NO), adenosine, prostaglandins, K^+, phosphate ions, and low oxygen (O_2) levels. Changes in concentration of any of these substances cannot explain autoregulation, however.
   (b) The **myogenic theory** proposes that vascular smooth muscle responds to wall tension, which is a function of pressure and wall radius according to the law of Laplace (see Chapter 11 III B 2 b). An increase in arterial pressure initially stretches the smooth muscle fibers. In response to this initial stretching, the vascular smooth muscle contracts and returns the wall tension to control levels that can only be achieved with a smaller vessel radius. The narrowed lumen represents an increased resistance and compensates for the higher arterial pressure, returning the blood flow to control levels.
   (2) **Reactive hyperemia** is a phenomenon that occurs after the occlusion of the artery to an organ or tissue.
   (a) When the occlusion is resolved, the blood flow exceeds the control level with

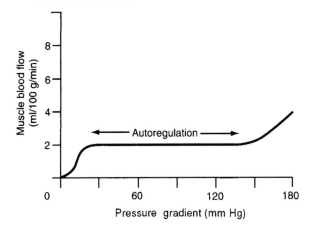

FIGURE 12-1. Autoregulation of blood flow. Note that blood flow remains relatively constant over a wide range of pressures. This may be accomplished only by changing the resistance to flow through the particular vascular bed in proportion to the change in pressure gradient.

a magnitude and duration that depends on the duration of the occlusion (Figure 12-2).

    (b) A metabolic mechanism that controls blood flow to tissues appears to cause reactive hyperemia.

  b. Pulsation dampening. The arterioles convert the pulsatile flow in the arteries to a steady flow in the capillaries.

C. **Microcirculation.** This involves a **meshwork** of vessels less than 100 μm in diameter.

  1. Components. The microcirculation is composed of **metarterioles, arterioles, capillaries,** and **postcapillary venules.** In some tissues (especially in the skin, where they are involved in thermoregulation), there are short, low-resistance connections between the arterioles and the veins called **arteriovenous shunts.**

    a. Metarterioles are relatively high-resistance conduits between arterioles and veins.

    b. Capillaries arise directly from arterioles or metarterioles. A cuff of smooth muscle cells called the **precapillary sphincter** surrounds the origin of capillaries in some tissues.

    c. Postcapillary venules, which measure 20–60 μm in diameter, are the **most permeable part** of the microcirculation.

  2. Cross-sectional area. The many capillaries that arise from each arteriole and metarteriole provide the microcirculation with a total cross-sectional area of 0.4–0.5 m².

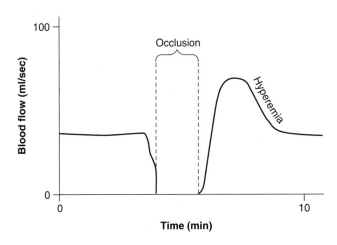

FIGURE 12-2. Hyperemia, or increased blood flow, which occurs after a period of ischemia. The hyperemic response increases and magnitude and duration if the period of occlusion is prolonged.

a. **Blood flow velocity** averages 0.3–0.4 mm/sec in the capillaries as a result of the large cross-sectional area. The velocity varies widely—within short periods of time, it can range from 0–1 mm/sec within the same capillary.

b. **Vasomotion** refers to the changes in capillary blood flow caused by constriction and dilation of regional arterioles.

  (1) Under basal conditions, 1%–10% of the capillaries are operational at any given time.

  (2) At times of high metabolic activities, significantly more capillaries carry blood simultaneously, enhancing the delivery of O_2 and metabolites to the tissues.

3. **Structure.** The **endothelial structure** of the capillaries varies in different organs depending on the function of the particular tissue.

  a. **Fenestrations.** In organs where transport of fluids is paramount [e.g., the renal glomeruli and the gastrointestinal (GI) tract], **large (2000–20,000 nm) transcellular openings** (fenestrations) exist in the endothelial cells.

  b. **Blood–brain barrier.** The microcirculatory endothelium of the brain does not exhibit fenestrations and possesses a complete basement membrane that retards or prevents the transfer of many substances between the blood and the brain.

4. **Endothelial functions.** The endothelium of the vascular system appears to be an **active metabolic tissue** that plays a major role in the **control of blood flow** in many organs.

  a. The endothelium responds to substances called **kinins** (e.g., **bradykinin, lysyl-bradykinin**) that **produce arteriolar dilation** and **increase capillary permeability.**

   (1) The kinins are formed from a precursor called a **kininogen** by a protease called **plasma kallikrein.**

   (2) The kinins are enzymatically inactivated by **kininase I** and **kininase II.** Kininase II is identical to **angiotensin-converting enzyme (ACE).**

  b. **Endothelium-derived relaxing factor** has been identified as NO (see Chapter 3 III C 2 a). NO has a **continuous vasodilating effect** in blood vessels with an intact endothelium.

   (1) **NO** is **continually released** from the endothelium by a number of compounds, including acetylcholine, and several polypeptides, including bradykinin.

   (2) Any injury to the endothelium reduces the amount of NO that is released.

  c. **Endothelins** represent a family of polypeptides that have diverse roles in many different organs. In the vascular system, they produce an initial vasodilation followed by a potent and long-lasting vasoconstriction. They also have positive inotropic and chronotropic effects on the myocardium. Endothelins exert their effects by activating specific receptors.

5. **Function: exchange.** The microcirculation provides a total surface area of approximately 700 m^2 for exchange between the circulatory system and the interstitial compartment. **Exchange of substances** occurs primarily in the capillaries and postcapillary venules. **The major mechanisms of exchange are diffusion and filtration (bulk flow).**

  a. **Diffusion** (see Chapter 1 III A) is the **principal mechanism** of microvascular exchange.

   (1) Molecules such as O_2, CO_2, water (H_2O), and glucose rapidly achieve equilibrium across the microvascular endothelium.

   (2) Larger molecules (e.g., albumin) cross the endothelial barrier very slowly or not at all.

  b. **Filtration (bulk flow).** A **hydrostatic pressure difference** across the endothelium leads to filtration (i.e., passage of H_2O and solutes from capillaries into tissues). The presence of large molecules (e.g., proteins, especially albumin) in the blood creates **oncotic pressure,** which **counteracts filtration.**

   (1) The **Starling hypothesis** maintains that the balance between filtration and reabsorption of H_2O depends both on the difference in hydrostatic and oncotic pressures between the blood and the tissues and on the permeability of the vessel.

   (2) Figure 12-3 shows how intra- and extravascular factors affect filtration and reabsorption of fluid across the microcirculation. The **bulk flow of H_2O (Q_w)** is expressed as:

$$Q_w = K \cdot [(P_c - P_i) - (\pi_c - \pi_i)]$$

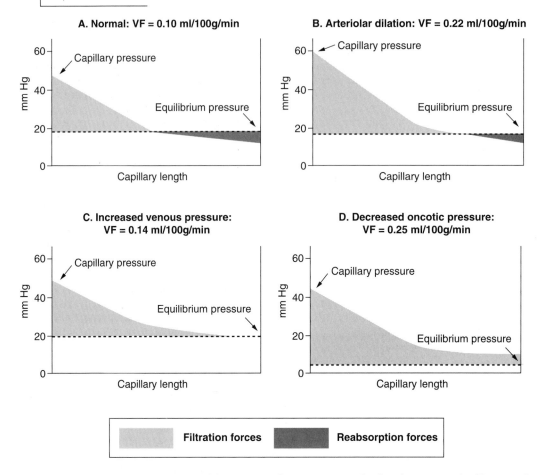

FIGURE 12-3. Schematic presentation of the intravascular pressures involved in determining the filtration of fluid across the microcirculation endothelium. The equilibrium pressure represents the pressure needed to balance the filtration and reabsorption forces. VF = volume filtered in ml/100 g tissue/min.

where K = the permeability–surface area coefficient, P_c = the hydrostatic capillary pressure, P_i = the hydrostatic interstitial pressure, π_c = the oncotic blood pressure, and π_i = the oncotic interstitial pressure.

(a) The **permeability–surface area coefficient (K)** depends on the number of microvessels receiving blood flow and the permeability of the vessels. Hypercapnia, hypoxia, NO, increased H^+ and K^+ concentrations, histamine, bradykinin, adenosine, and many other substances that result in vasodilation raise the value of K.

  (i) When the vessels are injured by hypoxia or inflammatory agents (e.g., histamine), permeability increases.

  (ii) Dilation of the arterioles, especially of the precapillary sphincters, raises the number of functional capillaries because a greater fraction of the arterial pressure is transmitted into a given capillary, and flow increases.

(b) The **hydrostatic capillary pressure** tends to force fluid out of the capillaries. Capillary pressure, which varies widely, is 30–45 mm Hg in most tissues; however, in the kidneys, the glomerular capillary pressure is 50–60 mm Hg. The hydrostatic capillary pressure depends on the arterial blood pressure, pre- and postcapillary resistance and, most importantly, venous pressure.

(i) In the presence of blood flow, the capillary pressure must always exceed the venous pressure.

(ii) **Contraction of the arteriolar smooth muscle** or precapillary sphincter may occlude the vascular lumen, causing the hydrostatic capillary pressure to equilibrate with the local venous pressure. A decrease in the capillary pressure (e.g., as in shock) tends to draw fluid from the tissues into the vascular system, which represents an **autoinfusion.**

(c) The **hydrostatic interstitial pressure** rises if the interstitial fluid volume increases (e.g., in the presence of edema). The higher hydrostatic interstitial pressure hinders additional fluid filtration from the capillaries. The value of the hydrostatic interstitial pressure in normal tissue is controversial but is considered to be slightly negative.

(d) The **oncotic pressure of blood** results from the osmotic pressure of blood proteins, which represent only a small fraction (0.005%) of the total osmotic pressure of blood. The normal oncotic pressure of blood is 25–27 mm Hg; this force tends to pull fluid into the capillaries.

(e) **Oncotic pressure of the interstitium.** Significant amounts of plasma proteins cross the endothelial barrier through either intercellular pores or fenestrae. Protein in the interstitial space generates a force that tends to pull fluid out of the vascular system. The effective oncotic pressure in the interstitium is estimated to range between 5–10 mm Hg in most tissues.

D. **Lymph vessels.** These vessels originate as closed endothelial tubes that are permeable to fluid and high–molecular-weight compounds.

1. Function. The lymphatic system represents the only mechanism for returning albumin and other interstitial macromolecules to the circulatory system. This system recovers approximately 200 g of protein daily that has been lost from the microcirculation. In addition, excess fluid is removed from the interstitium to maintain a **gel state.**

2. Mechanism

a. Lymphatic fluid is pumped out of the tissues by the contraction of the large lymph vessels and the contiguous skeletal muscles. The lymph vessels possess an extensive system of one-way valves that maintain flow toward the heart.

b. **Normal lymph flow** is approximately 2 L/day for the entire body. The **rate** of lymph flow varies in different organs and is highest in the GI tract and the liver.

E. **Veins.** The venous system is a low-resistance, low-pressure, highly distensible part of the vascular system. At normal pressures, the veins are approximately 20 times more compliant than the arteries. In comparable vessels, the veins provide a larger cross-sectional area than do the arteries.

1. Structure

a. The veins are relatively thin-walled structures that contain **small amounts of elastic tissue** and **smooth muscle.**

b. **Valves**

(1) The veins of the **dependent parts of the body** are equipped with a system of valves that **prevent the backflow of venous blood.**

(2) These valves also **support the column of blood** so that increases in capillary pressure in the dependent parts of the body (caused by hydrostatic pressure) are minimized.

2. Functions

a. **Reservoirs.** The veins serve as fluid reservoirs: 65%–75% of the circulating blood volume is in the veins at any one time. Normally, the veins are not fully distended. Therefore, small changes in pressure can cause large changes in volume (Figure 12-4).

b. **Conduits.** The systemic veins carry blood from the tissues to the right atrium, and the pulmonary veins collect blood from the lungs and return it to the left atrium.

(1) **Factors that enhance venous return**

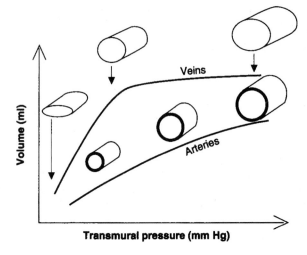

Volume (ml)

Veins

Arteries

Transmural pressure (mm Hg)

FIGURE 12-4. Pressure–volume relationship of arteries and veins. The slope of each line at any point represents compliance (distensibility). Note that the veins are much more compliant than the arteries at low pressures, because the veins are not completely distended at these pressures.

  (a) Venoconstriction is an extremely important mechanism involved in increasing cardiac output. The smooth muscle of the veins constricts in response to sympathetic stimulation, displacing blood toward the heart and raising the ventricular filling pressure.

  (b) Skeletal muscle pump. Contraction of skeletal muscle aids in venous return by compressing the veins between the contracting skeletal muscles.

  (c) Respiration. The normal negative intrathoracic (interpleural) pressure enhances venous return by increasing the pressure gradient between the heart and the peripheral vessels. **Inspiration** further amplifies the effect.

 (2) Factors that impede venous return

  (a) Standing causes approximately 500 ml of blood to shift from the pulmonary circulation to the dependent veins of the legs. The shift is caused by the hydrostatic pressure generated by the erect position. A reflex increase of sympathetic tone to the veins and heart usually compensates for the decreased circulating blood volume.

  (b) Positive end-expiratory pressure (PEEP) and the **Valsalva maneuver** impede venous return and produce a complex set of direct and reflex changes in the cardiovascular system (see also Chapter 20 IV B).

II. SPECIAL CIRCULATIONS

A. Coronary circulation

 1. Coronary arteries

  a. Superficial vessels. The major coronary vessels travel in the epicardium of the heart and subdivide, sending penetrating branches through the myocardium.

  b. Branches. The **penetrating branches** subdivide into **arcades** that distribute blood to the myocardium. Normally, the coronary arteries appear to function as **end arteries.** However, the presence of an arterial plaque or occlusion allows **anastomoses** between vessels to become functional.

 2. Veins

  a. Left ventricular venous drainage occurs primarily through the **coronary sinus.** The **thebesian veins** and **coronary–luminal vessels** (connections between the coronary vessels and the lumen of the heart) also return small amounts of blood to the left ventricle, contributing to an **anatomic shunt** effect [see Chapter 18 IV A 2 b].

  b. Right ventricular venous drainage occurs through the multiple **anterior coronary**

veins. The coronary–luminal connections carry a larger proportion of the flow in the right ventricle than in the left ventricle.

3. **Blood flow.** A continuous flow of blood to the heart is essential to maintain an adequate supply of O_2 and nutrients.
   a. **Normal coronary blood flow** represents approximately 5% of the resting cardiac output (250 ml/min), or approximately 60–80 ml blood/100 g tissue/min.
   b. **Coronary flow pattern.** During ventricular systole, myocardial wall tension increases and compresses the penetrating vessels, thus increasing the resistance to flow.
      (1) This extravascular compression produces a complex coronary flow pattern (Figure 12-5).
      (2) Maximal flow in the left coronary vessels usually occurs during isovolumic relaxation while the arterial pressure is still relatively high and the myocardium is relaxed.
   c. **Factors influencing coronary flow.** Coronary blood flow is characterized by a **supply–demand** relationship. The heart metabolizes all substrates in approximate proportion to their vascular concentration.
      (1) **Myocardial O_2 consumption** averages 6–8 ml O_2/100 g of tissue/min.
         (a) Normally, hemoglobin releases approximately 50% of its arterial O_2 content to the myocardium. In contrast, hemoglobin releases about 25% of its O_2 content for the body as a whole.
         (b) The coronary venous Po_2 is approximately 25–30 mm Hg under resting conditions and decreases during exercise or stress. During exercise, the cardiac O_2 consumption may increase five- to sixfold in well-trained athletes.
      (2) **Adenosine** is a major factor in production of coronary vasodilation during hypoxic states. Adenosine is derived from the degradation of adenosine monophosphate by 5′-nucleotidase. Release of adenosine into the myocardium produces an extremely strong vasodilator response.
      (3) **Sympathetic stimulation** increases the cardiac rate and contractility.
         (a) The resultant **increase in myocardial metabolic activity** leads to coronary va-

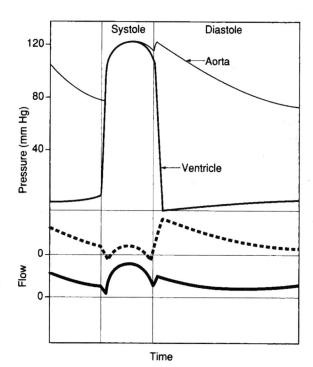

FIGURE 12-5. Diagram of the right coronary artery flow (*bold line*) and the left coronary artery flow (*dashed line*) associated with the left ventricular and aortic pressure pulses. Peak left coronary flow occurs at the end of the isovolumic relaxation, when extravascular coronary compression is low and the driving force (i.e., the aortic pressure) is high.

sodilation. If vasodilation is not adequate, the breakdown of adenosine triphosphate (ATP) will lead to the release of adenosine to enhance vasodilation.

(b) The coronary vessels contain both α and β receptors (see Chapter 3 III B 3). The α vasoconstrictor activity is rather weak, allowing the vasodilator (β) response to predominate.

B. **Cerebral circulation**

1. **Organization.** The **carotid arteries** are the major vessels supplying the brain in humans. The vertebral vessels supplement the carotid flow.

2. **Blood flow.** The brain relies on a continuous blood flow for adequate function. Interruption of blood flow for only 5–10 seconds causes a loss of consciousness, and circulatory arrest for only 3–4 minutes results in irreversible brain damage.

   a. **Normal cerebral blood flow** represents approximately 15% of the resting cardiac output (750 ml/min), or about 50–55 ml blood/100 g tissue/min.

   b. **Control of cerebral blood flow.** The brain is surrounded by a rigid skull, but vascular diameter can be altered in response to changing blood flow needs by a narrowing of the venous bed, which compensates for vasodilation on the arterial side.

      (1) **Cerebral autoregulation** is very effective in controlling blood flow over a range of arterial pressures (i.e., 80–180 mm Hg).

      (2) **CO_2 tension.** Moderate increases or decreases in CO_2 levels may double or halve the normal cerebral blood flow, respectively. Thus, CO_2 concentration is the major controller of cerebral blood flow.

      (3) **Neural control** of cerebral blood flow appears to be limited to the larger vessels and those located within the pia mater. Both sympathetic and parasympathetic neurons supply the cerebral vessels, and the role of these neurons remains unknown.

      (4) **Cushing reflex** is a systemic vasoconstriction in response to an increase in cerebrospinal fluid (CSF) pressure. The marked systemic hypertension helps maintain adequate blood flow to the brain in the presence of a high intracranial pressure. The reflex is initiated by the medullary centers, which activate when they become hypoxic as a result of limited blood flow.

C. **Skeletal muscle.** In an average adult man, 40%–50% of the total body weight is made up of skeletal muscle.

1. **Resting skeletal muscle** consumes about 20% of the resting O_2 consumption and receives about 20% of the cardiac output

   a. **Blood flow** in resting skeletal muscle varies from 1.5–6 ml/100 g tissue/min.

   b. **Red and white skeletal muscle.** Muscles composed primarily of red fibers receive a larger blood flow than those comprised mainly of white fibers.

2. **Exercising skeletal muscle**

   a. **Blood flow.** Exercising skeletal muscle receives approximately 80 ml blood/100 g tissue/min (a 15- to 20-fold increase over the resting state) and extracts approximately 80% of the O_2 from the arterial blood.

   b. The **release of metabolic products** from the muscle tissue during exercise results in a large increase in blood flow. These breakdown products include increased levels of CO_2, H^+, K^+, lactate, adenosine, and decreased O_2 levels.

   c. **Hemoglobin desaturation.** Even with the marked vasodilation that occurs during moderate to strenuous exercise, blood flow is inadequate to maintain adequate O_2 delivery to the cells.

   d. The **anaerobic threshold** is defined as the level of exercise that produces a significant rise in the level of lactic acid in the bloodstream. The anaerobic threshold occurs at an O_2 consumption that is approximately 60% of the maximal consumption for any individual.

D. **Fetal circulation.** Figure 12-6 shows the **circulatory pattern, blood flow,** and **hemoglobin saturation** in the fetus and the neonate, which differ in a number of significant ways.

A. Fetal circulation   **B. Neonatal circulation**

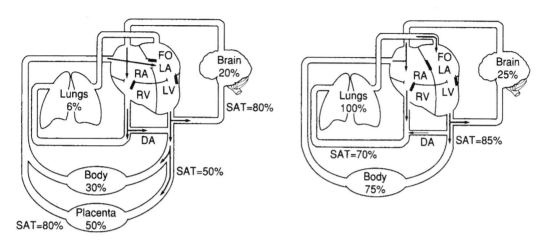

FIGURE 12-6. Fetal and neonatal circulatory patterns. Percentages within the organs indicate the percent of the total blood flow. (A) During fetal life, the two ventricles function in parallel as a result of the foramen ovale (FO) and the ductus arteriosus (DA). (*B*) Elimination of the placental circulation at birth almost doubles the systemic resistance, which increases the left atrial and ventricular pressures. Inflation of the lungs markedly reduces the pulmonary vascular resistance, lowering the right atrial and ventricular pressures. These pressure changes cause the foramen ovale to close and reverse the flow through the ductus arteriosus. LA = left atrium; LV = left ventricle; RA = right atrium; RV = right ventricle; SAT = hemoglobin saturation.

1. The **placenta** is a major organ in the fetus and **receives more than 50% of the combined output of both ventricles.**

2. At birth, marked changes occur in both the systemic and pulmonary circulations as the placental blood supply is lost. **Changes in pulmonary circulation** primarily result from a **90% decrease in pulmonary vascular resistance** as the lungs inflate after birth. The decreased resistance causes a **large drop in the afterload for the right ventricle** and **lowers the right atrial and ventricular pressures.**
   a. **Foramen ovale.** The drop in the right-sided pressures causes pressure in the left atrium to exceed the pressure in the right atrium. This pressure reversal causes the flap-like valve to close over the foramen ovale. The valve then normally fuses to the interatrial septum over the next few days.
   b. Closure of the foramen ovale prevents the right-to-left flow of venous blood and improves the oxygenation of the systemic arterial blood.

E. **Cutaneous circulation**

1. **Organization**
   a. **Cutaneous arterioles** form a dense network just under the dermis layer of the skin. These arterioles give rise to **metarterioles,** which subdivide into **capillary loops.** The **capillary loops** provide a large surface area for heat exchange. The venules form an extensive **subpapillary venous plexus.**
   b. **Arteriovenous anastomoses** are located in the distal parts of the extremities and the nose, lips, and ears. These vessels are wide, low-resistance connections that serve as shunts and allow blood to bypass the superficial capillary loops.

2. **Innervation** of the cutaneous vessels occurs through the sympathetic adrenergic system, which provides a tonic vasoconstrictor effect.
   a. The cutaneous arterioles and metarterioles have both α and β receptors. The arteriovenous anastomoses have only α receptors, however.

  b. The venous plexus has separate neural connections and can undergo marked venoconstriction, which minimizes the amount of blood in the skin.

3. Functions
  a. Nutrient supply. The metabolic rate of the skin is relatively small so that a minimal
  amount of blood flow to the skin can supply the nutritive functions.
  b. Temperature control. The major function of the cutaneous blood flow is to aid in the
  regulation of body temperature.
  (1) Heat conservation is accomplished by markedly diminishing the rate of blood
  flow to the skin. Body heat is preserved because less heat is dissipated to the environment.
  (2) Heat dissipation. When body temperature rises as a result of increased metabolic
  activity, the added heat load must be eliminated.
  (a) Vasodilation. The increased blood temperature stimulates centers in the hypothalamus that inhibit the normal tonic vasoconstrictor outflow to the cutaneous vessels and increase blood flow to the skin.
  (b) Radiation, conduction, and evaporation. The increased flow carries heat to
  the surface of the body, where it is dissipated by radiation, evaporation, and
  conduction to the environment. If the environmental temperature is higher
  than the body temperature, heat can only be dissipated by means of **evaporation of sweat;** under these conditions, radiation and conduction would cause
  the body to gain heat.

Case

**Twenty-four hours after birth, an infant exhibits peripheral cyanosis of the nail beds and
lips. A loud, continuous murmur is audible over the entire precordium. A chest x-ray
shows evidence of pulmonary congestion.**

  1. *What is the most likely diagnosis?*

DISCUSSION

This infant is suffering from patent ductus arteriosus (DA). The DA connects the descending aorta
and the pulmonary artery. Normally, the DA closes within a few hours after birth. Failure of the
DA to close provides a low-resistance path between the aorta and pulmonary artery. High flow
through the DA generates the continuous murmur, markedly reduces systemic blood flow, and
causes pulmonary congestion.

  2. *What treatment, other than surgery, might help this infant?*

DISCUSSION

Administration of aspirin may help close the patent DA. Aspirin, which blocks prostaglandin
production, leads to constriction of the smooth muscle in the wall that may eventually cause closure of the DA.

  3. *In what direction does blood usually flow through the DA in the fetus and newborn infant?*

DISCUSSION

During fetal life, the blood flows from the pulmonary artery into the descending aorta, because pressure in the pulmonary artery exceeds that in the aorta. Following birth, the direction of flow reverses; the pulmonary artery pressure decreases markedly as the pulmonary
vascular resistance falls. The aortic pressure rises as a result of an increased systemic vascular resistance due to the loss of the placental circulation.

Chapter 13

Cardiac Output and Venous Return

I. | **RELATIONSHIP BETWEEN CARDIAC OUTPUT AND VENOUS RETURN.** Over any significant period of time, venous return must equal cardiac output. For individuals at rest, the cardiac output and the venous return are approximately 5 L/min. A complicated interaction of neural, humoral, and physical factors determines the flow rate.

A. | **Vascular function curves** reflect the relationship between **venous return** and **venous pressure.** The heart removes blood from the veins and ejects it under higher pressure into the arteries, causing the arterial pressure to increase and the venous pressure to decrease. Thus, a higher cardiac output results in a lower venous pressure (Figure 13-1A).

1. **Mean circulatory pressure (MCP).** If the heart stops, blood continues to flow from the arteries to the veins for a few seconds until the pressures throughout the circulatory system equalize. The venous pressure is highest when the cardiac output (or venous return) is zero. This venous pressure is the MCP (see Figure 13-1A), and it varies with blood volume and the activity of the sympathetic nervous system (Figure 13-1B). **Sympathetic stimulation** causes the smooth muscle in the veins and arteries to contract, raising the MCP and shifting the vascular function curve to the right.

2. **Increased vascular resistance** causes a greater pressure drop between the arteries and the veins. This results in a lower venous pressure at any venous return and shifts the curve counterclockwise, as shown in Figure 13-1C.

B. | **Cardiac function curves** reflect the relationship between **venous pressure** and **cardiac output** (**Starling's law of the heart;** see Chapter 11 III A).

1. To summarize, an increase in venous pressure or preload produces a stronger contraction and a greater stroke volume.

2. Figure 13-1D depicts the normal cardiac function curve as well as the effects of sympathetic stimulation and ventricular failure (i.e., positive and negative inotropism).

C. | **Cardiovascular function curves.** Because both venous return and cardiac output depend on venous pressure, the normal curves from Figure 13-1A&D can be combined into one graph (Figure 13-2). The intersection of the curves for venous return and cardiac function is the only point where this system can function because cardiac output must equal venous return. Any change in cardiac contractility, blood volume, or vascular resistance will cause the operating point to shift, but **cardiac output and venous return will always be equal.** Exercise and congestive heart failure are just two of many conditions that can alter the operating point of the system.

1. **Exercise** (Figure 13-3A). The overall effect of exercise is an **increase in cardiac output that is proportional to the exercise intensity.** Sympathetic stimulation to the heart and vessels and the release of vasodilators from the skeletal muscle beds increase cardiac output.
   a. **Activation of the sympathetic system** increases ventricular contractility and heart rate, causing the cardiac output curve to shift to the left (i.e., to a higher level). Sympathetic stimulation also causes constriction of the venous smooth muscle, which increases the MCP.
   b. **Vasodilation,** which increases blood flow and provides more oxygen (O_2) and metabolites, occurs in the skeletal muscles. The vasodilation reduces the total peripheral resistance (TPR) or afterload, causing the vascular function curve to become steeper (see Figures 13-1C and 13-3A).

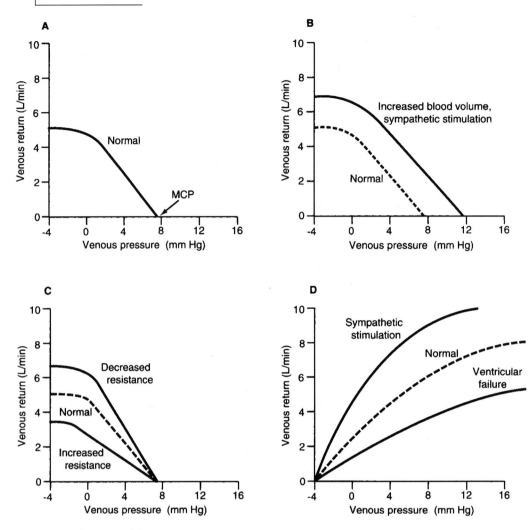

FIGURE 13-1. Vascular and cardiac function curves. In graphs *A* through *C,* venous pressure is the dependent variable but is plotted on the x-axis in contrast to the usual method of plotting the dependent variable along the y-axis. (*A*) Normal curve. Venous pressure decreases as venous return increases because the transfer of blood from the venous to the arterial system increases flow. When venous return (cardiac output) is zero, venous pressure is maximal and is referred to as the mean circulatory pressure (MCP). (*B*) Increased blood volume or sympathetic stimulation, which causes venous constriction, shifts the vascular function curve to the right and increases the MCP. (*C*) Changes in arteriolar resistance alter the slope of the vascular function curve. An increased resistance reduces the pressure transmitted through the microcirculation so that venous pressure is lower for any given flow rate. (*D*) Three cardiac function (Frank-Starling) curves demonstrate the effects of changes in contractility on the relationship between venous pressure and cardiac output.

2. **Congestive heart failure** (Figure 13-3B). This condition occurs when the output of one or both ventricles is not sufficient to supply the needs of the body. The **cardiac output** is limited by the weaker ventricle. Venous pressure increases behind the weaker ventricle, leading to edema that impairs function in other organs.
   a. **Etiology.** Causative factors include many different conditions that either lower contractile function (e.g., myocarditis, valvular heart disease) or raise the pressure or volume work. The primary defect in congestive heart failure is **decreased contractility** of the heart. The cardiac function curve shifts downward, **reducing cardiac output.**

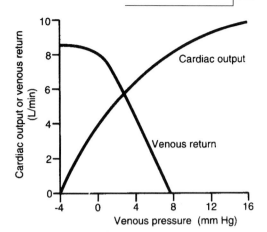

FIGURE 13-2. Vascular and cardiac function curves when superimposed. The only valid operating point on this graph is the intersection of the two curves, because this is the point where venous return equals cardiac output. In this graph, the cardiac output is 5 L/min, and the venous pressure is approximately 4 mm Hg.

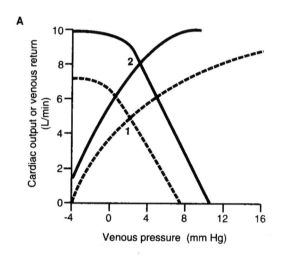

FIGURE 13-3. The effects of exercise and congestive heart failure on the vascular and cardiac function curves. (*A*) Exercise causes the vascular function curve to shift to the right and the cardiac function curve to shift to the left (upward), causing the operating point to shift from 1 to 2. (*B*) Congestive heart failure. Point 2 reflects the reduction in cardiac output from the normal level (1). Cardiac output returns toward normal (3) when the retention of fluids shifts the vascular function curve to the right.

b. **Increased blood volume.** The renin–angiotensin–aldosterone axis causes the kidneys to retain fluids and electrolytes. This increases the blood volume.
(1) The higher blood volume shifts the vascular function curve to the right, raising venous pressure, and **cardiac output returns toward normal (at the expense of an enlarged ventricle).**
(2) **Sympathetic stimulation** reflexly elevates heart rate and vascular resistance in an attempt to maintain the arterial pressure in the face of a reduced cardiac output.
c. **High venous pressure** produces edema. Left ventricular failure results in pulmonary edema, and right ventricular failure may lead to ankle swelling and fluid accumulation in the viscera.

II. MEASUREMENT OF CARDIAC OUTPUT.

The cardiac output averages 5 L/min in a normal man and 4.0 L/min in a woman. Measurement of this value involves use of either of the following techniques.

A. **The Fick principle,** which can be stated as:

$$CO = \frac{\dot{V}O_2}{(CaO_2 - C\bar{v}O_2)}$$

where CO = cardiac output, $\dot{V}O_2$ = O_2 consumption (ml/min), CaO_2 = arterial O_2 content, and $C\bar{v}O_2$ = mixed venous O_2 content.

1. **Measuring cardiac output**
   a. The O_2 consumption for the entire body equals the O_2 uptake from the lungs.
   b. **Arterial blood** can be sampled from any systemic artery.
   c. **Mixed venous blood** must be obtained either from the right ventricle or, preferably, from the pulmonary artery.

2. **O_2 consumption of organs** may be determined if the Fick principle is expressed as $\dot{V}O_2$ = $CO(CaO_2 - C\bar{v}O_2)$. The venous drainage from the specific organ must be sampled, and an independent measure of the arterial blood flow to the organ must be obtained. The arterial flow can be obtained by means of electromagnetic or Doppler flow probes.

B. **Indicator dilution method**

1. **Theory**
   a. **Volume.** If a suitable indicator is injected into an unknown volume of distribution, the volume can be estimated from the resultant indicator concentration:

$$V = A/c$$

where V = the volume of distribution, A = the injected amount of indicator, and c = the resultant indicator concentration.
   b. **Flow.** Similarly, the flow of a fluid (Q) can be measured by determining the time required for the mean concentration of the indicator to pass a given site:

$$Q = A/ (\bar{c} \cdot t)$$

where t = time and $\bar{c}$ = mean concentration of the indicator.

2. **Technique.** In the body, the indicator is injected instantaneously but is dispersed over time because of the different transit times between the injection and sampling sites. Usually, some recirculation of indicator occurs before passage of the indicator is complete. After the peak concentration is reached, the indicator concentration follows an exponential time course, so that the curve can be extrapolated to zero concentration, and the duration of the indicator passage (t) can be estimated (Figure 13-4).
   a. **Indicators** used for cardiac output measurement include Evans blue, Cardio-Green, hypertonic or hypotonic saline, ascorbate, and cold saline. Cold saline (thermodilution) is the most commonly used indicator in human cardiac output studies.

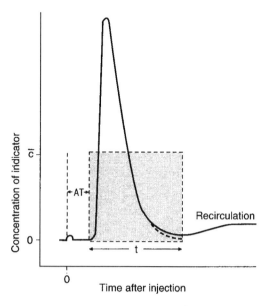

FIGURE 13-4. An indicator dilution curve that is used to measure cardiac output. AT = appearance time (i.e., the time required for the indicator to travel from the injection to the sampling site), $\bar{c}$ = mean indicator concentration for the first pass dye, and t = time for the indicator to pass the sampling site. Because some of the indicator will recirculate before all of the original indicator has passed, the curve must be extrapolated to zero (*dashed line*). The area of the *shaded rectangle* is equal to the area under the indicator curve. If $\bar{c}$ = 1 mg/L, t = 0.5 min, and a = 2.5 mg, then flow = 2.5/(1 · 0.5), or 5 L/min.

    b. Thermodilution uses a multilumened balloon catheter with a thermistor near the distal end (termed a **Swan-Ganz catheter** after its inventors).
      (1) The catheter is inserted into a peripheral vein and advanced into the central veins. The balloon is then inflated with air so that it carries the catheter along with the blood through the right ventricle into the pulmonary artery.
      (2) Cold saline is injected through a proximal opening of the catheter, which lies within the right atrium or ventricle. The saline mixes with the blood, and the temperature change of the blood is measured by the thermistor, which is downstream in the pulmonary artery.
      (3) Thermodilution has advantages because little or no recirculation of indicator occurs, withdrawal of blood is unnecessary for analysis of the indicator concentration, cold saline is relatively innocuous, and little temperature change occurs in the surrounding tissues.

Case

A 65-year-old retired businessman who has had hypertension for many years complains that extreme shortness of breath sometimes awakens him during the night. Going to the window and breathing fresh air relieves his breathing difficulty somewhat. He takes antihypertensive medication only when he "doesn't feel well." Because of discomfort when he lies flat, he has had to sleep on two or three pillows for the past few months. The man's heart rate is 96 beats/min, and his blood pressure is 160/105 mm Hg.

    1. *What is the cause of the shortness of breath?*

DISCUSSION

The man is short of breath because of pulmonary congestion and edema secondary to left ventricular failure. The decreased left ventricular function results in left ventricular distention, with elevation of the end-diastolic pressure. The increased pressure reflects back into the left atrium, pulmonary veins, and, eventually, the pulmonary capillaries. The elevated capillary pressure leads to pulmonary edema.

2. *Why does going to the window during the night bring relief?*

3. *What is the significance of sleeping on extra pillows?*

DISCUSSION

Standing, rather than the fresh air itself, results in a reduction in venous return that accounts for the relief obtained by going to the window. The decreased venous return and cardiac output relieve the pulmonary congestion, easing breathing and improving gas exchange.

The reason for the use of additional pillows involves the same principle cited previously, where standing results in improvement: Elevation of the head and thorax leads to a decrease in venous return. Respiratory discomfort that is aggravated by lying flat is referred to as orthopnea, and the severity of this condition is quantified by the number of pillows used by the patient. This man has "two-to-three pillow" orthopnea.

Chapter 14

Cardiovascular Control

I. **INTRODUCTION.** Control of blood volume and arterial pressure ensures that all of the organs receive sufficient blood flow.

II. **CONTROL OF BLOOD VOLUME** involves a complex interaction of neural, renal, and endocrine mechanisms.

A. **Neural regulation**

1. **Arterial (high-pressure) baroreceptors** are highly branched nerve endings located in the carotid sinus and the aortic arch that serve as **sensors** to detect increases in blood pressure.
   a. The arterial baroreceptors are stimulated by distention of the vessel walls; resultant nerve impulses are carried to the central nervous system (CNS) over the sinus and aortic nerves (branches of the glossopharyngeal and vagus nerves, respectively).
   b. Because the arterial baroreceptors are within the thoracic and cervical vascular systems, they detect changes in central vascular volume but not changes in the volume of the extracellular space. Standing causes fluid to shift from the thorax to the legs, which these receptors interpret as a decrease in the vascular volume.

2. **Atrial (low-pressure, stretch) baroreceptors** are located at the venoatrial junctions. These receptors are stimulated by stretch of the atrial walls caused by increased volume.

3. **Afferent impulses** from both high- and low-pressure receptors (see II A 2) are transmitted to the hypothalamus, where the neurohypophyseal cells are inhibited from releasing antidiuretic hormone (ADH) [Figure 14-1].

B. **Endocrine component**

1. **ADH.** When blood with an increased osmolality perfuses the brain, osmoreceptors located in the anterior hypothalamus detect the increased osmolality, prompting the release of ADH from the posterior pituitary (see Figure 14-1). ADH acts on the kidneys to increase the reabsorption of water from the distal convoluted tubule and especially from the collecting duct. Water retention occurs, diluting the solutes and returning the osmolality of the blood to normal.

2. The **renin–angiotensin–aldosterone system** (see Figure 14-1) is the primary regulator of electrolytes within the body. A decrease in the mean blood pressure or a decrease in the pulse pressure within the kidney causes the juxtaglomerular cells of the nephron to release the **enzyme renin** into the plasma.
   a. **Renin** reacts with a plasma protein called **angiotensinogen** to form the decapeptide **angiotensin I. Angiotensin-converting enzyme (ACE),** located on the endothelial surface of many organs (particularly the pulmonary vasculature), converts angiotensin I to angiotensin II (an octapeptide).
   b. **Angiotensin II** is one of the most **potent vasoconstrictive agents** known. Angiotensin II acts directly on the arterioles by **constricting vascular smooth muscle,** which raises blood pressure. In addition, angiotensin II **causes the release of aldosterone** from the zona glomerulosa of the adrenals.
   c. **Aldosterone** causes the distal tubule of the kidney to reabsorb electrolytes (primarily Na^+) and obligated water. The increased fluid reexpands circulating blood volume, which also tends to increase blood pressure (see Figure 14-1).

3. **Atrial natriuretic peptide** (ANP) has been found as storage granules in certain myocardial cells of the left and right atria. ANP, along with natriuretic factors from other

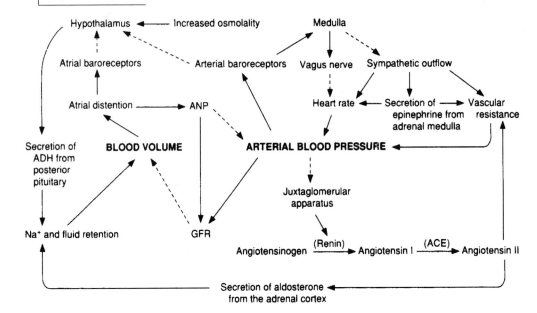

FIGURE 14-1. Major factors involved in cardiovascular control. *Solid lines* indicate an increase in the parameter or a stimulatory effect; *dashed lines* indicate a decrease or an inhibitory. Note that there are a large number of negative feedback loops that control both blood volume and arterial blood pressure. ACE = angiotensin-converting enzyme; ADH = antidiuretic hormone; ANP = atrial natriuretic peptide; GFR = glomerular filtration rate.

sources, is released into the circulation when the atria are distended by increases in blood volume.

   a. Natriuresis. ANP dilates afferent arterioles in the kidney and may relax mesangial cells (increasing the filtration area of the glomerulus). Both actions increase the glomerular filtration rate (GFR), enhancing the excretion of Na^+ and water and lowering blood volume and pressure in the arterial system (see Figure 14-1).

   b. Vasodilation. In addition to being a generalized vasodilator, ANP reduces the response to various vasoconstrictors.

III. CONTROL OF ARTERIAL PRESSURE

A. **Baroreceptor response.** Input from the baroreceptors provides information regarding the heart rate, the rate of change in blood pressure (related to ventricular contractility), and pulse pressure to the cardiovascular control centers in the CNS.

   1. The arterial baroreceptors generate a **receptor potential** in response to pressure-induced distention of the vascular walls. The receptor potential has **two distinct components.**

      a. The **dynamic receptor response** is the initial receptor potential, which is proportional to the rate of change in arterial pressure.

      b. The **static receptor response** is proportional to the new steady pressure and continues without adaptation as long as the pressure is maintained.

   2. **Afferent action potentials** (APs) are generated by the receptor potentials and are carried over the sinus and aortic nerves in response to increasing arterial blood pressure.

   3. The **baroreceptor or moderator reflex** is a reflex slowing of the heart via the vagus nerve and a withdrawal of sympathetic tone to the arterioles. This results in cardiac slowing, vasodilation, and a return of the blood pressure toward the set point.

    a. The **AP frequency** is linearly related to the increase in arterial pressure over a wide range.

    b. The **carotid sinus nerve** exhibits the **greatest sensitivity;** it responds to pressures that vary from approximately 50–160 mm Hg (Figure 14-2).

       (1) **Carotid sinus massage** is used clinically to interrupt paroxysmal atrial tachycardia by inducing a vagally mediated slowing of the heart.

       (2) **Stokes-Adams syndrome.** An increased sensitivity of the carotid sinus is seen in some elderly individuals who experience syncope as a result of vagally mediated sinus arrest, which causes a prolonged period of ventricular asystole.

B. **Central nervous system (CNS)**

   1. Medulla

    a. **Pressor** and **depressor areas** are located in the lateral and medial portions, respectively, of the reticular formation. The **depressor response** results from the **withdrawal of vasoconstrictor influence,** rather than an active vasodilation.

    b. The **cardioaccelerator** and **cardioinhibitory centers** are also located in the reticular formation. These centers send impulses to the heart over the cardiac sympathetic and vagal nerves, respectively.

   2. Hypothalamus

    a. The effects of **temperature changes** on the hypothalamic centers are relayed to the medulla, which causes the vessels of the skin to constrict (heat conservation) or to dilate (heat dissipation).

    b. **Emotional stresses** influence heart rate and blood pressure by impulses relayed from the hypothalamus to stimulate or inhibit the medullary centers.

   3. Cortex. Stimulation of various areas of the motor cortex leads to complex motor responses that include appropriate cardiovascular adjustments.

    a. **Biofeedback** can be used by patients to control heart rate and blood pressure. This use emphasizes the control the higher centers can exert on the autonomic nervous system (ANS).

    b. **Fight or flight response,** a complex set of responses, increases cardiac output and raises blood pressure in anticipation of flight or physical defense.

C. **Autonomic nervous system (ANS)** [see also III B 2, 3]

   1. Sympathetic nervous system. Most of the sympathetic nerves to blood vessels exhibit tonic activity that induces approximately 50% of the maximal **vasoconstrictor activity.** Thus, vasoconstriction or vasodilation is produced by increasing or decreasing sympathetic neural activity.

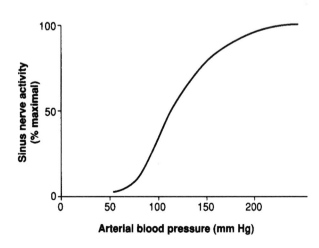

FIGURE 14-2. The effect of altering arterial blood pressure on the activity of the carotid sinus nerve. The increased sinus nerve activity in response to increasing blood pressure causes central reflexes that inhibit vasoconstriction and produce bradycardia.

a. **Innervation.** The organs are supplied by sympathetic fibers, which originate at a segmental level.

(1) Sympathetic **preganglionic fibers** exit the CNS through the ventral root and proceed to the paravertebral chain of ganglia, where they synapse with the **postganglionic cells** of the sympathetic system. Sympathetic postganglionic fibers also innervate some exocrine glands and sweat glands.

(2) The **stellate ganglion** supplies **postganglionic sympathetic nerve fibers** to the heart.

(3) **All** of the **preganglionic sympathetic fibers** are **cholinergic,** but **postganglionic sympathetic fibers** may be **either adrenergic or cholinergic.**

b. **Receptors.** The sympathetic nervous system contains α and β **receptors.** In the cardiovascular system, the α and β receptors have the following effects:

(1) **α Receptors** are stimulated most strongly by epinephrine and norepinephrine. Stimulation of the α receptors causes **vasoconstriction.**

(2) **β Receptors** are strongly stimulated by isoproterenol and less stimulated by norepinephrine. Pharmacologic agents are available that can stimulate or block the actions of both types of β receptors.

(a) **Activation of the β_1 receptors,** which are located in the **myocardium** (not the coronary arteries), results in positive inotropic and chronotropic responses.

(b) **Stimulation of β_2 receptors,** which are located in other body tissues, leads to bronchodilation or vasodilation.

2. **Parasympathetic nervous system.** The primary effect of this system, which arises from the cranial and sacral outflows of the CNS, on cardiovascular function is to slow the heart rate. Impulses conducted by the vagus nerve affect the sinoatrial and atrioventricular (AV) nodes and directly reduce atrial contractility. Marked efferent activity over the vagus nerve may result in extensive slowing of the heart, sinus arrest, AV nodal block, or a combination of these three conditions.

Case

A 72-year-old man is unconscious with a laceration on the back of the head when his wife finds him in the bathroom at 3 A.M. When she asks what happened, he says that he had gotten up to urinate and had difficulty starting his stream. He cannot remember anything else until he regained consciousness, when his wife was shaking him. Examination reveals no loss of motor power or sensation, and the man is oriented to time and place.

1. *What is the most likely cause of the loss of consciousness?*

DISCUSSION

No evidence of any heart or brain injury is apparent, so the most likely cause is a reflex effect initiated by straining during difficult urination. Straining or performing a Valsalva maneuver raises arterial blood pressure that stimulates the baroreceptors. Stokes-Adams syndrome represents ventricular slowing or arrest secondary to stimulation of the baroreceptors.

2. *What physiologic response is involved?*

DISCUSSION

A Valsalva maneuver, which markedly increases both intrathoracic and intra-abdominal pressures, may initiate the baroreceptor reflex. In this case, the patient is attempting to increase intra-abdominal pressure to begin urination. The higher intrathoracic pressure is transmitted to the arterial system, thus stimulating the baroreceptors. Afferent impulses from the baroreceptors cause reflex slowing or stoppage of the heart, resulting in hypotension, cerebral ischemia, and loss of consciousness.

Chapter 15

Cardiovascular Responses to Stress

I. **EXERCISE.** The effects of exercise on the cardiovascular system are discussed in tandem with the effects of exercise on the respiratory system (see Chapter 20 I).

II. **SHOCK** is a condition characterized by inadequate delivery of oxygen and nutrients to critical organs [e.g., the heart, brain, liver, kidneys, gastrointestinal (GI) tract].

A. **Types of shock**

1. **Low resistance shock** occurs when neural reflexes or toxic substances cause excessive vasodilation within the vascular system.

   a. **Primary shock (syncope, fainting, loss of consciousness)** is usually caused by a reflex that produces arteriolar and venous dilation, which causes peripheral pooling of blood or cardiac slowing. Fainting is most commonly provoked by **pain, stress, fright, or heat.**

   b. **Anaphylactic shock** occurs when a generalized antigen–antibody reaction takes place in patients who are sensitized to certain antigens, resulting in severe vasodilation.

   c. **Other causes of low resistance shock** include endocrine failure (e.g., as in Addison's disease or myxedema), severe hypoxia, drug overdose, and trauma to the nervous system.

2. **Hypovolemic shock** is caused by a low blood volume and may result from a number of disorders.

   a. **Septic shock** occurs when gram-negative septicemia or endotoxins cause hypotension. Gram-negative sepsis increases the permeability of the microvasculature, facilitating the movement of fluid into the tissues and intensifying the hypotension.

   b. **Hemorrhagic shock** occurs as a result of external or internal blood loss caused by ruptured vessels (e.g., from trauma). The typical sequence of changes that occurs during acute blood loss is summarized in Figure 14-1.

   c. **Dehydration shock.** Fluid loss from the GI tract (diarrhea or vomiting), kidneys (diabetes mellitus, diabetes insipidus, or excessive use of diuretics), or skin (burns, sweating, or exudation) can dehydrate the body and reduce the circulating blood volume.

3. **Cardiogenic shock** occurs when cardiac output is markedly decreased as a result of **depression of cardiac function.** Myocardial infarction, myopathy, or an abnormally slow or fast ventricular rate may cause this type of shock.

4. **Obstructive shock** occurs when cardiac output is reduced as a result of a **mechanical impediment to left or right ventricular filling.** Massive pulmonary emboli, tension pneumothorax, positive end-expiratory pressure (PEEP) respiration, and cardiac tamponade can all lead to obstructive shock.

B. **Symptoms of shock** initially are agitation and restlessness, which later progress to lethargy, confusion, and coma.

C. **Physical signs of shock** depend on the stage of shock and the severity of the dysfunction.

1. The **initial stage** of shock is characterized by a moderate reduction in cardiac output secondary to venous pooling, fluid loss, or a negative inotropic effect on the heart.

   a. Generally, **compensatory reflexes** maintain the blood pressure at normal or low-normal levels.

   b. These reflex adjustments result in an **increased heart rate, a rise in sympathetic discharge,** and a **marked increase in peripheral resistance.** The increased resistance is

selective in that the renal, skeletal muscle, and visceral beds undergo vasoconstriction, but the blood flow to essential organs (e.g., brain and heart) is maintained.

2. The **second stage** of shock occurs after a loss of blood volume of 15%–25%. It is characterized by **intense arteriolar vasoconstriction,** which is usually not adequate for maintenance of normal blood pressure.

3. The **third stage** of shock occurs when small additional losses of blood or cardiac function reduce blood flow to critical body organs. If this state persists, the inadequate blood flow causes **widespread tissue injury** from hypoxia. This rapidly progresses to what is termed **irreversible shock,** which is **fatal.**

D. **Treatment of shock** requires establishing an adequate blood flow to all body tissues.

1. **Approaches** include raising the circulating blood volume (if depleted) or improving ventricular function.

2. **Evaluation of shock** involves the use of a Swan-Ganz catheter, which can provide information regarding cardiac output and pulmonary wedge pressure. These data can be used to evaluate cardiac pump function and the extracellular fluid volume.

III. **HYPERTENSION** refers to an elevation of **arterial pressure** beyond the normal range. This increased pressure leads to damage to the heart and other organs because of the added stress to the blood vessels.

A. **Pulmonary artery hypertension** occurs when **pulmonary vascular resistance increases.** Pulmonary hypertension is commonly associated with exposure to high altitudes or pulmonary disease. **Idiopathic pulmonary hypertension** refers to pulmonary artery hypertension that results from an unknown cause.

B. **Systemic hypertension** is generally considered to be a systolic pressure of over 140 mm Hg and a diastolic pressure of over 90 mm Hg.

1. **Essential hypertension** comprises more than 90% of all cases of hypertension. The cause of this type of hypertension is unknown.

2. **Systolic hypertension** with a wide pulse pressure may be caused by various malformations or conditions that decrease the compliance of the aorta (e.g., aging) or increase the cardiac output or stroke volume of the left ventricle.

3. **Secondary hypertension** may develop as the result of a variety of conditions such as chronic **renal disease** or **endocrine dysfunction** (e.g., Cushing's syndrome, primary hyperaldosteronism, pheochromocytoma, acromegaly). **Coarctation of the aorta,** another cause, is important to diagnose because it can be cured surgically.

C. **Effects of hypertension** may include **left ventricular failure, atherosclerosis,** and **renal damage.** Such renal injury eventually causes **renal failure.**

Case

A man receives blunt trauma to the abdomen in an automobile accident. Thirty minutes after the accident, he is confused and very sweaty, with a heart rate of 110 beats/min and blood pressure of 100/65 mm Hg. Examination reveals a rigid abdomen and left upper quadrant pain.

1. *What is the most likely cause of the abdominal problem?*

2. *What leads to development of the rigid abdomen?*

DISCUSSION

This man has probably suffered a ruptured spleen. The spleen, a highly vascular organ, bleeds profusely on rupture. The loss of blood leads to shock (i.e., inadequate blood flow to major body organs).

The rigid abdomen results from accumulation of blood in the abdominal cavity. The blood is irritating to the peritoneum, resulting in reflex contraction of the abdominal muscles and a "board-like" abdominal wall.

> **3.** *What does the confusion signify?*
>
> **4.** *What accounts for the sweating?*

DISCUSSION

The confusion, an early sign of shock, results from deficient blood flow to the brain. The brain and other organs experience ischemic hypoxia because of inadequate blood flow and oxygen delivery.

Sweating, as well as increased heart rate, is an indicator of marked sympathetic outflow. The sympathetic discharge is a reflex response from low blood pressure.

$$\frac{q}{\alpha} = \alpha$$

PART III. CARDIOVASCULAR PHYSIOLOGY

STUDY QUESTIONS

1. In a recumbent person, the greatest difference in blood pressure exists between the

(A) ascending aorta and brachial artery
(B) saphenous vein and right atrium
(C) femoral artery and femoral vein
(D) pulmonary artery and left atrium
(E) arteriolar and venous ends of a capillary

2. A patient with coronary artery disease undergoes coronary arteriography, which reveals a 50% decrease in the lumen diameter of the left anterior descending coronary artery. For any arteriovenous pressure gradient, the flow through this artery (compared with normal) decreases by a factor of

(A) 2
(B) 4
(C) 8
(D) 12
(E) 16

3. Evaluation of a patient's left ventricular function involves use of a Swan-Ganz catheter that is advanced into a small branch of the pulmonary artery and wedged in place. Pulmonary artery wedge pressure is 15 mm Hg. Cardiac output, measured by thermodilution, is 4.5 L/min. Arterial blood pressure is 110/65 mm Hg (mean pressure of 76), and right ventricular pressure is 20/0 mm Hg. Which one of the following variables can be used on the abscissa (x-axis) of a Frank-Starling curve to evaluate left ventricular function?

(A) Cardiac output
(B) Pulmonary artery wedge pressure
(C) Mean arterial pressure (MAP)
(D) Stroke volume
(E) Right ventricular end-diastolic pressure (VEDP)

4. Which one of the following events is specifically seen on a standard 12-lead EKG?

(A) Sinoatrial (SA) node depolarization
(B) Atrioventricular (AV) node depolarization
(C) Bundle of His depolarization
(D) Bachmann's bundle depolarization
(E) Atrial muscle depolarization

5. The greatest resting arteriovenous difference in O_2 content is found in the

(A) liver
(B) skeletal muscle
(C) heart
(D) kidney
(E) lung

6. In a study of the carotid sinus reflex, a fellow classmate vigorously massages the area over the carotid sinus. Which one of the following events might be expected to result from this exercise?

(A) An increase in aortic blood pressure and heart rate
(B) A decrease in heart rate and aortic pressure
(C) A decrease in blood pressure and an increase in heart rate
(D) An increase in respiratory rate and depth
(E) A decrease in respiratory rate and depth

7. The rate of lymph flow in humans is approximately

(A) 10−20 L/day
(B) 1−2 L/day
(C) 100−200 ml/day
(D) 10−20 ml/hr
(E) 1−2 ml/hr

velocity of shortening

8. An increase in systemic blood pressure leads to which one of the following effects?

(A) An increase in the velocity at which blood is ejected from the left ventricle
(B) An increase in cardiac output
(C) An increase in the residual volume of blood in the left ventricle ↑ESV
(D) A decrease in the time it takes for the left ventricular wall to develop peak tension
(E) A decrease in the maximal wall tension developed in the left ventricular muscle

9. Distribution of blood flow is regulated primarily by the

(A) capillaries
(B) arterioles — smooth muscle
(C) venules
(D) arteriovenous anastomoses
(E) postcapillary venules

10. A decrease in heart rate with an unchanged stroke volume and peripheral resistance causes an increase in

(A) arterial diastolic pressure
(B) arterial systolic pressure
(C) cardiac output
(D) arterial pulse pressure
(E) mean arterial pressure (MAP)

11. The time from the upstroke of the carotid artery pulse to the incisura (dicrotic notch) is a measure of the period of

(A) atrial diastole
(B) ventricular ejection
(C) reduced ventricular filling
(D) rapid ventricular filling
(E) ventricular isovolumic relaxation

12. A patient has an abnormally slow heart rate. An EKG reveals no P waves in any lead, which indicates blockage of impulses from which one of the following structures?

(A) Sinoatrial (SA) node
(B) Bundle of His
(C) Purkinje fibers
(D) Left bundle branch
(E) Ventricular muscle

13. The pulmonic valve normally closes after the aortic valve because the

(A) diameter of the pulmonary artery is less than that of the aorta
(B) right ventricular contraction begins after left ventricular contraction
(C) velocity of ejection in the right ventricle is less than that in the left ventricle
(D) diastolic pressure in the pulmonary artery is less than that in the aorta
(E) leaflets of the pulmonic valve are stiffer and harder to close compared with those of the aortic valve

14. Which one of the following mechanisms is most important for maintaining an increased blood flow to skeletal muscle during exercise?

(A) An increase in aortic pressure
(B) An increase in α-adrenergic impulses
(C) An increase in β_1-adrenergic impulses
(D) Vasoconstriction in the splanchnic and renal areas
(E) Vasodilation within the skeletal muscle secondary to the effect of local metabolites

15. During diastole, blood flow into the ventricles sometimes produces

(A) a first heart sound (S_1)
(B) a second heart sound (S_2)
(C) a third heart sound (S_3)
(D) an ejection click
(E) an ejection-type murmur

16. Increasing the preload of cardiac muscle

(A) reduces the ventricular end-diastolic pressure (VEDP)
(B) reduces the peak tension of the muscle
(C) decreases the initial velocity of shortening
(D) decreases the time it takes the muscle to reach peak tension
(E) increases the ventricular wall tension

17. The atria contribute most to ventricular filling during which one of the following cardiac rhythms?

(A) Atrial flutter
(B) Atrial fibrillation
(C) Sinus tachycardia
(D) Sinus bradycardia
(E) Ventricular tachycardia

18. A patient receives an injection of epinephrine to counter an asthma attack. Which one of the following events will occur?

(A) The mean arterial pressure (MAP) will decrease
(B) The cardiac output will decrease
(C) The stroke volume will increase
(D) The ventricular end-diastolic volume (VEDV) will increase
(E) The arterial pulse pressure will decrease

19. Which of the following conditions leads to decreased ventricular end-diastolic pressure (VEDP) and increased aortic diastolic pressure?

(A) Myocardial tissue damage
(B) Increased arteriolar resistance
(C) Decreased ventricular contractility
(D) Increased heart rate
(E) Increased central venous pressure

20. Second heart sound (S_2) occurs during which interval of the cardiac cycle?

(A) Atrial contraction
(B) Isovolumic contraction
(C) Rapid ventricular ejection
(D) Reduced ventricular ejection
(E) Isovolumic relaxation

21. Achievement of maximal ventricular volume occurs during which interval of the cardiac cycle?

(A) Atrial contraction
(B) Isovolumic contraction
(C) Rapid ventricular ejection
(D) Reduced ventricular ejection
(E) Isovolumic relaxation

22. Which of the following factors is responsible for regulation of capillary filtration rate?

(A) Functional hyperemia
(B) Histamine
(C) Hypertension
(D) CO_2 tension (P_{CO_2})
(E) Capillary pressure

23. Which of the following factors is responsible for elevation of arterial diastolic pressure?

(A) Functional hyperemia
(B) Histamine
(C) Hypertension
(D) CO_2 tension (P_{CO_2})
(E) Capillary pressure

ANSWERS AND EXPLANATIONS

1. The answer is C [Figure 9-3; Chapter 12 I B]. In a recumbent person, the greatest difference in blood pressure exists between the femoral artery and vein, because the largest pressure drop in the vascular system (40–50 mm Hg) occurs as blood passes through the systemic arterioles.

2. The answer is E [Chapter 9 III B 2]. The effect of vessel radius on flow is so powerful because the flow rate is directly proportional to the fourth power of the radius (Poiseuille's law). Thus, decreasing the radius by half reduces the flow to one-sixteenth of the normal value.

3. The answer is B [Chapter 11 III A 1 a]. The x-axis usually represents the independent variable; for the Frank-Starling mechanism, this is the factor that defines the length of the sarcomere. In the intact heart, the sarcomere varies in length as a function of the ventricular end-diastolic volume (VEDV) or the ventricular end-diastolic pressure (VEDP). Because of the negligible resistance offered by the pulmonary veins, the VEDP is equivalent to the pulmonary artery wedge pressure.

4. The answer is E [Chapter 10 IV D 1 a]. Atrial muscle depolarization is seen as the P wave on a standard electrocardiogram (EKG). An EKG does not reveal depolarization of the sinoatrial (SA) node, atrioventricular (AV) node, bundle of His, or Bachmann's bundle, because the mass of tissue involved is too small to cause a deflection on the EKG.

5. The answer is C [Chapter 12 II A 3 c (1)]. The greatest resting arteriovenous difference in O_2 content is found in the heart. Under resting conditions, the heart removes approximately half of the O_2 from the blood, which results in an O_2 tension of approximately 27 mm Hg.

6. The answer is B [Chapter 14 II A 1 a, III A 2 b (1); Figure 14-1]. Externally applied pressure and increased arterial blood pressure both stimulate the high-pressure baroreceptors. The afferent impulses from the carotid sinus are carried over the glossopharyngeal nerve, where they stimulate the cardioinhibitory and depressor centers, leading to cardiac slowing and a decreased sympathetic tone to the vascular system. The result is decreased aortic blood pressure.

7. The answer is B [Chapter 12 I D 2 b]. The rate of lymph flow is approximately 1–2 L/day. Although this rate seems high, it is quite low compared with the flow through the entire vascular system. The rate of blood flow is approximately 8000 L/day. Thus, approximately 99.98% of the blood flow returns to the heart via the veins, leaving only 0.02% of the blood flow to be returned to the heart via the lymphatics.

8. The answer is C [Chapter 11 IV A; Figure 11-7B]. An increase in the systemic pressure (i.e., the afterload that the ventricle must overcome) reduces the velocity of shortening of the contractile elements in the muscle. A rise in afterload also limits the extent of muscle shortening, which results in a decreased stroke volume and, consequently, an increased residual volume. The time it takes for the left ventricular wall to develop peak tension is prolonged, because the velocity of contraction is reduced, and the peak tension is increased. Wall tension is a product of ventricular pressure and volume. Because pressure and volume are increased, wall tension also is higher in the presence of an increased afterload.

9. The answer is B [Chapter 12 I B 2 a]. The arterioles often are referred to as the stopcocks of the circulation because they act as valves to restrict or enhance blood flow to different tissues and organs.

10. The answer is D [Chapter 9 IV B 3 b]. The arterial pulse pressure increases when the heart rate decreases, and the stroke volume and peripheral resistance remain constant. The reduced cardiac output, in tandem with the constant peripheral resistance, causes the mean arterial pressure (MAP) to decline.

11. The answer is B (Chapter 11 II A 2 b (3) (a), B 1 b]. The upstroke of the carotid artery pulse and the incisura (dicrotic notch) indicate the beginning and end, respectively, of ventricular ejection.

12. The answer is A [Chapter 10 III A; IV D 1 a]. The sinoatrial (SA) node is the normal pacemaker of the heart. The depolarization of the SA node cannot be seen on the electrocardiogram (EKG) because of the small mass of tissue involved, but normally, SA node depolarization spreads to the atrial muscle. The depolarization of the atrial muscle is seen on the EKG as the P wave. The bundle of His, Purkinje fibers, left bundle branch, and ventricular muscle lie below the atria and normally do not cause depolarization of the atria.

13. The answer is C [Chapter 11 II A 2 b (5) (a)]. The onset of right ventricular ejection precedes left ventricular ejection, and right ventricular ejection continues after left ventricular ejection ends; therefore, the aortic valve must close first. The major components of the second heart sound (S_2) are the A_2 (produced by the closure of the aortic valve) and the P_2 (produced by the closure of the pulmonic valve). During inspiration, the P_2 is delayed and the A_2 occurs slightly earlier (i.e., the interval between the closure of the aortic and pulmonic valves is lengthened). This sequence can be appreciated during auscultation of the heart and is referred to as normal splitting of the S_2. If there is a delay in left ventricular activation, as in left bundle branch block, the A_2 may follow the P_2 and, during inspiration, the interval between these events is shortened. This is termed paradoxical splitting of the S_2.

14. The answer is E [Chapter 12 II C 2 b]. Vasodilation in active skeletal muscles, prompted by the release of metabolic products, reduces the resistance to flow and results in an increased blood flow. A decrease in total peripheral resistance (TPR) occurs because skeletal muscle represents approximately 50% of total body weight in the normal adult. Therefore, this vasodilation more than compensates for the increased resistance in tissues such as the gastrointestinal (GI) tract, kidneys, and skin.

15. The answer is C [Chapter 11 II A 3 b (3)]. The third heart sound (S_3) occurs during mid-diastole when the ventricular wall becomes tense toward the end of the rapid filling phase.

16. The answer is E [Chapter 11 III A 1 a, B 2 b (1)]. Increasing the cardiac muscle preload increases the ventricular wall tension. A rise in both end-diastolic pressure and volume (VEDP and VEDV, respectively) is synonymous with an increased preload. The higher preload causes a more forceful ventricular contraction, which results in an increase in the peak pressure generated by the ventricle as well as an increase in the stroke volume. This intrinsic property of the myocardium is termed the Frank-Starling mechanism. The increased preload results in an increased velocity of shortening, but because the peak pressure increases, the time to peak pressure usually remains constant under these conditions.

17. The answer is C [Chapter 11 II A 1 b (1)]. Atrial contribution to ventricular filling is most effective at fast heart rates when atrial contraction is coordinated. At slow heart rates ventricular filling ceases because end-diastolic and venous pressures equilibrate.

18. The answer is C [Chapter 9 IV B 1 a–c; Chapter 14 III C 1 b (1), (2)]. The overall effect of epinephrine, which is both an α- and β-adrenergic mediator, is stimulation of β receptors in the myocardium so that contractility and heart rate increase. In addition, the α-adrenergic action increases peripheral resistance. Both cardiac output and aortic pressure rise as a result of these combined effects, and pulse pressure typically increases due to the elevated stroke volume.

19. The answer is D [Chapter 11 II A 3 c (2) (a)]. An increased heart rate increases cardiac output and reduces VEDP, because both ventricular filling time and central venous pressure are reduced. An increase in cardiac output as the primary event decreases central venous pressure and increases aortic diastolic pressure. Because the heart pumps blood from the venous to the arterial side of the circulation, an increased cardiac output means that an additional volume of blood is transferred from the venous to the arterial system, which raises the pressure in the arteries and lowers the pressure in the veins.

20. The answer is E [Chapter 11 II A 2 b (4), 3 a]. The second heart sound (S_2) signals the beginning of ventricular relaxation (diastole), the first stage of which is isovolumic relaxation. The S_2 occurs when the semilunar valves close, stopping the backward flow of blood in the aorta and producing vibrations in the tissues.

21. The answer is A [Chapter 11 II A 1 a, b]. Contraction of the atria, late in diastole, increases ventricular volume so that it reaches a maximum. Ventricular filling begins as soon as the atrioventricular (AV) valves open in diastole and depends on the rate of venous return. The increased filling caused by atrial contraction is particularly important at fast heart rates, because the time for ventricular filling is abbreviated as a result of the shortened diastolic interval.

22. The answer is E [Chapter 12 I C 5 b]. Of the factors listed, capillary pressure is most closely associated with the capillary filtration rate. According to the Starling hypothesis, the capillary pressure and interstitial fluid oncotic pressure are direct determinants of the capillary filtration rate. Capillary pressure is counteracted by the oncotic pressure of the blood and the tissue pressure.

23. The answer is C [Chapter 15 III B]. An elevated arterial diastolic pressure reflects increased resistance in the systemic circulation and therefore is a more important indicator of hypertension [or the mean arterial pressure (MAP)] than is systolic pressure, which is largely determined by the stroke volume. High arterial diastolic pressure leads to vascular changes in certain organs. Arterial hypertension characteristically especially affects the kidneys and eyes.

PART IV

RESPIRATORY PHYSIOLOGY

Joseph Boyle, III

Chapter 16

Respiratory Mechanics and Gas Exchange

I. INTRODUCTION

A. **Functions of the respiratory system**

1. The **primary role** of the respiratory system is to maintain a constant internal environment by providing oxygen (O_2) for metabolic needs and excreting carbon dioxide (CO_2).
   a. **External respiration** involves the mechanics of lung ventilation, the transfer of gas across the respiratory membrane, and the transport of gas by the blood to and from the body cells. This section deals primarily with aspects of external respiration.
   b. **Internal respiration** is concerned with intracellular oxygen utilization through metabolic transformations and is generally considered the province of biochemistry.

2. **Secondary roles** of the respiratory system include:
   a. Aiding in acid–base balance
   b. Defending the body against inhaled particles (e.g., bacteria, pollen)
   c. Acting as a filter to prevent clots from entering the systemic circulation
   d. Regulating various hormonal and humoral concentrations by means of the pulmonary capillary endothelium

B. **Properties of air**

1. **Composition.** Air is a mixture of gases, primarily nitrogen (N_2) and O_2, with a variable amount of water (H_2O) vapor, a negligible quantity of CO_2, and a small amount of inert gases. **Dry atmospheric air** is approximately 79% N_2 and 21% O_2.

2. **Atmospheric (barometric) pressure** is the gas pressure exerted by the air.
   a. As temperature increases, so does the velocity of molecular movement, which increases the gas pressure if the volume occupied by the gas is constant (**Charles' law**). The pressure exerted by gas molecules can be measured using a **barometer.**
   b. Atmospheric pressure decreases as altitude increases. **Standard atmospheric pressure is 760 mm Hg at sea level,** 380 mm Hg at 18,000 feet [0.5 atmospheres (atm)], and 190 mm Hg at 34,000 feet (0.25 atm).

3. **Partial pressure.** In a mixture of gases, each gas exerts its own partial pressure (tension). The sum of the partial pressures of all gases in a mixture equals the total barometric pressure (**Dalton's law**). According to Dalton's law, partial pressure equals the fraction of that gas present times the total pressure.
   a. The **partial pressure of N_2 (PN_2)** is 600 mm Hg at sea level ($760 \cdot 0.79 = 600$).
   b. The **partial pressure of O_2 (PO_2)** is 160 mm Hg at sea level ($760 \cdot 0.21 = 160$).

II. LUNG VOLUMES AND CAPACITIES

A. The amount of gas in the lungs can be divided into various fractions with specific functions: four **nonoverlapping fractions of the maximal lung volume** and four **capacities** that are **combinations of** two or more of the **lung volumes.** Figure 16-1 shows how these volumes and capacities are organized and how they are dependent on the upper, lower, and equilibrium limits of the respiratory system. The pressure–volume relationships of the respiratory system determine the sizes of the various lung volumes.

B. Lung volumes

1. The **tidal volume (VT)** is the volume of gas inspired or expired with each breath. The normal tidal volume is **500 ml (0.5 L).**

2. The **inspiratory reserve volume (IRV)** is the additional volume that can be inspired above the tidal volume. Normally about 3.0 L, the IRV may be invaded if the tidal volume must be increased (e.g., during exercise).

3. The **expiratory reserve volume (ERV)** is the volume of gas that can be forcefully expired after a normal expiration. Normally about 1.3 L, the ERV also may be invaded when the tidal volume is increased.

4. The **residual volume (RV)** is the volume of gas that remains in the lungs after a maximal expiration. The RV, normally about 1.2 L, prevents complete collapse of the airways and the alveoli. The reopening of collapsed alveoli requires extremely large pressures to overcome surface tension forces.

C. Lung capacities

1. The **total lung capacity (TLC)** is the volume of gas in the lungs after a maximal inspiration. The TLC equals the sum of the four lung volumes.

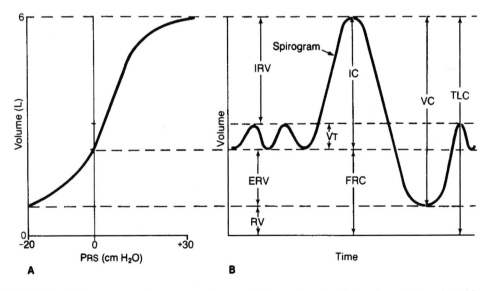

FIGURE 16-1. (*A*) A pressure–volume curve of the respiratory system. Residual volume (RV) and total lung capacity (TLC) are limited by the decreased compliance of the system, as indicated by the reduced slope of the curve at both extremes of volume. Functional residual capacity (FRC) is determined by the volume at which the transrespiratory pressure (PRS) is zero. (*B*) A spirogram showing two normal tidal volumes (VT), a maximal inspiratory effort followed by a maximal expiratory effort, [termed a vital capacity (VC) maneuver] and the return to a normal Vt. This tracing can be used to define all of the subdivisions of lung volume. ERV = expiratory reserve volume; IRV = inspiratory reserve volume; IC = inspiratory capacity.

2. The **vital capacity (VC)** is the maximal volume of gas that can be expired after a maximal inspiration.

3. The **inspiratory capacity (IC)** is the **sum of the tidal volume and the IRV** and is the maximal volume that can be inspired after a normal expiration.

4. The **functional residual capacity (FRC)** is the **sum of the RV and the ERV** and represents the equilibrium or resting volume of the respiratory system. The FRC is a reservoir of gas remaining in the lungs after a normal expiration that allows oxygenation of the blood between breaths. The FRC (or any lung capacity containing the RV) must be measured using a dilution or plethysmographic method.

   a. The **dilution method** is a widely applied physiologic principle using an indicator to measure the size of various volumes. **To determine the FRC,** an indicator gas that can be readily detected (e.g., helium) is placed in a spirometer. For example:

      (1) If the total volume of gas in the spirometer is 3 L and 20% of the gas is helium, then there is 0.6 L of helium in the spirometer. If a person begins to breathe from this spirometer at the end of a normal expiration, then the FRC is measured. The spirometer volume is maintained at 3 L by the addition of O_2.

      (2) After the subject breathes in and out of the spirometer for several minutes, the helium equilibrates between the lungs and the spirometer. If the fraction of helium is now found to be 10% of the total gas volume, then:

      $$F_1 \cdot V_{sp} = F_2 (V_{sp} + FRC)$$

      where F_1 = initial fraction of helium, V_{sp} = total volume of gas in the spirometer, F_2 = fraction of helium following equilibration, and FRC = functional residual capacity. Solving for FRC yields:

      $$FRC = F_1 \cdot V_{sp}/F_2 - V_{sp} = 0.2 \cdot 3/0.1 - 3 = 3 \text{ L}.$$

   b. The **plethysmographic method** uses the principles of **Boyle's law** and an airtight chamber or plethysmograph to measure lung volume. Measurement of the pressure changes within the chamber and the airways allows calculation of the **thoracic gas volume (TGV).** The TGV and the FRC measured by indicator dilution may vary under certain conditions.

III. VENTILATION OF THE LUNGS depends on the frequency and depth of breathing.

A. **Minute ventilation ($\dot{V}E$)** is the volume of air inspired *or* expired per minute, which equals the tidal volume (VT) multiplied by the respiratory rate or frequency (f): $\mathbf{\dot{V}E = VT \cdot f}$. The tidal volume at rest averages 500 ml (0.5 L), and the normal respiratory rate is 12–15 breaths/min; therefore, the normal minute ventilation is **6–7.5 L/min.**

B. **Dead space ventilation ($\dot{V}D$)** is the portion of the minute ventilation that fails to reach the area of the lungs involved in gas exchange.

1. The **anatomic dead space (VD)** is the volume of gas that occupies the airways, which are called the conducting zone. The conducting zone does not participate in gas exchange because of the thickness of the airway walls.

   a. The dead space ventilation is a function of the anatomic dead space and the frequency (f): $\dot{V}D = VD \cdot F$. The anatomic dead space contains approximately 150 ml (0.15 L) of gas; therefore, dead space ventilation equals approximately **2.25 L/min.**

   b. **Functions** of the anatomic dead space

      (1) **Conditioning of air**

         (a) During nasal breathing, the inspired gas is **warmed to body temperature** and **saturated with H_2O vapor** (i.e., 100% relative humidity) by the time it reaches the trachea. Mouth breathing or a tracheostomy allows cool, dry air to reach the lower airways, which can lead to tissue damage.

   (b) The addition of H_2O vapor to the inspired air dilutes the O_2 and N_2 concentrations slightly.
   (2) Removal of foreign material. Foreign particles and vapors are removed by impaction or filtration, or they are dissolved on the moist surfaces.
   (a) These particles are carried in the mucus that is propelled upward by the cilia of the respiratory epithelium.
   (b) Foreign material in the inspired gas (e.g., cigarette smoke, smog) can stimulate irritant receptors in the airways, which causes coughing, increased secretion of mucus, and hypertrophy of the mucous glands. Prolonged breathing of air that contains foreign materials can cause chronic bronchitis.

2. Alveolar dead space. In healthy people, the anatomic dead space represents the entire dead space, but in patients with lung disease, some alveoli do not receive any blood flow and therefore do not participate in gas exchange. These alveoli form the alveolar dead space.

3. The **total (physiologic) dead space** includes the anatomic dead space and the alveolar dead space. There are several methods of **measuring the total dead space.**
   (a) Bohr's method is used to measure the total dead space by determining CO_2 tensions in the expired and alveolar gases: $V_D = V_T \cdot (1 - P_{ECO_2}/P_{ACO_2})$, where P_{ECO_2} and P_{ACO_2} represent CO_2 tensions in mixed expired and alveolar gases, respectively. End-tidal samples of expired gases, theoretically, represent pure alveolar gas. An increase in the dead space lowers the CO_2 tension in the mixed expired gas. Thus, the lower the mixed expired CO_2 tension, the greater the ratio of dead space to minute ventilation.
   (b) Fowler's method of determining the dead space uses expired N_2 as an indicator. The subject inspires a VC of 100% O_2, and the expired N_2 is measured during the subsequent expiration [see Chapter 18 IV C 3 b (3)]. This method has limited applications, because in people with severe pulmonary disease, the various phases are distorted and difficult to recognize.

C. | **Alveolar ventilation ($\dot{V}_A$)** is the volume of gas that participates in the exchange of O_2 and CO_2 per minute. Alveolar ventilation, which equals the minute ventilation minus the dead space ventilation ($\dot{V}_A = \dot{V}_E - \dot{V}$), averages **4.5–5 L/min.** Adequate alveolar ventilation is critical because it determines O_2 and CO_2 tensions in the lungs (see Chapter 18 II).

1. Alveolar CO_2 tension (P_{ACO_2})
   a. The alveolar CO_2 tension is determined by the **ratio** of the **rate of CO_2 production ($\dot{V}_{CO_2}$) [L/min] to alveolar ventilation ($\dot{V}_A$) [L/min]:** $P_{ACO_2} = K_1 \cdot \dot{V}_{CO_2}/\dot{V}_A$, where K_1 is a constant (863 at sea level).
   (1) Figure 16-2 depicts the effect of varying alveolar ventilation on the arterial CO_2 tension (P_{aCO_2}) at rest and at an increased metabolic rate.
   (2) The alveolar and arterial CO_2 tensions are essentially equal because of the high diffusibility of CO_2. The presence or absence of O_2 has no direct effect on the alveolar CO_2 tension.
   b. Normally, the alveolar CO_2 tension is very closely regulated to a value of 40 ± 4 mm Hg. Regulation of this tension is important, because changes in CO_2 tension alter pH, which affects the rates of many enzymatic reactions.
   (1) Hypocapnia. An increase in alveolar ventilation (i.e., hyperventilation) with a constant rate of CO_2 production results in decreased alveolar CO_2 tension. The reduced CO_2 tension in the body leads to **respiratory alkalosis.**
   (2) Hypercapnia. An alveolar ventilation that is inadequate for the metabolic rate (i.e., hypoventilation) results in a rise in alveolar CO_2 tension, which, if it exceeds 45 mm Hg, is termed hypercapnia. This condition results in **respiratory acidosis.** Hypercapnia can lower the O_2 tension in the alveoli by displacing the O_2.

2. Alveolar O_2 tension (P_{AO_2}). O_2 is continually removed from the alveoli by diffusion into the pulmonary capillary blood. Inspiration brings fresh air into the alveoli, which normally maintains the alveolar O_2 tension at about 100 mm Hg.

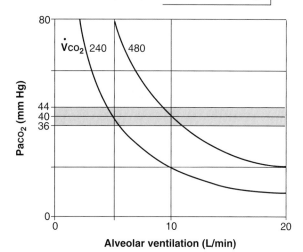

FIGURE 16-2. The graph depicts the effect of changing the alveolar ventilation on arterial CO_2 tension ($PaCO_2$). Note that a doubling of the CO_2 production ($\dot{V}CO_2$) requires a doubling of the alveolar ventilation to maintain the normal $PaCO_2$ (*shaded region*), and that a reduction of the alveolar ventilation by 50% doubles the $PaCO_2$.

   a. The alveolar O_2 tension is calculated using the **alveolar gas equation:**

$$PAO_2 = (PB - 47) \cdot FIO_2 - PaCO_2/R + K$$

   where PB = barometric pressure; 47 = H_2O vapor pressure at body temperature; FIO_2 = fraction of O_2 in the inspired gas; $PaCO_2$ = alveolar CO_2 tension; R = ratio of volume of CO_2 produced ($\dot{V}CO_2$) to volume of O_2 consumed ($\dot{V}O_2$) per minute, generally assumed to be 0.8; and K_2 = a constant that is relatively small and generally ignored. Therefore, at sea level, $PAO_2 = (760 - 47) \cdot 0.21 - 40/0.8$, or approximately 100 mm Hg.
   b. The alveolar O_2 tension is affected by changes in the barometric pressure (e.g., mountain climbing, diving), the fraction of O_2 inspired, and the alveolar CO_2 tension. The alveolar O_2 tension at sea level can be raised above 600 mm Hg by administering 100% O_2 through a mask. Prolonged use of high O_2 concentrations can lead to lung damage (see Chapter 20 V B).

IV. RESPIRATORY MECHANICS refers to the study of forces involved in altering **lung volume.** These factors include the forces generated by the respiratory muscles to inflate and deflate the respiratory system, the forces that impede volume changes (i.e., resistance and elastance), and the determinants of lung volume and its distribution within the lungs.

A. **Pleural space.** The **visceral** and **parietal pleura** are continuous membranes that, together, line the **pleural sac.** The pleural sac is only a potential space, because normally the two pleural membranes abut each other and enclose only a small amount of pleural fluid.

   1. The **pleural fluid** acts as a lubricant and causes the visceral and parietal pleura to adhere to one another.

   2. The **pleural membranes** function much the same way as two wetted glass slides; the slides move back and forth readily but are difficult to separate.

   3. Normally, the **pleural space** does not contain any gas, but gas can enter the pleural space (pneumothorax) from a rupture of the lung or a penetrating wound of the chest wall (see Chapter 20 VI).

B. **Muscles that produce volume change.** The lungs are passive structures that follow movements of the chest wall. The respiratory system always returns to its equilibrium (resting) position when the muscles are relaxed and the airways are open. Thus an inspiratory or expiratory force must be applied to the respiratory system to increase or decrease lung volume from the equilibrium position.

1. **Inspiration** is an active process, normally produced by contraction of the **inspiratory muscles** (negative-pressure breathing). Use of a respirator to inflate the respiratory system produces positive pressure (positive-pressure breathing).

   a. **Inspiratory muscles**

      (1) The **respiratory diaphragm,** the major muscle of inspiration, is a dome-shaped sheet of muscle that separates the thoracic and abdominal cavities.

      (a) The diaphragm acts similarly to a piston; contraction of the muscle causes the dome of the diaphragm to descend, enlarging the volume of the thoracic cavity inferiorly (Figure 16-3).

      (b) **Diaphragmatic contraction lifts the lower ribs.** The abdominal organs support the diaphragmatic dome, which acts as a fulcrum while the diaphragm originates from the lower ribs. The ribs are angled downward so that contraction of the diaphragm elevates the lower ribs, causing thoracic expansion laterally and anteriorly. This is referred to as a **bucket** or **pump handle effect.**

      (2) **External intercostal muscle** (see Figure 16-3) contraction also elevates the ribs, causing lateral and anterior enlargement of the thorax.

      (3) The **accessory muscles** (sternomastoid and other strap muscles of the neck) lift the clavicles and the sternum, helping to elevate the ribs and enlarge the thorax. The accessory muscles are activated only when there is increased respiratory demand (i.e., during exercise).

   b. **Inspiratory force** is generated by contraction of the inspiratory muscles, which **expands the gas volume** within the respiratory system.

      (1) **Boyle's law** states that the product of pressure and volume is a constant. Thus, if the volume of a structure containing a constant number of gas molecules is increased, the pressure will decrease.

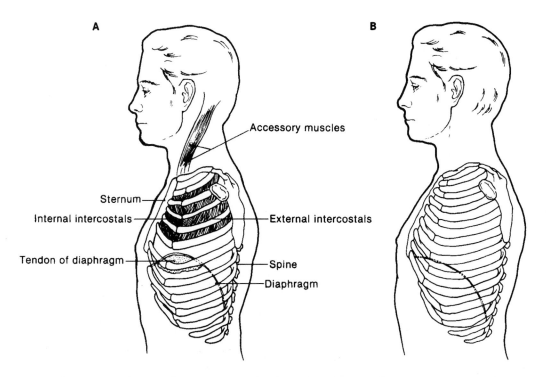

FIGURE 16-3. (*A*) The thorax and respiratory muscle relationships during end-expiration. (*B*) Maximal inspiration. Note the flattening of the diaphragm and the more horizontal position of the ribs denoting the increased volume of the thorax.

(a) At the beginning of inspiration, the lungs contain gas at atmospheric pressure. Contraction of the inspiratory muscles enlarges the thorax and expands the gas in the respiratory system. The increase in volume causes the gas pressure in the lungs to decrease below atmospheric pressure.

(b) A pressure less than atmospheric pressure is termed a **negative pressure,** and a pressure greater than atmospheric pressure is called a **positive pressure.** A **negative alveolar pressure** causes gas to flow from the atmosphere into the airways.

(c) **Maximal inspiratory pressure** is achieved by fully contracting the inspiratory muscles at a low lung volume when the airways are closed. This procedure is called a **Müller maneuver.** The maximal inspiratory pressure that can be generated is about -80 to -100 cm H_2O (Figure 16-4).

(2) **Normal inspiration** requires alveolar pressures of only -3 to -5 cm H_2O to produce adequate gas flow (see Figure 16-4). Normal individuals possess a tremendous reserve of inspiratory force that can be used to increase respiration during exercise or in the presence of pulmonary disease.

(3) **Impaired inspiratory force** may be caused by various neurologic or muscular diseases (e.g., muscular dystrophy, poliomyelitis) that interfere with the ability of muscles to contract. An inadequate inspiratory force leads to a lowered ventilation, which decreases O_2 and increases CO_2 levels (i.e., **respiratory failure**). Patients in respiratory failure require mechanical respirators to maintain adequate ventilation (see Chapter 20 IV).

2. **Expiration** is a **passive process** during quiet, normal breathing (**eupnea**). During inspiration, the respiratory system is inflated above its resting volume (e.g., such as when a balloon is blown up). During relaxation (release of the neck of the balloon), the **elastic forces** generated by the inflation compress the gas in the respiratory system, and gas flows out of the respiratory system until it returns to its **resting volume.**

a. **Expiratory muscle** contraction is required when respiration is increased during exercise or in the presence of severe respiratory disease. Contraction of expiratory muscles is also necessary to achieve lung volumes below the normal resting volume.

(1) The **rectus abdominus muscle** reduces lung volume by pulling down on the lower ribs and compressing the abdominal contents, forcing the diaphragm upward and decreasing the volume of the thoracic cavity.

(2) The **internal intercostal muscles,** which originate from the lower ribs posteriorly and insert on the upper ribs more anteriorly (see Figure 16-3). Contraction of these muscles lowers the ribs and decreases thoracic volume.

b. **Expiratory muscle force** compresses the gas in the respiratory system, increasing the alveolar pressure.

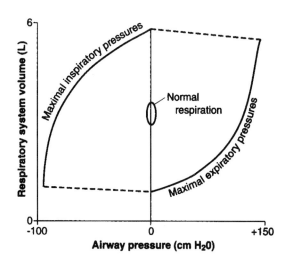

FIGURE 16-4. The *outer loop* represents the maximal pressure–volume relationships of the respiratory system. A subject inhales or exhales as forcefully as possible into a gauge after altering lung volume. If no gas escapes, there is no airflow, so that the gauge pressure is the same as the pressure in the alveoli. Note that maximal inspiratory pressures occur at low lung volumes, when the inspiratory muscles are at optimal length. Maximal expiratory pressures occur at maximal lung volumes. The *inner loop* represents the pressure and volume changes that occur during a normal respiratory cycle.

(1) Maximal expiratory pressure is achieved by fully contracting the expiratory muscles with the lungs completely inflated and the glottis or airway closed.

   (a) The **Valsalva maneuver,** which is commonly performed when lifting heavy objects or when defecating, involves maximal expiration against a closed airway.

   (b) Normally, the **maximal expiratory pressure** that can be achieved is $+100–150$ cm H_2O (see Figure 16-4).

(2) Normal expiration is **passive.** The inspiratory muscles gradually relax to provide a slow and controlled expiration. Many neuromuscular diseases may cause **impaired expiratory force;** however, because expiration is normally passive, a weakness of the expiratory muscles is not as critical as a weakness of the inspiratory muscles.

C. **Respiratory cycle** (Figure 16-5)

1. Alveolar pressure (PA). The **rate of gas flow** into or out of the lungs depends primarily on the pressure gradient between the alveoli and the atmosphere (i.e., **transairway pressure**).

   a. The highest gas flow rates occur when the pressure difference between the alveoli and the atmosphere is greatest. Conversely, when the alveolar pressure is zero (i.e., equal to atmospheric pressure), the gas flow is also zero (see Figure 16-5).

   b. Because the alveolar pressure is negative during inspiration and positive during expiration, the direction of gas flow reverses.

2. Interpleural (pleural) pressure (PPL)

   a. The interpleural pressure varies with the volume of the respiratory system and the action of the respiratory muscles.

   (1) Equilibrium volume. When the respiratory muscles are completely relaxed and the airways are open, the interpleural pressure is about -5 cm H_2O, and the lungs contain 2–2.5 L of gas.

   (a) The **chest wall** exerts an inspiratory force that tends to increase lung volume.

   (b) The **lungs** are distended and generate an elastic or recoil force that opposes the force generated by the chest wall.

   (c) These two opposing forces are equal but in opposite directions and are exerted across the pleural space, generating a **negative interpleural pressure.** Because of the balanced forces, the pressure difference across the respiratory system is zero. The volume of gas in the lungs represents the **equilibrium volume of the respiratory system,** or the **FRC.** The FRC is the lung volume at the end of a normal (eupneic), relaxed expiration (see II C 4).

   (2) During inspiration, the interpleural pressure becomes progressively more negative (see Figure 16-5) as lung volume increases. In addition, the negative alveolar pressure is transmitted to the interpleural space, making the interpleural pressure

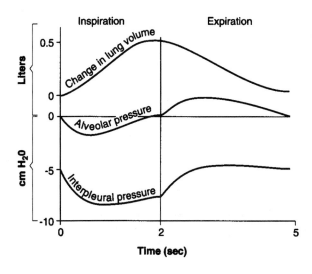

FIGURE 16-5. Pressure and volume changes during the respiratory cycle. The alveolar pressure (PA) is negative during inspiration, creating the gradient that produces gas flow. At the end of inspiration, when gas flow ceases, the PA is zero. During expiration, the elastic forces or contraction of the expiratory muscles compresses the gas in the lungs, and the PA becomes positive, creating a gradient for expiratory flow. The interpleural pressure (PPL) becomes progressively more negative during inspiration to increase the transpulmonary pressure so that the lungs can accommodate the tidal volume. During expiration, the PPL returns to its initial level.

even more negative during inspiratory flow. The change in interpleural pressure, from the beginning to the end of inspiration, measures the increased elastance generated by the inspired volume. This pressure change is used to calculate the **dynamic lung compliance** (see Figure 16-18).

 (3) **During expiration,** the interpleural pressure returns to its resting level. Normally, the interpleural pressure remains negative, but with forced expirations it can become positive.

 b. The interpleural pressure can be estimated by measuring the intrathoracic esophageal pressure, because the interpleural pressure and the internal pressure of the relaxed esophagus are equal.

 3. **Volume changes during the respiratory cycle**
  a. The volume changes that occur in the lungs during various breathing maneuvers can be measured using a **spirometer** (Figure 16-6A). This instrument consists of an in-

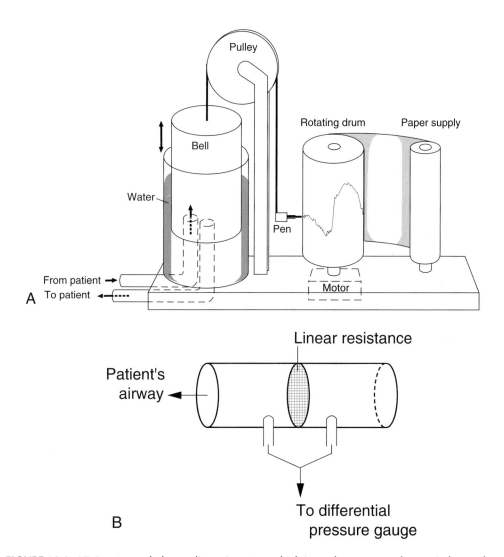

FIGURE 16-6. (*A*) A water-sealed recording spirometer, which is used to measure changes in lung volume. (*B*) Pneumotachygraph. A simple device that measures velocity of gas through a tube by means of a linear resistance screen and the pressure difference generated by flow. The flow signal is integrated as a function of time to yield volume.

TABLE 16-1. The General Gas Law

The general gas law is stated as

$$\frac{P_1 \cdot V_1}{T_1} = \frac{P_2 \cdot V_2}{T_2}$$

To convert gas volumes from spirometer to body conditions, the general gas law is used in the following form:

$$V_1 = \frac{V_2 (P_2 - PH_2O) \, T_1}{(P_1 - 47) \, T_2}$$

Where V_1 = gas volume in the body; V_2 = gas volume in the spirometer; P_1 = barometric pressure; P_2 = standard pressure (760 mm Hg); T_1 = body temperature (310°K); T_2 = room temperature (°K); PH_2O = water vapor pressure at room temperature; and 47 = water vapor pressure at body temperature.

To identify the conditions for different lung volumes, the following definitions are used:

ATPS = atmospheric temperature, pressure, saturated (conditions in a spirometer)

BTPS = body temperature, pressure, saturated (gas volumes in the body)

STPD = standard temperature (0°C), pressure (760 mm Hg), dry (used to express O_2 and CO_2 volumes for metabolic equivalence)

verted, airtight bell that is counterbalanced over a pulley so that it moves freely. The patient is connected to the spirometer (or some other device to measure changes in lung volume) by a mouthpiece and two tubes that contain one-way valves to minimize the dead space of the equipment. Expired gas is collected under the bell and inspired gas is withdrawn from the spirometer; usually, the expired gas is freed of CO_2 by means of a chemical absorbent. Records of the respiratory volume changes are made on a rotating drum or kymograph.

b. A **pneumotachygraph** can also be used to measure the velocity of gas flow into or out of the lungs (Figure 16-6B). The velocity signal is integrated electronically to give a volume signal.

c. **Conversion to BTPS conditions (Table 16-1).** Most spirometers use a water seal to prevent the escape of gas, which means that the gas in the spirometer is at room temperature and saturated with H_2O vapor [i.e., at **ATPS conditions** (see Table 16-1)].

(1) Spirometer gas occupies a different volume than it did in the body because of the change in the temperature and the amount of H_2O vapor.

(2) Any gas volume within the body must be expressed in terms of BTPS conditions. This volume can be calculated using the **general gas law,** which is a combination of Boyle's and Charles' laws, as shown in Table 16-1.

V. **TRANSMURAL PRESSURE–VOLUME RELATIONSHIPS.** The **elastic properties** of the respiratory system and its components are defined by the relationship between the **transmural pressure** of a structure and the **gas volume** within the respiratory system. Elastic properties must be studied under static conditions (i.e., no flow).

A. The **transmural pressure (PTM)** [literally, "the pressure across the wall"] is the difference in pressure between the inside (P_{in}) and the outside (P_{out}) of any structure ($PTM = P_{in} - P_{out}$) [Figure 16-7]. The **equilibrium volume** of a structure is defined as the volume it contains when the transmural pressure is zero (i.e., when **$P_{in} = P_{out}$**).

1. A **positive PTM ($P_{in} > P_{out}$),** a distending force, tends to raise the volume above the equilibrium volume.

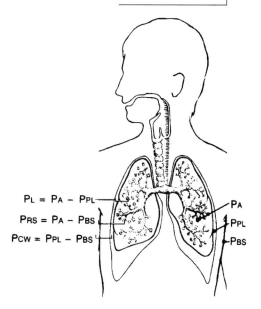

FIGURE 16-7. Schematic diagram of the components of the respiratory system and the locations used to define the transmural pressures of the different structures. P_A = alveolar pressure; P_{PL} = interpleural pressure; P_{BS} = pressure at the body surface (usually the atmospheric pressure); P_L = transpulmonary pressure; P_{CW} = transthoracic pressure; P_{RS} = transrespiratory pressure (relaxation pressure).

$P_L = P_A - P_{PL}$

$P_{RS} = P_A - P_{BS}$

$P_{CW} = P_{PL} - P_{BS}$

P_A

P_{PL}

P_{BS}

2. A **negative P_{TM} ($P_{in} < P_{out}$)** tends to deflate a structure below its equilibrium volume.

B. The **transpulmonary pressure (P_L)** is the transmural pressure **across the lungs** ($P_L = P_A-P_{PL}$; see Figure 16-7).

 1. Lung volume. The lung is a passive structure whose volume is determined by the transpulmonary pressure.

 a. Maximal volume. The lung volume increases curvilinearly as the transpulmonary pressure increases until a limiting volume is reached (P_L = approximately 20–30 cm H_2O; Figure 16-8A). The limiting volume is determined by the complex arrangement of collagen fibers in the interstitium of the lung.

 b. The **pulmonary equilibrium volume** is normally less than 10% of the maximal lung volume (see Figure 16-8A).

 2. Inflation and deflation of the lungs

 a. Compliance (distensibility) is the change in volume of a structure (ΔV) for each unit change in pressure (ΔP). Compliance is an indication of how easily a structure can be stretched or inflated (see also VI A).

 b. Elastance is the retractive (recoil) force generated by the distention of any structure (see also VI B).

 c. Relationship between compliance, elastance, and transmural pressure. If a rubber band is stretched, the force needed to lengthen the rubber band is the transmural pressure, and the recoil of the rubber is the elastance. The thicker (i.e., less compliant) the rubber band, the greater the recoil force generated by any increase in length. Therefore, **compliance (C) and elastance (E) are inversely related (C = 1/E).**

 (1) Inflation of the lungs occurs when transpulmonary pressure exceeds recoil forces and an open airway is present. The lungs increase in volume until the elastance force balances the transpulmonary pressure and the volume becomes constant.

 (2) Equilibrium. When a distensible structure has a constant volume or length, the elastance force and the transmural pressure are equal but in opposite directions; in other words, the system is at equilibrium.

C. The **transthoracic pressure (P_{CW})** is the **transmural pressure across the chest wall** ($P_{CW} = P_{PL} - P_{BS}$; see Figure 16-7), where P_{BS} equals pressure at the body surface. Normally, the P_{BS} is the atmospheric pressure.

A. Lungs

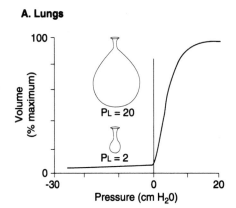

B. Chest wall

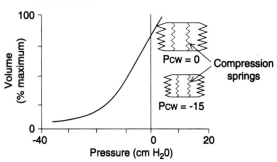

C. Lungs and chest wall

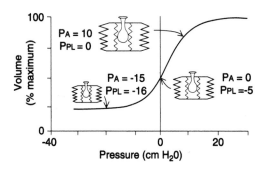

D. Lungs, chest wall, and respiratory system

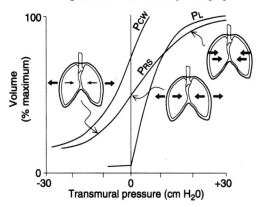

FIGURE 16-8. (*A*) Pressure–volume curve for the lungs, which are represented as a simple balloon whose volume depends on the interpleural pressure (PPL). The equilibrium volume of the lung is defined as the volume when the transpulmonary pressure (PL) equals zero. (*B*) Pressure–volume curve for the chest wall (PCW), which is represented as a bellows with internal compression springs. Note that the equilibrium volume for the chest wall is about 80% of the maximal volume, and that the curve is located largely on the negative side of the zero pressure axis. A negative PPL is necessary to lower the volume in this system. (*C*) Pressure–volume curve for the entire respiratory system, which is represented by the combination of the balloon and bellows. Note that the curve is sigmoid-shaped and that the equilibrium volume lies near mid-lung volume. This equilibrium volume represents the normal end-expiratory volume for the respiratory system. PA = alveolar pressure. (*D*) Superimposed pressure–volume curves for the lungs, chest wall, and respiratory system (PRS). The PTM for each structure is used to plot the respective curve; alternatively, the PTM for the lungs and chest wall may be algebraically summed to generate the respiratory system pressure–volume curve. The relative size and direction of the arrows indicates the forces involved at various points on the respiratory system pressure–volume curve.

1. **Expansion force.** In adults, the chest wall functions like a bellows that contains compression springs. The equilibrium volume of the chest wall is about 80% of maximal volume (Figure 16-8B).

2. At a lung volume less than the chest wall equilibrium volume, the transthoracic pressure is negative (PPL < PBS), because the chest wall is trying to reach its equilibrium volume.

D. The **transrespiratory pressure (PRS)** is the **transmural pressure across the entire respiratory system** (PRS = PA − PBS; see Figure 16-7).

1. The **respiratory system pressure–volume curve** is often referred to as a **relaxation pressure–volume curve** because of the method used to obtain it.
   a. The sigmoid-shaped relaxation pressure–volume curve is steepest in the middle and almost flat at both high and low lung volumes (Figure 16-8C). Normally, the respiratory system functions near the middle of the curve, where the system is most distensible.
   b. The respiratory system consists of the chest wall and lungs; therefore, the relaxation pressure–volume curve results from summation of the elastic properties of these structures (PRS = PL + PCW; Figure 16-8D).

2. **Respiratory system volumes**
   a. The **equilibrium volume of the respiratory system** occurs at about 40% of the maximal lung volume (see Figure 16-8D). This volume, which is also referred to as the **FRC,** represents the normal end-expiratory volume of the respiratory system.
   b. The **maximal volume** that the respiratory system can achieve is termed the **TLC.** Decreases in either compliance or the strength of the inspiratory muscles reduce the TLC.
   c. **RV** is present after a maximal expiration.
      (1) Reduced compliance at low volumes and the strength of the expiratory muscles determine the RV.
      (2) Closure of the airways or the increasing rigidity of the chest wall at low lung volumes reduce compliance. Early closure of the airways occurs when disease (e.g., bronchitis, emphysema) leads to airway narrowing and when the aging process or emphysema diminishes lung recoil.

VI. COMPLIANCE AND ELASTANCE

A. **Compliance.** In Figure 16-8, the slopes of the pressure–volume curves reflect the compliance of the various structures.

1. The **normal compliance** of the human lungs is about **0.2 L/cm H_2O** at FRC. The amount of gas inspired with each breath (i.e., the **tidal volume)** is about 500 ml (0.5 L). Thus, the transpulmonary pressure must increase by about 2.5 cm H_2O to "stretch" the lungs so they take up the normal tidal volume.

2. **Decreased compliance** of the lungs can be caused by lung diseases (e.g., tuberculosis, silicosis) that produce scarring or fibrosis of the lungs, destruction of functional lung tissue, or both.
   a. Reduced compliance produces a condition termed **restrictive lung disease (RLD).** Patients with RLD must generate greater-than-normal forces to expand the lungs.
   b. **Functional lung tissue.** The compliance of any system is dependent on its size (e.g., the amount of functional lung tissue). Thus, compliance is not a good measure of absolute distensibility.
      (1) **Example:** If a patient's lung compliance is 0.2 L/cm H_2O, then both lungs together are able to expand 0.2 L for each cm H_2O change in transpulmonary pressure. Assuming equal compliance in both lungs, each lung will take up 0.1 L of gas. If the patient undergoes a pneumonectomy, the compliance will be only 0.1 L/cm H_2O, even though the remaining lung is unchanged.
      (2) **Specific compliance (C_{sp})** is the compliance adjusted for volume: $C_{sp} = \Delta V/ (\Delta P \cdot V)$, which is the fractional change in volume per unit change in pressure.

       (a) Specific compliance is a measure of the **absolute distensibility of a structure.** For instance, the specific compliances of mice and elephants are nearly identical, but the lung compliances vary by several orders of magnitude.

       (b) If the patient in VI A 2 b (1) had an initial lung volume of 2 L, then the specific compliance prior to the pneumonectomy would equal 0.1 cm H_2O^{-1} (0.2/2). After the pneumonectomy, the lung volume is one-half the original value, but the specific compliance remains the same: 0.1 cm H_2O^{-1} (0.1/1).

  3. Increased compliance is produced by the pathologic processes that occur in **emphysema** as well as from the **aging process.**

    a. Alveolar septa, which provide some of the retractive force in the lungs, are destroyed in both conditions, but emphysema causes a much more extensive loss of septa than the normal aging process.

    b. In emphysema, there is a marked increase in airspace size as a result of the loss of many contiguous alveolar walls, a loss of alveolar surface area, and a reduction in the retractive forces of the lungs. These changes lead to abnormalities in gas exchange, in the pulmonary circulation, and in ventilation of the lungs (see Chapter 18 III C 3).

B. **Elastance.** The **recoil (retractive) forces** in the lungs are generated by both **tissue** (e.g., smooth muscle, elastin, collagen) and **surface forces.**

  1. Tissue forces. The lung contains large amounts of **collagen** and **elastin,** but the role of these connective tissue fibers in generating elastic (retractile) forces in the lungs is not fully understood.

  2. Surface forces (Figure 16-9) are generated at the alveolar surface.

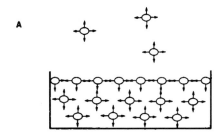

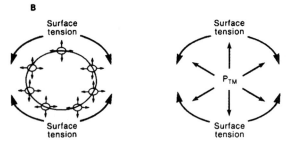

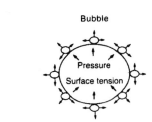

FIGURE 16-9. (*A*) Schematic representation of the intermolecular forces for molecules in the gas phase, at the surface, and in the bulk phase of a liquid. Note that surface molecules have an unbalanced force that tends to pull them into the liquid. (*B*) Surface forces in a hollow sphere, or an alveolus, generate retractive forces. (*C*) To maintain a constant volume in any structure, the transmural pressure (P_{TM}) must counterbalance the total retractive forces.

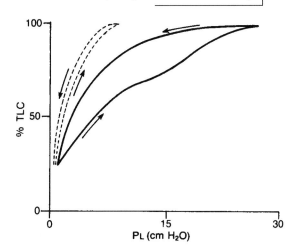

FIGURE 16-10. Pressure–volume loops for isolated lungs when filled with saline (*dotted line*) or air (*solid line*), showing the volume change as a percent of the total lung capacity (TLC). The arrows indicate the direction of volume change. Note the significant increase in the pressure that is required during inflation with air. PL = transpulmonary pressure.

    a. Alveolar surface. A phase change occurs between the alveolar gas and the surface of the alveolar membrane. A surface force (tension) is generated because of the unbalanced attraction of the liquid molecules at the surface. This force tends to minimize the surface area of the interface (i.e., it is an elastance force).

    b. Pulmonary recoil. Surface forces contribute to the total pulmonary recoil forces and increase the tendency of the lungs to deflate. An increased transmural pressure is necessary to counteract the effects of the surface forces.

        (1) Filling the lungs with a liquid (e.g., saline) will, theoretically, eliminate the surface forces so that only the tissue forces produce recoil. Figure 16-10 shows the results of such an experiment. Compared with air-filled lungs, fluid-filled lungs have markedly reduced recoil forces, leading to the conclusion that surface forces play a major role in generating elastance forces in the lungs.

        (2) Law of Young-Laplace. The transmural pressure of a structure depends on both the radius and surface (wall) tension.

            (a) Variable wall tension (Figure 16-11). The pressure inside the balloon is equal

$$P_{TM} = \frac{2 \cdot T}{r} \quad \therefore \quad \frac{T_1}{r_1} = \frac{T_2}{r_2} \quad \text{if P is constant.}$$

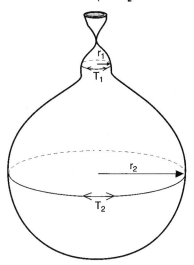

FIGURE 16-11. Demonstration of Laplace's Law. In an inflated balloon, the internal pressure is equal throughout. The structure is in equilibrium because the wall tension (T) varies in areas with different radii (r). The T:r ratio is a constant value. The neck of the balloon is collapsible (small r, low T), and the body of the balloon is rigid (large r, high T). PTM = transmural pressure.

throughout, but the wall tension varies directly with the radius of curvature. For example, the neck of the balloon (which has a small radius) is very collapsible (low wall tension), but the body of the balloon is more rigid (i.e., the wall tension is higher). The balloon is **stable** because the wall tension varies to counteract the differences in the radii at different points.

(b) Constant surface tension. Most **liquids** have a constant surface tension. Bronchoalveolar lavage fluid, derived from the lungs, has a variable surface tension that depends on the extent and rate of compression. The fluid contains pulmonary surfactant that allows it to achieve a surface tension approaching 0 dynes/cm.

3. Alveolar stabilization

a. Pulmonary surfactant is a complex substance that lines the alveolar surface and markedly decreases surface tension.

(1) Source and composition (Table 16-2). Pulmonary surfactant is formed by type II alveolar cells, which are cuboidal cells located in the corners of the alveoli. It is stored in **lamellar bodies** within the type II alveolar cells.

(a) Four unique proteins have been identified in surfactant: SP-A, SP-B, SP-C, and SP-D. SP-A and SP-D are hydrophilic proteins, and SP-B and SP-C are strongly hydrophobic proteins.

(b) Phospholipids, particularly **dipalmitylphosphotidylcholine (DPPC),** are strong **surface-active agents.**

(i) A **surface balance** is used to measure surface tension. It allows the surface area to be varied while preventing any loss of surface-active material. The surface tension initially decreases when surface-active agents are added to H_2O. Reduction of the surface area compresses the surface molecules and further lowers the surface tension (Figure 16-12).

(ii) Surface balance studies comparing pure DPPC and pulmonary surfactant (obtained by lung lavage) reveal significant differences between the two materials. Various roles have been assigned to the components of surfactant, especially the proteins.

(2) Functions

(a) Reducing surface tension. The primary function of pulmonary surfactant is to lower surface tension, which increases the compliance of the lungs, thereby decreasing the work of respiration. The low surface tension also facilitates the reopening of collapsed airways and alveoli.

(b) Increasing alveolar radius. Surfactant fills irregularities in the alveolar surface, which increases the mean alveolar radius. The increased radius reduces the

TABLE 16-2. Composition of Pulmonary Surfactant

Component		Percent Composition
Lipids		85%
DPPC	63.75%	
Neutral lipid	7.65%	
Cholesterol	5.95%	
Phosphatidylethanolamine	5.10%	
Sphingomyelin, lecithin	2.55%	
Proteins		13%
Other		2%

DPPC = dipalmitylphosphotidylcholine.

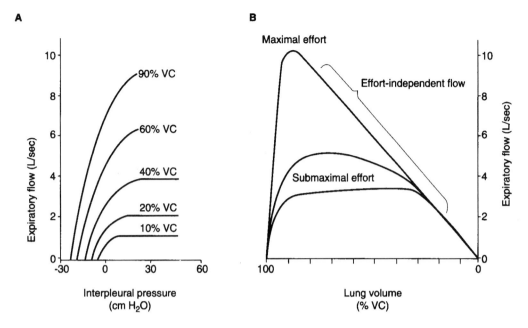

FIGURE 16-13. (*A*) Isovolume flow diagram. At volumes less than 80% of total lung capacity, the expiratory flow rate is constant at any lung volume. The flow rate is independent of effort as measured by the interpleural pressure. VC = vital capacity. (*B*) Flow–volume loop. The flow curve labeled maximal effort represents maximal flow rate and cannot be exceeded, because the flow rate at any volume is constant (as indicated in *A*). The maximal flow rate at each volume depends on the state of the airways and the lung parenchyma and provides important diagnostic information. %VC = percent vital capacity.

A. **Driving force for flow.** In Figure 16-13A, note that the expiratory flow rate remains constant at each lung volume, but the interpleural pressure varies over a large range (i.e., flow is independent of effort). The pressure gradient that produces flow under these conditions is no longer the **transairway pressure** (i.e., the alveolar pressure minus the mouth pressure)—instead, it is the **transpulmonary pressure,** which is a function of lung volume. This change in the driving pressure occurs as a result of the presence of a **flow-limiting segment** in the airways that is caused by the negative transmural airway pressure. This narrowing of the airways is referred to as dynamic compression of the airways.

B. **Dynamic compression of the airways** (Figure 16-14) occurs during forced expiration and limits the flow rate during the terminal 80% of expiration. The amount of dynamic compression depends on several variables that alter **radial traction** (Figure 16-15), which represents the dilating force exerted by alveolar septa on the outside of the airway walls.

1. **Lung volume** is the most powerful modulator of airway diameter. Any increase in lung volume will enhance the **radial traction,** thus dilating the airways.

2. **Decreased compliance (increased elastance)** [as in RLD] increases radial traction and expands the airways. Thus, patients with RLD are able to achieve relatively high flow rates for their lung volumes.

3. **Decreased elastic recoil** (as in aging or emphysema), which may be caused by destruction of alveolar septa, results in a marked loss of radial traction. This produces very compressible airways and substantial increases in airways resistance, especially during forced expiration.

4. **Pressure drop.** Increased airway resistance, caused by obstructive lung disease, increases the pressure drop along the small peripheral airways. This loss of pressure pro-

Eupneic expiration

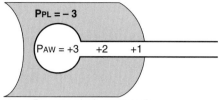

$PL = +3 - (-3) = 6cm\ H_2O$

Forced expiration

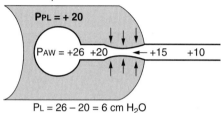

$PL = 26 - 20 = 6\ cm\ H_2O$

FIGURE 16-14. Schematic representation of the flow-limiting segment in an airway during forced expiration. Note that the pressures within the airways decrease because of resistance forces during flow. During eupneic expiration, the Ptm of the airways is positive, which distends the airways. During a forced expiration, the pressure decrement in the airways is steeper because of the increased flow rate. The PTM becomes negative (as indicated by the arrows), which narrows the airways, increases airway resistance, and limits the expiratory flow rate. PPL = interpleural pressure; PAW = airway pressure; PL = transpulmonary pressure.

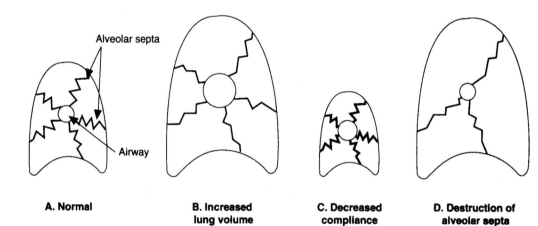

FIGURE 16-15. Various factors that may alter the radial traction forces on the airway walls, which help to keep the airways open. (A) Normal. (B) Increased lung volume is the most powerful factor in the expansion of airway diameter. Greater volume leads to dilation of airways by increasing the radial traction exerted by the alveolar septa. (C) Decreased compliance in restrictive lung disease reduces lung volume. The increased elastance forces support the airways and dilate them, compared with lungs of the same volume in normal individuals. (D) Destruction of alveolar septa (as in emphysema and aging) diminishes airway wall support, narrowing the lumen and creating high airway resistance.

duces a greater compressive effect on the airways, leading to further narrowing and even greater reduction in the rate of gas flow at any given lung volume.

C. **Flow–volume curves.** Much information can be obtained about pulmonary mechanics by recording flow rate as a function of lung volume (Figure 16-16). Figure 16-17 shows flow–volume curves for normal individuals and for patients with restrictive lung disease and obstructive lung disease.

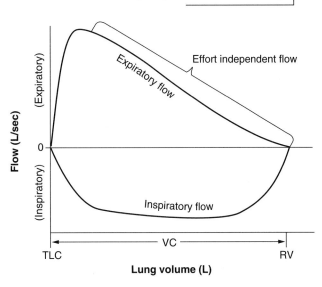

FIGURE 16-16. A normal maximal flow–volume curve showing both inspiratory and expiratory portions. Vital capacity (VC) is indicated by the length of the loop along the x-axis, with total lung capacity (TLC) and residual volume (RV) at the extremes. Effort-independent flow, which is produced by dynamic compression of the airways during a forced expiration, occupies most of the expiratory limb of the loop.

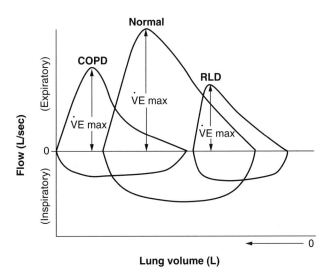

FIGURE 16-17. Maximal flow–volume curves for normal individuals and for patients with obstructive and restrictive lung disease. Note how the total lung capacity, residual volume, and maximal flow rates change in each of the three different situations. (See Figure 16-16 for position of lung volumes.) COPD = chronic obstructive pulmonary disease; RLD = restrictive lung disease.

IX. THE WORK OF RESPIRATION equals the change in pressure that is needed to inflate the lungs multiplied by the change in volume (Figure 16-18).

A. Work (pressure–volume) loops. The work of inflating the lungs can be evaluated by plotting the change in lung volume versus the interpleural pressure (Figure 16-19A–C). The **area** of the rectangle ($\Delta P \cdot \Delta V$) has the units of work (kg · m) and is proportional to the O_2 utilized by the respiratory muscles. If either the respiratory resistance increases or the compliance decreases, the respiratory work will increase and therefore, the respiratory muscles will use more O_2 to overcome the added load.

B. Normal work of breathing. Normally, the work of breathing represents **2%–3% of the resting O_2 consumption.** Because expiration is a passive process, all of the work of breathing is done during inspiration.

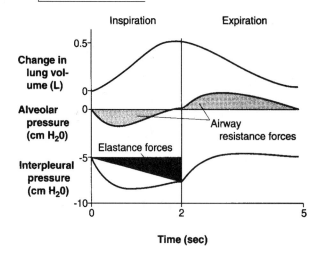

FIGURE 16-18. A graphic representation of the events of the respiratory cycle with the airway resistance and elastance forces identified (see also Figure 16-5). Increased resistance or increased elastance causes proportional increases in these areas. Thus, patients with obstructive lung disease (i.e., high airway resistance) must generate much higher transairway pressure gradients during inspiration and expiration, whereas patients with restrictive disease must generate more negative interpleural pressures at the end of inspiration to maintain normal respiratory activity.

C. **Minimal work of breathing.** The minimal work for respiration is a function of airway resistance and respiratory system compliance (Figure 16-20A). Airway resistance rises as flow rates increase at high rates of breathing, and elastance forces increase with increases in tidal volume. All species of animals use the combination of tidal volume and respiratory rate that requires the minimal work of respiration. How the brain establishes this combination is not known.

1. **RLD.** Patients with RLD (i.e., reduced compliance) must increase their elastance work to breathe. The elastance work can be minimized by reducing the tidal volume.
   a. **Work loop** (see Figure 16-19B). In RLD, patients must generate greater inspiratory effort to overcome their greater elastance forces. The interpleural pressure becomes more negative at the end of inspiration so that the total work of breathing is increased.
   b. **Compensatory mechanisms.** Elastance work can be minimized by **breathing rapidly and shallowly** (Figure 16-20B). The tidal volume is decreased, but the increased respiratory rate ensures adequate ventilation of the lungs.

2. **Obstructive lung disease.** Patients with obstructive lung disease must increase their resistance work to overcome airways resistance.
   a. **Work loop** (see Figure 16-19C). The width of the work loop is increased because increased pressures are necessary to generate inspiratory and expiratory gas flow.
   b. **Compensatory mechanisms.** Resistance work can be minimized by **breathing more slowly and deeply** (see Figure 16–20B). This prolongs the time of expiration, which reduces the pressure gradient necessary to generate gas flow. The increased tidal volume compensates for the decreased respiratory rate so that a normal alveolar ventilation is maintained.

D. **Respiratory failure.** The respiratory muscles, just like any skeletal muscles, can become fatigued if exposed to a high workload for a long time. If the respiratory muscles cannot generate sufficient force, then pulmonary ventilation decreases, reducing the supply of O_2 to the body and impairing the excretion of CO_2 (Figure 16-21). Respiratory failure is indicated by hypercapnia, not hypoxia.

X. PULMONARY FUNCTION TESTS

A. **Vital capacity (VC).** Measurement of VC under different conditions is the most commonly performed pulmonary function test.

1. The **slow VC** is used to evaluate the size of the lungs (see Figure 16-1). The VC can be

A. Normal

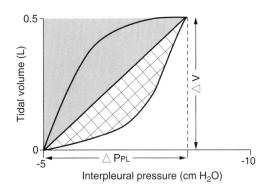

B. Restrictive lung disease

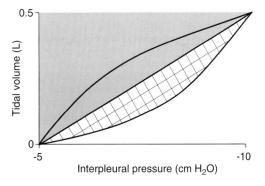

FIGURE 16-19. The work of ventilating the lungs can be evaluated by plotting the change in lung volume [i.e., tidal volume (VT)] against the interpleural pressure (PPL) during breathing. The resultant work loop is inscribed counterclockwise; the peak of the loop represents the end of inspiration. (*A*) Normal. The slope of a line drawn from the beginning to the end of inspiration represents the compliance of the lungs and bisects the loop into inspiratory (lower) and expiratory (upper) segments. The *cross-hatched area* denotes the resistance work during inspiration. The *shaded triangle* represents the stored elastic energy that is present at end-inspiration. This stored energy can compress the alveolar gas and create expiratory gas flow. The total area represented by $\Delta V \cdot \Delta PPL$ is proportional to the work that must be performed by the respiratory muscles. (*B*) Restrictive lung disease (RLD). Patients with RLD must overcome significantly higher elastance forces as indicated by the increased area of the *shaded triangle* if the VT remains in the normal range. (*C*) Obstructive lung disease. Patients with obstructive lung disease must generate increased pressure gradients to produce adequate air flows. The more negative alveolar pressure is transmitted to the PPL, causing the work loop to broaden significantly. If the work loop extends beyond the y-axis, it indicates active contraction of the expiratory muscles. This contraction supplements the stored elastic energy.

C. Obstructive lung disease

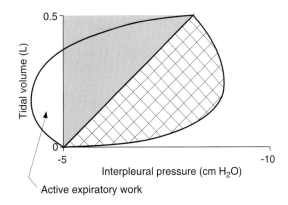

Active expiratory work

decreased by either reducing the TLC (restrictive disease) or by increasing the RV (obstructive disease) [see Figure 16-20].

2. The **forced vital capacity (FVC)** is used to evaluate the resistance properties of the airways and the strength of the expiratory muscles. The FVC is obtained by performing a VC maneuver as rapidly as possible into a recording spirometer (Figure 16-22A).
    a. The **forced expiratory volume in 1 second (FEV$_1$)** represents the volume expired in

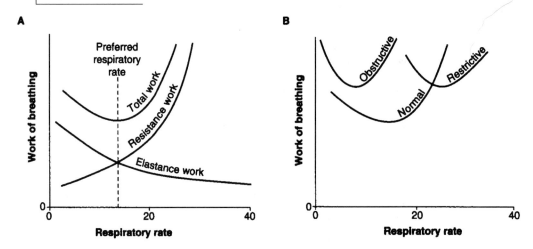

FIGURE 16-20. Determinants of an optimal breathing rate. (A) Variation in the different components of the work of breathing at a constant level of alveolar ventilation. At low respiratory rates, the tidal volume (VT) is increased to maintain a constant ventilation. Larger tidal volumes require greater distention of the lungs, and the elastance component of work is increased. Higher respiratory rates increase the velocity of flow through the airways, increasing the resistance component of work. Thus, for a given ventilation, there is a minimal work of breathing that is determined by a specific combination of tidal volume and respiratory rate. Normally, this optimal combination for humans occurs at a rate of 12–15 breaths/min and a tidal volume of about 0.5 L. (B) Total work of breathing curves reflect the compensatory mechanisms used by patients with obstructive or restrictive lung disease. Patients with obstructive pulmonary disease minimize their work of breathing by decreasing the respiratory rate, which minimizes the resistance component of respiration. Patients with restrictive disease minimize their respiratory work by decreasing tidal volume (to minimize the elastance component) and increasing their respiratory rate (to maintain a normal alveolar ventilation). The minimal respiratory work for patients with obstructive or restrictive lung disease is higher than normal, but it is optimal for the existing pathophysiologic conditions.

the first second of an FVC (see Figure 16-22A). The FEV_1 is the most commonly used screening test for airway disease.
(1) The FEV_1 is actually a flow rate; its units are L/sec.
(2) Because flow equals the driving pressure divided by resistance, the FEV_1 varies inversely as a function of the airway resistance and directly as a function of the maximal expiratory pressure. Therefore, patients with obstructive lung disease or expiratory muscle weakness have a low FEV_1 (Figure 16-22B).

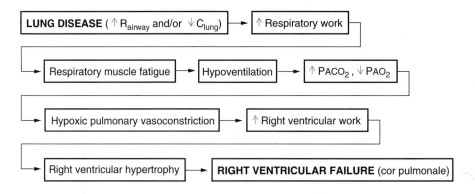

FIGURE 16-21. Typical sequence of events that occurs in respiratory failure. R_{airway} = airway resistance; C_{lung} = lung compliance; P_{ACO_2} = alveolar CO_2 tension; P_{AO_2} = alveolar O_2 tension.

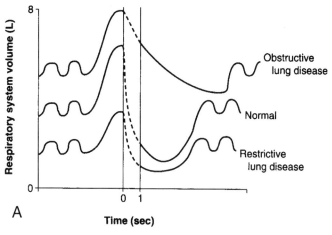

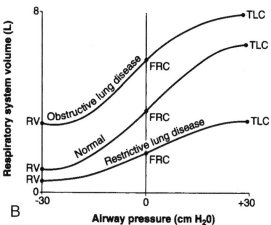

FIGURE 16-22. (*A*) Spirogram of a forced vital capacity (FVC) maneuver in normal individuals and in patients with obstructive and restrictive lung disease. The forced expiratory volume in 1 second (FEV$_1$) is indicated by the *dashed* portion of each curve. (*B*) Typical changes in pressure–volume relationships that occur in obstructive and restrictive lung diseases. Note the effect of changes in the position and slope of the curves (compliance) on total lung capacity (TLC), forced residual capacity (FRC), and residual volume (RV). The vital capacity (VC) in each patient is the difference between the TLC and RV.

b. The **FEV$_{1\%}$** is the percent of the VC expired in 1 second [i.e., FEV$_{1\%}$ = (FEV$_1$/FVC) · 100]. Normally, the FEV$_{1\%}$ is greater than 75%–80% of the FVC.

    (1) Patients with **restrictive lung disease** have a reduced VC but are able to achieve relatively high flow rates; therefore, their FEV$_{1\%}$ exceeds 80% (Table 16-3; see Figure 16-22A).

    (2) Patients with **obstructive lung disease** have low flow rates as a result of high airway resistance; consequently, their FEV$_{1\%}$ is abnormally low (see Figure 16-22A and Table 16-3).

TABLE 16-3. Effects of Lung Disease on the Forced Vital Capacity

	Resistance	FVC	FEV$_1$	FEV$_1$ (%)
Normal	. . .	. . .	. . .	> 80%
Restrictive	↓	↓	↓	> 80%
Obstructive	↑	↓	↓	< 80%

FEV$_1$ = forced expiratory volume in 1 second; FEV$_1$ (%) = percent of forced vital capacity in 1 second; FVC = forced vital capacity.

B. **Maximal expiratory pressure.** Measuring the maximal expiratory pressure allows physicians to determine whether the cause of a low expiratory flow rate is increased airway resistance or weakness of the expiratory muscles.

  1. **Method.** The maximal expiratory pressure is measured by having the patient expire as forcefully as possible into a pressure gauge.
     a. Because there is no airflow under these conditions, the pressure generated in the alveoli is transmitted without loss to the airway opening.
     b. If flow occurs, the pressure at the mouth is less than alveolar pressure as a result of the resistance decrement during flow.

  2. **Interpretation**
     a. Patients with a **high airway resistance** can generate normal expiratory pressures of approximately 100 cm H_2O.
     b. Patients with **expiratory muscle weakness** generate a lower expiratory pressure (see IV B 2).

C. **Maximal voluntary ventilation (MVV).** The MVV, which results in the highest rate of ventilation for any condition, represents the maximal volume of gas that an individual can breathe. This test stresses all of the mechanical factors of breathing and becomes abnormal with increases in airway resistance, reduced compliance, or decreased respiratory muscle force. The largest deficiency of this test is its dependence on patient complete cooperation; the results vary with the degree of cooperation.

  1. **Method.** The patient breathes as rapidly and deeply as possible while the volume changes are recorded. The test is carried out for 12 seconds, and the results are expressed in L/min.

  2. **Interpretation.** Results should be compared to predicted values based on age, height, and sex. A normal value for a young adult man is approximately 200 L/min.

Case

A 61-year-old man has suffered a partial transection of the spinal cord at C5 as a result of a skiing accident. Initially he is placed on a respirator, but eventually it is removed. When he is not on the respirator, he experiences occasional episodes of dyspnea.

The patient's pulmonary function tests are shown in the following table.

  1. *Why is the functional residual capacity (FRC) completely normal?*

  2. *Why is the forced expiratory volume in 1 second (FEV$_1$) decreased?*

Test	Units	Patient Value	Percent Predicted
Total lung capacity (TLC)	L	6.41	90%
Vital capacity (VC)	L	3.0	60%
Functional residual capacity (FRC)	L	3.65	100%
Residual volume (RV)	L	3.4	150%
FEV$_1$	L/sec	2.0	65%
Maximal inspiratory pressure	mm Hg	50	62%
Maximal expiratory pressure	mm Hg	30	29%

FEV$_1$ = forced expiratory volume in 1 second.

DISCUSSION

The FRC is determined only by the static elastic properties of the respiratory system. Because these properties do not depend on any muscle strength, they are not affected by loss of neural input, and the FRC is normal.

The FEV_1 is a flow rate, and as such it is dependent on the ratio of the driving force or maximal expiratory pressure to the airway resistance. The driving force is greatly reduced secondary to the spinal transection, and the airway resistance is presumably normal, which lowers the FEV_1.

> **3.** *Why is the maximal inspiratory pressure better preserved than the maximal expiratory pressure?*

DISCUSSION

The maximal inspiratory pressure is much higher than the maximal expiratory pressure because the transection at C5 has interrupted only part of the outflow of the phrenic nerve (C3–C5). The phrenic nerve innervates the diaphragm, the major inspiratory muscle. Most of the nerves that innervate the expiratory muscles, which originate in the lower thoracic and lumbar regions of the spinal cord, have lost their upper motor neurons as a result of the cervical transection.

Chapter 17

Gas Diffusion and Transport

I. **INTRODUCTION.** For oxygen (O_2) to cross the respiratory membrane, it must first dissolve in the tissues, then diffuse into the plasma of the pulmonary capillaries.

A. **Henry's law** defines the **volume of gas that will dissolve in any liquid:**

$$C_x = \alpha_x \cdot P_x$$

where C_x = volume of gas "x," α_x = its solubility (Bunsen) coefficient, and P_x = its partial pressure. Gas molecules dissolve in liquids the same way that sugar dissolves in coffee. To know how much sugar is dissolved, one needs to know how many scoops were put in (e.g., the partial pressure) as well as the size of the scoops (e.g., the solubility coefficient).

1. **Partial pressure.** The amount of any **gas dissolved in a liquid increases as a function of the partial pressure.**
   a. There are **no limits on the amount of gas that can be dissolved over physiologic ranges of gas tensions.**
   b. **Gas content versus partial pressure**
      (1) The **partial pressure** of the gas in a liquid represents the pressure it would exert in the gas phase. The units of partial pressure are mm Hg. **At equilibrium,** the partial pressure in the liquid equals the partial pressure in the gas phase. **In the absence of equilibrium,** the partial pressure in the liquid is less than in the gas phase.
      (2) The **gas content** represents the **volume** of the gas per unit volume of liquid that is present. The units of gas content are volume of gas/volume of solvent (e.g., ml/L, ml/dl, and so on).

2. **Solubility.** The solubility of a gas is a major determinant of the number of molecules present. A higher solubility **increases the rate of diffusion,** because this indicates the presence of an increased number of molecules.
   a. The **solubility coefficient** is a **constant** for each gas "x" that equates gas content and partial pressure.
   b. Increasing the temperature reduces the solubility of gases (Table 17-1).
   c. **Carbon dioxide (CO_2) is about 24 times more soluble than O_2** at body temperature.

II. **DIFFUSION** is the movement of individual molecules from areas of higher concentration to areas of lower concentration by random motion (see also Chapter 1 III A). The blood must be exposed to a gas tension for a finite time for gas to equilibrate between the gas and liquid phases. The time required for equilibration is a function of the contact area between the liquid and the gas (surface area), the solubility and diffusion properties of the gas, and the diffusion gradient. Normally, the blood spends about 0.75 second in the pulmonary capillaries of the lungs.

A. **The rate of pulmonary gas diffusion** (i.e., the volume of gas per minute that crosses the alveolar–capillary membrane) is determined by several factors as defined by **Fick's Law** of diffusion:

$$\dot{V}gas = PC - PA \cdot \frac{D \cdot A}{d}$$

1. The **partial pressure of the gas in the alveoli** (PA)

TABLE 17-1. Solubility Coefficients for Gases Important to Respiratory Physiology

	Solubility Coefficient (ml gas/ml saline/mm Hg gas tension)			
Temperature (°C)	O_2	N_2	CO_2	CO
0	0.049	0.024	1.71	0.035
20	0.032	0.016	0.90	0.023
37	0.024	0.012	0.58	0.019

2. The **partial pressure of the gas in the pulmonary capillary** (PC)

3. The **diffusion coefficient** of the gas (D) is a function of the molecular weight (diffusion is inversely related to the square root of the molecular weight), solubility in a particular solvent, and absolute temperature (310°K, normal body temperature).

4. The **dimensions of the alveolar–capillary membrane** [i.e., the diffusion distance (d) and the total surface area (A) for exchange]
   a. The **diffusion distance** is the average thickness of the alveolar–capillary membrane (Figure 17-1). Pulmonary edema or an increase in the thickness of the interstitium increases the diffusion distance and retards diffusion.
   b. The **surface area** of the respiratory membrane averages 80–100 m² in the normal adult. The large surface area and the small distance between the alveolar gas and the pulmonary capillary blood normally allow rapid equilibration.

B. **Diffusing capacity (DL).** DL is defined as the volume of gas absorbed by the lungs per minute (V̇) per mm Hg partial pressure gradient. DL is derived from Fick's Law.

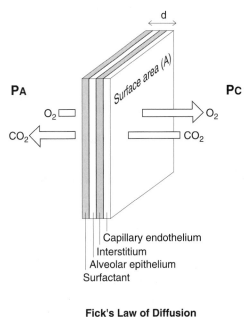

Capillary endothelium
Interstitium
Alveolar epithelium
Surfactant

Fick's Law of Diffusion

$$\dot{V} \text{ gas} = (PA - PC) \bullet \frac{D \bullet A}{d}$$

FIGURE 17-1. The alveolar–capillary membrane is multilayered but on average is only 0.5 μm (0.00002 inch) thick. The arrows indicate the direction of diffusion of O_2 and CO_2. V̇ = volume of gas transferred per minute; PA = alveolar gas tension; PC = pulmonary capillary gas tension; D = diffusion coefficient; d = thickness of membrane; A = surface area of membrane.

1. The **diffusion properties of the lungs** are evaluated by measuring the diffusing capacity.

$$DL = \frac{\dot{V}}{(PA - PC)}$$

Currently, the diffusing capacity of the lungs is measured using a single-breath technique and a dilute concentration (about 0.01%) of carbon monoxide (CO).

a. **Diffusing capacity of the lungs for CO (DLCO)**

   (1) The dilute CO mixture and the high affinity of hemoglobin for CO ensure that the pulmonary capillary CO tension (PCCO) is close to zero during the test (unless the subject is a smoker or exposed to high atmospheric CO levels). Utilizing CO simplifies the methodology, because the pulmonary capillary PCO is essentially zero and does not need to be measured.

   (2) The **normal value of the DLCO** is approximately **30 ml/min/mm Hg.**

b. The **diffusing capacity (calculated) of the lungs for O$_2$ (DLO$_2$)** is about **25 ml/min/mm Hg.**

2. **Factors affecting the diffusing capacity of the lungs.** Theoretically, the diffusing capacity of the lungs is proportional to the surface area of the lungs divided by the distance of the diffusion path. Actually, the transfer process is a function of both the diffusion properties of the system (i.e., the **membrane component**) and the rate of the chemical reaction with hemoglobin (i.e., the **blood component**). Each of these factors represents a resistance to gas transfer, and normally these resistances are about equal.

a. The **membrane component.** Pulmonary diseases affect the process of diffusion by reducing the exchange surface area (e.g., emphysema, which destroys the alveolar septa), increasing the diffusion distance (e.g., interstitial lung disease, pulmonary edema), or reducing the partial pressure gradient for the diffusion of gases (e.g., ventilation–perfusion abnormalities).

b. The **blood component depends** on the **chemical reaction time** and the **amount of hemoglobin** in the pulmonary capillaries.

   (1) An increased amount of hemoglobin in the pulmonary capillaries enhances the transfer of gases. Anemic patients have a reduced diffusing capacity.

   (2) Exercise increases the diffusing capacity to 60–75 ml O$_2$/min/mm Hg by increasing blood flow, which recruits more pulmonary capillaries and increases the surface area for exchange.

C. Equilibration

1. **O$_2$**

a. **Diffusion of O$_2$.** The normal alveolar PO$_2$ is 100 mm Hg, whereas the blood entering the pulmonary capillary normally has a PO$_2$ of 40 mm Hg. After dissolving in the alveolar–capillary membrane, the O$_2$ molecules diffuse into the plasma, raising the plasma O$_2$ tension. O$_2$ then diffuses into the red blood cell (RBC), where combination with hemoglobin takes place.

b. **Equilibration time.** Normally, enough O$_2$ diffuses across the respiratory membrane so that the blood O$_2$ tension and the alveolar O$_2$ tension equalize in about **0.25 second** (Figure 17-2).

2. **CO$_2$**

a. **Diffusion of CO$_2$** occurs **from the pulmonary capillary blood to the alveoli.** The average CO$_2$ tension in the pulmonary capillary blood is 46 mm Hg, as opposed to 40 mm Hg in the alveoli. Although the CO$_2$ diffusion gradient is only one tenth of the O$_2$ diffusion gradient, CO$_2$ diffuses almost 20 times more rapidly than O$_2$.

b. **Equilibration time.** It is estimated that the time required for the blood CO$_2$ tension and the alveolar CO$_2$ tension to equalize is also approximately 0.25 second.

3. **Factors affecting gas exchange.** Pulmonary gas exchange is determined by either perfusion or diffusion properties of the system (Figure 17-3).

a. **Perfusion-limited gas exchange** occurs when **equilibration takes place** between the

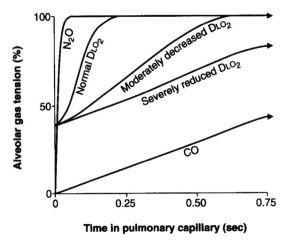

FIGURE 17-2. Pulmonary capillary gas tensions as a percentage of the alveolar gas tension. The red blood cells spend an average of 0.75 second in the pulmonary capillaries at rest. Normally, equilibration occurs between alveolar gas and pulmonary capillary blood within 0.25 second. If the normal diffusing capacity of the lung for O_2 (DL_{O_2}) is diminished, the equilibration time is prolonged or is never achieved. Carbon monoxide (CO) equilibration is slow, because it is administered in very low concentrations and the blood can combine with large volumes of the gas. Nitrous oxide (N_2O) equilibrates rapidly between alveolar gas and blood, because it is relatively insoluble in the blood and only small amounts of N_2O produce a rapid rise in gas tension.

alveolar gas and the pulmonary capillary blood (i.e., increased O_2 uptake can only be achieved by increasing blood flow).

   (1) Normally the transfer process is perfusion-limited. After equilibration, the net transfer of O_2 ceases until the capillary blood is replaced by new unsaturated venous blood.

   (2) Transit time. The average RBC spends approximately 0.75 second in the pulmonary capillary. If equilibration occurs in 0.25 second, then no further gas transfer normally takes place for the last 0.50 second of transit through the pulmonary capillary. This time provides a **safety margin** that ensures adequate O_2 uptake

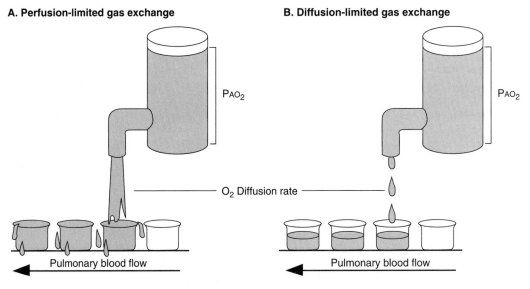

A. Perfusion-limited gas exchange

B. Diffusion-limited gas exchange

PA_{O_2}

PA_{O_2}

O_2 Diffusion rate

Pulmonary blood flow

Pulmonary blood flow

FIGURE 17-3. Perfusion- and diffusion-limited gas exchange. (*A*) In perfusion-limited gas exchange, the blood is equilibrated (as symbolized by the full beakers) so that the only method of increasing gas uptake is to increase pulmonary blood flow (by moving more beakers through the system). (*B*) In diffusion-limited gas exchange, the blood is not equilibrated (i.e., the beakers are not full) so that the diffusion rate must be increased to improve gas exchange. The diffusion rate can be increased by raising the alveolar O_2 tension (PA_{O_2}) and increasing the driving force for diffusion.

during periods of stress (e.g., exercise, exposure to high altitudes) or impaired diffusion.

   b. Diffusion-limited gas exchange occurs whenever **equilibration does not take place** between the alveolar and pulmonary gas tensions. Increasing the diffusion gradient [e.g., by raising the fraction of inspired O_2 (FIO_2)] is one way to treat diffusion-limited gas exchange.

   (1) CO exchange is diffusion-limited, which is why measurement of the $DLCO$ is an effective means of evaluating the diffusion properties of the respiratory system.

   (2) Clinical significance

   (a) Many pulmonary diseases reduce the rate of O_2 transfer (see Figure 17-2). Diffusion-limited gas exchange is one cause of **arterial hypoxia.**

   (b) Disease processes or **significant increases in altitude reduce the alveolar O_2 tension,** which in turn reduces the diffusion rate.

III. O_2 TRANSPORT

A. **Hemoglobin. O_2 combines reversibly with the four iron atoms of hemoglobin and converts deoxyhemoglobin into oxyhemoglobin.** The **driving force** for the chemical reaction between hemoglobin and O_2 is the **O_2 tension in the pulmonary capillaries.** The normal alveolar O_2 tension (PAO_2) is 100 mm Hg; this represents the upper limit for the O_2 tension in the body.

1. Hemoglobin saturation is the percent of hemoglobin that is combined with O_2. The percent saturation is the average saturation for the entire population of hemoglobin molecules in the blood.

   a. Each hemoglobin molecule can combine with as many as **four O_2 molecules.** If all of the sites on the hemoglobin molecule are occupied by O_2, then the molecule is 100% saturated.

   b. The hemoglobin saturation depends on the O_2 tension (PO_2) [Figure 17-4].

   c. The **loading (association) zone** of the hemoglobin saturation curve is the **plateau** that occurs above O_2 tensions of approximately 60 mm Hg (see Figure 17-4).

   (1) Arterial hemoglobin saturation. The O_2 tension of arterial blood is normally 85–100 mm Hg, which results in an arterial hemoglobin saturation of 96%–98% (Figure 17-5).

   (2) The loading zone provides a **margin of safety,** because the alveolar O_2 tension can be reduced substantially, yet the hemoglobin saturation remains quite high. This allows people to climb mountains to moderate altitudes or to suffer from various pulmonary diseases without experiencing a significant decrease in the arte-

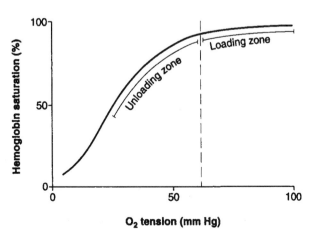

FIGURE 17-4. Hemoglobin saturation with O_2 as a function of the O_2 tension of the blood. In the pulmonary capillaries the hemoglobin is exposed to an O_2 tension of approximately 100 mm Hg, and the reversible, chemical combination between O_2 and hemoglobin occurs. When the hemoglobin reaches the systemic capillaries, the low O_2 tension in the tissues causes O_2 to diffuse from the blood into the tissues.

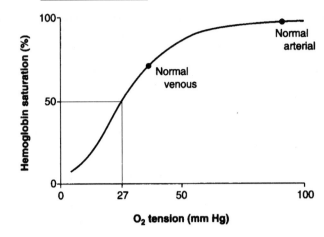

FIGURE 17-5. Arterial hemoglobin saturation. The normal arterial O_2 tension is about 95 mm Hg, which produces a hemoglobin saturation of approximately 98%. After O_2 is released to the tissues, the average venous O_2 tension is 40 mm Hg, which is equivalent to a hemoglobin saturation of 75%. The normal P_{50} (i.e., the O_2 tension that produces a 50% saturation of hemoglobin with O_2) is shown.

rial **hemoglobin saturation,** even though the arterial O_2 tension decreases substantially under these conditions.

- **d.** The **unloading (dissociation) zone** of the hemoglobin saturation curve is the **steep portion** of the curve that occurs at O_2 tensions below 60 mm Hg (see Figure 17-4).
  - **(1)** The unloading zone allows **hemoglobin to release large amounts of O_2 in response to relatively small changes in O_2 tension.** This property keeps the O_2 tension in the capillary blood relatively high so that the diffusion gradient for O_2 is maintained.
  - **(2)** O_2 **tension in the tissues** is very low (metabolism consumes O_2), causing O_2 to diffuse from blood to tissue.
- **e.** **Mixed venous hemoglobin saturation** represents the O_2 level in the pulmonary venous blood. The **mixed venous O_2 tension is about 40 mm Hg,** which is equivalent to a hemoglobin saturation of **75%** (see Figure 17-5). This represents the average value for the entire body. The O_2 tension in the venous blood varies from organ to organ as a function of the ratio of blood flow to O_2 consumption in each tissue.

2. Hemoglobin affinity for O_2 is **inversely related** to the **P_{50},** which is the O_2 tension that produces a 50% saturation of hemoglobin with O_2.
- **a.** The normal **P_{50}** for arterial blood is **27 mm Hg** (Figure 17-6; see Figure 17-5). Hemoglobin is an allosteric enzyme that reacts with O_2, and the affinity between hemoglobin and O_2 can be altered by various ligands.

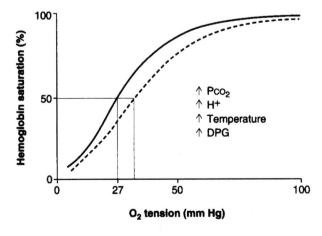

↑ P_{CO_2}
↑ H^+
↑ Temperature
↑ DPG

FIGURE 17-6. Results of increasing the P_{CO_2}, H^+ concentration, temperature, or diphosphoglycerate (DPG) concentration on P_{50} of hemoglobin (*dashed line*). The increased P_{50} indicates a reduced affinity of hemoglobin for O_2. This means that O_2 is released more readily, which raises the tissue O_2 tension. Decreases in these parameters cause the opposite effects.

b. Physiologic alterations in P_{50} (see Figure 17-6) are produced by changes in temperature and the concentration of CO_2, H^+, and other ligands [e.g., diphosphoglycerate (DPG), adenosine triphosphate (ATP), adenosine diphosphate (ADP), and other organic phosphates].

c. The **Bohr effect** refers to the change in P_{50} that is caused by an increase in PCO_2.

d.Decreased P_{50} (i.e., **increased hemoglobin affinity**) means that O_2 combines more readily with hemoglobin. A decreased P_{50} is an obvious benefit in the lungs because it enhances the hemoglobin saturation with O_2.

e. Increased P_{50} (i.e., **decreased hemoglobin affinity**) causes hemoglobin to release O_2 more readily at the tissue level. The increase in the P_{50} maintains the O_2 tension of the blood, which improves the diffusion gradient of O_2 from the blood to the tissues.

3. The **O_2 capacity** is the maximal amount of O_2 that can be carried in the blood by hemoglobin.

a. The O_2 capacity equals the hemoglobin concentration (in g/dl of blood) multiplied by 1.34 ml O_2/g (Table 17-2). Only the **functional hemoglobin concentration** is used to calculate the O_2 capacity.

b. The normal hemoglobin concentration is 12–15 g hemoglobin/dl blood, so that the **normal O_2 capacity** is **20.1 ml/dl** (or 20.1 vol%).

4. The **O_2 content** is the total volume of O_2 that is carried in the blood. Normally, the arterial blood carries approximately 20 ml O_2/dl, and hemoglobin carries about 98.5% of this O_2. The remaining 1.5% is dissolved in the plasma.

a. The amount of dissolved O_2 depends only on the O_2 tension in the blood. The **hemoglobin O_2** varies with the hemoglobin concentration, the O_2 tension, and the P_{50} of the hemoglobin (Figure 17-7; see Figure 17-6).

b. The **normal mixed venous O_2 content C$\bar{v}o_2$)** is approximately **15 vol%** at a tension of 40 mm Hg.

(1) Mixed venous blood represents the **weighted average of blood flow and O_2 consumption throughout the body.**

(2) The **venous O_2 content** from different organs varies widely. For example, the heart usually has a low venous O_2 content, but the kidney, which receives approximately 25% of the cardiac output, has a high venous O_2 content.

B. | **Factors that alter functional hemoglobin**

1. Carboxyhemoglobin, which is formed when CO combines with hemoglobin, imparts a typical **cherry-red color** to the skin and mucous membranes. CO binds to the same site on the hemoglobin molecule as O_2 but has about 200 times the affinity for hemoglobin than O_2.

a. Effects of CO

(1) CO decreases the functional hemoglobin concentration. Essentially, **CO poisoning** is a form of **acute-onset anemia** but it also causes a significant decrease in the P_{50} (see Figure 17-7). Because of the extreme affinity of CO for hemoglobin, a CO tension **(PCO) of only 0.5 mm Hg inactivates 50% of the hemoglobin** (Figure 17-8).

TABLE 17-2. Key Equations

O_2 capacity (ml/dl) = [Hb] · 1.34

O_2 content (ml/dl) = HbO_2 + dissolved O_2

$$\text{Hb saturation (\%)*} = \frac{O_2 \text{ content} - \text{dissolved } O_2}{O_2 \text{ capacity}} \cdot 100$$

Hb = hemoglobin; [Hb] = hemoglobin concentration; HbO_2 = oxyhemoglobin.

*The P_{50} is the O_2 tension that produces 50% Hb saturation with O_2.

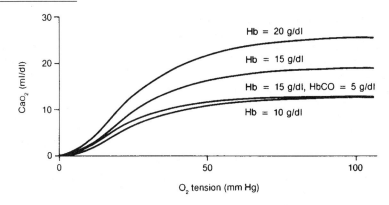

FIGURE 17-7. O_2 content of arterial blood (CaO_2) as a function of O_2 tension and hemoglobin (Hb) concentration. The arterial O_2 content varies according to the O_2 tension and the P_{50}, which have different values throughout the body. Note that carbon monoxide (HbCO) not only reduces O_2 content, it also reduces the P_{50}.

  (2) CO lowers the tissue O_2 tension by decreasing the O_2 content and the P_{50} for O_2. The shift in the P_{50} moves the hemoglobin dissociation curve to the left, which lowers the tissue O_2 tension even further (see Figure 17-7).

 b. Treatment of CO poisoning. Dissociation of CO from hemoglobin occurs slowly at normal O_2 tensions, requiring 8–12 hours. **Administration of 100% O_2** speeds the dissociation of CO from hemoglobin. In addition, about 1.5 vol% of O_2 are dissolved in the plasma at high O_2 tension, which significantly increases the O_2 delivery to the body (see III C).

2. Methemoglobin is formed when **hemoglobin iron** is oxidized from the **ferrous (Fe^{2+})** to the **ferric (Fe^{3+}) state.** Methemoglobin is incapable of carrying O_2 and has a bluish color that can impart a cyanotic hue to tissues.

 a. Hemoglobin is continuously oxidized to methemoglobin at a slow rate within the RBC. Many drugs and foods (e.g., nitrites, phenacetin, fava beans) can produce an increased oxidation of hemoglobin iron, especially in people who have a genetic deficiency of glucose-6-phosphate dehydrogenase.

 b. Methemoglobin is converted back to functional hemoglobin by reducing compounds that are produced in the RBC by metabolic reactions.

3. Abnormal hemoglobin molecules occur as genetic variants and have either **abnormal physical characteristics** (as in sickle cell anemia) or **abnormal affinities for O_2.**

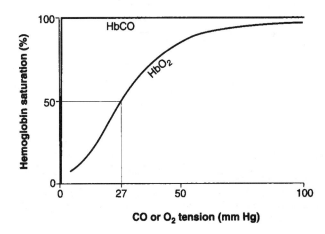

FIGURE 17-8. Hemoglobin saturation curves for both O_2 (HbO_2) and CO (HbCO). Note that the carboxyhemoglobin curve lies along the y-axis, which indicates extremely high affinity of hemoglobin for CO. The P_{50} for CO is about 0.5 mm Hg.

a. **Sickle cell hemoglobin (hemoglobin S)** becomes very insoluble in the deoxygenated state, causing the molecules to precipitate in the RBCs.

b. These hemoglobin S crystals give the sickled RBCs their characteristic, bizarre shape. The sickle cells are rigid and exhibit a higher viscosity to flow, causing them to lodge in capillaries. The absent or reduced blood flow results in ischemic damage to many different organ systems in affected individuals.

C. **O_2 delivery** represents the amount **of O_2 that is presented to body cells per minute** and is equal to the arterial O_2 content multiplied by the cardiac output. For the entire body, the normal arterial O_2 content is 195 ml/L, and the cardiac output is 5–5.5 L/min. Thus, the **normal O_2 delivery to the entire body** is about **1 L/min.**

1. **Decreased arterial O_2 content** may lead to inadequate O_2 delivery and tissue hypoxia (see Chapter 20 II C 1,3). The body effectively compensates for decreases in arterial O_2 content by increasing cardiac output.

2. **Decreased cardiac output** occurs secondary to many cardiac diseases. **Compensatory mechanisms** include **increased RBC production,** which is not an effective compensatory mechanism because the higher hematocrit increases blood viscosity and the ventricular afterload. These effects tend to reduce the cardiac output further.

IV. **CO_2 TRANSPORT.** CO_2 is the usual end-product of oxidative metabolism. CO_2 diffuses out of the cells and into the capillary blood, raising the CO_2 tension of the capillary and venous blood to levels 5–6 mm Hg higher than the arterial P_{CO_2}. CO_2 is transported in the blood in **several different forms.**

A. **Physically dissolved CO_2** accounts for approximately 5% of the total CO_2 in the blood.

B. **Carbaminohemoglobin** refers to CO_2 that combines with terminal amino (NH_3) groups on blood proteins, especially hemoglobin. Approximately 5% of the CO_2 is carried as carbamino compounds.

C. **Bicarbonate (HCO_3^-).** Approximately 90% of the CO_2 enters the RBC, where in the presence of **carbonic anhydrase,** it rapidly reacts with water to form **carbonic acid** (Figure 17-9).

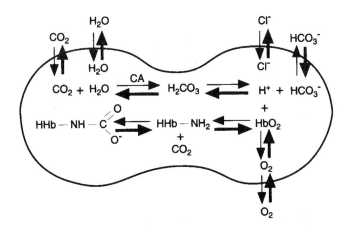

FIGURE 17-9. The chloride shift in a red blood cell (RBC). CO_2 tension increases in the blood as it passes through the systemic capillaries (*thin arrows*), causing CO_2 to diffuse into the RBC where it is quickly hydrated by carbonic anhydrase (CA). The hydrogen ion (H^+), derived from the dissociation of carbonic acid (H_2CO_3), is buffered by hemoglobin (HHb). CO_2 also combines with the amino terminal (NH_2) of hemoglobin, giving rise to carbaminohemoglobin (HHb–$NHCOO^-$). Bicarbonate (HCO_3^-) diffuses out of the RBC and is replaced by chloride (Cl^-). In the pulmonary capillaries, these reactions are reversed (*thick arrows*).

1. **Plasma HCO₃⁻.** The carbonic acid dissociates into HCO_3^- and hydrogen (H^+) ions. The HCO_3^- diffuses into the plasma, and the H^+ is buffered by the deoxygenated hemoglobin, which is a weaker acid than oxyhemoglobin. Although HCO_3^- is formed within the RBCs, most of the CO_2 is carried in the plasma as HCO_3^-.

2. **Chloride shift.** After the HCO_3^- is formed in RBCs, it diffuses out of the cells (see Figure 17-9). Because the RBC membrane is relatively impermeable to cations, as HCO_3^- diffuses out of the cell, the chloride ion (Cl^-) diffuses from the plasma into the red cell to replace the HCO_3^-.

D. The **Haldane effect** refers to the ability of deoxygenated blood to carry more CO_2 than oxygenated hemoglobin (Figure 17-10). The Haldane effect is a way of buffering the CO_2 molecule, which has the potential to form carbonic acid after being hydrated.

Case

A 55-year-old man who has smoked two packs of cigarettes a day for 40 years has had a chronic cough for many years that is productive of yellowish sputum. Laboratory tests reveal: arterial PO_2, 55 mm Hg; PCO_2, 48 mm Hg; and hemoglobin concentration, 18 g/dl. The transdermal hemoglobin saturation averages 85% during an examination.

1. *What is the O_2 capacity, and what does it indicate?*

DISCUSSION

The O_2 capacity is calculated from the hemoglobin concentration: O_2 capacity (ml/dl) = [Hgb] · 1.34 = 18 g/dl · 1.34 = 24.12 ml/dl (see Table 17-2). This value represents the maximal amount of O_2 carried by hemoglobin in this patient (i.e., when hemoglobin is 100% saturated).

2. *What is the O_2 content, and is this value more or less than normal?*

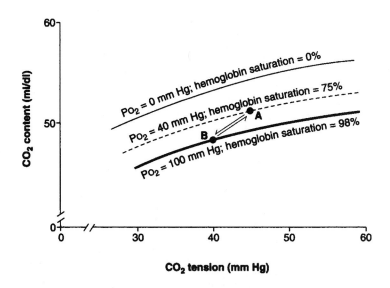

FIGURE 17-10. CO_2 dissociation curves, which demonstrate the role of the Haldane effect in the transport of CO_2. Note that the CO_2 content of blood varies depending on the hemoglobin saturation with O_2. Points A and B represent the normal CO_2 tension in the tissues and arteries, respectively. PO_2 = oxygen tension.

DISCUSSION

O_2 content (ml/dl) = O_2 capacity · % saturation (neglecting the amount of dissolved O_2) = 24.12 · 0.85 = 20.5 ml/dl. This value represents the actual amount of O_2 combined with hemoglobin. In this patient, the O_2 content is actually greater than normal, although he is still suffering from arterial hypoxia, whose definition is based on O_2 tension, not content. The decreased O_2 tension is detrimental to O_2 delivery, because the diffusion gradient between the blood and the tissues is reduced.

3. *What is the alveolar–arterial gradient, and what is its significance?*

DISCUSSION

The alveolar–arterial gradient is the difference in O_2 tension between the alveolar gas and the arterial blood. This gradient is increased, indicating the presence of lung disease. This patient's condition is typical of an individual with chronic obstructive lung disease secondary to cigarette smoking.

Chapter 18

Ventilation, Perfusion, and Gas Exchange

I. **INTRODUCTION.** Alveolar ventilation and pulmonary blood flow (perfusion) are not evenly distributed throughout the lungs. This uneven distribution affects alveolar and pulmonary capillary gas tensions, which alter the rate of diffusion and gas exchange of oxygen (O_2) and carbon dioxide (CO_2).

II. **DISTRIBUTION OF PULMONARY BLOOD FLOW.** Pulmonary blood flow varies throughout the lungs because of the relatively low vascular pressures, the distensibility of the vasculature, and the hydrostatic effects of gravity.

A. **Pulmonary blood flow.** The entire blood flow from the right ventricle is distributed to the pulmonary blood vessels. Because right- and left-sided output are necessarily equal, the pulmonary blood flow **equals the cardiac output (approximately 5 L/min at rest).**

B. **Pulmonary blood pressure**

1. **Pulmonary artery pressure** is much **lower than the pressure in the aorta, because the resistance to blood flow in the pulmonary circulation is about one tenth of that in the systemic circulation.** In the pulmonary artery, the normal systolic and diastolic pressures are approximately 20 mm Hg and 10 mm Hg, respectively.

2. **Hydrostatic pressure** (P_h) is caused by the weight of a column of fluid that is exposed to gravity [see Chapter 9 III A 2 b (1)].
   a. **The hydrostatic pressure adds to or subtracts from the potential energy (pressure) at levels below or above the zero reference plane, respectively.** The zero reference plane is at the level of the right atrium, which is approximately at the middle of the lungs.
   b. **Example.** Assume that the lungs are 40 cm from base to apex, the zero reference level is in the middle of the lungs, the mean pulmonary artery pressure is 20 cm H_2O, and the blood density is 1 g/cm³.
      (1) Under these conditions, the blood pressure is sufficient to lift the column of blood to a height of 20 cm above the right atrium, which is just to the apex of the lung.
      (2) If the pulmonary artery pressure decreases to 16 cm H_2O, then the top 4 cm of the lung is not perfused, because the pressure is inadequate to raise the column of blood to that height.
      (3) In the supine or prone positions, the lung is less affected by gravity; therefore, hydrostatic effects are minimized.

3. **Perfusion zones of the lung** depend on the relationships between alveolar, pulmonary artery, and pulmonary venous pressures (Figure 18-1).
   a. **Zone 1** is any region of the lung that does not receive blood flow. This occurs if the regional pulmonary artery pressure is less than the alveolar pressure **(Pa < PA).** Under these conditions, the pulmonary capillaries are collapsed (see Figure 18-1). Zone 1, which can be altered by the factors described in Table 18-1, **does not exist in normal lungs.**
   b. **Zone 2** occurs where the pulmonary artery pressure exceeds the alveolar pressure, which exceeds the pulmonary venous pressure **(Pa > PA > Pv).**
      (1) In this region, the driving force for blood flow is the arterial–alveolar pressure gradient, not the arteriovenous gradient. This condition is known as the **waterfall ef-**

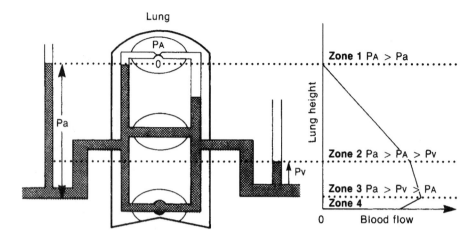

FIGURE 18-1. The effect of hydrostatic pressure and level on the distribution of pulmonary blood flow in a vertical lung. Pulmonary blood flow depends on the relationship between pulmonary artery pressure (Pa), alveolar pressure (PA), and pulmonary venous pressure (Pv). (Adapted from West JB, et al: Distribution of blood flow in the isolated lung: relation to vascular and alveolar pressure. *J Appl Physiol* 19:713, 1964.)

        fect, because changes in the downstream pressure, or the venous pressure, do not alter blood flow.*

    (2) The **driving force for blood flow increases** down zone 2, because the effective pulmonary artery pressure increases 1 cm H_2O for each centimeter descent from the apex of the lung. The alveolar pressure remains constant, however, and thus flow increases linearly from the top to the bottom of zone 2 (see Figure 18-1).

  c. **Zone 3** occurs when the pulmonary artery pressure exceeds the pulmonary venous pressure, which exceeds the alveolar pressure **(Pa > Pv > PA).** This condition occurs near the bottom of the lungs. The increased hydrostatic pressure in this zone causes distention and recruitment of both arteries and veins. Both distention and recruitment of blood vessels decrease the resistance to blood flow (Figure 18-2) so that blood flow increases down zone 3.

  d. **Zone 4** represents a zone of reduced blood flow and is an abnormal condition (see

TABLE 18-1. Conditions That Alter Perfusion Zone 1

Factors That Expand Zone 1	Factors That Reduce Zone 1
Decreased pulmonary artery pressure (e.g., circulatory shock, high "G" forces)	Increased pulmonary artery pressure (e.g., fluid or blood infusion, elevation of legs)
Increased alveolar pressure (e.g., positive end-expiratory pressure)	Reduced hydrostatic effect (e.g., placement in supine position)
Occlusion of blood vessels (e.g., pulmonary embolism)	

*The pulmonary artery pressure is the upstream height of the stream, the alveolar pressure represents the top of the waterfall, and the venous pressure is the bottom of the waterfall. The flow rate depends on the difference in elevation (pressure) between the upstream site and the top of the waterfall. Changes in venous pressure alter the height of the waterfall but do not influence the overall flow rate through the system until the venous pressure exceeds the alveolar pressure; at this point, the flow conditions represent zone 3.

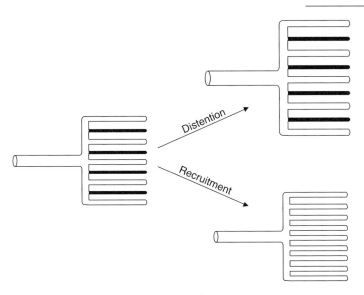

FIGURE 18-2. Schematic diagram depicting the difference between distention and recruitment in the pulmonary vasculature. Both mechanisms reduce the pulmonary vascular resistance and increase blood flow in the affected areas. Distention and recruitment occur in the dependent portions of the lungs where there is an increase in the hydrostatic pressure.

Figure 18-1). Zone 4 is present when pulmonary venous pressure is abnormally high (e.g., as a result of left ventricular failure or mitral stenosis) or when pulmonary edema produces fluid accumulation around the blood vessels. This edema, termed **vascular cuffing,** increases vascular resistance and reduces local blood flow.

C. **Factors that alter pulmonary blood flow**

1. **Alveolar hypoxia** (i.e., low alveolar O_2 tension) produces **hypoxic pulmonary vasoconstriction (HPV),** a local response that occurs only in hypoxic areas and is potentiated by hypercapnia and acidosis.
   a. **Function.** HPV is an important mechanism for **balancing blood flow and ventilation.** It results in increased pulmonary vascular resistance in hypoxic areas of the lung.
      (1) The increased resistance reduces blood flow to the hypoxic area and shifts blood flow to better ventilated pulmonary regions that have a higher alveolar O_2 tension. Thus, HPV tends to match the amount of pulmonary blood flow to the alveolar ventilation. This matching is not perfect, however (see IV A 1).
      (2) HPV is thought to result from decreased formation and release of nitric oxide (NO) by the pulmonary vascular endothelium in hypoxic areas. NO is a potent vasodilator, so vasoconstriction occurs in its absence. Recall that hypoxia, hypercapnia, and acidosis produce vasodilation in the systemic circulation rather than vasoconstriction, as in the pulmonary circulation.
   b. **Generalized alveolar hypoxia** occurs throughout the lung during hypoventilation or low inspired P_{O_2} (e.g., exposure to altitudes > 5000–7000 feet). Under these conditions, HPV increases the total pulmonary vascular resistance, which leads to **pulmonary hypertension.** Pulmonary hypertension increases the work of the right ventricle, resulting in right ventricular hypertrophy, right axis deviation (RAD), and, eventually, right ventricular failure.

2. **Changes in lung volume** markedly alter the pulmonary vascular resistance.
   a. **Pulmonary vascular resistance is minimal when the lung volume is close to functional residual capacity (FRC) and increases at both higher and lower lung volumes** (Figure 18-3A).

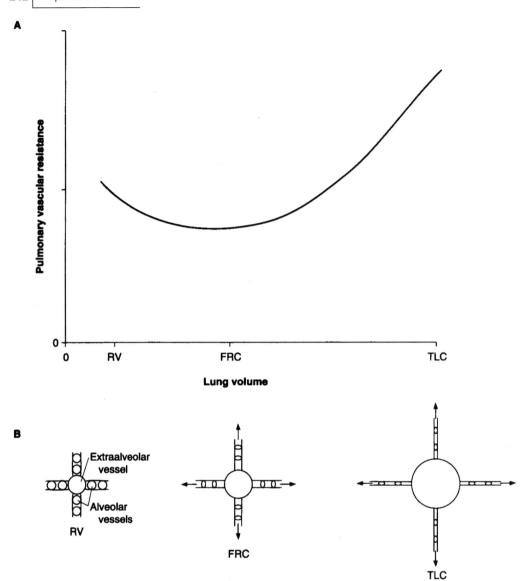

FIGURE 18-3. (*A*) The relationship between vascular resistance and lung volume, which shows a minimal value near the normal working lung volume, the functional residual capacity (FRC). (*B*) The effects of changes in lung volume on the alveolar vessels (i.e., the septal capillaries) and the extra-alveolar vessels. When volume increases, radial traction (as indicated by the *arrows*) puts tension on the septa, which, in turn, dilates the extra-alveolar vessels. The dilation decreases the flow resistance in these vessels. However, when the septa are stretched, the alveolar vessels (i.e., the septal capillaries) are compressed, which increases capillary flow resistance at high lung volumes. RV = residual volume; TLC = total lung capacity.

      b. The effect of lung volume on pulmonary vascular resistance is complex, because two different categories of blood vessels are involved.

          (1) The **extra-alveolar vessels** are the **larger distributing arteries and veins** in the lungs.

              (a) These vessels are dilated at high lung volumes because of the radial traction exerted on their walls by the alveolar septa (Figure 18-3B).

              (b) The increased diameter reduces the flow resistance in these vessels.

    (2) The **alveolar vessels, usually pulmonary capillaries,** are located in the alveolar septa and are compressed by the enlarged alveoli at high lung volumes (see Figure 18-3B). During inspiration, the capillary vascular resistance increases while the larger vessels dilate, increasing their contained blood volume.

3. Pulmonary diseases (e.g., emphysema, pulmonary emboli) that obstruct or destroy pulmonary vessels can further **alter the pattern of blood flow,** resulting in a more uneven distribution of blood flow.

III. **DISTRIBUTION OF VENTILATION.** Alveolar ventilation, like pulmonary blood flow, is not evenly distributed throughout the lungs. The distribution of alveolar ventilation is **dependent on the interpleural pressure (PPL) gradient, the time constant of the lung, and closure of the airways.**

A. The **interpleural pressure gradient** is caused by the effects of gravity on the lung within the intact thorax.

    1. The **cause of the interpleural pressure gradient** is incompletely understood, but it is believed that the lung behaves as if it were a low-density fluid (because of its gas content) when it is exposed to gravity.

      a. The **density of the normal lung** is about 0.25–0.30 g/cm³, which produces a hydrostatic pressure difference of 7.5–10 cm H_2O between the apex and the base of a vertical lung.

      b. The **interpleural pressure** in a standing adult increases from about -10 cm H_2O at the apex of the lung to about -2 cm H_2O at the base (Figure 18-4A).

    2. Effects

      a. The **regional lung volume** varies with changes in interpleural pressure because changes in interpleural pressure alter the transpulmonary pressure, or PL (the other determinant is alveolar pressure) [PL = PA − PPL].

        (1) Because the alveolar pressure is zero throughout the lung under static conditions, the transpulmonary pressure varies from 2 cm H_2O at the base to 10 cm H_2O at the apex of the vertical lung (see Figure 18-4A).

        (2) The difference in transpulmonary pressure and lung volume causes **the apex and the base to function at very different points on the lung compliance curve** (Figure 18-4B).

      b. The **tidal volume** (VT) is unevenly distributed in the vertical lung because of the variation in compliance in different sections of the lung.

        (1) In a vertical lung, most of the tidal volume goes to the base of the lung when inspiration starts at FRC (Figure 18-4C).

        (2) There is a linear reduction in regional tidal volume from base to apex under these conditions (Figure 18-5). The tidal volume is much more evenly distributed in supine individuals, because the hydrostatic effect on interpleural pressure is reduced.

B. The **time constant of the lung** is the **product of airway resistance (R)** and **lung compliance (C).**

    1. Function. The time constant establishes the rate of acinar volume change.

      a. The **acinus** is the functional unit of the lung; it consists of a respiratory bronchiole and all of the alveolar ducts and alveoli distal to it. The acinus **fills and empties exponentially.**

      b. For each time constant, the volume changes 63% toward the equilibrium value (Figure 18-6A).

      c. In the healthy lung, all acini have essentially equal time constants.

    2. In the diseased lung, some areas have low compliance, and other areas have high airway resistance, which can cause markedly unequal time constants. This results in a wide variation in regional alveolar ventilation, which produces large differences in the regional alveolar O_2 tension. This can markedly interfere with gas exchange in the diseased lung.

A. Transpulmonary pressure

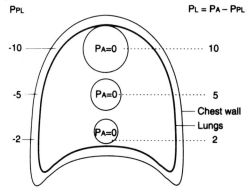

B. End-expiratory phase

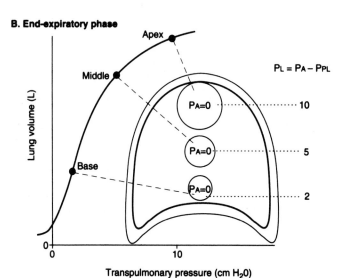

C. End-inspiratory phase

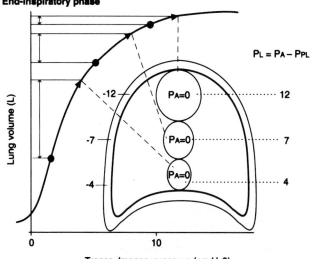

FIGURE 18-4. (*A*) Diagram showing a gradient of about 8 cm H_2O in the interpleural pressure (PPL) between the apex and the base of the vertical lung. This gradient causes the regional transpulmonary pressure (PL) to vary from 2–10 cm H_2O between the base and the apex of the lung, respectively. This change in transmural pressure causes a marked difference in the extent of inflation between the base and apex of the lung. (*B*) End-expiratory phase. The correlation between the PL and the extent of lung inflation is shown. The PL for the base and the apex of the lung place these regions on much different regions of the pressure–volume curve. The base of the lung is poorly inflated but located on a high-compliance segment of the pressure–volume diagram. The apex is almost maximally inflated and located on a low-compliance segment. (*C*) End-inspiratory phase. The *points* on the pressure–volume curve indicate the pressure–volume coordinates at end-expiration, and the *arrowheads* indicate the pressure–volume coordinates at end-inspiration. The *thin arrows* along the y-axis show the volume change in the three regions that occurs with inspiration. Most of the tidal volume goes to the base of the lung because it is very distensible; conversely, very little of it reaches the apex because of its low compliance. PA = alveolar pressure.

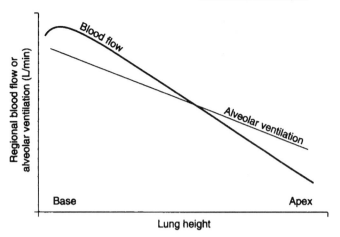

FIGURE 18-5. The distribution of pulmonary blood flow and alveolar ventilation in different regions of the vertical lung. Note that blood flow (perfusion) exceeds ventilation at the base, but ventilation exceeds blood flow at the apex. Because of these relationships, the ventilation–perfusion ratio ($\dot{V}A/\dot{Q}C$) is less than 1 at the base of the lungs and greater than 1 at the apex.

a. **In obstructive lung disease, the time constant is increased** as a result of the high airway resistance. This leads to a **slower rate of acinar filling and emptying** (Figure 18-6B).

   (1) **Dynamic lung compliance (CL_{dyn})** is the ratio of the tidal volume to the change in interpleural pressure that occurs during the respiratory cycle.

      (a) In obstructive lung disease, the CL_{dyn} is reduced compared with the static lung compliance. The low CL_{dyn} occurs because the lung has not fully inflated as a result of the prolonged time constant.

      (b) **Frequency-dependent compliance** occurs when dynamic lung compliance decreases as respiratory rate increases. In the presence of lung acini with increased time constants, the extent of lung filling varies as a function of inspiratory time (see Figure 18-6B). Patients with frequency-dependent compliance

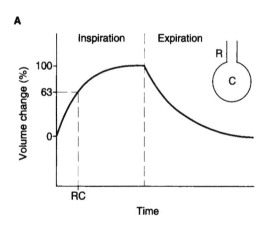

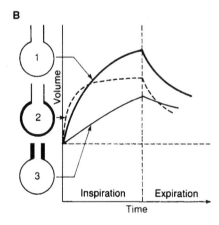

FIGURE 18-6. (A) The acinus can be modeled by a balloon and a tube; the balloon provides compliance (C), and the tube provides airway resistance (R). In such a unit, the volume change occurs exponentially and the rate of filling is determined by the time constant (R · C). The time constant RC is defined as the time required for the unit to reach 63% of its maximal volume. (B) Models of acini showing the effects of (1) normal compliance and resistance, (2) decreased compliance, and (3) increased resistance on the time course of filling. A decreased compliance results in rapid filling but a reduction in volume change. When airway resistance is increased, the acini fill slowly, and the volume change depends on the duration of inspiration as well as the compliance.

can reduce respiratory work by breathing more slowly. The longer respiratory cycle provides additional time for pulmonary inflation and deflation to occur.

(2) Intrinsic positive end-expiratory pressure (PEEP). Patients with high airway resistance frequently do not deflate their lungs to FRC at the end of expiration, and the additional lung volume keeps the alveolar pressure from reaching zero. Thus, these patients function with an alveolar pressure that remains positive at end-expiration. This added pressure enhances the gradient for expiratory air flow [see Chapter 20 IV A 2 a].

  b. Restrictive diseases reduce the time constant because of the decreased compliance. This results in areas of the lung that change volume rapidly but undergo smaller volume changes than normal (see Figure 18-6B). This decreased alveolar ventilation reduces regional alveolar PO_2 and leads to abnormal gas exchange.

C. **Airway closure** alters regional alveolar ventilation and increases the work of breathing, because high pressures must be developed to reopen the closed airways. **Early airway closure** occurs when airways close prematurely (i.e., at a higher volume than predicted for a person's age and sex).

  1. Cause. Airway closure occurs when the regional transpulmonary pressure is reduced to a critical level.

    a. Any process that narrows the airway lumen leads to early airway closure and maldistribution of alveolar ventilation.

    b. Inflammation, excess mucus production, contraction of bronchial smooth muscle, or **loss of radial traction on the airways** are common causes of early airway closure.

  2. Detection of airway closure. The **single-breath nitrogen (N_2) test** can be used to detect airway closure.

    a. Method. In this test, an individual expires to residual volume (RV), inspires 100% O_2 to total lung capacity (TLC), and, finally, expires slowly and steadily to RV. The N_2 tension in the expired gas is measured during the second expiration.

      (1) At RV, the base of the lungs is almost completely deflated, but the apex is moderately inflated with gas containing 80% N_2.

      (2) After inspiring 100% O_2 to TLC, the base contains almost no N_2, and the apex contains significant amounts of N_2.

      (3) During the subsequent expiration, when basal airways begin to close, only gas from the more apical regions continues to be expired, which has a higher N_2 tension. This generates the inflection that causes phase 4 of the N_2 trace (Figure 18-7).

    b. Terminology

      (1) The **closing volume** is the portion of the vital capacity that remains in the lungs when airway closure begins.

      (2) The **closing capacity** is the closing volume plus the RV.

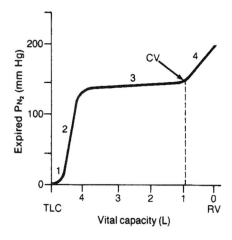

FIGURE 18-7. Record of a single-breath N_2 test. The tracing shows the expired N_2 tension (PN_2) following an inspiratory vital capacity of 100% O_2. The numbers indicate the different phases of the record. Phase 1 is pure dead space gas, phase 2 is a mixture of dead space and alveolar gas, phase 3 (alveolar plateau) represents pure alveolar gas, and phase 4 indicates the onset of airway closure [closing volume (CV)]. TLC = total lung capacity; RV = residual volume.

IV. **THE VENTILATION–PERFUSION RATIO ($\dot{V}A/\dot{Q}C$)** is the ratio of the alveolar ventilation to the pulmonary blood flow. The $\dot{V}A/\dot{Q}C$ at the acinar level determines the regional alveolar O_2 and CO_2 tensions, and therefore, is critical in determining the gas exchange in each acinus of the lung (Figure 18-8). Ventilation–perfusion imbalances may result from any pulmonary or cardiovascular disease that alters the normal regional distribution of ventilation or perfusion (see Figure 18-5). Such imbalances are by far the most common cause of arterial hypoxia.

A. Variations in the ventilation–perfusion ratio

1. **Normal $\dot{V}A/\dot{Q}C$.** The most efficient gas exchange occurs when the $\dot{V}A/\dot{Q}C$ is **approximately 1.** Normally **alveolar ventilation is 4.5–5.0 L/min,** and the **cardiac output** is approximately **5 L/min,** so that overall, the $\dot{V}A/\dot{Q}C$ is about 0.9.
   a. **When the $\dot{V}A/\dot{Q}C$ is 0.9–1.0,** the alveolar O_2 tension is about 100 mm Hg and the alveolar CO_2 tension is about 40 mm Hg (Figure 18-9). These gas tensions would equilibrate with the pulmonary capillary blood.
   b. **Normally, the $\dot{V}A/\dot{Q}C$ varies from about 0.6 at the base to about 3 at the apex** of the lung. This relatively narrow range impairs gas exchange only slightly, but in the presence of pulmonary disease, the $\dot{V}A/\dot{Q}C$ can vary from zero to infinity.

2. **A low $\dot{V}A/\dot{Q}C$ is caused either by inadequate ventilation or excessive blood flow** to an area of the lung. Either condition causes the **alveolar O_2 tension to decrease.**
   a. **A physiologic shunt** is present when the $\dot{V}A/\dot{Q}C$ is **greater than zero but less than one.** Under these conditions, there is a low alveolar O_2 tension, which causes a low PO_2 and hemoglobin saturation in the blood leaving this area of the lungs. When this blood mixes with blood from better ventilated areas, it produces a decrease in the overall arterial O_2 tension and content.
   b. An **anatomic shunt** occurs when the $\dot{V}A/\dot{Q}C$ **equals zero** (see Figure 18-9).
      (1) When an area of the lungs receives no ventilation ($\dot{V}A/\dot{Q}C = 0$), the alveolar O_2 tension rapidly decreases until it equals the O_2 tension in the mixed venous blood. Therefore, no further gas exchange occurs. The presence of an anatomic shunt means that true venous blood is mixing with oxygenated blood.
      (2) An anatomic shunt may be **intra-** or **extrapulmonary.** An extrapulmonary anatomic shunt may result from **congenital cardiac malformations** (e.g., atrial or ventricular septal defect with right-to-left blood flow).
   c. **Measurement of shunted blood**
      (1) The **shunt equation** can be used to measure the fraction of shunted blood.

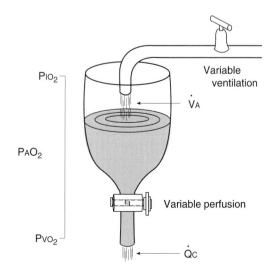

FIGURE 18-8. The ratio of alveolar ventilation ($\dot{V}A$) to capillary perfusion ($\dot{Q}C$) determines the local O_2 tension in the lungs (PAO_2). Increasing the alveolar ventilation raises the alveolar O_2 tension, which adds more O_2 to each unit of blood. Eventually, the alveolar O_2 tension stabilizes at a higher level when outflow of O_2 equals inflow. Increasing the blood flow lowers the alveolar O_2 tension, because more O_2 is removed. Eventually, the O_2 tension stabilizes at a new lower value. The alveolar O_2 tension is limited on the low end by the mixed venous blood (PVO_2) and on the high end by the inspired O_2 tension (PIO_2).

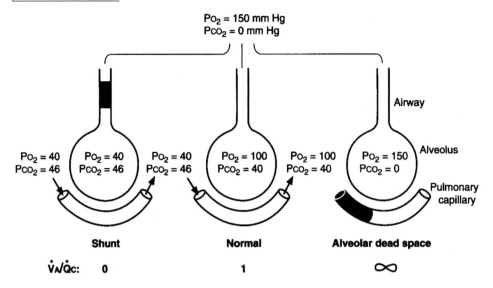

FIGURE 18-9. The three-compartment model of gas exchange. The three lung units, comprised of a pulmonary capillary and an alveolus, all receive the same inspired gas and mixed venous blood gas concentrations. The *blackened areas* indicate blockage sites. The unit on the *left,* an anatomic shunt unit, receives no ventilation. Therefore, its ventilation–perfusion ratio ($\dot{V}A/\dot{Q}C$) equals zero. No gas exchange takes place; the blood leaving the unit has the same mixed venous concentration as that entering. The unit on the *right,* which represents alveolar dead space, receives no blood flow. Therefore, its $\dot{V}A/\dot{Q}C$ is infinity. Again, there is no gas exchange and the alveolar gas has the same composition as the inspired gas. The unit in the *center* receives ventilation and blood flow in equal proportions, so the alveolar gas and pulmonary venous blood have normal gas concentrations. Areas of the lung with values of $\dot{V}A/\dot{Q}C$ less than one but greater than zero have gas concentrations between the normal and the shunt units. Lung regions with high values of $\dot{V}A/\dot{Q}C$ have gas concentrations between the normal and the alveolar dead space units. PCO_2 = carbon dioxide tension; PO_2 = oxygen tension.

$$\dot{Q}s/\dot{Q}t = (CiO_2 - CaO_2)/(CiO_2 - C\bar{v}O_2)$$

where $\dot{Q}s/\dot{Q}T$ = fraction of shunted blood (i.e., the shunt flow divided by the total flow); CiO_2 = ideal O_2 content (present in the pulmonary capillaries), which is dependent on the alveolar O_2 tension); CaO_2 = arterial O_2 content; and $C\bar{v}O_2$ = mixed venous O_2 content.

   (2) **Sample calculation.** A patient is found to be cyanotic, and subsequent studies reveal a hemoglobin concentration of 16 g/dl, an arterial O_2 content of 19 ml/dl, and a venous O_2 content of 14 ml/dl. Assuming that the alveolar O_2 tension is normal and that the pulmonary capillary blood has a normal saturation of 97%, then the $CiO_2 = 16 \cdot 1.34 \cdot 0.97$, or 20.8 ml/dl. Substituting in the equation gives: $\dot{Q}s/\dot{Q}T = (20.8 - 19)(20.8 - 14)$, or 0.26. Thus, 26% of the patient's cardiac output is being shunted.

d. Differentiating between anatomic and physiologic shunts

   (1) **Administration of 100% O_2** to a patient with a significant anatomic shunt does not raise the arterial O_2 tension above 500 mm Hg, because the shunted blood is never exposed to the high alveolar O_2 tension.

   (2) In contrast, when 100% O_2 is administered to a patient with a physiologic shunt (i.e., a ventilation–perfusion imbalance), the arterial O_2 tension exceeds 500 mm Hg. **Normal individuals** have an anatomic shunt consisting of **less than 5% of their cardiac output.**

3. A high $\dot{V}A/\dot{Q}C$ is caused either by **excessive ventilation** or **inadequate blood flow** to an area of the lung.

   a. In areas of the lung where the $\dot{V}A/\dot{Q}C$ exceeds one, the **alveolar and capillary O_2 ten-**

sions are **high** but the **O$_2$ uptake is minimal.** This is true because very little O$_2$ is added to the blood because of the plateau of the O$_2$–hemoglobin dissociation curve (see Figure 17-4).

b. Alveolar dead space

   (1) Alveolar dead space ventilation is the excess ventilation that raises the V̇A/Q̇C and the alveolar O$_2$ tension above normal. It is considered wasted ventilation, because it produces little O$_2$ uptake.

   (2) **If the blood flow to an area of the lung is zero** (i.e., **V̇A/Q̇C equals infinity**), then there is no gas exchange in these alveoli, and all of this ventilation represents alveolar dead space ventilation (see Figure 18-9).

   (3) **Total dead space.** Alveolar dead space ventilation contributes, along with the anatomic dead space, to the total (physiologic) dead space. Unless the minute ventilation is increased, an increase in alveolar dead space results in CO$_2$ retention and hypoxia.

   (4) **In the typical patient with increased alveolar dead space,** the initial hypercapnia stimulates the respiratory centers, increasing the minute ventilation so that the CO$_2$ tension returns to normal, but the hypoxia remains due to the effects of a physiologic shunt.

B. The **O$_2$–CO$_2$ diagram** (Figure 18-10) is **one method of visualizing the effects of ventilation–perfusion alterations on the blood gas tensions.**

1. **The ideal gas point** represents the mean value of the O$_2$ and CO$_2$ tensions for all alveoli.

2. **R is the ratio of the volume of CO$_2$ released per minute** (V̇CO$_2$) to the volume of O$_2$ absorbed per minute (V̇O$_2$). Both gas and blood phases have R lines that intersect at the V̇A/Q̇C line.

3. **Total dead space** is represented on the gas R line as the mixed expired gas point (E). Increasing dead space causes E to move further away from the ideal point (i.e., toward the inspired gas point).

4. **Shunt flow** causes the point representing the arterial blood gas composition to move along the blood R line toward the mixed venous point.

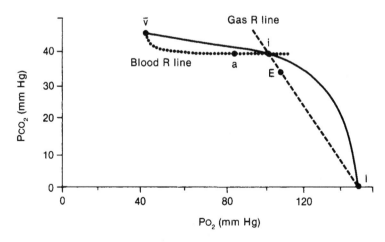

FIGURE 18-10. The O$_2$–CO$_2$ diagram. The solid line, the ventilation–perfusion line, is defined by three points that represent the mixed venous blood composition (*point v̄*), the composition of the ideal pulmonary capillary blood (*point i*), and the inspired gas composition (*point I*). The arterial blood gas composition (*point a*) is determined by the ratio of shunt flow to cardiac output; the mixed-expired gas composition (*point E*) is determined by the ratio of the dead space to the tidal volume. The blood R line (*dotted line*) and the gas R line (*dashed line*) intersect at the ventilation–perfusion line. PCO$_2$ = carbon dioxide tension; PO$_2$ = oxygen tension.

A

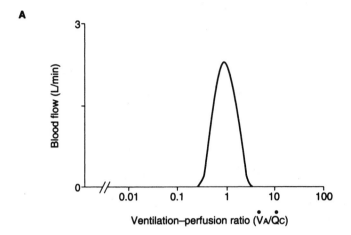

B

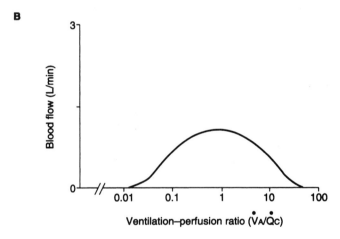

C

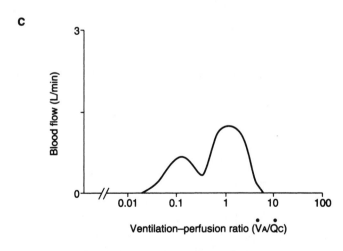

FIGURE 18-11. Various distributions of the ventilation–perfusion ratio ($\dot{V}_A/\dot{Q}_C$). The *ordinate* represents the blood flow for each value of the ratio, and the *abscissa* shows the ratio on a log scale. (*A*) Normal. The mean $\dot{V}_A/\dot{Q}_C$ is 1 and the standard deviation of the population is 0.2, giving a variation of 0.6–3 for the $\dot{V}_A/\dot{Q}_C$. (*B*) An increased standard deviation of the acinar population causes a wider distribution of values, which results in a severe physiologic shunt and alveolar dead space. (*C*) A bimodal distribution, which can be caused by a focal disease, indicates two separate populations of acini. A decrease in the overall mean $\dot{V}_A/\dot{Q}_C$ would produce hypercapnia and hypoxia in the arterial blood.

5. Note that there can be a marked reduction in O_2 tension with only a minimal rise in the CO_2 tension as one proceeds along the blood R line. This is typical of the blood gas values obtained from patients with ventilation–perfusion abnormalities.

C. **Distribution of ventilation–perfusion ratios.** The lungs are comprised of one or more populations of acini with different values of V̇A/Q̇C. In normal lungs, there is only one population of acini represented by a log-normal distribution curve with a range that covers approximately one decade of ventilation–perfusion values (Figure 18-11A). Patients with a ventilation–perfusion imbalance may have either a single mode of distribution with a much wider range of values than normal (Figure 18-11B) or multiple modes of distribution (Figure 18-11C).

1. **Single mode of distribution.** The mean V̇A/Q̇C for any lung is determined by the overall level of alveolar ventilation and the cardiac output.
   a. If all of the acini in the lung had the same V̇A/Q̇C, then there would be no physiologic shunting or alveolar dead space. This condition could be modeled by one acinus that received all of the ventilation and all of the blood flow; however, this is obviously an unrealistic model.
   b. A population of acini with varying values of V̇A/Q̇C (see Figure 18-11A) is a more realistic model. Thus, even in the normal lung, shunts and dead space are present.

2. **Multiple modes of distribution** represent populations of acini with **varying values of** V̇A/Q̇C that are produced by disease processes. Each of these populations may generate a physiologic shunt or alveolar dead space. The further any V̇A/Q̇C is from the ideal value, the more severe the effect on overall gas exchange.

Case

A 28-year-old woman who works as an administrative assistant has a routine chest radiograph that reveals bilateral apical densities. The woman, who does not know whether she has had any previous chest films, is admitted for evaluation.

On examination, she is a well-developed black female in no distress. The history and physical examination are all within normal limits except for cyanosis of the mucous membranes. Pulmonary function tests are within normal limits. Blood gas analysis reveals:

	PaO_2 (mm Hg)	$PaCO_2$ (mm Hg)	Hemoglobin Saturation (%)	Hemoglobin Concentration (g/dl)
Breathing air	62	38	82	16.1
Breathing 100% O_2	98	42	95	

Pulmonary artery angiograms reveal bilateral apical connections between the pulmonary artery and pulmonary veins (pulmonary arteriovenous anastomoses).

1. *What has produced the arterial hypoxia in this patient?*

DISCUSSION

This patient has congenital, bilateral pulmonary arteriovenous anastomoses, which represent a source of an anatomic shunt. Pulmonary artery blood, normally only 75% saturated, is being added to the well-oxygenated pulmonary venous blood through these vascular connections.

2. *What proportion of the cardiac output is shunt flow?*

DISCUSSION

The amount of shunt flow can be calculated using the shunt equation: $\dot{Q}s/\dot{S}_T = (Ci_{O_2} - Ca_{O_2})/Ci_{O_2} - C\bar{v}_{O_2})$. In this patient, $Ci_{O_2} = O_2$ capacity + dissolved $O_2 = 16.1 \cdot 1.34 + 673 \cdot 0.003 = 21.6 + 2.0 = 23.6$ ml O_2/dl. $Ca_{O_2} = O_2$ capacity $= 21.6 \cdot 0.75 = 16.2$. $\dot{Q}s/\dot{S}_T = (23.6 - 20.5)/(23.6 - 16.2) = 3.1/7.4 = 0.42$. In this patient, 42% of the right ventricular output is going through the arteriovenous anastomosis, producing an anatomic shunt of that extent.

3. *Under what circumstances can the P_{CO_2} be low in the setting of a low arterial O_2 tension?*

DISCUSSION

By definition, a physiologic shunt is caused by acini with values for $\dot{V}A/\dot{Q}c$ that are low but greater than zero. These acini are ventilated so that administering 100% O_2 produces a maximal alveolar P_{O_2} of normally about 670 mm Hg. This high P_{O_2} is reduced slightly by the normal anatomic shunt, but usually, the arterial P_{O_2} remains above 500 mm Hg.

Chapter 19

Respiratory Control

I. CENTRAL NERVOUS SYSTEM (CNS) MECHANISMS

A. **Introduction.** The respiratory muscles are **typical skeletal muscles** requiring electrical stimulation from the CNS.

    1. Innervation of the respiratory muscles is provided via somatic nerves. The major inspiratory muscle, **the diaphragm, is innervated by the phrenic nerve,** which arises from C3–C5 levels of the spinal cord.

    2. Dual pathway. The phrenic nerve is activated by either **voluntary (i.e., corticospinal) or involuntary tracts.** This dual pathway allows voluntary control of breathing during activities such as talking, singing, and swimming, in addition to involuntary control, which allows humans to breathe without conscious effort.

B. **Medullary centers**

    1. Function. The automatic, involuntary, basic rhythm of respiration is generated within the medulla. Respiration continues as long as the medulla and the spinal cord are intact.

    2. Mechanism. Two nuclei act as oscillators to generate the basic rhythm. These cells, called the **dorsal respiratory group (DRG)** and the **ventral respiratory group (VRG),** discharge rhythmically. These pons, hypothalamus, reticular activating system (RAS), and the cerebral cortex as well as afferent activity in the vagus, glossopharyngeal, and somatic nerves influence both the DRG and VRG (Figure 19-1).

        a. The **DRG** lies within the **nucleus of the tractus solitarius.** The DRG cells are primarily **inspiratory cells** (i.e., they discharge during inspiration).

            (1) Function. The DRG may be the **primary rhythm generator** for respiration, because the activity in these cells gradually increases during inspiration (see Figure 19-1).

            (2) Pattern. The electrical activity of this center rises to a crescendo during inspiration and then rapidly disappears.

        b. The **neurons of the VRG** are active during both inspiration and expiration; however, expiratory activity does not activate the expiratory muscles during normal respiration (eupnea), because expiration is normally passive (see Figure 19-1).

C. **Pontine centers.** The **pneumotaxic center (PNC)** and the **apneustic center (APN)** both modify the activity of the medullary respiratory centers.

    1. APN

        a. Function. Efferent outflow from the APN stimulates the DRG and enhances inspiration.

        b. Mechanism. The **APN increases the tidal volume and the duration of inspiration,** resulting in a deeper and more prolonged inspiratory effort. The APN is normally inhibited by **impulses carried by the vagus nerves** and also by the activity of the **pneumotaxic center.** Bilateral vagotomy and destruction of the pneumotaxic center remove two inhibitory influences on the APN and lead to prolonged periods of inspiration [i.e., **apneusis or apneustic breathing** (see Figure 19-5)].

    2. PNC

        a. Function. The PNC **inhibits the ANC.**

        b. Mechanism. Stimulation of the PNC shortens inspiration, leading to a shallower and more rapid respiratory pattern.

D. **Reticular activating system (RAS).** The RAS stimulates the respiratory centers to increase respiratory drive. During sleep, RAS activity diminishes, decreasing respiratory drive, which diminishes alveolar ventilation and results in a slight elevation of arterial CO_2 tension.

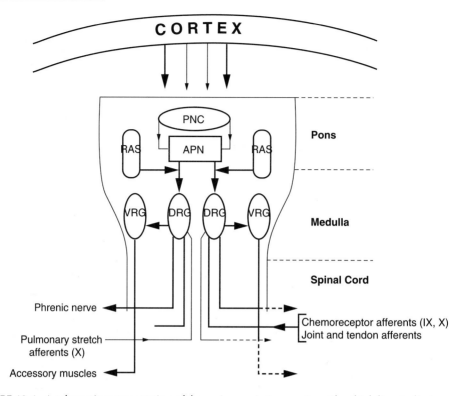

FIGURE 19-1. A schematic representation of the major respiratory centers. The *thick lines* indicate stimulation or increased output. The *thin lines* indicate inhibition or decreased output. The *thick dashed* lines indicate symmetrical functions on the other side of the body. PNC = pneumotaxic center; APN = apneustic center; RAS = reticular activating system; DRG = dorsal respiratory group; VRG = ventral respiratory group; IX = glossopharyngeal nerve; X = vagus nerve.

E. Central chemoreceptors are cells that lie just beneath the ventral surface of the medulla; they respond to the hydrogen ion (H+) concentration in the surrounding interstitial fluid (Figure 19-2).

1. **Mechanism**
   a. **Charged ions** do not readily cross the **blood–brain barrier.** Ion pumps in the choroid and pia arachnoid membranes regulate the ionic composition of the cerebrospinal fluid (CSF).
   b. **CO_2** readily crosses the blood–brain barrier, because it is a small, very soluble, uncharged molecule. The hydration and subsequent dissociation of CO_2 into H+ and bicarbonate ions (HCO_3^-) alter the H+ concentration in the CSF and brain tissues. An **increase in CSF CO_2 (H+) stimulates respiration,** whereas a decrease in CSF CO_2 (H+) inhibits respiration.

2. **Approximately 85% of the resting (basal), chemical drive of respiration** results from the stimulatory effect of CO_2 (H+) on the central chemoreceptors.

II. PERIPHERAL CHEMORECEPTOR MECHANISMS

A. **Peripheral chemoreceptors** are located in the carotid and aortic bodies. These receptors **respond to lowered O_2 tensions, increased CO_2 tensions, and increased H+ concentrations in the arterial blood.** The peripheral chemoreceptors are the **only sites that detect changes in Po_2.**

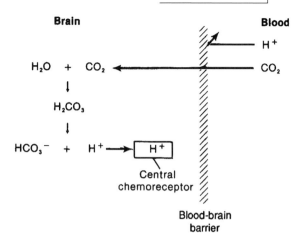

FIGURE 19-2. The effects of the blood–brain barrier on the transport of charged ions (e.g., H^+) and the diffusibility of CO_2. CO_2 can readily cross the blood–brain barrier, and it serves as a source of H^+ to stimulate the central chemoreceptors.

1. **Function.** The afferent impulses from the chemoreceptors stimulate the DRG, which leads to an **increased rate and depth of respiration.**

2. **Mechanism**
   a. **O_2 tension.** The peripheral chemoreceptors receive a tremendous blood flow for their size and thus can be considered to **monitor the dissolved O_2, or Po_2, rather than its total content.**
      (1) The increased alveolar ventilation that occurs secondary to hypoxia "blows off" CO_2, decreasing CO_2 concentration in the body fluids. The loss of this volatile acid produces **respiratory alkalosis,** which, in turn, inhibits the respiratory drive. Over the course of several days, ion transport from the meningeal tissues reduces the CSF HCO_3^-. This removes the inhibitory alkalotic influence, so that respiration continues to increase during the first several days of exposure to acute hypoxia.
      (2) The kidneys also counteract the inhibitory effect of alkalemia on ventilation during this period by excreting HCO_3^-. The respiratory response to hypoxia continues to increase as the braking effect of alkalosis is removed. As ventilation increases, the hypoxia is ameliorated (see Chapter 16 III C 1).
   b. **O_2 content.** Decreases in the O_2 content of blood caused by anemia, methemoglobinemia, or CO poisoning do not stimulate the peripheral chemoreceptors, because the O_2 tension, which is determined by the amount of dissolved O_2, remains normal.
   c. **CO_2 tension.** Elevated CO_2 tension also stimulates the peripheral chemoreceptors, but the major effect of CO_2 is on the central chemoreceptors.
   d. **H^+ concentration.** An **increased H^+ concentration** caused by the addition of fixed acids (e.g., lactate, acetoacetate, butyrate) to the blood **stimulates the peripheral chemoreceptors so that ventilation increases.** The increased alveolar ventilation lowers the CO_2 tension and also produces a **respiratory alkalosis** (see II A 2 c).

B. Other receptors

1. **Stretch receptors** located in the **small airways** are stimulated by inflation of the lungs, which initiates the **Hering-Breuer (inspiratory inhibitory) reflex.** The afferent limb of this reflex is carried over the vagus nerve (see Figure 19-1). This reflex is not very powerful in adult humans, but occurs in newborns and in some animal species.

2. **Irritant receptors,** which are located in the **large airways,** are stimulated by smoke, noxious gases, and particulates in the inspired air.
   a. These receptors initiate **reflexes** that cause **coughing, bronchoconstriction, mucus secretion,** and **breath-holding** (i.e., **apnea**).
   b. **Chronic exposure** to inhaled irritants (e.g., in smog, industrial atmospheres, or cigarette smoke) may lead to chronic **bronchitis,** one of the causes of obstructive lung disease.

3. J receptors, which are located in the **pulmonary interstitium** at the level of the pulmonary capillaries, are stimulated by distention of the pulmonary vessels and certain chemicals or drugs. These receptors initiate **reflexes** that cause **rapid, shallow breathing (tachypnea).**

4. Chest wall receptors detect the force generated by the respiratory muscles during breathing. If the force required to distend the lungs becomes excessive, the sensation of **dyspnea (difficulty in breathing)** develops.

III. DYSFUNCTION OF RESPIRATORY CONTROL

A. **Tests of respiratory control. Gases containing different amounts of O_2 or CO_2 can be administered to evaluate the respiratory drive of the respiratory system.**

1. Increasing the CO_2 tension of inspired gas raises the arterial CO_2 tension and should stimulate the chemoreceptors, leading to an increase in the minute ventilation (Figures 19-3 and 19-4). Hypercapnia is enhanced by a decrease in O_2 tension, so that the respiratory response is much greater than with either stimulus alone (see Figure 19-3).

2. Patients vary in their response to this test, depending on the sensitivity of their chemoreceptors, the activity of the RAS, the work of breathing, and the lung volume.

3. Marked blunting or elimination of the respiratory response occurs as a result of the use of drugs such as morphine, barbiturates, and cocaine (Figure 19-5).

B. **Abnormal respiratory patterns.** Changes in the environment or diseases affecting the respiratory system, cardiovascular system, or brain can produce various respiratory patterns (Figure 19-6).

1. Cheyne-Stokes respiration is an abnormal respiratory pattern that occurs with depression of the brain that results from disease, drug overdose, congestive heart failure, and hypoxia. Cheyne-Stokes respiration is characterized by periods of waxing and waning tidal volumes separated by periods of apnea.

2. Biot's breathing is another type of periodic breathing that consists of one or more large tidal volumes separated by periods of apnea. The condition occurs in many diseases that produce brain damage (e.g., diseases that increase the intracranial pressure, meningitis).

3. Kussmaul's respiration is rapid, deep breathing often seen in patients suffering from diabetic ketoacidosis. It occurs as the body tries to compensate for metabolic acidosis by increasing the rate of CO_2 excretion.

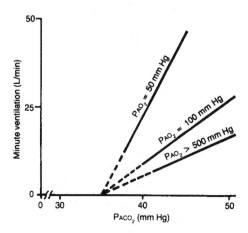

FIGURE 19-3. CO_2 response curves obtained at alveolar O_2 tensions (P_{AO_2}) of 50, 100, and more than 500 mm Hg. P_{ACO_2} = alveolar CO_2 tension.

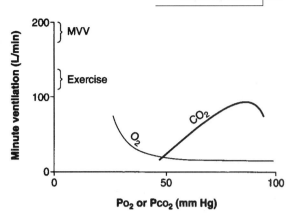

FIGURE 19-4. Ventilatory response to several different respiratory stimuli. The highest level of ventilation is achieved by voluntary increases in respiratory rate and tidal volume [i.e., as takes place during maximal voluntary ventilation (MVV)]. This level of ventilation can only be maintained for a short time. The maximal level of ventilation that can be sustained for a significant period of time is approximately 66% of the MVV. Chemical factors that affect respiration (e.g., O_2 and CO_2 tensions of the blood) are less powerful influences on ventilation.

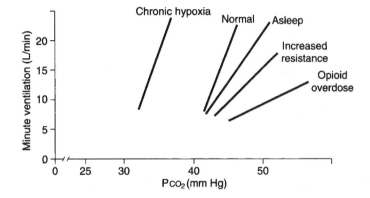

FIGURE 19-5. The effect of various conditions on CO_2 response curves. PCO_2 = carbon dioxide tension.

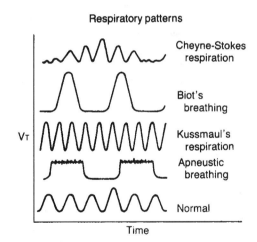

FIGURE 19-6. Illustration of various breathing patterns. V_T = tidal volume.

4. **Ondine's curse** involves the **loss of automatic respiratory control with destruction of the involuntary neural pathways.** Patients with this condition can breathe only by conscious effort and, therefore, cannot sleep without the aid of a mechanical respirator.

5. **Sleep apnea syndromes** have been recognized as disorders of respiratory control that affect a large portion of the population, especially middle-aged and elderly men. Many

sleep centers have been established to study patients by recording physiologic parameters (e.g., respiratory and eye movements, airflow, electroencephalographic data, and hemoglobin saturation) during sleep.

a. Obstructive sleep apnea occurs when inspiration is prevented by transient blockage of the airway.

    (1) Causes

        (a) Loss of muscle tone. Some individuals experience a marked loss of muscle tone in the **pharyngeal muscles** during **rapid eye movement (REM) sleep,** which causes partial or complete **obstruction of the oropharynx** during inspiration. The negative inspiratory pressure in the airway causes the hypopharynx to collapse, preventing airflow even though strong inspiratory muscle contractions occur (Figure 19-7).

        (b) Obesity. The association of sleep apnea with extreme obesity is referred to as the Pickwickian syndrome.

    (2) Clinical signs

        (a) Partial airway obstruction causes snoring, because the inspired air causes the soft tissues to vibrate.

        (b) The **hypoxia** that develops with complete airway obstruction awakens patients so that muscle tone is reestablished and the obstruction is relieved. Episodes may occur hundreds of times each night, and each one can produce a **marked drop in the hemoglobin saturation of the arterial blood.** The person awakens unrested because of the **poor sleep pattern.** Frequently, these people fall asleep at work, in lectures, or even while eating because of the lack of restful nighttime sleep.

    (3) Treatment may involve the use of an **oropharyngeal appliance** to keep the airway open or a **positive-pressure nasal mask** to overcome the negative pressure in the hypopharynx. In severe cases, **surgery** may be required to remove some of the soft tissue to maintain an open airway. Patients with extreme cases of obstructive sleep apnea may require a **tracheostomy** to bypass the airway obstruction.

b. Nonobstructive (central) sleep apnea refers to a complete absence of rhythmic activity from the respiratory centers. Obviously, there is no respiratory muscle contraction because the neural impulses are absent (see Figure 19-7).

    (1) These periods of apnea, which may last 30–60 seconds, produce a marked drop in arterial hemoglobin saturation.

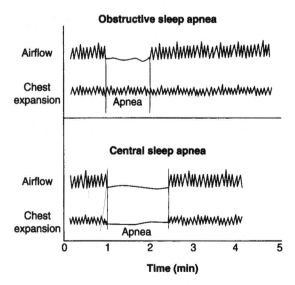

FIGURE 19-7. Simulated records of air flow and chest movements in patients with sleep apnea syndrome. *Upper panel.* Obstructive sleep apnea is caused by occlusion of the pharyngeal airways. Although the patient contracts the inspiratory muscles, generating chest movement, the airway obstruction prevents air flow. *Lower panel.* Central sleep apnea is caused by the absence of phrenic nerve impulses; therefore, the inspiratory muscles do not contract, and no chest movement is visible.

(2) Affected persons and some of their family members have been shown to have a
decreased chemoreceptor sensitivity to O_2 and CO_2.

(3) Central sleep apnea syndrome has been proposed as one of many possible causes
of **sudden infant death syndrome (SIDS; crib death).**

Case

**A 38-year-old employee of an electric utility company complains that he often falls asleep
during the day. He notes that for the past 2 years he has experienced increasing shortness
of breath and bluish coloration of the skin.**

**Physical examination indicates that the man is markedly overweight, and he appears
cyanotic. Laboratory evaluation reveals: hematocrit, 59%; an arterial P_{O_2}, 32 mm Hg; and
arterial P_{CO_2}, 85 mm Hg. Pulmonary function tests are all within normal limits.**

1. *Is this patient's arterial hypoxia a result of lung disease or hypoventilation?*

DISCUSSION

To answer this question, the alveolar–arterial P_{O_2} difference must be calculated. An abnormal
value indicates the presence of lung disease, while a normal value indicates the absence of lung
disease; the hypoxia results from hypoventilation alone. The alveolar P_{O_2} is calculated using the
alveolar gas equation (see Chapter 16 III C 2): $P_{AO_2} = (760 - 47) \cdot 0.21 - 85/0.8 = 44$ mm Hg.
The alveolar–arterial gradient is 44–32, or 12 mm Hg, which is within normal limits. The hypoxia is due entirely to hypoventilation.

2. *What is the association between the obesity and the hypoventilation?*

3. *What is the term for the combination of massive obesity and hypoventilation?*

DISCUSSION

The obesity produces a decreased thoracic compliance simply because of the additional weight
that the respiratory muscles must move to inflate the lungs. The decreased compliance eventually increases the work of the respiratory muscles, leading to respiratory muscle fatigue. Alveolar
ventilation decreases secondary to the fatigue, resulting in the buildup of CO_2. The term for this
combination of hypoventilation and obesity is the Pickwickian syndrome.

4. *How can this individual's condition be improved?*

DISCUSSION

Treatment must be based on weight loss. With a decrease in body weight, the patient's alveolar
ventilation should gradually return to normal. As ventilation normalizes, the blood gas values
will also return to normal.

Chapter 20

Respiratory Responses to Stress

I. EXERCISE

A. Introduction. The effects of exercise on the cardiorespiratory system have generated significant interest because of the current concern with **physical conditioning and prevention of cardiovascular disease.** Exercise is also frequently used to evaluate the cardiovascular and respiratory systems (i.e., as a **stress test**).

1. **Specificity.** Endurance (aerobic) training produces different effects in the skeletal muscles than weight training. Training effects are specific for the particular muscle groups involved; **only aerobic exercises produce cardiovascular conditioning.**

2. **Aerobic training** increases the availability of oxygen to the skeletal muscle cells, leading to **increased O_2 delivery** to the body cells.
   a. Muscles conditioned by endurance training exhibit increases in capillary density, myoglobin concentration, glycogen, and mitochondrial enzymes of the citric acid cycle.
   b. The mitochondrial enzymes allow the conservation of muscle glycogen by facilitating the breakdown of long-chain fatty acids, which serve as an alternate energy source during exercise.

B. Cardiovascular responses are summarized in Figure 20-1.

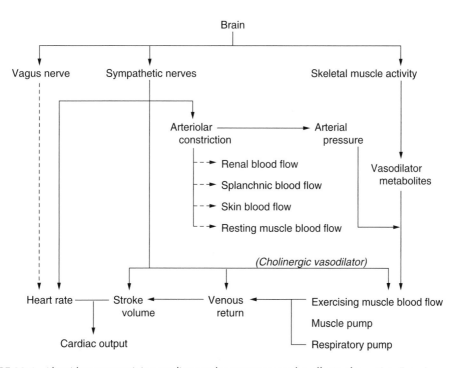

FIGURE 20-1. Algorithm summarizing cardiovascular responses to the effects of exercise. Exercise requires the coordination of many different systems by the central nervous system as well as local regulation of vascular resistance and blood flow.

1. **Heart rate** increases linearly with the work rate up to a maximum, which is determined by the subject's age. The **maximal heart rate (HR$_{max}$)** is approximately equal to 210 − [0.65 · age (years)], and is unaffected by conditioning.

2. **Optimal cardiovascular conditioning** requires attaining a heart rate of 60%–70% of the maximum for 20–30 minutes three to four times a week for at least 3 months.

3. **Stroke volume.** Endurance training increases the stroke volume of the heart by increasing the ventricular end-diastolic volume. Thus, conditioned athletes can maintain any level of cardiac output at a lower heart rate than nonconditioned individuals.

4. **Maximal cardiac output** is greater in conditioned athletes than in deconditioned individuals (e.g., 30–35 L/min in olympic-class runners, as compared with 15 L/min in deconditioned adults).

5. **Anaerobic threshold (AT)** is defined as **the level of activity that produces an elevation of blood lactate levels, which results from a shift from aerobic to anaerobic metabolism.** The AT occurs at higher levels of activity in conditioned athletes than in deconditioned individuals.
   a. The AT occurs at approximately **60% of the maximal exercise level,** regardless of the level of physical fitness.
   b. The onset of the AT in **cardiac patients** occurs at low levels of activity because the cardiac output is low. These patients reach maximal heart rates at much lower levels of exercise than healthy individuals (Figure 20-2).

C. **Respiratory responses in normal individuals** (Figure 20-3)

1. The **minute ventilation increases linearly** along with the work rate (O$_2$ consumption) until the AT is reached. Above the AT, minute ventilation increases more steeply as the work rate increases, because the lactic acid that is generated imposes an additional respiratory drive.
   a. **Endurance (aerobic) training increases the maximal minute ventilation** that is achieved during exercise but does not improve the maximal voluntary ventilation.
   b. **Respiratory muscle training.** The maximal duration of exercise is limited by fatigue of the respiratory muscles in both conditioned and nonconditioned individuals. Specific training of the respiratory muscles allows one to increase the duration and intensity of exercise.

2. **CO$_2$ output increases linearly** with the work rate until the AT is reached. Above the AT, the

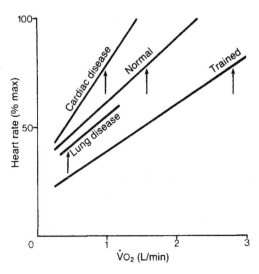

FIGURE 20-2. The effect of training, heart disease, and lung disease on the heart rate response to endurance (aerobic) exercise. *Vertical arrows* mark the onset of the anaerobic threshold, which occurs at about 60% of the maximal exercise level for every individual. $\dot{V}O_2 = O_2$ utilization.

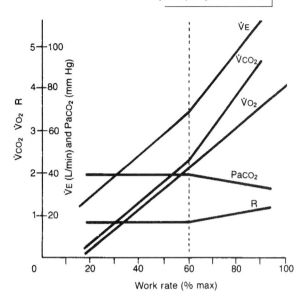

FIGURE 20-3. The effects of exercise on respiratory parameters of gas exchange. The *dashed line* indicates the onset of the anaerobic threshold. $\dot{V}_E$ = minute ventilation; $\dot{V}_{CO_2}$ = CO_2 excreted in the expired gas (L/min); $\dot{V}_{O_2}$ = O_2 utilization (L/min); Pa_{CO_2} = arterial CO_2 tension; R = respiratory exchange ratio.

CO_2 output increases more steeply because of the increased respiration. The arterial CO_2 tension declines as the body stores are depleted, because excretion exceeds production.

3. **O_2 consumption increases linearly** with the work rate and is exactly dependent on the work performed.
   a. The O_2 consumption does not decrease with training at any workload (i.e., training does not improve the body's efficiency unless muscle coordination is improved by practice).
   b. Conditioning produces a 5%–20% increase in the maximal O_2 consumption, because the cardiac output increases and the arteriovenous O_2 difference widens at the maximal exercise level.

4. The **alveolar–arterial O_2 gradient** normally remains at 5–10 mm Hg during moderate levels of exercise, but widens slightly beyond the AT because the alveolar O_2 tension increases. Arterial O_2 tension may decline slightly due to the marked desaturation of venous blood and the presence of an anatomic shunt.

5. The **respiratory exchange ratio** equals the ratio of expired CO_2 divided by the O_2 consumption ($\dot{V}_{CO_2}/\dot{V}_{O_2}$). At work levels above the AT, the respiratory exchange ratio exceeds 1, but normally never exceeds 1.25 even at maximal levels of exercise. The conversion of bicarbonate to carbonic acid during the buffering of lactic acid increases the amount of CO_2 that is liberated by the lungs, and therefore increases the respiratory exchange ratio.

D. **Respiratory responses to exercise in patients with lung disease**

1. In patients with **chronic obstructive pulmonary disease,** the ability to exercise is limited, primarily because of the onset of severe **dyspnea.**
   a. The heart rate does not reach the minimal level necessary to achieve cardiovascular conditioning. The AT occurs at very low levels of exercise because O_2 uptake is impaired (see Figure 20-2).
   b. Exercise training has only slight benefits, which seem to relate primarily to desensitization to dyspnea. It is worthwhile to train the respiratory muscles in these patients.

2. In patients with **moderately or severely reduced diffusing capacity of the lungs,** exercise may cause the arterial O_2 tension to decrease (Figure 20-4). These patients may **switch from perfusion-limited gas exchange at rest to diffusion-limited gas exchange during exercise.**

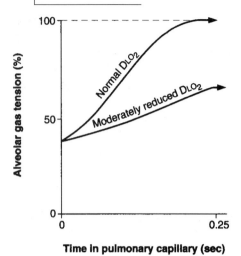

FIGURE 20-4. Effects of exercise on the diffusion process in the lungs. Normally, the red blood cell spends 0.75 second in the pulmonary capillary, but during exercise, this time is reduced to 0.25 second. During exercise, individuals with normal diffusing capacities are still able to achieve equilibration between the alveolar gas and the pulmonary capillary blood, in spite of the abbreviated transit time. In fact, in healthy people, exercise increases the diffusing capacity to approximately three times the resting value because the capillary blood volume increases and additional capillaries are perfused as a result of the increased pulmonary artery pressure and cardiac output. On the other hand, patients with a moderately reduced diffusing capacity may be unable to achieve equilibration during exercise (resulting in a decreased arterial O_2 tension) because of the reduced transit time. DLO_2 = diffusing capacity of the lungs for O_2.

II. **HYPOXIA** is defined as an **inadequate O_2 supply to the body tissues.** The entire body or a localized region may be affected. Disease processes can severely limit the O_2 supply anywhere between the atmosphere and the body's cells (Figure 20-5). Hypoxia occurs "downstream" of the limitation (i.e., toward the cells); a normal O_2 tension may be present "upstream" (i.e., toward the environment).

A. **Symptoms of hypoxia** depend on the **rapidity** and the **severity of the decrease in O_2 tension,** the tissues that are involved, and the effectiveness of the body's compensatory mechanisms.

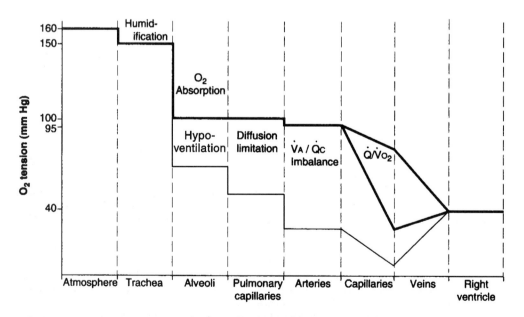

FIGURE 20-5. The oxygen cascade. Normally, the transfer of O_2 along the pathway from the atmosphere to the tissues produces several small decrements in the O_2 tension. A large change in O_2 tension occurs when the blood in the systemic capillaries releases O_2 to the tissues; the amount of O_2 that is released depends on the tissues' metabolic rate and the rate of blood flow. The *thick lines* represent the normal O_2 tension for a subject at sea level. The *thin lines* represent an estimate of the changes in O_2 tension that can be caused by diseases. $\dot{V}A/\dot{Q}C$ = ventilation–perfusion ratio; $\dot{Q}/\dot{V}O_2$ = blood flow–O_2 consumption ratio.

1. **Fulminant hypoxia** occurs within seconds after exposure to an **arterial O_2 tension of less than 20 mm Hg** (e.g., as occurs if an aircraft loses cabin pressure above 30,000 feet and no supplemental O_2 is available). **Unconsciousness** occurs in as few as 15–20 seconds, and **brain death** may follow in 4–5 minutes.

2. **Acute hypoxia** is produced by exposure to **arterial O_2 tensions of 25–40 mm Hg** (e.g., as would occur at altitudes of 18,000–25,000 feet).
   a. **Symptoms** of acute hypoxia are very similar to the effects of ethyl alcohol; they include **lack of coordination, slowed reflexes, slurred speech, overconfidence,** and, eventually, **unconsciousness.**
   b. **Coma** and **death** can occur in minutes to hours if the compensatory mechanisms of the body are not adequate.

3. **Chronic hypoxia** is produced by exposure to **arterial O_2 tensions of 40–60 mm Hg** (e.g., as would occur at altitudes of approximately 10,000–18,000 feet) for extended periods of time. Most clinical causes of hypoxia are in this category. Patients with chronic hypoxia may be **bedridden** or limited to a chair, because respiratory or cardiac disease prevents them from increasing the O_2 supply to the tissues.
   a. **Symptoms** of chronic hypoxia, which are similar to those of **severe fatigue,** include **dyspnea** (difficulty breathing) and **shortness of breath.**
   b. **Respiratory arrhythmias** (e.g., **Cheyne-Stokes breathing**) can occur in patients with chronic hypoxia, especially during sleep, which can contribute to the hypoxic state.

B. Signs of hypoxia

1. **Cyanosis** is the **bluish color** of tissue caused by the presence of more than 5 g of deoxyhemoglobin/dl in the capillary blood. The coloration is most readily seen in the nail beds, lips, mucous membranes, and earlobes, but it may not be recognized because of skin pigmentation or poor lighting. Cyanosis is **not a reliable sign of hypoxia.**
   a. **Anemic patients** may never develop cyanosis, even though they are extremely hypoxic because of an inadequate hemoglobin concentration. In contrast, **patients with polycythemia** [see II D 1 b (1)] may be cyanotic as a result of a high concentration of hemoglobin, even though their tissues are adequately oxygenated.
   b. **Methemoglobin,** with its slate-gray color, can also impart a bluish color to tissues.

2. **Tachycardia** occurs as a peripheral chemoreceptor reflex response to the low arterial O_2 tension. (see Chapter 17 III C).

3. **Tachypnea** (i.e., **rapid breathing**) and **hyperpnea** (i.e., **deep breathing**) are also reflex responses to hypoxia that are activated by the arterial chemoreceptors.

C. Types of hypoxia (Table 20-1)

1. **Arterial hypoxia** (Figure 20-6A) results from **inadequate oxygenation of the arterial blood,** caused by breathing gas with a low O_2 tension or by one or more of **four pathophysiologic mechanisms** (see Table 20-1).
   a. **Hypoventilation** occurs when the **alveolar ventilation is not adequate** to blow off the CO_2 that is produced. The inadequate alveolar ventilation reduces both the alveolar and arterial O_2 tensions, and it increases the alveolar and arterial CO_2 tensions. **Hypercapnia** is pathognomonic of hypoventilation.
   b. **Diffusion limitation** results from a reduction in the diffusing capacity of the lung secondary to pulmonary disease that prevents an equilibration between the O_2 tension in the alveoli and the pulmonary capillaries (see Chapter 17 II B 2 a).
   c. **Physiologic shunts [ventilation–perfusion ratio ($\dot{V}A/\dot{Q}C$) imbalances]** produce low O_2 tensions in areas of the lung with low $\dot{V}A/\dot{Q}C$ ratios.
      (1) **Ventilation–perfusion imbalance is by far the most common cause of hypoxia.**
      (2) Administration of 100% O_2 to affected patients can correct the hypoxia, because the O_2 flushes the N_2 from the alveoli, and the alveolar O_2 tension, even in low ventilation–perfusion areas, eventually exceeds 650 mm Hg at sea level.
   d. **Anatomic shunts** are characterized by the mixing of true venous blood and arterial (oxygenated) blood, which dilutes the normal O_2 concentration (see Chapter 18 IV A

TABLE 20-1. Differentiating Types of Hypoxia

Type of Hypoxia	PaO$_2$	PaCO$_2$	P$\bar{v}$O$_2$	PaO$_2$ During Exercise	Effect of 100% of O$_2$
Arterial hypoxia					
Hypoventilation	↓	↑*	↓	↓↑	↑ PaCO$_2$
Diffusion limitation	↓	Normal	↓	↓↓*	PaO$_2$ > 600 mm Hg
Physiologic shunt	↓	↓↑	↓	↑↓	PaO$_2$ > 600 mm Hg
Anatomic shunt	↓	Normal	↓	↑↓	PaO$_2$ < 500 mm Hg*
Hypokinetic hypoxia	Normal	Normal	↓*	↑↓	↑ dissolved O$_2$
Anemic hypoxia	Normal	Normal	↓*	Normal	↑ dissolved O$_2$
Histotoxic hypoxia	Normal	Normal	↑*	Normal	↑ dissolved O$_2$

PaCO$_2$ = arterial CO$_2$ tension; PaO$_2$ = arterial O$_2$ tension; P$\bar{v}$O$_2$ = mixed venous O$_2$ tension; ↑ = increased; ↓ = decreased; ↑↓ = variable; * = critical determinant.

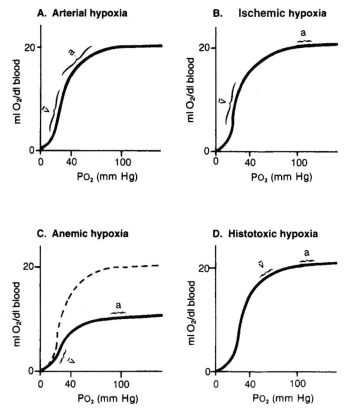

FIGURE 20-6. O$_2$–hemoglobin dissociation curves illustrating the four types of hypoxia. Note that the effects of 7.5 g/dl of hemoglobin are indicated on the anemic hypoxia curve (*curve C*) as the *solid line,* and the normal curve (as would be produced by 15 g/dl of hemoglobin) is indicated as the *dashed line.* The arterial O$_2$ tension is below normal only in arterial hypoxia (*curve A*), but the mixed venous blood point is below normal in all cases except in histotoxic hypoxia (*curve D*), where it is increased. a = arterial point; $\bar{v}$ = mixed venous point; PO$_2$ = O$_2$ tension.

2 b). The arterial O_2 tension is reduced in proportion to the fraction of the cardiac output that is shunted. **Normal individuals** have an **anatomic shunt** consisting of **less than 5% of their cardiac output.**
   (1) Causes
      (a) Some of the **coronary blood** enters the chambers of the left heart through the **thebesian veins** and **coronary–luminal connections.**
      (b) **Bronchial venous blood** drains into the pulmonary veins and lowers the O_2 tension.
      (c) **Pathologically,** an anatomic shunt may result from **congenital cardiac malformations** or from blood flow through **atelectatic areas** of the lungs.
   (2) Diagnosis. The presence of an anatomic shunt can be diagnosed by administering **100% O_2.** Patients with a significant anatomic shunt have an arterial O_2 tension less than 500 mm Hg while breathing 100% O_2 at sea level.

2. **Ischemic hypoxia** (ischemia) is caused by an **inadequate blood flow.**
   a. The reduced blood flow may involve either the **entire body** (e.g., as in congestive heart failure), **or** only a **localized area** of the body (e.g., as in arteriosclerosis). **Arteriosclerosis,** the most common cause of arterial obstruction, occurs when deposits of cholesterol and other lipids in the endothelium narrow the vessel lumen. The narrowing increases the local vascular resistance, which severely reduces or completely blocks the blood flow.
      (1) Ischemic hypoxia represents a decreased O_2 delivery to the body or a particular organ or tissue. Depending on the site and the severity of the blood flow reduction, ischemia can result in an infarct or dysfunction to any body organ or tissue.
      (2) Detection. The low O_2 tension decreases the amount of adenosine triphosphate (ATP) available for cellular processes, leading to cellular damage and the release of various cellular constituents such as enzymes into the circulation. **Measurement of isoenzymes** is frequently used clinically as an index of the type and extent of tissue damage.
   b. The **arterial O_2 tension** and content may be normal, but because of inadequate blood flow, the tissues withdraw large amounts of O_2 from the capillary blood, so that the **venous O_2 content is markedly reduced** (Figure 20-6B). However, measuring venous blood from various organs is not generally feasible. The blood flow from the affected organ may not be sufficient to abnormally lower the oxygen saturation of the mixed venous blood.

3. **Anemic hypoxia** is caused by an **insufficient amount of functional hemoglobin** (see Chapter 17 III A 3 a).
   a. The decrease in functional hemoglobin may be caused by deficiency of essential nutrients (e.g., iron, vitamin B_{12}), or it may result from blood loss or abnormal amounts of methemoglobin or carboxyhemoglobin.
   b. Patients with anemic hypoxia have a **reduced O_2 capacity** and, consequently, **a decreased O_2 content.** However, the arterial O_2 tension remains normal (Figure 20-6C).

4. **Histotoxic hypoxia** is caused by the **inactivation of certain metabolic enzymes** (e.g., **cytochromes**) and by **chemical poisons** (e.g., **cyanide**). If the tissues are unable to use O_2, the venous O_2 tension and content are high (Figure 20-6D).

D. **Physiologic responses to chronic hypoxia**

1. **Compensatory mechanisms.** The body has many ways to compensate for decreases in the O_2 supply.
   a. **Accommodation** refers to the **immediate reflex adjustments** of the **respiratory and cardiovascular systems** to hypoxia.
      (1) Hyperventilation occurs secondary to stimulation of the peripheral chemoreceptors by low O_2 tension in the arterial blood.
         (a) The increased ventilation **reduces the alveolar CO_2 tension, which raises the alveolar O_2 tension proportionately.**
         (b) The reduced CO_2 tension causes a respiratory **alkalosis,** which, in turn, low-

ers the respiratory drive. The respiratory drive continues to increase during this time as the alkalosis is corrected.

    (2) Tachycardia increases O_2 delivery to the tissues by increasing cardiac output. In humans who go to high altitudes, the cardiac output returns to normal after several weeks.

    (3) The **diphosphoglycerate (DPG) concentration** increases in response to hypoxia and alkalosis. The increased DPG concentration raises the P_{50} of hemoglobin, which helps maintain the tissue O_2 tension at slightly higher levels than it would be otherwise (see Chapter 17 III A 2 a).

  b. Acclimatization refers to **changes in the body tissues** in response to **long-term exposure** to hypoxia.

    (1) Polycythemia is an increased number of red blood cells (RBCs)/μl of blood (> 5.5 million). The higher number of RBCs results in an above-normal elevation of both hemoglobin and hematocrit. Polycythemia secondary to tissue hypoxia results from the release of **renal erythropoietic factor,** which acts on a plasma globulin to form **erythropoietin.** This stimulates the production of erythrocytes by the bone marrow. The increased number of RBCs allows each unit of blood to carry additional O_2, which compensates for the decreased O_2 tension.

    (2) Pulmonary hypertension occurs secondary to the generalized hypoxic pulmonary vasoconstriction (HPV). The increased pulmonary artery pressure causes a more even distribution of the pulmonary blood flow, which can improve gas exchange. However, the elevated pulmonary artery pressure can induce cor pulmonale if the hypoxia is sufficiently severe.

    (3) Responses at cellular and tissue levels

      (a) Oxidative enzyme concentrations increase within the mitochondria of many tissues, which allows more rapid generation of ATP via oxidative phosphorylation.

      (b) Mitochondrial density increases within cells, which reduces the diffusion distance and provides more sites for O_2 utilization.

      (c) Capillary density increases in skeletal and cardiac muscle, which reduces the diffusion distance from the blood into the cells.

    (4) Lifelong exposure to hypoxia causes additional alterations that appear to improve the body's tolerance of low O_2 levels.

      (a) A **decreased respiratory drive** is present in individuals exposed to hypoxia for prolonged periods. The reduced drive leads to higher CO_2 tensions and lower O_2 tensions, but it diminishes the work of respiration, which reserves more O_2 for use by other skeletal muscles.

      (b) An **increased total lung capacity (TLC)** and **diffusing capacity** of the lung occur in high-altitude natives compared to their sea-level counterparts. The increase in TLC is evidenced by the enlarged chest that high-altitude natives develop.

2. Clinical syndromes caused by high altitude

  a. Acute mountain sickness (AMS) occurs in many individuals who are exposed to altitudes in excess of 9000–10,000 feet above sea level.

    (1) Symptoms of AMS are typical of those for acute hypoxia (e.g., fatigue, shortness of breath, confusion, loss of appetite).

    (2) Risks

      (a) In some individuals, **cerebral** or **pulmonary edema** occurs if the hypoxia is not treated.

      (b) Exercise should be **limited** during the first several days at high altitude, because it can lead to severe pulmonary edema. The edema is caused by the combination of HPV and an elevated cardiac output.

    (3) Treatment involves increasing the O_2 tension, either by administering supplemental O_2 or, preferably, by removal to a lower altitude.

  b. Chronic mountain sickness (Monge's disease) occurs in some long-term residents of high altitudes who develop extreme polycythemia, cyanosis, malaise, fatigue, and exercise intolerance. These individuals must be removed to a lower altitude to prevent rapid development of fatal pulmonary edema.

III. **BIRTH** is the most traumatic event that the respiratory system must withstand during the entire life span of an individual.

A. **Perinatal respiration**

1. In the **fetus,** the airways are filled with **pulmonary fluid,** which keeps the respiratory system at approximately functional residual capacity (FRC).

2. Following birth, the fluid must be drained and absorbed from the airways while inflation of the airspaces is maintained. Because of the high viscosity of the pulmonary fluid, newborns must generate very high interpleural pressures to initiate breathing (Figure 20-7).

B. **Physiologic responses to birth**

1. **Normal surfactant** is essential for maintaining lung inflation because pulmonary surfactant lowers the alveolar surface tension, which decreases the retraction forces in the lung and enhances the absorption of fluid by the pulmonary capillaries [see Chapter 16 VI B 3 a (2)]. The low surface tension stabilizes the alveoli and allows the lung volume to increase steadily during the first few days and weeks of life (see Figure 20-7).

2. The transport mechanisms in the alveolar epithelium change from fluid secretion to fluid reabsorption. The decreased fluid content of the lungs improves diffusion of gases by reducing the diffusion distance.

IV. **MECHANICAL VENTILATION.** In several situations (e.g., drug-induced depression of respiratory centers, paralysis of respiratory muscles, ineffective pump function of thorax, respiratory muscle fatigue secondary to excessive work of breathing), **hypoventilation** results in CO_2 retention. **Positive-pressure respiration** may be used to normalize alveolar ventilation and the arterial CO_2 tension.

A. **Intermittent positive pressure** applied to the airways can increase alveolar ventilation to reduce the CO_2 level in the body. Administration typically involves a respirator that delivers regulated volumes of gas under positive pressure. Inflation results from the positive pressure within the airways, and deflation occurs when the positive pressure is removed (Figure 20-8).

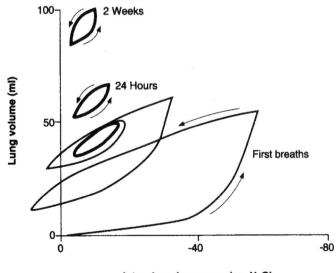

FIGURE 20-7. Work loops demonstrating the changes that occur in lung volume over the first several weeks after birth. Note the marked negativity of the interpleural pressure that is required to generate the first breath. This large pressure gradient is necessary to displace the pulmonary fluid and overcome the surface forces so that a gas volume may be established in the lungs. There is a progressive increase in gas volume in the lungs as the pulmonary fluid is absorbed and alveolar development continues. The *arrows* indicate the direction of volume change.

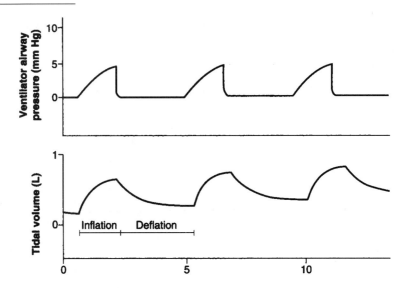

FIGURE 20-8. A record of airway pressure changes (*upper panel*) and the resultant change in lung volume (*lower panel*) that is produced by positive-pressure ventilation. The increase in lung volume is dependent on the peak airway pressure and the compliance of the respiratory system. Deflation (i.e., expiration) occurs when the positive airway pressure decreases. Note that the decrease in lung volume requires a significant time, which is dependent on the patient's airway resistance.

B. **Respirators** are used to provide positive pressure to the airways to ensure adequate ventilation, administer supplemental O_2, and provide **positive end-expiratory pressure (PEEP)** to help maintain alveolar inflation.

   1. **PEEP** increases lung volume by increasing the transmural pressure of the respiratory system. The increase in alveolar volume helps **stabilize the alveoli, reinflate atelectatic regions of the lung,** and **reduce pulmonary edema.**

      a. **Reduction of edema.** This occurs because the increased alveolar pressure opposes the filtration forces across the capillary wall [see Chapter 12 I C 5 b (1)].

      b. **Respiratory distress syndrome (RDS).** Patients with RDS have disorders of surfactant function resulting in atelectasis, edema, and hemorrhage in different areas of their lungs. Although the use of supplemental O_2 and PEEP has lowered the mortality rate of RDS, this disease is still associated with high mortality.

      c. **Intrinsic PEEP ("auto-peep")**

         (1) **Definition.** The lungs of patients with a high airway resistance may not deflate to the equilibrium volume (i.e., normal FRC) because of low expiratory flow rates. Under these conditions, the alveolar pressure remains positive at the end of expiration. Consequently, the lung volume rises (part of each tidal volume is retained) until the alveolar pressure has increased sufficiently to expel the entire tidal volume (Figure 20-9). Lung volume is now well above the normal FRC.

         (2) **Recourse.** Decreasing the respiratory rate or reducing the time for inflation provides a longer time for deflation to occur. The additional time may be sufficient to allow the lungs to deflate to their equilibrium volume and eliminate "auto-peep."

C. **Risks**

   1. **Barotrauma.** The increased tidal volumes produced by ventilators can overdistend segments of the lung, causing **laceration of tissues** and **leakage of air out of the alveolar spaces (Figure 20-10).**

      a. Laceration of the visceral pleura with leakage of gas into the pleural space is termed **pneumothorax.** This condition results in lung collapse (see VI).

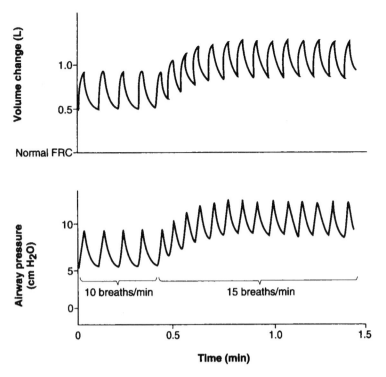

FIGURE 20-9. Effect of increasing the respiratory rate on intrinsic positive end-expiratory pressure (PEEP). Note that the lung volume has not stabilized at the end of expiration, indicating that the respiratory system has not achieved its equilibrium volume [i.e., functional residual capacity (*FRC*)]. The increased lung volume creates PEEP. An increased respiratory rate shortens the time allotted for expiration (i.e., lung deflation), further increasing the lung volume and end-expiratory pressure.

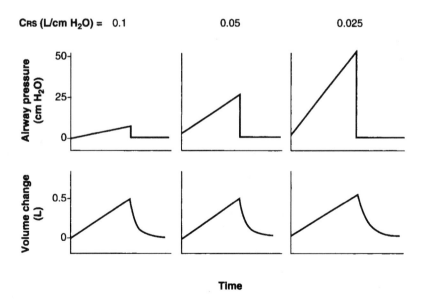

FIGURE 20-10. Graphic depiction of the pressures generated during lung inflation in patients with varying respiratory system compliance (CRS). As the compliance is reduced, the airway pressure progressively increases. The tidal volume (VT) in each example is 0.5 L and the maximal pressure (assumed to be due only to elastance forces) is equal to VT/CRS. If the compliance varies in different areas of the lungs, those areas with high compliance may become overdistended. Overdistention can result in tissue damage, tearing or laceration of the tissues, and air leakage into the pleural space or interstitial lung tissues.

    b. The high pressures in the lungs can also force gas into the interstitium where it can dissect its way to the mediastinum and, from there, to the subcutaneous tissues, causing **subcutaneous emphysema.**

  2. Reduced cardiac output. One of the biggest disadvantages of PEEP is that it raises the intrathoracic pressure, which reduces the venous return. The **reduced cardiac output** causes a **decreased O$_2$ delivery, which is detrimental to tissue oxygenation.**

D. **Common modes of positive-pressure respiration**

  1. Controlled ventilation is used when complete takeover of the ventilatory functions of the respiratory system is necessary (Figure 20-11). This type of ventilation is required when all ventilatory function has been lost (i.e., complete paralysis, severe drug overdose). The patient is connected to the ventilator, and the respiratory rate and tidal volume are set by the physician.

  2. Assisted ventilation is used in conscious patients who are capable of initiating an inspiratory effort. An initial negative airway pressure, which is generated by the inspiratory muscles, triggers the ventilator to deliver a tidal volume under positive pressure (see Figure 20-11).

V. **O$_2$ TOXICITY.** O$_2$ in high concentrations is injurious to the body. Two types of O$_2$ toxicity are recognized: **hyperbaric toxicity,** which affects the **central nervous system (CNS),** and **normobaric toxicity,** which affects the **lungs.**

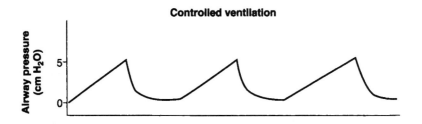

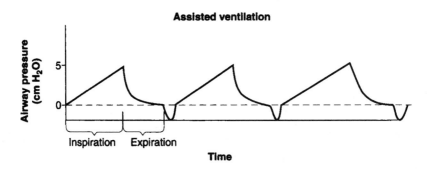

FIGURE 20-11. Controlled and assisted modes of positive-pressure ventilation. In controlled ventilation, the tidal volume and respiratory rate are set by the physician. Controlled ventilation is used to ventilate patients with no intrinsic function of the respiratory neuromuscular system. Assisted ventilation requires the patient to trigger the ventilator. The trigger is the negative airway pressure that is generated by the patient's initial effort to inspire. Assisted ventilation is used to augment the patient's inspiratory effort if the respiratory muscles are weakened or fatigued as the result of a disease process.

A. **Hyperbaric (CNS) O$_2$ toxicity** requires exposure to a minimum of 1.5–2.0 atmospheres (atm) of O$_2$ tension (Figure 20-12).

    1. Causes. Obviously, hyperbaric O$_2$ toxicity only occurs during diving or hyperbaric (pressures > 1 atmosphere) chamber operations. The high O$_2$ tension results in inactivation of several sulfhydryl-containing enzymes within the brain.

    2. Effects. CNS O$_2$ toxicity is evidenced by an increased irritability of nerves and muscles that eventually leads to grand mal seizures. Because of the danger of convulsions during scuba diving, it is unlawful to use 100% O$_2$ to refill scuba tanks for the general public.

B. **Normobaric (pulmonary) O$_2$ toxicity** requires exposure to a minimum of 0.5 atm of O$_2$ tension for 18–24 hours (see Figure 20-12).

    1. Causes. Administration of supplemental O$_2$ for long periods of time can produce pulmonary O$_2$ toxicity.

    2. Effects. The high O$_2$ tension destroys the type II cells that produce surfactant, resulting in pulmonary edema, areas of atelectasis, and hemorrhage. The gas exchange functions of the lungs are impaired, and the arterial O$_2$ levels decline. To maintain arterial oxygenation at viable levels, the alveolar O$_2$ tension is increased, which leads to further damage to the lung tissue. This vicious cycle frequently occurs in patients with RDS, who may require external artificial oxygenators or even lung transplants to sustain gas exchange.

VI. **PNEUMOTHORAX** is the presence of **air in the pleural space.** Humans have a complete mediastinum; therefore, a pneumothorax is typically **unilateral** because the two pleural sacs do not communicate.

A. **Causes.** Laceration or rupture of a lung, traumatic penetration of the chest wall, or rupture of the esophagus can permit air to enter the pleural space because the normal interpleural pressure is negative.

B. **Effects.** The presence of air in the pleural space **uncouples the affected lung from the ipsilateral chest wall.**

    1. As the volume of the pneumothorax increases, the interpleural pressure becomes less negative. The decreased negativity of the interpleural pressure causes the transmural pressure for both the chest wall and the lungs to decrease.

    2. Figure 20-13 shows that the chest wall expands and the lungs deflate along their respective pressure–volume curves. The difference in volume between the chest wall and the lungs represents the volume of gas in the pleural space.

FIGURE 20-12. Typical dose–duration curves demonstrating the threshold for hyperbaric [central nervous system (CNS)] O$_2$ toxicity and normobaric (pulmonary) O$_2$ toxicity. The asymptotes for the CNS effects are 15 minutes and 1.5 atm, and the asymptotes for the pulmonary effects are 18 hours and 0.5 atm. The asymptotes represent the minimal values that produce the effects. Theoretically, the administration of 0.4 atm (40% F$_{IO_2}$ at sea level) is safe for an infinite period of time, but administration of more than 50% F$_{IO_2}$ at sea level eventually produces O$_2$ toxicity in the lungs.

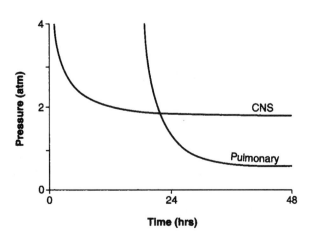

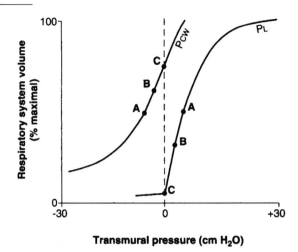

FIGURE 20-13. Pressure–volume curves for the chest wall (PCW) and the lungs (PL). *Point A* on each curve represents the normal condition, where the interpleural pressure is −5 cm H_2O so that PL = 5 cm H_2O and PCW = −5 cm H_2O. Both points occur at the same respiratory system volume and all of the gas is contained within the lungs. The presence of a simple pneumothorax causes the interpleural pressure to decrease to about −3 cm H_2O, so that PL = 3 cm H_2O and PCW = −3 cm H_2O. The volume of gas in the lungs has decreased to *point B on the PL curve* but the total gas within the respiratory system is indicated by *point B on the PCW curve.* The volume of gas in the interpleural space is given by the difference between points B on the two curves. *Point C* on each curve reflects the volume of gas within the chest wall and lungs, respectively, if the interpleural pressure increases to zero. A tension pneumothorax results in a positive interpleural pressure, which causes the chest wall to exceed its equilibrium volume and the lung to reach its minimal volume.

C. **Types of pneumothorax**

1. **Simple pneumothorax** occurs when the **air leak** into the pleural space **seals** and the patient is left with one partially collapsed lung and an expanded chest wall on the affected side. This condition can be detected by physical examination or by radiograph.
   a. **Treatment.** If the patient is having respiratory difficulty, a simple pneumothorax can be treated by needle aspiration.
   b. **Resorption.** If the patient is not having respiratory difficulty, the pneumothorax can be allowed to resorb.
      (1) **Diffusion gradient.** Gas in the pleural space or in tissues is slowly absorbed. The total gas tension in the veins is approximately 50 mm Hg less than the atmospheric pressure, and this diffusion gradient causes the slow absorption of gas pockets within the body.
      (2) **Rate of resorption.** Normally, the pneumothorax is absorbed at the rate of about **1% per day.**

2. **Tension pneumothorax.** At times, the site of gas entry into the pleural space acts as a **one-way valve,** letting gas into the pleural space with each breath. Under these conditions, the interpleural pressure slowly increases. Eventually, the interpleural pressure becomes positive and the vascular pressure gradient responsible for venous return is gradually eliminated.
   a. **Diagnosis**
      (1) The positive pressure causes **venous distention** that **can be noted in the jugular veins.**
      (2) A high pressure in one hemithorax causes the mediastinum to shift to the contralateral side. The **shifted mediastinum can be detected by physical examination.**
   b. **Treatment.** A tension pneumothorax presents an **acute emergency** because the cardiac output rapidly decreases and the patient goes into low cardiac output shock.

Treatment requires that the positive intrathoracic pressure be relieved, which can be accomplished by **needle aspiration.**

Case

A 55-year-old woman complains of shortness of breath and a chronic productive cough that is worse in the morning. She expectorates several cups of yellowish sputum each day. She admits to having smoked two packs of cigarettes a day for 35 years. Physical examination is normal except for some expiratory wheezes heard posteriorly in both lungs.

The hemoglobin concentration is 17.6 g/dl. The pulmonary function tests are shown in the following table.

Test	Units	Patient Value	Percent Predicted
Total lung capacity (TLC)	L	5.4	106
Vital capacity (VC)	L	2.5	60
Functional residual capacity (FRC)	L	3.2	120
Residual volume (RV)	L	2.9	140
FEV_1	L/sec	1.1	50
Arterial PO_2	mm Hg	56	
Arterial PCO_2	mm Hg	39	

FEV_1 = forced expiratory volume in 1 second; PCO_2 = CO_2 tension; PO_2 = O_2 tension.

1. *What type of lung disease is present?*

DISCUSSION

These findings are most typical of obstructive lung disease. The increase in residual volume (RV) and functional residual capacity (FRC) provides a mechanism for minimizing the increase in airway resistance through the effect of radial traction. The decreased forced expiratory volume in 1 second (FEV_1) results from an increased airway resistance, which is synonymous with obstructive airway disease.

2. *What is the most likely cause of the arterial hypoxia?*

3. *Why is the arterial PCO_2 normal and the arterial PO_2 reduced?*

DISCUSSION

The arterial hypoxia is caused by ventilation–perfusion imbalance at the acinar level of the lungs. Typically, the spectrum of values of the ventilation–perfusion ratio ($\dot{V}a/\dot{Q}c$) is much wider than normal but does not include an increase in anatomic shunt flow ($\dot{V}a/\dot{Q}c = 0$). Ventilation–perfusion imbalance is by far the most common cause of hypoxia in individuals with lung disease.

The arterial PCO_2 is normal, because the $\dot{V}a/\dot{Q}c$ is increased in some parts of the lungs and decreased in others. The increased ventilation–perfusion regions represent alveolar dead space. To compensate, the minute ventilation is greater than normal.

4. *What is a reasonable estimate of the arterial O_2 content in this patient?*

DISCUSSION

The hemoglobin saturation is approximately 85%. This value can be obtained by understanding that arterial hemoglobin saturation is between 75% (P_{O_2} = 40 mm Hg) and 95% (P_{O_2} = 90 mm Hg), or about 85%. Arterial O_2 content = O_2 capacity · hemoglobin saturation = 17.6 · 1.34 · 0.85 = 20.0 mg/dl. This patient, who has a normal O_2 content but a reduced O_2 tension, is suffering from arterial hypoxia because of the low arterial P_{O_2}.

PART IV.   RESPIRATORY PHYSIOLOGY

STUDY QUESTIONS

1. A 62-year-old man is known to have chronic lung disease and hypercapnia. He needs a major operation to remove an intestinal tumor. To ensure that he has adequate alveolar ventilation while being anesthetized, which of the following should be available?

(A) Tank of 100% O_2
(B) Tank of 95% O_2, 5% CO_2
(C) Mechanical respirator
(D) Cardiac defibrillator
(E) Electrocardiograph

2. Maximal inspiratory gas flow occurs when the

(A) lung volume approaches total lung capacity (TLC)
(B) lung volume approaches residual volume (RV)
(C) alveolar pressure is most negative
(D) interpleural pressure is approximately −5 cm H_2O
(E) abdominal muscles are maximally contracted

3. The diffusion coefficient of O_2, as compared with that of CO_2, is

(A) greater because O_2 combines with hemoglobin
(B) less because O_2 is less soluble
(C) greater because of a higher pressure gradient
(D) less because of the lower molecular weight of O_2
(E) essentially the same

4. Which of the following regarding the transmural pressure for the lungs is true?

(A) It is always negative
(B) It is equal to the interpleural pressure minus the atmospheric pressure ($P_{PL} - P_B$)
(C) It is equal to the interpleural pressure minus the alveolar pressure ($P_{PL} - P_A$)
(D) It is equal to the alveolar pressure minus the interpleural pressure ($P_A - P_{PL}$)
(E) It is independent of lung volume when the muscles are relaxed

5. Airway resistance can be reduced by

(A) increasing vagal impulses to the lungs
(B) administering a β-adrenergic blocking drug
(C) decreasing the radial traction exerted by lung tissue
(D) performing a maximal forced expiration
(E) increasing lung volume

6. A reduction of arterial O_2 tension is typical of which one of the following?

(A) Anemia
(B) CO poisoning
(C) Moderate exercise
(D) Cyanide poisoning
(E) Hypoventilation

7. Which one of the following statements regarding the compliance of the respiratory system is true?

(A) It is greater than the compliance of the chest wall
(B) It is greater than the compliance of the lungs
(C) It is equal to the compliance of the chest wall
(D) It is equal to the compliance of the lungs
(E) It is less than the compliance of the chest wall

8. During the effort-independent portion of a forced vital capacity (FVC) maneuver, the expiratory flow rate

(A) varies as a function of the interpleural pressure
(B) is limited by compression of the airways
(C) depends on the alveolar pressure
(D) is maximal for that individual
(E) is constant

9. A lack of normal surfactant, as occurs in infants with respiratory distress syndrome (RDS), results in

(A) increased lung compliance
(B) stabilization of alveolar volume
(C) increased retractive force of the lungs
(D) reduced alveolar–arterial O_2 tension difference
(E) decreased filtration forces in the pulmonary capillaries

10. During inspiration, as the diaphragm contracts, the pressure in the interpleural space becomes

(A) equal to zero
(B) more positive
(C) more negative
(D) equal to the pressure in the alveoli
(E) equal to the pressure in the atmosphere

11. The volume of gas in the lungs at the end of a normal expiration is referred to as the

(A) residual volume (RV)
(B) expiratory reserve volume (ERV)
(C) functional residual capacity (FRC)
(D) inspiratory reserve volume (IRV)
(E) total lung capacity (TLC)

12. The major area of airway resistance during breathing is located in the

(A) oropharynx
(B) trachea and large bronchi
(C) intermediate-sized bronchi
(D) bronchioles < 2 mm in diameter
(E) alveoli

13. A patient with restrictive lung disease (RLD) typically has

(A) an increased forced expiratory volume in 1 second (FEV_1) and a normal lung compliance
(B) a decreased FEV_1 and an increased lung compliance
(C) a decreased FEV_1 and a decreased lung compliance
(D) an increased FEV_1 and an increased lung compliance
(E) an increased FEV_1 and a decreased lung compliance

14. The volume of N_2 dissolved in body fluids is greatest while breathing which of the following gas mixtures?

(A) Air at sea level
(B) Air at an altitude of 15,000 feet
(C) 20% O_2, 20% N_2, 60% He, while scuba diving at 2 atm of pressure
(D) 20% O_2, 30% N_2, 50% He, while scuba diving at 2 atm of pressure
(E) 20% O_2, 10% N_2, 70% He, while scuba diving at 5 atm of pressure

15. Increasing the tidal volume while keeping everything else constant increases the

(A) dead space ventilation
(B) functional residual capacity (FRC)
(C) inspiratory capacity
(D) alveolar ventilation
(E) alveolar CO_2 tension

16. Which of the following statements regarding the fraction of O_2 in inspired (tracheal) gas is true?

(A) It equals 0.25 at sea level
(B) It decreases as a function of altitude
(C) It varies as a function of the weather
(D) It is less than the fraction of O_2 in the atmosphere
(E) It equals the fraction of O_2 in the alveoli

17. Which one of the following statements regarding the CO_2 tension in mixed expired gas is true?

(A) It is greater than the alveolar CO_2 tension
(B) It is less than the alveolar CO_2 tension
(C) It is equal to the alveolar CO_2 tension
(D) It is equal to the atmospheric CO_2 tension
(E) It is greater than the CO_2 tension in venous blood

18. Alveolar ventilation is equal to the

(A) dead space ventilation
(B) tidal volume times respiratory rate
(C) minute ventilation
(D) minute ventilation minus dead space ventilation
(E) CO_2 production/min

19. A reduction in local alveolar ventilation is associated with

(A) an increase in regional pulmonary blood flow
(B) a decrease in regional alveolar CO_2 tension
(C) a decrease in regional alveolar O_2 tension
(D) an increase in regional tissue pH
(E) an increase in capillary hemoglobin saturation

20. The following figure shows two ventilatory patterns: one normal and the other abnormal. Which experimental maneuver listed below will create the abnormal pattern?

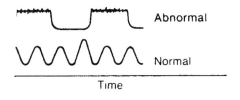

(A) Midpons transection with vagi intact
(B) Transection of the brain stem between the pons and medulla
(C) Midpons transection with vagi cut
(D) Transection rostral to the pons with vagi cut
(E) Transection rostral to the pons with vagi intact

21. The major sign of hypoventilation is

(A) cyanosis
(B) increased airway resistance
(C) hypercapnia
(D) dyspnea
(E) hypoxia

22. Which of the following statements regarding the normal alveolar CO_2 tension is true?

(A) It is equal in all alveoli
(B) It is highest at the base of vertical lungs
(C) It is directly proportional to the inspired O_2 tension
(D) It is directly proportional to the alveolar ventilation
(E) It is equal to 46 mm Hg

23. Hypercapnia affects respiration primarily by stimulating the

(A) carotid and aortic bodies
(B) receptors
(C) central (medullary) chemoreceptors
(D) arterial baroreceptors
(E) hypoglossal nerve

24. The vital capacity (VC) is the sum of the

(A) residual volume (RV), tidal volume, and expiratory reserve volume (ERV)
(B) RV, tidal volume, and inspiratory reserve volume (IRV)
(C) RV, ERV, and IRV
(D) ERV, IRV, and tidal volume
(E) functional residual capacity (FRC) and inspiratory capacity

25. The venous O_2 tension is higher than normal in which one of the following conditions?

(A) Cyanide poisoning
(B) Exercise
(C) Decreased cardiac output
(D) Anemia
(E) CO poisoning

26. The respiratory system is at the equilibrium position in all of the following conditions EXCEPT

(A) at the end of a normal expiration
(B) when the transrespiratory pressure is zero
(C) when lung recoil is balanced by chest wall expansion
(D) when lung volume is at residual volume (RV)
(E) when the respiratory muscles are relaxed and the airway is open

27. All of the following can reduce vital capacity (VC) EXCEPT

(A) decreased total lung capacity (TLC)
(B) increased residual volume (RV)
(C) weakness of the inspiratory muscles
(D) weakness of the expiratory muscles
(E) decreased alveolar surface tension

Questions 28–32 are based on the following graph, which shows a normal respiratory cycle followed by a maximal inspiration, a maximal forced expiration, and another normal respiratory cycle.

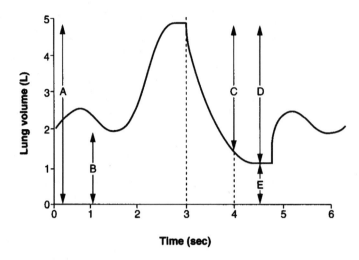

28. Select the lettered arrow that corresponds to vital capacity (VC)
29. Select the lettered arrow that corresponds to forced expiratory volume in 1 second (FEV$_1$)
30. Select the lettered arrow that corresponds to functional residual capacity (FRC)
31. Select the lettered arrow that corresponds to total lung capacity (TLC)
32. Select the lettered arrow that corresponds to residual volume (RV)

ANSWERS AND EXPLANATIONS

1. The answer is C [Chapter 16 III C 1 b (2); Chapter 20 II C 1 c (2), IV B]. The only treatment option that provides ventilation is the respirator. Administering supplemental O_2 may correct the hypoxia, but to correct hypercapnia, the lungs must be adequately ventilated. The patient certainly does not need extra CO_2, because he is hypercapnic. Neither the defibrillator nor the electrocardiograph will aid in ventilating the alveoli.

2. The answer is C [Chapter 16 IV C 1 a, 2 a (1)]. The driving force for gas flow is the alveolar pressure; during normal breathing, negative pressures cause inspiratory flow, and positive pressures cause expiratory flow. It is the ratio of alveolar pressure to airway resistance that determines the actual flow of gas. As lung volume approaches either total lung capacity (TLC) or residual volume (RV), much of the muscle force is expended in overcoming the low compliance of the respiratory system. When the lung volume is in mid-range, alveolar pressure may be either positive or negative depending on muscle activity. The abdominal muscles are expiratory muscles and, when contracted, generate positive alveolar pressures and expiratory flow if the airways are open.

3. The answer is B [Chapter 17 II A 3, C 2 a]. O_2 is much less diffusible than CO_2 in the lungs. The diffusion coefficient concerns the movement of molecules in solution and is determined by the molecular weight and the solubility of the substance. O_2 has a lower molecular weight than CO_2, but is also about 25 times less soluble. The increased diffusibility of CO_2 is important because there is a gradient of only approximately 5 mm Hg to cause CO_2 to diffuse from the pulmonary capillary blood to the alveoli.

4. The answer is D [Chapter 16 IV A, B]. In the lungs, the transmural pressure is the transpulmonary pressure, which equals the alveolar pressure minus the interpleural pressure ($PA − PPL$). The transmural pressure simply represents the pressure across the wall of a hollow organ and is defined as the inside pressure minus the outside pressure. In humans, the interpleural pressure is estimated by measuring the esophageal pressure, because the esophagus is a flaccid tube that essentially traverses the pleural space. The interpleural pressure in animal experiments usually is measured by inserting a needle into an intercostal space and connecting it to a pressure gauge. The transmural pressure across the chest wall (i.e., transthoracic pressure) equals the interpleural pressure minus the pressure at the body surface, which is usually equal to the atmospheric pressure ($PPL − PB$). The lung is a passive, elastic structure so that any change in lung volume produces a change in the transmural pressure.

5. The answer is E [Chapter 16 VII A 2 b (2), VIII B 1]. Increases in lung volume produce a mechanical force (i.e., radial traction) that acts on the airway walls, dilating the airways and reducing resistance. Radial traction is one of the most powerful factors that can alter airway resistance. The aging process can diminish radial traction, contributing to the higher airway resistance often seen in older individuals. Increasing vagal impulses to the lungs or administering a β-adrenergic blocking drug increases airway resistance by narrowing the airways: β-adrenergic blockers inhibit adrenergic substances (e.g., epinephrine) that act as bronchodilators, and stimulating the vagus nerve produces active contraction of bronchial smooth muscle. A forced expiration increases airway resistance, because the positive interpleural pressure compresses the large intrathoracic airways, creating a high-resistance, flow-limiting segment.

6. The answer is E [Chapter 17 III B 1; Chapter 20 II C 1 a, 4; Figure 20-6]. Hypoventilation can lead to arterial hypoxia, which is distinguished from other types of hypoxia by a low arterial O_2 tension and hypercapnia. In anemia and CO poisoning, the O_2 content (i.e., amount of O_2 carried by hemoglobin) is decreased, but the O_2 tension (i.e., amount of O_2 dissolved in plasma) is unaffected. In these disorders, the tissue or venous O_2 tension is reduced as a consequence of the inadequate O_2 delivery. Moderate exercise should not affect the arterial O_2 tension in a normal person.

7. The answer is E [Chapter 16 V D 1 b; Figure 16-8D]. The compliance of the respiratory system (CRS) is determined by the compliance of the lungs (CL) and the chest wall (CCW) and can be calculated as $1/CRS = 1/CL + 1/CCW$. Because of the need to add reciprocals, the compliance of the respiratory system always is less than the compliance of either of its parts.

8. The answer is B [Chapter 16 VIII B]. Dynamic compression of the airways occurs during forced expiration and limits the flow rate during the terminal 80% of expiration [i.e., effort-independent portion of a forced vital capacity (FVC) maneuver]. The driving force for expiration during the effort-independent period is the transpulmonary pressure, which is a function of lung volume. The term indicates that flow is independent of effort and that changes in expiratory force do not alter the flow rates. Therefore, the expiratory flow rate neither varies as a function of the interpleural pressure nor depends on the alveolar pressure, because these values are altered by expiratory effort. The expiratory flow rate is not maximal, because maximal flow can be achieved only when lung volume is just below total lung capacity (TLC).

9. The answer is C [Chapter 16 VI B 3 a (2)–(3)]. The lack of normal surfactant produces a high alveolar surface tension, which increases the retractile force of the lungs, resulting in a high transmural pressure. The high transmural pressure means that the lungs are less distensible, and the alveoli tend to collapse because of the increased surface forces. In addition, the increased alveolar surface tension decreases the interstitial pressure, which increases the filtration forces across the pulmonary capillaries and leads to edema. The edema and atelectasis cause an abnormal range of values of the ventilation–perfusion ratio ($\dot{V}A/\dot{Q}C$), which impairs gas exchange. The alveolar–arterial O_2 tension difference is a good measure of the gas exchange capabilities of the lungs; this difference increases in the presence of ventilation–perfusion or diffusion abnormalities.

10. The answer is C [Chapter 16 IV C 2 a (1); Figure 16-5]. Contraction of the inspiratory muscles expands the chest wall, increasing the transpulmonary pressure and making the interpleural pressure more negative. The chest wall expansion also expands the gas in the lungs, because the visceral and parietal pleurae are coupled by the interpleural fluid. The expansion of the alveolar gases decreases the alveolar pressure, which causes the gas to flow into the respiratory system through open airways.

11. The answer is C [Chapter 16 II B 4]. The functional residual capacity (FRC) is the volume of gas in the lungs at the end of a normal expiration. Because expiration is passive, the lung volume decreases during expiration until the equilibrium volume (i.e., FRC) is reached. The equilibrium volume represents the volume of a distensible structure when the transmural pressure (i.e., the pressure inside minus the pressure outside) is zero. The residual volume (RV) is the volume of gas in the lungs following a maximal expiration. The expiratory reserve volume (ERV) is the volume of gas that can be forcefully expired after a normal expiration, and the inspiratory reserve volume (IRV) is the additional volume of gas that can be inspired over the tidal volume. The total lung capacity (TLC) is the volume of gas in the lungs after a maximal inspiration.

12. The answer is C [Chapter 16 VII A 2 a (2), b]. The highest resistance to airflow occurs in the intermediate-sized bronchi because of the high airflow velocity in these segments. The airway tree develops such that each generation of airways is only slightly smaller in diameter than the parent airways. Thus, there is almost an exponential increase in cross-sectional area proceeding toward the periphery of the lung. Because of this relationship, the linear velocity of gas molecules decreases markedly as these molecules approach the terminal bronchioles. Therefore, very little pressure is required to achieve this velocity (i.e., there is a low resistance). Direct measurements indicate that bronchioles less than 2 mm in diameter represent less than 10% of the total airway resistance.

13. The answer is C [Chapter 16 IX C 1, X A 2 a–b; Figure 16-22]. By definition, patients with restrictive lung disease (RLD) have reduced lung compliance, and, typically, a reduced forced expiratory volume in 1 second (FEV_1) because of the reduced vital capacity (VC). These patients typically can expire a larger fraction of their own VC in 1 second because of the greater radial traction that results from the decreased compliance. Thus, these patients have a high FEV_1%, which is the ratio of the FEV_1 to the VC. The increased radial traction reduces airway resistance in the lungs. These patients have no difficulty breathing at high frequencies because of the low airway resistance and usually choose a high rate of respiration coupled with a reduced tidal volume to minimize the work of breathing.

14. The answer is A [Chapter 17 I A]. Among these choices, the volume of N_2 dissolved in the body fluids is greatest when breathing air at sea level. Henry's law states that the volume of gas dissolved in a liquid equals the partial pressure of the gas times the solubility coefficient. Because the partial pressure of N_2 at an altitude of 15,000 feet would be less than the partial pressure of N_2 at sea level, the amount of N_2 dissolved in the tissues also would be less. The N_2 tension when breathing air at sea level is 0.79 atm. Gas equilibration in the body requires approximately 12 hours after any change in pressure and occurs at different rates in different tissues. For N_2, equilibration takes the longest in the fatty tissues because of the high N_2 solubility and the low blood flow to this type of tissue. Scuba diving at 2 atm while breathing a gas with 20% N_2 provides 0.4 atm of N_2 tension. The other two scuba conditions yield N_2 tensions less than 0.79 atm as well.

15. The answer is D [Chapter 16 II B–C, III C]. If the respiratory rate, dead space, and ventilation–perfusion ratio ($\dot{V}A/\dot{Q}C$) remain constant, then an increase in tidal volume raises the minute and alveolar ventilation. Because the dead space ventilation equals the dead space volume times the respiratory rate, increasing the tidal volume has no effect on the dead space ventilation. The functional residual capacity (FRC) is not altered, and the inspiratory capacity is reduced by increases in tidal volume. Alveolar CO_2 tension is reduced by an increased alveolar ventilation because the increased ventilation washes out CO_2 from the alveoli.

16. The answer is D [Chapter 16 I B, III C 2 a]. The fraction of O_2 in inspired gas is less than the fraction of O_2 in the atmosphere, because nasal breathing adds water vapor to inspired air, which decreases the O_2 content of the air by the time it reaches the trachea. The fraction of O_2 in the air is constant from sea level to several hundred thousand feet altitude and equals 0.21. However, the O_2 tension decreases with increased altitude, because the total pressure declines as one ascends. The partial pressure of any gas is given by the product of the mole fraction of the gas and the total or barometric pressure. Alveolar gas is diluted by the addition of CO_2 from the blood, so that the fraction of O_2 in the alveoli is less than that in the trachea.

17. The answer is B [Chapter 16 III B 3]. Mixed expired gas has a lower CO_2 tension than alveolar gas because it is a mixture of alveolar and dead space gas. The composition of this gas varies depending on the ratio of dead space ventilation to alveolar ventilation. This fact can be used to determine the dead space–tidal volume ratio:

$$VD/VT = 1 - PECO_2/PACO_2$$

where VD/VT = dead space–tidal volume ratio; $PECO_2$ = CO_2 tension of mixed, expired gas; and $PACO_2$ = CO_2 tension of alveolar gas.

The CO_2 tension in venous blood is higher than that in alveolar gas, which is why CO_2 diffuses from the pulmonary capillaries into the alveoli.

18. The answer is D [Chapter 16 III C]. Alveolar ventilation equals the minute ventilation minus the dead space ventilation. Minute ventilation is the volume of gas expired per minute, which is equal to the product of tidal volume times respiratory rate. Not all of the minute ventilation reaches the gas exchange region of the lungs; some remains in the conducting system.

19. The answer is C [Chapter 18 IV A 2]. A decrease in local (i.e., regional) alveolar ventilation decreases the influx of gas to that region of the lung, so that, transiently, more O_2 is absorbed, and less CO_2 is flushed out. Consequently, in the affected area of the lung, the alveolar O_2 tension declines and the alveolar CO_2 tension increases. The hypoxia, hypercapnia, and resultant local acidosis cause hypoxic pulmonary vasoconstriction (HPV), which results in a decrease in pulmonary blood flow to the affected area of the lungs. The decrease in local O_2 tension reduces the hemoglobin saturation of the blood that leaves this area of the lung. These changes represent the effects of a low ventilation–perfusion ratio ($\dot{V}A/\dot{Q}C$) on gas exchange in a localized area of the lung.

20. The answer is C [Chapter 19 I C 1; Figure 19-6]. This pattern of breathing is called apneustic breathing, or inspiratory breath-holding, which occurs when the inhibitory influences from both the periphery (via the vagus nerves) and the pneumotaxic center (PNC) are interrupted. The PNC lies in the rostral pons, and the apneustic center (ANC) [which enhances inspiratory drive] lies in the caudal pons. The vagus nerve carries impulses from stretch receptors in the airways that tend to inhibit inspiration after a certain threshold of tidal volume is exceeded.

21. The answer is C [Chapter 16 III C 1 b (2); Chapter 20 II B 1, C 1 a]. Hypercapnia is pathognomonic of hypoventilation, because the alveolar CO_2 tension is determined primarily by the alveolar ventilation. Cyanosis may be present with hypoventilation, but it is a sign (and not a very good one) of hypoxia, not hypoventilation. Both an increased airway resistance and dyspnea may be symptoms of airway disease, but neither is characteristic of hypoventilation.

22. The answer is B [Chapter 18; Figure 18-5]. The normal alveolar CO_2 tension is highest at the base of the lungs, because it varies inversely as a function of the ventilation–perfusion ratio ($\dot{V}_A/\dot{Q}_C$) and the alveolar ventilation. The $\dot{V}_A/\dot{Q}_C$ is low at the base of the lungs because blood flow exceeds ventilation. Therefore, CO_2 delivery to the lungs via the pulmonary blood flow is high, and the alveolar ventilation is insufficient to lower it to normal. The O_2 tension varies reciprocally with the CO_2 tension. In an individual inspiring air at sea level, the sum of the two gas tensions cannot exceed 150 mm Hg, which is the inspired O_2 tension, because the remaining gas fraction is occupied by N_2, which is not utilized by the body. Normally, the average alveolar CO_2 tension is maintained at 40 mm Hg to maintain the pH of body fluids in the normal range.

23. The answer is C [Chapter 19 I E]. Approximately 85% of the effect of CO_2 on the respiratory drive is mediated through the central (medullary) chemoreceptors; only 15% of the effect comes from the carotid and aortic bodies (i.e., peripheral chemoreceptors). CO_2 readily crosses the blood–brain barrier, but charged ions (e.g., H^+) do not. The hydration and subsequent dissociation of CO_2 into H^+ and HCO_3^- after it crosses the blood–brain barrier increases the H^+ concentration in the cerebrospinal fluid (CSF) and the brain tissues,

stimulating respiration. J receptors, arterial baroreceptors, and the hypoglossal nerve are not affected by changes in CO_2.

24. The answer is D [Chapter 16 II C; Figure 16-1]. The vital capacity (VC) consists of the expiratory reserve volume (ERV), the inspiratory reserve volume (IRV), and the tidal volume. It is the maximal amount of gas that can be expired after a maximal inspiration. Residual volume (RV), the fourth primary subdivision of lung volume, is not included in the VC; it is the small volume of gas that remains in the lungs after a maximal expiration. The RV prevents complete collapse of the alveoli.

25. The answer is A [Chapter 20 II C 4]. Cyanide poisoning causes the venous O_2 tension to be higher than normal, because the tissue oxidative enzymes are inactivated by cyanide and the cells utilize less O_2. Therefore, less O_2 diffuses out of the blood in the systemic capillaries, leaving a greater amount in the venous blood. During exercise, the tissues remove more O_2 from the capillary blood, which decreases the venous O_2 tension. A decreased cardiac output, anemia, and CO poisoning all reduce the O_2 delivery to tissues so more O_2 than normal is extracted from the capillary blood, and the venous O_2 tension declines.

26. The answer is D [Chapter 16 V C 1]. At residual volume (RV), the chest wall has a strong tendency to expand because it is far from its equilibrium position, which is about 80% of total lung capacity (TLC). At the same time, the recoil force of the lungs is reduced, because the RV is close to the equilibrium position of the lung. As a result of these unequal forces, either the expiratory muscles must be contracting to hold the respiratory system at that level, or the glottis must be closed to prevent gas from entering the airways. If the glottis is closed and the respiratory muscles are relaxed, then the strong expansion force of the chest wall causes the gas in the airways to expand. The alveolar gas pressure becomes less than atmospheric, and the transrespiratory pressure is negative.

27. The answer is E [Chapter 16 II B 4, C 1, VI B 3 a (2) (a), X A 1–2]. A decreased alveolar surface tension increases lung compliance, resulting in an increased total lung capacity (TLC) and an increased vital capacity (VC).

The VC equals the TLC minus the residual volume (RV), so either a decrease in TLC or an increase in RV can reduce the VC. Expanding the lungs to the normal TLC requires a strong inspiratory muscle force. Thus, weakness of the inspiratory muscles decreases the TLC. Similarly, expiratory muscle force is required to decrease the lung volume to the normal level of the RV. A decrease in expiratory muscle force can result in an increase in the RV.

28. The answer is D [Chapter 16 II C 2; Figure 16-1] The vital capacity (VC, indicated by the arrow labeled *D*) is the maximal volume of gas that can be expired after a maximal inspiration. The VC equals the sum of the tidal volume, the inspiratory reserve volume (IRV), and the expiratory reserve volume (ERV).

29. The answer is C [Chapter 16 X A 2 a; Figure 16-22]. The forced expiratory volume in 1 second (FEV_1) is the volume of gas that can be expired in 1 second during a maximal forced expiration. The forced expiration begins at the third second on the graph; the volume expired

1 second later is indicated by the arrow labeled *C*.

30. The answer is B [Chapter 16 II C 4; Figure 16-1]. The functional residual capacity (FRC, indicated by the arrow labeled *B*) is the reservoir of gas that remains in the lungs after a normal expiration. This gas buffers the changes in the O_2 and CO_2 tensions in the blood that traverses the capillaries between inspirations.

31. The answer is A [Chapter 16 II C 1; Figure 16-1]. The total lung capacity (TLC, indicated by the arrow labeled *A*) represents the amount of gas in the lungs after a maximal inspiration.

32. The answer is E [Chapter 16 II B 4; Figure 16-1]. The residual volume (RV, indicated by the arrow labeled *E*) is the amount of gas in the lungs after a maximal expiration. The RV cannot be removed from the lungs, because the chest wall becomes rigid, preventing further reduction of lung volume. In older individuals, the RV is set by closure of the airways, which prevents further emptying of the lungs.

PART **V**

RENAL PHYSIOLOGY

John Bullock

Chapter 21

Overview of Renal Function and Structure

I. FUNCTIONS

A. Maintenance of homeostasis (Table 21-1)

1. **Regulation of extracellular fluid (ECF) volume and composition.** The kidneys precisely balance the intake, production, excretion, and consumption of many organic and inorganic compounds via the conservation and excretion of water and solutes.
   a. **Intake of water and electrolytes**
      (1) **Ingested.** The gastrointestinal (GI) system is the primary source for the normal intake of water and electrolytes.
      (2) **Metabolically produced**
         (a) The **oxidation of food** provides a secondary but important source of **water.** The ordinary mixed diet leads to the production of approximately 300 ml of metabolic water per day, mostly from the oxidation of fat.
         (b) Metabolism also produces **urea,** a nontoxic product of protein metabolism; **uric acid,** the end product of purine metabolism; and **creatinine,** an endogenous anhydride of muscle creatine.
   b. **Excretion of water and solutes**
      (1) **Amounts excreted**
         (a) Normally, the kidneys excrete 1000–1500 ml/day of hypertonic urine. Along with the water, the kidneys must excrete about 600 mOsm/day of urinary solute, principally in the form of urea and salts of Na^+ and K^+.
            (i) The lower limit of urine dilution is 50 mOsm/kg H_2O. This requires an obligatory urine volume of 12 L/day (i.e., 600 mOsm/day ÷ 50 mOsm/kg H_2O).
            (ii) The upper limit of urine concentration is 1200 mOsm/kg H_2O. This requires an obligatory urine volume of 0.5 L/day (i.e., 600 mOsm/day ÷ 1200 mOsm/kg H_2O). This is the minimum volume of urine needed to excrete the daily urinary solute at maximum concentration.
         (b) About 100 ml of fluid together with 5 mEq each of sodium are excreted in the feces per day.
      (2) **Metabolic losses.** A nonperspiring young man in a basal metabolic state loses approximately 30 ml of water/hr by insensible perspiration. This, together with water loss from the lungs, constitutes the **insensible water loss,** which can range between 700 and 1000 ml/day, depending on body surface area and metabolic rate. **Sensible sweat** is a hypotonic solution with a Na^+ concentration ranging from 30 to 70 mEq/L of water.

2. **Acid–base homeostasis** (see Chapter 37)

TABLE 21-1. Daily Input and Output of Water and Sodium

	H$_2$O (ml/day) Normal	Prolonged, heavy exercise	Na$^+$ (mEq/day) Normal
INPUT			
Fluids ingested (water and food)*	2100	Variable	150
From metabolism (primarily fat metabolism)	200	200	...
Total input	2300	Variable	150
OUTPUT			
Insensible (skin)	350	350	25
Insensible (lungs)	350	650	...
Sweat†	100	5000	5
Feces	100	100	5
Urine	1400	500	115
Total output	2300	6600	150

*This represents the total intake resulting from drink (about 1300 ml) and food (about 800 ml).

†Sodium concentration of sweat ranges from 30–80 mEq/L.

B. Hormonogenesis

1. **Renin.** The formation and release of renin, which is a major component of the renin–angiotensin–aldosterone mechanism, allows the kidneys to regulate blood pressure by exerting control over fluid volume (see Chapter 14 II B 2).

2. **Renal erythropoietic factor (REF, erythropoietin).** The formation and release of REF increases the number of circulating erythrocytes.
   a. **Function.** REF is the primary regulator of red blood cell (RBC) formation in the bone marrow and is often produced in response to arterial hypoxia, hypokinetic hypoxia, and anemic hypoxia (see Chapter 20 II D 1 b). REF is the primary stimulus of erythropoiesis.
   b. **Source.** The peritubular capillary endothelial cells may be the major site of renal erythropoietin synthesis. In fetuses and neonates, the liver is the primary source of REF.
   c. **Clinical relevance.** The anemia in the setting of renal failure is primarily due to the impairment in erythropoietin production.

C. Vitamin D$_3$ activation. Dietary vitamin D$_3$ must undergo two hydroxylations in order to be useful to the body. The first step is performed by the liver. The final hydroxylation, performed by the kidneys, converts vitamin D$_3$ to its most biologically active form (1,25-dihydroxycholecalciferol) by the action of 1α-hydroxylase, a mitochondrial enzyme found in the cells of the proximal tubule.

D. Gluconeogenesis. The kidney acquires the important ability to synthesize and secrete glucose produced from noncarbohydrate sources (e.g., glutamine) only in unusual circumstances such as prolonged starvation and chronic respiratory acidosis.

1. The proximal tubule is the major site of renal gluconeogenesis.

2. The renal cortex utilizes pyruvate, lactate, citrate, α-ketoglutarate, glycine, and glutamine as gluconeogenic substrates.

3. The deamination of glutamine and glutamate serves the dual purpose of gluconeogenesis and ammonium ion formation.

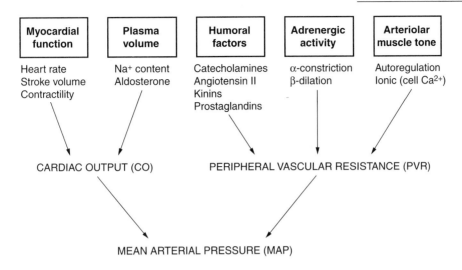

FIGURE 21-1. Physiologic determinants of mean arterial blood pressure (MAP).

E. **Regulation of blood pressure** (Figure 21-1). The kidneys play a critical role in the long-term maintenance of blood pressure by virtue of their regulation of blood volume, which is mediated through Na$^+$ balance.

1. **An increase in blood volume leads to increased excretion of Na$^+$ and H$_2$O,** which tends to correct the increase in blood (plasma) volume. The converse of this statement is also true.

2. The **Na$^+$ content of the body** can only be constant if renal Na$^+$ excretion balances net dietary input.

3. Changes in **Na$^+$ content** produce parallel changes in ECF volume, blood volume, and arterial pressure. The stability of arterial blood pressure is a function of Na$^+$ balance.

4. The primary determinants of **mean arterial pressure (MAP)** are cardiac output (CO) and peripheral vascular resistance (PVR), as indicated in the following expression:

$$MAP = CO \times PVR$$

   a. Cardiac output is determined by plasma volume, stroke volume, heart rate, and myocardial contractility.

   b. PVR is a function of the balance of humoral vasoconstrictor and vasodilator factors, adrenergic activity, and the intrinsic smooth muscle tone of the arterioles.

   c. The four integrated systems for the maintenance of blood pressure are:

   (1) Arterial baroreceptor reflex

   (2) Renal regulation of plasma volume by the aldosterone effect on **Na$^+$ content**

   (3) The renin–angiotensin II–aldosterone system

   (4) Vascular autoregulation of myogenic tone

II. **STRUCTURE** (Figure 21-2). The kidneys are paired organs that are located retroperitoneally in the upper dorsal region of the abdominal cavity. Each human kidney is composed of approximately 1 million nephrons, is about the size of a fist, and weighs approximately 150 g.

A. **Nephron** (Figure 21-3)

1. **Components.** This basic functional unit of the kidney is composed of a glomerulus, with its associated afferent and efferent arterioles, and a renal tubule.

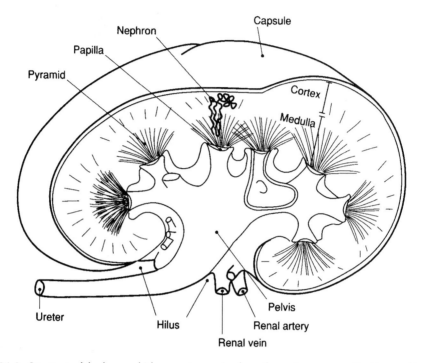

FIGURE 21-2. Structure of the human kidney, cut away to show the various zones. (Redrawn with permission from Marsh DJ: *Renal Physiology*. New York, Raven, 1983, p 37.)

   a. **Glomerulus** (Figure 21-4). The glomerulus consists of an expanded, invaginated bulb **(Bowman's capsule),** which houses a **tuft of 20–40 capillary loops.**
   b. **Renal tubule** (see Figure 21-3)
      (1) **Bowman's capsule** forms the beginning of the renal tubule. Its epithelium is an attenuated layer that is about 4 μm thick.
      (2) **Proximal tubule.** The proximal tubule consists of a convoluted segment and a straight segment (pars recta).
      (3) **Loop of Henle.** The loop of Henle consists of the **thin descending limb** and the **thin and thick segments of the ascending limb.**
      (4) **Cortical segments.** The **distal convoluted tubule,** the **connecting tubule,** and the **cortical collecting duct** comprise the three cortical segments.
      (5) **Medullary collecting duct.** The medullary collecting duct carries the final urine to the renal pelvis and ureter.

2. **Types of nephrons**
   a. **Cortical nephrons** comprise approximately 85% of the nephrons in the kidney and have glomeruli located in the renal cortex. These nephrons have **short loops of Henle,** which descend only as far as the outer layer of the renal medulla.

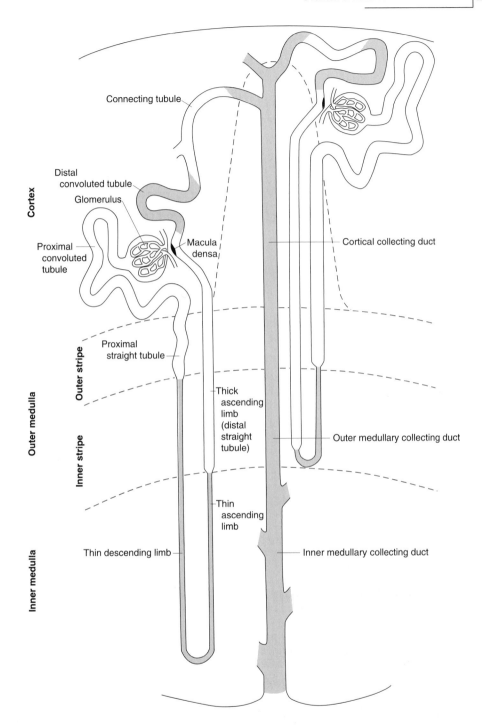

FIGURE 21-3. Detail of the functional unit of the kidney showing a cortical (superficial) nephron on the *right,* and a juxtamedullary nephron on the *left. Shaded areas* delineate tubule and collecting duct segments. The macula densa can be seen at the junction of the thick ascending limb and the distal convoluted tubule. Collectively, the distal convoluted tubule, connecting tubule, cortical collecting duct, and medullary collecting duct are known as the distal nephron. (Redrawn with permission from Windhager EE (ed): Renal physiology VII. In *Handbook of Physiology,* sect 8. Published for the American Physiological Society, New York, Oxford University Press, 1992, p 2443.)

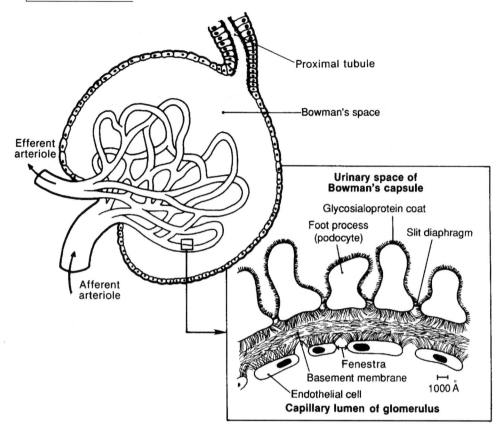

FIGURE 21-4. Organization of the glomerulus. The afferent arteriole forms a capillary plexus, which then fuses to form the efferent arteriole. The outer lining of the glomerulus, called Bowman's capsule, is continuous with the proximal tubule. (Reprinted from Marsh DJ: *Renal Physiology.* New York, Raven Press, 1983, p 41.) **Inset:** Glomerular capillary wall in cross-section. The luminal surface is covered by fenestrated endothelial cells. The basement membrane has a middle lamina densa surrounded by lamina rara interna and externa. Overlying this are the foot processes of epithelial cells, separated by small slit diaphragms. The endothelium, basement membrane, and filtration slits contain negatively charged proteoglycans (glycoproteins) because of the sialic and dicarboxylic amino acid residues. (Illustration by Nancy Lou Gahan Markris. Reprinted from Brenner BM, Beeuwkes R III: The renal circulations. *Hosp Pract* 13:35–46, 1978.)

    b. Juxtamedullary nephrons begin at the junction of the cortex and the medulla of the kidney. Juxtamedullary nephrons have **long loops of Henle,** which penetrate deep into the medulla and sometimes reach the tip of the renal papilla. These nephrons are important in the **countercurrent system,** by which the kidneys concentrate urine.

B. **Renal blood vessels**

    1. Renal arteries. Each kidney receives a renal artery, which is a major branch from the aorta.

      a. Afferent and efferent arterioles

        (1) Afferent arterioles. Each renal artery subdivides into progressively smaller branches, and the smallest branches give off a series of afferent arterioles.

          (a) Each afferent arteriole contributes to the tuft of capillaries that protrudes into Bowman's capsule.

          (b) The capillary endothelium is **fenestrated** and has an **incomplete basement membrane.** These features minimize resistance (allowing plasma filtration) and act as a sieve (allowing retention of plasma proteins and blood cells).

(2) Efferent arterioles. The capillaries within Bowman's capsule come together and form a second arteriole, the efferent arteriole, which divides shortly after to form the peritubular capillaries that surround the various portions of the renal tubule.

b. **Peritubular capillaries** differ in organization depending on their association with different nephrons.

(1) The efferent arterioles of **cortical nephrons** divide into peritubular capillaries that connect with other nephrons, forming a rich meshwork of microvessels. This meshwork functions to remove water and solutes that have diffused from the renal tubules.

(2) The efferent arterioles of **juxtamedullary nephrons** form the **vasa recta.** The vasa recta descend with the long loops of Henle into the renal medulla and return to the area of the glomerulus, forming capillary beds at different levels along the loop of Henle.

2. **Renal veins** are formed from the confluence of the peritubular capillaries and exit the kidney at the **hilus.** The pattern of the renal venous system is similar to that found in the end arterial system, except for the presence of multiple anastomoses between veins at all levels of the venous circulation.

III. RENAL BLOOD FLOW

A. **Rate.** Renal blood flow is approximately **1200 ml/min (400 ml/100 g tissue/min).** Under basal conditions, the total renal blood flow is approximately **20% of the resting cardiac output.** During exercise, sympathetic tone to renal vessels increases and shunts renal blood flow to the skeletal muscles.

B. **Significance.** In addition to supplying O_2 and metabolic substrates to the kidneys, a large renal blood flow is required to produce a high glomerular filtration rate (GFR) for the excretion of metabolic by-products (e.g., urea, uric acid, creatinine).

1. **O_2 requirements.** In terms of O_2 consumption, the kidney is ranked second to the heart. Renal O_2 consumption is approximately **6 ml/100 g tissue/min.**

a. **Arteriovenous O_2 difference.** The difference between the arterial and venous O_2 content in the human kidney is approximately 1.5 ml/dl of blood, which is the smallest arteriovenous O_2 difference of the major organ systems.

b. **Relationship to renal blood flow.** The kidneys are unique in that changes in blood flow are accompanied by parallel changes in O_2 consumption. Renal O_2 consumption correlates best with the active reabsorption of Na^+, but a significant fraction is also required for H^+ secretion via the H^+–ATPase pumps.

(1) A decline in blood flow is usually associated with a decrease in the GFR, which leads to a decrease in the filtered load of NaCl to be reabsorbed.

(2) Because tubular reabsorption of Na^+ is the major determinant of renal O_2 consumption, the metabolic demand for O_2 consumption is reduced when renal blood flow is lowered. Unlike other organs, where the blood flow is related to the O_2 requirements of the organ, in the kidney, the O_2 consumption is a function of blood flow.

2. **GFR.** The high blood flow to the kidney reflects the need to supply fluid (i.e., plasma) for filtration. The excretion of urea, the primary end-product of protein catabolism, is dependent on the GFR and renal blood flow.

IV. KEY EQUATIONS

A. **Renal physiology equations** (Table 21-2)

B. **Acid–base equations** (Table 21-3)

TABLE 21-2. Renal Physiology Equations

Clearance	$C = \dfrac{U_x \cdot \dot{V}}{P_x}$	(ml/min)
Osmolal clearance	$C_{osm} = \dfrac{U_{osm} \cdot \dot{V}}{P_{osm}}$	(ml/min)
Free-water clearance	$C_{H_2O} = \dot{V} - C_{osm}$	(ml/min)
Free-water reabsorption	$-C_{H_2O} = T^c{}_{H_2O} = C_{osm} - \dot{V}$	(ml/min)
Clearance ratio	$CR = \dfrac{C_x}{C_{in}} = \dfrac{U_x \cdot \dot{V}}{GFR \cdot P_x}$	(no units)
Glomerular filtration rate	$GFR = \dfrac{U_{in} \cdot \dot{V}}{P_{in}} = C_{in}$	(ml/min)
Effective renal plasma flow (Fick)	$ERPF = \dfrac{U_{PAH} \cdot \dot{V}}{P_{PAH}}$	(ml/min)
True renal plasma flow	$TRPF = \dfrac{ERPF}{E}$	(ml/min)
Extraction ratio (E)	$E = \dfrac{A_{PAH} - V_{PAH}}{A_{PAH}}$	(no units)
Renal blood flow	$RBF = \dfrac{P_{aorta} - P_{RV}}{R}$	(ml/min)
Renal blood flow	$RBF = \dfrac{RPF}{1 - Hct}$	(ml/min)
Renal blood flow (Fick)	$RBF = \dfrac{\text{Excretion of X}}{A_x - V_x} = \dfrac{\dot{E}}{A_x - V_x}$	(ml/min)
Renal blood flow (Fick)	$RBF = \dfrac{\dot{V}_{O_2}}{A_{O_2} - V_{O_2}}$	(ml/min)
Filtration fraction	$FF = \dfrac{GFR}{RPF} = \dfrac{C_{in}}{C_{PAH}}$	(no units)
Filtered load	$\dot{F} = GFR \cdot P_x$	(mg/min)
Amount filtered	$\dot{F} = C_{in} \cdot P_x$	
Filtered load	$\dot{F} = C_{cr} \cdot P_{cr}$	
Amount reabsorbed	$\dot{R} = \dot{F} - \dot{E}$	(mg/min)
Reabsorption rate	$\dot{R} = (GFR \cdot P_x) - (U_x \cdot \dot{V})$	
Amount secreted	$\dot{S} = \dot{E} - \dot{F}$	(mg/min)
Secretion rate	$\dot{S} = (U_x \cdot \dot{V}) - (GFR \cdot P_x)$	
Amount excreted (Excretion rate)	$\dot{E} = \dot{F} + \dot{S} - \dot{R}$	(mg/min)
Fractional excretion	$FE_x = \dfrac{\dot{E}}{\dot{F}}$	(no units)
(see Clearance ratio)		

TABLE 21-2. Renal Physiology Equations (*Continued*)

$$FE_x = \frac{U_x \cdot \dot{V}}{GFR \cdot P_x} = \frac{C_x}{C_{in}}$$

Fractional reabsorption	$FR_x = \dfrac{\dot{R}}{\dot{F}}$	(no units)
	$FR_x = \dfrac{(GFR \cdot P_x) - (U_x \cdot \dot{V})}{GFR \cdot P_x}$	
Dilution principle	$V = \dfrac{\text{Mass}}{\text{Concentration}}$	(ml)
Intracellular fluid volume	ICFV = Total body water − ECFV	(ml)
Interstitial fluid volume	ISFV = ECFV − PV	(ml)
Net filtration pressure	$NFP = P_{GC} - COP_{GC} - P_{BC}$	(mm Hg)
Glomerular filtration rate	$GFR = K_f \cdot NFP$	(ml/min)
Filtration coefficient	$K_f = L_P \cdot S$	(ml/min/mm Hg)

TABLE 21-3. Acid–Base Equations

Logarithmic (Briggsian)		
	$[H^+] = \text{antilog}(9 - pH)$	
	$pH = 9 - \log[H^+]$	
Henderson Equation (nonlogarithmic)		
PCO_2 in mm Hg	$[H^+] = 24\,\dfrac{PCO_2}{[HCO_3^-]}$	(nEq/L;nM/L)
$[HCO_3^-]$ in mEq/L	$[HCO_3^-] = 24\,\dfrac{PCO_2}{[H^+]}$	
	$PCO_2 = \dfrac{[H^+]\,[HCO_3^-]}{24}$	
Net acid excretion (NAE)	$(TA + NH_4^+) - HCO_3^-$	(mEq/day)
	$[(U_{TA} \cdot \dot{V}) + (U_{NH_4} + \dot{V})] - (U_{HCO_3}^- \cdot \dot{V})$	

Concentration units: mM/L · valence (mEq/L); mM/L · # particles formed in solution (mOsm/L)

Case

A man has suffered a significant blood loss over 20 minutes. At the end of this period, **his arterial blood pressure has fallen from 100 mm Hg to 70 mm Hg, and his heart rate has increased from 70 beats/min to 140 beats/min. His hematocrit is 36%, and his skin is cold.**

    1. *How might you describe the renal responses to volume depletion due to hemorrhage?*

DISCUSSION

The decrease in blood pressure as a result of the blood loss is detected by the carotid sinus and aortic arch, as well as by other baroreceptors in the veins, atria, and afferent arteriole. This fall in pressure decreases the firing rate of the baroreceptors via the ninth (IX) and tenth (X) cranial nerves to the cardiovascular centers in the brain stem, which respond by sympathetic outflow to the heart and vascular smooth muscle. Sympathetic stimulation of the renal arterioles by both the renal nerves and epinephrine from the adrenal medulla causes both renal afferent and efferent arteriolar constriction, which decreases renal blood flow.

In addition, these reflexes decrease the glomerular filtration rate (GFR) to a lesser degree. When sympathetic tone is increased, both afferent and efferent arterioles receive sympathetic innervation and constrict, but not to the same extent. The decline in GFR is less than the fall in renal blood flow because the efferent arterioles lie distal to the glomerulus. Therefore, an increase in resistance **raises** glomerular capillary pressure; this is just the opposite of the effect of afferent arteriolar constriction. Thus, sympathetically induced afferent and efferent arteriolar constriction have **opposing** effects on glomerular capillary pressure—hence, GFR—but additive (parallel) effects on renal vascular resistance—hence, renal blood flow. Because renal blood flow decreases relatively more than GFR, the filtration fraction (FF) [GFR/renal plasma flow] increases.

The renal vasoconstriction contributes to the rise in total peripheral resistance, which contributes to the restoration of arterial blood pressure toward normal. Vasoconstriction also helps raise arterial blood pressure by increasing the retention of Na^+ and water via stimulation of the renin–angiotensin II–aldosterone axis and antidiuretic hormone (ADH) secretion.

The second major regulator of renal blood flow and GFR is angiotensin II via its two major actions—Na^+ and H_2O retention—together with vasoconstriction of both the afferent and efferent arterioles. Because the diameter of the efferent arteriole is smaller, the increase in efferent arteriolar resistance is much greater. The net effect of angiotensin II is a reduction in renal blood flow and an **elevation** in the hydrostatic pressure in the glomerular capillary, which tends to maintain GFR when the renin–angiotensin–aldosterone axis is activated.

    2. *What is the effect of hemorrhage on the plasma oncotic pressure?*

DISCUSSION

Hemorrhage does not immediately alter plasma protein concentration, because all components are lost in equivalent proportions. However, it lowers venous pressure, and, in turn, capillary hydrostatic pressure. The change in Starling forces reduces or stops filtration of fluid out of the capillaries, which leads to partial restitution of blood volume from the interstitial space as the fluid enters the capillaries. Thus, immediately following blood loss, the proportion of red cell volume to plasma volume (hematocrit) in the vascular compartment is unchanged. However, the hematocrit falls over several hours as the red cells are diluted by the fluid moving from the interstitial fluid (ISF) space into the intravascular space.

The entry of protein-free fluid from the interstitium lowers the plasma protein concentration, which tends to raise GFR. This response is inappropriate because Na^+ conservation, not Na^+ loss, is a proper response to hemorrhage. It is important to appreciate that the decreased arterial pressure and increased sympathetic outflow to the afferent arterioles causes the glomerular capillary hydrostatic pressure to fall to a greater degree than the plasma oncotic pressure falls.

Chapter 22

Body Fluids

I. **WATER CONTENT AND DISTRIBUTION.** The two major fluid compartments are the intracellular fluid (ICF) and extracellular fluid (ECF) volumes.

A. **Total body water (TBW)** constitutes 55%–60% of the body weight in young men and 45%–50% of the body weight in young women. The lower percentage in women largely is due to the relatively greater amount of adipose tissue in women than in men. Body water is inversely related to body fat.

1. **Distribution.** Approximately one-third of the TBW is in the ECF compartment, and the remaining two-thirds is in the ICF compartment (Table 22-1). TBW is distributed as follows:
   a. Muscle (50%)
   b. Skin (20%)
   c. Other organs (20%)
   d. Blood (10%)

2. **Lean body mass (LBM).** Although the percentage of TBW declines with advancing age and with obesity, the percentage for any individual (regardless of gender) remains a constant 70% of that individual's LBM (fat-free mass).* Based on this constant relationship, the amount of body fat can be determined as:

$$\text{Body fat (\%)} = 100 - \frac{\text{percentage of TBW}}{0.7}$$

and the LBM can be estimated as:

$$\text{LBM (kg)} = \frac{\text{TBW (L)}}{0.7}$$

B. **Extracellular fluid (ECF).** The ECF compartment has several subcompartments.

1. **Plasma** volume, the fluid portion of the blood, represents approximately 25% of the ECF.
   a. **Blood volume,** which occupies approximately 80 ml/kg of body weight (8%) can be obtained from the plasma volume and the hematocrit:

   $$\text{Blood volume (L)} = \text{plasma volume (L)} \cdot \frac{100}{(100 - \text{hematocrit})}$$

   b. **Plasma volume,** then, can be calculated from the blood volume and the hematocrit:

   $$\text{Plasma volume (L)} = \text{blood volume (L)} \cdot \frac{(100 - \text{hematocrit})}{100}$$

2. **Interstitial fluid (ISF) [milieu interieur]** surrounds all cells except blood cells and includes lymph, which constitutes 2%–3% of the total body weight. On average, the ISF represents approximately 15% of the total body weight and 75% of the ECF. Edema is the palpable swelling produced by expansion of the ISF volume.

3. **Transcellular fluid** volume is about 1 L in most humans and occupies approximately 15 ml/kg of body weight (1.5%).
   a. This ECF subcompartment represents fluid in the lumen of structures lined by epithelium and includes digestive secretions; sweat; cerebrospinal fluid (CSF); pleural, peri-

---

*LBM is defined as 15% bone, 10% fat, and 75% tissue.

TABLE 22-1. Distribution of Body Water in a Young, 70–kg Man

| | | Percent | | |
| | Volume | Body | Lean Body | Body |
Compartment	(L)	Weight*	Mass	Water
Total body water (TBW)	42[†]	60[‡]	70	100
Extracellular fluid (ECF)	14	20	24	33
Plasma	3.5	5	6	8
Interstitial fluid	10.5	15	18	25
Intracellular fluid (ICF)	28	40	46	67

[†]20-40-60 rule: ECF (20%) + ICF (40%) = TBW (60%).
[†]Total body water is 35 L in a young 70-kg woman.
[‡]Body water accounts for 50% and 70% of the total body weight of a young 20-kg woman and a 5-kg neonate, respectively.

toneal, synovial, intraocular, and pericardial fluids; bile; and luminal fluids of the gut, thyroid, and cochlea.
   (1) Gastrointestinal (GI) luminal fluid constitutes about half of the transcellular fluid and occupies approximately 7.4 ml/kg of body weight.
   (2) CSF occupies approximately 2.8 ml/kg of body weight.
   (3) Biliary fluid volume is approximately 2.1 ml/kg of body weight.
  b. When the transcellular fluid compartment is unusually large, as in certain pathologic conditions (e.g., pleural effusions, ascites), it is referred to as the **third space** because this fluid is not readily exchangeable with the rest of the ECF.

C. **Intracellullar fluid (ICF).** The volume of the ICF compartment varies but usually constitutes 30%–40% of the body weight. This is the larger of the two major fluid compartments.

II. VOLUME MEASUREMENT IN THE MAJOR FLUID COMPARTMENTS

A. **Indicator dilution principle** (see also Chapter 13 II B). The volume of water in each fluid compartment can be measured by the indicator dilution principle. This principle is based on the relationship among the amount of a substance injected intravenously (A), the volume in which that substance is distributed (V), and the final concentration attained (c).

1. Equation. The equation for this relationship, based on the definition of concentration (c), is

$$c = \frac{A}{V} \text{ or } V = \frac{A}{c}$$

where V is the volume (in ml or L in which the quantity, A (in g, kg, or mEq), is distributed to yield the concentration, c (in g/ml or L or in mEq/ml or L).

Example. If 25 mg of glucose are added to an unknown volume of distilled water and the final concentration of glucose after mixing is 0.05 mg/ml, then the volume of solvent is

$$V = \frac{25 \text{ mg}}{0.05 \text{ mg/ml}} = 500 \text{ ml}$$

2. Application. Volume measurement by the dilution principle requires that the introduced substance be distributed evenly in the body fluid compartment being measured.

   a. The solute may leave the compartment through one of the following mechanisms:

     (1) Excretion in the urine or transfer to another compartment where it exists in a different concentration

     (2) Metabolism of the solute

     (3) Vaporization of the solute from the skin and respiratory tract

   b. The amount of substance lost from the fluid compartment, then, is subtracted from the quantity administered:

$$V = \frac{A \text{ administered} - A \text{ removed}}{c}$$

Example. A 60-kg woman is infused with 1 millicurie (mCi) of tritium oxide (^3H_2O). After 2 hours, 0.4% of the administered dose is lost in the urine and by vaporization from the skin and respiratory tract. The radioactivity of a plasma sample is measured by liquid scintillation spectrometry and indicates a concentration of 0.03 mCi/L of plasma water. Because the concentration of ^3H_2O throughout the body fluids should be the same as in plasma after the equilibration, the TBW can be calculated as

$$V = \frac{A \text{ infused} - A \text{ excreted}}{c}$$

$$= \frac{1 \text{ mCi} - (1 \text{ mCi} \cdot 0.004)}{0.03 \text{ mCi/L}}$$

$$= \frac{0.996}{0.03}$$

$$= 33.2 \text{ L}$$

  3. Markers. Regardless of compartment, desirable markers share **four qualities:**

   a. They are **measurable.**

   b. They **remain in the compartment being measured.**

   c. They **do not alter water distribution** in the compartment being measured.

   d. They are **nontoxic.**

  4. ^3H_2O is an unstable isotope and the substance of choice for measuring TBW. It is a weak beta emitter with a **biologic half-life** of 10 days but a **physical half-life of 12 years.** Other substances used to measure TBW include:

   a. Antipyrine and *N*-acetyl-4-amino antipyrine (NAAP), which rarely are used

   b. Deuterium oxide (^2H_2O), which is a stable isotope

   c. Urea and thiourea

B. **Extracellular fluid (ECF) volume**

  1. Plasma volume is measured using either of **two dilution methods.**

   a. The first method uses **substances that neither leave the vascular system nor penetrate the erythrocytes.** Such substances include:

     (1) Evans blue dye (T-1284)

     (2) Radioiodinated human serum albumin (RISA), which slowly leaks out of the circulation into the ISF

     (3) Radioiodinated gamma globulin and fibrinogen, which generally do not leak out of the bloodstream

   b. The second method is based on the fact that the radioisotopes of phosphorus (^{32}P), iron ($^{55,59}Fe$), and chromium (^{51}Cr) penetrate and bind to erythrocytes. The **tagged cells** are injected intravenously, and their volume of distribution is measured. Plasma volume is then calculated from the measured erythrocyte volume and hematocrit.

   c. Substances used to measure the ECF volume are of two types:

     (1) Saccharides such as inulin, sucrose, raffinose, and mannitol

     (2) Ions such as thiosulfate, thiocyanate, and the radionuclides of sulfate (SO_4^{2-}), chloride (Cl^-), bromide (Br^-), and Na^+

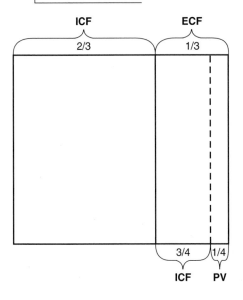

FIGURE 22-1. Distribution of water in a 70-kg adult man. The intracelluar-to-extracellular fluid volume ratio (ICF:ECF) is 2:1, and the interstitial fluid–to–plasma volume ratio (ISF:PV) is 3:1.

2. **ISF volume** cannot be measured directly, because no substance is distributed exclusively within this compartment. To measure the ISF volume, the capillary membranes must be permeable to a substance injected intravenously, which becomes distributed throughout the ECF and not exclusively in the interstitium. Therefore, the ISF volume is determined as the **difference between ECF volume and plasma volume.**

C. **Intracellular fluid (ICF) volume** cannot be measured directly by dilution, because no substance is confined exclusively to this compartment after intravenous injection of a marker substance. The ICF volume is obtained by subtracting the ECF volume from the TBW.

III. **DISTURBANCES OF VOLUME AND CONCENTRATION OF BODY FLUIDS** (Figures 22-1 and 22-2; Table 22-2) Because **aldosterone** regulates the **volume** of body fluid compartments and **antidiuretic hormone (ADH)** regulates the **concentration** of the body fluids, these two hormones attempt to reestablish normal volumes and concentrations by increasing or decreasing their secretion.

TABLE 22-2. Steady-State Changes in Volume and Osmolal Concentration of Body Fluids (ECF)

Type of Change	Volume (L)		Osmolality (mOsm/kg H$_2$O)	
	ICF	ECF	ICF	ECF
Contraction (dehydration)				
Isosmotic	0	↓	0	0
Hypersomotic	↓	↓	↑	↑
Hyposomotic	↑	↓	↓	↓
Expansion (overhydration)				
Isosmotic	0	↑	0	0
Hyperosmotic	↓	↑	↑	↑
Hyposmotic	↑	↑	↓	↓

The changes in volume and osmolality refer to the ECF compartment in the new steady-state.
ECF = extracellular fluid; ICF = intracellular fluid.

A. | Terms and general concepts

1. **Volume.** The general clinical terms for volume abnormalities are **dehydration** and **over-hydration.** Both conditions are associated with a change in ECF volume.

2. **Concentration. Osmolarity** refers to the number of solute particles per liter of solution, and **osmolality** refers to the number of solute particles per kilogram of water.
   a. The **tonicity** of a solution is related to the effect of the concentration of the solution on the volume of a cell (e.g., erythrocytes).
      (1) Isotonic solutions do not change the volume of the cell.
      (2) Hypotonic solutions cause a cell to swell, and if sufficiently dilute, to burst (lyse).
      (3) Hypertonic solutions cause a cell to shrink (undergo crenation).
   b. The adjectives **isosmotic, hyperosmotic,** and **hyposmotic** refer to the osmolar concentration of the ECF in its new steady-state and are used to describe changes in volume (i.e., dehydration, overhydration).

3. **Osmosis** (see Chapter 1 III B) determines the distribution of body water in the ECF and ICF compartments. When considering effective osmoles, osmotic equilibrium is achieved primarily by water movement. **Note** that although the cell membrane is permeable to Na^+ and K^+, both these ions are able to function as effective osmoles because they are restricted to their respective body fluid compartments by the Na^+–K^+–ATPase pump in the plasma membrane.

B. | Approach. A three-step method can be used to evaluate possible changes in volume and concentration.

1. **Identify the change in volume and osmolal concentration of the ECF.**
   a. Volume changes determine the state of hydration (i.e., the volume of **solvent** added to or removed from the ECF).
   b. Osmolal changes determine the type of hydration (i.e., the amount of **solute** that has been added to or removed from the ECF). All states of hydration (volume and osmolal concentration) are expressed in terms of ECF.

2. **Determine the direction of osmotic equilibrium.** Water diffuses from a region of lower solute concentration to a region of higher solute concentration.

3. After observing the water shift between the ICF and ECF, if any, **analyze the effect of water diffusion on the volume and concentration changes on the ECF and then on the ICF.**

C. | Units of concentration of body fluids. The **concentrations of body fluids** are relatively dilute.

1.
$$mEq/L = mmol \times valence$$
   (1) For example, 142 mEq/L of Na^+ = 142 mmol/L $\times$ 1.
   (2) For Ca^{2+}, 2.5 mmol/L = 5 mEq/L $\div$ 2.
$$mmol/L = mEq \div valence$$
   (3)
$$mOsm/Kg = mmol/L \times n$$
   where n is the number of dissociable particles per molecule (milliosmolality). For glucose, 300 mOsm/kg = 300 mOsm $\times$ 1. It should be noted that equation **(3)** is precise if the units mmol/L refer to mmol/L of **water** instead of mmol/L of **solution,** because 1 L of water equals 1 kg of water but 1 L of **solution** may contain less than 1 kg of water.

D. | Dehydration

1. **Definition.** Dehydration is a clinical state characterized by physical signs, which can be separated into two groups (Table 22-3), interstitial volume signs and plasma volume signs. This condition is caused by a decrease in ECF volume, specifically by the loss of Na^+ [i.e., a decrease in Na^+ content (negative Na^+ balance)].

TABLE 22-3. Physical Signs of Dehydration

Decreases in Interstitial Volume	Decreases in Plasma Volume
Decreased skin turgor ("tenting") and decreased tongue turgor	Increased heart rate
	Flat neck veins (patient supine) [low central venous pressure]
Soft and sunken eyeballs	
Dry mucous membranes	Increased arterial pulse
Dry cool skin	Decreased blood pressure (severe cases)
Sunken fontanelles (in infants)	Increased hematocrit

   2. Detection. Only a physical examination can diagnose dehydration. No clinical laboratory test can detect this state. Signs of dehydration include the following (see Table 22-3):
   a. Reduced urine flow. Decreased plasma volume leads to decreased perfusion pressure of organs including the kidneys, which, in turn, leads to decreased urine flow.
   b. Increased urine osmolality
   c. Decreased body weight due to fluid loss

   3. Treatment. Therapy requires Na^+ replacement for volume repletion.
   a. Intravenous fluids are usually provided as isotonic solutions.
   b. Oral therapy with dilute, glucose-containing NaCl solutions provides for more efficient intestinal Na^+ absorption.

   4. Dehydration (volume contraction) states (see Figure 22-2A)
   a. Isosmotic dehydration
      (1) Causes. Hemorrhage, plasma exudation through burned skin, and GI fluid loss (e.g., vomiting, diarrhea) lead to isosmotic dehydration.
      (2) Description
         (a) Initially, fluid is lost from the plasma and then is replaced from the interstitial space. No major change occurs in the osmolality of the ECF; therefore, no fluid shifts into or out of the ICF compartment.
         (b) Finally, the volume of the ECF is reduced with no change in osmolality.
   b. Hyperosmotic dehydration
      (1) Causes. Water deficits caused by decreased intake, diabetes insipidus (neurogenic or nephrogenic), diabetes mellitus, alcoholism, administration of lithium salts, fever, and excessive evaporation from the skin through heavy loss of sweat (e.g., heavy exercise), which is hypotonic, result in hyperosmotic dehydration.
      (2) Description
         (a) Initially, fluid is lost from the plasma, which becomes hyperosmotic, causing a fluid shift from the ISF to the plasma.
         (b) The rise in ISF osmolality causes fluid to shift from the ICF back to the ECF.
         (c) Finally, the ECF and ICF volumes both are decreased, and the osmolality of both major fluid compartments is increased.
   c. Hyposmotic dehydration
      (1) Causes. Causes include renal loss of NaCl because of adrenal insufficiency [e.g., primary hypoadrenocorticalism (Addison's disease)].
      (2) Description
         (a) Initially, loss of NaCl causes loss of water (solute diuresis). This is followed by water retention (water intoxication) with a continued loss of NaCL.
         (b) A net loss of NaCL in excess of water results in a decreased osmolality of the ECF and a subsequent shift of fluid from the ECF to the ICF compartment.
         (c) Finally, the ECF volume is decreased, the ICF volume is increased, and the osmolality of both major fluid compartments is decreased.

E. **Overhydration (volume expansion) states** (see Figure 22-2B)

   1. Isosmotic overhydration

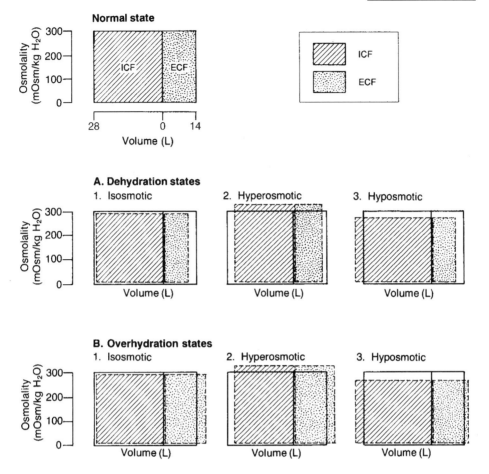

FIGURE 22-2. A Darrow-Yannet diagram representing the volume (*abscissa*) and osmolality (*ordinate*) of the intracellular and extracellular fluid (ICF and ECF) compartments in a 70-kg man. The area of each fluid compartment rectangle represents the total milliosmoles of solutes in that compartment. In all diagrams, the normal state is indicated by *solid lines,* and the shifts from normality are indicated by *dashed lines.* (Reprinted from Valtin H: *Renal Function: Mechanism Preserving Fluid and Solute Balance in Health,* 2nd edition. Boston, Little, Brown, 1983, p 272.)

    a. Causes. Edema and oral or parenteral administration of a large volume of isotonic NaCl (150 mmol/L) cause isosmotic overhydration.

    b. Description. Isosmotic overhydration is characterized by an overall expansion of the ECF volume with no change in the osmolality of the ICF and ECF compartments together with no change in ICF volume.

2. Hyperosmotic overhydration

    a. Cause. Oral or parenteral intake of large amounts of hypertonic fluid causes hyperosmotic overhydration.

    b. Description

        (1) Oral intake of large amounts of salt or intravenous infusion of a hypertonic saline solution leads to an increase in the plasma osmolality.

        (2) The rise in plasma osmolality causes water to shift from the interstitium into the plasma, thereby initially increasing plasma volume.

        (3) Concomitantly, the increase in plasma salt concentration causes NaCl to diffuse into the interstitium. The net result is an increase in the osmolality of the ECF.

        (4) The increase in the osmolality of the ECF causes water to flow out of the ICF, which eventually decreases the volume of the ICF and increases the volume of the ECF. The osmolality of both major fluid compartments is increased.

3. Hyposmotic overhydration

  a. Causes. Ingestion of a large volume of water and renal retention of water due to the syndrome of inappropriate antidiuretic hormone secretion (SIADH) are causes of hyposmotic overhydration.

  b. Description

  (1) Initially, water enters the plasma, causing a decline in the plasma osmolality, a shift of water into the interstitial space, and a decrease in the ISF osmolality.

  (2) The decrease in ISF osmolality causes water to shift from the ECF to the ICF compartment.

  (3) Finally, the ECF and ICF volumes increase and the osmolality of both major fluid compartments decreases.

F. Clinical applications

  1. Hypotonicity. This condition, in which body fluids are excessively dilute, occurs when the intake of electrolyte-free water exceeds free-water loss. Patients who exhibit hypotonicity always have hyponatremia.

  a. Because glucose is rapidly metabolized, the administration of glucose (dextrose) solutions is physiologically equivalent to the administration of distilled water. The primary indication for the use of dextrose solutions is to provide free water to replace insensible losses, correct hypernatremia due to a water deficit, or provide calories (1 g of glucose is the caloric equivalent of 4 kcal).

  b. One liter of an isosmotic glucose solution is distributed:

  (1) 670 ml (67%) in the ICF

  (2) 330 ml (33%) in the ECF, with 250 ml (25%) in the ISF and 80 ml (8%) in the plasma

  c. All solutions containing only permeant solutes (e.g., urea) must be regarded as hypotonic regardless of their osmolality. Therefore, for such solutions, osmolality and tonicity are not interchangeable terms.

  d. Solutions of impermeant solutes (e.g., NaCl solution) are osmotically effective. Therefore, for such solutions, osmolality and tonicity are interchangeable terms.

  2. Hypertonicity. This condition, in which cells are dehydrated, results from the loss of water or from the addition of solute.

  a. When caused by a water deficit or by the addition of Na^+ salts, hypertonicity is accompanied by hypernatremia.

  b. In diabetic ketoacidosis, glucose is confined to the extracellular space. It becomes an impermeant solute and, therefore, an effective osmole that causes water diffusion into the ECF and hyponatremia by dilution.

G. Darrow-Yannet diagram (see Figure 22-2). This diagram can simplify the clinical analysis of fluid balance. Important characteristics of the diagram include the following:

  1. The state of hydration is denoted in terms of the ECF volume.

  2. The ECF volume does *not* necessarily correlate with the plasma Na^+ concentration. Alterations in Na^+ balance result in changes in ECF volume, not in plasma Na^+ concentration or plasma osmolality. Plasma Na^+ concentration can be used as a measure of three pieces of information.

  a. Plasma $[Na^+]$ is a good index of P_{osm} (plasma osmolality), not the total amount of osmotically active solute either in the body or in the TBW.

  b. Plasma Na^+ concentration is a measure of concentration, not volume.

  c. Plasma Na^+ concentration is an index of water metabolism, not Na^+ metabolism.

  3. The ICF volume varies inversely with the plasma Na^+ concentration.

  4. Osmoregulation (i.e., osmolality of ECF) is maintained by ADH (vasopressin), which regulates (increases) free-water reabsorption by the collecting ducts.

  5. Volume regulation (i.e., size of ECF) is maintained by aldosterone, which regulates (increases) the amount of Na^+ reabsorbed by the collecting ducts.

6. Hypernatremia represents hyperosmolality and, in most instances, hyponatremia represents hyposmolality. One exception occurs with hyperglycemia when the plasma [Na$^+$] is lowered by the osmotic effect of elevated glucose in diabetic ketoacidosis.
   a. Hypernatremia is usually a sign of relative or absolute water deficit (dehydration), not Na$^+$ overload.
   b. Hyponatremia is usually a sign of water excess (overhydration), not Na$^+$ deficit.

7. Water flows from the compartment of lower osmolality (solute concentrations) to that of higher osmolality (solute concentration) until the osmotic pressures are equivalent. Because water is in osmotic equilibrium across the capillary wall and the cell membranes, measuring plasma osmolality also provides a measure of the osmolality of the ECF and ICF. The ICF and ECF are in osmotic equilibrium.

8. Because plasma membranes are relatively impermeable to Na$^+$ and Cl$^-$, sodium is an effective osmole between the ISF and ICF. However, sodium is not an effective osmole between the plasma and the ISF because of the high Na$^+$ permeability (low reflection coefficient) of the capillary membranes.

9. The major difference between the composition of the ISF and that of the plasma is that the plasma contains significantly more protein.

H. Osmoregulation versus volume regulation (Table 22-4)

1. Plasma osmolality is determined by the ratio of solutes (primarily Na$^+$ salts) and water (Table 22-5). The **Na$^+$ concentration** is regulated primarily by ADH.

2. ECF volume is determined primarily by the **absolute amount** (volume × Na$^+$ concentration), which, in turn, is regulated by aldosterone.

IV. IONIC COMPOSITION OF BODY FLUIDS (Table 22-6)

A. General considerations

1. **Ions** constitute approximately 95% of the solutes in the body fluids.

2. The sum of the concentrations (in mEq/L) of the **cations** equals the sum of the concentrations (in mEq/L) of the **anions** in each compartment, making the fluid in each compartment **electrically neutral.**

TABLE 22-4. Differences Between Osmoregulation and Volume Regulation

Characteristic	Osmoregulation	Volume Regulation
What is being sensed	Plasma osmolality	Effective circulating volume
Sensors	Hypothalamic osmoreceptors	Carotid sinus
		Afferent arteriole
		Atria
Effectors	ADH	Renin–angiotensin–aldosterone system
	Thirst	Sympathetic nervous system
		Natriutretic peptides, including ANP and urodilatin
		Pressure natriuresis
		ADH
What is affected	Water excretion	Urinary sodium excretion
	Water intake (via thirst)	

ADH = antidiuretic hormone; ANP = atrial natriuretic peptide.

TABLE 22-5. Osmotic and Volume Effects of Addition of NaCl, Water, Saline, and Glucose

Substance Added	Plasma Osmolality	Plasma Sodium Concentration	Extracellular Volume	Intracellular Volume
NaCl (hypertonic)	↑	↑	↑	↓
Water	↓	↓	↑	↑
Isotonic NaCl*	0	0	↑	0
Isosmotic Glucose	0	↓	↑	↑

*150 mM/L of 0.9% NaCl. After the infusion of 1 liter of isotonic saline the ISF volume increases by 750 ml and the plasma volume increases by 250 ml.

   3. Physicians rely on the changes in electrolyte concentrations in the ECF compartment, particularly in the plasma, in the diagnosis and treatment of patients with fluid or electrolyte imbalances, or both.

B. **Electrolyte concentrations in urine** (see Table 22-6)

   1. In a 70-kg man on an average diet, solute balance requires the renal excretion of metabolic wastes and excess dietary salt that total approximately 600 mOsm/day.

TABLE 22-6. Electrolyte Concentration of Body Fluids

Ion	(mg/L)	Plasma (mEq/L H_2O*)	Plasma (mmol/L H_2O*)	Interstitial Fluid (mEq/L H_2O*)	ICF (mEq/L H_2O*)	Urine (mEq/L)
Cations						
NA^+	3266	153	153	147	10	50–130
K^+	156	5.4	5.4	4	145	20–170
Ca^{2+}	50	2.7	1.35	2.4	<1	2–12
Mg^{2+}	27	1.9	0.95	1.8	27	5–18
NH_4^+	...	...	...	...	...	30–50
Total cations	3499	163	160.7	155.2	182	107–380
Anions						
Cl^-	3692	111	111	114	10	50–130
HCO_3^-	1464	26.2	26.2	30	10	...
Phosphate$^+$	104	1	0.55	1	80	20–40
Sulfate$^-$*	16	1.1	0.55	1	20	...
Proteinate$^-$	65,000	17.2	1.23	1	62	30–45
Organic acids	175	6.5	3.2	8.2	...	20–50§
Total anions	70,451	163	142.7	155.2	182	120–265
Total electrolytes	73,950	326	303.4	310.4		

   At the pH of body fluids, the proteins have multiple charges per molecule (average valence of -15). Hence, the ICF has more total charges than does the ECF. The total concentration of cations in each compartment must equal the total concentration of anions in each compartment when expressed in mEq/L. Determining the solute concentration in urine is of limited value because of the high variability of urine volume.
   ECF = extracellular fluid; ICF = intracellular fluid.
   *Concentration per liter of water; to convert to concentration per liter of plasma, multiply by 0.93.
   †HPO_4^{2-} (ECF, ICF): $H_2PO_4^-$ (urine).
   ‡As free sulfur.
   §Assuming average valence of -2.

2. However, water balance requires a much more variable renal water excretion. Simultaneous balance is accomplished by varying the osmolality of the urine (U_{osm}) relative to that of plasma, with the product remaining constant. In humans, the following relationship holds true:

$$U_{osm} \times \dot{V} = 600 \text{ mOsm/day}$$

where U_{osm} is urine osmolality in mOsm/kg H_2O and $\dot{V}$ is urine flow in L/day.

   a. Division of both sides of this equation by plasma osmolality (P_{osm}; about 300 mOsm/kg H_2O) gives the osmolal clearance (C_{osm}):

$$C_{osm} = \frac{V_{osm} \times \dot{V}}{P_{osm}}$$

$$= \frac{600}{300} = 2 \text{ L/day}$$

   b. C_{osm} represents the flow of isotonic urine required for the obligatory solute excretion.
   c. Because humans can maximally concentrate urine to about 1200 mOsm/kg H_2O, the necessary minimum flow rate of urine is about 0.5 L/day.

4. In normal individuals, urinary Na^+ excretion approximately equals dietary intake ($\approx$140 mEq/day).

C. Cations

1. The **monovalent cations** Na^+ and K^+ are the predominant cations of the ECF and ICF compartments, respectively. Essentially all of the body K^+ is in the exchangeable pool, whereas only 65%–70% of the body Na^+ is exchangeable. Only the exchangeable solutes are osmotically active.

2. The **divalent cations** Mg^{2+} and Ca^{2+} exist in body fluids in relatively low concentrations. Almost all of the body Ca^{2+} (in bone) and most of the body Mg^{2+} (in bone and cells) is nonexchangeable. After K^+, Mg^{2+} is the main cation of the ICF. After Na^+, Ca^{2+} is the main cation of the ECF.

D. Anions. The chief anions of the body fluids are Cl^-, bicarbonate (HCO_3^-), phosphates, organic ions, and polyvalent proteins.

1. Organic phosphates, proteins, and organic ions are the predominant anions in the ICF.
2. Cl^- and HCO_3^- are the predominant anions in the ECF.

Case 1

After running several miles, a man drinks 3 L of pure H_2O to replace the fluid lost by sweating. It is determined that his sweat has a Na^+ concentration of 75 mEq/L. Use the figure to help determine the answers to the following questions.

a. Water/electrolyte depletion

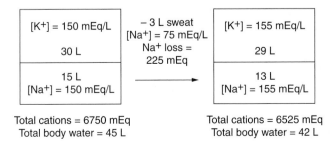

b. Water repletion

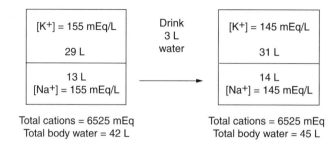

$$[K^+] = 155 \text{ mEq/L}$$

29 L

13 L
$$[Na^+] = 155 \text{ mEq/L}$$

Drink
3 L
water

$$[K^+] = 145 \text{ mEq/L}$$

31 L

14 L
$$[Na^+] = 145 \text{ mEq/L}$$

Total cations = 6525 mEq
Total body water = 42 L

Total cations = 6525 mEq
Total body water = 45 L

    1. *What is the volume of the man's intracellular fluid (ICF) and the extracellular fluid (ECF), and what is the concentration of K^+ and Na^+ in the ICF and ECF? (For purposes of simplicity, the kidney is assumed to play no role.)*

DISCUSSION

At the end of exercise the man is dehydrated (hyperosmotic dehydration) because sweat is a hypotonic solution. The replacement of the lost fluid with 3 L of water is distributed with 2 L in the ICF and 1 L in the ECF, resulting in an overall increase in the ICF volume and a decrease in the ECF volume compared to the preexercise level. The cation concentrations are also decreased.

    2. *Will the man continue to be thirsty after drinking the water?*

DISCUSSION

Because his ECF volume remains reduced, the man continues to be thirsty. It is important to appreciate that replacing the volume without solute leads to hyposmotic dehydration. Therefore, to replace the ECF, it is necessary to replace the lost electrolyte because Na^+ (and its attendant anions) determines the volume of the ECF. Furthermore, the volume of distribution of isotonic saline is the ECF volume, and the volume of distribution of water is the total body water (TBW).

Case 2

A 45-year-old woman who had previously been in good health suddenly developed abdominal cramps, nausea, vomiting, and diarrhea. Thirty-six hours after the onset of symptoms, when the cramps and diarrhea had subsided but the vomiting persists, she enters the hospital.

    At the time of hospitalization, she weighs 60 kg (usual 62 kg) and has a temperature of 37°C. Her blood pressure is 100/60 mm Hg (supine), her heart rate is 92 beats/min, and her respiration rate is 18/min. Her neck veins are not visible when she is supine. While sitting, her blood pressure is 70/20 mm Hg, with an increase in heart rate to 105 beats/min. Her abdomen is distended, and she has active bowel sounds.

    1. *What does this information indicate?*

DISCUSSION

The initial low blood pressure with postural hypotension, flat neck veins, and elevated hematocrit are consistent with an acute depletion of fluid (blood) volume. The weight loss and medical history suggest Na^+ and water loss from the gastrointestinal (GI) tract. The distended abdomen suggests some "third space" sequestration of saline to the transcellular fluid of the gut.

Laboratory tests reveal hematocrit, 50% (usual 40%); white blood cell (WBC) count, 10,500/μL; serum Na^+, 135 mEq/L; K^+, 3.5 mEq/L; Cl^-, 98 mEq/L; HCO_3^-, 24 mEq/L; glucose, 85 mg/dl; blood urea nitrogen (BUN), 35 mg/dl; creatinine, 1.2 mg/dl; and albumin, 3.6 g/dl. Urine volume is not recorded, but she voids several times.

The woman is placed on nasogastric suction and started on intravenous fluids. Over the next 24 hours she receives 6 L of half-isotonic saline (Na^+ concentration, 77 mEq/L), with each liter containing 60 mEq of KCl. Urine output is 2200 ml, and nasogastric suction is 1500 ml. The next day, her laboratory values are hematocrit, 39%; serum Na^+, 134 mEq/L; K^+, 3.5 mEq/L; Cl^-, 98 mEq/L; HCO_3^-, 25 mEq/L; glucose, 95 mg/dl; BUN, 20 mg/dl; and creatinine, 1.0 mg/dl. Blood pressure is 110/70 mm Hg without postural fall, and her neck veins are visible. Her abdomen is less distended. She weighs 63 kg (gain of 3 kg).

> **2.** *What do the laboratory data suggest?*

DISCUSSION

The common denominator in all hypovolemic disorders is diminution of the effective circulating volume. The decline in effective circulating volume sets in motion the cascade of events mediated by the neurohumoral effector systems that lead to vasoconstriction, tachycardia, antinatriuresis, and antidiuresis. The loss of Na^+ by hemorrhage or in fluids via the skin, gastrointestinal (GI) tract, or kidney leads to contraction of the plasma and interstitial volumes. Thus, the depletion of Na^+ is almost essential for hypovolemia.

It is important to appreciate that the hematocrit does not increase as a result of water depletion, because there is a proportionate loss from red blood cells (RBCs) and plasma. The only criterion needed for the diagnosis of water depletion is hypernatremia.

The normal serum Na^+ and glucose concentrations indicate no osmolar disturbance, while the normal serum HCO_3^- suggests the absence of an acid–base imbalance. The postural changes in blood pressure and heart rate are the most sensitive signs of depletion of the extracellular fluid (ECF). The hormonal response to hypovolemia includes increased antidiuretic hormone (ADH) and angiotensin II (aldosterone) secretion, both of which bring about repletion of the plasma volume.

The loss of isotonic fluid from the ECF is another consideration. This loss increases the plasma concentration (oncotic pressure) and decreases the capillary hydrostatic pressure, slowing filtration from the capillaries. As a result, there is a tendency to shift fluid into the intravascular compartment, leading to a disproportionate loss from the interstitial fluid (ISF). This attenuates the reduction of plasma volume.

Chapter 23

Overview of Renal Tubular Function

I. INTRODUCTION

A. The constancy of the body's internal environment is maintained, in large part, by the continuous functioning of its roughly 2 million nephrons. As blood passes through the kidneys, the nephrons clear the plasma of some substances (e.g., urea) while simultaneously retaining other, essential substances (i.e., water).

1. **Substances to be excreted** are removed by **glomerular filtration** and **renal tubular secretion** and passed into the urine.

2. **Substances that the body needs** are retained by **renal tubular absorption** (e.g., Na^+, HCO_3^-) and returned to the blood by **reabsorptive processes** (Figure 23-1).

B. **Glomerular filtration** is the initial step in urine formation.

1. The plasma that traverses the glomerular capillaries is filtered by the highly permeable **glomerular membrane,** and the resultant fluid, the **glomerular filtrate,** is passed into Bowman's capsule.

2. The term **glomerular filtration rate (GFR)** refers to the volume of glomerular filtrate formed each minute by all of the nephrons in both kidneys.

C. The terms **renal tubular secretion** and **renal tubular reabsorption** refer to the **direction of transport,** not to differences in the underlying mechanisms of transport.

1. **Secretion** refers to the transport of solutes from the peritubular capillaries into the tubular lumen (i.e., it is the **addition of a substance to the filtrate**).

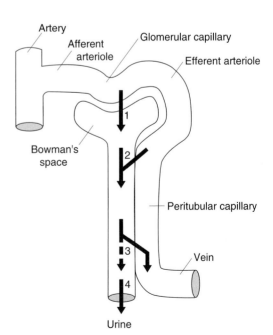

FIGURE 23-1. Filtration, secretion, and reabsorption. The amount excreted (*4*) equals the sum of the amounts filtered (*1*) and secreted (*2*) minus the amount reabsorbed (*3*).

2. Reabsorption denotes the active transport of solutes and the passive movement of water from the tubular lumen into the peritubular capillaries (i.e., it is the **removal of a substance from the filtrate**).

II. RENAL CAPILLARY MEMBRANE TRANSPORT

A. **Filtration** is the bulk transport of a fluid with its dissolved small solutes across the glomerular membrane. This solute transport mechanism, a passive process, is called solvent drag, or convection. It involves the transport of water and solute via transmembrane pathways, or pores.

1. A **hydrostatic pressure difference** between the glomerular capillaries and Bowman's capsule promotes filtration (see also Chapter 12 I C 5 b). On the other hand, some anions (HPO_4^{2-}) and cations (Ca^{2+} and Mg^{2+}) bind to plasma proteins to a significant extent; however, it is the **ionized concentration** which affects their rate of filtration. For example, approximately 50% of the total plasma calcium is bound to plasma proteins. Therefore, the rate of Ca^{2+} filtration is about 50% of the rate calculated from the product of the GFR and the **total** plasma calcium concentration. (This product is the filtered load of Ca^{2+}.)

2. Because there are **no concentration gradients for inorganic ions, glucose, amino acids,** and **inulin,** the concentrations in plasma and the ultrafiltrate in Bowman's space are the same.

3. The **filtered load** (i.e., the amount of solute transported across the glomerular membranes per unit time) is proportional only to the GFR and to the forces that affect filtration, namely differences in hydrostatic and oncotic pressure as well as **ionized concentration.** Mathematically, the filtered load is equal to the GFR times the plasma concentration of the solute.

B. **Simple diffusion** is the principal mode of transport in the interstitial space and within cells. For an ion, the driving force for diffusion consists of two gradients: a concentration gradient and an electric (voltage) gradient.

C. **Fenestrated** capillaries are found in association with secretory and reabsorptive epithelia. The endothelia of most of the exchange vessels in the kidney [except for the descending vasa recta (DVR)] are **fenestrated.**

III. RENAL EPITHELIAL TRANSPORT. The transport mechanisms of the proximal tubule are used as the basis for this discussion. Table 23-1 provides an overview of the transport mechanisms throughout the tubular segments of the nephron.

TABLE 23-1. Overview of Renal Transepithelial Transport

Carriers			
Pumps	**Symporters**	**Antiporters**	**Channels**
$3Na^+ - 2K^+ - ATPase$	$Na^+ - Glucose$	$Na^+ - H^+$	Na^+
$3H^+ - ATPase$	$Na^+ - Amino\ acid$	$Na^+ - NH_4^+$	K^+
$H^+ - K^+ - ATPase$	$2Na^+ - HPO_4^{2-}$	$3Na^+ - Ca^{2+}$	Cl^-
$Ca^{2+} - ATPase$	$Na^+ - 3\ HCO_3^-$	$Cl^- - HCO_3^-$	Ca^{2+}
	$Na^+ - 2Cl^- - K^+$		
	$K^+ - Cl^-$		

A. **Basolateral (abluminal) membrane transport systems** (Figure 23-2A)

1. **Primary active transport.** Na^+ transport through the basolateral membrane is mediated principally by the **Na+–K+–ATPase pump,** which transports Na^+ against an electrochemical potential from the cell interior and **maintains a low intracellular Na^+ concentration** (Figure 23-2B). Active transport of Na^+ (efflux) across all cells of the body consumes 30%–50% of the energy derived from metabolism in most cells.

2. **Facilitated diffusion,** which involves the passive transport of a substance by a protein carrier from a region of higher concentration to a region of lower concentration, translocates glucose from the intracellular fluid across the membrane to the interstitial fluid (ISF) [see Figure 23-2B].

B. **Apical (luminal or adluminal) membrane transport systems.** The apical surface of the renal epithelium of the proximal tubule differs from the other cell membranes in that simple diffusion plays almost no role in the transport of Na^+, K^+, Cl^-, H^+, glucose, or amino acids. The movement of Na^+ across the luminal membrane (influx) is favored by the electrochemical gradient, but the bulk of Na^+ transport is mediated by specific membrane transport proteins, not by simple diffusion. The apical surface possesses two transport mechanisms for Na^+.

1. A **diffusion** mechanism is available for Na^+ to pass through the tight junction in association with Cl^-. Most of the Cl^- that is reabsorbed never enters the cell but is reabsorbed by paracellular transport (see Figure 23-2B).

2. **Carrier-mediated (secondary active) transport.** The transport of Na^+ down its gradient provides energy for active (uphill) transport of other solutes (e.g., glucose, amino acids). There are two types of Na^+-dependent transport mechanisms (see Figure 23-2B).

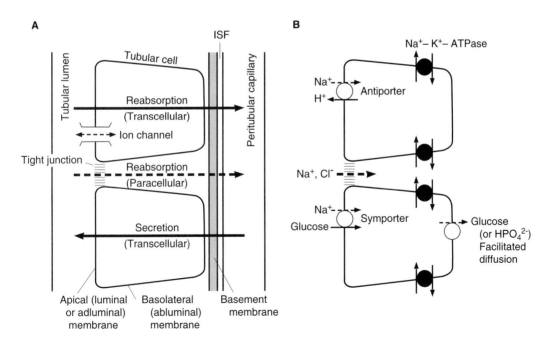

FIGURE 23-2. (*A*) Major modalities of renal transport. (*B*) Transport systems of the proximal tubule. Pumps (*solid circles*), carriers (*open circles*) and channels (*slanting parallel lines*) are important renal transport mechanisms. Diffusion takes place through channels, and facilitated diffusion is represented by *carriers with single dashed arrows. Dashed arrows* represent downhill transport (i.e., transport along a concentration gradient) and *solid arrows* represent uphill transport (i.e., transport against a concentration gradient). Movement of both solute and water from the interstitial fluid into the capillaries occurs by bulk flow.

  a. **Cotransport (symport)** denotes the transport of two substances by a protein carrier in the **same direction.**
  b. **Countertransport (antiport)** defines the transport of two substances by a protein carrier in **opposite directions.**

C. **Transepithelial transport.** The differences between apical and basolateral membrane properties account for the transepithelial transport of all solutes, which can occur via the transcellular or the paracellular pathway (see Figure 23-2A).

1. The **transcellular pathway** is used for **active transepithelial transport.** Approximately two-thirds of **proximal** Na^+ reabsorption is active and transcellular. Na^+ transport is primarily transcellular and carrier-mediated. The $Na^+–H^+$ antiporter is the main determinant of proximal Na^+ and water reabsorption.

2. The $Na^+–K^+–ATPase$ pump indirectly provides the energy that allows virtually all of the transport proteins to translocate filtered solutes passively. This pump has several important functions.
  a. It actively transports reabsorbed Na^+ from the tubular cell into the systemic circulation via the peritubular capillaries.
  b. It maintains a low intracellular Na^+ concentration that allows luminal Na^+ to continue entering the cell down a concentration gradient.
    (1) Na^+ influx across the proximal tubular lumen is linked to the cotransport (symport) of other solutes (see Table 23-1).
    (2) Na^+ entry also occurs by countertransport (antiport). The carrier promotes both Na^+ reabsorption and H^+ secretion into the lumen leading primarily to HCO_3^- reabsorption (see Table 23-1).
  c. It contributes to the development of a cell interior negative potential by promoting net loss of cations.
  d. It regulates cell volume.

3. The proximal tubule primarily carries out the nearly isosmotic reabsorption of two-thirds to three-fourths of the glomerular filtrate.

4. Water reabsorption results from differences in osmolarity between lumen and ISF created by the reabsorption of solute.

5. The **paracellular (intercellular) pathway,** which follows the lateral intercellular spaces, is used for **passive transepithelial transport.** Approximately one-third of total proximal Na^+ and water reabsorption occurs passively by paracellular transport through the tight junctions. This type of transport requires an electrochemical gradient for the substance in the reabsorptive direction and tight junctions that are permeable to the substance (solute or water).
  a. **Paracellular pathway for Cl^- reabsorption in the proximal tubule**
    (1) As water moves out of the tubule secondary to Na^+ reabsorption, the increase in luminal Cl^- concentration acts as a driving force for paracellular Cl^- reabsorption by diffusion.
    (2) Active transport of Na^+ leaves the luminal membrane negatively charged with respect to the ISF. This transtubular voltage gradient constitutes a second driving force for paracellular Cl^- reabsorption by diffusion.
  b. A **paracellular pathway for K^+** exists in the interspaces of the proximal tubule and the thick segment of the ascending limb of the loop of Henle.

Case

A functionally anephric male patient receives an infusion of 3 L of isotonic NaCl and 3 L of 5% dextrose in water (D_5W). Before the infusion, his initial plasma Na^+ concentration is 140 mEq/L, but after the infusion, it falls to 130 mEq/L.

1. *How do the intracellular fluid (ICF) and extracellular fluid (ECF) volumes change? (Assume that no fluid or electrolyte loss occurs during the infusion and that the initial fluid balance is normal.)*

DISCUSSION

Because the D5W solution is isosmolar to plasma, and glucose is rapidly metabolized, 3 L of solute-free water remains. **Therefore, isosmotic glucose is a hypotonic solution.** The water distributes between the ICF and the ECF in proportion to the original volumes (i.e., 2 L enter the ICF, and 1 L remains in the ECF). The isotonic saline solution would remain in the ECF, increasing its volume by 3 L.

Compartment	NaCl	D$_5$W	Total
ICF	0	2	2 L
ECF	3	1	4 L

2. *If the man weighed 70 kg before the infusion, how much does he weigh after the infusion?*

DISCUSSION

The man now weighs 76 kg [70 kg + 6 L (kg)].

3. *What is the actual volume of the ICF after the infusion of 3 L of isosmotic dextrose? Use the change in plasma Na$^+$ concentration for this calculation.*

DISCUSSION

The ICF volume after the isosmotic dextrose infusion is 15 L; the 3-L infusion increases the volume of the ECF by 1 L. To perform this calculation, the starting volumes of the ICF and ECF must be determined. Because the man weighs 70 kg, his total body water (TBW) is about 60% of his body weight, or 42 L, which is distributed in a 2:1 ratio between the ICF and ECF. Therefore, before the infusion, the ICF volume is 28 L, and the ECF volume is 14 L. In addition, it must be understood that the plasma osmolality reflects the ICF volume (inverse relationship). The **amount** of Na$^+$ in the ECF before the infusion is 140 mEq/L × 14 L, or 1960 mEq. After the saline infusion, the Na$^+$ concentration is 130 mEq/L. Solving for x:

$$140 \text{ mEq/L } (14 \text{ L}) = 130 \text{ mEq/L } (X)$$

$$X = \frac{1960}{130} = 15 \text{ L}$$

Thus, the infusion of isosmotic dextrose has increased the volume of the ECF by 1 L.

ADDITIONAL DISCUSSION

The volume of distribution of isotonic NaCl is only in the ECF volume, whereas the volume of distribution of solutions that have water without NaCl (e.g., D5W) is TBW. Thus, solutions containing permeant solutes or metabolizable solutes (glucose) are distributed throughout the TBW.

Considering that the ECF volume is about 20% of TBW, a given volume of isotonic NaCl expands the ECF volume more effectively than a comparable volume of D_5W.

Colloid-containing solutions are used in emergent settings because a given volume of plasma or blood expands the plasma volume three to five times more effectively than an equal volume of saline. Na^+ has a lower reflection coefficient across capillary membranes than across cellular membranes. Because glucose is rapidly metabolized to CO_2 and H_2O, the administration of glucose (dextrose) is physiologically equivalent to the administration of distilled water.

Chapter 24

Renal Clearance

I. **INTRODUCTION. Clearance,** which emphasizes the excretory function of the kidney, forms the basis for the quantitative evaluation of renal function.

A. Definitions

1. **Renal clearance** of a given substance is the **ratio of the renal excretion rate of the substance to its concentration in the blood plasma.** This ratio is expressed as:

$$C_x = \frac{U_x \cdot \dot{V}}{P_x}$$

where C_x = clearance of the substance (ml/min), U_x = concentration of the substance in urine (mg/ml), P_x* = concentration of the substance in plasma (mg/ml), and $\dot{V}$ = volume of urine output per minute (ml/min).

a. An increase in the plasma concentration of a substance leads to an increase in its rate of excretion, and the clearance remains unchanged.

b. Clearance is the virtual volume of plasma from which a substance is completely removed and excreted into the urine per unit time.

2. **Clearance** is the volume of plasma from which a substance is removed from plasma per unit time to provide the amount of that substance excreted by the urine in the same time period. This relationship is demonstrated by a simple rearrangement of the clearance equation:

$$C_x \cdot P_x = U_x \cdot \dot{V}$$

Clearance and urinary excretion rate ($U_x \cdot \dot{V}$) of a substance are not identical, because increasing the plasma concentration of a substance leads to an increased rate of excretion; the clearance remains unchanged.

B. **Units.** Clearance is expressed in ml/min:

$$C_x = \frac{U_x \cdot \dot{V}}{P_x} = \frac{(mg/ml)\ (ml/min)}{(mg/ml)} = ml/min$$

C. **Tubular transport processes** (Figure 24-1). Although clearance quantitates the net process used by the kidney to transport a substance from and into the plasma, **it does not define the actual transport mechanism.** Substances can be cleared by **filtration, tubular secretion,** or a **combination** of these processes.

1. The **magnitude of the tubular clearance** depends on the plasma concentration and the tubular transport capacity (Tm) for reabsorption or secretion. (The phenomenon of tubular transport capacity is discussed in more detail in Chapter 27 I.)

2. In general, renal transport occurs in three ways:
   a. **Glomerular filtration**
   b. **Reabsorption** from the tubular fluid back into the blood
   c. **Secretion** from the blood into the tubular lumen

3. Clearance can define the transport process only on a **net basis.** For example, suppose

---

*Plasma concentrations rather than whole blood concentrations are used in calculations of renal clearance, because only the plasma is cleared by filtration.

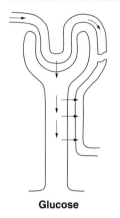

Glucose

Glucose is completely
reabsorbed. Plasma
clearance: 0

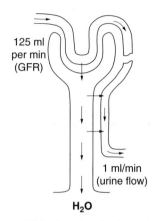

125 ml
per min
(GFR)

1 ml/min
(urine flow)

H₂O

Water is reabsorbed very
nearly completely (99%).
Plasma clearance: 1 ml/min.

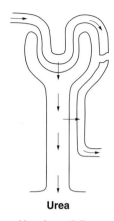

Urea

Urea is partially
reabsorbed. Plasma
clearance: 75 ml/min

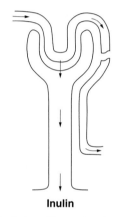

Inulin

Inulin is neither reabsorbed
nor excreted by the tubules.
Plasma clearance: 125 ml/min
(GFR).

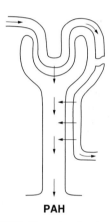

PAH

PAH is filtered at the glomerulus
and secreted into the tubules so
that only a small amount leaves
the kidney in the renal veins.
Plasma clearance (nearly equals
plasma flow): 700 ml/min.

FIGURE 24-1. Renal clearance of various substances, with diagrams of nephrons with afferent and efferent glomerular vessels and a tubular capillary. The arrows show the direction of movement of each substance under discussion, and their length is a measure of the relative amount that is moving. In the diagram for H_2O, the volume of plasma passing into the kidney is 700 ml/min, the volume of filtrate formed at the glomerulus is 125 ml/min, and the volume eliminated as urine is 1 ml/min. Because the 700 ml of plasma flowing through the glomerulus each minute carries the red blood cells (RBCs), the volume of blood flowing through the kidneys is 1200 ml/min. GFR = glomerular filtration rate; PAH = *para*-aminohippuric acid.

that the amount of substance X filtered ($\dot{F}$) is 10 mg/min, the amount reabsorbed ($\dot{R}$) is 8 mg/min, and the amount secreted ($\dot{S}$) is 5 mg/min. Calculating the amount excreted ($\dot{E}$) in mg/min:

$$\dot{E} = \dot{F} + \dot{S} - \dot{R} = 10 + 5 - 8 = 7 \text{ mg/min}$$

a. This result indicates that on a **net basis,** 30% of filtered substance X has been re-absorbed. A substantial rate of secretion can be overlooked.

FIGURE 24-2. Clearances of several substances plotted against their plasma concentrations. There are two types of substances with reference to the clearance of inulin: substances with clearances below that for inulin are filtered and reabsorbed (e.g., glucose), and substances with clearances above that for inulin are filtered and secreted [e.g., *para*-aminohippuric acid (PAH)]. Units of plasma concentrations vary over a wide range so that values on the abscissa are relative only. Note that the ordinate is interrupted, and PAH clearance at low plasma concentration is greater than 600 ml/min. (Reprinted from Bauman JW Jr, Chinard FP: Measurement of renal integrity. In *Renal Function: Physiological and Medical Aspects.* St. Louis, CV Mosby, 1975, p 43.)

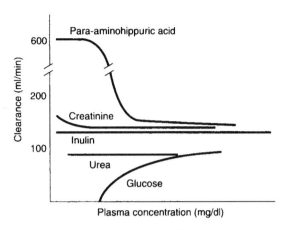

b. Note that clearance makes use of the transport processes of filtration and secretion. Reabsorption decreases clearance and, therefore, clearance and reabsorption are inversely related.

II. APPLICATIONS. The concept of clearance can be applied to tubular function.

A. Inulin clearance

1. Inulin, a fructopolysaccharide that does not occur naturally in the body, can be used in a **test for determining renal function** (functional renal mass).
   a. **As a measure of glomerular filtration rate (GFR)**
      (1) **Inulin clearance** (C_{in}) is a measure of GFR because the volume of plasma completely cleared of inulin per unit time equals the volume of plasma filtered per unit time (i.e., $C_{in} = GFR$). The following characteristics of inulin account for this quality.
         (a) Inulin is only **freely filtered.** Because no inulin is secreted or reabsorbed, all excreted inulin must come from the plasma.
         (b) Inulin is **biologically inert** and **nontoxic.**
         (c) Inulin is **not bound to plasma proteins,** and it is **not metabolized to another substance.**
      (2) Although inulin is used most commonly, **other substances** can measure GFR. The most frequently used agents include mannitol, sorbitol, sucrose (intravenous), iothalamate, radioactive cobalt-labeled vitamin B_{12}, ^{51}Cr-labeled edetic acid (EDTA), and radioiodine-labeled Hypaque. (Endogenous creatinine clearance is used clinically as an estimate of GFR, as discussed in II B, because a small amount of creatinine is secreted in humans.)
   b. **As an indicator of plasma clearance mechanisms.** A comparison of the clearance of a given substance (C_x) with the clearance of inulin (C_{in}) provides information about the renal transport processes used to remove the substance from plasma (Figure 24-2).
      (1) When C_x **equals** C_{in}, excretion is by **filtration alone.** Therefore, the mass of the substance excreted in the urine per unit time equals the mass of the substance filtered during the same time:

$$U_x \cdot \dot{V} = C_{in} \cdot P_x{}^*$$

      (2) When C_x **is less than** C_{in}, excretion is by filtration and reabsorption. In this case,

---

*The mass filtered per unit time (also called the **amount filtered** or **filtered load**) is equal to GFR · P_x (or $C_{in} \cdot P_x$) and is expressed in mg/min (see Chapter 27 I B).

the mass of the substance excreted in the urine is less than the mass of the substance filtered during that time:

$$U_x \cdot \dot{V} < C_{in} \cdot P_x$$

(3) When C_x **is greater than** C_{in}, excretion is by filtration and secretion. In this case, the mass of the substance excreted in the urine is greater than the mass of the substance filtered during the same time.

$$U_x \cdot \dot{V} > C_{in} \cdot P_x$$

2. **Clearance ratios.** The clearance ratio is the ratio of the clearance of any substance (C_x) to the clearance of inulin (C_{in}).
   a. **Interpretation**
      (1) C_x/C_{in} **= 1.** A ratio of 1 indicates that the amount of the substance excreted per unit time equals the amount of the substance filtered in the same time:

$$U_x \cdot \dot{V} = C_{in} \cdot P_x$$

   (a) A clearance ratio of 1 indicates that, **on a net basis,** the substance is **neither reabsorbed nor secreted** and, therefore, is **only filtered.**
   (b) Substances with clearance ratios close to 1 include mannitol, sorbitol, thiosulfate, ferricyanide, iothalamate, vitamin B_{12}, and sucrose (intravenous).
      (2) C_x/C_{in} **< 1.** A clearance ratio of less than 1 demonstrates that the amount of the substance excreted per unit time is less than the amount filtered per unit time:

$$U_x \cdot \dot{V} < C_{in} \cdot P_x$$

   (a) A clearance ratio of less than 1 indicates that, on a net basis, the substance undergoes reabsorption.
   (b) Substances with clearance ratios of less than 1 include glucose, xylose, and fructose.
      (3) C_x/C_{in} **> 1.** A clearance ratio that is greater than 1 indicates the net excretion of the substance over time is greater than the quantity filtered over time:

$$U_x \cdot \dot{V} > C_{in} \cdot P_x$$

   (a) A clearance ratio of more than 1 represents **net secretion** of the substance into the lumen; therefore, the substance is cleared by **filtration and secretion.**
   (b) Substances with clearance ratios greater than 1 include *para*-aminohippuric acid (PAH), phenol red, iodopyracet, certain penicillins, and creatinine (in humans).
   b. **Tubular fluid-to-plasma (TF/P) concentration ratio.** A comparison of the tubular fluid (TF) solute concentration to the plasma (P) solute concentration is called the TF/P concentration ratio. The TF/P concentration ratio is not compared to that of inulin and is, therefore, a single ratio.
      (1) This ratio **measures the tubular solute concentration along the nephron,** which is a function of solute transport (i.e., reabsorption or secretion) as well as water reabsorption (Figure 24-3).
      (2) TF/P solute concentration ratios also can represent **total solute concentration** rather than the concentration of a single solute. When measuring the total solute concentration, the TF/P or urine-to-plasma (U/P) ratio is expressed in terms of osmolality (osmolarity) and can be interpreted as follows.
      (a) When TF_{osm}/P_{osm} **= 1 or** U_{osm}/P_{osm} **= 1,** the tubular fluid or urine is isosmotic with respect to plasma. When $(TF/P)_x = 1$, the reabsorption of solute is commensurate with the reabsorption of water and, therefore, the solute concentration in the TF does not change.
         (i) If a freely filtered solute has a TF/P ratio of 1 in Bowman's space, no net reabsorption or secretion has occurred.
         (ii) Sodium has a TF/P concentration ratio of 1 along the proximal tubule, indicating isosmotic reabsorption.
      (b) When TF_{osm}/P_{osm} **or** U_{osm}/P_{osm} **< 1,** the tubular fluid or urine is hyposmotic

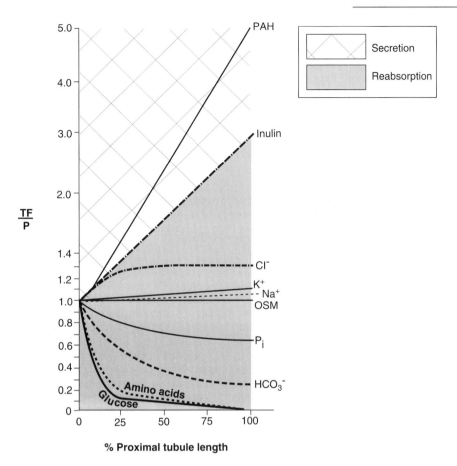

FIGURE 24-3. Transport of various solutes along the length of the proximal tubule. TF/P = tubular fluid-to-plasma concentration ratio for a particular solute. The TF/P concentration ratio for inulin rises to approximately 3 at the end of the proximal tubule, indicating water reabsorption (because inulin is not reabsorbed). Along the initial portion of the proximal tubule, there is little Cl^- reabsorption, so the TF/P concentration ratio rises as a result of the reabsorption of water. Bicarbonate (HCO_3^-) reabsorption lowers the TF/P concentration ratio for HCO_3^- to approximately 0.2 at the end of the proximal tubule, indicating that the concentration of HCO_3^- in the tubular fluid is approximately 5 mmol/L, or 20% of its concentration in plasma. Glucose and amino acids are reabsorbed rapidly, so that at 25% of the proximal tubular length, their concentrations in the tubular fluid decline to approximately 10% of their concentrations in the glomerular filtrate (or plasma), as shown by the TF/P ratio of 0.1. OSM = osmolarity or osmolality (i.e., the total concentration of all solutes in the tubular fluid); PAH = *para*-aminohippuric acid; P_i = inorganic phosphate. (Modified from Brenner B, Coe FL, Rector FC: Transport functions of renal tubules. In *Renal Physiology in Health and Disease*. Philadelphia, WB Saunders, 1987, p 33.)

    with respect to plasma. When $(TF/P)_x < 1$, the reabsorption of solute is greater than the reabsorption of water, causing the concentration in the TF to fall below that in plasma. Examples include glucose, HCO_3^-, and HPO_4^{2-}.

(c) **When TF_{osm}/P_{osm} or $U_{osm}/P_{osm} > 1$,** the tubular fluid or urine is hyperosmotic with respect to plasma. When $(TF/P)_x > 1$, reabsorption of solute is less than water reabsorption (Cl^-), net secretion of solute into the tubule (PAH) has occurred, or only water reabsorption without solute reabsorption or secretion has occurred (e.g., with inulin).

(d) **Example.** States of hydropenia (dehydration) lead to antidiuretic hormone (ADH) secretion. This, in turn, leads to increased water reabsorption and an elevation of U_{osm}, which has an upper limit in humans of about 1400 mOsm/kg. With a P_{osm} of about 300 mOsm/kg, this is equivalent to a maximal U_{osm}/P_{osm} of approximately 4.7.

B. **Creatinine clearance.** Although inulin clearance can be used to measure GFR, in clinical practice it is more common to determine the 24-hour endogenous creatinine clearance as an estimate of GFR. Creatinine clearance determinations do not require administration of exogenous creatinine because creatinine is a product of muscle metabolism.

1. **Creatinine clearance** has a normal range of 80–110 ml/min per 1.73 m² body surface area (estimated average body surface area of a 25-year-old human) and declines with age in healthy individuals. Because creatinine clearance is an index of GFR, it reflects the normal decline in GFR with age.

2. **Plasma creatinine concentration** remains remarkably constant through life, averaging 0.8–1.0 mg/dl in the absence of renal disease. Estimates of renal function tend to rely on serum **creatinine concentration** rather than **creatinine clearance.**
   a. Because a small amount (10%–20%) of creatinine enters the urine by secretion, the creatinine clearance exceeds the clearance of inulin by the same amount.
   b. The colorimetric determination of plasma creatinine involves interfering substances, leading to the overestimation of plasma creatinine concentration by 10%–20%. This error makes up for the slight increase in creatinine clearance caused by secretion of these substances. Therefore, the creatinine clearance is a reasonably accurate estimate of GFR.
   c. Using serum creatinine concentration as a basis for drug dosages can lead to drug overdose, especially in elderly individuals. Overdose is a particularly serious risk with drugs that are cleared primarily by renal mechanisms (e.g., digoxin, aminoglycoside antibiotics). The dosages for these drugs frequently are based on serum creatinine concentration, although it is incorrect to do so. To avoid this error, patient age should be considered together with measurements of creatinine clearance and blood levels of the drug. Drug dosages should be adjusted to the 30%–40% decrease in GFR that normally occurs in individuals 30–80 years old.

3. **Urinary creatinine excretion.** Because creatinine clearance normally declines with age and plasma creatinine concentration does not, the decline in clearance is attributed to a parallel decrease in the excretion rate of creatinine.
   a. The decline in creatinine clearance is not due to a decreased tubular secretion of creatinine, because the clearance ratio of creatinine to inulin is a quite constant 1.2, about 120% of inulin clearance. Thus, urinary creatinine excretion exceeds the amount filtered, because approximately 20% of the urinary creatinine is derived from tubular secretion by the secretory pathway in the proximal tubule.
   b. The plasma creatinine concentration varies inversely with GFR (Figure 24-4), and the product of GFR and plasma creatinine concentration is constant. Thus, a fall in GFR may be the earliest clinical sign of renal disease (i.e., a decline in functional renal mass).
   c. The decline in creatinine excretion with age is due to a primary decline in renal function and a secondary decline in muscle mass.
      (1) The decline in GFR is due to declines in renal plasma flow and cardiac output as well as renal tissue mass. (Decreased GFR is the most clinically significant renal functional deficit occurring with age.)
      (2) The decline in creatinine excretion with a decline in muscle mass over time accounts for the relatively constant plasma creatinine concentration in healthy individuals. Excreted creatinine is proportional to the phosphocreatine content of muscle and, therefore, excretion rate of creatinine can be an estimate of muscle mass.

Case

A woman with two equally functional kidneys has a creatinine clearance of 140 L/day and a plasma creatinine concentration of 1.0 mg/dl. She plans to donate a kidney to a relative with renal failure.

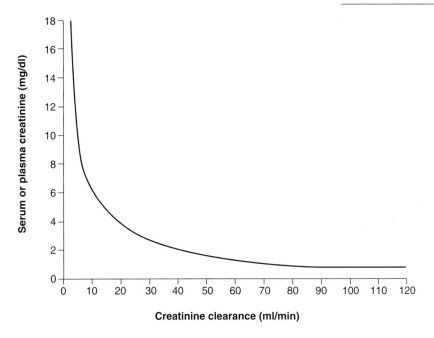

FIGURE 24-4. Serum or plasma creatinine concentration as a function of creatinine clearance.

A blood sample and a 24-hour urine collection were taken immediately after the surgery to remove the kidney.

1. *What changes would occur in the (1) creatinine concentration, (2) creatinine clearance, and (3) creatinine excretion rate immediately following the unilateral nephrectomy?*

DISCUSSION

1. Because creatinine continues to be produced from muscle at a constant rate, it begins to accumulate in the body, and the **plasma creatinine concentration** rises. When the plasma creatinine concentration reaches twice its original value (2 mg/dl), the rate of creatinine excretion equals its production rate. For a short time, this higher concentration will remain at this steady state value. This higher creatinine concentration initially occurs because the rate of filtration (and thus the rate of excretion) is less than the rate of production. (Eventually, however, at a new steady state, the filtered load of creatinine again equals the rate of production.) According to the following equation:

Presurgery:

$$P_{cr} = \frac{U_{cr} \cdot \dot{V}}{C_{cr}} = \frac{1400}{140} = 10 \text{ mg/L} = 1 \text{ mg/dl}$$

Postsurgery:

$$P_{cr} = \frac{U_{cr} \cdot \dot{V}}{C_{cr}} = \frac{1400}{70} = 20 \text{ mg/L} = 2 \text{ mg/dl}$$

2. Immediately following unilateral nephrectomy, **creatinine clearance** would fall by half—from a normal value of 140 L/day to 70 L/day.

3. The rate of creatinine excretion would also decrease by one-half—from 1400 mg/day (140 L/day × 10 mg/L) to 700 mg/day (70 L/day × 10 mg/L). It is imperative to note from the clearance equation the rate of creatinine excretion is determined by the creatinine clearance multiplied by the plasma concentration of creatine. There is a short transient period during which the rate of creatinine production exceeds the rate of creatinine excretion. The resultant rise in plasma creatinine concentration causes a proportionate increase in filtered load and thus in excretion until a new steady state is reached with the elevated plasma creatinine concentration.

2. *How would the filtered load of creatinine change immediately following the unilateral nephrectomy?*

DISCUSSION

The filtered load of creatinine [glomerular filtration rate (GFR) $\cdot$ P_{cr}] is equal to the rate of excretion ($U_{cr} \cdot \dot{V}$), which is equal to the rate of production (≈ 1.8 g/day). The filtered load of creatinine does not change immediately following the nephrectomy in spite of a decline in creatinine clearance (GFR):

Presurgery:

$$\text{Filtered creatinine} = 10 \cdot 140 = 1400 \text{ mg/day}$$

Postsurgery:

$$\text{Filtered creatinine} = 20 \cdot 70 = 1400 \text{ mg/day}$$

ADDITIONAL DISCUSSION

Creatinine is a metabolic waste product with a constant plasma concentration (0.8–1.0 mg/dl) when renal function, dietary protein intake, and muscle mass are stable. Because it is an endogenous substance, derived almost entirely from the catabolism of muscle creatinine and creatine phosphate, it does not require infusion. It is eliminated from the body almost exclusively via the kidneys. Creatinine clearance or plasma creatinine concentration is used to measure glomerular filtration rate (GFR). Creatinine is cleared by filtration and, to a small degree, by secretion, and therefore, it is not a perfect marker for GFR. The measurement of creatinine clearance requires only a single blood sample and a timed (24-hour) urine collection. Total urinary excretion of creatinine is equal to the filtered load of creatinine plus the amount secreted.

The donor's remaining kidney will undergo hypertrophy (i.e., the remaining nephrons will become larger), leading to an increase in the filtered load and excretion rate of creatinine. As the excretion rate increases, the creatinine clearance also increases, and the plasma creatinine concentration decreases. In time, the creatinine clearance of the remaining kidney will approach that of one of the original kidneys, resulting in a decline in the plasma creatinine concentration and creatinine clearance. As the excretion rate increases, the creatinine clearance rises, leading to a fall in plasma creatinine concentration.

Chapter 25

Glomerular Filtration and Renal Blood Flow

I. GLOMERULAR FILTRATION

A. **Physical factors affecting glomerular filtration.** Hydrostatic and oncotic pressures play a role. Fluid movement is proportional to the permeability and to the balance between hydrostatic and oncotic (osmotic) forces across the glomerular membrane. When hydrostatic pressure exceeds oncotic pressure, filtration occurs. Conversely, when oncotic pressure exceeds hydrostatic pressure, reabsorption occurs. The GFR is proportional to the sum of Starling forces that exist across the capillaries $[(P_{cap} - P_{Bow}) - \sigma(COP_{cap} - COP_{Bow})]$ multiplied by the filtration coefficient, K_f.

1. The term **effective filtration pressure (EFP)** refers to the **net driving forces** for water and solute transport across the glomerular membrane. EFP is a function of two variables: (1) the **hydrostatic pressure gradient** driving fluid **out** of the glomerular capillary and into Bowman's capsule, and (2) the **colloid osmotic pressure gradient** bringing fluid **into** the glomerular capillary (Figure 25-1). Using these variables, EFP is expressed as:

$$EFP = (P_{cap} - P_{Bow}) - COP_{cap}$$

where $(P_{cap} - P_{Bow})$ = the outward forces promoting filtration and COP_{cap} = the inward forces opposing filtration. The colloid osmotic pressure in Bowman's capsule (COP_{Bow}) is not expressed in this equation because the glomerular filtrate normally contains little protein.

2. The **reflection coefficient (σ)** describes the selectivity of a membrane with regard to solute and solvent. This coefficient denotes the fraction of solute that is rejected (reflected) at the membrane under conditions of ultrafiltration in the absence of a concentration gradient; the reflected fraction sets up an osmotic gradient that opposes filtration.

3. The **filtration coefficient (K_f)**, the product of hydraulic (water) permeability of the glomerular membranes (L_p) and the surface area (S), is expressed in ml/min/Hg.

4. The **glomerular filtration rate (GFR)** is equal to the EFP multiplied by the filtration coefficient: $GFR = K_f \cdot EFP$.
   a. The filtration coefficient normally equals approximately 12.5 ml/min/mm Hg.
   b. The EFP, which can be determined from the normal values for P_{cap} (45 mm Hg), P_{Bow} (10 mm Hg), and COP_{cap} (25 mm Hg), normally equals about 10 mm Hg.
   c. The **normal GFR** for both kidneys is approximately 125 ml/min per 1.73 m² of body surface area, or a daily GFR of 180 L/day!

B. **Morphologic factors affecting glomerular filtration** (Figure 25-2)

1. **Capillaries.** The glomerular capillaries are derived from the afferent arterioles.
   a. The endothelial cells contain fenestrae, which are large capillary openings that have a high hydraulic permeability. In adult humans, the majority of fenestrae lack a diaphragm, unlike the peritubular capillaries.
   b. In the kidney, the resistance to flow across the arterioles constitutes 85% of renal vascular resistance. The remaining 15% is attributed to the peritubular capillaries and renal veins.

2. **Mesangial cells.** These cells are attached to the glomerular basement membrane (GBM).
   a. Mesangial cells maintain the structural integrity of the glomerular tuft against high pressures inside both the glomerular capillaries and the glomerular mesangium.
   b. Mesangial cells possess receptors for angiotensin II, vasopressin [antidiuretic hor-

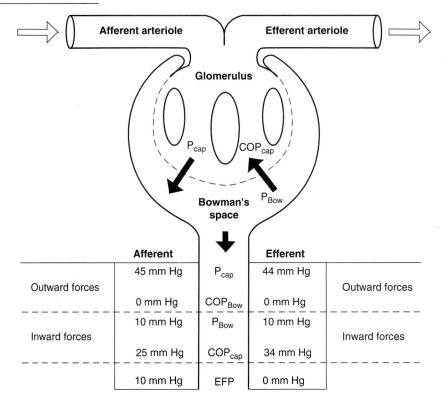

	Afferent		Efferent	
	45 mm Hg	P_{cap}	44 mm Hg	
Outward forces				Outward forces
	0 mm Hg	COP_{Bow}	0 mm Hg	
	10 mm Hg	P_{Bow}	10 mm Hg	
Inward forces				Inward forces
	25 mm Hg	COP_{cap}	34 mm Hg	
	10 mm Hg	EFP	0 mm Hg	

FIGURE 25-1. Model of a glomerular capillary and the Starling forces across the filtration barrier. The effective filtration pressure (EFP) is the net outward force and is calculated as the difference between the outwardly and inwardly directed forces (*dark arrows*). When the hydrostatic pressure forces exceed the colloid oncotic (osmotic) pressure forces, outwardly directed filtration results. COP_{Bow} = Bowman's capsule oncotic pressure; COP_{cap} = capillary oncotic pressure; P_{Bow} = Bowman's capsule hydrostatic pressure; P_{cap} = capillary hydrostatic pressure; *light arrows* = direction of blood flow. (Modified and redrawn with permission from Berne RM and Levy MN: *Physiology,* 3rd ed. St. Louis, CV Mosby, 1993, p 735.)

mone (ADH)], insulin, insulin-like growth factor (IGF), and interleukin-1 (IL-1). In addition, mesangial cells can synthesize prostaglandins.

  c. The mesangium is composed of two types of cells:

    (1) Cells containing microfilaments that exhibit contractile activity. These cells participate in the regulation of capillary filtration by altering filtration surface area and, therefore, the filtration coefficient K_f.

    (2) Macrophages and monocytes that move in and out of the mesangium. These cells can ingest tracer molecules as well as macromolecules and immunocomplexes.

3. GBM. This structure serves as the structural backbone of the glomerular tuft.

  a. The GBM is composed primarily of type IV collagen, sialoglycoproteins (laminin, fibronectin), and proteoglycans (mainly heparan sulfate).

  b. The GBM has a negative charge that constitutes a charge barrier to filtration through electrostatic repulsion. This charge is attributed mainly to polyanionic proteoglycans (heparan sulfate).

4. Epithelial cells. These cells are attached to the GBM.

  a. The visceral cells (podocytes) have long cytoplasmic processes called foot processes (pedicles) with the cell bodies suspended in the urinary space. A thin membrane (slit diaphragm) closes the pores between the foot processes (slit pores).

  b. The parietal cells form an epithelial lining around Bowman's capsule, facing the urinary space.

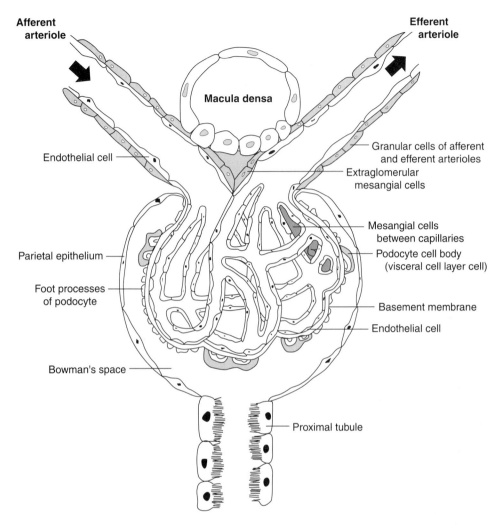

FIGURE 25-2. Anatomy of the glomerulus and the juxtaglomerular apparatus. (Modified from Koushanpour E, Giebisch W: *Renal Physiology: Principles, Structure, and Function,* 2nd ed. Berlin, Springer-Verlag, 1986.)

C. **Ultrafiltrate formation** (Figure 25-3)

1. **Capillary exchange area and filtration coefficient.** The filtration coefficient of the glomerulus is 50–100 times greater than that of a muscle capillary. The **total glomerular capillary exchange area** is estimated to be 1.6 m², of which 2%–3% is available for filtration. Thus, the filtration surface measures between 500 and 800 cm².

2. **Systemic filtration rate.** Approximately 20 L of fluid are filtered daily from the systemic capillaries. Of this, approximately 18 L/day are reabsorbed in the venular ends of the capillaries, and the remaining 2 L/day represent lymph flow. (However, **diffusional exchange** across the entire systemic capillary bed is about 80,000 L/day!)

3. **GFR.** Approximately 180 L of fluid are filtered daily from the glomerular capillaries. Therefore, the transtubular flow of fluid out of the glomerular capillaries (GFR = 180 L/day) far exceeds the filtration from systemic capillaries (20 L/day).

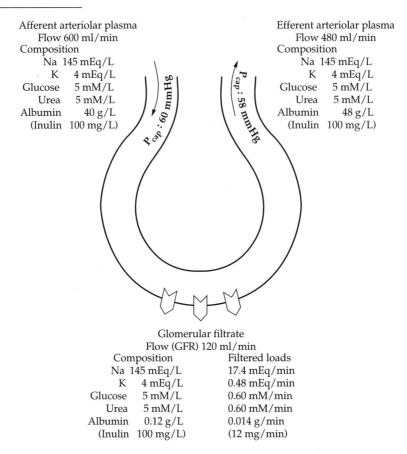

Afferent arteriolar plasma
Flow 600 ml/min
Composition
Na 145 mEq/L
K 4 mEq/L
Glucose 5 mM/L
Urea 5 mM/L
Albumin 40 g/L
(Inulin 100 mg/L)

P_{cap} : 60 mmHg

P_{cap} : 58 mmHg

Efferent arteriolar plasma
Flow 480 ml/min
Composition
Na 145 mEq/L
K 4 mEq/L
Glucose 5 mM/L
Urea 5 mM/L
Albumin 48 g/L
(Inulin 100 mg/L)

Glomerular filtrate
Flow (GFR) 120 ml/min

Composition		Filtered loads
Na	145 mEq/L	17.4 mEq/min
K	4 mEq/L	0.48 mEq/min
Glucose	5 mM/L	0.60 mM/min
Urea	5 mM/L	0.60 mM/min
Albumin	0.12 g/L	0.014 g/min
(Inulin	100 mg/L)	(12 mg/min)

FIGURE 25-3. The fluid in Bowman's space resembles a nearly ideal ultrafiltrate of plasma. The oncotic pressure is higher than that in the systemic circulation because of the removal of protein-free filtrate in the glomerulus.

4. **Filtration fraction (FF).** Given that the GFR is about 120 ml/min and renal plasma flow is about 600 ml/min, only about 20% of the renal plasma flow is actually filtered (FF) into Bowman's space.
   a. The FF is the ratio of GFR to the renal plasma flow, or the ratio of inulin (or creatinine) clearance to that of *para*-aminohippuric acid (PAH) clearance.
   b. Changes in FF are primarily induced by changes in efferent arteriolar resistance. With a renal plasma flow of 600 ml/min, 80% (480 ml/min) of the FF continues through the glomerulus into the peritubular capillaries, and it returns to the systemic circulation via the renal vein (see Figure 25-3).

II. RENAL BLOOD FLOW.
Although the major determinant of the GFR is the hydrostatic pressure within the glomerular capillaries, the renal blood flow through the glomeruli has an effect on the GFR. When the rate of renal blood flow increases, so does the GFR.

A. Renal circulation

1. The vascular resistance of the kidneys is very low, and these organs receive about 20% of the cardiac output, which amounts to a blood flow of 1000–1200 ml/min.

2. Renal blood flow per 100 g of kidney weight (300 g) amounts to about 400 ml/100 g of tissue. (Table 25-1)

TABLE 25-1. Blood Flow and Oxygen Consumption of Various Organs*

Region	Mass (kg)	Blood Flow		Arteriovenous Oxygen Difference (ml/L)	Oxygen Consumption		Resistance (R units)		Percentage of Total	
		ml/min	ml/100 g/min		ml/min	ml/100 g/min	Absolute	Per kg	Cardiac Output	Oxygen Consumption
Liver	2.6	1500	57.7	34	51	2.0	3.6	9.4	27.8	20.4
Kidneys	0.3	1260	420	14	18	6.0	4.3	1.3	23.3	7.2
Brain	1.4	750	54	62	46	3.3	7.2	10.1	13.9	18.4
Skin	3.6	462	12.8	25	12	0.3	11.7	42.1	8.6	4.8
Skeletal muscle	31	840	2.7	60	50	0.2	6.4	198.4	15.6	20.0
Heart muscle	0.3	250	84	114	29	9.7	21.4	6.4	4.7	11.6
Rest of body	23.8	336	1.4	129	44	0.2	16.1	383.2	6.2	17.6
Entire body**	63	5400	8.6	46	250	0.4	1.0	63.0	100.0	100.0

*In a 63-kg adult with a mean arterial blood pressure of 90 mm Hg and an O_2 consumption of 250 ml/min. R units are mm Hg/ml/sec.

**The lung is the only organ to receive the entire cardiac output.

3. The kidneys are unique in that changes in blood flow are accompanied by **parallel** changes in oxygen consumption, with the arteriovenous oxygen difference remaining the same. This occurs because a change in renal blood flow generally is accompanied by a parallel change in GFR, and, therefore, in the reabsorption of solutes.

    a. The arteriovenous oxygen content difference is approximately 1.5 ml/100 ml of blood (1.5 ml O_2/dl) and is the lowest for any organ; therefore, renal blood flow is very high relative to the oxygen needs of the kidney.

    b. Solute reabsorption, in turn, requires oxygen for energy, with as much as 75%–85% of the renal oxygen consumption being used for active reabsorption of ions, particularly Na^+ and active secretion of other ions (e.g., H^+).

4. Renal arterial plasma flow is **greater** than renal venous plasma flow because of the formation of glomerular filtrate. Therefore, renal arterial plasma flow is equal to the **sum** of renal venous plasma flow and urine flow.

5. Renal oxygen consumption is directly proportional to the amount of Na^+ reabsorbed (Figure 25-4).

    a. The oxygen consumption of the kidney is about 400 μm O_2/100 g, which amounts to 4%–8% of the whole body oxygen consumption.

    b. Under physiologic conditions, there is a consistent linear relationship between renal blood flow and renal oxygen consumption.

    c. The linear relationship between renal blood flow and O_2 utilization is coincidental to changes in GFR and filtered Na^+ load, reflecting a direct relationship between tubular Na^+ reabsorption and oxygen consumption.

    d. About 20% of the oxygen consumption (about 100 μm O_2/min/100 g of kidney) is used for basal metabolic needs. About 28 mEq of Na^+ are reabsorbed per millimole of O_2 consumed.

    e. In an individual with a hematocrit of 40%, the **renal plasma flow** is about 600 ml/min (see Figure 25-3).

        (1) Approximately 20%, or 120 ml/min, enters Bowman's space and constitutes the GFR.

        (2) About 80%, or 480 ml/min, escapes filtration and perfuses the renal peritubular capillaries and vasa recta. Approximately 80% of the renal blood flow perfuses the cortex, and the remaining 20% perfuses the medulla.

    f. The metabolic demand of the kidney is determined by blood flow, whereas the opposite is true for other organs with significant metabolic regulation.

        (1) Not all Na^+ reabsorbed by the kidney is transported by an energy-requiring pathway.

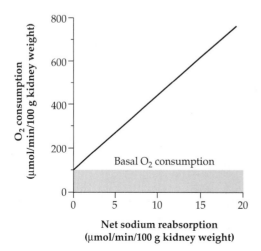

FIGURE 25-4. Relationship between tubular sodium reabsorption and oxygen consumption by the kidney. The primary determinant of oxygen consumption above basal levels is the rate of sodium reabsorption. The darker hatched area represents the normal ranges of sodium reabsorption and oxygen consumption. (Adapted from Windhager EE: Renal metabolism. In *Renal Physiology*, Oxford University Press, 1992, p 2267.)

(2) Approximately 60% of the Na$^+$ reabsorption in the **entire** kidney occurs by active transport.

B. **Autoregulation of arterial pressure** [Figure 25-5; see also Chapter 12 I B 2 a (1)]. Intrarenal mechanisms such as autoregulation keep the GFR relatively constant despite changes in renal arterial pressure and prevent fluid delivery from exceeding the reabsorptive capacity of the collecting tubules.

1. Over a wide range of renal arterial pressures (i.e., 90–190 mm Hg), the GFR and renal blood flow remain quite constant. This intrinsic phenomenon observed in the renal capillaries also occurs in the capillaries of muscles and is termed autoregulation. However, intrarenal autoregulation is virtually absent at mean arterial blood pressures below 70 mm Hg.
   a. Autoregulation has been observed to persist after renal denervation, in the isolated perfused kidney, in the transplanted kidney, after adrenal demedullation, and even in the absence of erythrocytes.
   b. Autoregulation of renal blood flow is necessary for the autoregulation of GFR.

2. Intrarenal autoregulation probably is mediated by changes in preglomerular (afferent) arteriolar resistance. The major factors that determine blood flow (Q) are a pressure gradient (ΔP) and resistance (R):

$$Q = \frac{\Delta P}{R}$$

It becomes clear that to maintain a constant blood flow with a concomitant increase in renal perfusion pressure (ΔP), there must be a commensurate increase in renal vascular resistance.

C. Arteriolar resistance (Figure 25-6)

1. **Effects of changes in arteriolar resistance** (Table 25-2)
   a. The **afferent arteriole** has a larger diameter than the efferent arteriole and is the major site of autoregulatory resistance. When resistance is altered in the afferent arterioles, the GFR and renal blood flow change in the same direction. Therefore, **changes in afferent arteriolar resistance do not affect the FF** (see I C 4).
   (1) **Constriction** of the afferent arteriole **decreases both** the renal plasma flow and the GFR.

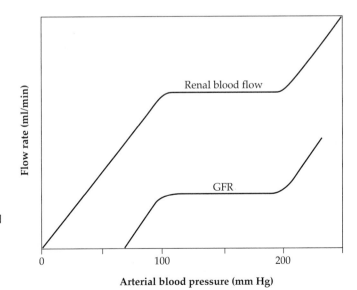

FIGURE 25-5. Relationships between arterial blood pressure and renal blood flow and glomerular filtration rate (GFR). Autoregulation of blood flow and GFR is maintained as blood pressure changes from 90 to 190 mm Hg.

A. Constriction of a vessel

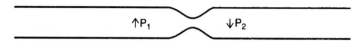

$\uparrow P_1$ $\downarrow P_2$

B. Constriction of afferent arteriole ($\downarrow$ RPF, $\downarrow$GFR)

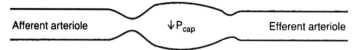

Afferent arteriole $\downarrow P_{cap}$ Efferent arteriole

C. Constriction of efferent arteriole ($\downarrow$ RPF, $\uparrow$GFR)

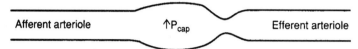

Afferent arteriole $\uparrow P_{cap}$ Efferent arteriole

FIGURE 25-6. Relationship between arteriolar resistance, glomerular filtration rate (GFR), and renal plasma flow (RPF). (*A*) If flow is constant, vasoconstriction results in an increase in hydrostatic pressure proximally (P_1) and a fall in hydrostatic pressure distally (P_2). (*B*) Constriction of the afferent arteriole reduces both the renal plasma flow and the GFR without affecting the filtration fraction. (*C*) Constriction of the efferent arteriole also reduces the renal plasma flow, but the glomerular hydrostatic pressure (P_{cap}) increases, leading to an increase in filtration fraction.

> **(a)** An increase in vascular resistance proximal to the glomeruli leads to a decrease in renal plasma flow.
> **(b)** A decrease in hydrostatic pressure within the glomerular capillaries leads to a decrease in GFR.
> **(2) Dilation** of the afferent arteriole increases both the renal plasma flow and the GFR.
> **(a)** A decrease in vascular resistance proximal to the glomeruli leads to an increase in renal plasma flow.

TABLE 25-2. Effects of Changes in Renal Vascular Resistance With a Constant Renal Perfusion

Renal Arterial Vascular Resistance Afferent	Efferent	P_{GC} (mm Hg)	GFR (ml/min)	RPF (mm/min)	Filtration Fraction	P_{PTC} (mm Hg)
$\uparrow$	...	$\downarrow$	$\downarrow$	$\downarrow$	No change	$\downarrow$
$\downarrow$	...	$\uparrow$	$\uparrow$	$\uparrow$	No change	$\uparrow$
...	$\uparrow$	$\uparrow$	$\uparrow$	$\downarrow$	$\uparrow$	$\downarrow$
...	$\downarrow$	$\downarrow$	$\downarrow$	$\uparrow$	$\downarrow$	$\uparrow$

Note that GFR and RPF exhibit parallel shifts with changes in afferent arteriolar resistance but show divergent shifts with changes in efferent arteriolar resistance. Increases in vascular resistance always lead to a decline in RPF, and decreases in arteriolar resistance always lead to an increase in RPF. In the first two columns, upward arrows denote the effect of vasoconstriction, and downward arrows denote the effect of vasodilation. Note also the parallelism between P_{GC} and GFR.

GFR = glomerular filtration rate, P_{GC} = glomerular capillary hydrostatic pressure, P_{PTC} = peritubular capillary hydrostatic pressure, RPF = renal plasma flow.

(b) An increase in glomerular capillary perfusion pressure leads to an increase in GFR.

b. When resistance is altered in the **efferent arterioles,** the GFR and the renal plasma flow change in opposite directions. Therefore, **changes in efferent arteriolar resistance affect the FF.**

(1) Constriction of the efferent arteriole **decreases the renal plasma flow** and **increases the GFR.**

(a) An increase in vascular resistance distal to the glomeruli leads to a decrease in renal plasma flow.

(b) An increase in the hydrostatic pressure within the glomerular capillaries leads to an increase in GFR.

(c) Following an increase in efferent arteriolar resistance, the FF increases.

(2) Dilation of the efferent arteriole **increases the renal plasma flow and decreases the GFR.**

(a) A decrease in vascular resistance distal to the glomeruli leads to an increase in renal plasma flow.

(b) A decrease in the hydrostatic pressure within the glomerular capillaries leads to a decrease in GFR.

(c) Following a decrease in efferent arteriolar resistance, the FF decreases.

2. Factors affecting arteriolar resistance

a. Sympathetic stimulation

(1) In addition to the autoregulatory response to hypotension (i.e., vasodilation), the reflex increase in sympathetic tone results in both afferent and efferent arteriolar vasoconstriction and an increase in renal vascular resistance, together with a decrease in GFR.

(2) Conversely, the autoregulatory response to increases in renal arterial blood pressure (i.e., vasoconstriction) causes the reflex decrease in sympathetic tone, which results in renal arteriolar vasodilation and a decrease in renal vascular resistance, together with an increase in GFR.

b. Hormonal regulation

(1) Hormones that cause vasoconstriction, and thereby decrease renal blood flow and the GFR, include epinephrine, norepinephrine, angiotensin II, and adenosine. During hemorrhage, norepinephrine, epinephrine, and angiotensin II decrease the renal blood flow in an effort to conserve water.

(a) Norepinephrine elicits an intense vasoconstriction of the afferent and efferent arterioles.

(b) An increase in sympathetic activity increases the release of epinephrine and angiotensin II, enhancing vasoconstriction.

(c) Low concentrations of angiotensin II cause a predominant constriction of the efferent arteriole. At high concentrations of this vasoactive hormone, constriction of both the afferent and efferent arterioles occurs.

(2) Hormones that cause vasodilation, and thereby increase renal plasma flow and GFR, include the prostaglandins PGE_2 and PGI_2 (prostacyclin).

(a) Prostaglandins do not regulate renal blood flow or GFR in subjects who are in the basal state.

(b) During hemorrhage, prostaglandins are produced locally within the kidneys in response to sympathetic nerve activity and angiotensin II. These prostaglandins, which enhance blood flow, vasodilate both the afferent and efferent arterioles.

III. MEASUREMENT OF RENAL BLOOD FLOW/RENAL PLASMA FLOW

A. **Ohm's law** (see II B 2)

$$RBF = \frac{\Delta P}{R}$$

where ΔP = aortic pressure minus renal venous pressure.

B. **Fick principle.** The oxygen consumption ($\dot{Q}O_2$) of an organ is related directly to the rate of blood flow to that organ ($\dot{Q}$) and to the difference in oxygen content between the artery (RAO_2) and vein (RVO_2) of that organ.

$$\dot{Q} = \frac{\dot{Q}O_2}{RAO_2 - RVO_2}$$

where $RAO_2 - RVO_2$ is the renal arteriovenous oxygen content difference.

C. **Clearance of PAH** (Fick principle). The amount of a substance removed (excreted) by an organ (kidney) per unit time ($U_{PAH} \cdot \dot{V}$) is equal to the renal plasma flow multiplied by the arteriovenous difference in plasma PAH concentration:

$$U_{PAH} \cdot \dot{V} = RPF\,(a_{PAH} - v_{PAH})$$

Transposing gives:

$$RPF = \frac{U_{PAH} \cdot \dot{V}}{ao_2 - v_{PAH}}$$

1. At **low** plasma concentrations of PAH, all the PAH is excreted into the urine and none is returned to the circulation via the renal vein.

2. As a result, the venous PAH concentration is zero and can be eliminated. The equation now is the clearance equation for PAH, or:

$$C_{PAH} = RPF = \frac{U_{PAH} \cdot \dot{V}}{P_{PAH}}$$

3. Because PAH is not excreted by any organ other than the kidney, a sample from any peripheral vein can be used to measure plasma PAH concentration.

4. To convert renal plasma flow into renal blood flow, it is necessary to measure the hematocrit (Hct) ratio:

$$RBF = \frac{RPF}{1 - Hct}$$

5. Renal plasma flow calculated from the C_{PAH} is referred to as the effective RPF (ERPF) because only about 90% of the plasma PAH is extracted. Therefore, the ERPF underestimates true RPF by about 10%.
   a. To obtain the true RPF, it is necessary to divide the C_{PAH} by 0.9:

$$C_{PAH} = \frac{ERPF}{0.9} = \text{True RPF}$$

   b. To obtain true RBF it is necessary to divide true RPF by $(1 - Hct)$:

$$\text{True RBF} = \frac{\text{True RPF}}{(1 - Hct)}$$

D. **Renal blood flow can also be determined indirectly from the FF:**

$$FF = \frac{GFR}{RPF} = \frac{C_{in}}{C_{PAH}}$$

Transposing gives:

$$RPF = \frac{GFR}{FF}$$

It is again necessary to divide renal *plasma* flow by (1 − Hct) to calculate the renal *blood* flow.

Case

A 45-year-old woman with diabetic nephropathy has chronic renal failure, as indicated by a plasma creatinine concentration of 2.1 mg/dl and hypertension.

1. *What are possible treatment options?*

DISCUSSION

Possible treatment plans include administration of an angiotensin-converting enzyme (ACE) inhibitor, which primarily dilates the efferent arteriole, or another antihypertensive agent, which primarily dilates the afferent arteriole. Each treatment modality is equally effective in lowering systemic blood pressure.

2. *Which of these two treatment modalities is preferable?*

DISCUSSION

Intraglomerular hypertension has been thought to be a significant contributor to secondary glomerular injury, including diabetic nephropathy. However, treatment with an antihypertensive agent that dilates the afferent arteriole must be avoided. Because the afferent arteriole is upstream from the glomerulus, dilation of this vessel leads to an increase in glomerular capillary hydrostatic pressure, along with increases in the glomerular filtration rate (GFR), renal plasma flow, and peritubular capillary hydrostatic pressure. Thus, despite the decline in systemic hydrostatic pressure, the increased glomerular capillary pressure can be potentially deleterious and exacerbate the nephropathy.

An ACE inhibitor, which evokes dilation of the efferent arteriole, downstream from the glomerulus, also reduces the systemic blood pressure. The agent causes a decline in glomerular capillary pressure, a decrease in GFR, and increases in RPF and peritubular hydrostatic pressure. This fall in glomerular hydrostatic pressure reduces the potential for glomerular injury, making the ACE inhibitor the preferred treatment.

Chapter 26

Intrarenal Regulation of Effective Circulating Volume (ECV) and Sodium Balance: Autoregulation

I. REGULATION OF EFFECTIVE CIRCULATING VOLUME (ECV) [Table 26-1 and Figure 26-1]

A. Definitions

1. ECV is the volume of the extracellular fluid (ECF) in the arterial system ($\approx$ 0.7 L in a 70-kg man), which perfuses the tissues and is regulated by the arterial baroreceptors in the carotid sinus, aortic arch, and the glomerular afferent arterioles.

2. In the normal state, the **ECV varies directly with the ECF volume.**

3. The ECV is not a measurable and distinct body fluid compartment.

B. Role of sodium ion (Na^+): normal state

1. The regulation of Na^+ balance and the maintenance of ECV are closely related.
   a. Na^+ loading produces volume expansion.
   b. Na^+ loss leads to volume depletion.

2. In **ECF volume depletion, retention of renal Na^+ and H_2O is an appropriate response.**

C. Role of sodium ion (Na^+): abnormal state

1. In disorders that lead to **edema** (e.g., heart failure, cirrhosis, some cases of nephrotic syndrome), **renal retention of Na^+ and H_2O occur, despite the increased content of total body Na^+ and H_2O,** which is a paradoxical renal response. In edematous disorders, there must be a fluid compartment that is "underfilled," even in the presence of an expanded ECF volume and blood volume.
   a. This "underfilled" body fluid compartment, the ECV or **effective arterial blood volume (EABV),** is the primary determinant of Na^+ and H_2O balance.

TABLE 26-1. Effective Circulating Volume (ECV) Depletion Association With Expansion of Extracellular Fluid (ECF) Volume

Condition	ECV	ECV Volume	Plasma Volume	Na^+ Reabsorption	Plasma [Na^+]	Aldosterone	ADH
Na^+-depleted normal subject	↓	↓	↓	↑*	↓	↑	↑
Heart failure	↓	↑	↑	↑†	↓	↑	↑
Hepatic cirrhosis	↓	↑	↑	↑†	↓	↑	↑

*Na^+ content restored toward normal value.
†Paradoxical increase in total body weight.
Note that ECV depletion is the dominant stimulus for ADH and aldosterone secretion.
ADH = antidiuretic hormone.

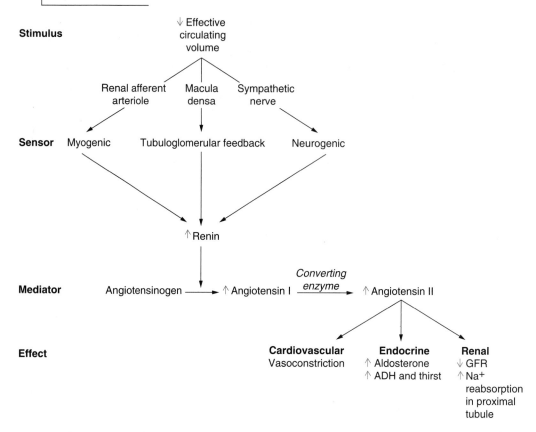

FIGURE 26-1. Hormonal regulation of renal function—the renin–angiotensin system. Afferent arteriolar resistance is affected by Na^+ delivery to and reabsorption of Na^+ by the macula densa region of the thick ascending limb of the loop of Henle. The afferent arteriole constricts (R_A increases) as Na^+ delivery increases. If the glomerular filtration rate (GFR) should rise, with a resultant increased NaCl delivery to the macula densa, NaCl reabsorption in this region secondarily increases. A signal generated by increased NaCl delivery transport by the macula densa cell increases R_A. The rise in R_A then reduces the glomerular capillary pressure, thus returning GFR and NaCl delivery to the loop of Henle to preexisting levels. This process, by which NaCl delivery to the macula densa region modulates GFR, is called tubuloglomerular feedback (TGF).

The two factors that modulate R_A—afferent arteriolar myogenic tone and TGF—also affect renin release. However, the changes are in opposite directions; an increase in afferent arteriolar pressure or macula densa NaCl delivery increases R_A but suppresses renin release. A third factor, sympathetic nerve activity, also controls R_A and renin release. The endocrine system regulates the circulating levels of angiotensin II but is an important regulator of systemic hemodynamics and adrenal function.

Angiotensin II has many cardiovascular, endocrine, and renal effects. It powerfully constricts vascular smooth muscle; increases adrenal releases and biosynthesis of aldosterone, which controls Na^+ reabsorption in the cortical collecting tubules; stimulates ADH release and thirst; and effectively regulates Na^+ transport directly in the early proximal tubule.

    b. In a 70-kg man, the total body water (TBW) is approximately 42 L, of which 0.7 (1.7% of TBW, or 1% of body weight) resides in the EABV.

    c. It is important to note that the TBW, ECF volume, interstitial fluid (ISF) volume and intravascular volume are **not** primary determinants of renal Na^+ and H_2O balance, because Na^+ and H_2O retention persist in edematous patients.

  2. In congestive heart failure and hepatic cirrhosis, the ECV may be independent of the ECF volume.

    a. Affected patients behave as if they were volume-depleted (decline in ECV), which induces a compensatory renal retention of Na^+ and H_2O, leading to increases in both plasma volume and ECF volume (see Table 26-1). These patients exhibit an **increase in total body Na^+ content, with a decline in Na^+ concentration.**

b. The decline in ECV leads to hyponatremia, which is indicative of severely impaired water excretion.

c. The elevation in intravascular pressure and decline in plasma osmolality following the increase in plasma volume results in the movement of retained fluid into the ISF compartment. This fluid accumulation is apparent as **edema.**

d. The depletion in ECV increases water reabsorption via the release of renin, angiotensin II, aldosterone, and antidiuretic hormone (ADH), which are the hypovolemic hormones. In normal subjects, the major determinant of renin secretion is Na^+ intake.

II. REGULATION OF RENAL SODIUM AND WATER EXCRETION

A. **Principle.** Multiple factors affect renal Na^+ and H_2O excretion and, therefore, the regulation of the ECV.

1. The distal nephron, particularly the collecting tubule, is the site at which the final qualitative changes in urinary excretion take place.
   a. Normal H_2O excretion is 1–1.5 L/day.
   b. Normal Na^+ excretion is 100–300 mEq/day.

2. The total reabsorptive capacity of the collecting tubules is limited.
   a. The collecting ducts contain a lower level of Na^+–K^+–ATPase activity than other nephron segments (except for the thin descending and thin ascending limbs of the loop of Henle).
   b. The distal nephron is relatively impermeable to the passive transcellular or paracellular movement of both H_2O (in the absence of ADH) and Na^+.

B. **Intrarenal processes prevent Na^+ and H_2O delivery from exceeding the limited reabsorptive capacity of the collecting tubules.**

1. **Autoregulation,** which maintains the glomerular filtration rate (GFR) in the presence of variations in renal arterial pressure
   a. Maintenance of GFR through the vascular smooth muscle tone of the afferent arteriole
   b. Tubuloglomerular feedback (TGF), which lowers the GFR if the NaCl load to the macula densa is increased

2. **Glomerulotubular balance (GTB),** which involves the increase of proximal and loop reabsorption of Na^+ if there is an elevation of GFR

III. AUTOREGULATION.
In this regulatory process, renal plasma flow/renal blood flow and GFR are maintained constant when the renal arterial pressure fluctuates between 90 and 190 mm Hg (see Figure 25-5). Autoregulation, which is present in other capillaries and also intrinsic to the kidney, occurs in denervated, perfused, and intact kidneys.

A. **Characteristics of autoregulation**

1. Because glomerular capillary pressure is an important determinant of GFR (see Table 25-2), changes in preglomerular (afferent arteriolar) resistance can regulate GFR.

2. GFR and renal plasma flow/renal blood flow are maintained in parallel and, therefore, autoregulation is mediated in large part by changes in afferent arteriolar tone. GFR and renal plasma flow/renal blood flow vary inversely with changes in efferent arteriolar resistance (see Table 26-1).

3. Renal autoregulation keeps the tubular load of water and electrolytes fairly constant and prevents Na^+ and filtrate delivery from exceeding the limited reabsorptive capacity of the collecting ducts.

TABLE 26-2. Glomerulotubular Balance (GTB)*

Condition	GFR (L/day)	Plasma [Na+] (mEq/L)	Ḟ (mEq/day)	Proximal Ṙ (67%)† (mEq/day)	Leaving Proximal (mEq/day)	Ḟ × 99.4%‡ (mEq/day)	Ė = Ḟ − Ṙ (mEq/day)
Normal	180	140	25,200	16,800	8400	25,049	151
+2% GFR	183.6	140	25,704	17,222	8482	25,550	154
Difference	+ 3.6	−	+ 504	+ 422	+ 82	+ 501	+ 3†

*Note that the 3% increment in GFR is approximately equivalent to the plasma volume. A 2% increase in GFR increases the amount of Na+ excreted by 2% (i.e., 151—154 mEq/day). Thus, the increase in the filtered load (Ḟ) of Na+ (504 mEq/day) is not all excreted. Rather, 99.4% of 504 mEq/day (501 mEq/day) is reabsorbed, resulting in a smaller loss of Na+ (≈ 3mEq/day). It is important that tubular reabsorption varies with the spontaneous changes that can occur in GFR in order to maintain the extracellular fluid volume and blood pressure.
†% of filtered load.
‡99.4% of filtered load.
Ė = amount of Na+ excreted, Ḟ = filtered load of Na+, Ṙ = amount of Na+ reabsorbed; GFR = glomerular filtration rate.

4. Autoregulation attenuates large changes in Na+ and H_2O excretion, ensuring that solute and fluid excretion remain relatively constant.

5. Autoregulatory responses maintain ECF volume and, in turn, blood pressure and adequate tissue perfusion.

B. **Myogenic hypothesis of autoregulation (see Figure 26-1)**

1. The afferent arterioles account for the largest part of preglomerular resistance; these vessels constrict in response to wall stretch produced by the distending forces of increased transmural pressure. The constrictive force matches the distending force, maintaining a constant blood flow. The development of wall tension by the resistance vessels is dependent on an increase in calcium influx.

2. The efferent arterioles do not contribute directly to the myogenic response. Efferent arteriolar constriction can result from renin–angiotensin II release, which contributes to the maintenance of GFR at reduced renal perfusion pressures.

3. The **law of Laplace** states that the force T (tension) is directly proportional to the product of pressure across the vascular wall (inside pressure minus outside pressure) and the radius (r) of the vessel [i.e., $T = (P_{in} − P_{out})r$].
   a. Assuming T is constant, changes in transmural pressure ($P_{in} − P_{out}$) result in inverse changes in vessel radius.
   b. When perfusion pressure decreases, transmural pressure also decreases, and vessel radius increases (dilation) to maintain constant wall tension.
   c. When perfusion pressure increases, the transmural pressure increases, and vessel radius decreases (constriction) to maintain constant tension.

4. Metabolic autoregulation of flow in the kidney is unlikely. In the kidney, metabolic demand is a function of blood flow, in contrast to some other organs, where various metabolic factors regulate blood flow.

C. **Tubuloglomerular feedback (TGF) and the macula densa**

1. **Control of vascular tone** (Figures 26-2 and 26-3; see Figure 26-1). TGF is another mechanism for the autoregulation of GFR that prevents excessive salt and water losses. The effector site of the TGF loop is the afferent arteriole.
   a. The **macula densa** consists of tubular epithelial cells located at the distal end of the cortical thick ascending limb of the loop of Henle, where tubular fluid is hypotonic. This structure functions as an intratubular chemoreceptor. The sensor site for TGF is

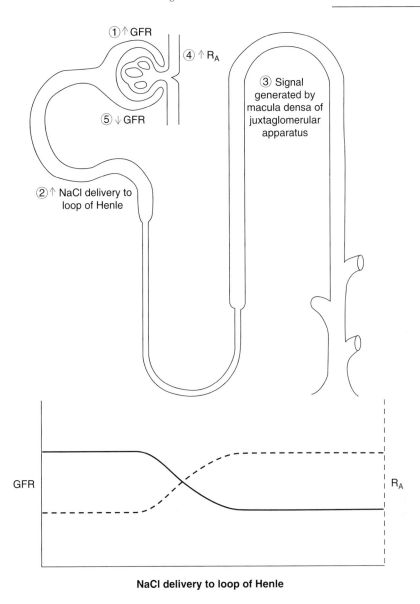

NaCl delivery to loop of Henle

FIGURE 26-2. Tubuloglomerular feedback (TGF) mechanism. An increase in GFR (1) increases NaCl delivery to the loop of Henle (2), which is sensed by the macula densa and converted to a signal (3) that increase R_A (4) which decreases GFR (5). JGA = juxtaglomerular apparatus; R_A = afferent arteriolar resistance. (Modified from Koeppen BM, Stanton BA: *Renal Physiology,* St. Louis, CV Mosby, 1992, p 44.)

the macula densa, which responds to changes in the delivery (concentration × flow rate) and subsequent reabsorption of NaCl.

b. The dissociation between changes in distal NaCl concentration and the TGF response caused by NaCl transport inhibitors indicates that the cells of the macula densa do **not** possess receptors sensitive to changes in **NaCl concentration.** A change in **NaCl transport** is the initiating event that leads to the vascular response.

    (1) At the macula densa, NaCl concentration is primarily a function of tubular flow rate.

    (2) The active NaCl transport by a water-impermeable epithelium results in the transformation of a flow signal into a change in salt concentration.

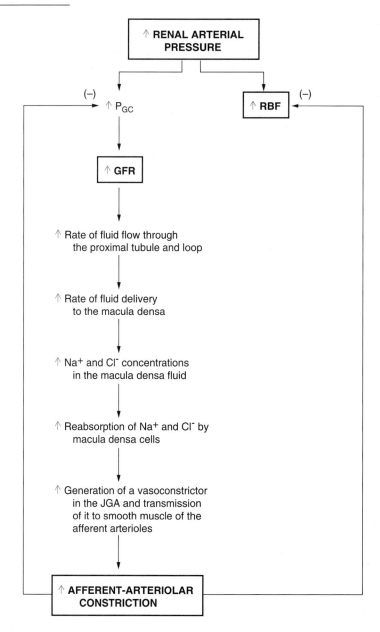

FIGURE 26-3. Tubuloglomerular feedback (TGF) contribution to autoregulation: regulation of GFR by tubular NaCl load. P_{GC} = glomerular capillary pressure; JGA = juxtaglomerular apparatus. (Modified from Vander AJ: Control of renal dynamics. In *Renal Physiology,* 4th edition. New York, McGraw-Hill, 1991, p 71.)

    c. The homeostatic effect of the TGF control system is maintenance of the composition of the tubular fluid in the region of the tubule around the macula densa.

    d. The macula densa is relatively impermeable to water and has a low Na^+–K^+–ATPase activity, which accounts for its low capacity for NaCl transport.

    e. NaCl transport initiated by NaCl uptake by the Na^+–Cl^-–K^+ cotransporter is a critical early step in TGF signal transmission.

        (1) The activity of this symporter is determined by a change in luminal Cl^- concentration.

      (2) This cotransporter is the major pathway for Cl⁻ reabsorption in the loop of Henle.
  f. TGF stimulation reduces glomerular capillary pressure and GFR in parallel.
  g. Adenosine is the suggested mediator of the TGF response.
      (1) This autocoid, which is locally synthesized by the juxtaglomerular cells, elicits vasoconstriction in the renal vasculature.
      (2) Therefore, it counteracts the elevation in renal arterial pressure.

2. Control of renin secretion (Figure 26-4; see Figure 26-1)

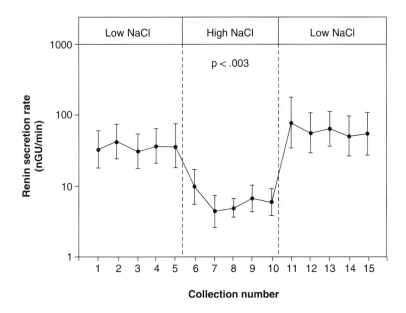

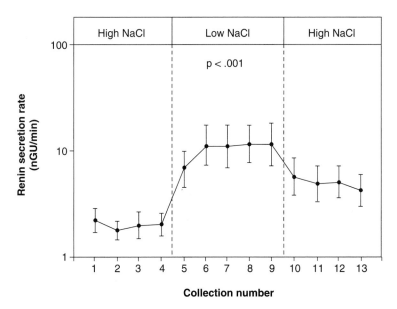

FIGURE 26-4. Macula densa–mediated changes in renin secretion. [Modified from Selin DW, Giebisch G (editors): Function of the juxtaglomerular apparatus. In *The Kidney: Physiology and Pathophysiology* (volume 1), New York, Raven Press, 1992, p 1278.]

  a. NaCl concentration is a more important determinant of renin release than NaCl delivery (NaCl concentration × flow rate).

   (1) When a luminal NaCl load (delivery) is reduced by 80% by decreasing tubular **NaCl concentration** at a constant flow rate, a large change in renin secretion (eightfold) occurs.

   (2) When a luminal NaCl load is reduced by 80% by **decreasing flow rate** at a constant NaCl concentration, a small increment in renin secretion (twofold) occurs.

  b. Increasing NaCl concentration at the macula densa suppresses renin secretion.

D. **Summary of macula densa function**

 1. Changes in NaCl concentration in the tubular fluid in the region of the macula densa induce **direct** changes in the smooth muscle tone of the afferent arteriole (TGF response).

 2. Changes in NaCl concentration at the macula densa have an inverse effect on the GFR (TGF response).

 3. Changes in NaCl concentration at the macula densa have an inverse effect on renin secretion from the granular cells.

IV. **GLOMERULOTUBULAR BALANCE (GTB): EFFECT ON REGULATION OF SODIUM AND WATER EXCRETION** (Table 26-2)

A. **Background and definitions**

 1. GTB describes a fundamental property of the kidney whereby tubular reabsorption is adjusted in proportion to GFR in order to minimize changes in ECF volume and, in turn, blood pressure.

 2. GTB minimizes changes in distal (collecting duct) delivery of Na^+ and fluid and acts to prevent fluid delivery from exceeding the reabsorptive capacity of the collecting tubules. The collecting ducts function most efficiently when the bulk of the filtrate is reabsorbed in the proximal tubule and loop of Henle, and the distal delivery is held relatively constant.

 3. The **fractional** tubular reabsorption of filtrate remains relatively constant despite changes in GFR.

 4. The **absolute** level of tubular reabsorption is directly related to the filtration rate (GFR).

B. **Proximal tubular regulation**

 1. Tubular reabsorption is related to changes in GFR rather than to the filtered load of Na^+. Note: The filtered load of Na^+ is the product of the plasma Na^+ concentration and GFR ($P_{Na^+} \times GFR$).

 2. When the filtered load of Na^+ is varied by changing GFR at **constant** plasma Na^+ concentration, the fractional reabsorption of Na^+ remains constant.

 3. When the filtered load of Na^+ is varied by changing plasma Na^+ concentration at constant GFR, large changes in fractional Na^+ reabsorption occur.

C. **Summary of glomerulotubular balance (GTB).** GTB balance is observed only when the filtered load of Na^+ is changed by varying the GFR. It is **not** observed when the filtered load of Na^+ is changed by varying the plasma Na^+ concentration.

Case

A 58-year-old overweight married homemaker is rushed to the emergency department because she experiences the sudden onset of severe shortness of breath. Because she is

markedly dyspneic, orthopneic, and cyanotic, she receives immediate treatment with oxygen and morphine sulfate before a further history is obtained.

While waiting for the woman's condition to improve, a physician conducts a quick examination which reveals a blood pressure of 240/120 mm Hg, a respiratory rate of 26 breaths/min, a heart rate of 120 beats/min, and temperature of 37°C. Cyanosis, neck vein distention, respiratory rales, and peripheral edema are evident. In addition, she is hyponatremic (130 mEq/L).

    1. *What is the diagnosis?*

DISCUSSION

The sudden dyspnea in the presence of severe pulmonary congestion, hypertension, and an enlarged heart suggest a cardiac emergency—congestive heart failure. The edema is due to an increase in venous pressure that produces a parallel rise in capillary hydraulic pressure.

    2. *What is the pathology of the edema, distended neck veins, and hypo-osmolality of the plasma in this patient?*

DISCUSSION

The major anasarca syndromes (congestive heart failure, hepatic cirrhosis, and nephrotic syndrome), which all result in massive edema, have the same mechanism for the positive Na^+ and H_2O balance. In these conditions, the extracellular fluid (ECF) expansion occurs in response to "underfilling" of the arterial compartment [i.e., diminished effective circulating volume (ECV), or effective arterial blood volume (EABV)], which produces excessive renal Na^+ and H_2O retention. Arterial "underfilling" is caused by: (1) a decrease in cardiac output in congestive heart failure due to incomplete ventricular emptying, known as systolic dysfunction, or inadequate ventricular relaxation, known as diastolic dysfunction; (2) peripheral arterial vasodilation in cirrhosis of the liver; and (3) diminished plasma colloid osmotic pressure in nephrotic syndrome, leading to contraction of intravascular volume.

    The signs and symptoms of NaCl excess are due to ECF volume expansion, and the excess fluid is the result of renal NaCl and H_2O retention. This renal response seems paradoxical, be-

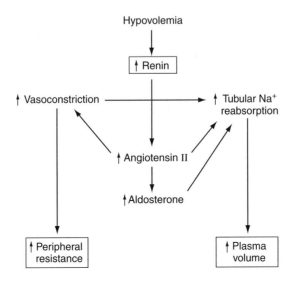

cause both the ECF and vascular volume in congestive heart failure patients is increased. However, the effective circulating volume (ECV) is decreased because of poor cardiac performance and a consequent fall in cardiac output. Therefore, the renal response is directed to increasing the ECV and thereby tissue perfusion. The decline in ECV stimulates the secretion of antidiuretic hormone (ADH) and reduces the delivery of tubular fluid to the diluting segment of the nephron (thick ascending limb of the loop of Henle), with a resultant decrease in water excretion. In most hypo-osmolal states, the water retention leading to an excess of water in relation to solute is the common denominator. This water retention results in hyponatremia, which essentially only occurs when there is a defect in water excretion.

However, it must be emphasized that there is an increase in Na^+ content. It is necessary to appreciate that Na^+ excretion determines the ECF volume, while water excretion controls the Na^+ concentration. This primary Na^+ retention accounts for the pulmonary and peripheral edema, together with the elevated jugular venous pressure, because affected patients are truly volume-expanded.

The renal retention of Na^+ and H_2O seen in the anasarca syndromes results from both a hypovolemia-induced fall in the glomerular filtration rate (GFR) and, more importantly, an increase in tubular reabsorption throughout the nephron. The initial decline in ECV affects the distal nephron as collecting tubular Na^+ reabsorption is enhanced, a response largely mediated by an increase in renin and aldosterone. The decline in the distal delivery of NaCl to the macula densa also leads to dilation of the afferent arteriole via the tubuloglomerular feedback (TGF) loop. As the congestive heart failure progresses, proximal reabsorption is also stimulated due to increased levels of angiotensin II and renal sympathetic neural tone.

Chapter 27

Renal Tubular Transport: Reabsorption and Secretion

I. PARAMETERS OF RENAL ACTIVE TRANSPORT

A. **Renal tubular transport maximum (Tm)** refers to the maximal amount of a given solute that can be transported (reabsorbed or secreted) per minute by the renal tubules.

1. **Definitions**
   a. The highest attainable rate of reabsorption, called the **maximum tubular reabsorptive capacity,** is designated **Tr.** Substances reabsorbed by an active carrier-mediated process that have a Tm include phosphate ion (HPO_4^{2-}), sulfate (SO_4^{2-}), glucose (and other monosaccharides), many amino acids, uric acid, and albumin, acetoacetate, β-hydroxybyrate, and α-ketoglutarate.
   b. The highest attainable rate of secretion is called the **maximum tubular secretory capacity** and is designated **Ts.** Substances that are secreted by the kidneys and that have a Tm include penicillin, certain diuretics, salicylate, *para*-amino-hippuric acid (PAH), and thiamine (vitamin B_1).
   c. The **threshold concentration** (i.e., the plasma concentration at which a solute begins to appear in the urine), is characteristic for a substance that is reabsorbed, and not for a substance which is secreted.

2. **Exceptions**
   a. Uric acid and urea are organic substances both reabsorbed and secreted by the kidney. K^+ and HCO_3^- are inorganic ions that are both reabsorbed and secreted by the kidney.
   b. Some solutes have no definite upper limit for unidirectional transport and, hence, have **no transport maximum.**
      (1) Reabsorption of Na^+ along the nephron
      (2) Secretion of K^+ by the distal tubules
      (3) HCO_3^- (no absolute transport maximum)

B. **Filtered load and excretion rate.** Reabsorption and secretion are not directly measured variables but are derived from the measurements of the amount of solute filtered (filtered load) and the amount of solute excreted (excretion rate).

1. **Definitions.** Capital letters with dots above them denote rate functions for various renal transport processes with units of mg/min.
   a. The **filtered load** is the amount of a substance entering the tubule by filtration per unit time and is mathematically equal to the product of the glomerular filtration rate (GFR) and the plasma concentration of the substance (P_x):

   $$\dot{F} = \text{Filtered load} = GFR \cdot P_x \ [(ml/min) \ (mg/ml) = mg/min]$$

   Because the GFR is equal to the clearance of inulin (C_{in}), the filtered load can be calculated as $C_{in} \cdot P_x$.
   b. The **excretion rate** is the amount of a substance that appears in the urine per unit time and is mathematically equal to the product of urine flow rate ($\dot{V}$) and the urinary concentration of the substance (U_x):

   $$\dot{E} = \text{Excretion rate} = U_x \cdot \dot{V} \ [(mg/ml) \ (ml/min) = mg/min]$$

   (1) **Secretion.** If the secretion rate exceeds the filtered load [or if the clearance of the substance (C_x) is greater than C_{in}], net tubular secretion of that substance has occurred. Thus, secretion ($\dot{S}$) is expressed as the excretion rate minus filtered load, or $\dot{S} = \dot{E} - \dot{F}$.

For secretion: $U_x \cdot \dot{V} > C_{in} \cdot P_x$ or $C_x > C_{in}$

(2) **Reabsorption.** If the filtered load exceeds the excretion rate (or if C_x is $< C_{in}$), net reabsorption of that substance has occurred. Thus, reabsorption ($\dot{R}$) is expressed as the filtered load minus excretion rate, or $\dot{R} = \dot{F} - \dot{E}$.

For reabsorption: $C_{in} \cdot P_x > U_x \cdot \dot{V}$, or $C_x < C_{in}$

2. **Calculation of transport maximum (Tr or Ts).** Transport maximum is the difference between the filtered load ($C_{in} \cdot P_x$) and the excretion rate ($U_x \cdot \dot{V}$). Tr and Ts, then, are expressed as:

$$Tr = C_{in} \cdot P_x - U_x \cdot \dot{V} \text{ (in mg/min)}; \ Tr = \dot{F} - \dot{E}$$

$$Ts = U_x \cdot \dot{V} - C_{in} \cdot P_x \text{ (in mg/min)}; \ Ts = \dot{E} - \dot{F}$$

    a. Tm pertains to solutes that are actively transported.
    b. Substances that are passively transported (urea) do not exhibit a Tm.

II. GRAPHIC REPRESENTATION OF RENAL TRANSPORT PROCESSES: RENAL TITRATION CURVES (Figure 27-1)

A. Construction of renal titration curves (glucose and PAH)

    1. A titration curve is constructed by plotting the following pairs of variables:
        a. The filtered load ($C_{in} \cdot P_x$) against the plasma concentration (P_x)
        b. The excretion rate ($U_x \cdot \dot{V}$) against P_x
        c. The difference between the filtered load and excretion rate (i.e., Tr or Ts) against P_x, which is the independent variable

    2. The plotted renal titration curve, therefore, can be used to estimate the plasma concentration (P_x) at which the renal tubular membrane carriers are fully saturated (Tm). This plasma concentration associated with the Tm is **not** the renal threshold.

    3. The Tm for glucose **and** PAH is given by the vertical distance between the linear range of excretion rate ($U_x \cdot \dot{V}$) and the filtered load ($C_{in} \cdot P_x$) [see Figure 27-1B].

B. Glucose transport: reabsorption

    1. Characteristics of glucose transport
        a. Glucose is an essential nutrient that is actively reabsorbed into the proximal tubule by a transport maximum-limited process. The transport maximum for glucose (Tm_G) is about 375 mg/min (about 2 mmol/min).
        b. Because the Tm_G is nearly constant and depends on the number of functional nephrons, it is used clinically to estimate the number of functional nephrons, or the tubular reabsorptive capacity (Tr).
        c. Glucose is transported from the early and late proximal tubular lumen by SGLT-2 and SGLT-1, respectively.

    2. Glucose titration curve. Figure 27-1A illustrates that glucose transport and excretion processes are functions of the plasma glucose concentration (P_G).
        a. Increasing the P_G results in a progressive linear increase in the filtered load ($C_{in} \cdot P_G$).
            (1) At a low P_G, the reabsorption of glucose is complete; hence, the clearance of glucose (C_G) is zero (see Figure 27-1C).
            (2) When P_G in humans reaches the renal threshold concentration of 180–200 mg/dl (10–11 mmol/L), glucose appears in the urine (glycosuria). Note that the threshold concentration is not synonymous with the P_G that completely saturates the transport mechanism, which is about 300 mg/dl. The appearance of glucose in the urine before the transport maximum is reached is termed **splay** and results from:
                (a) Heterogeneity in glomerular size, proximal tubular length, and numbers of carrier proteins for glucose reabsorption. For example, a nephron with a

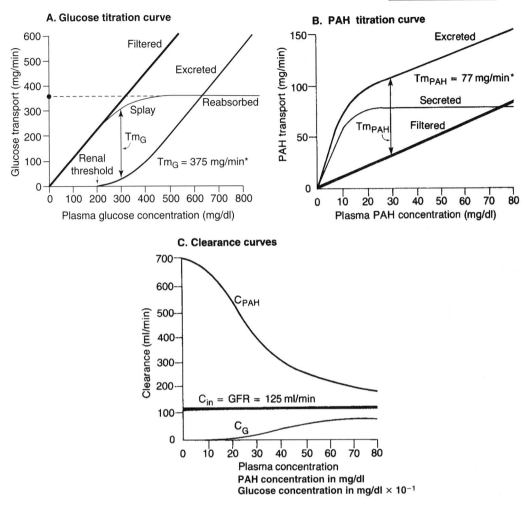

FIGURE 27-1. Relationships of renal titration curves and clearance curves to plasma concentration. The dependent variables [i.e., filtered load, excretion rate, maximum tubular reabsorptive capacity (Tm), and maximum tubular secretory capacity (Ts)] are plotted on the ordinate as a function of the independent variable [i.e., the plasma concentration of the substance (P_x)]. The splay (*curved portions*) observed in the glucose reabsorption and excretion curves (*graph A*) and the splay in the *para*-aminohippuric acid (PAH) secretion and excretion curves (*graph B*) are due to the kinetics of tubular transport and the heterogeneity of the nephron population in terms of number, length, and functional variations in transport. The clearance of glucose (C_G) increases and approaches the clearance of inulin (C_{in}) asymptotically as the plasma glucose concentration increases beyond the tubular transport maximum for glucose (Tm_G) [*graph C*]. Conversely, the clearance of PAH (C_{PAH}) declines and approaches the C_{in} asymptotically as the plasma PAH concentration increases above the tubular transport maximum for PAH (Tm_{PAH}) [*graph C*]. In *graph C*, the plasma PAH concentration is in mg/dl and the plasma glucose concentration is plotted as one-tenth of the actual concentration (i.e., mg/dl $\cdot$ 1.0^{-1}). * = per 1.73 m^2 body surface area. (Adapted from Selkurt EE: Renal function. In *Physiology*, 5th edition. Edited by Selkurt EE. Boston, Little, Brown, 1984, pp 424 and 429.)

    large glomerulus (i.e., a high filtered load), or a short proximal tubule (i.e., low reabsorptive capacity) will spill glucose into the urine at a lower P_G than predicted from the transport maximum for the whole kidney.

  (b) Variability in the transport maximum of the nephrons. For example, there is variability in the number of glucose carriers, the transport rates of the carriers, and the binding affinities of the carriers for glucose.

b. As the Tm_G is approached, the urinary excretion rate increases linearly with increasing P_G (first-order reaction kinetics).
  (1) When the Tm_G is reached, the quantity of glucose reabsorbed per minute remains constant and is independent of P_G (zero-order reaction kinetics).
  (2) When the Tm_G is exceeded, the C_G becomes increasingly a function of glomerular filtration. Therefore, the C_G approaches C_{in}, and the amount reabsorbed becomes a smaller fraction of the total amount excreted.

C. *Para*-aminohippuric acid (PAH) transport: secretion

1. Characteristics of PAH transport
  a. PAH, a weak organic acid, is actively secreted into the proximal tubule by a transport maximum-limited process. PAH is a foreign substance that is not stored or metabolized and is excreted virtually unchanged in the urine. By filtration and secretion, PAH is almost entirely cleared from the plasma in a single pass through the kidney, if the transport maximum for PAH (Tm_{PAH}) has not been reached. (The Tm_{PAH} in humans is about 80 mg/min.)
  b. Because approximately 10% of the plasma PAH is bound to plasma proteins, PAH is not entirely freely filterable, and the concentration of PAH in the plasma (P_{PAH}) is greater than that in the glomerular filtrate. However, PAH binding does not significantly diminish the effectiveness of tubular secretion.
  c. Because the Tm_{PAH} is nearly constant, it is used clinically to estimate Ts.

2. PAH titration curve. Figure 27-1B illustrates that the filtration and secretion of PAH are functions of the P_{PAH}. The amount of PAH excreted per minute ($U_{PAH} \cdot \dot{V}$) exceeds the amount filtered ($C_{in} \cdot P_{PAH}$) at any P_{PAH}.
  a. When the P_{PAH} is low (10 mg/dl), virtually all of the PAH is secreted, and PAH is almost completely cleared from the plasma by the combined processes of glomerular filtration and tubular secretion.
  b. When P_{PAH} is above 20 mg/dl, the transepithelial secretory mechanism becomes saturated, and the Tm_{PAH} is reached.
  c. When the Tm_{PAH} is reached, the quantity of PAH secreted per minute remains constant and is independent of P_{PAH}.
  d. When the Tm_{PAH} is exceeded, the C_{PAH} becomes progressively more a function of glomerular filtration; hence, the C_{PAH} approaches C_{in} (see Figure 27-1C), and the constant amount of PAH secreted becomes a smaller fraction of the total amount excreted.

3. PAH clearance (C_{PAH}) and renal plasma flow (Chapter 25 III C)
  a. Fick principle. According to the Fick principle, blood flow through an organ can be determined with the equation:

$$Q = \frac{R}{A_x - V_x}$$

  where Q = blood flow (ml/min), R = rate of removal (or addition) of a substance from (or to) the blood as it flows through an organ (in mg/min), A_x = concentration of the substance in the blood entering the organ (mg/ml), and V_x = the concentration of the substance in the blood leaving the organ (mg/ml).
  b. Because C_{PAH} **can be used to measure renal plasma flow,** the Fick principle equation can be modified to:

$$RPF = \frac{U_{PAH} \cdot \dot{V}}{A_{PAH} - V_{PAH}}$$

  where RPF = renal plasma flow (ml/min), $U_{PAH} \cdot \dot{V}$ = rate of PAH excretion (mg/min), and A_{PAH} and V_{PAH} = concentrations of PAH (in mg/ml) in the renal artery and the renal vein, respectively.
  (1) At low concentrations of PAH in arterial plasma, the renal clearance is nearly complete. Therefore, as a first approximation, the PAH concentration in renal venous plasma may be taken to be zero.

(a) Approximately 10%–15% of the total renal plasma flow perfuses nonexcretory (nontubular) portions of the kidney such as the renal capsule, perirenal fat, the renal medulla, and the renal pelvis; therefore, this plasma cannot be completely cleared of PAH by filtration and secretion.

(b) Because about 10% of the PAH remains in the renal venous plasma, the renal plasma flow calculated from C_{PAH} underestimates the actual flow by about 10%. Accordingly, the C_{PAH} actually measures the **effective renal plasma flow (ERPF):**

$$ERPF = \frac{U_{PAH} \cdot \dot{V}}{A_{PAH}} = C_{PAH}$$

(2) Because PAH is not metabolized or excreted by any organ other than the kidney, a sample from any peripheral vein can be used to measure arterial plasma PAH concentration, and the equation is written as:

$$ERPF = \frac{U_{PAH} \cdot \dot{V}}{P_{PAH}} = C_{PAH}$$

c. **Effective renal blood flow (ERBF)** is calculated from the relationship between plasma volume (PV), hematocrit (Hct), and blood volume (BV), as*

$$Blood\ volume = \frac{plasma\ volume \cdot 100}{(100 - hematocrit)}$$

and, therefore,

$$ERBF = \frac{ERPF \cdot 100}{(100 - hematocrit)}$$

d. **True renal plasma flow (TRPF)** can be determined if the extraction ratio (E) is known, where:

$$E = \frac{A_{PAH} - V_{PAH}}{A_{PAH}}, \text{ and } TRPF = \frac{ERPF}{E}; TRBF = \frac{TRPF \cdot 100}{(100 - hematocrit)}$$

III. RENAL TRANSPORT OF COMMON SOLUTES AND WATER (Table 27-1)

A. **General considerations** (see Figure 24-3)

1. **The proximal tubules reabsorb 60%–65% of the filtered Na$^+$, Cl$^-$, bicarbonate (HCO$_3^-$), and water and virtually all of the filtered K$^+$, HPO$_4^{2-}$, and amino acids.** In addition, glucose is reabsorbed almost completely by the proximal tubules and begins to appear in the urine when the renal threshold is exceeded (i.e., at approximately 200 mg glucose/dl arterial plasma, or 11 mmol/L). Eighty percent of the filtered HCO$_3^-$ is reabsorbed proximally.

2. Reabsorption of water is passive, and reabsorption of solutes can be passive or active; solute reabsorption generates an osmotic gradient, which causes the passive reabsorption of water (osmosis).

3. Two-thirds of Na$^+$ reabsorption occurs transcellularly mainly via the Na$^+$–H$^+$ countertransporter, whereas one-third is transported by the paracellular (intercellular) pathway by one of the following gradients:
   a. Electrodiffusion (e.g., electrorepulsion of Na$^+$ via the lumen-positive transepithelial voltage generated by the diffusion of Cl$^-$)

---

*In humans, the C_{PAH} is 600–700 ml/min and, when corrected to ERBF (assuming an Hct of 45%), is approximately 1100–1200 ml/min, which is about 20% of the resting cardiac output.:

TABLE 27-1. Daily Renal Transport of Electrolytes, Nonelectrolytes, and Water in a Normal Adult

Substance	Unit	Filtered Load ($\dot{F}$)	Amount Reabsorbed ($\dot{R}$)	Amount Secreted ($\dot{S}$)	Amount Excreted ($\dot{E}$)[†]	Filtered Load Reabsorbed [$\dot{R}/\dot{F}$] (%)
Na^+	mEq/day	25,200	25,050	. . .	150	99.4
Cl^-	mEq/day	18,000	17,850	. . .	150	99.2
HCO_3^-	mEq/day	4320	4318	. . .	2	99.9+
K^+	mEq/day	720	620	50	100	86.1
Ca^{2+}	mEq/day	540	530		10	98.1
	mmol/day	270	265	. . .	5	
HPO_4^{2-}	mEq/day	260	234		26	90
	mmol/day	144	130	. . .	14	
Urea*	mmol/day	870	460	. . .	410	52.9
Glucose	mmol/day	800	799.5	. . .	0.5	99.9+
Uric acid	mmol/day	50	49	4	5	98.0
Total solute	mmol/day	50,374	49,541.5	54	836.5	98.3
Water	ml/day	180,000	179,000	. . .	1000	99.4

*Urea diffuses into and out of parts of the nephron (i.e., it secreted and reabsorbed, respectively).
†The amount excreted ($\dot{E}$) = filtered load ($\dot{F}$) + amount secreted ($\dot{S}$) − amount reabsorbed ($\dot{R}$)
Amount filtered (filtered load) = GFR · P_x = $\dot{F}$
Amount reabsorbed = (GFR · P_x) − (U_x · $\dot{V}$) = $\dot{F}$ − $\dot{E}$
Amount secreted = (U_x · $\dot{V}$) − (GFR · P_x) = $\dot{E}$ − $\dot{F}$
Amount excreted = U_x · $\dot{V}$ = $\dot{E}$

   b. Diffusion along a concentration gradient (e.g., Cl^-)
   c. Bulk flow driven by a hydrostatic pressure gradient, which causes solute transport by convection
   d. Accumulation of solutes in the intercellular space, which also promotes water reabsorption by osmosis

4. The reabsorption of every substance, including water, is linked in some way to the operation of the Na^+–K^+–ATPase pump. No ATP-dependent **anion** pump has been found in the nephron.

5. The kidney plays a major role in Na^+ reabsorption to maintain the extracellular fluid (ECF) volume and, therefore, over time, to maintain blood pressure.

6. Most of the energy utilized by the kidney is used for active Na^+ reabsorption. However, not all reabsorption of Na^+ is active.
   a. For every mole of ATP, 20–30 Na^+ ions are reabsorbed.
   b. The reabsorption of 28 equivalents of Na^+ requires 1 mole of oxygen.

B. **Proximal reabsorption of sodium, chloride, and water** (Figures 27-2 and 27-3; see Chapter 23 III and Figure 24-3)

   1. Transcellular Na^+ reabsorption by the proximal tubule is a two-step process.
      a. Na^+ moves across the apical membrane down an electrochemical gradient established by the Na^+–K^+–ATPase pump.
      b. Na^+ moves across the basolateral membrane against an electrochemical gradient via the Na^+–K^+–ATPase pump.

   2. The main determinant of Na^+ (and H_2O) reabsorption in the early proximal tubule is the Na^+–H^+ antiporter, which has three major effects on proximal transport.

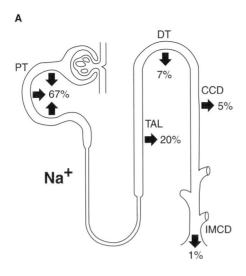

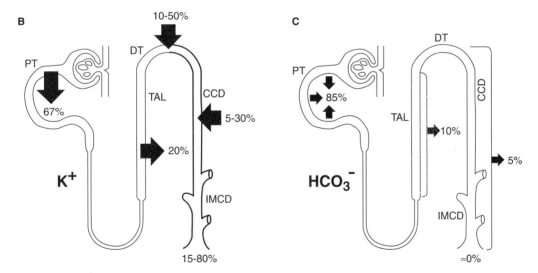

FIGURE 27-2. Segmental reabsorption of ions. (A)The kidneys reabsorb virtually all of the filtered load of Na^+. The major regulator for collecting duct Na^+ reabsorption is aldosterone. Chloride reabsorption occurs in parallel with Na^+. (B) Potassium excretion is determined by the rate of K^+ secretion by the distal tubule and collecting duct. K^+ secretion by these segments is stimulated by hyperkalemia, aldosterone, tubular flow rate, ADH, metabolic alkalosis, and $[Na^+]$ in the tubular fluid. The DT and CD have the dual capacity to reabsorb and secrete K^+. (C) Normally the entire filtered load of HCO_3^- is reabsorbed. The process of H^+ secretion achieves HCO_3^- reabsorption. *(continued)*

    a. It promotes both Na^+ reabsorption and active H^+ secretion into the lumen leading primarily to HCO_3^- reabsorption across the basolateral border via the 3 HCO_3^-/1 Na^+ carrier.

    b. The preferential absorption of Na^+ with HCO_3^- and water creates the concentration gradient for proximal passive (paracellular) reabsorption of Cl^-.

D

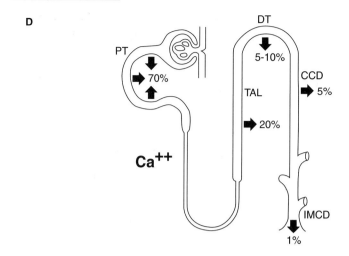

E

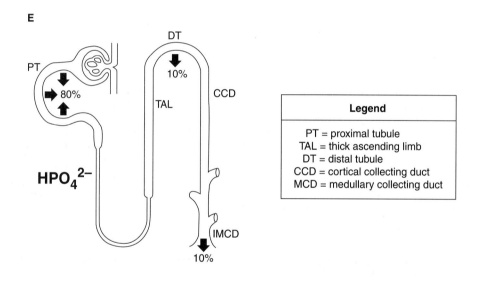

Legend
PT = proximal tubule
TAL = thick ascending limb
DT = distal tubule
CCD = cortical collecting duct
MCD = medullary collecting duct

FIGURE 27-2. (*continued*) (D) Plasma [Ca^{2+}] is regulated by parathyroid hormone (PTH) and 1,25-dihydroxyvitamin D_3. Calcium excretion by the kidneys is determined by the rate of Ca^{2+} reabsorption by the TAL, which is regulated mainly by PTH, which stimulates distal nephron Ca^{2+} reabsorption. (E) Plasma [HPO_4^{2-}] is regulated by PTH and 1,25-dihydroxyvitamin D_3. Renal $H_2PO_4^-$ excretion is determined mainly by the rate of proximal reabsorption. PTH inhibits HPO_4^{2-} reabsorption by the proximal tubule and enhances urinary $H_2PO_4^-$ excretion. (Modified from Koepper BM, Stanton, BA: *Renal Physiology.* Philadelphia, Mosby Yearbook, 1992, pp 98, 116, 126, 143, 149.)

    c. It promotes **active** Cl^- reabsorption by operating in parallel with the Cl^-–formate exchanger in the late proximal segment (Figure 27-4).

  3. Sodium is also cotransported across the luminal membrane of the early proximal segment with inorganic phosphate (HPO_4^{2-}) and organic molecules such as glucose, amino acids, and lactate.

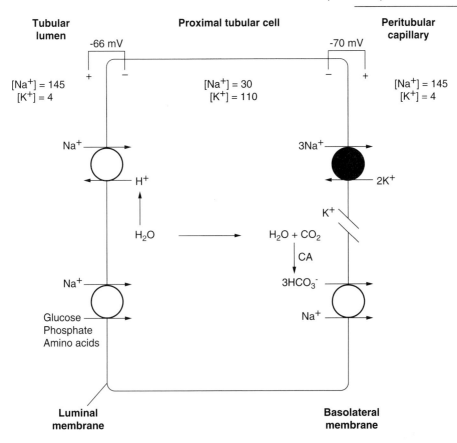

FIGURE 27-3. Schematic representation of the chemical and electrical gradients and some of the carrier-mediated mechanisms involved in proximal tubular solute transport. The low cell Na^+ concentration that is maintained by the $Na^+–K^+–ATPase$ pump in the basolateral membrane permits secondary active transport in which passive Na^+ entry into the cell is coupled by specific cotransporters to the uphill reabsorption of glucose, phosphate, and amino acids, or to the secretion of H^+. Units are mEq/L; CA represents carbonic anhydrase. (Modified from Rose BD: *Clinical Physiology of Acid–Base and Electrolyte Disorders,* 4th edition. New York, McGraw-Hill, 1994, p 71.)

4. In the early proximal tubule, the transepithelial potential difference is lumen-negative due to Na^+ reabsorption.

5. In the late proximal tubule, Na^+ is reabsorbed primarily with Cl^- across both the transcellular and paracellular pathways. Paracellular NaCl reabsorption occurs because of the concentration gradient created by the rise in tubular fluid Cl^- concentration.
   a. This Cl^- diffusion gradient provides for Cl^- reabsorption by bulk flow via the paracellular channel.
   b. Active reabsorption of Na^+ leaves the early proximal tubular lumen negative and provides a driving force for Cl^- reabsorption by electrodiffusion through charge repulsion.
   c. Transcellular Cl^- can be returned to the systemic circulation by a basolateral membrane $K^+–Cl^-$ cotransporter.

6. Most of the H^+, NH_4^+, organic anions (PAH), and organic cations (creatinine) are **secreted** by the proximal tubule.

7. Two-thirds of the filtered H_2O is reabsorbed proximally in response to a transtubular osmotic gradient established by solute (e.g., Na^+, Cl^-, Na^+-glucose) reabsorption.
   a. Two-thirds of the total proximal Na^+ and H_2O reabsorption occurs through the transcellular pathway.

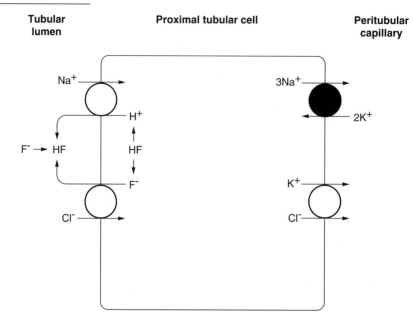

FIGURE 27-4. Role of filtered formate (F⁻) in active Cl⁻ reabsorption in the proximal tubule. The essential steps are transport of uncharged formic acid (HF) into the cell, formate secretion and Cl⁻ reabsorption via a formate–chloride exchanger, and recycling of formate into the cell as formic acid. Reabsorbed Cl⁻ is returned to the peritubular capillary by a KCl cotransporter in the basolateral membrane. (Modified from Rose BD: *Clinical Physiology of Acid–Base and Electrolyte Disorders,* 4th edition. New York, McGraw-Hill, 1994, p 74).

    b. One-third of the total proximal Na^+ and H_2O reabsorption occurs passively through the tight junction (paracellular pathway).

C. **Reabsorption of sodium by the loop of Henle** (Figure 27-5).

    1. About 20% of the filtered Na^+ and Cl^- and 15% of the filtered H_2O occurs in the loop of Henle, the exclusive site of H_2O reabsorption.

        a. Thin descending limb of the loop of Henle (DLH). Little reabsorption of Na^+ and Cl^- occurs here. Water reabsorption in the loop of Henle occurs exclusively in the thin descending segment.

        b. Thin ascending limb of the loop of Henle (ALH). Limited passive reabsorption of Na^+ and Cl^- occurs in this water-impermeable limb.

        c. Thick ALH

            (1) Na^+ movement across the apical membrane, which is mediated by the Na^+–$2Cl^-$–K^+ symporter, is not linked to organic solutes. This cotransporter, with the downhill movement of Na^+ and Cl^-, drives the uphill movement of K^+ influx.

            (2) This electroneutral symporter provides the major pathway for Cl^- reabsorption in this segment.

                (a) Cl^- delivery is rate-limiting, as NaCl transport increases directly with the tubular fluid Cl^- concentration.

                (b) K^+ is returned to the lumen for continued activation of the Na^+–$2Cl^-$–K^+ carrier and creates a lumen-positive potential difference.

            (3) About half of Na^+ reabsorption is transcellular and active, while the other half is paracellular and passive due to the lumen-positive potential created by K^+ efflux.

            (4) Sodium that enters the cell is returned to the systemic circulation by the primary active Na^+–$2Cl^-$–K^+ pump in the basolateral membrane.

            (5) Chloride exits the cell through selective Cl^- channels.

            (6) The thick ALH is water impermeable and paracellular transport of Na^+ occurs via the electrogenic effect of luminal K^+.

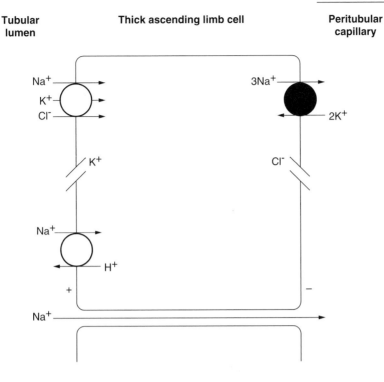

Tubular lumen	Thick ascending limb cell	Peritubular capillary

FIGURE 27-5. Schematic model of the major steps involved in NaCl transport in the medullary thick ascending limb of the loop of Henle. Entry into the cell occurs via a passive $Na^+–K^+–2Cl^-$ carrier in the luminal membrane. The energy for this process is indirectly provided by the $Na^+–K^+–ATPase$ pump in the basolateral membrane that maintains a relatively low cell Na^+ concentration. The return of reabsorbed Na^+ and Cl^- to the systematic circulation occurs via the $Na^+–K^+–ATPase$ pump and a Cl^- channel, respectively. Recycling of K^+ across the luminal membrane creates a lumen-positive potential that allows one-half of loop Na^+ reabsorption to occur passively via the paracellular route. (Modified from Rose BD: *Clinical Physiology of Acid–Base and Electrolyte Disorders,* 4th edition. New York, McGraw-Hill, 1994, p 106.)

> **(7)** Transcellular Na^+ reabsorption also occurs by $Na^+–H^+$ exchange, leading to HCO_3^- reabsorption.

D. **Reabsorption of sodium by the collecting duct** (Figure 27-6)

1. The collecting duct reabsorbs about 5% of the filtered NaCl, secretes variable amounts of K^+ and H^+, and reabsorbs 8%–17% of the water in response to the effect of antidiuretic hormone (ADH) on the medullary collecting duct.
   a. The collecting duct is water-impermeable in the absence of ADH.
   b. Na^+ enters the systemic circulation via the $Na^+–K^+–ATPase$ pump.
   c. Cl^- enters the bloodstream mainly via the paracellular route and is driven by the lumen-negative charge generated by the diffusional influx of Na^+ through Na^+-selective channels in the apical membrane.

2. **Collecting ducts** are composed of **two cell types.**
   a. **Principal cells,** which reabsorb Na^+ and water through apical membrane channels and secrete K^+ through luminal channels (see Figure 27-6)
   b. **Intercalated cells,** which can be further subdivided into two types
      (1) Alpha (A)-type cells, which secrete H^+ via a luminal $3H^+–ATPase$ pump, can also reabsorb K^+ via a luminal primary active $H^+–K^+–ATPase$ pump.
      (2) Beta (B)-type cells secrete HCO_3^- in alkalotic states via a luminal Cl^-/HCO_3^- exchanger.

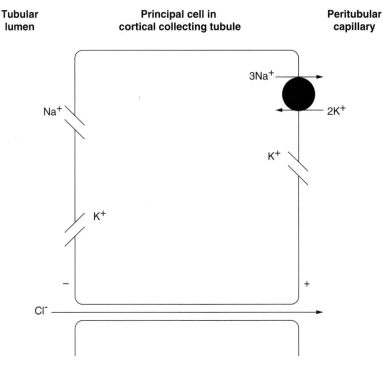

| Tubular lumen | Principal cell in cortical collecting tubule | Peritubular capillary |

FIGURE 27-6. Ion transport in the principal cell in the cortical collecting tubule. Luminal Na^+ enters the cell through a Na^+ channel in the luminal membrane. The lumen-negative voltage created by this movement of Na^+ then promotes either the secretion of K^+ or the reabsorption of Cl^- via the paracellular route. These cells also can reabsorb water in the presence of antidiuretic hormone (ADH). (Modified from Rose BD: *Clinical Physiology of Acid–Base and Electrolyte Disorders,* 4th edition, New York, McGraw-Hill, 1994, p 138.)

3. **Aldosterone** stimulates ionic transport in the principal cells of the cortical collecting ducts in three ways—by increasing:
   a. The number of luminal Na^+ conductive channels, enhancing the reabsorption of 3%–4% of the filtered Na^+ load
   b. The number of luminal K^+ conductive channels, leading to increased cellular K^+ concentration and secretion
   c. The number of Na^+–K^+–ATPase molecules in the basolateral membrane

4. **Aldosterone** also has a stimulatory effect on H^+ secretion by the synthesis of new electrogenic H^+–ATPase pumps, which are inserted into the luminal membrane of the intercalated A-cells.

E. **Mechanisms by which sodium reabsorption drives reabsorption of other substances.** Na^+ reabsorption:

1. Creates lumen-negative transtubular potential difference across the epithelium, which favors the paracellular reabsorption of anions (e.g., Cl^-) by diffusion

2. Creates transtubular osmolality differences, which favor reabsorption of water by osmosis. In turn, water reabsorption concentrates many luminal solutes (e.g., Cl^-, urea), thus favoring their reabsorption by diffusion.

3. Accomplishes reabsorption of many organic nutrients, as well as phosphate and Cl^-, by cotransport

4. Accomplishes secretion of H^+ (in the proximal tubule) by countertransport; these H^+ ions are required for the reabsorption of HCO_3^-. The Na^+–H^+ antiporter significantly af-

fects proximal transport (see III B 2). It should be noted that preferential reabsorption of HCO_3^- and H_2O creates favorable gradient for the passive reabsorption of Cl^-.

F. **Proximal potassium reabsorption** (Figure 27-7)

1. Almost all of the filtered K^+ is reabsorbed in the proximal tubule (67%) and the loop of Henle (20%), so that approximately 10% is delivered to the early distal tubule.

2. Proximal K^+ reabsorption can be reabsorbed in several ways. Paracellular (passive) transport involves:
   a. Diffusion along a concentration gradient accounts for 60% of proximal reabsorption
   b. Solvent drag with the bulk flow of water
   c. Active transport via the $Na^+–K^+–ATPase$ pump

3. It is unlikely that K^+ is actively reabsorbed across the proximal apical membrane.

4. Luminal fluid equilibrates with the low K^+ concentration in the interspace, which decreases K^+ concentration in the lumen below peritubular capillary levels.
   a. The apical membrane has K^+ conductance channels, which allow K^+ ions to leak into the lumen.
   b. Exit of K^+ ions from the interspace into the peritubular fluid is driven by the movement of fluid and K^+ (solvent drag) along the hydrostatic pressure gradient that normally develops along the interspace from luminal to basolateral end.

5. Three pathways for K^+ reabsorption, which exit across the basolateral membrane (see Figure 27-7)
   a. A conductive channel
   b. The $K^+–Cl^-$ cotransporter
   c. The $Na^+–K^+–ATPase$ pump

6. In the late proximal tubule, the transepithelial potential difference becomes lumen-positive and provides a favorable driving force for net K^+ reabsorption.

G. **Reabsorption of potassium by the loop of Henle**

1. The primary driving force for net K^+ reabsorption is ATP-driven active $Na^+–K^+$ exchange across the basolateral membrane.

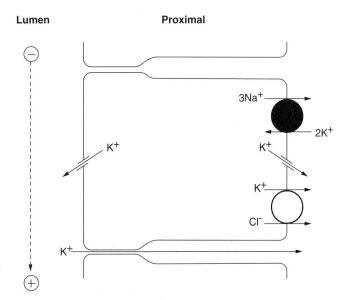

FIGURE 27-7. Proximal K^+ reabsorption occurs by three basolateral pathways: (1) a conductive channel; (2) a KCl cotransporter, and (3) the $Na^+–K^+–ATPase$ pump. [Modified from Seldin DW, Giebisch G (editors): Renal potassium excretion. In *The Kidney: Physiology and Pathophysiology,* 2nd edition (vol 2). New York, Raven Press, 1992, p 222.]

a. This pump generates the steep Na$^+$ gradient that provides energy for the influx of Na$^+$ across the apical membrane.

b. Entry of Na$^+$ is coupled to the entry of 1 K$^+$ and 2 Cl$^-$ by the Na$^+$–2Cl$^-$–K$^+$ cotransporter (see Figure 27-5).

2. Passive conductive pathways for K$^+$ exist in the apical and basolateral membranes.

a. There are also basolateral Cl$^-$ conductance pathways. Cl$^-$ conductance across the basolateral membrane is dominant over K$^+$ conductance.

b. The luminal K$^+$ conductance (efflux) and the basolateral Cl$^-$ conductance (efflux) generate diffusion potentials oriented with the cell interior negative to the ECF.

H. **Reabsorption and secretion of potassium by the collecting ducts**

1. Both the principal and the intercalated (A-type) cells regulate renal K$^+$ secretion and reabsorption, respectively by the cortical collecting duct (Figure 27-8; see Figure 27-6)
   a. Principal cells secrete K$^+$ via apical conductance channels.
   b. A-type intercalated cells actively secrete H$^+$ via the H$^+$–K$^+$–ATPase pump.

2. Active potassium uptake across the basolateral membrane is coupled to active Na$^+$ extrusion by the Na$^+$–K$^+$–ATPase pump. The H$^+$–ATPase pump, the Na$^+$–K$^+$–ATPase pump, and the Na$^+$ and K$^+$ conductive channels are activated by aldosterone.

3. K$^+$ enters the systemic circulation from the cortical collecting duct by diffusion through K$^+$ conductance channels.

4. The primary event in determining urinary K$^+$ excretion is K$^+$ secretion from the blood into the tubular fluid of the distal tubule and collecting duct, which involves two processes.
   a. Active potassium uptake across the basolateral membrane by Na$^+$–K$^+$–ATPase
   b. Diffusion of K$^+$ from the cell into the tubular fluid

I. Effect of potassium on acid–base balance (Figure 27-9). Changes in plasma [K$^+$] have important effects on acid-base balance and, conversely, changes in acid–base balance have important effects on plasma [K$^+$]. In the distal nephron, which has the capacity for both net secretion and net reabsorption of K$^+$, intracellular H$^+$ and K$^+$ behave as if they were competing with each other for secretion into the lumen (Table 27-2).

J. **Renal regulation of hydrogen ion balance** (see Table 27-2). To maintain a normal plasma [HCO$_3^-$], the kidney must secrete H$^+$ into the tubular lumen. The process of H$^+$ secretion and HCO$_3^-$ reabsorption occurs throughout the nephron, except in the DLH (see Figure 27-10).

1. **H$^+$ secretion** permits conservation of HCO$_3^-$ via reabsorption of filtered HCO$_3^-$ (i.e., HCO$_3^-$ reabsorption) and regeneration of HCO$_3^-$ by urinary net acid excretion (Figure 27-10).
   a. H$^+$ secretion into the tubular lumen occurs by active transport and is coupled to Na$^+$ reabsorption; for each H$^+$ secreted, one Na$^+$ and one HCO$_3^-$ are reabsorbed.
   b. The renal epithelium secretes approximately 4300 mEq (mmol) of H$^+$ daily.
   (1) Approximately 85% of the total H$^+$ secretion occurs in the proximal tubules by the Na$^+$–H$^+$ antiporter in the luminal membrane.
   (2) Approximately 10% of the total H$^+$ secretion occurs in the distal tubules; and about 5% occurs in the collecting ducts (type A intercalated cells). Secretion of H$^+$ in these segments of the nephron occurs mainly via the H$^+$–ATPase active secretory pump in the luminal membrane.
   (3) It is essential to appreciate that H$^+$ excretion can be quantitatively equated to the renal contribution of new HCO$_3^-$. Conversely, it is critical to understand that the urinary excretion of HCO$_3^-$ is equivalent to the addition of H$^+$ to the body.

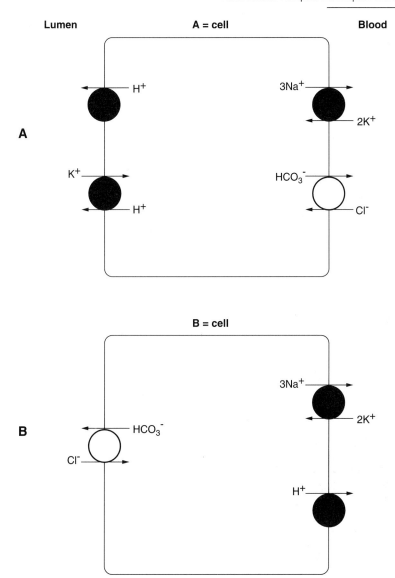

FIGURE 27-8. Mechanistic models for H$^+$ secretion (A-cell) and HCO$_3^-$ secretion (B-cell) by the intercalated cells of the collecting duct. *A cell:* H$^+$ ions are secreted into the lumen by the H$^+$–ATPase pump. Bicarbonate ion is then returned to the systemic circulation via the Cl$^-$–HCO$_3^-$ exchanger in the basolateral membrane. The favorable inward concentration gradient for Cl$^-$ provides the energy for HCO$_3^-$ reabsorption. H$^+$–K$^+$–ATPase pumps may also be present in the luminal membrane. *B cell:* HCO$_3^-$ is secreted into the lumen via the Cl$^-$–HCO$_3^-$ exchanger. The favorable inward concentration gradient for Cl$^-$ provides the energy for HCO$_3^-$ secretion.

    2. HCO$_3^-$ conservation. Reabsorption of HCO$_3^-$ alone cannot maintain normal acid–base balance. Therefore, the kidney is capable of generating new HCO$_3^-$ as well.
      a. HCO$_3^-$ reabsorption
        (1) Process (see Figure 37-1)
          (a) H$^+$ secreted into the tubular fluid combines with filtered HCO$_3^-$ to form carbonic acid (H$_2$CO$_3$):

$$H^+ + HCO_3^- \rightleftarrows H_2CO_3$$

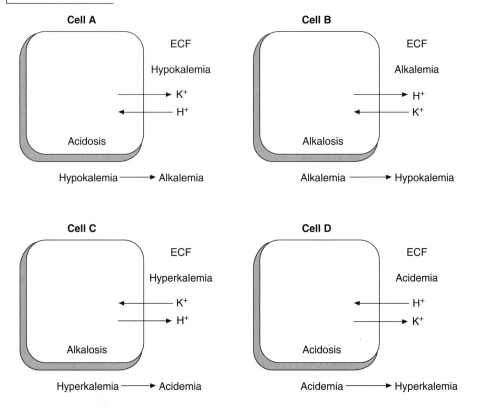

FIGURE 27-9. K$^+$–H$^+$ relationships. (*A*) Hypokalemia leads to alkalemia. During hypokalemic states, cellular K$^+$ enters the extracellular fluid (ECF) and H$^+$ enters the cell, leading to a state of relative intracellular acidosis and extracellular alkalemia. (*B*) Alkalemia leads to hypokalemia. During metabolic alkalosis, cellular H$^+$ enters the ECF and K$^+$ enters the cell, leading to a state of hypokalemia. (*C*) Hyperkalemia leads to acidemia. During hyperkalemic states, cellular H$^+$ enters the ECF and K$^+$ enters the cell, leading to a state of relative intracellular alkalosis and extracellular acidemia. (*D*) Acidemia leads to hyperkalemia. During a state of metabolic acidosis, cellular K$^+$ enters the ECF and H$^+$ enters the cell, leading to a state of hyperkalemia.

      (b) Luminal (brush border) carbonic anhydrase catalyzes the dehydration of
          H_2CO_3 into CO_2 and H_2O:

$$H_2CO_3 \underset{\longleftarrow}{\xrightarrow{\text{carbonic anhydrase}}} CO_2 + H_2O$$

          (i) The CO_2 that diffuses back across the luminal membrane adds to the intracellular CO_2 pool produced by metabolism.
          (ii) This intracellular CO_2 pool serves as a substrate for the formation of H_2CO_3 via intracellular carbonic anhydrase.
          (iii) The dissociation of this H_2CO_3 forms H$^+$ and HCO_3^-. The H$^+$ is secreted again into the lumen. The HCO_3^- is transported downhill across the basolateral membrane by a secondary active transport system (3 HCO_3^- − 1 Na$^+$ cotransporter).
      (c) Buffering of secreted H$^+$ by filtered HCO_3^- does not contribute to the urinary excretion of H$^+$. The CO_2 formed in the lumen from secreted H$^+$ returns to the tubular cell to form another H$^+$ and, therefore, **no net H$^+$ secretion occurs.**
    (2) **Effect of plasma [K$^+$] on HCO_3^- reabsorption.** Body K$^+$ stores influence HCO_3^- reabsorption. There is an inverse relationship between plasma [K$^+$] and proximal HCO_3^- reabsorption.

TABLE 27-2. Normal Renal Regulation of H^+ and HCO_3^-

Ion	$\dot{F}$ Filtered (mEq/day)	$\dot{R}$ Reabsorbed (mEq/day)	$\dot{S}$ Secreted (mEq/day)	$\dot{E}$ Excreted (mEq/day)	$\dot{R}/\dot{F}$ Filtered Load Reabsorbed (%)
HCO_3^-	4320	4318	None	2	99.9+
HPO_4^{2-}	260	240	None	20	92
NH_4^{+*}	None	. . .	. . .	40	. . .
H^+	<0.1	4315†	4375	58‡	. . .

*Secreted mainly as NH_3 and NH_4^+.
†98.6% of the secreted H^+ is reabsorbed daily.
‡Note that total H^+ excretion equals the sum of titratable acid (HPO_4^{2-}) and NH_4^+ minus urinary HCO_3^- concentration.

(a) **Hypokalemia.** A decrease in plasma $[K^+]$ leads to an increase in HCO_3^- reabsorption.
  (i) Hypokalemia is associated with **intracellular acidosis.**
  (ii) Hypokalemia provides a concentration gradient for K^+ to move out of the cell (see Figure 27-9A). In response to the efflux of K^+, both H^+ and Na^+ enter the cell to maintain electroneutrality.
  (iii) The increase in intracellular $[H^+]$ favors HCO_3^- reabsorption because HCO_3^- reabsorption depends on H^+ secretion.
(b) **Hyperkalemia.** An elevated plasma $[K^+]$ leads to a decreased HCO_3^- reabsorption.
  (i) Hyperkalemia is associated with **intracellular alkalosis.**
  (ii) In hyperkalemia, K^+ moves into the cell (see Figure 27-9C). In response to the K^+ uptake by the cells, H^+ and Na^+ leave the cells to maintain electroneutrality.
  (iii) Hyperkalemia tends to alkalinize the cell and reduce HCO_3^- reabsorption.
b. **HCO_3^- regeneration.** New HCO_3^- can be formed by two mechanisms that provide for the excretion of H^+.
  (1) **Nonbicarbonate buffering.** Most of the H^+ ions secreted in excess of those required for HCO_3^- reabsorption are buffered by nonbicarbonate buffers and subsequently excreted. Normally, the most important of these nonbicarbonate buffers is filtered **dibasic phosphate (HPO_4^{2-}).**
    (a) When secreted H^+ combines with HPO_4^{2-}, the formation of **monobasic phosphate ($H_2PO_4^-$, titratable acid)** takes place in the proximal tubule.
    (b) The excretion of $H_2PO_4^-$ is equivalent to HCO_3^- conservation and the addition of new HCO_3^- to the blood.
  (2) **Glutamine catabolism.** The kidneys can also add new HCO_3^- to the blood via the catabolism of glutamine, which results in the formation of two ammonium (NH_4^+) ions and two HCO_3^- ions.
    (a) The NH_4^+ can be secreted into the proximal lumen by the Na^+–NH_4^+ exchanger and is excreted. The NH_4^+ is produced within the proximal cells and not from the combination of luminal NH_3 with H^+ derived from carbonic acid.
    (b) The excretion of NH_4^+ is equivalent to the addition of HCO_3^- to the renal venous blood.
    (c) When the two NH_4^+ are metabolized by the liver, there is the formation of urea and two H^+.
    (d) To add HCO_3^- to the blood, the alpha-ketoglutarate anion must be metabolized to two HCO_3^-, removing the protons (which is equivalent to generating HCO_3^-), and the two NH_4^+ must be excreted in the urine.
    (e) The HCO_3^- is transported into the peritubular capillaries and constitutes new HCO_3^- formation.

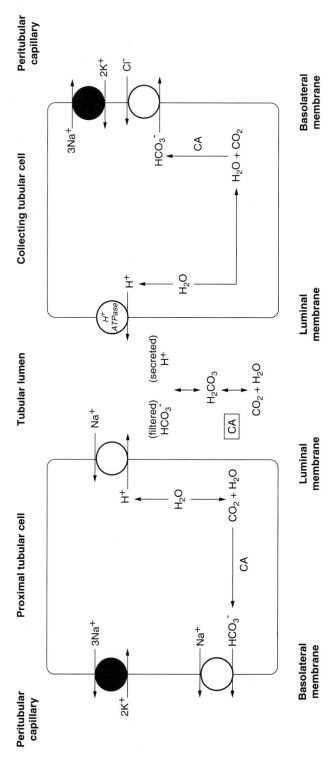

FIGURE 27-10. Major cellular and luminal events in bicarbonate reabsorption in the proximal tubule and the collecting tubules. Intracellular H_2O combines with CO_2 to form HCO_3^-, via a reaction catalyzed by carbonic anhydrase (CA). In the proximal tubule, the H^+ is secreted into the lumen by the Na^+-H^+ exchanger, whereas the HCO_3^- is returned to the systemic circulation primarily by a $Na^+-HCO_3^-$ cotransporter. These same processes occur in the collecting tubules, although they are respectively mediated by an active $H^+-ATPase$ pump in the luminal membrane and a $Cl^--HCO_3^-$ exchanger in the basolateral membrane. The secreted H^+ ions combine with filtered HCO_3^- to form carbonic acid (H_2CO_3) and then $CO_2 + H_2O$, which can be passively reabsorbed. This dissociation of carbonic acid is facilitated when luminal carbonic anhydrase (CA in *box*) is present, as occurs in the early proximal tubule. The net effect is HCO_3^- reabsorption, even though the HCO_3^- ions returned to the systemic circulation are not the same as those that were filtered. Although not shown, the collecting tubule cells also have $H^+-K^+-ATPase$ pumps in the luminal membrane that are primarily involved in K^+ reabsorption. (Modified from Rose BD: *Clinical Physiology of Acid–Base and Electrolyte Disorders*, 4th edition. New York, McGraw-Hill, 1994, p 305.)

3. **HCO$_3^-$ secretion.** All segments of the nephron normally reabsorb HCO$_3^-$, except for the **cortical collecting duct,** which, under conditions of normal acid–base balance or metabolic alkalosis, secretes HCO$_3^-$ from type B intercalated cells.

  a. The **collecting tubule** (i.e., the cortical, outer medullary, and inner medullary collecting ducts) consists of **two cell types:**

   (1) **Principal cells,** which reabsorb Na$^+$ and secrete K$^+$. These cells do not exhibit H$^+$ secretory activity.

   (2) **Intercalated cells** (see Figure 27-8)

      (a) **A-type intercalated cells secrete H$^+$** (i.e., reabsorb HCO$_3^-$). Because the luminal membranes of A-type intercalated cells contain H$^+$–K$^+$–ATPase pumps, they can also **reabsorb K$^+$.**

      (b) **B-type intercalated cells** differ from A-type intercalated cells in that the polarity of the membrane transporters is reversed, so that they **secrete HCO$_3^-$.**

         (i) H$^+$ ions are transported into the peritubular capillary by H$^+$–ATPase pumps located in the basolateral, rather than the luminal, membrane.

         (ii) HCO$_3^-$ ions, in comparison, are secreted into the tubular lumen by a Cl$^-$–HCO$_3^-$ exchanger located in the luminal, rather than the basolateral, membrane.

         (iii) The basolateral H$^+$–ATPase pump transports H$^+$ into the blood, where it combines with HCO$_3^-$, causing plasma [HCO$_3^-$] levels to decline and resulting in the excretion of HCO$_3^-$ in the urine.

  b. The HCO$_3^-$-secreting intercalated cell may play an important role in the excretion of HCO$_3^-$ during metabolic alkalosis.

4. **Total (net) acid excretion** (see Table 27-2)

  a. **Titratable acid.** Approximately 20 mEq (mmol) of H$^+$ per day are buffered by filtered HPO$_4^{2-}$ and excreted as H$_2$PO$_4^-$. The proximal tubule is the major nephron site for titratable acid formation.

  b. **Ammonia.** About 40 mEq (mmol) of H$^+$ per day are buffered by ammonia (NH$_3$) and excreted as ammonium (NH$_4^+$).

  c. The total amount of H$^+$ excreted daily by an individual on a normal diet equals the sum of titratable acid and NH$_4^+$ excreted, or about 60 mEq (mmol) of H$^+$ per day. Thus, only a minute concentration of **free** H$^+$ normally exists in the final urine despite the 4300 mEq (mmol) of H$^+$ secreted daily.

K. **Water reabsorption.** Water movement across membranes is determined by hydrostatic and osmotic pressure gradients. Water is reabsorbed passively by diffusing along an osmotic gradient, which primarily is established by the reabsorption of Na$^+$ and Cl$^-$.

1. **Proximal tubules**

  a. In humans, about 75%–80% of the reabsorption of filtered water occurs in the proximal tubule.

  b. The proximal reabsorption of water is invariant and involves no change in osmolality.

2. **Loop of Henle**

  a. Unlike the proximal tubule, the loop of Henle reabsorbs considerably more solute than water. Only about 5% of the reabsorption of filtered water occurs here (DLH).

  b. The tubular fluid entering the DLH always is **isosmotic,** regardless of the hydration state.

3. **Distal and collecting tubules**

  a. The distal and collecting tubular reabsorption of water occurs only in the presence of ADH. In the presence of a maximal ADH effect, 99% of the water is reabsorbed; in the absence of ADH, 88% of the water is reabsorbed.

  b. The tubular fluid entering the distal tubule always is **hyposmotic** to plasma, regardless of the hydration state. In the terminal distal tubule and the collecting ducts, the osmolality in the tubular fluid changes according to the water permeability of the tubule.

L. **Summary of hormonal determinants of NaCl and water metabolism** (Table 27-3)

TABLE 27-3. Hormones That Regulate NaCl and Water Reabsorption

Segment	Hormone	Effects on NaCl and Water Reabsorption
Proximal Tubule		
	Angiotensin II	↑ NaCl ↑ H_2O
	Glucocorticoids	↑ NaCl ↑ H_2O
Thick Ascending Limb		
	Aldosterone	↑ NaCl
	Vasopressin	↑ NaCl
Distal Tubule/Collecting Duct		
	Aldosterone	↑ NaCl ↑ H_2O
	Atrial natriuretic peptide	↓ NaCl ↓ H_2O
	Prostaglandins	↓ NaCl ↓ H_2O
	Vasopressin	↑ NaCl ↑ H_2O

Case

A 63-year-old man who is found on the street having a generalized seizure is brought to the emergency department. Previous history is significant for heavy alcohol consumption. Initial physical examination reveals recurrent generalized seizures; vital signs are temperature, 37.5°C; blood pressure, 115/55 mm Hg; heart rate, 44 beats/min; and respiratory rate, 20 breaths/min. The remainder of the examination, including an evaluation of neurologic function, is normal.

Urinalysis shows 4+ hemoglobin, 0–2 red blood cells (RBCs) and > 20 white blood cells (WBCs) per high-power field. Laboratory data reveal:

Plasma creatinine = 2.0 mg/dl

Blood urea nitrogen (BUN) = 18 mg/dl;

Serum electrolytes:

$[Na^+]$	128 mEq/L
$[K^+]$	9.1 mEq/L
$[Cl^-]$	98 mEq/L
$[HCO_3^-]$	8 mEq/L

Arterial blood gases:

pH	7.15
P_{CO_2}	24 mm Hg
P_{O_2}	78 mm Hg

The electrocardiogram (EKG) reveals tall peaked T waves, absent P waves, and widening of the QRS complex.

1. *What is the most life-threatening laboratory abnormality in the initial evaluation?*

DISCUSSION

Severe hyperkalemia (9.1 mEq/L) undoubtedly poses the greatest risk of sudden death due to cardiac dysrhythmia and/or circulatory arrest. The decreased heart rate suggests the possibility of an idioventricular rhythm. The absence of P waves indicates atrial standstill, the prolonged QRS complexes suggest intraventricular block, and the peaked T waves suggset hyperkalemia.

2. *What is the most likely pathogenesis of the hyperkalemia?*

DISCUSSION

The patient's history of alcoholism is consistent with low dietary K^+ intake, which predisposes the patient to hyperkalemia. He did not receive drugs that impair renal K^+ disposal [angiotensin-converting enzyme (ACE) inhibitors, K^+-sparing diuretics)] or extrarenal K^+ disposal (digitalis, β-blockers), or oral or parenteral K^+ supplementation.

The plasma creatinine is about two times normal (range, 0.8–1.0 mg/dl), while the BUN is only slightly above normal (range, 10–15 mg/dl). The elevated plasma creatinine concentration could be caused by simple retention due to renal failure or by the increased production of creatinine. The BUN and plasma creatinine levels vary inversely with the glomerular filtration rate (GFR), but BUN is a less useful reflection of GFR than plasma creatinine. However, renal failure (as measured by a reduction in GFR) results in elevated plasma concentrations of both urea and creatinine. Thus, in this patient, the elevations in plasma creatinine and K^+ concentration are not due to renal failure.

The increased level of plasma creatinine compared to BUN is most consistent with the release of muscle creatine and subsequent nonenzymatic conversion to creatinine as opposed to simple creatinine retention due to renal failure. The cause of the hyperkalemia is due to a large K^+ leakage from skeletal muscle due to generalized seizure-induced rhabdomyolysis. The presence of heme pigments in the urine, which is due to the urinary excretion of myoglobin, and the 0–2 RBCs is consistent with rhabdomyolysis.

3. *With respect to the hyperkalemia, how should this patient's condition be managed?*

DISCUSSION

The focus of immediate attention should be prevention of further episodes of generalized seizures and provision of adequate ventilation. Therapy for the hyperkalemia should include procedures aimed at (1) ameliorating the cardiac and skeletal muscle toxicity of hyperkalemia; (2) redistribution of elevated extracellular K^+ levels to the intracellular fluid (ICF); and (3) facilitating renal and extrarenal excretion of K^+. The intravenous administration of Ca^{2+} salts rapidly corrects abnormal tissue excitability. Insulin and glucose administration promote the uptake of K^+ from the extracellular fluid (ECF) to the ICF. Exchange resins can be given by enema to remove K^+ by an extrarenal route. $NaHCO_3$ administration results in the movement of K^+ into the cells in exchange for the efflux of H^+. Thus, the HCO_3^- would raise the plasma pH and increase the H^+–K^+ exchange across the cell membranes. Selective $β_2$-adrenergic agonists (albuterol) also increase cellular K^+ uptake. Lastly, dialysis (hemodialysis and peritoneal dialysis) are effective measures for extrarenal K^+ removal in hyperkalemia.

Chapter 28

Renal Concentration and Dilution of Urine: Antidiuretic Hormone (ADH) and Osmoregulation

I. FUNCTIONAL CONSIDERATIONS

A. **Purpose.** The kidney can alter the composition of the urine in response to the body's daily needs, thereby maintaining the osmolality of body fluids. When it is necessary to conserve body water, the kidney excretes urine with a high solute concentration. When it is necessary to rid the body of excess water, the kidney excretes urine with a dilute solute concentration.

B. **Role of antidiuretic hormone (ADH).** The principal regulator of plasma osmolality and urine composition is the hormone ADH. In the absence of ADH, the kidney excretes a large volume of dilute urine; when ADH is present in high concentration, the kidney excretes a small volume of concentrated urine.*

C. **Components of the concentrating and diluting system.** The formation of urine that is dilute (hyposmotic to plasma) or concentrated (hyperosmotic to plasma) is achieved by the countercurrent system of the nephron and capillaries (Figure 28-1).[†]

This system consists of the:

1. Descending limb of the loop of Henle (DLH)

2. Thin and thick segments of the ascending limb of the loop of Henle (ALH)

3. Medullary interstitium

4. Distal convoluted tubule

5. Collecting duct

6. Vasa recta, which are the vascular elements of the juxtamedullary nephrons [descending vas recta (DVR), ascending vasa recta (AVR)]

D. **Mechanisms of dilution and concentration.** The kidney forms a dilute urine in the absence of ADH. In the presence of ADH, the kidney forms a concentrated urine via the functioning of the **countercurrent multipliers** (i.e., the loop of Henle and collecting duct) and the **countercurrent exchangers** (i.e., the vasa recta). However, regardless of ADH, the fluid osmolality in the loop of Henle, vasa recta, and medullary interstitium always increases progressively from the corticomedullary junction to the papillary tip (see Figure 28-1D).

1. The **fundamental processes** involved in the excretion of a dilute or concentrated urine include (Table 28-1):
   a. Variable permeability of the nephron to the passive back-diffusion (reabsorption) of water along an osmotic gradient and of urea along its concentration gradient
   b. Passive reabsorption of NaCl by the thin segment of the ALH
   c. Active reabsorption of Na^+ by the thick segment of the ALH via the $Na^+–2Cl^-–K^+$ symporter and the $Na^+–K^+–ATPase$ pump

2. The **formation of hyperosmotic urine** involves the following steps:
   a. The medullary interstitium becomes hyperosmotic by the reabsorption of NaCl and urea by:

---

*In the presence of a maximal ADH effect, 99% of the water is reabsorbed; in the absence of ADH, 88% of the water is reabsorbed.

[†]Only the juxtamedullary nephrons, with their long loops of Henle, contribute to the medullary hyperosmolality.

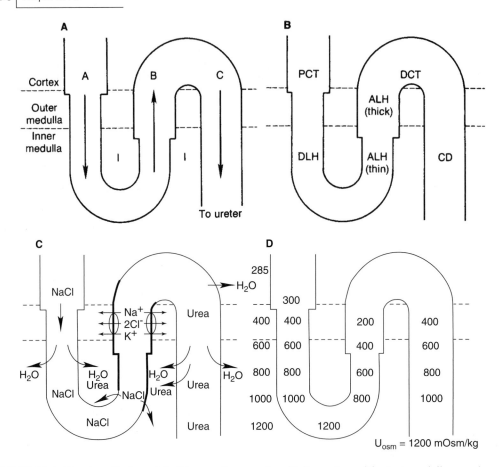

FIGURE 28-1. The three-limb model of the countercurrent multiplier system of the juxtamedullary nephron. *Model A* represents the directions of tubular flow (countercurrent). A = concentrating segment; B = diluting segment; C = collecting duct; and I = interstitium. *Model B* represents the major components of the nephron. PCT = proximal convoluted tubule; DLH = descending limb of the loop of Henle; ALH = ascending limb of the loop of Henle (thick and thin segments); DCT = distal convoluted tubule; and CD = collecting duct. *Model C* represents solute and solvent transfer. The *heavy line* in model C indicates water impermeability. *Model D* represents the vertical (longitudinal) and horizontal (transverse) osmotic gradients in the presence of antidiuretic hormone (ADH). U_{osm} = urine osmolality. (After Jamison R, Maffly RH: The urinary concentrating mechanism. *N Engl J Med* 295:1059–1067, 1976.)

    (1) Active transport of ions (Na^+, K^+, Cl^-) into the interstitium by the thick ALH
    (2) Active transport of ions from the collecting duct into the interstitial fluid (ISF) of the medulla
    (3) Simple diffusion and also by facilitated diffusion via a luminal membrane carrier in the inner medullary collecting duct
    (4) Simple diffusion of additional Na^+ and Cl^- into the interstitium from the thin ALH
  b. The urine entering the medullary collecting ducts equilibrates osmotically with the hyperosmotic interstitium, resulting in the excretion of a small volume of concentrated urine in the presence of ADH.

3. The final osmolality of the urine is determined by the permeability of collecting ducts to water.

4. The vascular loop (vasa recta) prevents the dissipation of the osmotic (hypertonic) "layering" in the interstitium (see III A–B).

TABLE 28-1. Permeability and Transport Characteristics of the Loop of Henle and Collecting Ducts

Segment	H_2O	Transport NaCl Passive	Transport NaCl Active	Urea[1] Passive
tDLH	H	O	L	L
tALH	O	H	No	M
TALH	O	M^2	Yes^3	O
CD	H (+ADH)	O	Yes^4	H (+ADH)*
	O (−ADH)			O (−ADH)

*Inner medullary collecting duct

ADH = antidiuretic hormone; ± ADH = in the presence or absence of ADH, respectively; CD = collecting duct; H = high permeability; L = low permeability; M = moderate permeability; O = impermeable; tALH = thin ascending limb of the loop of Henle; TALH = thick ascending limb of the loop of Henle; tDLH = thin descending limb of the loop of Henle.

Notes: (1) Denotes that the permeability of the inner medullary collecting duct is greater than that of the cortical and outer medullary collecting ducts. (2) Denotes that paracellular Na^+ reabsorption is due to lumen-positive potential created by K^+ efflux. Na^+ enters the paracellular pathway by electrorepulsion, **not** by bulk flow. (3) Denotes a luminal $Na^+–2Cl^-–K^+$ symporter; basolateral $Na^+–K^+–ATPase$ pump. (4) Denotes a luminal Na^+ conductive channel; basolateral $Na^+–K^+–ATPase$ pump.

II. COUNTERCURRENT MULTIPLIERS (see Figure 28-1)

A. General considerations

1. The countercurrent multiplier system is analogous to a three-limb model consisting of the two limbs of the loop of Henle, which are connected by a hairpin turn, and the collecting duct. The fluid flow through the three limbs is countercurrent (i.e., in alternating opposite directions; see Figure 28-1A).

2. The countercurrent multiplier process has two important consequences.
   a. At equilibrium in the presence of ADH, a maximal vertical (axial) gradient of 900 mOsm/kg is established between the corticomedullary junction (300 mOsm/kg) and the renal papillae (1200 mOsm/kg). This explains the origin of the term "countercurrent multiplier."
   b. At any given level in the renal medulla, the osmolality is almost the same in all fluids except that in the ALH. The fluid in the ALH is less concentrated than that in either the DLH or the interstitium and becomes hyposmotic to plasma (see Figure 28-1D).

B. Loop of Henle

1. The **DLH** is the **concentrating segment** of the nephron (Figure 28-2; see Figure 28-1C & D). The following characteristics of the DLH account for this:
   a. The DLH is highly permeable to water. Solute-free water leaves the DLH, causing the fluid in the DLH to become concentrated to a degree that is consistently higher than that of the fluid in the ALH.
   b. The DLH has a low permeability to NaCl and urea.
   c. The fluid in the DLH nearly attains the osmolality of the adjacent medullary interstitium. [The interstitial osmolality is maintained by solvent-free solute (NaCl) that is transported out of the ALH.]

2. The **ALH,** both the thick and thin segments, lead to dilution of the tubular fluid; however, it is the thick ALH that is defined as the "diluting segment," which is the site of free-water formation. Both segments are impermeable to water and both are permeable to NaCl. In addition, the thin segment of the ALH is moderately permeable to urea (see Table 28-1).

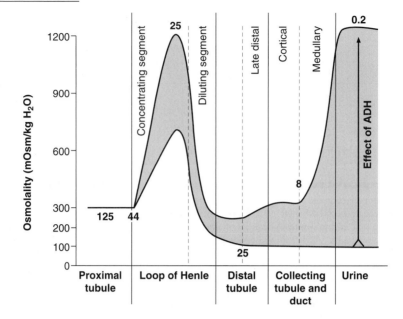

FIGURE 28-2. Axial profile of osmolality of the tubular fluid. Initially, the tubular fluid is isosmotic. In the descending limb of the loop of Henle (DLH), it increases in osmolality, and in the ascending limb of the loop of Henle (ALH), it decreases in osmolality. The tubular fluid enters the distal nephron hyposmotic to plasma, where it may become more hyposmotic [in the absence of antidiuretic hormone (ADH)], or hyperosmotic (under the influence of ADH). Numerical values indicate the approximate tubular flow rate in ml/min. (Modified with permission from Guyton AC: *Textbook of Medical Physiology,* 8th ed. Philadelphia, WB Saunders, 1991, p 312.)

   a. As fluid passes through the **thin segment** of the ALH, NaCl diffuses down its concentration gradient into the ISF. This contributes to the increased interstitial osmolality and renders the tubular fluid hyposmotic to the peritubular interstitium.
   b. The **thick segment** of the ALH actively transports Na^+ out of the lumen. The only active step in countercurrent multiplication is NaCl reabsorption in the thick ascending limb via the $Na^+–2Cl^-–K^+$ symporter.
   c. The active and passive transport of NaCl from the ALH (thick and thin segments, respectively) to the interstitium forms a horizontal osmotic gradient of up to 200 mOsm/kg between the tubular fluid of the ALH and the combined fluid of the interstitium and the DLH (see Figure 28-1D), leaving behind a smaller volume of hypotonic fluid rich in urea. This fluid flows into the distal convoluted tubule and the cortical and medullary collecting ducts.
   d. The fluid in the ALH becomes diluted by the net loss of NaCl in excess of the net gain of urea by diffusion. This efflux of NaCl causes the tubular fluid in the ALH to become hyposmotic and that in the ISF to become hyperosmotic.
   e. The fluid emerging from the ALH is always hyposmotic, approximately 100 mOsm/kg H_2O, because of a low NaCl concentration, regardless of the final urine osmolality (diuresis or antidiuresis).
   f. The reabsorption of NaCl by the loop of Henle allows for the separation of solute and water (free water), which is essential for the formation of hyposmotic urine.

C. **Simultaneous events in the interstitium**

   1. Fluid in the interstitium contains hyperosmotic concentrations of NaCl and urea.
   a. As the collecting ducts join in the inner medulla, they become increasingly perme-

able to urea (especially in the presence of ADH), allowing urea to flow passively along its concentration gradient into the interstitium (see Figures 28-1C and 28-2).

b. The increase in medullary osmolality causes water to move out of the adjacent tubules, the terminal collecting ducts, and the DLH.

c. It is important to appreciate that the medullary interstitium is hypertonic, not because its water content is lower (in fact, it is higher), but because its solute content is higher.

d. The principal solute that accounts for the high osmolality of medullary interstitium is urea; most of the remainder is accounted for by Na^+ and an accompanying anion, mainly Cl^-.

2. Water is reabsorbed in the last segment of the distal convoluted tubule and in the collecting duct in the cortex and outer medulla in the presence of ADH.

3. In the inner medulla, both water and urea are reabsorbed from the collecting duct (see Figure 28-1C).

a. Some urea reenters the ALH but at a **slower** rate than the efflux of NaCl.

b. This **medullary recycling of urea,** in addition to solute trapping by countercurrent exchange, causes urea to accumulate in large amounts in the medullary interstitium, where it osmotically abstracts water from the DLH and thereby concentrates NaCl in the DLH fluid. It is important to appreciate that urea is an effective osmole in the medullary interstitium.

D. **Collecting duct.** The cortical and upper medullary collecting ducts are relatively impermeable to water, urea, and NaCl (Figure 28-3 and III B 2).

1. The relative impermeability to water occurs in the absence of ADH.

2. The relative impermeability to NaCl permits the high interstitial concentration of NaCl to act as an effective osmotic gradient between the tubular fluid and the interstitium.

3. When the kidney forms concentrated urine, the collecting duct receives an isosmotic fluid from the distal tubule. The collecting duct becomes permeable to water, and the urine equilibrates with the hyperosmotic medullary interstitium, resulting in the excretion of a low volume, hypertonic urine.

4. If the collecting duct is impermeable to water (ADH absent), the dilute tubular fluid entering the collecting duct from the distal tubule remains hypotonic and is excreted as a higher volume, hypotonic urine.

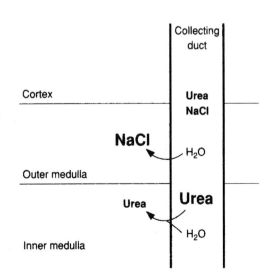

FIGURE 28-3. The differences between the relative NaCl and urea concentrations in tubular fluid and the interstitium are represented by *type size*. The high NaCl concentration in the outer medullary interstitium [which results from NaCl reabsorption in the thick segment of the ascending limb of the loop of Henle (ALH)] and the high urea concentration in tubular fluid (as a result of water reabsorption upstream), coupled with the different reflection coefficients for NaCl and urea (approximately 1 and < 1, respectively), favors water reabsorption in the outer medullary collecting duct, despite equal osmolalities on both sides of the tubular wall. At the outer–inner medullary junction, the urea permeability of the collecting duct increases so that urea diffuses into the interstitium, increasing the osmotic gradient for additional water reabsorption.

III. VASA RECTA AS COUNTERCURRENT EXCHANGERS.
The vasa recta function as countercurrent diffusion exchangers, increasing the efficiency of the concentrating mechanisms.

A. Anatomic and physiologic considerations (Figure 28-4)

1. The vasa recta are derived from the efferent arterioles of the juxtamedullary glomeruli and function to maintain the hyperosmolality of the medullary interstitium. The vasa recta are in juxtaposition with the loops of Henle.

2. These vessels are permeable to solutes and water and reach osmotic equilibrium with the medullary interstitium.

B. General functions

1. To supply oxygen and nutrients and remove carbon dioxide and metabolic end products

2. To preserve the axial (vertical) concentration gradient of NaCl and urea generated by the loop of Henle by maximizing the transport of solute between the arterial and venous capillaries
   a. As the blood flows down the DVR and encounters the progressively hypertonic interstitium, water is lost, and solutes to which the capillary is permeable (i.e., essentially all solutes except plasma protein) enter.

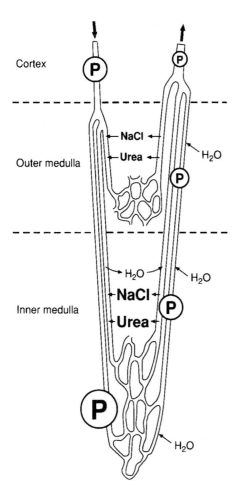

FIGURE 28-4. The vasa recta function to maintain the hyperosmolality of the medullary interstitium. NaCl and urea that have been reabsorbed from the loop of Henle and collecting tubule (respectively) accumulate in the medullary interstitium, where they are absorbed by the descending limb of the vasa recta and returned to the interstitium by the ascending limb of the vasa recta. This countercurrent exchange "traps" the solutes in the medullary interstitium. At the same time, water (H_2O) is removed from the descending vasa recta, increasing the plasma protein (P) concentration. In the ascending vasa recta, the oncotic pressure causes the capillaries to take in fluid. In this manner, water reabsorbed by the nephron is removed from the interstitium and returned to the general circulation. *Type size* indicates the relative concentration of each solute with respect to its location in the medulla, but not necessarily with respect to concentrations of other solutes. (Redrawn with permission from Jamison RL, Ghrig JJ Jr: Renal physiology VII. In *Handbook of Physiology*, edited by Windhager EE. Published for the American Psychological Society. New York, Oxford University Press, 1992, p 1268.)

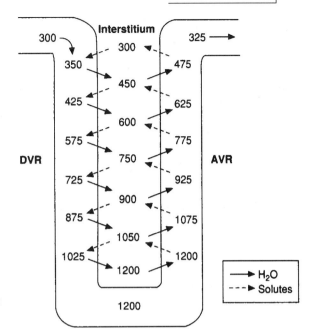

FIGURE 28-5. Countercurrent exchange in the vasa recta. Water and solute transport occur by diffusion. AVR = ascending vasa recta; DVR = descending vasa recta. (Modified and redrawn with permission from Vander AJ: *Renal Physiology,* 4th ed. New York, McGraw-Hill, 1991, p 108.)

    b. The reverse process occurs as blood leaves the medulla in the AVR; water is added and solutes are lost.

  3. To keep the concentrations of Na$^+$ and urea in the medullary interstitium high by keeping the blood flow slow

  4. To remove water added to the medullary interstitium from the DLH and the collecting ducts. The vasa recta return the NaCl and water reabsorbed in the loops of Henle and collecting ducts to the systemic circulation.

C. **Countercurrent exchange effects** (Figure 28-5)

  1. Na$^+$, Cl$^-$, and urea are passively reabsorbed from the ALH, diffuse across the ISF into the DVR, and are returned to the interstitium by the AVR.
    a. These solutes recirculate in the vasa recta capillary loops and increase the medullary osmolality.
    b. Na$^+$, Cl$^-$, and urea also recirculate in the loop of Henle.

  2. Water diffuses from the DVR across the ISF and into the AVR.* As a result, the cortex receives blood that is only slightly hypertonic to plasma (see Figure 28-5).

IV. **ROLE OF UREA.** The main function of urea in the countercurrent system is to exert an osmotic effect on the DLH, promoting the abstraction of water and raising the intraluminal concentration of NaCl (see Figures 28-1 and 28-3).

A. **Effect of ADH on urea concentration.** In the medulla, ADH enhances both water and urea permeabilities of the collecting duct.

  1. Urea diffuses into the thin segment of the ALH via secretion but is more concentrated in the fluid entering the distal convoluted tubule (concentrated in a smaller volume) than in

*Water is continually removed by the AVR.

the filtrate entering the proximal convoluted tubule. The thin segment of the ALH is less permeable to urea than to NaCl, and the thick segment of the ALH is impermeable to urea.

2. During **antidiuresis** (i.e., under the influence of ADH), the tubular concentration of urea in the cortical collecting duct increases as a result of urea-free water reabsorption from the cortical collecting duct into the outer medullary interstitium.

3. When the tubular fluid enters the urea-permeable inner medullary collecting duct, urea, along with water, diffuses into the medullary interstitium. There it is trapped by counter-current exchange in the vasa recta, resulting in a high urea concentration in the inner medulla.

4. Urea recirculates in the loops of Henle and the vasa recta. The vasa recta are permeable to urea, so that urea diffusing out of the papillary collecting duct is trapped in the medullary interstitium.
   a. Of the 1200 mOsm/kg of solute present in the renal papillary loop during **antidiuresis,** approximately one-half is NaCl and one-half is urea.
   b. During water **diuresis,** about 10% of the total medullary solute concentration is urea. The maximal urine osmolality (U_{osm}) cannot exceed that in the interstitium, and the ability to conserve water by excreting concentrated urine is reduced when the papillary concentration is reduced.

B. Effect of urea on urine osmolality

1. Urea increases urine osmolality via a **three-step process:**
   a. The high concentration of urea in the inner medullary collecting duct causes continued diffusion of urea out of the collecting duct and into the medullary interstitium.
   b. The interstitial urea supplied by the inner medullary collecting duct removes water from the DLH and causes the tubular NaCl concentration to increase above that in the interstitium, favoring the passive reabsorption of NaCl from the thin ascending limb.
   c. As water is reabsorbed from the urea-impermeable cortical and outer medullary collecting ducts, urea becomes the principal solute in tubular fluid entering the inner medullary collecting duct.

2. This process establishes the gradients for urea and NaCl in opposite directions: urea concentration in the collecting duct tubular fluid is higher than that in the interstitium, and the NaCl concentration in the collecting duct is lower than that in the interstitium (see Figure 28-3).
   a. These two concentration gradients for urea and NaCl are due to the higher reflection coefficient of the collecting duct for NaCl (approximately 1) than that for urea (< 1).
   b. Thus, despite equal osmolalities on both sides of the collecting tubules at the inner–outer medullary junction, the effective driving force for water transport favors water reabsorption.

V. MEASUREMENT OF RENAL WATER EXCRETION AND CONSERVATION (Figure 28-6)

A. Renal water excretion. The **quantitative** measure of the kidney's ability to excrete water is termed **free-water clearance.** U_{osm} is not an accurate estimate of the kidney's ability to dilute or concentrate urine.

1. General considerations
   a. Under most circumstances, water moves across epithelia primarily by convective, or bulk flow, which is the movement of water by a difference in osmolality. The water molecules move as an ensemble rather than as a consequence of the random movement of molecules.
   b. Free-water clearance denotes the volume of **pure** (i.e., solute-free) **water** that must be removed from, or added to, the flow of urine (in ml/min) to make it isosmotic with plasma.

A. Dilute urine (low ADH)

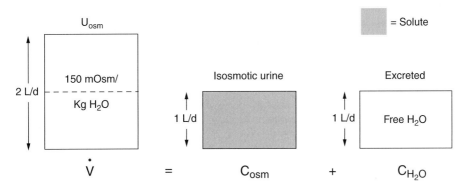

B. Concentrated urine (high ADH)

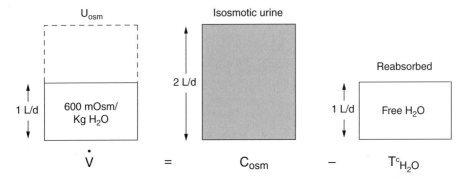

FIGURE 28-6. Block diagram showing relationship between urine volume ($\dot{V}$) and its two components; one containing all of the urinary solute in a solution isosmotic with plasma (osmolal clearance, C_{osm}) and one containing the volume of free-water that has been added to make the urine isosmotic with plasma (free-water clearance, C_{H_2O}) *or* the volume of free-water that has been reabsorbed (free-water reabsorption, $T^c_{H_2O}$) to make the urine isosmotic with plasma. ADH = antidiuretic hormone.

    (1) It is a measure of the ability of the kidneys to generate solute-free water.
    (2) It is not a true clearance, because no osmotically free water exists in plasma.

2. Measurement. Free-water clearance (C_{H_2O}) is calculated using the equation:

$$\dot{V} = C_{osm} + C_{H_2O}$$

$$C_{H_2O} = \dot{V} - C_{osm}$$

where

$$C_{osm} = \frac{U_{osm} \cdot \dot{V}}{P_{osm}}$$

Substituting for C_{osm}, the equation becomes:

$$C_{H_2O} = \dot{V} - \frac{U_{osm} \cdot \dot{V}}{P_{osm}}$$

where $\dot{V}$ = urine volume per unit time (ml/min); U_{osm} = urine osmolality; P_{osm} = plasma osmolality; and C_{osm} = osmolal clearance, which is the volume of plasma (in ml) completely cleared of osmotically active solutes that appear in the urine each minute.

    a. Therefore, **during water diuresis** (i.e., in a hydrated state and in the absence of ADH), the U_{osm} is less than the P_{osm} (hyposmotic urine), and the U_{osm}/P_{osm} ratio is less than 1. Therefore, **C_{H_2O}** is positive, indicating that water is being eliminated by the excretion of a large volume of dilute urine. The maximum free-water clearance in humans is 15–20 L/day (10–15 ml/min).

    b. Similarly, **during antidiuresis** (i.e., in a dehydrated state and in the presence of ADH), the U_{osm} is greater than the P_{osm} (hyperosmotic urine), and the U_{osm}/P_{osm} ratio is greater than 1. Therefore, **C_{H_2O}** is negative, indicating that water is being conserved by the excretion of a small volume of concentrated urine. (To avoid the use of the term "negative free-water clearance," the symbol $T^c_{H_2O}$ is used to denote **free-water reabsorption.** The superscript "c" signifies that net reabsorption occurs in the collecting tubule.)

3. Factors affecting free-water clearance (C_{H_2O}). Free-water clearance represents the volume of distilled water that must be **removed** from the urine (during diuresis) in order to render the urine isosmotic with plasma.

    a. Solute-free water is formed by NaCl reabsorption **without** water in the thick ALH (diluting segment).

    b. This water is then excreted by maintaining the impermeability of the collecting tubules to water (i.e., low ADH).

B. **Renal water conservation.** A quantitative measure of the ability of the kidney to reabsorb water is termed **free-water reabsorption.**

1. General considerations. Free-water reabsorption denotes the volume of free water reabsorbed per unit time, or, the amount of free water that must be removed from the urine by tubular reabsorption to make it hyperosmotic with plasma. Renal water conservation is dependent on:

    a. The formation and maintenance of the medullary osmotic gradient (i.e., a hyperosmotic interstitium to provide for water reabsorption by the collecting duct)

    b. Equilibration of the fluid (urine) in the collecting tubules with the hyperosmotic medullary interstitium

2. Measurement. Free-water reabsorption (**$T^c_{H_2O}$**) is calculated using the equation:

$$T^c_{H_2O} = C_{osm} - \dot{V}$$

where

$$C_{osm} = \frac{U_{osm} \cdot \dot{V}}{P_{osm}}$$

Note that the urine flow rate ($\dot{V}$) of hypertonic urine is by rearrangement:

$$\dot{V} = C_{osm} - T^c_{H_2O}$$

Therefore, **during antidiuresis** the U_{osm} exceeds P_{osm}, and the U_{osm}/P_{osm} ratio is greater than 1, indicating that the **$T^c_{H_2O}$** is positive. A positive $T^c_{H_2O}$ suggests that water is being conserved by the elimination of a small volume of concentrated urine.

3. Factors affecting free-water reabsorption ($T^c_{H_2O}$). Free-water reabsorption represents the volume of pure water that must be **added** to the urine (during antidiuresis) in order to make the urine isosmotic with plasma. Note: It is important to appreciate that C_{H_2O} is the volume of free-water **excreted** per unit time and that $T^c_{H_2O}$ is the volume of free-water **reabsorbed** per unit time.

    a. Formation and maintenance of a high medullary osmotic gradient

b. Equilibration of tubular fluid in the collecting ducts with the hyperosmotic medullary interstitium via increased water and urea permeability (i.e., high ADH)

C. **Urine.** Urine can be conceptualized as consisting of two virtual volumes.

1. One contains all the urinary solutes in an isosmotic solution (i.e., osmolal clearance, C_{osm}). Note: It is important to appreciate that the osmolality of all body fluids is compared to normal plasma.

2. The other contains the volume of solute-free water (pure water) that must be removed from, or added to, the urine to make it isosmotic to plasma.

D. **Antidiuresis and diuresis.** These two processes can be examined in terms of the volume of urine excreted per unit time ($\dot{V}$). Recall that $\dot{V}$ is the algebraic sum of osmolar clearance (C_{osm}) and either free-water clearance (C_{H_2O}) or free-water reabsorption (T^cH_2O).

1. **Antidiuresis** (i.e., a decrease in $\dot{V}$) can result from:
   a. Elevated secretion of ADH
   b. Water deprivation, which leads to an increase in plasma osmolality
   c. Reduced circulating blood volume

2. **Diuresis** (i.e., an increase in $\dot{V}$) can result from:
   a. Reduced secretion of ADH
   b. Reduced osmotic reabsorption of water, leading to increased solute-free water clearance and **water diuresis**
   c. Reduced solute reabsorption (primarily Na^+ with associated anions), leading to increased osmolar clearance and **osmotic diuresis**

E. **Calculations of free-water excretion or reabsorption** (see Figure 28-6)

1. **Dilute urine (low ADH)**
   a. Calculate osmolal clearance:

$$C_{osm} = \frac{U_{osm} \cdot \dot{V}}{P_{osm}}$$

$$= \frac{150 \times 2}{300} = 1 \text{ L/day}$$

   or the volume that contains all of the urinary solutes in a solution isosmotic with plasma.
   b. Calculate free-water clearance by the difference between urine volume ($\dot{V}$) and osmolal clearance (C_{osm}):

$$\dot{V} = C_{osm} + C_{H_2O}$$

$$C_{H_2O} = \dot{V} - C_{osm}$$

$$= 2 - 1 = 1 \text{ L/day}$$

   or the volume of pure water removed from the urine to make it isosmotic with plasma.

2. **Concentrated urine (high ADH)**
   a. Calculate osmolal clearance:

$$C_{osm} = \frac{U_{osm} \cdot \dot{V}}{P_{osm}}$$

$$= \frac{600 \cdot 1}{300} = 2 \text{ L/day}$$

or the volume that contains all of the urinary solutes in a solution isosmotic with plasma.

b. Calculate free-water reabsorption by the difference between urine volume ($\dot{V}$) and osmolal clearance (C_{osm}):

$$\dot{V} = C_{osm} + C_{H_2O}$$

$$C_{H_2O} = \dot{V} - C_{osm}$$

$$-C_{H_2O} = -\dot{V} + C_{osm}$$

$$\text{but } -C_{H_2O} = T^c{}_{H_2O}$$

$$\text{therefore } T^c{}_{H_2O} = C_{osm} - \dot{V}$$

$$= 2 - 1 = 1 \text{ L/day}$$

or the volume of pure water that must be added to the urine to make it isosmotic with plasma.

F. **Relationship between free-water clearance, urine volume, and osmolal clearance: a summary** (Figure 28-7)

1. With isosmotic urine (see Figure 28-7A), neither excretion nor reabsorption of solute-free water occurs.
   a. Solute-free water clearance (C_{H_2O}) = 0.
   b. Urine flow ($\dot{V}$) is equal to osmolal clearance (C_{osm}).

2. With hyposmotic urine (see Figure 28–7B), the urine is divided into two virtual volumes; one that contains solute that is isosmotic to plasma (C_{osm}) and a volume that is solute-free water (C_{H_2O}).
   a. Osmolal clearance (C_{osm}) is equal to solute-free water clearance (C_{H_2O}) [i.e., $C_{osm} = C_{H_2O}$].
   b. Urine flow rate ($\dot{V}$) is equal to the sum of osmolal clearance (C_{osm}) and free-water clearance (C_{H_2O}), (i.e., $\dot{V} = C_{osm} + C_{H_2O}$).

3. With hyperosmotic urine, $T^c{}_{H_2O}$ ($-C_{H_2O}$) [see Figure 28-7C] represents the volume of free-water that would have to be added to the urine to make it isosmotic to plasma.
   a. Urine volume ($\dot{V}$) is equal to the difference between osmolal clearance (C_{osm}), and free-water reabsorption.
   b. The osmolal clearance (C_{osm}) is equal to the sum of urine volume ($\dot{V}$) and free-water reabsorption ($T^c{}_{H_2O}$).

Case

A patient excretes 500 ml of urine in 24 hours at a concentration of 1200 mOsm/kg H_2O (600 mOsm/500 ml H_2O).

   1. *What is the volume of solute-free water reabsorption?*

DISCUSSION

To excrete 500 ml of urine containing 600 mOsm of solute, approximately 1.5 L of solute-free water must be reabsorbed:

$$C_{osm} = \frac{U_{osm} \cdot \dot{V}}{P_{osm}}$$

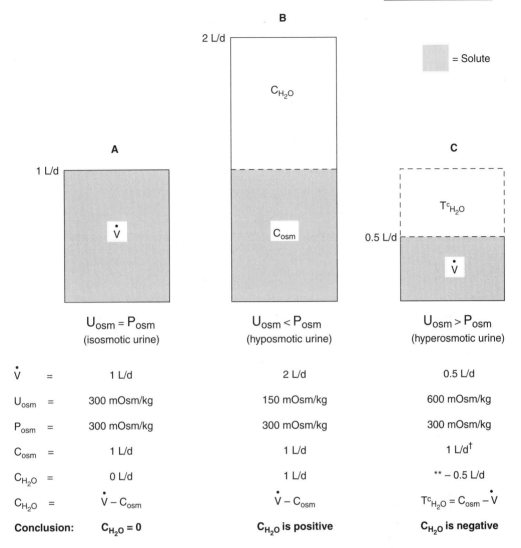

FIGURE 28-7. Relationship between free-water clearance (C_{H_2O}), urine volume ($\dot{V}$), and osmolal clearance (C_{osm}). C_{osm} is (1) the volume of urine needed to excrete solutes at the concentration of solutes in plasma, (2) the volume of urine that contains all the solutes in a solution that is isosmotic with plasma, and (3) the volume of pure water (distilled water) that has either been removed from a dilute urine (+C_{H_2O}) or added to a concentrated urine ($-C_{H_2O}$). $^*C_{osm} = U_{osm} \cdot \dot{V} / P_{osm}$; $^{\dagger}\dot{V} = C_{osm}$ 2 $T^c_{H_2O}$; $\therefore T^c_{H_2O} = C_{osm} - \dot{V}$

$$= \frac{1200\,(0.5)}{300} = 2\ \text{L/day}$$

$$T^c_{H_2O} = C_{osm} - \dot{V}$$

$$= 2 - 0.5 = 1.5\ \text{L/day}$$

Another way of analyzing this problem is based on the normal daily excretion of solute, which is about 600 mOsm/day [i.e., excretion rate ($\dot{E}$) = $U_{osm} \cdot \dot{V}$].

$$\dot{E} = U_{osm} \cdot \dot{V} = 600\ \text{mOsm/day}$$

Solving for $\dot{V}$:

$$\dot{V} = \frac{\dot{E}}{U_{osm}} = \frac{600}{1200} = 0.5 \text{ L/day}$$

Thus, it requires 500 ml to excrete the solute load of 600 mOsm. If the urine were isosmotic to plasma (300 mOsm/kg H_2O), 2 L would be necessary:

$$\dot{V} = \frac{\dot{E}}{U_{osm}}$$

$$= \frac{600}{300} = 2 \text{ L/day}$$

A patient excretes 6000 ml of urine containing 600 mOsm of solute (100 mOsm/kg H_2O) in 24 hours.

2. *What is the solute free-water clearance?*

DISCUSSION

Free-water clearance represents the volume of excess pure water excreted when the urine is dilute. A patient who excretes 6000 ml (6 L) of urine containing 600 mOsm (100 mOsm/kg H_2O) has eliminated 4000 ml (4 L) of free-water in excess of the volume needed to maintain normal plasma osmolality:

$$C_{osm} = \frac{U_{osm} \cdot \dot{V}}{P_{osm}}$$

$$= \frac{100\ (6)}{300} = 2 \text{ L/day}$$

$$C_{H_2O} = \dot{V} - C_{osm}$$

$$= 6 - 2 = 4 \text{ L/day}$$

Another way of analyzing this problem is based on the normal daily excretion of solute, which is 600 mOsm/day [i.e., excretion rate $(\dot{E}) = (U_{osm} \cdot \dot{V})$].

$$E = U_{osm} \cdot \dot{V} = 600 \text{ mOsm/day}$$

Solving for $\dot{V}$:

$$\dot{V} = \frac{\dot{E}}{U_{osm}} = \frac{600}{100} = 6 \text{ L/day}$$

Thus, it requires 6 L to excrete the solute load of 600 mOsm. If the urine were isosmotic to plasma (300 mOsm/kg H_2O), 2 L would be necessary:

$$\dot{V} = \frac{\dot{E}}{U_{osm}} = \frac{600}{300} = 2 \text{ L/day}$$

Caveat: In solving water balance problems it is first necessary to focus on the volume and osmolality of the urine to determine if the patient has a diuresis (excreting free-water) or an antidiuresis (reabsorbing free-water). Thus, the first patient is dehydrated and excreted a low volume (400 ml/day) of highly concentrated urine (1200 mOsm/kgH_2O) while the second patient is overhydrated and excreted a high volume (6 L/day) of dilute urine (100 mOsm/kgH_2O). In summary, patient 1 exhibited negative free-water clearance by reabsorbing 1.5 L of free-water per day. Patient 2 exhibited positive free-water clearance by excreting (4 L/day) of solute-free H_2O.

Chapter 29

Antidiuretic Hormone (ADH): Regulation of Body Fluid Osmolality

SYNTHESIS AND CHEMICAL CHARACTERISTICS

A. Antidiuretic hormone (ADH), also known as **vasopressin,** * is a **hypothalamic hormone** synthesized in the supraoptic and paraventricular nuclei in the **hypothalamus** (ventral diencephalon). These unmyelinated neurosecretory neurons synthesize, store, and secrete ADH.

1. The ADH-secreting neurons constitute the **supraopticohypophysial tract,** which terminates in the pars nervosa, or the posterior lobe of the pituitary gland (i.e., the neurohypophysis).
   a. ADH is stored (but not synthesized) in the pars nervosa.
   b. In the absence of a pars nervosa, the newly synthesized hormone still can be released into the circulation from the hypothalamus.

2. Because these **hypothalamoneurohypophysial neurons** produce hormones, they are known as **endocrine neurons** or **neuroendocrine cells.**
   a. Neurosecretory neurons are peptidergic neurons that conduct action potentials like all neurons, but, unlike ordinary neurons, synthesize and secrete peptide hormones.
   b. The hypothalamic nuclei that synthesize and secrete ADH are collectively called **magnocellular neurosecretory neurons.**
   c. ADH secretion is triggered by the depolarization of the supraopticohypophysial neurons, which causes Ca^{2+} influx, fusion of secretory granules with the cell membrane, and extrusion (exocytosis) of secretory products (ADH, oxytocin, and neurophysin).

B. ADH is a nonapeptide with a disulfide body.

C. The neurophysins are the physiologic **carrier proteins** for the intraneuronal transport of ADH and are released into the circulation with the neurosecretory products (ADH and oxytocin) without being bound to the hormone.

D. The **biologic half-life** of ADH is 16–20 minutes.

II. **CONTROL OF ADH SECRETION: STIMULI AND INHIBITORS** (Table 29-1)

A. **Stimuli.** The major stimuli for ADH secretion are hyperosmolality and effective circulating blood volume depletion (Figures 29-1, 29-2, 29-3, and 29-4).

---

*The term vasopressin denotes an excitatory action on the blood vessels, causing vasoconstriction of the arterioles and an increase in systemic blood pressure. This effect is observed only when relatively large quantities of vasopressin are released from the posterior lobe (e.g., during hemorrhage) or when pharmacologic amounts are injected. Therefore, the vasopressor effect usually is not considered to be a physiologic effect. The biologically active form of ADH in humans is **arginine vasopressin.**

TABLE 29-1. Factors that Influence Antidiuretic (ADH) Secretion in Humans

	Physiologic	Pathologic	Pharmacologic	Clinical
Stimuli	Hyperosmolality Upright posture (orthostatic hypotension) Exercise	Decrease in effective circulating blood volume (hemorrhage, nephrotic syndrome, cirrhosis, congestive heart failure) Hypothalamic disease Pulmonary disorders (e.g., pneumonia, tuberculosis) CNS disorders (e.g., stroke, meningitis, subdural hema- toma) Hypothyroidism †Na$^+$ deficiency Vasovagal reactions (syncope) Pain Nausea Emotional stress Diabetes mellitus (glucose)	Lithium Morphine (high doses) Barbiturates Nicotine Acetylcholine Diuretics* Isoproterenol* Nitroprusside* Trimethaphan* Histamine* Bradykinin* Angiotensin II Insulin 2-deoxy-D-glucose Cholinergic drugs β-Adrenergic agonists	Positive-pressure breathing
Inhibitors	Hyposmolality Recumbent posture	Diabetes insipidus Elevation of blood pressure‡ Hyposmolality SIADH	Norepinephrine§ Ethanol Caffeine Anticholinergic drugs CO$_2$ inhalation Morphine (low doses) Phenytoin Lithium	Infusion of solutions (hypervolemia) Negative- pressure breathing Weightlessness$^\|$

CNS = central nervous system; SIADH = syndrome of inappropriate ADH secretion.
*Stimulates ADH secretion by lowering blood pressure
†Inhibits ADH secretion by contracting extracellular fluid (ECF) volume
‡ADH secretion is normal in patients with uncomplicated essential hypertension
§Inhibits ADH secretion by raising blood pressure
$^\|$Due to a net shift of blood from the limbs to the abdomen and chest

1. **Osmotic stimuli (osmoregulation)**
   a. **Hyperosmolality.** Under usual conditions, a 1%–2% increase in plasma osmolality is the prime determinant of ADH secretion, and the most common physiologic factor altering the osmolality of the blood is water depletion or water excess. (In clinical medicine, volume deficits are much more prevalent than volume excesses.)
      (1) The osmoreceptors are **located in the anterior hypothalamus** and are distinct from the cells that synthesize ADH.
         (a) The osmoreceptors have the lowest **threshold** (i.e., they are most sensitive) to changes in the **osmolal concentration of plasma.**
         (b) **Stimulation** of these osmoreceptors causes **reflex secretion of ADH.**
      (2) Not all solutes (e.g., urea) stimulate the osmoreceptors, despite increasing plasma osmolality. Only those solutes to which cells are relatively impermeable increase the effective osmotic pressure, in response to which ADH is secreted.

A. Osmoregulation

B. Baroregulation

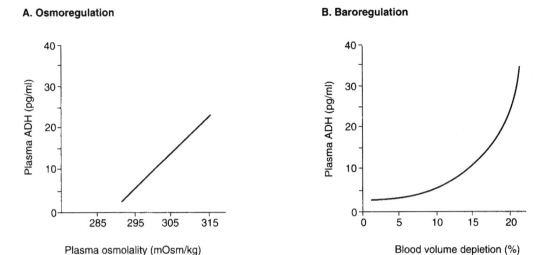

FIGURE 29-1. Stimulation of antidiuretic hormone (ADH) secretion in response to (*A*) increases in plasma osmolality (*B*) decreases in blood volume. In general, the plasma [Na$^+$] is the primary determinant of ADH release. Note that the osmoreceptor is extraordinarily sensitive and, therefore, has the primary role in mediating the ADH response to changes in water balance. In states of hypovolemia, however, the baroreceptor stimulus becomes dominant over the chemoreceptor stimulus. The plasma [Na$^+$] remains the primary osmotic determinant of ADH release.

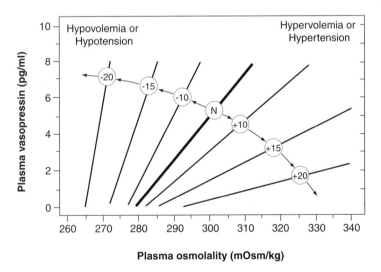

FIGURE 29-2. Effects of hemodynamic variables on the osmoregulation of vasopressin. Each *line* depicts the relationship of plasma vasopressin to plasma osmolality in the presence of varying levels of acute hypovolemia or hypotension (*left*) or hypervolemia or hypertension (*right*). Note that hemodynamic influences do not disrupt osmoregulation of vasopressin but hypovolemia is the dominant stimulus over plasma osmolality. Volume depletion not only potentiates the antidiuretic hormone (ADH) response to increases in osmolality but also can prevent the inhibition of ADH release normally induced by a fall in plasma osmolality. The *circled numbers* denote percentage change in volume or pressure. *Line N* refers to the normovolemic, normotensive subject. [Modified with permission from Seldin DW, Giebisch G (editors). Regulation of vasopressin secretion. In *The Kidney: Physiology and Pathophysiology*, 2nd edition. New York, Raven Press, 1992, p 1604.]

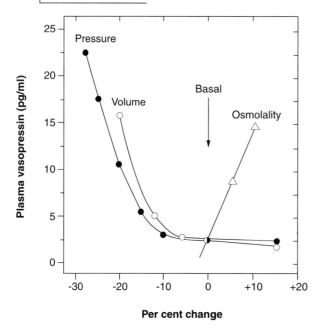

FIGURE 29-3. Comparative sensitivities of the osmoregulatory and baroregulatory mechanisms. Note that vasopressin secretion is much more sensitive to small changes in blood osmolality than volume. All points on the osmolality curve are associated with normovolemia, while all points on the pressure–volume curves are associated with isosmolality. Note that the vasopressin response to changes in blood volume is quantitatively and qualitatively similar to the response to blood pressure. [Modified with permission from Seldin DW, Giebisch G (editors): Regulation of vasopressin secretion. In *The Kidney: Physiology and Pathophysiology,* 2nd edition. New York, Raven Press, 1992, p 1602.]

    (a) Na$^+$ and mannitol. These substances, which cross the blood–brain barrier relatively slowly, **are potent stimulators of ADH release.** Because the plasma [Na$^+$] accounts for 95% of the effective osmotic pressure, the osmoreceptors normally function as plasma Na$^+$ receptors.

    (b) Glucose. Hyperglycemia is a **less potent stimulus** for ADH production and secretion than hypernatremia for the same level of osmolality. In uncontrolled diabetes mellitus, hyperglycemia is associated with insulin deficiency. In this setting, glucose acts as an effective stimulus for ADH.

  b. Volume disturbances. The control of ADH secretion by osmolality can be overridden by volume disturbances. For example, marked hyponatremia is tolerated to maintain circulating blood volume (see Figure 29-2).

2. Nonosmotic stimuli

  a. Hypovolemia (i.e., decreased effective circulating blood volume) is a more dominant stimulus to ADH release than hyperosmolality. A 10%–25% decrease in blood volume evokes ADH release. A 10% decrease in blood volume is sufficient to cause the release of enough ADH to participate in the immediate regulation of blood pressure. Contraction of blood volume without an alteration in the tonicity of body fluids may cause ADH release (see Figure 29-3 and Figure 29–4).

  b. Baroreceptors. Hemodynamic changes (i.e., changes in blood volume, pressure, or both) are mediated by autonomic afferents that arise in pressure (volume)-sensitive receptors in the atria, aortic arch, carotid sinus, great veins, and pulmonary vessels, and traject via the vagal and glossopharyngeal nerves to primary synapses in the nucleus tractus solitarius in the brain stem.

    (1) Changes in the rate of afferent discharge from these visceral afferent neurons affect the activity of the vasomotor center in the medulla. The **low-pressure (stretch) receptors** are the primary mediators of volume effects on ADH secretion.

    (2) From the synapses in the brain stem, postsynaptic fibers project to the region where the osmoreceptors are located (i.e., outside the blood–brain barrier in the circumventricular organs, primarily the organum vasculosum of the lamina terminalis).

    (3) Elevation of blood pressure inhibits the ADH-producing cells. Conversely, decreased blood pressure reduces the firing frequency of the baroreceptors, causing

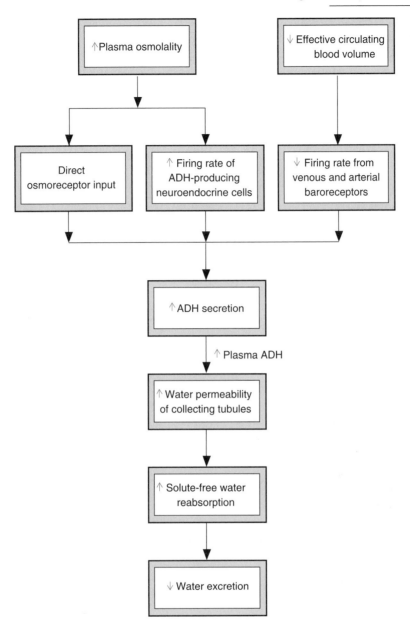

FIGURE 29-4. Pathways for antidiuretic hormone (ADH) secretion associated with plasma osmolality and circulating blood volume.

stimulation of ADH synthesis and release. The vasopressin response to changes in blood volume is similar in response to blood pressure.

(4) Baroregulation of ADH secretion can be a dominant stimulus, but it is not the physiologic regulator of ADH secretion (see Figure 29-4).

c. **Other nonosmotic stimuli of ADH release** (see Table 29-1)

B. Inhibitors

1. **Osmotic inhibitors.** Expansion of the intracellular volume of the osmoreceptors sec-

ondary to hyposmolality of the extracellular fluid (ECF) inhibits ADH secretion. **Water ingestion** contributes to hyposmolality of the ECF.

2. Nonosmotic inhibitors

a. Increased arterial pressure secondary to vascular or ECF volume expansion inhibits ADH release.

(1) Thus, ADH release is inhibited by increased tension in the left atrial wall, great veins, or great pulmonary veins secondary to increased intrathoracic blood volume due to hypervolemia, a reclining position, negative-pressure breathing, and water immersion up to the neck.

(2) In the recumbent position, the increase in central blood volume leads to an increase in left atrial pressure and inhibition of ADH release. During sleep, the production of a concentrated urine is by and large due to a reduction of blood pressure, which offsets the effect of reduced ADH secretion due to a change in body position.

b. Other nonosmotic inhibitors of ADH release (see Table 29-1)

III. ROLE IN REGULATION OF RENAL WATER EXCRETION

A. **Renal effects** (Figure 29-5)

1. The major physiologic role of ADH is the control of ECF osmolality, largely through its antidiuretic and concentrating effects.

2. ADH also affects ECF volume and blood pressure by its vasoconstrictive and antinatriuretic effects on the kidney.

3. ADH promotes solute-free water reabsorption (T^cH_2O) by increasing the luminal permeability to the transepithelial transport of water by the principal cells of the collecting duct.

4. The **major site of action** of ADH is the receptor in the basolateral membrane of the principal cells of the medullary collecting ducts, where ADH increases the permeability to water. The **membrane shuttle hypothesis** may explain the action of ADH:

a. The apical plasma membrane of the principal cell of the collecting duct has a low water permeability in the unstimulated (i.e., ADH-depleted) state, whereas the basolateral membrane is highly water-permeable.

b. Intracellular, membrane-bound vesicles that contain proteinaceous water channels migrate and fuse with the apical plasma membrane in response to ADH.

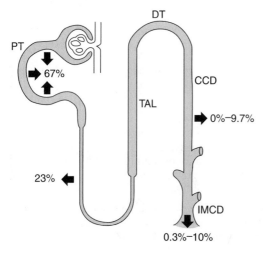

FIGURE 29-5. Segmental water reabsorption. The percentage of the filtered load of water reabsorbed by each nephron segment is indicated. The amount of water reabsorbed by the proximal tubule and the loop of Henle is relatively constant regardless of whether dilute or concentrated urine is excreted. The volume of water reabsorbed by the terminal portion of the distal tubule and the collecting duct is controlled by antidiuretic hormone (ADH). When ADH is absent, only a small volume of water is reabsorbed, and water excretion can reach 10% of the filtered load. Conversely, when ADH levels are maximal, a large volume of water is reabsorbed, and water excretion is less than 1% of the filtered load. PT = proximal tubule; TAL = thick ascending limb; DT = distal tubule; CCD = cortical collecting duct; IMCD = inner medullary collecting duct. [Modified with permission from Berne RM, Levy MN (editors): *Physiology,* 4th edition. St. Louis, Mosby, 1998, p 726.]

      c. Subsequently, apical membrane permeability (and thereby transcellular water permeability) increases, leading to the reabsorption of water.

    5. The water channels involved in the collecting duct response to ADH are the aquaporin-2 channels, which are inserted into the apical membrane.

    6. The movement of water across the basolateral membrane of the principal cell is mediated by aquaporin-3 and aquaporin-4.

C. Actions

    1. ADH, with its effect on increased water reabsorption, leads to the production of urine with a decreased volume and increased osmolality. A typical diet can be associated with a daily urinary solute excretion of 600–800 mOsm/day.

    2. In the absence of ADH (diabetes insipidus), urine volumes can be as high as 12–15 L/day. Therefore, ADH is responsible for the reabsorption of about 9%–10% of the reabsorption of water from the glomerular filtrate (180 L/day).

    3. In addition, ADH decreases renal medullary blood flow.

D. Extrarenal effects.
In addition, ADH stimulates the release of **adrenocorticotropic hormone (ACTH)** from the anterior lobe of the pituitary gland. ACTH plays a relatively small role in controlling aldosterone secretion (see Chapter 31 III A 1).

IV. ANTIDIURETIC HORMONE (ADH)-RELATED DISTURBANCES (Table 29-2)

A. Syndrome of inappropriate ADH secretion (SIADH).
SIADH leads to **water intoxication** (overhydration, or a dilution syndrome) [see Table 29-2].

    1. Etiology. SIADH is characterized by an excessive or inappropriate secretion of ADH from the posterior lobe or from an ectopic (nonhypothalamic) source such as a malignant tumor (e.g., bronchogenic carcinoma). This syndrome is not caused by excessive water intake.

    2. Clinical characteristics. Excessive secretion of ADH has the following effects when water is ingested:

        a. Water retention occurs, leading to expansion of the blood and ECF volumes.

        b. Hypernatriuria (i.e., increased urinary excretion of Na^+) and **hyponatremia** are present because aldosterone secretion is suppressed.

TABLE 29-2. Effects of Antidiuretic Hormone (ADH) Excess (SIADH) and Deficiency (Diabetes Insipidus) on Membrane Permeability

	Diabetes Insipidus	SIADH
Permeability of the collecting ducts to water	↓	↑
Urine flow	↑	↓
Urine osmolality	↓	↑
ECF volume	↓	↑
ECF osmolality	↑	↓
ECF sodium concentration	↑	↓
ICF volume	↓	↑
ICF osmolality	↑	↓

ADH = antidiuretic hormone; ECF = extracellular fluid; ICF = intracellular fluid; SIADH = syndrome of inappropriate antidiuretic hormone (secretion).

    c. Edema. Hyposmolality (i.e., decreased serum osmolality) results from increased water retention and urinary loss of Na^+. (It is the increased ADH secretion despite the presence of hyposmolality that is inappropriate.) The low plasma osmolality causes water to shift into the interstitial space (edema), and as the osmolality of that space decreases, there is a further shift of water into the ICF.

    d. Increased urine osmolality. This results because of the decreased urinary excretion of water and continued excretion of Na^+.

        (1) The U_{osm} exceeds the P_{osm}, and the urinary $[Na^+]$ exceeds 20 mEq/L.

        (2) **If water intake is restricted,** water retention does not occur, and the excessive ADH has no effect on the plasma $[Na^+]$. Edema does not occur because the increase in volume suppresses aldosterone secretion and increases Na^+ excretion.

  3. Therapy. SIADH is treated with demeclocycline, a tetracycline that blocks the effect of ADH on the kidney. Demeclocycline, lithium carbonate, amphotericin B, and methoxyflurane anesthesia may cause nephrogenic diabetes insipidus.

B. **Diabetes insipidus** (see Table 29-2)

  1. Etiology. Diabetes insipidus is characterized by a complete or partial **failure** of either **ADH secretion [central (neurogenic) diabetes insipidus]** or **the renal response to ADH (nephrogenic diabetes insipidus).**

  2. Clinical characteristics. Regardless of the cause, diabetes insipidus is characterized by a decrease in renal water reabsorption by the collecting ducts.

    a. Polyuria. Decreased water reabsorption results in a diuresis of dilute urine (up to 3–20 L/day). In nephrogenic diabetes insipidus, urine output is directly related to the volume of water delivered to the collecting ducts.

    b. Polydipsia. Because of the stimulation of thirst and increased water intake (polydipsia), most patients with diabetes insipidus maintain water balance with a near-normal plasma $[Na^+]$.

  3. Diagnosis. Diabetes insipidus is confirmed in polyuric patients by the demonstration of insignificant antidiuresis or by the production of hypertonic urine following water restriction or hypertonic saline infusions. Hypertonic hypernatremia is the hallmark of diabetes insipidus.

    a. A response to injected vasopressin documents the diabetes insipidus as neurogenic.

    b. Lack of a response to vasopressin is indicative of nephrogenic diabetes insipidus.

  4. Therapy

    a. Neurogenic diabetes insipidus

        (1) **Hormonal therapy** involves administration of ADH as **vasopressin tannate** or **nasal lysine vasopressin.**

        (2) **Nonhormonal therapy** for neurogenic diabetes insipidus includes administration of **oral hypoglycemic agents** (e.g., chlorpropamide), **thiazide diuretics with sodium restriction, carbamazepine,** and **clofibrate.** A major side effect of chlorpropamide therapy is hypoglycemia, a common problem with hypopituitarism.

    b. Nephrogenic diabetes insipidus. Thiazide diuretics also are quite effective in treating nephrogenic diabetes insipidus, which does not respond to treatment with vasopressin injection or chlorpropamide. Thiazides are effective in treating diabetes insipidus because they inhibit Na^+ reabsorption in the diluting segment (i.e., the thick ALH). Therefore, U_{osm} does not fall below 300 mOsm/kg, and urine volume can be reduced by 50%. (Urine osmolality can be increased sixfold from a minimum of 50 mOsm/kg.)

Case

A 35-year-old woman involved in a motor vehicle accident is brought to the hospital in a comatose state. Her husband states that she has no known medical problems and takes no medication. Physical examination reveals deep coma and a skull fracture; blood pressure

is normal, and a jugular venous pulse with reduced skin turgor. The initial laboratory tests were all normal, with a [Na$^+$] of 140 mEq/L.

The next day, urine output increased to about 220 ml/hour (polyuria). A review of her chart shows that the urine output has been rising progressively since admission. The repeat laboratory values are:

Plasma Chemistries		Urine Chemistries	
[Na$^+$]	148 mEq/L	[Na$^+$]	22 mEq/L
[K$^+$]	4.2 mEq/L	[K$^+$]	19 mEq/L
[Cl$^-$]	108 mEq/L		
[HCO$_3$$^-$]	26 mM/L		
Glucose	119 mg/dl		
BUN	18 mg/dl		
Creatinine	1.2 mg/dl		
P$_{osm}$	318 mOsm/kg H$_2$O	U$_{osm}$	67 mOsm/kg H$_2$O

BUN = blood urea nitrogen.

1. *What is the most likely cause of this patient's hypernatremia?*

DISCUSSION

Hypernatremia represents hyperosmolality, and it can result from water loss or Na$^+$ retention. However, in the clinical setting, osmolality (tonicity) disorders are almost always due to changes in water balance. To cause hypernatremia, water loss must occur in excess of solute loss. Thus, the only criterion needed for the diagnosis of water depletion is an elevated Na$^+$ concentration (or osmolality). Free-water can be lost from the skin, respiratory tract, and in dilute urine. The latter requires either decreased secretion of antidiuretic hormone (ADH) [central, or neurogenic, diabetes insipidus] or end-organ resistance to ADH (nephrogenic diabetes insipidus). The hematocrit does not increase in water depletion, because of a proportional loss of water from red blood cells (RBCs) and plasma.

The combination of hypernatremia and dehydration (poor skin turgor) characterizes this patient's imbalance as hyperosmotic dehydration. Her water deficit could be due either to decreased ingestion or increased excretion, but the examination is consistent with the latter. Dehydration resulting from decreased water intake would produce a low urine volume with a high urine osmolality. Conversely, this patient has a high urine volume with a low urine osmolality, despite the high plasma osmolality. These data are consistent with excessive free-water clearance due to defective renal conservation, known as diabetes insipidus.

2. *How could the etiology of this hypernatremia be established?*

DISCUSSION

The clinical and laboratory data are highly suspicious of diabetes insipidus of central origin (neurogenic), given the history of head trauma causing a skull fracture. This diagnosis could be corroborated by measuring plasma arginine vasopressin (AVP) together with plasma and urine osmolalities and repeating these tests following administration of exogenous AVP. Initially, the observation of a low plasma AVP concentration with high plasma osmolality and low urine osmolality, with a significant increase in urine osmolality after AVP injection is strongly suggestive of neurogenic diabetes insipidus.

The diagnosis could be confirmed with a water deprivation test (dehydration test), which gives the following results:

    a. Normal: $U_{osm} > 800$ mOsm/kg, little or no increase in U_{osm} after ADH administration, and increase in plasma AVP after dehydration

    b. Neurogenic diabetes insipidus: $U_{osm} < 300$ mOsm/kg H_2O that is substantially increased after ADH administration, and nondetectable plasma AVP in response to water deprivation

    c. Nephrogenic diabetes insipidus: $U_{osm} = 300–500$ mOsm/kg H_2O, little or no increase in U_{osm} in response to ADH administration, and significant increase in plasma AVP in response to dehydration

    d. Polydipsia: $U_{osm} > 500$ mOsm/kg H_2O, little or increase in U_{osm} after ADH administration, and significant increase in plasma AVP in response to water deprivation

    3. *What are the symptoms and signs of hypernatremia?*

DISCUSSION

The symptoms of hypernatremia (hyperosmolality) are primarily neurologic. Lethargy, weakness, irritability, seizures, coma, and death can occur in severe cases. Symptoms are related to the movement of water out of the brain cells down the osmotic gradient created by the rise in the effective plasma osmolality. This decrease in brain volume causes rupture of the cerebral veins, resulting in hemorrhaging and neurologic dysfunction, which may be irreversible. A lumbar puncture may reveal blood in the cerebrospinal fluid (CSF).

    4. *What are the major therapeutic modalities for diabetes insipidus?*

DISCUSSION

In neurogenic diabetes insipidus, the ability to form a concentrated urine can be restored by exogenous administration of ADH or a congener and drugs such as chlorpropamide, an oral hypoglycemic agent, which enhances NaCl reabsorption in the thick ascending limb of the loop of Henle (ALH) and promotes an increase in the water permeability of the collecting duct. The polyuria of nephrogenic diabetes insipidus is treated paradoxically with a thiazide diuretic together with a low-sodium, low-protein diet. The volume depletion produced by the diuretic enhances the proximal NaCl and water reabsorption resulting in a decreased delivery of water to the collecting tubules (the site of ADH action); therefore, less water is excreted.

Chapter 30

Aldosterone: Regulation of Body Fluid Volume

I. SYNTHESIS, SECRETION, AND INACTIVATION

A. Synthesis

1. Aldosterone is a C-21 (21 carbon atoms) corticosteroid that is synthesized in the outermost area of the adrenal cortex, the **zona glomerulosa. Adrenocorticotropic hormone (ACTH), angiotensin II,** and **increased plasma [K$^+$]** stimulate the biosynthesis of aldosterone.

2. Aldosterone represents less than 0.5% of the corticosteroids, and as all of the corticosteroids, it is stored in very small quantities. However, aldosterone is the major **mineralocorticoid** in humans.

3. The **circulatory half-life** of aldosterone is about 30 minutes in humans during normal activity.

4. **Cholesterol (esterified)** is the precursor for steroidogenesis and is stored in the cytoplasmic lipid droplets in the adrenocortical cells. (Free plasma cholesterol appears to be the preferred source of cholesterol for corticosteroid synthesis.)

B. Secretion. Most of the secreted aldosterone is bound to **albumin,*** with a lesser amount bound to **corticosteroid-binding globulin (CBG; transcortin).** CBG preferentially binds **cortisol,** which is a **glucocorticoid.**

C. Inactivation. Aldosterone is metabolized mainly in the liver, where more than 90% of this corticosteroid is inactivated during a single passage.

1. Most aldosterone inactivation is by **saturation (reduction)** of the double bond in the A-ring.

2. The major metabolite is **tetrahydroaldosterone,** most of which is conjugated with glucuronic acid at the carbon-3 position of the A-ring. The resultant **glucuronides** are more polar and, therefore, more water-soluble, making them readily excreted by the kidney.

II. PHYSIOLOGIC EFFECTS. Aldosterone has the primary function of promoting Na$^+$ retention. In addition, it enhances K$^+$ and H$^+$ secretion (Figure 30-1).

A. Conservation of Na$^+$

1. Aldosterone stimulates electrogenic Na$^+$ reabsorption in the connecting segment of the distal tubule and in the cortical collecting tubules (distal nephron).

2. Of the amount of filtered Na$^+$ (25,000 mEq/day), only 1%–2% (250–500 mEq or 6000–12,000 mg/day) are actively reabsorbed via an aldosterone-dependent mechanism in the distal nephron.†

3. Aldosterone also promotes Na$^+$ reabsorption in the epithelial cells of the sweat glands, salivary glands, and the gastrointestinal mucosa of the descending and sigmoid colon (distal colon).

4. By restricting the renal excretion of Na$^+$, which is the main determinant of plasma osmolality, aldosterone regulates the extracellular fluid (ECF) volume. Therefore, **aldos-**

---

*Protein-bound hormones are biologically inactive.
†Filtered load refers to the amount of Na$^+$ in the glomerular filtrate and not in the distal nephron.

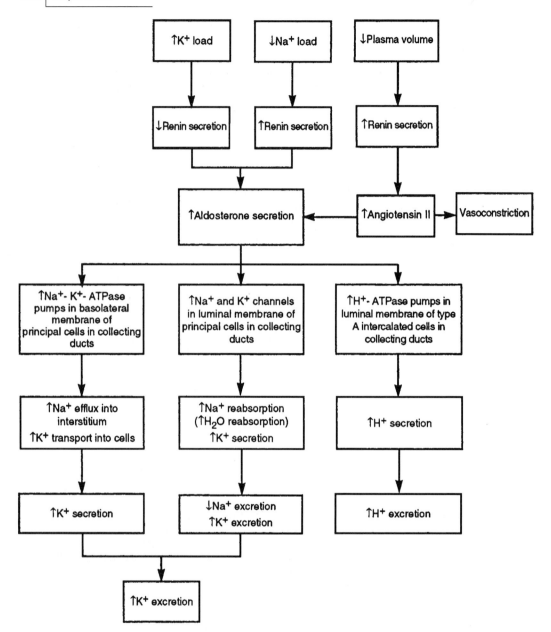

FIGURE 30-1. Effects of aldosterone on Na$^+$, K$^+$, and H$^+$ balance.

terone regulates the **total body Na$^+$ content,** while antidiuretic hormone (ADH) regulates the **plasma Na$^+$ concentration.**

B. **Secretion and excretion of K$^+$** (see Chapter 27 III F, G, H, and Figures 27-7 and 27-9)

  1. Aldosterone promotes K$^+$ secretion as a secondary effect of its action on Na$^+$ reabsorption.

  a. In the distal nephron, the linked Na$^+$ reabsorption–K$^+$ secretion is referred to as the **distal Na$^+$–K$^+$ exchange process.**

  b. Although K$^+$ appears to be secreted in exchange for Na$^+$, the distal secretion of K$^+$ is only indirectly related to Na^+ reabsorption. Distal Na^+ reabsorption is linked to the secretion of both K^+ and H^+.*

    c. Aldosterone increases the $[K^+]$ in sweat glands and saliva.

2. Stimulation of K^+ excretion greatly depends on dietary Na^+, as indicated by a lack of K^+ excretion after aldosterone administration in animals with Na^+-deficient diets.

3. More than 75% of the K^+ excreted in the urine is attributed to distal K^+ secretion.

    a. Excess aldosterone secretion causes a decline in the urinary Na^+/K^+ concentration ratio (from a normal value of about 2), because it decreases Na^+ excretion and increases K^+ excretion.

    b. Elevated aldosterone release increases the plasma Na^+/K^+ concentration ratio (from a normal value of 30) due to the increased excretion of K^+. Aldosterone can cause an isotonic expansion of the ECF volume with no change in the plasma $[Na^+]$ or a hypertonic expansion of the ECF volume with a rise in the plasma $[Na^+]$. In any case, the total amount of body Na^+ is increased.

C. Water excretion and ECF volume regulation

1. The effect of aldosterone on water excretion is not important physiologically, as aldosterone treatment fails to correct the impaired water excretion by patients with hypofunctional adrenal glands (due to Addison's disease or adrenal insufficiency) and by patients who have undergone adrenalectomy.

2. Aldosterone has no direct effect on the glomerular filtration rate (GFR), renal plasma flow, or renin production; however, by stimulating Na^+ reabsorption aldosterone causes water retention, and the resultant expansion of the ECF volume then leads to an increase in GFR and renal plasma flow and a decrease in renin production.

3. A high circulating aldosterone level is a common finding in edema and is due primarily to the increased aldosterone secretion induced by the depletion of the effective circulating blood volume (see Chapter 26 I A–C).

    a. It is unlikely that the plasma $[Na^+]$ is a major regulator of aldosterone secretion because the plasma $[Na^+]$ during Na^+ depletion is normal in humans.

      (1) Hyponatremia often is a consequence of ADH secretion and is accompanied by an increase in the ECF volume, which tends to suppress rather than stimulate aldosterone secretion. When ADH and water are given to Na^+-depleted individuals, aldosterone secretion falls despite a fall in plasma $[Na^+]$.

      (2) By and large, hyponatremia in the clinical setting is due to **excess body Na^+** caused by a decreased effective blood volume. The low blood volume leads to an increase in ADH secretion and aldosterone secretion which, in turn, lead to edema. **Over 90% of the cases of hyponatremia should be treated by restriction of NaCl and water.**

    b. Therefore, it is the volume of the ECF rather than the plasma $[Na^+]$ that influences aldosterone secretion in most circumstances.

D. Effects of aldosterone: cortical collecting duct (see Figure 30-1)

1. Transport of Na^+ (electrogenic) down its electrochemical gradient in the principal cells of the cortical collecting tubules

    a. Aldosterone causes insertion of new Na^+ luminal conductive channels.

    b. New $Na^+–K^+–ATPase$ molecules are inserted into the basolateral membrane resulting in the stimulation of active Na^+ extrusion into the interstitium.

    c. Sodium (hyponatremia) intake remains a major determinant of renin secretion.

      (1) A normal daily dietary salt intake is between 100 and 250 mEg per day.

      (2) This dietary salt intake corresponds to 2.3 to 5.7g Na^+ or 6 to 15g of NaCl.

      (3) Obligatory salt losses occur through sweat, stool, and urine.

---

*Na^+ transport in the proximal tubule is not associated with K^+ or H^+ exchange processes.

2. Increased intracellular K^+ concentration via the Na^+–K^+–ATPase pumps in the principal cells

   a. Insertion of luminal K^+ channels that promotes K^+ efflux against its electric gradient

   b. Increase in intracellular K^+ concentration in the tubular cells that promotes K^+ secretion

3. Promotes insertion of new electrogenic proton translocating ATPases into the luminal membrane of the A-type intercalated cells.

E. **Aldosterone and acid–base balance.** Aldosterone affects acid–base balance through its control of K^+ secretion. As stated above, aldosterone promotes increased distal tubular secretion and, therefore, **excretion** of K^+. Aldosterone also promotes the excretion of H^+ and NH_4^+ (see Chapter 27 III I and Figure 27-9).

1. **Hyperaldosteronemia** (i.e., increased aldosterone secretion) is one cause of K^+ depletion, a condition termed **hypokalemia.**

   a. Hypokalemia is characterized by an increase in intracellular $[H^+]$, which favors distal tubular secretion of H^+ over K^+ and results in **metabolic alkalosis.**

   b. Conversely, if metabolic alkalosis is the primary event, there is a decrease in intracellular $[H^+]$. This results in an increase in distal tubular intracellular $[K^+]$, which favors increased urinary loss of K^+ over H^+ and results in **hypokalemic metabolic alkalosis** (as occurs in hyperaldosteronemia).

2. **Hypoaldosteronemia** (i.e., decreased aldosterone secretion) is one cause of excess K^+, a condition termed **hyperkalemia.**

   a. Hyperkalemia is characterized by an increase in intracellular $[K^+]$, which favors distal tubular secretion of K^+ over H^+ and results in **metabolic acidosis.**

   b. On the other hand, when metabolic acidosis is the primary event, there is an increase in intracellular $[H^+]$. This results in an increase in distal tubular intracellular $[H^+]$, which favors increased secretion of H^+ over K^+ and results in **hyperkalemic metabolic acidosis** (as occurs in hypoaldosteronemia).

3. **Hypokalemia** causes the following conditions:

   a. **Impaired renal concentrating ability** leads to the formation of hyposmotic urine and polyuria that is resistant to ADH.

   b **Reduced carbohydrate tolerance** leads to a decline in insulin secretion.* As a rule, fasting hyperglycemia is not present with reduced insulin secretion.

III. **CONTROL OF ALDOSTERONE SECRETION** (Tables 30-1 and 30-2). At least three well-defined mechanisms control aldosterone secretion: ACTH, plasma $[K^+]$, and the renin–angiotensin system.

A. **Extrarenal control mechanisms.** The following mechanisms cause the release of aldosterone by direct action on the adrenal cortex:

1. **Hypothalamic–hypophysial–adrenocortical axis.** Under normal conditions, ACTH is not a major factor in the control of aldosterone synthesis or secretion. However, the pituitary gland plays an important role in the maintenance of the growth and biosynthetic capacity of the zona glomerulosa.

   a. **ACTH,** also known as **corticotropin,** is a 39-amino-acid polypeptide that supports steroidogenesis in the zona glomerulosa (Figure 30-2). ACTH enhances aldosterone production by stimulating the early biosynthetic pathway (i.e., the 20,22-desmolase enzyme complex that catalyzes the conversion of cholesterol to pregnenolone). ACTH also plays a minor role in mediating the diurnal rhythmic secretion of all of the corticosteroids.

   b. **Corticotropin releasing hormone (CRH),** a hypothalamic **hypophysiotropic** polypeptide, is made up of 41 amino acid residues. CRH is secreted into the hypophysial por-

---

*The reduction in carbohydrate tolerance due to hypokalemia occurs in only about half of patients with elevated plasma aldosterone.

TABLE 30-1. Factors that Regulate Renin and Aldosterone Secretion

	Intrarenal				Extrarenal	
	−Volemia		Intraluminal [Na$^+$]		Plasma [K$^+$]	
Hormone	**Hypo-**	**Hyper-**	**Depletion**	**Loading**	**Depletion**	**Loading**
Renin	↑	↓	↑	↓	↑	↓
Aldosterone	↑	↓	↑	↓	↓	↑
		←——Nonosmotic——→			←——————Osmotic——————→		
		(Baroreceptor)			(Chemoreceptor)	

tal system and causes release of ACTH from the pituitary gland. Because CRH secretion is regulated by higher brain centers (e.g., the limbic system), these centers play a role in Na$^+$ balance.

(1) Hypophysectomized patients and those with pituitary insufficiency exhibit normal aldosterone secretion on a moderate salt intake; however, these individuals demonstrate a suboptimal aldosterone response to Na$^+$ restriction.

TABLE 30-2. Regulators of NaCl and Water Reabsorption

Renal Sympathetic Nerves

(↑ Activity: ↓ NaCl Excretion)

- ↓ GFR
- ↑ Renin secretion
- ↑ Proximal tubule and thick ascending limb of Henle's loop NaCl reabsorption

Renin–Angiotensin–Aldosterone

(↑ Secretion: ↓ NaCl Excretion)

- ↑ Angiotensin II levels stimulate proximal tubule NaCl reabsorption
- ↑ Aldosterone levels stimulate thick ascending limb of the loop of Henle and collecting duct NaCl reabsorption
- ↑ ADH secretion

Atrial Natriuretic Peptide

(↑ Secretion: ↑ NaCl Excretion)

- ↑ GFR
- ↓ Renin secretion
- ↓ Aldosterone secretion
- ↓ NaCl reabsorption by the collecting duct
- ↓ ADH secretion

ADH

(↑ Secretion: ↓ H$_2$O and NaCl Excretion)

- ↑ H$_2$O reabsorption by the collecting duct
- ↑ NaCl reabsorption by the thick ascending limb of the loop of Henle
- ↑ NaCl reabsorption by the collecting duct

ADH = antidiuretic hormone; GFR = glomerular filtration rate.

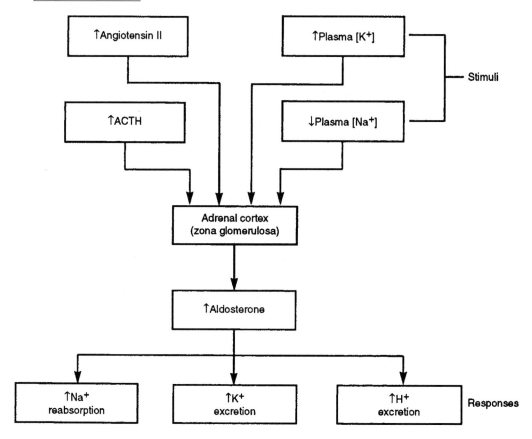

FIGURE 30-2. Angiotensin II and hyperkalemia, the two physiologic stimuli for aldosterone secretion, are more potent stimuli than adrenocorticotropic hormone (ACTH) and hyponatremia. Na^+ reabsorption and the secretion (and excretion) of K^+ and H^+ are the major responses to aldosterone secretion. The principal and intercalated cells of the collecting ducts are the primary target cells of aldosterone–Na^+ reabsorption and K^+ excretion take place at the principal cells, and H^+ excretion occurs in the type A intercalated cells. ACTH and hyperkalemia are extrarenal stimuli; hyponatremia and angiotensin II are intrarenal stimuli.

    (2) Normal individuals injected chronically with ACTH show an acute rise in aldosterone secretion followed by a return to control level or below in 3–4 days, despite ACTH administration over a period of 7–8 days.

    (3) When aldosterone is administered for several days to normal individuals, the kidney "escapes" from the Na^+-retaining effect but not from the K^+-excreting effect. The escape phenomenon prevents the appearance of edema in individuals treated with aldosterone for prolonged periods and in patients with primary aldosteronism.

2. Hyperkalemia. A 1% increase in plasma $[K^+]$ (< 0.1 mEq/L) can stimulate the synthesis and release of aldosterone by a direct action on the zona glomerulosa (see Figure 30-2). In the anephric human, K^+ appears to be the major regulator of aldosterone even though aldosterone levels are low.

    a. This release probably occurs by the depolarization of the glomerulosa cell membrane by the elevated plasma $[K^+]$.

    b. Stimulation of aldosterone secretion by K^+ loading is limited by the simultaneous reduction in renin release.

    c. K^+ stimulates an early step in the biosynthetic pathway for aldosterone synthesis.

    d. K^+ loading increases the width of the zona glomerulosa layer in experimental animals; prolonged aldosterone administration results in atrophy of this layer due to depressed renin secretion.

3. **Hyponatremia.** Hyponatremia can increase aldosterone secretion, but a very large reduction in plasma Na^+ concentration is needed; therefore, a physiologic role of hyponatremia is unlikely.
   a. A 10% decrease in plasma $[Na^+]$ also appears to stimulate the synthesis and release of aldosterone directly at the level of the zona glomerulosa (see Figure 30-2).
   b. However, this effect usually is overridden by changes in the effective circulating volume. Thus, aldosterone secretion is increased in the hyponatremic patient who is volume-depleted but is reduced in the hyponatremic patient who is volume-repleted.

B. **Intrarenal control mechanism.** Aldosterone secretion also is regulated by the renin–angiotensin system, the major component of which is the **juxtaglomerular apparatus.** The renin–angiotensin–aldosterone system is also regulated by the sympathetic nervous system.

1. **Anatomy of the juxtaglomerular apparatus** (Figure 30-3). The juxtaglomerular apparatus is a combination of specialized tubular and vascular cells located at the vascular pole where the afferent and efferent arterioles enter and leave the glomerulus. The juxtaglomerular apparatus is composed of **three cell types.**
   a. **Juxtaglomerular cells** are specialized **myoepithelial** (modified vascular smooth muscle) cells located in the **media** of the afferent arteriole, which synthesize, store, and release a proteolytic enzyme called **renin.** Renin is stored in the granules of the juxtaglomerular cells.
      (1) The juxtaglomerular cells are **baroreceptors** (tension receptors) and respond to changes in the transmural pressure gradient between the afferent arteriole and the interstitium. They are innervated by sympathetic nerve fibers.
      (2) These vascular "volume" receptors monitor renal perfusion pressure and are stimulated by hypovolemia, or decreased renal perfusion pressure.
   b. **Macula densa** cells are specialized renal tubular epithelial cells located at the transition between the thick segment of the ascending limb of the loop of Henle (ALH) and the distal convoluted tubule (see Figure 30-3). They are not innervated.
      (1) These cells are in direct contact with the mesangial cells, in close contact with the juxtaglomerular cells, and contiguous with both the afferent and efferent arterioles as the tubule passes between the arterioles supplying its glomerulus of origin.
      (2) The macula densa cells are characterized by prominent nuclei in those cells on the side of the tubule that is in contact with the mesangial and vascular elements of the juxtaglomerular apparatus.
      (3) The macula densa cells function as **chemoreceptors** and are stimulated by a decreased NaCl load. This inverse relationship between NaCl concentration and renin release provides a reasonable explanation for the clinical problems involv-

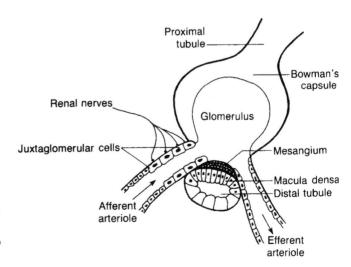

FIGURE 30-3. The anatomic components of the juxtaglomerular apparatus. (Reprinted from Yates FE, et al: The adrenal cortex. In *Medical Physiology,* 14th edition. Edited by Mountcastle VB. CV Mosby, 1980, p 1590.).

ing a decreased filtered load of Na^+ and Cl^- in association with increased renin release.

    (4) In summary, the initiating signal for macula densa control of renin secretion is a change in NaCl transport rate via the luminal $Na^+–2Cl^-–K^+$ cotransporter whose activity is determined by a change in luminal NaCl concentration.

    (5) Because the cotransporter has a higher affinity for Na^+ than Cl^-, it is most likely that the luminal Cl^- concentration is the most critical signal.

  c. **Mesangial cells** also are referred to as the **polkissen** (asymmetrical cap) and are the interstitial cells of the juxtaglomerular apparatus. Mesangial cells are in contact with both the juxtaglomerular cells and the macula densa cells. A decreased intraluminal Na^+ load, Cl^- load, or both in the region of the macula densa stimulates the juxtaglomerular cells.

2. Role of the sympathetic nervous system. The sympathetic nervous system plays an important role in the control of renin release via the **renal nerves.**

  a. The juxtaglomerular cells of the afferent arterioles are innervated directly by the sympathetic postganglionic fibers (unmyelinated). In the absence of renal nerves, the renal response to Na^+ depletion is attenuated.

  b. Circulating catecholamines (i.e., epinephrine and norepinephrine) and stimulation of the renal nerves produce vasoconstriction of the afferent arterioles, which causes renin release by a decrease in perfusion pressure.

    (1) This renin response caused by catecholamines and renal nerve stimulation is mediated via the β_1-adrenergic receptor and can be elicited by the synthetic sympathomimetic amine, **isoproterenol,** which is a β-agonist.

    (2) Renal denervation and β_1-adrenergic receptor blockade by **propranolol** inhibit the release of renin.

  c. Renal innervation is not a requisite for renin release because the denervated kidney can adapt to a variable salt intake.

  d. In humans, assuming an upright posture increases renal sympathetic activity, which produces renal arteriolar vasoconstriction and an increase in renin release. Thus, the sympathetic nervous system, by modulating the secretion of renin, has an **indirect effect on aldosterone secretion.**

3. Role of renin: stimuli for release (Table 30-3)

  a. Renin has a circulatory half-life of 40–120 minutes in humans. The common denominator for renin release by the intrarenal mechanism is a decrease in the effective circulating blood volume, which is induced by:

    (1) Acute hypovolemia associated with hemorrhage, diuretic administration, or salt depletion

    (2) Acute hypotension associated with ganglionic blockade or a change in posture (postural hypotension)

    (3) Chronic disorders associated with edema (e.g., cirrhosis with ascites, congestive heart failure, nephrotic syndrome)

  b. Renin release is increased by K^+ depletion, epinephrine, norepinephrine, isoproterenol, and standing.

4. Role of renin: inhibition of renin secretion

  a. Renin release is inhibited by angiotensin II, angiotensin III, ADH, hypernatremia, hyperkalemia, and atrial natriuretic peptide (ANP).

  b. **K^+ loading** leads to the inhibition of renin release and to the direct stimulation of the glomerulosa cells to secrete aldosterone. In contrast to its effect on normal individual, aldosterone administration to patients with heart failure, cirrhosis with ascites, or nephrosis causes Na^+ retention without K^+ excretion, because of greater proximal reabsorption of Na^+ with less Na^+ available for the distal exchange with K^+.

5. Angiotensin synthesis

  a. Renin is secreted into the bloodstream, where it combines with the renin substrate, angiotensinogen, which is an α_2-globulin synthesized in the liver.

    (1) Renin is not saturated with its substrate in normal plasma; the same amount of renin generates more angiotensin I if the substrate concentration is increased above normal.

TABLE 30-3. Factors Regulating Renin Secretion

Factor	Effect
Renal perfusion pressure	
Increase	Inhibit
Decrease	Stimulate
Sodium chloride delivery at the macula densa	
Increase	Inhibit
Decrease	Stimulate
Angiotensin II	Inhibit
Plasma electrolytes	
Potassium	Inhibit
Calcium	Inhibit
Prostaglandins (PGI$_2$)	Stimulate
Sympathetic nervous system	
β-Adrenergic stimulation	Stimulate
α-Adrenergic stimulation	Inhibit
Natriuretic factors	
Dopamine	Inhibit
Atrial natriuretic hormone	Inhibit
Other factors	
Vasopressin	Inhibit
Adrenocorticotropic hormone	Stimulate

    (2) Oral contraceptives increase plasma angiotensinogen concentration and decrease plasma renin concentration.
  b. The only physiologic effect of renin is to convert **angiotensinogen** to the biologically inactive decapeptide, angiotensin I.
  c. **Angiotensin I** is converted primarily in the lung by pulmonary endothelial cells to the physiologically active octapeptide, angiotensin II (Figure 30-4).
    (1) The enzyme that forms angiotensin II is a peptidase (dipeptidyl carboxypeptidase) called angiotensin-converting enzyme (ACE). It is found chiefly in pulmonary tissue and to a lesser degree in renal tissue and blood plasma.
    (2) The converting enzyme is identical to kininase II, which converts the nonapeptide vasodilator, bradykinin (kallidin-9), to inactive peptides, thereby diminishing the circulating levels of a vasodepressor substance and enhancing the vasoconstrictive action of angiotensin II.
  d. **Angiotensin II,** with a circulatory half-life of 1–3 minutes, has several important physiologic actions (Figure 30-5).
    (1) It functions as the tropic hormone for the zona glomerulosa and stimulates the secretion (and synthesis) of aldosterone (see Figure 30-2). Angiotensin II is the **aldosterone-stimulating hormone.**
    (2) It is a potent **local vasoconstrictor (vasopressor)** of the renal arterioles at low plasma concentrations; at higher concentrations, angiotensin II exerts a general vasopressor effect on the smooth muscle cells of arterioles throughout the cardiovascular system, leading to an elevation of systemic mean arterial blood pressure.
      (a) Angiotensin II stimulates the secretion of ADH and ACTH.
      (b) Angiotensin II stimulates thirst, which leads to increased fluid consumption. It also stimulates the release of epinephrine and norepinephrine from the adrenal medulla.

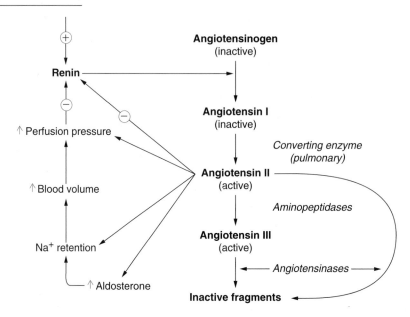

FIGURE 30-4. Components of the renin–angiotensin–aldosterone system, stimuli for renin secretion: ↓ macula densa NaCl, ↓ blood volume, ↓ perfusion pressure, ↑ β₁-adrenergic activity, and ↑ prostaglandins (PGI₂).
+ = indicates stimulation; − = indicates inhibition.

(3) Angiotensin II is inactivated by two angiotensinases (peptidases), and it can be converted to angiotensin III, which is a heptapeptide and a very potent stimulator of aldosterone secretion. Angiotensin III is not an effective vasoconstrictor in contrast to angiotensin II.

(4) Renin, converting enzyme, angiotensinogen, and angiotensin II have been found in brain tissue.

6. **Plasma renin activity and plasma renin concentration. Plasma renin activity** is defined as the rate of angiotensin I formation when plasma renin acts on **endogenous substrate. Plasma renin concentration** is measured when **exogenous substrate** is added to plasma to saturate the enzyme and increase the velocity of angiotensin I formation to a maximal rate.

a. Oral contraceptive administration is known to increase plasma renin activity and aldosterone secretion via a marked increase in renin substrate concentration, whether the woman is normotensive or hypertensive prior to the therapy.

b. As a result of the increased angiotensin II formation, plasma renin concentration is suppressed. Thus, the increase in plasma renin activity in this situation occurs without an increase in renin concentration.

c. Oral contraceptives are a cause of hypertension in women through this mechanism.

IV. ALDOSTERONISM refers to a condition of excessive aldosterone secretion (Table 30–4).

A. **Primary hypoaldosteronism** (Conn's syndrome)

1. **Etiology.** Primary hyperaldosteronism results from a tumor of the **zona glomerulosa.**

2. **Characteristics** of primary hypoaldosteronism include:

a. Elevated plasma (and urinary) aldosterone

b. Hypertension due to Na⁺ and water retention

c. Hypokalemic alkalosis with a K⁺ excretion rate of greater than 40 mEq/day*

---

*Hypokalemia is not always concomitant with hypermineralocorticoidism (e.g., in 11β-hydroxylase deficiency).

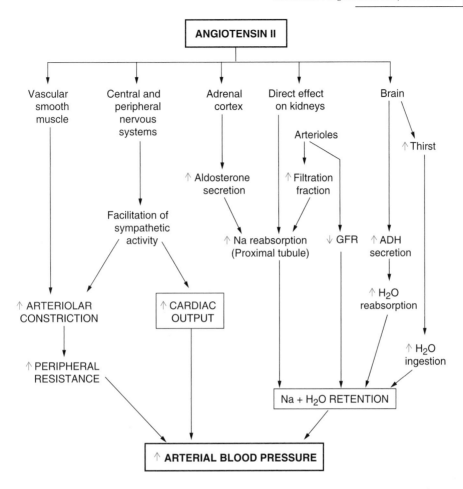

FIGURE 30-5. Summary of those angiotensin-mediated actions that facilitate fluid retention and elevate the arterial blood pressure. The arrow connecting "Na and H_2O retention" to "arterial blood pressure" represents a simplified shortcut—of course, fluid retention affects arterial blood pressure only by altering cardiac output and peripheral resistance. (Modified with permission from Vander AJ: *Renal Physiology*, 4th edition. New York, McGraw-Hill, 1991, p 138.)

    d. Decreased levels of angiotensin and renin
    e. Decreased hematocrit due to the expansion of the plasma volume
    f. Polyuria and dilute urine due to secondary nephrogenic diabetes insipidus
    g. Absence of peripheral edema
    h. Decreased plasma colloidal osmotic (oncotic) pressure due to ECF expansion

B. **Secondary hyperaldosteronism**

    1. Etiology. Secondary hyperaldosteronism is caused by the following extra-adrenal factors:
      a. Dietary therapy, which is the most common cause
      b. Extravascular loss of Na^+ and water, which is associated with edema (due to such underlying factors as nephrosis, cirrhosis, and congestive heart failure), an increase in the total ECF volume, and a loss of effective blood volume
      c. Hyperreninism caused by a tumor of the juxtaglomerular cells
      d. Renovascular disease (e.g., renal artery stenosis)

    2. Characteristics. Secondary hypoaldosteronism is characterized by edema and Na^+ retention. Urinary K^+ excretion is not increased because there is a reduced flow of fluid

TABLE 30.4 Pathophysiologic Effects of Aldosterone Excess and Deficiency

	Primary Hyperaldosteronism	Primary Hypoaldosteronism (Primary Adrenal Insufficiency)	Secondary Hyperaldosteronism (Congestive Heart Failure)
Total body sodium	↑	↓	↑
ECF volume	↑	↓	↑
Plasma volume	↑	↓	↑
Blood pressure	↑	↓	↑*
Plasma potassium concentration	↓	↑	No Change
Blood (plasma) pH	↑	↓	↑
Edema (yes or no)	No	No†	Yes
Plasma renin activity	↓	↑	↑

*Variable.
†Cerebral edema.
ECF = extracellular fluid.

into and through the distal segments of the nephron. This low fluid flow reduces K^+ secretion and offsets the stimulating effect of aldosterone. Also, with decreased Na^+ and water delivery to the distal tubule, the quantity of K^+ (and H^+) secreted in the urine is limited. Additional characteristics of secondary hyperaldosteronism include:
  a. Increased plasma (and urinary) aldosterone
  b. Hypertension with edema (due to Na^+ retention and water accumulation in the interstitial fluid compartment) and a decrease in plasma volume
  c. Hypokalemic alkalosis
  d. Increased angiotensin and plasma renin activity*
  e. Peripheral edema

3. Chronic licorice ingestion in excessive amounts can mimic aldosteronism, because licorice contains the salt-retaining substance, glycyrrhizinic acid. Patients with this condition present with:
  a. Hypertension and hypokalemic alkalosis
  b. Suppressed plasma renin levels
  c. Reduced aldosterone secretion due to chronic volume expansion

V. ALDOSTERONE ANTAGONISM: SPIRONOLACTONE

A. **Renal effects.** Spironolactone is a steroidal aldosterone antagonist, which competitively blocks the Na^+-retaining and K^+-excreting effects that aldosterone exerts on the distal nephron. As a result, spironolactone leads to an increase in urinary Na^+ excretion and a decrease in K^+ excretion. This antagonist is efficacious only in the presence of aldosterone or another mineralocorticoid; spironolactone is without effect in adrenalectomized individuals.

B. **Blood pressure effect.** Because the drug enhances Na^+ diuresis, spironolactone is effective in potentiating the action of many antihypertensive drugs whose dosage should be reduced in its presence.

---

*The elevated renin level is the characteristic that differentiates secondary aldosteronism from the primary form.

C. | **Clinical application.** Spironolactone is useful in the differential diagnosis of primary and secondary hyperaldosteronism.

1. If both plasma [K^+] and blood pressure are returned to normal with spironolactone, primary hyperaldosteronism is suspected.

2. If spironolactone causes the plasma [K^+] to return to normal without the antihypertensive effect, secondary hyperaldosteronism is suspected.

Exercise

Renovascular Hypertension

Renal arterial stenosis leads to renal arterial ischemia because of the resultant decline in renal arterial perfusion pressure. The response to the stenosis is the stimulation of renin secretion from the juxtaglomerular cells which is a protease that converts angiotensinogen into angiotensin I. The angiotensin-converting enzyme (ACE) from the pulmonary endothelial cells converts the decapeptide (angiotensin I) to the bioactive octapeptide (angiotensin II). It is this peptide hormone that exerts multiple effects that ultimately involve the regulation of fluid volume and electrolyte balance, which, in turn, regulate blood pressure. The two major effects of angiotensin II include: (1) systemic arteriolar vasoconstriction, both directly and by enhancing the release and effect of norepinephrine; and (2) promotion of Na^+ reabsorption, both directly from the proximal tubule and through the stimulation of aldosterone secretion. Aldosterone enhances Na^+ reabsorption in the cortical collecting tubules, leading to volume expansion with a resultant hypertension. The type of hypertension described here is referred to as renovascular, or renoprival, hypertension caused by hyperaldosteronism.

1. *Is this pathology a primary or secondary hyperaldosteronism?*

DISCUSSION

Because the lesion leading to the aldosteronism is outside of the adrenal(s), this represents secondary hyperaldosteronism.

2. *Summarize the disease entities that should be considered in the differential diagnosis of patients with aldosterone excess.*

DISCUSSION

Salt and water retention, leading to extracellular fluid (ECF) volume expansion in the absence of edema, are observed in primary aldosteronism, while edema is a concomitant of secondary aldosteronism. Both types of patients also develop hypertension, hypokalemia, and metabolic alkalosis. The laboratory data separate mineralocorticoid hypertensive patients into four groups, according to the plasma levels of renin and aldosterone:

a. High renin–high aldosterone: caused by (1) hypersecretion of a renin tumor or hyperplasia of the juxtaglomerular cells, and (2) renal arterial stenosis or intrarenal vascular disease

b. Low renin–high aldosterone: caused by (1) a tumor of the adrenal gland (primary aldosteronism), (2) bilateral adrenal hyperplasia, and (3) adrenal carcinoma

c. Low renin–low aldosterone: caused by (1) chronic exogenous administration of corticosteroids, (2) licorice abuse, (3) swallowing of chewing tobacco extracts, and (4) adrenogenital syndromes (11-hydroxylase and 17-hydroxylase deficiencies)

d. Low renin–variable aldosterone: caused by (1) adrenocorticotropic hormone (ACTH) excess and/or (2) Cushing's syndrome (hypercortisolism)

3. *What is the expected effect of elevated aldosterone secretion on Na^+, K^+, and H^+ concentrations in plasma?*

DISCUSSION

Aldosterone does not raise the plasma Na^+ concentration, because there is a commensurate retention of water in the collecting tubules if antidiuretic hormone (ADH) is present. If ADH is absent, the ensuing small elevation in plasma Na^+ concentration stimulates ADH release and thirst, which also leads to water retention. Aldosterone promotes both K^+ and H^+ secretion and excretion leading to hypokalemia and alkalosis (hypokalemic alkalosis).

4. *What are major effects brought about by the effect of aldosterone on plasma K^+ concentration?*

DISCUSSION

Hypokalemia leads to muscle weakness, cramping, myalgias, myolysis, paresis, and paralysis. Hypokalemia alters cardiac excitability by hyperpolarizing the resting membrane potential. Hypokalemia also decreases membrane permeability to K^+ ions, prolonging the duration of the action potential, because K^+ efflux is responsible for rapid repolarization. Furthermore, pacemaker activity is increased, because spontaneous depolarization is caused by a decline in K^+ conductance (fall in K^+ efflux). Other cardiac effects of hypokalemia include increased risk of digitalis toxicity, flat or inverted T waves, depressed ST segments, and prominent U waves. Hypokalemia also causes structural myocardial damage and constriction of arterioles.

5. *What is the acid–base state of the patient with renovascular hypertension?*

DISCUSSION

Because aldosterone promotes K^+ secretion by the principal cells and H^+ secretion by the intercalated (A-type) cells of the collecting duct, there is an increased excretion of these two ions and a resultant hypokalemic metabolic alkalosis.

6. *How can the physician differentially diagnose primary and secondary hyperaldosteronemia?*

DISCUSSION

Renin secretion is reduced by an autonomous adrenal adenoma (primary aldosteronism), probably due to the volume expansion induced by Na^+ (and water) retention. In contrast, renin release is enhanced by volume depletion (or renal ischemia), and the increased formation of angiotensin II is responsible for secondary hyperaldosteronemia. Furthermore, edema is a characteristic of secondary hyperaldosteronism, not primary hyperaldosteronism.

Chapter 31

Atrial Natriuretic Peptide (ANP)

I. **INTRODUCTION.** Atrial natriuretic peptide (or factor) [(ANP), (ANF)] refers to a group of polypeptides produced by the atrial muscle cells. ANP exerts a hormonal influence on the kidney, which results in changes in intrarenal hemodynamics through its effects on fluid volume, electrolyte (Na^+) balance, and blood pressure homeostasis.

II. **SYNTHESIS**

A. In mammals, ANP is synthesized, stored, and released from **atrial cardiocytes.** The secretory activity of these cells is evidenced by the presence of membrane-bound storage granules with electron-dense cores.

B. The ANP group is comprised of peptides that have molecular weights ranging from approximately 2500 to 13,000 daltons and lengths ranging from 21 to 73 amino acid residues. All are derived from a common 126-amino-acid precursor called **pro-ANP (atriopeptigen),** which is the predominant form of ANP in the atrium.

C. In humans, ANP is synthesized in a **prepro** (i.e., **pre-atriopeptigen**) form containing 151 amino acid residues.

D. The predominant circulating form of ANP is the 28-amino-acid peptide.

III. **SECRETION.** Stimuli for ANP release include atrial distention (hypervolemia), epinephrine, arginine vasopressin antidiuretic hormone, acetylcholine, and a high Na^+ **diet.**

IV. **PHYSIOLOGIC EFFECTS OF ANP** (Figures 31–1 and 31–2)

A. **Renal and adrenal responses**

1. **An increased glomerular filtration rate (GFR)** is associated with constriction of the efferent arteriole, which increases the glomerular hydrostatic pressure. It is important to note that ANP induces relaxation (dilation) of precontracted renal arteries.

2. **Dilation of the afferent arteriole** and vasoconstriction of the efferent arteriole increases the hydrostatic pressure in the glomerular capillary.

3. **Natriuresis** (i.e., increased urinary Na^+ excretion) occurs primarily as a result of the increase in GFR.
   a. Due, in part, to increased glomerular capillary hydrostatic pressure
   b. Relaxation of mesangial cells leading to increase in the glomerular ultrafiltration coefficient, K_f, and, in turn, to increased GFR
   c. ANP antagonizes the angiotensin II-induced increment in proximal tubular Na^+ and water reabsorption
   d. Inhibition of solute (Na^+) and water reabsorption in the medullary collecting duct

4. **Inhibition of aldosterone secretion.** ANP blocks aldosterone secretion that is pre-stimulated by Na^+ depletion, angiotensin II, adrenocorticotropic hormone, K^+, and cyclic adenosine 3′5′-monophosphate.

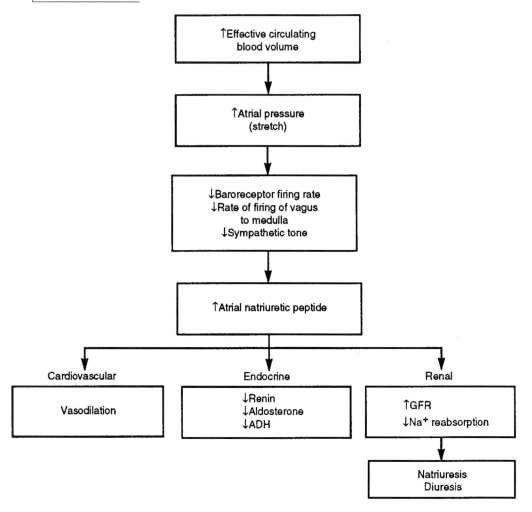

FIGURE 31-1. Activation of atrial natriuretic peptide (ANP) via low-pressure baroreceptors in the atria (especially the left atrium) leads to cardiovascular, endocrine, and renal effects. *ADH* = antidiuretic hormone; *GFR* = glomerular filtration rate.

    5. Inhibition of renin secretion occurs via the increase in NaCl delivery to the macula densa or the increase in hydrostatic pressure at the juxtaglomerular apparatus due to afferent arteriolar vasodilation with efferent arteriolar vasoconstriction.

B. **Cardiovascular effects**

    1. Decreases in mean systemic arterial blood pressure occur due to vasorelaxation or suppression of renin secretion and decreased peripheral resistance caused by inhibition of sympathetic tone.

    2. Reduction in cardiac output occurs due to a fall in heart rate and contractility.

    3. ANP can increase, decrease, or have no effect on renal blood flow.

        a. There is a vasodilatory effect on renal blood vessels that are preconstricted with angiotensin II, norepinephrine, or vasopressin.

        b. The diuretic effect of ANP is not dependent on changes (increase) in renal blood flow.

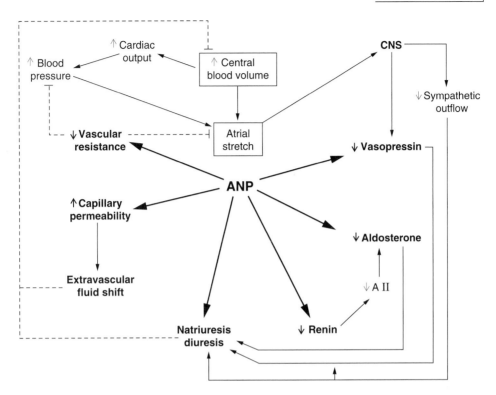

FIGURE 31-2. Schematic representation of the regulation of atrial natriuretic peptide (or factor)[ANP(ANF)] secretion, its major target organ actions, and its interrelationship with reflex inhibition of central sympathetic outflow during expansion of central blood volume. *Dashed lines* indicate probable negative feedback signals. Although unproved, it is likely that ANP-induced inhibition of aldosterone and renin release, natriuresis, and extravascular fluid shifts occur at near physiologic concentrations of the hormone. The latter two effects, by diminishing venous return to the heart, would provide negative feedback signals for ANP secretion. Inhibition of vasopressin release and decreased vascular resistance are probably not major effects under normal physiologic conditions. Antagonism of vasoconstrictor action is probably significant in certain pathologic states, and the resultant decrease in vascular resistance would tend to counter the rise in blood pressure due to increased cardiac output and might also have negative feedback effects on atrial stretch. *A II* = angiotensin II.(Reprinted with permission from Windhager EE (ed): *Handbook of Physiology,* vol II, section 8. Renal Physiology, Chart 33, Atrial Natriuretic Factor. New York, Oxford University Press, 1992, p 1632.)

Exercise

Atrial natriuretic peptide (ANP), stored in the atrial myocytes, is released into the circulation in response to stretching (volume receptors) of the atria. This release of ANP promotes increased natriuresis by hemodynamic and hormonal mechanisms. The hemodynamic effects include (1) increased glomerular filtration rate (GFR) (the increased Na^+ filtered load promotes natriuresis) and (2) medullary blood flow (Na^+ reabsorption is depressed, and urinary Na^+ excretion increases). The hormonal effects include direct reduction of aldosterone secretion and indirect suppression of aldosterone secretion via inhibition of renin release and subsequent depression of angiotensin II secretion. These hormonal effects decrease Na^+ reabsorption and promote urinary Na^+ excretion. Conversely, diminution of extracellular fluid (ECF) volume provides negative feedback that suppresses the release of ANP, which results in Na^+ retention.

What effect will each of the following conditions have on the release of ANP?

    1. *Ingestion of a Na+ load (e.g., potato chips) without water*

2. *Ingestion of a water load, which is normally rapidly excreted without a change in the extracellular fluid (ECF) volume*

3. *An intravenous infusion of isotonic saline*

4. *Marked diarrhea in which the plasma Na$^+$ concentration remains normal (isosmotic dehydration)*

5. *Congestive heart failure*

Discussion

1. An Na$^+$ load without water will cause both volume expansion and an elevation in the plasma Na$^+$ concentration and, therefore, plasma osmolality. As a result atrial natriuretic peptide (ANP) and antidiuretic hormone (ADH) secretion will rise, and aldosterone secretion will fall.

2. A water load is rapidly excreted, because the resultant fall in plasma osmolality will diminish ADH release, resulting in the excretion of dilute urine. In this setting ANP and aldosterone secretion will not change.

3. Isotonic NaCl will expand volume without affecting osmolality. Thus, ANP levels will rise, and aldosterone and ADH levels will fall.

4. Isosmotic volume depletion will enhance the secretion of aldosterone and ADH and diminish the release of ANP.

5. Although there is a decline in the **effective** circulating volume (effective arterial blood volume), patients who have congestive heart failure have a greater extracellular fluid (ECF) volume. Even though the patients retain Na$^+$ and are vasoconstricted, the increased cardiac filling pressures lead to the release of ANP.

PART V

STUDY QUESTIONS

1. The following renal function data were obtained for substance x:

Urine flow rate = 90 ml/hr

Urine concentration of
substance $\times$ (U_x) = 480 mg/ml

Plasma concentration of
substance $\times$ (P_x) = 6 mg/ml

What is the clearance of substance x?

(A) 12 ml/min
(B) 100 ml/min
(C) 120 ml/min
(D) 240 ml/min
(E) 480 ml/min

2. The renal transport maximum (Tm) for a substance is defined as the maximal

(A) glomerular filtration rate (GFR)
(B) urinary excretion rate
(C) tubular reabsorption or secretion rate
(D) renal clearance rate
(E) amount of a substance filtered by the glomeruli per minute

3. Of the renal systems available for the excretion of H^+, which is the one with the greatest activity?

(A) H^+ secretion
(B) Monobasic phosphate (NaH_2PO_4) excretion
(C) Sulfate (SO_4^{2-}) excretion
(D) Titratable acid excretion
(E) NH_4^+ excretion

4. When the secretion of para-aminohippuric acid (PAH) reaches the renal tubular transport maximum (Tm), a further increase in plasma PAH concentration causes its clearance to do which of the following?

(A) Increase in proportion to its plasma concentration
(B) Approach glucose clearance asymptotically
(C) Remain constant
(D) Approach inulin clearance asymptotically
(E) Increase in proportion to the glomerular filtration rate (GFR)

5. Which one of the following statements regarding Na^+ transport is correct?

(A) Active transport of Na^+ across all cells consumes most of the energy derived from cellular metabolism.
(B) The Na^+ concentration is highest in the intracellular fluid (ICF).
(C) Na^+ reabsorption across proximal tubular cells is mainly active and transcellular.
(D) The Na^+ concentration gradient provides energy for the cotransport of H^+.
(E) The transport of Na^+ across the apical membrane of the nephron is an active transport process.

6. The renal threshold for a solute denotes the

(A) maximum filtration rate
(B) maximum reabsorption rate
(C) plasma concentration at which a solute begins to appear in the urine
(D) maximum secretion rate
(E) maximum tubular secretory capacity (Ts)

7. Which one of the following conditions causes a decrease in the extracellular fluid (ECF) volume, an increase in the intracellular fluid (ICF) volume, and a decrease in the osmolar concentration of both compartments?

(A) Hyperosmotic dehydration
(B) Hyposmotic dehydration
(C) Isosmotic dehydration
(D) Hyperosmotic overhydration
(E) Hyposmotic overhydration

8. Which of the following substances has the lowest renal clearance?

(A) Glucose
(B) Urea
(C) Inulin
(D) Creatinine
(E) Para-aminohippuric acid (PAH)

9. Stimulation of renin secretion will increase the

(A) K^+ concentration in the blood
(B) volume of the extracellular fluid (ECF)
(C) hematocrit
(D) plasma colloid oncotic pressure
(E) H^+ concentration in the blood

10. Given a glomerular filtration rate (GFR) of 125 ml/min, a plasma glucose concentration of 400 mg/100 ml, a urine glucose concentration of 75 mg/ml, and a urine flow rate of 2 ml/min, what is the renal tubular transport maximum (Tm) for glucose?

(A) 300 mg/min
(B) 350 mg/min
(C) 400 mg/min
(D) 500 mg/min
(E) 550 mg/min

11. Which one of the following factors best explains an increase in the glomerular filtration rate (GFR)?

(A) Increased arterial plasma oncotic pressure
(B) Increased hydrostatic pressure in Bowmans capsule
(C) Increased glomerular capillary hydrostatic pressure
(D) Decreased net filtration pressure
(E) Vasoconstriction of the afferent arteriole

12. Measurements taken after an intravenous injection of inulin indicate that the substance appears to be distributed throughout 30% to 35% of the total body water (TBW). This finding suggests that inulin most likely is

(A) excluded from the cells
(B) distributed uniformly throughout the TBW volume
(C) restricted to the plasma volume
(D) neither excreted nor metabolized by the body
(E) not freely diffusible through capillary membranes

13. A patient is inadvertently given 2 L of isotonic saline (0.9% NaCl) over a 4-hour period of time. This infusion should cause an increase in

(A) antidiuretic hormone (ADH)
(B) plasma oncotic pressure
(C) angiotensin II
(D) atrial natriuretic factor
(E) aldosterone

14. Which one of the following conditions is associated with an increase in the secretion of atrial natriuretic peptide?

(A) Weightlessness
(B) Hemorrhage
(C) Hypovolemia
(D) Hypotension
(E) A reduction in effective circulating volume

Questions 15–19

Questions 15–19 are based on the following figure.

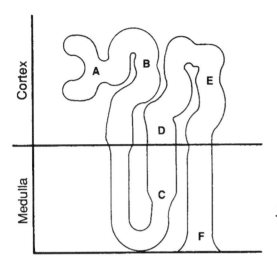

15. Tubular fluid is always hyposmotic at which of the lettered sites?

16. The tubular fluid-to-plasma (TF/P) ratio for glucose is 1.0 at this site.

17. The urea concentration is highest at this site.

18. The urine osmolality (U_{osm}) can reach 1200 to 1400 mOsm/L at this site.

19. The macula densa is closest to this site.

Questions 20–22

For each of the the following substances, select the appropriate lettered tubular fluid-to-plasma (TF/P) curve on the graph here.

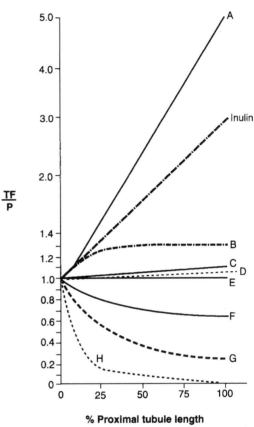

20. Inorganic phosphate (P_i)

21. Glucose

22. Glycine

Questions 23–26

The following graph shows the proximal tubular secretion of *para*-aminohippuric acid (PAH) versus the plasma concentration of PAH. In these questions, assume that all the plasma flows through the nephron vasculature and that the glomerular filtration rate (GFR) and the filtration fraction (FF) are normal.

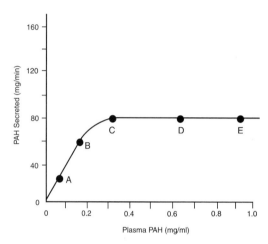

23. Which of the following points corresponds to the lowest clearance of *para*-aminohippuric acid (PAH)?

(A) A
(B) B
(C) C
(D) D
(E) E

24. Which of the following points is associated with the greatest renal venous *para*-aminohippuric acid (PAH) concentration?

(A) A
(B) B
(C) C
(D) D
(E) E

25. Which of the following points represents the highest excretion rate of *para*-aminohippuric acid (PAH)?

(A) A
(B) B
(C) C
(D) D
(E) E

26. Which of the following points corresponds to the greatest concentration in Bowman's capsule?

(A) A
(B) B
(C) C
(D) D
(E) E

27. At plasma concentrations of glucose higher than those associated with the transport maximum ($\approx$ 300 mg/dl), which of the following statements is correct?

(A) The clearance of glucose is zero
(B) The excretion rate of glucose equals the filtered load of glucose
(C) The reabsorption rate of glucose equals the filtered load of glucose
(D) The excretion rate of glucose increases with increasing plasma glucose concentrations
(E) Renal venous glucose concentration equals the renal arterial glucose concentration

28. The reabsorption of glucose from the renal tubular lumen into the cells

(A) depends on the presence of Na^+ in the filtrate
(B) occurs against an electrochemical gradient
(C) is a primary active transport process
(D) is inhibited by the simultaneous transport of *para*-aminohippuric acid (PAH)
(E) occurs mainly in the distal tubule

29. Use of the Fick principle and the following data allow for the calculation of the renal blood flow (in ml/min).

Indicator concentration (renal artery): 0.2 mg/ml
Indicator concentration (renal vein): 0.05 mg/ml
Urine minute volume: 1.5 ml/min
Indicator concentration (urine): 80 mg/ml

Which of the following values is correct?

(A) 400
(B) 600
(C) 800
(D) 1000
(E) 1200

30. After severe hemorrhage, a man's blood pressure drops to 50/35 mm Hg, his heart rate increases from 70 to 140 beats/min, and his pulse is weak. Immediately following infusion of 3 L of plasma, his blood pressure rises to 100/70 mm Hg, and his heart rate slows to 90 beats/min. As a result of the infusion of plasma, which one of the following is decreased?

(A) Cardiac output
(B) Stroke volume
(C) Peripheral vascular resistance (PVR)
(D) Plasma oncotic pressure
(E) Glomerular filtration rate (GFR)

Questions 31–32

The following table shows changes in the glomerular filtration rate (GFR) and in the filtration fraction (FF) in various conditions.

	A	B	C	D	E
GFR	↑	↓	↓	↑	↑
FF	↑	↑	No change	↓	No change

31. Which column summarizes the changes in GFR and FF that occur with increased afferent arteriolar resistance?

(A) A
(B) B
(C) C
(D) D
(E) E

32. Which column summarizes the changes in GFR and FF that occur with increased efferent arteriolar resistance?

(A) A
(B) B
(C) C
(D) D
(E) E

33. The following data were obtained from a patient:

Plasma	Urine
Inulin concentration: 1 mg/ml	Inulin concentration: 150 mg/ml
Concentration of substance X: 2 mg/ml	Concentration of substance X: 100 mg/ml
	Urine flow rate: 1 ml/min

Assuming that substance X is freely filtered, which one of the following statements is correct?

(A) There is net secretion of X.
(B) There is net reabsorption of X.
(C) The clearance of X can be used to measure glomerular filtration rate (GFR).
(D) There is both reabsorption and secretion of X.
(E) The clearance of X is greater than the clearance of creatinine.

34. Reabsorption of filtered bicarbonate

(A) contributes to the excretion of titratable acid
(B) is reduced during a state of acidosis
(C) is accomplished by the net secretion of Na^+
(D) requires carbonic anhydrase
(E) is usually lower than Na^+ reabsorption

35. Which of the following solutions has the highest osmolal concentration?

(A) 300 millimolar sucrose solution
(B) 300 milliosmolar sucrose solution
(C) 300 millimolar NaCl solution
(D) 300 milliosmolar NaCl solution
(E) 400 millimolar urea solution

36. Renal autoregulation explains changes in resistance to blood flow without the involvement of the nervous system. The major site of autoregulatory resistance changes is the

(A) renal artery
(B) interlobular artery
(C) afferent arteriole
(D) efferent arteriole
(E) peritubular capillary

Questions 37–40

Questions 37–40 are based on the diagrams below, which represent the volumes and osmolarities of the extracellular (ECF) and intracellular (ICF) fluid compartments in a normal subject (*solid lines*). The height of the rectangles denotes osmolarity, and the width represents volume. The dashed lines indicate change in the osmolarity and/or volume of the intracellular and extracellular compartments. For each of the procedures or disease states that follows, select the lettered diagram that best describes the changes that would result.

37. Infusion of 500 ml of an isotonic NaCl solution

38. Infusion of 1 L of a 300 mmol/L saline solution

39. Drinking 1 L of tap water

40. Chronic elevated secretion of antidiuretic hormone (ADH)

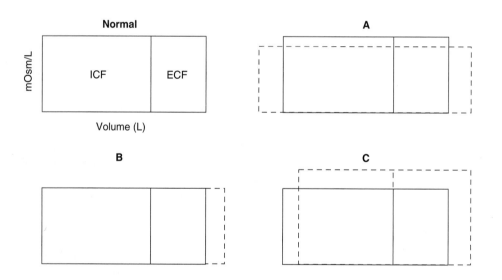

41. Which of the following statements regarding osmosis is correct?

(A) Osmotic pressure gradients are proportional to the concentration gradient of permeable ions.
(B) Osmosis is the new movement of water from an area of high osmolarity to one of low osmolarity.
(C) Osmotic pressure is decreased by the $Na^+–K^+–ATPase$ pump.
(D) Water usually flows against its concentration gradient.
(E) The osmotic pressure gradient is zero when all molecules are permeable.

Questions 42–45

Questions 42–45 are based on the following figure. Select the correct lettered region on the diagram of the nephron.

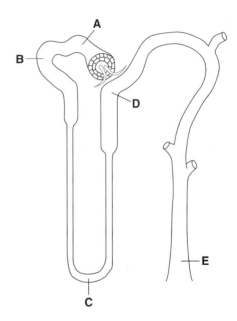

42. The point that represents the lowest tubular fluid-to-plasma (TF/P) concentration ratio for inulin.

43. The point that represents the lowest TF_{osm}/P_{osm} ratio in a well-hydrated individual.

44. The point that represents the highest TF concentration of *para*-aminohippuric acid (PAH).

45. The site of the highest TF glucose concentration.

46. The following data were obtained from an experimental animal. Which of the following is the net filtration pressure in mm Hg?

	Afferent Arteriole	Bowman's Space
Glomerular capillary hydrostatic pressure (mm Hg)	60	14
Oncotic pressure (mm Hg)	21	0

(A) 0
(B) 7
(C) 25
(D) 39
(E) 46

47. Which of the following statements correctly describes glucose reabsorption by the kidney?
(A) Secondary active cotransport at the luminal membrane
(B) Below the renal threshold, the filtered load, and the reabsorption rate are different
(C) Glucose is actively transported across the basolateral membrane
(D) Renal glucose transport is Na^+-independent
(E) Renal glucose transport is an electroneutral process

48. A normal 60-kg person has an extracellular fluid (ECF) volume of 12.8 L, a blood volume of 4.3 L, and a hematocrit of 40%. His body is 57% water by weight. The plasma volume (Evans blue space) [in L] is approximately

(A) 2.0
(B) 2.3
(C) 2.6
(D) 3.0
(E) 3.3

49. Which of the following is the effective renal blood flow (ml/min) using the following values?

Plasma [PAH]: 0.2 mg/ml
Urine [PAH]: 48 mg/ml
Urine flow rate: 2.0 ml/min
Hematocrit: 40%

(A) 120
(B) 240
(C) 300
(D) 480
(E) 800

50. Which of the following proximal tubular processes is linked to the reabsorption of Na^+?
(A) Active proton reabsorption
(B) Bicarbonate reabsorption
(C) Active reabsorption of chloride
(D) Establishment of a lumen-negative transepithelial potential
(E) The efflux of K^+ through luminal conductive channels

51. A woman runs a marathon in 90°F heat and replaces the 3 L of sweat lost by drinking 3 L of distilled water. Compared to her pre-exercise condition, she has

(A) decreased total body water (TBW)
(B) hypernatremia
(C) decreased hematocrit
(D) decreased plasma osmolality
(E) increased intracellular osmolality

52. Which of the following statements that refers to the glomerulus is correct?

(A) It filters Na^+ mainly by diffusion.
(B) It contains no active transport systems that produce an important effect on the composition of filtrate.
(C) It produces a filtrate with a lower concentration of amino acids than found in plasma.
(D) It produces a filtrate with a higher concentration of urea than found in plasma.
(E) It does not contain fenestrated capillaries.

53. Which of the following increases formation of both antidiuretic hormone (ADH) and angiotensin?

(A) Increased blood urea nitrogen (BUN) concentration
(B) Decreased BUN concentration
(C) Increased effective circulating volume (ECV)
(D) Decreased ECV
(E) Decreased plasma Na^+ concentration

54. In the figure showing five renal transport systems for various ions and a nonelectrolyte (glucose), which of the following transport processes is an example of secondary active transport (cotransport) only in the proximal tubule?

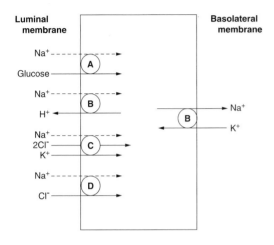

(A) A
(B) B
(C) C
(D) D
(E) E

55. Which of the following causes an increase in both glomerular filtration rate (GFR) and renal plasma flow?

(A) Hyperproteinemia
(B) A ureteral stone
(C) Dilation of the afferent arteriole
(D) Dilation of the efferent arteriole
(E) Constriction of the efferent arteriole

56. Which of the following can increase the percentage of fluid reabsorbed by the proximal tubule?

(A) Aldosterone
(B) Angiotensin II
(C) An increase in peritubular capillary pressure
(D) Antidiuretic hormone (ADH)
(E) A decrease in oncotic pressure in the peritubular capillaries

57. Which of the following would be expected to cause a reduction in glomerular filtration rate (GFR)?

(A) A reduction in mean arterial pressure (MAP) from 100 mm Hg to 95 mm Hg
(B) A marked reduction in plasma protein concentration
(C) A decrease in sympathetic outflow to the afferent arteriole
(D) An increase in glomerular capillary hydrostatic pressure
(E) Complete ureteral obstruction

58. Following the intravenous administration of 1 L of 5% glucose, which of the following will occur?

(A) The extracellular fluid (ECF) volume will increase by about 330 ml.
(B) The intersitial fluid volume will increase by about 80 ml.
(C) The ECF volume will increase by about 670 ml.
(D) The ECF volume will increase by about 1 L.
(E) The intracellular fluid (ICF) volume will remain unchanged.

59. According to the myogenic theory of autoregulation, an elevation in renal perfusion pressure immediately causes

(A) a reduction in extravascular (interstitial) hydrostatic pressure
(B) a reduction in transmural pressure in the afferent arteriole
(C) a reduction in intravascular hydrostatic pressure
(D) an increase in afferent arteriolar radius followed by afferent arteriolar vasoconstriction
(E) a reduction in afferent arteriolar wall tension

60. In a micropuncture study, the tubular fluid-to-plasma ratios (TF/Ps) for substance X and inulin are determined at three locations.

	TF_x/P_x	TF_{in}/P_{in}
Bowman's capsule	1	1
End of proximal tubule	6	3
End of collecting duct	240	120

On the basis of these data, you can conclude that substance X

(A) is reabsorbed in the collecting duct
(B) shows a net secretion in the proximal tubule
(C) shows a net secretion in the loop of Henle
(D) is not secreted nor reabsorbed by the tubule
(E) is reabsorbed at a higher rate than water in the proximal tubule

61. Effective circulating volume (ECV)

(A) is part of the extracellular fluid
(B) is in the venous system
(C) is independent of Na^+ intake
(D) can be measured by the dilution principle
(E) is constant with changes in the extracellular fluid (ECF) volume

62. In the capsular fluid of Bowman's space, the concentration of all but which of the following is equal to its plasma concentration?

(A) Glucose
(B) Sodium
(C) Urea
(D) Protein bound calcium
(E) Potassium

63. The dashed lines in the figures of net transport in the nephron represent the vascular and urinary routes followed by various substances.

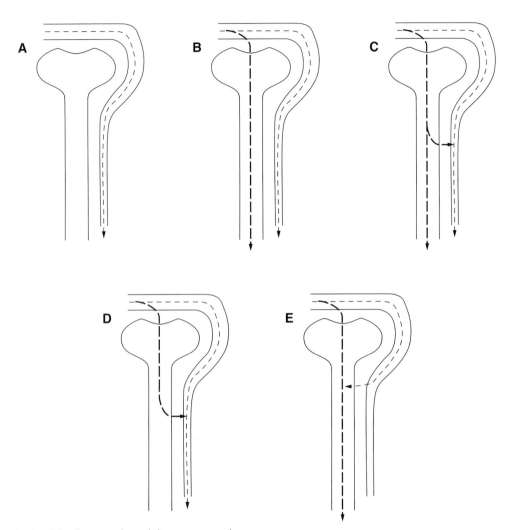

Which of the five renal models represents the clearance of *para*-aminohippuric acid (PAH) at high plasma PAH concentrations?

(A) A
(B) B
(C) C
(D) D
(E) E

64. Approximately one-third of the proximal Na^+ reabsorption occurs through the paracellular pathway. The primary driving force for this passive reabsorption of Na^+ in the late proximal tubule is

(A) a higher luminal than peritubular hydrostatic pressure
(B) a higher luminal than peritubular Na^+ concentration
(C) a lumen-positive transepithelial voltage created by paracellular Cl^- transport
(D) a lower interstitial fluid than luminal oncotic pressure
(E) operation of the Na^+–H^+ countertransporter

65. A reduction in the effective circulating volume (ECV)

(A) leads to increased Na^+ excretion
(B) is observed in congestive heart failure
(C) does not cause edema
(D) leads to increased water excretion
(E) causes reduction in renin secretion

1. The answer is C [Chapter 24 I A 1]. The renal clearance of a substance (C_x) is defined as the ratio of the renal excretion rate of the substance to its concentration in the blood plasma. Thus, the renal clearance is an empiric measure of the volume of plasma that contains the same amount of the substance as is excreted in urine in 1 minute. The clearance equation is:

$$C_x = \frac{U_x \cdot \dot{V}}{P_x}, \text{ where}$$

U_x and P_x are the urinary and plasma concentration of substance $\times$ in mg/ml, respectively; $\dot{V}$ is the urine flow rate in ml/min; and

C_x is the clearance of substance $\times$ in ml/min. Using the data given:

$$C_x = \frac{480 \text{ mg/ml} \cdot 1.5 \text{ ml/min}}{6 \text{ mg/ml}} = 120 \text{ ml/min}$$

Notice that the units of concentration cancel out, leaving the units for clearance as ml/min.

2. The answer is C [Chapter 27 I A 1 a,b]. Renal tubular transport maximum (Tm) is defined as the upper limit for the unidirectional rate of active transport—either reabsorptive or secretory—depending on the direction of solute transport. The units for transport maximum are mg/min. Thus, there is a maximal rate of reabsorption called maximum tubular reabsorptive capacity (Tr) and a maximal rate of secretion called maximum tubular secretory capacity (Ts). Tubular maxima vary with the substance involved. Renal reabsorption of glucose and secretion of para-amino-hippuric acid (PAH) are examples of actively transported solutes exhibiting tubular transport maxima. An example of a substance that is not transport-maximum limited is the reabsorption of Na^+ along the nephron. Tubular maximum is the difference between the filtered load and the rate of excretion of a solute. The glomerular filtration rate (GFR) is defined as the volume of plasma filtered per minute (ml/min), whereas clearance is the virtual volume of plasma from which a substance is removed per minute (ml/min).

3. The answer is E [Chapter 27 III J 4]. The concentration of free H^+ at a urinary pH

above 4.4 is negligible; therefore, acid must be excreted in a buffered form. The two main urinary buffers are dibasic phosphate (HPO_4^{2-}) and ammonia (NH_3). The amounts of secreted H^+ excreted bound to ammonia and phosphate are measured as ammonium (NH_4^+) and titratable acid, respectively. The sum of ammonium and titratable acid minus the amount of excreted bicarbonate (HCO_3^-) equals net acid excretion, which normally is approximately 1 mEq/kg body weight per day. Ammonia (ammonium) production occurs primarily in the proximal tubule, and it represents the major adaptive mechanism available to the kidney for the increased excretion of H^+ during states of acidosis. In contrast, the phosphate buffer enters the tubular lumen by glomerular filtration. The normal kidney excretes titratable acid (20 mEq H^+ per day). Approximately 4300 mEq of H^+ must be excreted per day to accomplish the reabsorption of 4300 mEq of HCO_3^-. In this process, most of the secreted H^+ is reabsorbed in the form of water. Sulfate (SO_4^{2-}) in combination with ammonium forms a neutral salt [$(NH_4)_2 SO_4$], which makes the tubular urine less acidic.

4. The answer is D [Chapter 27 II C; Figure 27-1C]. At low plasma concentrations of para-aminohippuric acid (PAH), PAH is almost completely cleared from the plasma by a combination of glomerular filtration and tubular secretion. When plasma concentrations of PAH are elevated beyond 30 mg/dl, the secretory mechanism becomes saturated, and the tubular transport maximum (Tm) is reached. As the tubular secretory mechanism becomes saturated and is exceeded by progressive increases in plasma PAH concentration, the clearance of PAH declines and becomes more a function of glomerular filtration. Because inulin clearance is essentially equal to the glomerular filtration rate (GFR), the PAH clearance asymptotically approaches the inulin clearance. Thus, the amount of PAH secreted becomes a smaller fraction of the total amount of PAH excreted. The clearance of PAH is always greater than the clearance of inulin, because some PAH is always secreted.

5. The answer is C [Chapter 23 III C; Figure 23-2]. Most of the proximal reabsorption of Na^+ occurs by active transport and is transcellular. The transcellular pathway consists of the apical and basolateral membranes. The Na⁺-K⁺-adenosine triphosphatase pump in all cell membranes is responsible for active Na⁺ transport (efflux) and active K⁺ transport (influx). This enzyme maintains the low intracellular Na⁺ concentration and the high extracellular Na⁺ concentration. Active Na⁺ transport consumes 30% to 50% of the energy derived from metabolism in most cells. Although the influx of Na⁺ from the tubular lumen to the proximal tubular cell is in the direction favored by the electrochemical potential, this transport is mediated by specific membrane carrier proteins and not by simple diffusion. These membrane proteins couple the active movement of other solutes to the passive movement of Na⁺. Examples include Na⁺-glucose, Na⁺-amino acid symporters, and an Na⁺-H⁺ antiporter. In each case, the potential energy released by the downhill transport of Na⁺ is used to power the uphill transport of the other substance. These transport systems are referred to as Na⁺-coupled, secondary active transport processes. It is essential to understand that reabsorption includes not only Na⁺ influx from the tubular lumen but also active transport of Na⁺ out of the cell into the bloodstream.

6. The answer is C [Chapter 27 I A 1 c, B 1 a]. The renal threshold for a substance denotes the plasma concentration at which the solute begins to appear in the urine. It is not the plasma concentration that completely saturates the transport mechanism either for reabsorption or secretion. When the plasma concentration of a solute exceeds the renal threshold, the amount of that solute transported through the nephron exceeds the tubular transport maximum (Tm), and the solute appears in the urine in increasing amounts. The filtered load is the amount of a substance entering the tubule by filtration per unit time.

7. The answer is B [Chapter 22 III B 4 b; Figure 22-2]. Hydration states are named in terms of the extracellular fluid (ECF) compartment. Overhydration, or fluid and salt retention, results from excessive influx of water and NaCl. Dehydration, or fluid and salt depletion, usually involves both ECF and intracellular fluid (ICF). The volume of the ECF compartment is determined by the Na⁺ content of the body, not by the Na⁺ concentration of the plasma. The situation described in the question represents a state of dehydration because of the

contraction of the ECF volume. Because the solute concentration of the ECF is also decreased, there is hyposmotic dehydration (e.g., as occurs with excessive salt loss in primary adrenal insufficiency). A net loss of salt in excess of water loss leads to hyposmolality of the ECF and causes water to shift from the ECF to the ICF. Thus, the volume of the ECF is decreased, the volume of the ICF is increased, and the osmolality of both is decreased.

8. The answer is A [Chapter 24 II A 1 b (2), 2 a (2) (b)]. Renal clearance can be measured for any solute present in the plasma and excreted by the kidney; clearance best represents the rate of elimination of a substance from the plasma by the kidney. If the kidney removes a substance (e.g., inulin) from the plasma by filtration only, the tubular clearance will be zero and the excretion rate will be proportional to the plasma concentration. If the clearance involves filtration and either tubular reabsorption or secretion, then clearance depends on the plasma concentration and the tubular transport capacity for reabsorption or secretion. Thus, clearance is higher for substances that are filtered and secreted than for substances that are filtered and reabsorbed. The lowest clearance is observed with substances that are completely reabsorbed, such as glucose. Approximately 50% of the filtered urea is reabsorbed. Creatinine and para-aminohippuric acid (PAH) are filtered and secreted, which increases their clearance compared with inulin.

9. The answer is B [Chapter 30 III B 5; Figure 30-4]. The only known physiologic effect of renin is to cause the formation of angiotensin I from its plasma substrate, angiotensinogen. Angiotensin I, in turn, appears to serve only a specific substrate for angiotensin converting enzyme (ACE). ACE is a peptidase that converts angiotensin I to angiotensin II, which does have significant biologic activity. Angiotensin II exerts a potent vasoconstrictive action on the vascular smooth muscle of peripheral arterioles, which causes an increase in the mean arterial blood pressure. It also stimulates the release of aldosterone from the zona glomerulosa of the adrenal cortex, causing an increase in the extracellular fluid (ECF) volume through increased active reabsorption of Na⁺ by the collecting ducts. The increased ECF volume accounts for the decreased concentration of K⁺, decreased hematocrit, and decreased plasma colloid oncotic pressure. Aldosterone also acts on the distal tubule and collecting duct to increase the net reabsorption of Na^+ in exchange for the secretion of K^+ and H^+. Thus, aldosterone tends to produce hypokalemia and metabolic alkalosis.

10. The answer is B [Chapter 27 I B 1–2]. The algebraic difference between filtered load and amount excreted determines which of the two processes is used by the kidney to excrete a substance. In the case of glucose, the amount excreted is less than the amount filtered, which is consistent with reabsorption. Using the data given, the transport maximum (Tm) for glucose is found to be 350 mg/min:

Tm = amount filtered–amount excreted

$$= C_{in} \cdot P_G - U_G \cdot \dot{V}$$

$$= (125 \text{ ml/min} \cdot 4 \text{ mg/ml}) - (75 \text{ mg/ml} \cdot 2 \text{ ml/min})$$

$$= 500 \text{ mg/min} - 150 \text{ mg/min}$$

$$= 350 \text{ mg/min, where}$$

C_{in} = inulin clearance

P_G = concentration of glucose in plasma

U_G = concentration of glucose in urine

$\dot{V}$ = volume of urine output per minute

All substances that are reabsorbed or secreted have a transport maximum.

11. The answer is C [Chapter 25 I A 1, II; Figure 25-6] The major determinant of the glomerular filtration rate (GFR) is the hydrostatic pressure within the glomerulus. An increase in glomerular capillary hydrostatic pressure is a major force that drives fluid out of the glomerular capillary and into Bowman's capsule. In glomerular capillaries, the net movement of fluid is primarily out of the capillaries, whereas in systemic capillaries, the change in the balance of Starling forces is such that net movement out of the capillaries is nearly balanced by net return of fluid into the vessels. Increases in the plasma oncotic pressure, hydrostatic pressure in Bowman's space, and afferent arteriolar resistance decrease the GFR, as does a decrease in the effective filtration pressure (EFP).

12. The answer is A [Chapter 22 I A-B; II A 3, B]. The extracellular fluid (ECF) volume constitutes approximately one-third of the total body water (TBW), or approximately 12 to 19 L. This compartment includes two subcompartments separated by the capillary membrane: blood plasma (intravascular fluid) and interstitial fluid. The ECF volume is measured with a test substance that does not penetrate the cells. Therefore, it has become common to measure the volume distribution of a specific substance and refer to it as, for example-the inulin space-if the test substance is inulin. All substances used to measure the ECF volume must cross capillaries and distribute at the same concentration in plasma and interstitial fluid.

13. The answer is D [Chapter 31]. The infusion of 2 L of isotonic NaCl will expand the extracellular fluid (ECF) by 2 L, of which 750 ml will enter the intracellular fluid (ICF). The plasma volume will then expand by 250 ml. This volume increases the stretch on the atrial receptors, leading to the secretion of atrial natriuretic peptide [or factor (ANP, ANF)]. ANP (ANF) will activate those mechanisms to restore the volume to normal through the excretion of NaCl and water.

14. The answer is A [Chapter 31]. In the state of weightlessness mobilization of blood occurs from the extremities to the abdomen and thorax. This redistribution causes a stretch on the atrial receptors and secretion of atrial natriuretic peptide (ANP). All of the other factors listed have the commonality of reduced blood volume and, therefore, are negative signals for ANP secretion.

15. The answer is C [Chapter 28 II A 2 b; Figure 28-1D]. The solute concentration in the ascending limb of the loop of Henle (ALH, site C) is less than that in any segment of the descending limb. The tubular fluid leaves the ascending limb at a lower concentration than it had when it entered the descending limb. Thus, the fluid presented to the distal tubule is always hyposmotic, regardless of the body's state of hydration.

16. The answer is A [Chapter 23 II A 2]. Ultrafiltration separates water and nonprotein constituents (the "crystalloids") of plasma from the blood cells and protein macromolecules (the "colloids"). Except for proteins and lipids, the concentrations of crystalloids (e.g., Na^+, glucose) in the plasma and Bowman's capsule (site A) are nearly the same.

17. The answer is E [Chapter 28 IV]. The wall of the ALH is relatively impermeable to water. Therefore, NaCl in this segment is reabsorbed to the virtual exclusion of water, a process that renders the medullary and papillary interstitium hyperosmotic to plasma. The medullary interstitial osmolality is higher in antidiuresis than diuresis, due to urea and NaCl. Thus, the highest osmolality exists in the papillary interstitium. With continued reabsorption of water, urea becomes even more concentrated at the terminals of the collecting ducts (site E).

18. The answer is E [Chapter 28 IV B]. During dehydration with maximal antidiuretic hormone (ADH) secretion, the urine-to-plasma osmolality ratio (U_{osm}/P_{osm}) approaches 4 to 1 (at site E) because of the increased free-water reabsorption.

19. The answer is C [Chapter 30 III B 1 b]. The macula densa is located at the junction of the thick segment of the ALH and the distal convoluted tubule (site C).

20. The answer is F [Chapter 24 II A 2 b; Figure 24-3]. Under normal conditions, inorganic phosphate (P_i) reabsorption occurs mainly in the proximal tubule. The intraluminal phosphate concentration along the proximal tubule is lower than that in the plasma filtrate, with a mean of approximately 0.7 times the plasma concentration [i.e., a tubular fluid-to-plasma (TF/P) concentration ratio close to 0.7 (curve F)].

21. The answer is H [Figure 24-3]. The rate of urinary glucose excretion always is less than the rate of glucose filtration at the glomerulus. Thus, there is a net reabsorption of glucose that occurs solely in the proximal tubule. The TF/P concentration ratio for glucose falls to a value of 0.1, indicating that 90% of the filtered glucose is reabsorbed in the early portion (first quarter) of the proximal tubule (curve H). The filtered glucose is reabsorbed by an active, carrier-mediated process with transport maximum-limited characteristics.

22. The answer is H [Figure 24-3]. Like glucose, glycine (an amino acid) is transported from the tubular fluid into the proximal tubular cell by specific carrier molecules that also combine with Na^+. Thus, glycine transport is a Na^+-coupled, secondary active transport process. The TF/P concentration ratio for amino acids also falls to a value of 0.1, indicating that approximately 90% of the filtered glycine is reabsorbed in the initial 25% of the proximal tubule (curve H). The active reabsorption of amino acids also involves a transport maximum-limited process.

23. The answer is E [Chapter 25]. At high plasma concentrations of *para*-aminohippuric acid (PAH), the transepithelial secretory mechanism becomes saturated, and the transport maximum for PAH is exceeded. When this occurs, the C_{PAH} becomes progressively reduced and the C_{PAH} asymptotically approaches the C_{in}. Therefore, the lowest C_{PAH} is associated with point E.

24. The answer is E [Chapter 25]. With high plasma concentrations of *para*-aminohippuric acid (PAH), C_{PAH} declines continuously. As the C_{PAH} falls, the amount of secreted PAH becomes a smaller fraction of the filtered load of PAH and greater amounts of PAH remain in the plasma, beginning with the renal venous system.

25. The answer is E [Chapter 25]. With this secretion curve for *para*-aminohippuric acid (PAH), it is necessary to visualize the curves for the filtered load and excretion rate. It is important to appreciate that with the secretory process, the excretion rate curve is higher than the filtered load curve. Both of these curves increase linearly as a function of PAH concentration. Therefore, point E is associated with the highest point on the PAH excretion curve.

26. The answer is E [Chapter 25]. As the plasma concentration of *para*-aminohippuric acid (PAH) increases, the amount of filtered PAH increases. The concentration of PAH in Bowman's space approximates the plasma concentration of PAH, so point E is associated with the highest concentrations of PAH in the plasma and Bowman's capsule.

27. The answer is D [Chapter 25]. When the renal threshold for glucose is exceeded, the clearance of glucose is no longer zero (i.e., glucose begins to appear in the urine). Now the amount filtered is higher than the amount reabsorbed; some excretion occurs. Furthermore, as the plasma glucose concentration rises, the excretion rate of glucose also increases. However, the renal venous glucose concentration of glucose is never equal to the renal arterial glucose concentration, because the kidney continues to reabsorb glucose at all plasma glucose concentrations. This reabsorption reduces the renal venous concentration of glucose.

28. The answer is A [Chapter 25]. Glucose reabsorption in the proximal nephron is a Na^+-dependent process as it is in all epithelial cell transport. Thus, this transport system is called the Na^+-glucose symporter (cotransporter), which is a secondary active transport system meaning that the immediate source of energy for transport is the Na^+ concentration gradient. Of course, the low intracellular Na^+ concentration depends on the basolateral Na^+–K^+–ATPase primary active transport system. Thus, the downhill influx of Na^+ drives the uphill transport of glucose. This transport process is electrogenic, because transport of a cation (Na^+) with a neutral substance (glucose) occurs.

29. The answer is C [Chapter 25]. The Fick principle basically states that the rate of uptake of a substance by an organ is equal to the rate at which the substance is removed from the bloodstream. Under these conditions, the rate at which the substance is removed from the bloodstream is equal to the blood flow (rate) times the difference between the concentration of the blood entering the organ (arterial) and the concentration of the blood leaving the organ (venous), or blood flow ($C_a - C_v$), where BF is blood flow and C_a and C_v are the arterial and venous plasma concentrations, respectively.

$$U_x \cdot \dot{V} = BF\,(C_a - C_v)$$

$$80 \cdot 1.5 = BF\,(0.2 - 0.05)$$

$$= 800 \text{ ml/min}$$

30. The answer is C [Chapter 21]. The infusion of 3 L of plasma has raised the cardiac output and increased the blood pressure, leading to a reduction in sympathetic stimulation evoked through the baroreceptor reflex. The hemorrhage caused a loss of effective circulat-

ing volume (ECV) and therefore a drop in cardiac output. The fall in sympathetic outflow reduced the heart rate and total peripheral resistance (TPV). The reduced firing frequency of impulses to the cardiovascular centers in the brain stem led to an increase in sympathetic tone, and this higher sympathetic discharge caused an increase in peripheral vascular tone, heart rate, and myocardial contractility. There is no change in plasma oncotic pressure following the infusion of plasma.

31. The answer is C [Chapter 26]. The glomerular filtration rate (GFR) and renal plasma flow (renal blood flow) change in parallel with changes in afferent arteriolar resistance; therefore, the filtration fraction (FF) remains constant. With increased afferent arteriolar resistance, there is a reduction in glomerular capillary hydrostatic pressure, and, in turn, a reduction in GFR.

32. The answer is A [Chapter 26]. With changes in efferent arteriolar resistance, the glomerular filtration rate (GFR) and renal plasma flow (renal blood flow) change in opposite directions and, therefore, the filtration fraction (FF) changes. Therefore, with increased efferent arteriolar resistance, there is an increase in glomerular capillary pressure and, in turn, an increase in GFR. An increase in efferent arteriolar resistance leads to a decline in renal plasma flow (renal blood flow). Because of these changes in GFR and renal plasma flow (renal blood flow), an increase in the FF now occurs.

33. The answer is B [Chapter 23]. It is necessary to determine the clearance of a reference substance such as inulin, which is filtered but not reabsorbed or secreted. Then the clearance of inulin can be compared to the clearance of another substance to identify the net renal process for transport.

$$C_{in} = \frac{150 \cdot 1}{1} = 150 \text{ ml/min}$$

$$C_x = \frac{100 \cdot 1}{2} = 50 \text{ ml/min}$$

Because the clearance of substance X is less than the clearance of inulin, substance X must be freely filtered and is also reabsorbed (on a net basis).

34. The answer is D [Chapter 27]. There is no proximal luminal transporter for HCO_3^-. Instead, the Na^+–H^+ countertransporter secretes H^+ into the lumen, and it combines with HCO_3^- in the filtrate and forms carbonic acid (H_2CO_3). This volatile acid dehydrates by the catalytic action of luminal (brush border) carbonic anhydrase to form CO_2 and H_2O. These two substances diffuse into the proximal cell, where the intracellular carbonic anhydrase hydrates the CO_2 to reform carbonic acid which dissociates into H^+ and HCO_3^-. The HCO_3^- is transported across the basolateral membrane by the 3 HCO_3^-–1 Na^+ cotransporter. Normally, there is complete reabsorption of filtered HCO_3^- by the nephron in which there is no net gain or loss of HCO_3^-.

35. The answer is C [Chapter 22]. Osmolal concentration includes the concentration of all solutes, whether or not they are effective osmoles. Osmolal concentration should not be confused with osmotic pressure, which is a function of osmotically effective solutes. It is necessary to convert millimolar into milliosmolar (L) concentrations according to the relationship:

$$mOsm/L \text{ or } mOsm/Kg\ H_2O = mmol/L \times n$$

where n equals the number of particles formed in solution. The hypertonic solution in answer C is equivalent to:

$$mOsm/L = 300\ mmol/L \times 2$$

$$= 600\ mOsm/L\ solution$$

$$= 600\ mOsm/Kg\ H_2O$$

36. The answer is C [Chapter 26]. The major site of autoregulatory resistance is at the level of afferent arteriole. For this reason, the glomerular filtration rate (GFR) and renal plasma flow (renal blood flow) change in parallel; between 90 and 180 mm Hg of renal arterial pressure, no change in GFR and renal plasma flow (renal blood flow) occurs.

37. The answer is B [Chapter 22]. The infusion of an isotonic NaCl solution expands the extracellular fluid (ECF) only by 500 ml. Again, concentration should always be converted into mOsm/kg H_2O, which in this case is 300 mOsm/kg H_2O. This infusion leads to isosmotic overhydration.

38. The answer is C [Chapter 22]. Conversion of 300 millimolar to the equivalent value in milliosmolars yields 600 mOsm/kg H_2O.

$$300\ mmol/L \times n = 300\ mmol/L \times 2$$

$$= 600\ mOsm/Kg\ H_2O$$

This is a hypertonic (hyperosmotic) solution, which raises the extracellular fluid (ECF) volume and osmolar concentration, creating an osmotic gradient for water to leave the intracellular fluid (ICF) and enter the ECF. This results in the reduction in ICF volume, which increases the osmolar concentration of the ICF. At osmotic equilibrium, this condition is hyperosmotic overhydration.

39. The answer is A [Chapter 22]. Drinking 1 L of tap water increases the intracellular fluid (ICF) volume by 667 ml and the extracellular fluid (ECF) volume by 333 ml. However, the osmolar concentrations are both reduced; the final state is hyposmotic overhydration.

40. The answer is A [Chapter 22]. With chronic elevation of antidiuretic hormone (ADH), syndrome of inappropriate antidiuretic hormone secretion (SIADH) occurs. This condition is equivalent to water retention (increased free-water reabsorption), which expands and dilutes both major fluid compartments, leading to hyposmotic overhydration.

41. The answer is E [Chapter 23]. Osmotic pressure is proportional to the number of particles per volume of solvent, not the type, valence, or weight of the particle. However, the solute must be unable to cross the cell membrane (i.e., have a high reflection coefficient). Thus, Na^+ is an effective osmole between the interstitial fluid (ISF) and the intracellular fluid (ICF), and urea is an ineffective osmole because it is a permeant solute with a low reflection coefficient. In summary, the osmotic pressure gradient is proportional to the concentration gradient of the impermeant solutes.

Water moves from a region of lower solute concentration to a region of higher solute concentration, or from a region of higher water concentration to a region of lower water concentration. Although the cell membrane is actually permeable to Na^+ and K^+, these ions act as effective osmoles because they are restricted to their respective compartments by the Na^+–K^+–ATPase pump in the cell membrane.

42. The answer is A [Chapter 24]. The lowest concentration of inulin in the tubular fluid is in Bowman's space. Therefore, this is the site for the lowest tubular fluid-to-plasma (TF/P) concentration ratio for inulin.

43. The answer is D [Chapter 24]. Because all the filtered inulin is excreted, the highest concentration of inulin is in the collecting duct. The TF/P concentration ratio for inulin may be as high as 100, because water is continuously reabsorbed along the nephron except in the thin and thick segments of the ascending limb of the loop of Henle. The concentration of inulin in the tubular fluid is an excellent index of water reabsorption.

Regardless of the state of hydration, the tubular fluid leaving the thick segment of the ascending limb of the loop of Henle is always hyposmotic ($\approx$ 100 mOsm/kg H_2O). Therefore, the tubular fluid-to-plasma (TF/P) osmolality ratio is lowest at this site than anywhere else along the nephron.

44. The answer is E [Chapter 24]. *Para*-amino-hippuric acid (PAH) is both filtered and secreted by the proximal tubule; it is not reabsorbed. Therefore, all the PAH that is filtered and secreted into the tubules remains there and becomes increasingly more concentrated by the reabsorption of water along the nephron.

45. The answer is A [Chapter 24]. The highest glucose concentration exists in Bowman's space, because glucose at plasma concentrations (< 180 mg/ml) is completely reabsorbed by the proximal tubule. Therefore, the highest tubular fluid-to-plasma concentration ratio (TF/P) equals 1.

46. The answer is C [Chapter 26]. It is necessary to subtract the inward forces (plasma oncotic pressure plus the hydrostatic pressure in Bowman's space) from the outward forces (afferent arteriolar capillary hydrostatic pressure plus the oncotic pressure in Bowman's capsule). Outward forces: 60 + 0 = 60 mm Hg. Inward forces: 21 + 14 = 35 mm Hg. Outward forces minus inwards forces: 60 − 35 = 25 mm Hg.

47. The answer is A [Chapter 27]. Glucose reabsorption takes place by secondary active transport (synport) linked to Na^+ influx at the proximal luminal membrane. All of the glucose in the filtered load is reabsorbed when the carriers are not saturated (i.e., the filtered load equals the amount reabsorbed). The plasma concentration at which glucose begins to saturate some carriers and appear in the urine is the renal threshold. The renal threshold does not correspond to the transport maximum (Tm) Because glucose is transported with Na^+, this transport process is electrogenic. The Na^+–K^+–ATPase pump maintains the Na^+ gradient across the luminal membrane; it is the Na^+ gradient that drives the luminal transport of glucose, but the Na^+-pump uses ATP to extrude Na^+ from the cell. Glucose leaves the proximal cell by facilitated diffusion.

48. The answer is C [Chapter 22]. The relationship between blood volume (BV) and plasma volume (PV) is:

$$BV = \frac{PV}{1} - \text{hematocrit}$$

$$PV = BV\,(1 - \text{hematocrit})$$

$$= 4.3 \times 0.6 = 2.58 \text{ L}$$

The other answer choices are distractors.

49. The answer is E [Chapter 26]. Renal blood flow is determined by first determining the renal plasma flow by calculating the clearance of *para*-aminohippuric acid (PAH):

$$C_{PAH} = \frac{U_{PAH} \cdot \dot{V}}{P_{PAH}}$$

$$= \frac{48 \cdot 2.0}{0.2} = \frac{96}{0.2}$$

$$RBF = \frac{RPF}{1 - Hct} = \frac{480}{0.6} = 800 \text{ ml/min}$$

50. The answer is B [Chapter 27]. The reabsorption of Na^+ down its electrochemical gradient energizes the proximal secretion of H^+ (i.e., the Na^+–H^+ antiporter). The secreted H^+ combines with HCO_3^- to form carbonic acid by association and CO_2 and H_2O by the enzymatic action of carbonic anhydrase. The absorbed (reabsorbed) CO_2 combines with H_2O

intracellularly, forming H^+ and HCO_3^-. The H^+ is secreted, and the HCO_3^- enters the interstitium via the 3 HCO_3^-–Na^+ cotransporter. The protons are reabsorbed in the form of H_2O. The paracellular transport of Na^+ is not linked to the Na^+–H^+ antiporter and represents Na^+ diffusion in response to the positive transepithelial voltage gradient created by the paracellular transport of Cl^- along a concentration gradient. K^+ efflux through conductive channels occurs in the thick ascending limb of the loop of Henle (ALH) and in the collecting ducts.

51. The answer is D. [Ch 22 Case Figure 1 a, 1b] The marathon runner loses 3 L of a hypotonic solution (sweat), which consists of water and electrolytes, leading to hyperosmotic dehydration. The distribution of the additional 3 L of water is intracellular fluid (ICF) [2 L] and extracellular fluid (ECF) [1 L] into the ECF. This dilutes both the ICF and ECF. There is no decrease in total body water (TBW), but there is a decrease in total electrolyte content, as well as an increase in hematocrit because the plasma volume remains reduced after the addition of 3 L of water.

52. The answer is B [Chapter 26]. Transport of fluid and small solutes across the fenestrated glomerular capillary membrane occurs by bulk flow inasmuch, because there are no concentration gradients for filterable solutes and no carrier-mediated transport systems in the glomerulus.

53. The answer is D [Chapter 21]. A fall in the effective circulating volume evokes secretion of antidiuretic hormone (ADH) and formation of angiotensin II. Urea is an ineffective osmole because it has a low reflection coefficient. Permeant solutes do not contribute to osmotic pressure and do not stimulate ADH secretion. Increased effective circulating volume (ECV) does not stimulate secretion of aldosterone or ADH; however, volume depletion causes the secretion of both of these hormones. Formation of angiotensin II in hypovolemic states enhances aldosterone secretion. In normal individuals, both the plasma renin activity and aldosterone vary inversely with dietary Na^+ intake. Decreased plasma Na^+ concentration (hyponatremia) increases renin secretion and, therefore, angiotensin II formation, but inhibits ADH secretion.

54. The answer is A [Chapter 23]. Of the luminal transport systems shown, only the Na^+–glucose symporter exists solely in the proximal tubule. The Na^+–H^+ antiporter is found in the proximal tubule and the thick ascending limb of the loop of Henle, the Na^+–Cl^-–K^+ symporter is located in the thick segment of the ascending limb of the loop of Henle, and the Na^+–Cl^- symporter is found in the distal tubule. The basolateral Na^+–K^+–ATPase pump exists in all tubular segments.

55. The answer is C [Chapter 26]. Hyperproteinemia causes in an increase in plasma oncotic pressure and a resultant decline in glomerular filtration rate (GFR). A ureteral stone would cause a severe reduction in GFR. The dilation of the afferent arteriole would increase glomerular capillary hydrostatic pressure and, therefore, the GFR as well as increase the renal plasma flow (renal blood flow). Dilation of the efferent arteriole would lead to a fall in glomerular capillary pressure and a resultant decline in GFR. The efferent arteriolar dilation would increase renal plasma flow (renal blood flow). Constriction of the efferent arteriole would lead to an increase in glomerular capillary pressure, an increase in GFR, and a decline in renal plasma flow (renal blood flow).

56. The answer is B [Chapter 27]. Aldosterone promotes distal nephron (connecting tubule and cortical connecting tubule) Na^+ reabsorption, whereas angiotensin II promotes proximal Na^+ reabsorption by activation of the Na^+–H^+ antiporter. It must be understood that Na^+ reabsorption also promotes water reabsorption via the osmotic gradient created by Na^+ reabsorption. Forces that reduce fluid reabsorption are increased capillary (peritubular) hydrostatic pressure and a reduction in capillary (peritubular) oncotic pressure. Antidiuretic hormone (ADH) promotes water (solute-free) reabsorption in the medullary collecting duct.

57. The answer is E [Chapter 21]. A blockade downstream in the nephron exerts an increase in hydrostatic pressure proximal to the small decrease in blood pressure has minimal effects on glomerular capillary hydrostatic pressure and filtration, primarily because of renal autoregulation. In contrast, a large drop in blood pressure produces a drop in glomerular capillary pressure and filtration. The reduced renal perfusion pressure together with an increase in sympathetic neural activity results in vasoconstriction of both afferent and efferent arterioles. This decrease leads to a greater decline in renal blood flow (renal plasma flow) than glomerular filtration rate (GFR) and an increase in filtration fraction (GFR/renal plasma flow). A decrease in plasma oncotic pressure reduces a force opposing filtration. A decrease in sympathetic neural outflow dilates the afferent arteriole, leading to a rise in glomerular capillary pressure and filtration.

58. The answer is A [Chapter 22]. The isosmotic glucose (5% glucose) is distributed 667 ml to the intracellular fluid (ICF) and 333 ml to the extracellular fluid (ECF), with 250 ml entering the interstitial fluid (ISF) and 80 ml remaining in the plasma. However, because glucose is a permeant solute in a metabolic sense, the glucose is metabolized to CO_2 and H_2O, leading to the subsequent fall in the osmolarity of both the ICF and ECF. Thus, isosmotic glucose administration is an excellent way to expand the ICF (with water) **without** administering water, which would cause hemolysis. Furthermore, glucose provides calories; 1 L of 5% dextrose adds 250 kcal (5 kcal/g of dextrose). Therefore, in a strict sense, isosmotic glucose is a hypotonic solution because glucose is a permeant solute that is metabolized.

59. The answer is D [Chapter 26]. The law of Laplace states that the force on a blood vessel wall, called tension, is directly proportional to the pressure across the vessel wall (transmural pressure) and to the radius of curvature of the vessel wall. Because in a cylinder one radius of curvature is infinite (or zero), the law can be stated as: $T = \Delta Pr$, where ΔP is the inside minus the outside pressure. Because the notion of autoregulation requires that the tension T remain constant, the change in pressure and radius of the vessel are inversely related.

It should be noted that changes in pressure difference are due to the intravascular pressure, because the extravascular pressure [interstitial fluid (ISF) pressure] is constant. Thus, when the transmural pressure is increased, the vessel vasoconstricts to maintain the constant tension in the vessel wall, and ultimately, constant pressure and flow in the blood vessel (afferent arteriole).

60. The answer is B [Chapter 24]. The tubular fluid-to-plasma (TF/P) concentration ratio for substance X is greater than 1 at the end of the proximal tubule. Two explanations are possible: (1) solute reabsorption has occurred but was less than was the reabsorption of water, or (2) net secretion of the solute has taken place in the proximal tubule (choice B).

61. The answer is A [Chapter 26]. The effective circulating volume (ECV) is a component of the extracellular fluid (ECF) volume, specifically the volume of the ECF in the arterial system. Therefore, the ECV varies directly with the ECF volume. It can also be defined as the pressure perfusing the arterial baroreceptors. The Na^+ content is the major determinant of ECV, because the Na^+ salts act to hold water within the extracellular space. The ECV cannot be measured by the dilution principle and can only be estimated as about 1.7% of total body water.

62. The answer is D [Chapter 27]. The concentration of all solutes **other than macromolecules (plasma protein) and protein-bound solutes (e.g., Ca^{2+}, HPO_4^{2-})** is the same in both the plasma and the filtrate in Bowman's space.

63. The answer is C [Chapter 24]. At high plasma concentrations (> 20 mg/dl), *para*-aminohippuric acid (PAH) is filtered and partially secreted, because at such concentrations, it has saturated the proximal carrier proteins. A higher percentage of the filtered PAH remains in the systemic circulation.

64. The answer is C [Chapter 27]. The positive transepithelial voltage gradient created by the paracellular transport of Cl^- in the late proximal tubule causes the electrodiffusion (electrorepulsion) of Na^+ out of the tubular fluid through the intercellular (paracellular) pathway.

65. The answer is B [Chapter 26]. In some pathologic states (e.g., congestive heart failure), the effective circulating volume (ECV) may be independent of the extracellular fluid (ECF) volume, the plasma volume, or even cardiac output. In congestive heart failure, there is a decrease in ECV because a primary decrease in cardiac output lowers the pressure at the level of the baroreceptors. This decline in pressure and flow, in turn, induces compensatory fluid (and Na^+) retention by the kidney, leading to expansion of the ECF volume. The net result is ECV depletion with increases in both the plasma and total ECF volumes. In one sense, this increase in volume in congestive heart failure can improve cardiac contractility and raise the cardiac output and systemic blood pressure. However, the elevation in intravascular pressure in congestive heart failure can be maladaptive, because it promotes fluid movement out of the vascular space, potentially leading to edema. It is imperative to appreciate that a decline in ECV leads to a paradoxical Na^+ retention because it is the effective arterial blood volume that is "underfilled."

PART VI

ACID–BASE PHYSIOLOGY

John Bullock

Chapter 32

Acid Production and Elimination: An Overview

I. **INTRODUCTION.** Although the body produces large amounts of acid in two forms [i.e., carbonic (volatile) and noncarbonic (nonvolatile, or fixed) acids], body fluids are maintained in an alkaline state (pH = 7.4). Most of the hydrogen ion (H^+) is formed as an end product of metabolism. The pathways for acid removal include the kidneys, lungs, and gastrointestinal (GI) tract.

A. **Sources of H^+.** The greatest source of H^+ is the **carbon dioxide (CO_2)** produced as one of the end products of the oxidation of glucose and triglyceride during **oxidative metabolism.** Unfortunately, the proton donor–acceptor terminology of Brønsted does not allow for the classification of CO_2 as an acid, but CO_2 functions as the single most important weak acid in the body fluids. Thus, CO_2 is an acid (H^+) generator.

1. Anaerobic metabolism of carbohydrates yields nonvolatile acids.

2. Aerobic metabolism of fats and proteins also yields nonvolatile acids, such as β-hydroxy-butyric acid (a ketoacid), sulfuric acid, and phosphoric acid.

3. Intracellular aerobic metabolism of carbohydrates, fats, and proteins yield CO_2, which is the anhydride of carbonic acid, a volatile acid.

B. **Three processes** are available **for maintaining the hydrogen ion concentration within normal limits:**

1. Combination of H^+ with a blood buffer (e.g., HCO_3^- or hemoglobin) or an intracellular buffer (e.g., organic or inorganic phosphate)

2. Reduction of carbonic acid (H_2CO_3) by elimination of CO_2 via pulmonary ventilation (see III)

3. Reduction of noncarbonic acid by renal elimination of H^+

II. **ACID INTAKE AND URINARY ACID.** In addition to reclaiming (reabsorbing) virtually all of the filtered HCO_3^+, the kidney must excrete an amount of acid equal to that generated by endogenous acid production, which varies with the dietary intake of exogenous acid-generating foods.

A. **Western diets,** which are high in protein, generate between 40 and 80 milliequivalents (mEq) of H^+ per day in the form of nonvolatile (noncarbonic, or fixed) acid. The renal tubules cannot generate a hydrogen ion concentration gradient between tubular urine and blood of more than 3 pH units (i.e., a pH lower than 4.4, which is equivalent to a urine-to-blood [H^+] gradient of 1000:1). The concentration of free H^+ at a urinary pH above 4.4 is negligible; thus, the acid must be excreted in buffered (combined) form.

1. There is no term for free H^+ in the urine, even at a minimal pH of 4.4, because the free H^+ concentration is trivial.

2. At a pH of 4.4, each liter of urine has $10^{-4.4}$ mol/L of free H^+ (0.04 mmol/L).
   a. More than 99% of renal acid excretion occurs in the form of H^+ bound to buffers.
   b. Renal H^+ excretion is assessed by measuring urinary titratable acidity and ammonium.

3. Considering a net acid production of approximately 80 mEq/day, if net acid excretion in a patient with a urine pH of 4.4 occurred exclusively as free urinary H^+ because of the absence of urinary buffers, a daily urine output of more than 1800 L would be required to maintain acid-base balance.

B. The **two main urinary buffers** are HPO_4^{2-} (dibasic phosphate) and NH_3 (ammonia).

1. The amounts of secreted H^+ excreted bound to NH_3 and HPO_4^{2-} are measured as NH_4^+ (ammonium) and titratable acid ($H_2PO_4^-$), respectively.

2. The sum of NH_4^+ excretion ($U_{NH4}^+ \times \dot{V}$)* and titratable acidity ($U_{H_2PO_4}^- \times \dot{V}$) minus the amount of HCO_3^- ($U_{HCO3}^- \times \dot{V}$) equals net acid secretion, which normally is approximately 1 mEq per kilogram body weight per 24 hours (U = urine concentration; $\dot{V}$ = rate of urine formation).

C. The great bulk of **HCO_3^- reabsorption** occurs in the proximal tubule and is Na^+-dependent, whereas the **excretion** of acid (i.e., the regeneration of HCO_3^-) is to a large extent a distal nephron event and mainly Na^+-independent.

III. CARBONIC ACID (H_2CO_3).

Because CO_2 can be formed from H_2CO_3 and, in turn, CO_2 can be eliminated by the lungs, H_2CO_3 is called a **volatile acid.**

A. **The oxidation of most carbohydrates and triglycerides does not generate acid.** The CO_2 combines with H_2O to form H_2CO_3, and thereby prevents acidemia by eliminating CO_2 by pulmonary ventilation.

B. **Conditions where the oxidation of glucose and fat do lead to acid formation** include:

1. Lactic acid formation from the oxidation of carbohydrates during hypoxic states

2. Ketoacid generation from the oxidation of fats in uncontrolled diabetes mellitus

C. **Hydration-dehydration: dissociation-association reaction.** For every H_2CO_3 molecule that has its H^+ taken up by a buffer, one HCO_3^- appears in the blood. These HCO_3^- ions are distributed between the erythrocytes and plasma. Excess fluid intake (hydration) reduces the $[HCO_3^-]$, which causes a corresponding increase in $[H^+]$ if the CO_2 tension(P_{CO_2})is constant. This noncarbonic acidosis is corrected more rapidly by the renal excretion of excess water than by the renal secretion of the apparent excess of H^+. Dehydration has the opposite effect.

1. $$CO_2 + H_2O \underset{\text{dehydration}}{\overset{\text{hydration}}{\rightleftharpoons}} H_2CO_3 \underset{\text{association}}{\overset{\text{dissociation}}{\rightleftharpoons}} H^+ + HCO_3^-$$

2. $H^+ + HCO_3^- + Na^+$ buffer $\rightleftharpoons H \cdot$ buffer $+ Na^+ + HCO_3^-$

D. **CO_2 production.** CO_2 is the **chief product of metabolism** and represents the greatest portion of acid continuously eliminated from the body by the lungs.

1. Most CO_2 in the body is produced from the decarboxylation reactions of the tricarboxylic (citric) acid cycle.

---

*Ammonium secretion per se does not generate HCO_3^-, but it preserves cations and prevents urea (and H^+) from forming in the liver from the ammonium.

2. HCO_3^- is an excellent buffer for noncarbonic acid added to the blood by diet, metabolism, and disease. However, the HCO_3^- buffer system plays no role in the buffering of carbonic acid.

3. More CO_2 than HCO_3^- is produced metabolically in the body. However, the extracellular fluid (ECF) contains a preponderance of the HCO_3^- form.

4. Under basal conditions, with a respiratory exchange ratio of 0.82, the average adult produces approximately 300 L (13.5 mol) of CO_2 per day (Table 32-1).

5. The lungs and kidneys are the principal routes for eliminating protons and maintaining normal $[HCO_3^-]/S \times Pco_2$ ratios.

    a. During one day, the equivalent of 20 to 40 L of 1 N acid (20,000–40,000 mEq H^+) are eliminated via the lungs, or, more correctly, the amount of CO_2 produced in a day in a normal individual is potentially capable of forming 20 to 40 equivalents of H^+.

    b. During a 24-hour period, the equivalent of 50 to 150 ml of 1 N acid (50–150 mEq H^+) is excreted via the kidneys.

6. CO_2 must also be removed from the blood by the lungs at a rate of 200 ml/min during resting conditions. With a resting cardiac output of 5 L/min, 40 ml of CO_2 must be added to each liter of blood per minute (i.e., 5 L/min $\times$ 40 ml/L = 200 ml/min).

7. Metabolic production does not constitute a net gain of H^+, because all H^+ ions generated via these reactions as blood passes through the tissues are re-incorporated into water.

E. **Buffering of H_2CO_3** is primarily by the intracellular **nonbicarbonate buffers** (i.e., proteins, organic and inorganic phosphate, hemoglobin). Buffering occurs mostly in the erythrocytes, where the hemoglobin buffer system is quantitatively the most important intracellular buffer.

IV. **NONCARBONIC ACIDS cannot be converted to CO_2** and, therefore, are called nonvolatile (or fixed) acids. Because noncarbonic acids do not form a volatile end product, they must be buffered until they are excreted by the kidneys. Noncarbonic acids are derived from three sources: diet, intermediary metabolism, and stool HCO_3^- loss (Table 32-2).

A. **Diet.** A high-protein diet accounts for the formation of more acids than bases.

    1. Foodstuffs such as glucose and triglyceride are not acids in body fluids but are converted to CO_2 during their metabolism. Much of this CO_2 is hydrated to form H_2CO_3, which then dissociates into H^+ and HCO_3^-.

    2. A vegetarian diet produces an excess of alkali, which must be excreted by the kidneys as HCO_3^-.

B. **Intermediary metabolism.** The primary source of noncarbonic acid in humans is the metabolism of exogenous protein. The body produces H^+ daily from the catabolism of proteins such as phosphoproteins and methionine, which are metabolically equivalent to phosphoric and sulfuric acids, respectively (Table 32-3).

TABLE 32-1. CO_2 Production under Basal Conditions*

Time Elapsed	Volume (L)	Molarity	
		(mmol)	(mol)
1 minute	0.2	9	9×10^{-3}
1 hour	12.0	540	0.54
1 day	300	13,500	13.5

*Data for a respiratory exchange ratio of 1.0.

TABLE 32-2. Sources of Noncarbonic (Nonvolatile) Acids in Humans

Source	Amount (mEq/day)	Noncarbonic Acid
Diet	30	Phosphoproteins, sulfur-containing amino acids, chloride salts
Intermediary metabolism	30	Ketoacids, lactic acid
Stool loss	30	Loss of HCO_3^-

1. Most **neutral amino acids** are metabolized in the liver by their conversion into glucose or triglycerides and energy [adenosine triphosphate]. There is no net generation of acid in this setting as:

$$\text{amino acid}^\circ \rightarrow \text{glucose}^\circ \text{ (or triglyceride}^\circ\text{)} + \text{urea}^\circ$$

2. **Sulfuric acid** is produced from the catabolism of sulfur-containing neutral amino acids (i.e., methionine, cysteine, cystine). These amino acids are converted into a proton (H^+) and an SO_4^{2-} anion as:

$$\text{Methionine}^\circ \text{ (or cysteine}^\circ\text{)} \rightarrow \text{glucose}^\circ \text{ (or triglyceride}^\circ\text{)} + \text{urea}^\circ + 2\,H^+ + SO_4^{2-}$$

Sulfuric acid is initially buffered in the ECF by HCO_3^- as:

$$H_2SO_4 + 2\,NaHCO_3 \rightarrow Na_2SO_4 + 2H_2CO_3 \rightarrow 2H_2O + CO_2$$

The excess H^+ must still be excreted by the kidneys to prevent progressive depletion of HCO_3^- and other buffers as well as development of metabolic acidosis.

3. **Hydrochloric acid** is formed from the catabolism of a cationic amino acid (i.e., arginine,

TABLE 32-3. Metabolic Production of Noncarbonic Acids and Alkali from the Diet

Dietary Source	Production of		Quantity Produced (mEq/day)	
	Acid	Alkali	Acid	Alkali
Carbohydrate	0	0	0	0
Fat	0	0	0	0
Amino acids				
Sulfur-containing*	H_2SO_4		70	
Cationic†	HCl		135	
Anionic‡		HCO_3^-		100
Organic anions§		HCO_3^-		60
Phosphate	$H_2PO_4^-$		30	
Net acid production			75††	

*Cysteine and methionine (neutral amino acids)
†Lysine, arginine, and histidine
‡Aspartate and glutamate
**Acetate, citrate, gluconate, lactate, and malate
§Nonvolatile acid production from 100 g protein per day is approximately 100 mmol (or mEq) per day plus 30 mmol per day of H^+ from phosphate. Because metabolism of organic anions yields 60 mmol of HCO_3^- per day, the net acid production is about 70 mmol (or mEq) per day, or about 1 mmol H^+ per day per kilogram of body weight.

lysine, some histidine residues) through the conversion into a proton (H^+) and a chlorine (Cl^-) anion as:

a. Arginine$^+$ · Cl^- → glucose° (or triglyceride°) + urea° + H^+ + Cl^-

b. Lysine$^+$ · Cl^- → CO_2° (or triglyceride°) + urea° + H^+ + Cl^-

4. Phosphoric acid is formed when the phosphoproteins (phosphoesters) are hydrolyzed as:

$$R \cdot H_2PO_4 + H_2O \rightarrow ROH + 0.8\ HPO_4^{2-}/0.2\ H_2PO_4^- + 1.8\ H^+$$

Phosphoric acid cannot be further metabolized to CO_2 and H_2O. Thus, the elimination of this acid and the H^+ that it yields can only be accomplished by the kidneys.

5. The metabolism of foodstuffs is a significant source of noncarbonic acids:

  a. Lactate is produced from the anaerobic metabolism of glucose or glycogen.

   (1) Excessive production of lactic acid during heavy exercise or hypoxia can transiently increase noncarbonic acid production. This excess must be buffered until it is excreted or metabolized to CO_2 and H_2O.

   (2) Although most organs generate lactic acid, the skeletal muscle, erythrocytes, and skin produce the largest amount. (Liver, kidney, and muscle can convert lactic acid to HCO_3^-.)

   (3) Tissue hypoxia leads to **hyperlacticemia,** which reduces the plasma [HCO_3^-] and increases the anion gap. The increment in the anion gap is a measure of serum lactate. Clinical conditions associated with tissue hypoxia include cardiac arrest, shock, severe cardiac failure, and severe hypoxemia.

   (4) Alkalosis stimulates glycolysis and generates lactic acid, which occurs mainly through activation of phosphofructokinase. Respiratory alkalosis is a more effective stimulus for glycolysis, because CO_2 more readily crosses cellular membranes.

  b. Acetoacetic acid and β-hydroxybutyric acid are products of triglyceride metabolism.

   (1) These **ketone bodies** are noncarbonic acids produced by normal subjects during fasting. Upon eating, acetoacetic and β-hydroxybutyric acids are further catabolized to CO_2 and H_2O.

    (a) Excess ketone bodies associated with insulin-dependent diabetes mellitus are excreted by the kidneys, accounting for ketonuria.

    (b) Clinically more important is the acidosis of uncontrolled diabetic ketoacidosis, when accumulated acetoacetic acid and β-hydroxybutyric acids in the ECF produce coma and death.

   (2) The conversion of acetoacetic acid to β-hydroxybutyric acid is catalyzed by β-hydroxybutyric dehydrogenase.

   (3) The β-hydroxybutyrate-acetoacetate ratio is usually approximately 3:1. Acetoacetic acid can be converted to acetone by nonenzymatic decarboxylation. Acetone is excreted via the lungs and kidneys, with a small component being metabolized to glucose.

  c. Phosphoric acid is produced from the metabolism of phosphoproteins.

  d. Uric acid is produced from the metabolism of nucleoproteins.

  e. Acetic acid (vinegar) functions transiently as a noncarbonic acid because humans can convert it rapidly to CO_2 and H_2O.

6. Buffering of noncarbonic acids. In contrast to the bicarbonate buffer system, which can buffer only noncarbonic acids, the nonbicarbonate buffer systems can buffer both noncarbonic and carbonic acids.

  a. The plasma bicarbonate system is quantitatively the most important buffer in the ECF for noncarbonic acids.

  b. When noncarbonic acids are being buffered in the erythrocytes, more than 60% of the buffering occurs by the hemoglobin and more than 30% by the bicarbonate system in the erythrocytes. Approximately 10% of the buffer capacity in erythrocytes is attributed to the organic phosphate esters.

  c. The bodily response to mineral acids (e.g., HCl) is different in that lactic acid is distributed throughout the body water and is metabolized, whereas mineral acids are confined to the ECF and are buffered and excreted without being metabolized.

C. | Stool HCO_3^- loss

1. The diet also contains organic cationic and anionic salts that may be metabolized to yield noncarbonic acids and bases (HCO_3^-). Organic anions metabolized in the body to HCO_3^- include acetate, citrate, and—in the presence of insulin—the anions of the ketoacids.

2. Digestive processes result in the loss of 20 to 40 mmol of alkali in the stool, a loss equivalent to the addition of nonvolatile acid in the body.

Exercise

Describe the relationship between the tissue production of acids and the renal excretion of acids.

DISCUSSION

The tissue production of acids results from the intermediary metabolism of energy-containing substances. Oxidation of carbohydrates can result in the formation of lactic and pyruvic acids; degradation of fatty acids from triglycerides produces ketoacids; oxidation of sulfur-containing amino acids generates sulfuric acid; and the degradation of nucleic acids produces phosphoric acid. The cellular release of these acids generates H^+ and anions. The H^+ will reduce extracellular HCO_3^-, whereas the anion will bind the Na^+ previously bound to the HCO_3^-. The amount of reduced HCO_3^- will be identical to the amount of fixed acids—both organic and inorganic. To maintain acid-base balance, the kidney must fully reclaim (reabsorb) the filtered HCO_3^- as a first step in the excretion of the acid load. This is because H^+ excretion is equivalent to the addition of new HCO_3^- to the blood. However, the complete reabsorption of HCO_3^-, although critical, does not help at all in the renal excretion of the metabolically generated acids.

As a second step, the kidney must regenerate the HCO_3^- neutralized in the tissues by exchanging the cation (usually Na^+) bound to the filtered anion (organic or inorganic) for secreted H^+, thus producing titratable acid. Excretion of H^+ by the kidney with the concomitant maintenance of Na^+ (and $K+$) balance is accomplished by the production within the kidney of an organic cation (NH_4^+) that can be excreted with the filtered anion.

Chapter 33

Metabolic Origin of Alkali (Bases)

I. **AMINO ACIDS AND OTHER ORGANIC IONS** (see Table 32-3). The metabolism of foodstuffs does not always acidify the body fluids; some foodstuffs have an alkalinizing action. For example, the large amounts of organic acids ingested with fruit (e.g., lactate, isocitrate, citrate) alkalinize the fluids because these organic ions are metabolized to CO_2 and H_2O, a process that involves consumption of H^+.

A. **Daily production.** Between 40 and 60 mmol of inorganic and organic acids that are not derived from CO_2 are produced daily. Approximately half of the metabolically produced acids are neutralized by bases in the diet, but the remainder must be neutralized by the buffer systems of the body.

B. In contrast to the production of H^+ from sulfur-containing amino acids and cationic amino acids, the metabolism of anionic amino acids (i.e., glutamate, aspartate) results in the production of HCO_3^- (see Table 32-3).*

C. The hepatic metabolism of the other dietary anions by oxidation contributes to the **formation of HCO_3^-** as:

$$Citrate^- + 4.5\ O_2 \rightarrow 5\ CO_2 + 3\ H_2O + HCO_3^-$$

The metabolism of dietary organic ions (e.g., citrate) results in the production of approximately 60 mmol/day of HCO_3^-.

II. **AMMONIUM EXCRETION AND REGULATION OF ACID-BASE BALANCE**

A. **The kidney increases the HCO_3^- content of the body through its ability to metabolize glutamine and excrete NH_4^+.**

1. The excretion of the two ammonium ions produced by the proximal tubule of the kidney plays no direct role in removing protons: NH_4^+ is merely a side product in the formation of α-ketoglutarate.

2. Net H^+ loss occurs when NH_4^+ is excreted primarily by substituting for protons on the Na^+-H^+ exchanger on the luminal membrane of the proximal tubule. H^+ is also removed when α-ketoglutarate is metabolized to the neutral end product glucose or CO_2.

3. If glutamine catabolism is to be an HCO_3^- generating process, the NH_4^+ liberated during the conversion of glutamine to either CO_2 and water or glucose must be excreted (Figures 33-1, 33-2).

B. The **HCO_3^- ion** formed by the proximal tubule is transported across the basolateral membrane to the extracellular fluid (ECF), where it restores HCO_3^- that was neutralized by systemic metabolic acid production.

1. The **NH_4^+ ions** formed by the proximal tubule are actively secreted into the luminal fluid and are excreted via the urine.

2. If the NH_4^+ is not excreted and returned to the ECF, it is incorporated into the urea by

---

*The consumption of the H^+ ions by glutamate and lactate is equivalent to the production of new HCO_3^- in the body.

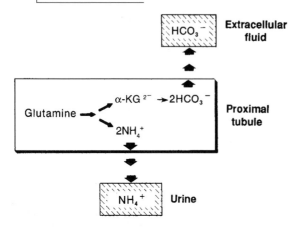

FIGURE 33-1. Formation and active secretion of NH_4^+ by the proximal tubules. Most of the NH_4^+ excreted in the urine is produced by the proximal tubular cells and is mainly from glutamine. Urea formation in the liver is quantitatively the most important disposal route for ammonia, and glutamine serves as a nontoxic storage and transport form of ammonia. α-KG $^{2-}$ = α-ketoglutarate. [Reprinted from Seldin DW, Giebisch G (eds): New concepts in renal ammonium excretion. In *The Regulation of Acid-Base Balance.* New York, Raven, 1989, p 170.]

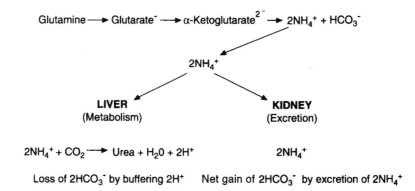

FIGURE 33-2. Glutamine is metabolized by the kidneys, and NH_4^+ is excreted in the urine. At the same time HCO_3^- is returned to the systemic circulation to replenish the HCO_3^- that is lost in the titration of nonvolatile acids. The formation of new HCO_3^- by this reaction depends on the ability of the kidney to excrete NH_4^+ in the urine. If NH_4^+ is not excreted in the urine but instead enters the systemic circulation, it will titrate plasma HCO_3^-, thus negating the process of new HCO_3^- generation.

the liver. If this occurs, the two H+ ions liberated during urea synthesis neutralize the two HCO_3^- ions produced from the oxidation of glutamine, and there is no net gain of HCO_3^- (see Figure 33-2).

C. Salient aspects of renal HCO_3^-

1. The "new" HCO_3^- added to the ECF in association with NH_4^+ excretion is actually produced in the proximal tubule from the metabolism of α-ketoglutarate formed from the deamination and deamidation of glutamine.

2. The addition of HCO_3^- to the renal venous blood requires the metabolism of the α-ketoglutarate anion, which removes protons and is a process equivalent to generating "new" HCO_3^- ions.

3. The NH_4^+ must be excreted in the urine; otherwise, it would return via the renal veins to the liver, where it would be converted to urea plus 2 H+ (see Figure 33-2).

4. New HCO_3^- (regenerated HCO_3^-)* is also produced in the tubular cells by the excre-

---

*HCO_3^- regeneration is also termed acid excretion because the kidney excretes various conjugate acids as part of the HCO_3^--producing process.

tion of titratable acid ($H_2PO_4^-$) formed proximally and distally by the secretion of protons that are buffered by HPO_4^{2-}

Exercise

It is commonly thought that acids such as citric, lactic, and ascorbic acids tend to acidify the blood and urine. Why is this a common misconception?

DISCUSSION

Citric acid in such juices as grapefruit juice exists mainly in its anionic form, particularly in its Na^+ and K^+ salts. Citrate and lactate anions are metabolized to bicarbonate and tend to alkalinize the blood and urine. Alkalinization occurs even though the pH of the juice is low, because bicarbonate generation exceeds the free protons formed by the dissociation of the acids. For example, a liter of juice with a pH of 4 has only 0.1 mmol (10^{-4} mol/L) of H^+ ions. However, alkalinization will occur whenever the quantity of organic anions exceeds the quantity of free protons.

   Clinically, vitamin C (ascorbic acid) is occasionally prescribed to acidify the urine. Vitamin C can be commercially prepared in the form of the dissociated anion ascorbate and is then metabolized to bicarbonate, thus alkalinizing the urine. Even the protonated form, ascorbic acid, does not lower the urine pH as much as expected. The dissociation of the acid has an acidifying effect, but the metabolism of the ascorbate to bicarbonate has an alkalinizing effect. Acidification will only occur to the extent that ascorbate is excreted unmetabolized.

Chapter 34

The Hydrogen Ion and pH

I. **FUNDAMENTAL CHEMISTRY** (Table 34-1). H^+ is a proton (i.e., a hydrogen atom without its orbital electron); H^+ in aqueous solution exists as a hydrated proton called the hydronium ion, or H_3O^+. pH refers to the negative Briggsian logarithm of the H^+ concentration. The gain and loss of protons constitutes acid-base chemistry. The currently accepted model of acid-base relationships is that proposed by Brønsted.

A. An **acid** is a substance that acts as a proton donor.

B. A **base** is a substance that accepts protons (i.e., H^+) in solution. Thus, bicarbonate ion (HCO_3^-), phosphate ion (HPO_4^{2-}), ammonia (NH_3), and acetate ion (CH_3COO^-) all are bases.

C. Some substances are nearly equally divided between the acidic and basic forms at the normal H^+ concentration of the body. For example, the imidazole side groups of hemoglobin undergo the following reaction:

$$HHb \rightleftharpoons H^+ + Hb^-$$

The acid, deoxyhemoglobin (HHb), dissociates to form H^+ and the conjugate base Hb^-. HHb and Hb^- occur in approximately equal concentrations in blood cells.

II. **CONCEPT OF pH AND H^+ CONCENTRATION** (Table 34-2)

A. **H+ concentration is expressed in two different ways,** either directly as $[H^+]$ or indirectly as **pH.** (The symbol $[H^+]$ refers to H^+ concentration in mol/L or Eq/L.) The relationship between $[H^+]$ and pH can be expressed as:

1. $pH = \log_{10} \dfrac{1}{[H^+]}$

2. $pH = -\log_{10} [H^+]$

3. $[H^+] = 10^{-pH}$

TABLE 34-1. Important Buffer Acids at Physiologic $[H^+]$

Proton Donor (Conjugate Acid)*		Proton (H^+)		Proton Acceptor (Conjugate Base)*
$(CO_2)H_2CO_3$	$\rightleftharpoons$	H^+	+	HCO_3^-
$H_2PO_4^-$	$\rightleftharpoons$	H^+	+	HPO_4^{2-}
$H \cdot Protein$	$\rightleftharpoons$	H^+	+	$Proteinate^-$
$HHbO_2$	$\rightleftharpoons$	H^+	+	HbO_2^-
HHb	$\rightleftharpoons$	H^+	+	Hb^-

*A conjugate acid can be an anion or a cation; a conjugate base usually is an anion; HCO_3^-, a conjugate base, also can be an acid; ammonia is a neutral base (NH_3).

TABLE 34-2. Relationship between pH and [H⁺]

pH	[H⁺] (nEq/L)
7.70	20
7.40 (plasma)	40
7.30 (CSF)	50
7.10 (ICF)	80
7.00	100
6.90	126

CSF = cerebrospinal fluid; ICF = intracellular fluid.

B. **pH is a dimensionless number** and should be treated as such; it should not be referred to in concentration units or as "pH concentration." In fact, the quantity whose logarithm determines the pH is a volume per equivalent, which is the inverse of concentration. Thus, pH could be correctly conceptualized as a logarithmic expression of the volume required to contain 1 equivalent of H^+. In human plasma at pH 7.4 [i.e., [H⁺] of 40×10^{-9} mol (Eq)/L or 40 nmol (nEq)/L], that volume is 25 million liters!

C. Because pH is the logarithmic expression of [H⁺], it permits a graphic representation of a wide range of [H⁺] values. (It is important to note that **pH and [H⁺] are inversely related.**) Another advantage of the pH concept is that when the pK′ of a buffer system is known, it is immediately possible to determine the effective pH range of the buffer.*

D. **A disadvantage of the pH system** is that it both inverts and uses the logarithmic scale to express [H⁺]. For example, it is not immediately apparent that a decrease in pH from 7.4 to 7.1 represents a doubling of the [H⁺] from 40 nmol/L to 80 nmol/L.

III. H⁺ CONCENTRATION OF BODY FLUIDS (Figure 34-1; Table 34-3)

A. **Blood and plasma.** Regarding [H⁺], the body fluid compartment most studied is arterial blood plasma. The term **blood pH** always refers to **plasma pH** (7.4), which is higher than the intracellular pH of the erythrocyte (7.2).

1. In normal individuals, the [H⁺] is approximately 40 nmol (nEq)/L, which is equivalent to pH 7.4. The range of [H⁺] that is compatible with life is 20 to 126 nEq/L, which is equivalent to a pH range of 7.7 to 6.9.

2. In normal individuals at rest, the pH of mixed venous blood is 7.38 compared with 7.41 for arterial blood because of the uptake of CO_2 by blood as it perfuses the tissues.

3. The [H⁺] of plasma is very small compared with that of other ions in plasma (e.g., the plasma Na^+ concentration is approximately 142 million nmol/L, and the K^+ concentration is approximately 4 million nmol/L).

B. **Cerebrospinal fluid (CSF)** is essentially a bicarbonate buffer with a negligible concentration of protein (between 2×10^{-2} g/dl and 4×10^{-2} g/dl) or other nonbicarbonate buffers.

1. The arterial pH (7.4) is higher than that of CSF (7.32), because the CO_2 tension (PCO_2) is approximately 48 mm Hg in the CSF and approximately 40 mm Hg in the arterial blood (see Figure 34-1).

---

*K = the ionization or dissociation constant; pK = the negative logarithm of K (-log K) and is equal to the pH at which half of the acid molecules are dissociated and half are undissociated; pK′ = the apparent pK (see IV B 1).

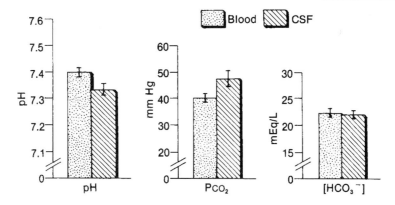

FIGURE 34-1. Comparison of the relationship between pH, CO_2 tension (PCO_2), and [HCO_3^-] in arterial blood and cerebrospinal fluid (CSF) in normal adult humans. Each vertical bar represents ±1 SD. (Reprinted from Seldin DW, Giebisch G (eds): Acid-base balance in specialized tissues: central nervous system. In *The Regulation of Acid-Base Balance.* New York, Raven, 1989, p 109.)

2. Generally, it is possible to characterize acid-base disturbances precisely in terms of the blood data; however, the extracellular changes do not always reflect the intracellular changes. Also, acid-base alterations in arterial blood may produce similar or opposite changes in the CSF depending on whether the blood [H^+] changes are due to respiratory or metabolic abnormalities.
   a. An **increase in arterial CO_2 tension (respiratory acidosis)** leads to a parallel rise in the CSF CO_2 tension, with a resulting increase in the [H^+] of both arterial blood and CSF.
   b. A **decrease in arterial CO_2 tension (respiratory alkalosis)** leads to a parallel decline in CSF CO_2 tension, with a resulting decrease in the [H^+] of both arterial blood and CSF.

TABLE 34-3. H^+ Concentration ([H^+]) and pH of Biologic Fluids

Fluid	pH	[H^+] (nEq/ or nmol/L)*	[H^+] (Eq/L or mol/L)
Pure water	7.0	100	1×10^{-7}
Blood			
Normal mean	7.40	40	3.98×10^{-8}
Normal range	7.36–7.44	44–36	$4.36 \times 10^{-8} - 3.63 \times 10^{-8}$
Acidosis (severe)	6.9	126	1.26×10^{-7}
Alkalosis (severe)	7.7	20	2.00×10^{-8}
CSF (normal range)	7.36–7.44	44–36	$4.36 \times 10^{-8} - 3.63 \times 10^{-8}$
Pure gastric juice (normal)	1.0	100,000,000	1×10^{-1}
Urine			
Normal average	6.0	1000	1×10^{-6}
Maximum acidity	4.5	31,600	3.16×10^{-5}
Maximum alkalinity	8.0	10	1×10^{-8}
ICF (muscle)	6.8	158	1.58×10^{-7}

CSF = cerebrospinal fluid; ICF = intracellular fluid. (Adapted from Brobeck JR (ed): Regulation of hydrogen ion concentration in body fluids. In *Best and Taylor's Physiological Basis of Medical Practice,* 10th ed. Baltimore, Williams & Wilkins, 1979, pp 5–13.)

*n = nano- = 10^{-9}. Thus, 100 nEq/L = 100×10^{-9} Eq/L, where nEq = nmol of a monovalent ion.

c. An **increase in arterial [H+](metabolic acidosis)** stimulates ventilation, lowering the CO_2 tension of the arterial blood and CSF, resulting in CSF alkalosis and blood acidosis.

d. A **decrease in arterial [H+](metabolic alkalosis)** decreases ventilation, raising the CO_2 tension of the arterial blood and CSF, which results in CSF acidosis and blood alkalosis.

IV. HENDERSON–HASSELBALCH EQUATION

A. **Significance.** Acid–base balance is maintained primarily through the control of two organ systems. The lungs control the CO_2 tension through the regulation of alveolar ventilation, and the kidneys control the HCO_3^- concentration ($[HCO_3^-]$). The classic description of the acid-base state is based on the Henderson–Hasselbalch equation, which is an expression of three variables (pH, PCO_2, and $[HCO_3^-]$ and two constants (pK' and S).

B. **Definition of parameters.** The Henderson–Hasselbalch equation could functionally be written as:

$$pH = pK' + \log \frac{kidneys}{lungs^*} \qquad (1)$$

However, the equation is expressed more usefully as:

$$pH = pK' + \log \frac{[HCO_3^-]}{S \cdot PCO_2} \qquad (2)$$

or, using specific values for pK' and S (defined in IV B 1 and 2), as:

$$pH = 6.1 + \log \frac{[HCO_3^-]}{0.03 \cdot PCO_2} \qquad (3)$$

From equation (3) it is clear that the value of arterial pH depends on the ratio of $[HCO_3^-]$ to $S \cdot PCO_2$, not on the individual value of each variable. In clinical medicine, pH, CO_2 tension, and $[HCO_3^-]$ can be measured directly. However, with equation (3) any one of the variables can be calculated if the other two are known.

1. **pK** is defined as the negative logarithm of the [H+] at which half the acid molecules are undissociated and half are dissociated. When equimolar concentrations of weak acid and conjugate base exist, the pH value equals the pK (i.e., the log of 1 is 0).

a. The **actual dissociation constant (K)** for carbonic acid (H_2CO_3) in dilute aqueous solution at 38°C is 1.6×10^{-4} mol/L (pK = 3.8). Thus, H_2CO_3 is almost completely dissociated in the body where [H+] = 4×10^{-8} mol/L, and it exists in quantities that are too small to be analyzed (i.e., 2.4×10^{-4} mEq/L). The formation and dissociation of H_2CO_3 is expressed as:

$$\begin{array}{c} CO_2 \\ alveolar \\ gas \end{array} \rightleftharpoons \begin{array}{c} CO_2 \\ plasma \end{array} + H_2O \quad \underset{500:1}{\overset{\text{carbonic anhydrase}}{\rightleftharpoons}} \quad H_2CO_3 \underset{4000:1}{\rightleftharpoons} H^+ + HCO_3^- \qquad (4)$$

At equilibrium there are approximately 500 mmol of CO_2 for every 1 mmol of H_2CO_3 and approximately 4000 mmol of H_2CO_3 for every 1 mmol of H+. Because of the presence of carbonic anhydrase, equilibrium between CO_2 and H_2CO_3 is rapid and constant.[†]

b. Because the denominator of equation (3) is increased by a factor of 500, the **apparent dissociation constant (K')** for the CO_2/HCO_3^- buffer system in plasma at 38°C is cor-

---

[*]The kidneys primarily regulate $[HCO_3^-]$, the numerator; the lungs mainly regulate CO_2 tension, the denominator.
[†]Carbonic anhydrase is found in erythrocytes, gastric parietal cells, renal tubular cells, pancreatic and pulmonary tissue, bone, and the eye; it is not found in muscle, peripheral nerves, or skin.

respondingly smaller (8×10^{-7} mol/L, or 800 nmol/L), and the **apparent pK (pK')** for this same buffer pair is correspondingly larger (6.1). As a rule, the optimal buffer region of a buffer pair system is within a range of ± 1 pH units of its pK value.

c. It is important to note that, because CO_2 increases $[H^+]$, as shown in equation (4), it is considered an acid even though it is an acid **anhydride.** Thus, dissolved CO_2 is present as a potential H^+ donor, and its concentration is proportionate to the true donor, H_2CO_3. For these reasons, it is more meaningful to characterize acid-base disturbances in terms of the CO_2/HCO_3^- buffer system instead of the H_2CO_3/HCO_3^- system. For all practical purposes, the H_2CO_3/HCO_3^- buffer pair can be considered to be composed of HCO_3^- (conjugate base) and dissolved CO_2 (conjugate "acid").

2. **S** is defined as the solubility constant for CO_2 in plasma at 38°C and is equal to 0.03 mmol/L/mm Hg. S represents the solubility constant between CO_2 and CO_2 tension. For blood plasma at 38°C, the amount of dissolved CO_2 is expressed as:

$$\text{dissolved } CO_2 = 0.03 \cdot P{CO_2}^*$$

where CO_2 = the millimoles of dissolved CO_2 per liter of plasma. At an arterial PCO_2 of 40 mm Hg, the CO_2 concentration ($[CO_2]$) is expressed more usefully as:

$$0.03 \text{ mmol/L/mm Hg} \cdot 40 \text{ mm Hg} = 1.2 \text{ mmol/L}$$

Multiplying the solubility constant (0.03) by milliliters of CO_2 per millimole (22.3 ml/mmol) yields a solubility constant of 0.67 ml/L/mm Hg for CO_2 in plasma. At this solubility constant and at a CO_2 tension of 40 mm Hg, the concentration of dissolved CO_2 is expressed as:

$$0.67 \text{ ml/L/mm Hg} \cdot 40 \text{ mm Hg} = 26.8 \text{ ml/L}^\dagger$$

3. **$[HCO_3^-]$** denotes the bicarbonate ion concentration, which is expressed in millimolarity rather than molarity. The normal value of $[HCO_3^-]$ in plasma is 24 mmol (mEq)/L.

4. From equation (4) it is essential to appreciate that CO_2 is not only an H^+ generator but also an HCO_3^- generator.
   1. Note that when CO_2 is added to body fluids it is the H^+ concentration that increases, with little change in the HCO_3^- concentration.
   2. The ratio of HCO_3^- concentration (24×10^{-3} mol/L) to H^+ concentration (4×10^{-8} mol/L) is equal to 24×10^{-3} M $\div$ 4×10^{-8} M, or 6×10^5 to 1, or 600,000 to 1.
   3. Therefore, the addition of CO_2 to a solution has a much greater effect on the dilute concentration of H^+ compared with a lesser effect on the much higher concentration of HCO_3^-.

C. Calculations with the Henderson–Hasselbalch equation

1. **Traditional calculation of pH.** pH in normal arterial plasma = 7.4; normal CO_2 tension = 40 mm Hg, and normal $[HCO_3^-]$ = 24 mmol/L (or 24 mEq/L). Applying the Henderson-Hasselbalch equation, pH is calculated as:

$$pH = 6.1 + \log \frac{[HCO_3^-]}{0.03 \cdot PCO_2}$$

$$= 6.1 + \log \frac{24 \text{ mmol/L}}{0.03 \cdot 40 \text{ mm Hg}}$$

$$= 6.1 + \log \frac{24 \text{ mmol/L}}{1.2 \text{ mmol/L}}$$

$$= 6.1 + \log 20$$

$$= 7.4$$

---

*This amounts to approximately 5% of the total amount of CO_2 carried in the arterial blood.

2. Simple calculation of [H$^+$] and pH
a. Conversion of pH to [H$^+$]:a close approximation
(1) Equation. The [H$^+$] in plasma is expressed in nanomoles per liter. The equation for [H$^+$] now becomes:

$$\log [H^+] - 9 = - pH \text{ or } [H^+] = \text{antilog} (9 - pH)$$

(2) Examples (see Table 34-2)
(a) At pH 7.4:

$$[H^+] = \text{antilog} (9 - 7.4)$$
$$= \text{antilog} 1.6$$
$$= 39.6 \text{ nmol/L}$$

(b) At pH 6.9:

$$[H^+] = \text{antilog} (9 - 6.9)$$
$$= \text{antilog} 2.1$$
$$= 126 \text{ nmol/L}$$

b. Conversion of [H$^+$] to pH
(1) Equation. The [H$^+$] in plasma is expressed in nanomoles per liter. The equation for pH is:

$$pH = 9 - \log [H^+]$$

(2) Examples (see Table 34-2)
(a) At [H$^+$] = 40 nmol/L:

$$pH = 9 - \log 40$$
$$= 9 - 1.6$$
$$= 7.4$$

(b) At [H$^+$] = 126 nmol/L:

$$pH = 9 - \log 126$$
$$= 9 - 2.1$$
$$= 6.9$$

V. HENDERSON EQUATION

A. **Use of the Henderson equation.** This equation provides a simple means for converting pH to [H$^+$], because CO$_2$ tension and [HCO$_3$$^-$] will have been provided. Additionally, this equation provides a simple **arithmetic estimate** of [HCO$_3$$^-$], because the value of [H$^+$] often will have been approximated from the pH value reported by the laboratory.

B. **Calculations with the Henderson equation.** The Henderson equation represents the non-logarithmic (arithmetic) method of determining [H$^+$] [HCO$_3$$^-$] or P$CO_2$ as:

$$[H^+] = K' \frac{P_{CO_2}}{[HCO_3^-]} \text{ or } [HCO_3^-] = K' \frac{P_{CO_2}}{[H^+]} \text{ or } P_{CO_2} = \frac{[H^+][HCO_3^-]}{24}$$

1. A value for K' is derived by converting the apparent pK for carbonic acid (6.1) into a dissociation constant (expressed in nanomoles per liter) and multiplying that value by the solubility constant for CO$_2$ in plasma at 38°C (i.e., 0.03). K' has a value of 800 nmol/L [see IV B 1 (a)], which, when multiplied by 0.03, equals 24.

2. Using normal values for CO_2 tension, $[H^+]$, and $[HCO_3^-]$, the Henderson equation is applied as:

$$[H^+] = 24 \; \frac{P_{CO_2} \; (mm \; Hg)}{[HCO_3^-] \; (mmol/L)}$$

$$= 24 \; \frac{40}{24} = 40 \; nmol/L$$

Similarly,

$$[HCO_3^-] = 24 \; \frac{P_{CO_2} \; (mm \; Hg)}{[H^+] \; (nmol/L)}$$

$$= 24 \; \frac{40}{40} = 24 \; mmol/L$$

Additionally,

$$P_{CO_2} = \frac{[H^+] \cdot [HCO_3^-]}{24}$$

$$= \frac{40 \cdot 24}{24} = 40 \; mm \; Hg$$

Exercises

1. *Describe the two notations used to quantitate the acidity of a solution with a pH of 7.4.*

2. *How is one scale of acidity converted to the other one?*

3. *Does the proton concentration contribute significantly to the maintenance of electroneutrality of body fluids?*

4. *What is the major difference between expressing acidity in nanomoles per liter and pH units?*

5. *Is the pH of body fluids regulated by a direct physiologic control of H^+ concentration?*

6. *How do the approximately 2 mEq/L of arteriovenous difference of plasma $[HCO_3^-]$ relate to the 15,000 mEq/day of volatile acid production?*

DISCUSSION

1. A solution that contains $10^{-7.4}$ mol/L of H^+ (i.e., $10^{1.6} \times 10^{-9}$ mol/L) has a pH of 7.4. Note that $10^{-7.4}$ mol/L is equivalent to 40×10^{-9} mol/L or, 40 nmol/L.

2. To convert pH values to nanomoles per liter, first subtract the pH value from 9.00 and then obtain the antilog; that is, nanomoles per liter = antilog $(9 - pH)$. To convert nanomoles per liter to pH, first obtain the log of nanomoles per liter and then subtract the result from 9, that is, $pH = 9 - \log [H^+]$.

3. No. The proton concentration is infinitesimally small compared with the concentration of major ions in body fluids (Na^+, Cl^-); therefore, it contributes little to the maintenance of electroneutrality.

4. The major difference is that the expression of acidity in nanomoles per liter uses an

arithmetic scale, whereas the notation of pH uses a logarithmic scale. When acidity is expressed in pH units, due to the logarithmic scale, it becomes difficult to conceptualize the quantitative changes. For example, a change in pH from 7.4 to 7.1 represents an increase in H^+ concentration from 40 nanomoles per liter to 80 nmol/L, that is, a twofold increase. The Henderson-Hasselbalch equation is simply the logarithmic form of the Henderson equation.

Most individuals can tolerate a pH as low as 7.1 (80 nmol/L) and as high as 7.7 (20 nmol/L) in their extracellular fluid, a 100% and a 50% decrease in H^+ concentration, respectively. However, a 50% change in the Na^+ concentration of plasma in either direction is not compatible with life.

5. No. Acidity is regulated by altering the levels of the components that determine $[H^+]$, namely P_{CO_2} and HCO_3^- concentrations. The unique characteristic of the CO_2/HCO_3^- buffer pair lies in the ability of the lungs to eliminate the volatile acid H_2CO_3 as nonionizable CO_2.

6. The product of arteriovenous difference of plasma $[HCO_3^-]$ per liter of blood and the cardiac output in liters per minute yields the CO_2 production in millimoles per minute. This value, multiplied by 1440 min/day, provides the daily production in millimoles or milliequivalents. Thus, 2 mEq/L $\times$ 5 L/min of cardiac output $\times$ 1440 min/day = 14,400 mEq/day (ca. 15,000 mEq/day).

Chapter 35

Body Buffer Systems

I. **BUFFER SYSTEMS.** A buffer is a solution consisting of a weak acid and its conjugate base. Buffering is the primary means by which large changes in $[H^+]$ are minimized.

A. Types of body buffer systems

1. **Blood buffers** (Table 35-1)
   a. It is important to note that the blood buffers are not solely plasma buffers, but that hemoglobin, HCO_3^-, and phosphate are found in erythrocytes and act as important blood buffers.
      (1) In blood, the chief H^+ acceptor is HCO_3^-, which exists in a concentration of 20–30 mEq/L.
      (2) H^+ acceptor is available in the hemoglobin system, where reduced hemoglobin (deoxyhemoglobin) is a stronger base than oxyhemoglobin (i.e., deoxyhemoglobin has a stronger capacity to combine with H^+).
      (3) The hemoglobin buffer system is quantitatively as important as the bicarbonate buffer system.
   b. The major buffer anions of whole blood—HCO_3^-, protein, and hemoglobin—have a total concentration of approximately 48 mEq/L.
   c. With the bicarbonate and hemoglobin systems taken together, 5 L of blood of a normal adult have sufficient buffer capacity to combine with almost 150 millimoles (mmol) of protons (150 ml of 1 N HCl) before the pH of body fluids becomes dangerously acidic.

2. **Tissue buffers.** The major buffer capacity of the body is not in the blood but in the H^+ acceptors found in other tissues, principally in the muscle and in bone. These tissues can neutralize about five times as much acid as the blood buffers.
   a. **Muscle**
      (1) Since skeletal muscle represents about half of the cellular mass, most intracellular buffering presumably occurs in muscle.
      (2) For any individual, the body HCO_3^- concentration averages 13 mEq/kg body weight. Muscle cells contain HCO_3^- at a concentration of about 12 mEq/L, and most other cells contain it at higher concentrations. The intracellular fluid (ICF) and extracellular fluid (ECF) compartments each contain about 50% of the total body HCO_3^-.
   b. **Bone** plays an important role in buffering H^+.
      (1) The total body store of bone carbonate is about 50 times the amount of HCO_3^- in the ICF and ECF compartments together. Bone carbonate appears to be the predominant source of base for neutralizing excess noncarbonic acid in the ECF. Indeed, it has long been recognized that chronic noncarbonic acidosis causes bone dissolution (resorption) through the loss of calcium carbonate ($CaCO_3$). The early carbonate release is in the form of sodium carbonate (Na_2CO_3).
         (a) Bone carbonates amount to a total of approximately 35,000 mEq in an adult and they contribute significantly to the buffering capacity of the body. The H_2CO_3/HCO_3^- buffer system provides about 700 mEq of HCO_3^- to neutralize an equally large acid load.
         (b) It has been estimated that about 40% of the buffering of an acute acid load occurs in the bone.
      (2) Bone contains about 80% of the total CO_2 (including CO_3^{2-}, HCO_3^-, and CO_2) in the body. About two-thirds of this CO_2 is in the form of CO_3^{2-} complexed with Ca^{2+}, Na^+, and other cations located in the lattice of the bone crystals. The other

TABLE 35-1. Whole Blood Buffers

Buffer Type	Buffering Capacity of Whole Blood (%)
Bicarbonate	
Plasma	35
Erythrocyte	18
Total bicarbonate	53
Nonbicarbonate	
Hemoglobin and oxyhemoglobin	35
Plasma proteins	7
Organic phosphate	3
Inorganic phosphate	2
Total nonbicarbonate	47

Adapted from Brobeck JR (ed): Regulation of hydrogen ion concentration in body fluids. In *Best and Taylor's Physiological Basis of Medical Practice,* 10th ed. Baltimore, Williams & Wilkins, 1979, pp 5–14.

third consists of HCO_3^- and is located in the hydration shell of the hydroxyapatite crystal, an inorganic compound found in the matrix of bone and teeth.

B. **Distribution of body buffer systems in major compartments**

1. **Blood,** in regard to its buffering activity, usually is considered as a whole rather than in terms of its components. Blood buffers are described here in terms of separate compartments (i.e., plasma and erythrocytes) for didactic purposes only.
    a. **Important concepts**
        (1) Whole blood is an excellent buffering system for noncarbonic acids because of its nonbicarbonate buffers as well as its bicarbonate buffer system.
        (2) More than 90% of the blood's capacity to buffer carbonic acid is attributed to the hemoglobin buffer system. Thus, the nonbicarbonate buffer in the erythrocyte is quantitatively more important than the bicarbonate buffer in that compartment. The bicarbonate buffer system remains quantitatively important, however, in the erythrocyte (see Table 35-1).
            (a) The bicarbonate buffer system does not function as a buffer for carbonic acid.
            (b) The nonbicarbonate buffer systems can buffer both noncarbonic and carbonic acids.
    b. **Buffer capacity of blood components**
        (1) **Plasma,** which contains three buffer systems, has a considerable capacity for buffering noncarbonic acids but a much smaller capacity for buffering carbonic acid.
            (a) **Bicarbonate buffer system** (HCO_3^-/H_2CO_3 or HCO_3^-/CO_2). This buffer exists in a concentration of 24 mmol/L of plasma. When **noncarbonic acid** is added to normal plasma, more than 75% of the buffering capacity of plasma is due to the HCO_3^-/CO_2 system. Most of the remaining buffering of noncarbonic acid involves the plasma protein buffers and, to a small degree, the phosphate buffer system. Again, the HCO_3^-/CO_2 system plays no role in the buffering of carbonic acid.
            (b) **Nonbicarbonate buffer systems**
                (i) **Plasma protein** ($Protein^-/H \cdot Protein$). Plasma is a salt solution containing 7% protein, which exists as polyanions at the pH of plasma. Plasma protein H^+ acceptors exist in a concentration of about 1.1 mmol/L of plasma and account for less than one-sixth of the total buffering capacity of whole blood.
                (ii) **Inorganic orthophosphate** ($HPO_4^{2-}/H_2PO_4^-$). Because this buffer system

exists in a concentration of only 0.66 mmol/L of plasma, it contributes little to the total buffering activity of plasma.* At a plasma pH of 7.4, the concentration ratio of $HPO_4^{2-}/H_2PO_4^-$ is 4:1. Therefore, 80% of the inorganic phosphate exists as disodium phosphate, and 20% is in the form of monosodium phosphate. The $HPO_4^{2-}/H_2PO_4^-$ system is a major elimination route for H^+ via the urine, which has a relatively high phosphate content.

(2) **Erythrocytes.** Although the blood contains other cells, the erythrocyte is the only important cellular component of the blood buffer system. The erythrocyte contains four buffer systems.

- (a) **Bicarbonate buffer system.** The HCO_3^-/CO_2 system exists in a concentration of 15 mmol/L of erythrocytes, compared to a concentration of 21 mmol/L and 25 mmol/L of whole blood and plasma, respectively.
- (b) **Nonbicarbonate buffer systems**
  - (i) **Hemoglobin buffers** (Hb^-/HHb and $HbO_2^-/HHbO_2$) [see II]. One L of **erythrocytes** contains 334 g (5.1 mmol) of hemoglobin. One L of **whole blood** contains 150 g (2.3 mmol) of hemoglobin.
  - (ii) **Organic phosphate.** Although the erythrocyte contains a significant amount of organic phosphate buffer, this amount is quantitatively small compared to the bicarbonate and hemoglobin buffer concentrations in the erythrocyte.
  - (iii) **Inorganic orthophosphate.** The $HPO_4^{2-}/H_2PO_4^-$ system exists in a concentration of 2 mmol/L of erythrocytes.

2. **Interstitial fluid (including lymph)**
   - a. **Bicarbonate buffer system.** The HCO_3^-/CO_2 system is quantitatively the most important buffer of noncarbonic acid. The $[HCO_3^-]$ of the interstitial fluid is 27 mmol/L, which is similar to, or about 5% higher than, the $[HCO_3^-]$ of plasma. It is important to consider that, in humans, the interstitial fluid volume is about three times that of plasma; therefore, the total capacity of the interstitial fluid to buffer noncarbonic acid is considerably greater than that of the total blood volume to buffer these acids. **On a per unit of volume basis,** however, **the interstitial fluid has nearly the capacity of plasma to buffer noncarbonic acids.**
   - b. **Nonbicarbonate buffer system.** The $HPO_4^{2-}/H_2PO_4^-$ system exists in a concentration of 0.7 mmol/L of interstitial fluid; therefore, this compartment has little capacity to buffer carbonic acid. The interstitial fluid is essentially free of protein.

3. **Intracellular fluid** (ICF; excluding erythrocytes)
   - a. **Bicarbonate buffer system.** The ICF contains only about 12 mmol of HCO_3^-/L in skeletal and cardiac muscle.
   - b. **Nonbicarbonate buffer systems.** Protein and organic phosphate compounds exist in quantitatively significant amounts in the ICF, giving this compartment the capacity to effectively buffer both noncarbonic and carbonic acids as well as alkali. The ICF concentrations of these major buffer anions are:
     - (1) $HPO_4^{2-}/H_2PO_4^-$ (skeletal muscle) = 6 mmol/L
     - (2) $Protein^-/H \cdot Protein$ (skeletal muscle) = 6 mmol/L
     - (3) Organic anions (skeletal muscle) = 84 mmol/L

II. | HEMOGLOBIN: AN "EXTRACELLULAR" BUFFER

A. | **Important concepts.** Although hemoglobin is found intracellularly, it is more conventionally regarded as extracellular and, therefore, part of the extracellular buffer system because:

---

*The pK' of the acid form (i.e., $H_2PO_4^-$) is 6.8. With this pK', the $HPO_4^{2-}/H_2PO_4^-$ system would be a more effective buffer than the HCO_3^-/CO_2 system (pK' = 6.1) if it were present in an appreciable concentration. Many of the organic phosphate compounds found in the body have pK' values within half of a pH unit from 7.0.

    1. Hemoglobin is confined to the erythrocyte, which is a cellular component of the ECF.

    2. Hemoglobin is readily available for the buffering of extracellular acids.

    3. Hemoglobin is the primary nonbicarbonate buffer of the blood.

B. **Hemoglobin as a buffer.** Like all proteins, hemoglobin is a buffer. At pH 7.2 (i.e., the pH of normal arterial erythrocytes), the buffering action of hemoglobin is due mainly to the imidazole groups of the histidine residues.

    1. The titration curves of deoxyhemoglobin and oxyhemoglobin in Figure 35-1 illustrate the basis for the ability of hemoglobin to neutralize H^+ formed subsequent to the diffusion of CO_2 into the erythrocyte. Most of the H^+ is buffered by hemoglobin and most of the HCO_3^- diffuses into the plasma.*

    2. Oxyhemoglobin dissociates more completely than does deoxyhemoglobin, and, as a result, deoxyhemoglobin produces less H^+ at a given pH than does oxyhemoglobin, which is a stronger acid. Thus, hemoglobin becomes a more effective buffer when CO_2 and, hence, H^+ are added from the tissues. This is important because the diffusion of CO_2 from the tissues to the capillary blood is accompanied by the simultaneous reduction of oxyhemoglobin (Chapter 17 III).

    3. As the uptake of CO_2 depends on H^+ acceptors, this increase in H^+ acceptors in the form of deoxyhemoglobin facilitates the uptake and buffering of the H^+ generated by the hydration of CO_2 and the dissociation of H_2CO_3. As a result of these reactions, CO_2 is converted into HCO_3^- within the erythrocyte.

        a. For each mmol of oxyhemoglobin that is reduced, about 0.7 mmol of H^+ can be taken up and, consequently, 0.7 mmol of CO_2 can enter the blood without a change in pH (see Figure 35-1, *point A* to *point C*).

        b. A reaction that causes no change in $[H^+]$ (or pH) is called **isohydric buffering.**

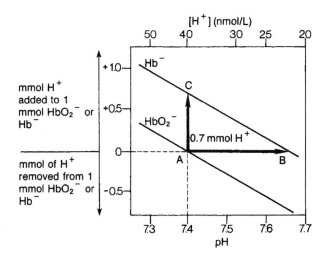

FIGURE 35-1. Titration curves of oxyhemoglobin (*HbO₂⁻*) and deoxyhemoglobin (*Hb⁻*), illustrating the importance of hemoglobin as a buffer. The complete deoxygenation of 1 mmol of HbO_2^- to liberate 1 mmol of O_2 results in the neutralization of 0.7 mmol of H^+ without a change in pH. *Arrow AC* indicates the amount of H^+ that can be added during the reduction of hemoglobin without causing a pH change. *Arrow AB* represents the pH change that would occur if the oxyhemoglobin at pH 7.4 was completely reduced. The reduction of HbO_2^- to Hb^- would cause a large increase in pH if CO_2 and, hence, H^+ were not added simultaneously to the system. Reduction of hemoglobin denotes the O_2-free state without a change in the valence of iron. (Adapted from White A, et al: Hemoglobin and the chemistry of respiration. In *Principles of Biochemistry,* 5th ed. New York, McGraw-Hill, 1973, p 843.)

*The buffer capacity of nonbicarbonate buffers is dependent primarily on the hemoglobin concentration.

4. **Respiratory exchange ratio (RER).** When the body is at rest, the rate of O_2 consumption ($\dot{V}o_2$) under standard conditions is 250–350 ml/min, and the rate of CO_2 production ($\dot{V}co_2$) is 200–250 ml/min. (The dot over the symbol V denotes **volume per unit time.**) RER represents the ratio of CO_2 production to O_2 consumption. Normally, on a mixed diet, the O_2 consumption exceeds the CO_2 production, and the RER is less than 1.
   a. The metabolic RER equals the **molar ratio** of CO_2 production rate to the corresponding O_2 consumption rate by metabolizing tissues.
   b. If the RER rate is 0.7, then, for 1 mmol of O_2 consumed, 0.7 mmol of CO_2 is produced, which, when converted to H_2CO_3, yields 0.7 mmol of H^+ upon dissociation.
   c. The complete deoxygenation of 1 mmol of oxyhemoglobin to liberate 1 mmol of O_2 results in the neutralization of 0.7 mmol of H^+ without a change in pH. Thus, all of the H^+ produced when the RER is 0.7 can be buffered by deoxyhemoglobin with no change in pH (see Figure 35-1).

5. At pH 7.2, about 84% of the deoxyhemoglobin is in the form of HHb, whereas only about 23% of the oxyhemoglobin is in the form of $HHbO_2$. Of the total oxyhemoglobin that causes O_2 to form deoxyhemoglobin:
   a. 23% was already combined with H^+,
   b. 16% will not combine with H^+, and
   c. 61% will take up H^+ before a pH decrease occurs.

6. CO_2 entering the erythrocytes rapidly undergoes two reactions.
   a. CO_2 is hydrated to form H_2CO_3, a reaction that is catalyzed by carbonic anhydrase in the erythrocyte. The H_2CO_3 dissociates to form HCO_3^- and H^+, which is buffered primarily by the hemoglobin buffers. Much of the HCO_3^- formed within the erythrocyte diffuses into the plasma in exhange for Cl^-.
   b. CO_2 combines with the amino groups of deoxyhemoglobin to form carbaminohemoglobin. The carbaminohemoglobin dissociates to a carboxylate anion and H^+, which is buffered primarily by the hemoglobin buffers. In summary:

$$Hb \cdot NH_2 + CO_2 \rightleftharpoons Hb \cdot NHCOO^- + H^+$$

7. The unloading of O_2 from oxyhemoglobin to the tissues causes the formation of deoxyhemoglobin that is better able to tie up the H^+ produced by the simultaneous uptake of CO_2. The loss of O_2 from hemoglobin facilitates the uptake of CO_2 in the form of carbaminohemoglobin by the erythrocytes. Oxyhemoglobin contains about 0.1 mmol and deoxyhemoglobin about 0.3 mmol of carbaminohemoglobin per mmol.

Exercise

1. *What is the so-called isohydric principle?*
2. *What is the relative importance of the buffering compartments (ICF and ECF)?*

DISCUSSION

1. The isohydric principle establishes that the acid/base ratio of all the different buffer pairs (e.g., H_2CO_3/HCO_3^-, $H_2PO_4^-/HPO_4^{2-}$, $H^+ \cdot protein/proteinate^-$) is altered in a parallel manner in response to a change in $[H^+]$ of the solution. Evaluation of the ratio of a single buffer pair allows for the prediction of the ratio of the other pairs in the solution. The law of mass action is defined in the following formula for the case of $[H^+]$:

$$[H^+] = K_a \frac{[HA]}{[A^-]}$$

If several buffers are in solution, the relationships among the buffer pairs are as follows:

$$[H^+] = K_{a1} \frac{[H_2CO_3]}{[HCO_3^-]} = K_{a2} \frac{[H_2PO_4^-]}{[HPO_4^{2-}]} = K_{a3} \frac{[H^+ \cdot \text{Protein}]}{[\text{Proteinate}^-]}$$

where K_{a1}, K_{a2}, and K_{a3} are respective dissociation constants for each buffer pair. Since the buffer pair considered in clinical practice is $[H_2CO_3]/[HCO_3^-]$, we use the following formula:

$$[H^+] = 24 \frac{P_{CO_2}}{[HCO_3]}$$

which is the Henderson equation.

2. In metabolic disturbances, the ECF HCO_3^- system plays a key role. In contrast, buffering during respiratory disturbances is mostly intracellular (because non-bicarbonate buffers have a high intracellular concentration. Bone plays a clear role in metabolic acidosis. Quantitatively, it has been estimated that when a fixed acid load (HCl) is infused into the bloodstream of a mammal, about half of the total-body buffering occurs in the ECF with the other half taking place in the ICF and bone. Thus, the regulation of pH is a dynamic balancing act between processes that alter $[HCO_3^-]$ and P_{CO_2} and pathways that return them to their normal values. This interplay of opposing processes is the essence of acid-base physiology.

Chapter 36

Respiratory Regulation of Acid-Base Balance

I. INTRODUCTION. It is not immediately apparent that the actual quantities of CO_2 and O_2 transported in the blood are far greater than the amounts of these gases in physical solution, because these gases are transported mainly in the form of chemical derivatives. Furthermore, it is even less apparent that there is far more total CO_2 than O_2 in every liter of blood. At the level of the lung, the HCO_3^- combines with the potential protons (i.e., the protons associated with $HHbO_2$) to produce HbO_2^- and H_2CO_3, resulting in the elimination of the protons as CO_2 and water.* Thus, free H^+ never appear to any appreciable extent but are in the form of HHb or H_2CO_3. **The entire respiratory cycle can be regarded as an exchange of a HCO_3^- for a HbO_2^-,** with the HCO_3^- transported from the tissues to the lungs and the HbO_2^- transported to the tissues from the lungs (see Chapter 17 III).

II. BLOOD FORMS OF CO_2

A. **CO_2 is transported in three forms.** However, H_2CO_3 ultimately must be converted to CO_2 to be eliminated through the lungs.

1. HCO_3^- accounts for 90% of the total CO_2 in plasma.

2. Carbamino compounds (i.e., carbamates of hemoglobin and protein) represent the combination of CO_2 with free NH_2 groups of blood proteins according to the equation:

$$R \cdot NH_2 + CO_2 \rightleftharpoons R \cdot NHCOO^- + H^+$$

About 5% of the CO_2 normally carried in arterial blood is in the form of carbamino compounds (carbamates).

3. A small amount of CO_2 gas (5%) is physically dissolved in plasma and also hydrated as H_2CO_3. Also, approximately 500 mmol of CO_2 exist for every 1 mmol of H_2CO_3 (see Chapter 34 IV B 1 a).

B. It is important to recognize that the term "bicarbonate" is used interchangeably with the term "total CO_2 combining power" or "total CO_2." This must never be confused with the term "partial pressure of CO_2," which is the PCO_2 of the arterial blood gas measurement.

1. The laboratory report does not say $[HCO_3^-]$. Rather, it says "total CO_2" or "carbon dioxide" or maybe just "CO_2" (with no "P").

2. Clinical laboratories typically measure $[HCO_3^-]$ indirectly by means of a technique that produces carbon dioxide gas. They add strong acid to the plasma sample, and protons from the acid react with plasma HCO_3^-, as:

$$HCO_3^- + H^+ \rightarrow H_2O + CO_2$$

   a. For each millimole of HCO_3^- in the plasma, 1 mmol of CO_2 is liberated.
   b. The concentration of CO_2 is then determined by an electronic sensor. It is this concentration that is reported as "CO_2" or "total CO_2."

3. Total CO_2 content = $[HCO_3^-]$ + $[CO_2]$ dissolved + $[H_2CO_3]$ in mmols per liter.

C. In blood with an arterial O_2 tension of 100 mm Hg and a mixed venous O_2 tension of 40

---

*$HhbO_2$ and HbO_2^- are forms of oxygenated hemoglobin and constitute a buffer pair, where the protonated form, $HHbO_2$, is the conjugate acid and the unprotonated form, HbO_2^-, is the conjugate base.

mm Hg, there are 200 ml O_2/L and 150 ml O_2/L of arterial and mixed venous blood, respectively. However, the arterial CO_2 tension and mixed venous CO_2 tension are associated with 480 ml CO_2/L and 520 ml CO_2/L of arterial and mixed venous blood, respectively.

III H_2CO_3 AND OTHER CO_2-FORMING ACIDS

A. Source

1. The oxidation of glucose and triglyceride leads to the formation of CO_2, much of which is hydrated to H_2CO_3. H_2CO_3, in turn, dissociates into H^+ and HCO_3^-.

2. CO_2 and water are the most abundant end products of metabolism.
   a. Lactic acid, a noncarbonic acid, normally is metabolized to CO_2 and water.
   b. The ketone bodies, β-hydroxybutyric acid and acetoacetic acid, also are noncarbonic acids, which are produced primarily by the liver during fasting. On reingestion, these acids that have accumulated are further catabolized to CO_2 and water by the extrahepatic tissues.

B. Elimination

1. Respiration accounts for the greatest portion of acid eliminated continuously from the body.

2. The lungs eliminate H_2CO_3 in the dehydrated (anhydrous) form of CO_2. Indeed, the unique property of the CO_2/HCO_3^- buffer system lies in the ability of the lungs to eliminate undissociated H_2CO_3 as nonionizable CO_2.

C. Buffering of H_2CO_3. Because CO_2 readily penetrates cellular membranes, H_2CO_3 is buffered by the entire body.

1. Most of the buffering of H_2CO_3 occurs via the nonbicarbonate buffer systems within erythrocytes. The H^+ derived from the dissociation of H_2CO_3 is buffered primarily by the hemoglobin buffer system.

2. The erythrocyte bicarbonate buffer and the plasma bicarbonate buffer play no role in the buffering of H_2CO_3.

3. Although HCO_3^- is an effective buffer for noncarbonic acids, it cannot buffer H_2CO_3, because the combination of H^+ with HCO_3^- results in the regeneration of H_2CO_3 as:

$$H_2CO_3 + HCO_3^- \rightarrow HCO_3^- + H_2CO_3$$

Exercise

The H_2CO_3/HCO_3^- has several unique characteristics that make it a valuable buffer system. Describe some of these characteristics.

DISCUSSION

1. One characteristic that makes the H_2CO_3/HCO_3^- system valuable is that the size of this buffer system is large enough to provide approximately 600 mEq of HCO_3^- to neutralize an equally large acid load.

2. It is necessary to be reminded that the $[H^+]$ is determined by the ratio of the components of the buffer pair (HA/A^-)—for example, the ratio of $H_2PO_4^-$/HPO_4^{2-} or the ratio of H_2CO_3/HCO_3^-. An acid load typically diminishes the denominator and increases the numerator of this ratio to the same degree. Thus, with most buffer systems, the ratio is changed by both a decrease in the denominator and by an increase in the numerator.

Although this concept is true for most buffer systems including the HPr/Pr^- and $H_2PO_4^-/HPO_4^{2-}$, the H_2CO_3/HCO_3^- is an exception. Since the numerator (H_2CO_3) is in equilibrium with a gas (CO_2) and therefore does not accumulate, the change in $[H^+]$ is exclusively the result of a decrease in the denominator. This release of the volatile acid form of the buffer pair from the solution greatly increases the buffer value of the system.

3. Another characteristic of the H_2CO_3/HCO_3^- system relates to the physiologic mechanisms that are readily available to (a) minimize the change in the respiratory (CO_2) or metabolic (HCO_3^-) component that was primarily altered (e.g., lactic acidosis induces a decrease in pH that inhibits lactic acid production via glycolysis); (b) tend to preserve the ratio of the buffer pair by altering the concentration of the other component in the same direction (e.g., HCl-induced depletion of HCO_3^- results in a prompt decrease in PCO_2, the respiratory response to acidemia (hyperventilation).

4. Carbon dioxide can be formed from H_2CO_3 and, in turn, CO_2 can be eliminated by the lungs, making H_2CO_3 a volatile acid. The kidneys can regulate $[HCO_3^-]$. Hence, two organ systems can regulate the two members of the HCO_3^- buffer system ($[HCO_3^-]$ and CO_2) independently.

Chapter 37

Renal Regulation of Acid-Base Balance

I. OVERVIEW

A. Normal acid-base conditions met by the kidneys

1. The kidneys are responsible for ridding the body of metabolically produced noncarbonic acids.

   a. Among these are sulfuric and phosphoric acids and smaller amounts of hydrochloric, lactic, uric, β-hydroxybutyric, and acetoacetic acids.

   b. About half of these metabolically produced acids are neutralized by base in the diet. The other half must be neutralized by buffer anion systems of the body. Of those noncarbonic acids buffered in the extracellular fluid, 97%–98% are buffered by reacting with HCO_3^-.

2. Type of diet is a major determinant of the daily acid-base conditions that must be regulated by the kidneys.

   a. High-protein diets contain large amounts of sulfur in the form of sulfhydryl groups. The sulfur is oxidized to sulfate ion (SO_4^{2-}), a process that tends to lead to metabolic acidosis.

   b. Vegetarian diets are associated with large intakes of lactate and acetate, and the metabolites of these anions tend to lead to metabolic alkalosis.

B. Kidney function

1. The primary role of the kidneys in acid-base regulation is to conserve major cations and anions in the body fluids. To maintain the total quantities and concentrations of the major electrolytes within normal limits, the kidneys perform two major functions.

   a. The kidneys stabilize the standard HCO_3^- pool by obligatory reabsorption (mainly by the proximal tubule) and by controlled reabsorption of filtered HCO_3^- (by the distal and collecting tubules).

   b. The kidneys excrete a daily load of 40–80 mEq of metabolically produced noncarbonic acid.* This represents a H^+ excretion of about 1 mEq/kg of body weight/day.

      (1) In most cases, 25% of this noncarbonic acid (10–30 mEq/day) is excreted in the form of titratable acid (see IV).

      (2) About 75% (30–50 mEq/day) is excreted in the form of acid combined with ammonia to form **ammonium** (i.e., NH_4^+; see V).

      (3) The normal urinary ratio of NH_4^+ to **titratable acid** is between 1 and 2.5.

2. The major sites of urine acidification are the distal and collecting tubules.

   a. Essentially all the H^+ within the tubular lumen is from the tubular secretion of H^+ generated by metabolism. There is no significant contribution of H^+ from the glomerular filtrate, which accounts for less than 0.1 mmol of H^+ per day.

   b. Since the lowest pH attainable in urine is 4.4 (i.e., a $[H^+]$ of 40×10^{-6} Eq/L) and the plasma $[H^+]$ is 40×10^{-9} Eq/L, the kidney can cause a 1000-fold $[H^+]$ gradient between plasma and urine.

3. An important difference between the acidification of urine and free H^+ excretion is that the ability to reduce urinary pH (acidification) does not reveal a great deal about the amount of **free** H^+ excreted. This is because most of the H^+ that is excreted occurs in association with an anion (mostly as $H_2PO_4^-$) or in combination with ammonia (as NH_4^+).

---

*In normal individuals in Western countries, a net of 40–80 mEq of noncarbonic acid is excreted daily.

4. Most secreted H^+ is used to bring about HCO_3^- reabsorption and therefore is not excreted.

II. BASIC ION EXCHANGE MECHANISMS (Figures 37–1; 37–2)

A. **Transport of Na^+.** Entry of Na^+ into the luminal (adluminal) membrane of the tubular cell is operationally linked to the secretion of H^+ into the tubular lumen. (It is a cation-exchange process that maintains intracellular electroneutrality.)

1. Although the movement of Na^+ across the luminal membrane is favored by the electrochemical gradient, the transport is mediated by specific membrane transport proteins (i.e., it is carrier-mediated) and is *not* by simple diffusion.

2. Secretion of H^+ is active in that it occurs against an electrochemical gradient.

3. The process of H^+ secretion and HCO_3^- reabsorption occurs throughout the nephron, with the exception of the descending limb of the loop of Henle.

4. The Na^+-H^+ antiporter is the major mechanism for H^+ secretion in the proximal tubule and thick ascending limb of the loop of Henle. This antiporter system is termed "secondary active" transport because the energy is derived from the Na^+ concentration gradient and not directly from the hydrolysis of adenosine triphosphate (ATP).

5. The Na^+-H^+ antiporter exchanges one Na^+ for one H^+ and, therefore, is electroneutral.

B. **Active transport of Na^+.** Subsequent to the downhill transport of Na^+ across the luminal membrane, Na^+ is actively reabsorbed across the basolateral (abluminal) membrane into the peritubular capillary in association with HCO_3^- that was formed within the cell. The

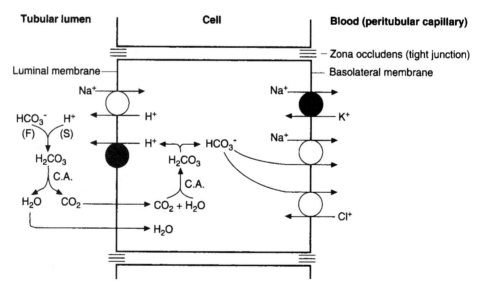

FIGURE 37-1. Major cellular and luminal processes in HCO_3^- reabsorption in the proximal tubule. The proximal nephron accounts for the largest fraction of HCO_3^- reabsorption, and it occurs by secondary active transport (antiport) via the Na^+-H^+ exchanger rather than by direct reabsorption. The secreted H^+ reacts with filtered HCO_3^- to form carbonic acid, which is dehydrated to CO_2 and H_2O, both of which diffuse into the cell. Note that the secreted H^+, which combined with HCO_3^- in the lumen, is not excreted. Whether H^+ are secreted by a Na^+-H^+ exchanger or by a H^+ pump at the luminal membrane, the filtered HCO_3^- will be converted to H_2CO_3 and subsequently to CO_2 and H_2O. *C.A.* = carbonic anhydrase; ● = H^+- or Na^+-K^+-adenosine triphosphatase (ATPase) pump; ○ = protein carrier; *F* = filtered; *S* = secreted.

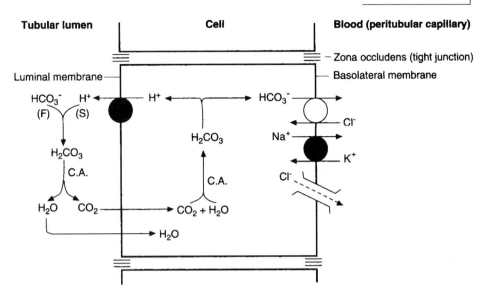

FIGURE 37-2. H^+ secretion and HCO_3^- reabsorption in the type A intercalated cell of the collecting tubules. Unlike the proximal tubule, the collecting duct lacks luminal carbonic anhydrase (C.A.). ● = adenosine triphosphatase (ATPase) pump; ○ = protein carrier; ⇌ = channel; F = filtered; S = secreted.

secretion of 1 mol of H^+ leads to the reabsorption of 1 mol of Na^+ and 1 mol of HCO_3^- in the peritubular blood.

1. H^+ for secretion originates from the hydration-dissociation reaction within the tubular cell [see Chapter 34 IV B 1 a, equation (4)].

2. H^+ secretion exceeds H^+ excretion; the amount of H^+ excreted in the form of free H^+ is negligible.

3. The net effect of H^+ secretion is to facilitate the transfer of HCO_3^- from tubular lumen to tubular cell.

4. It is probable that H^+ secretion along the entire tubule is mediated by an active transport process.

III. **REABSORPTION OF HCO_3^-** (see Figures 37–1; 37–2). The filtered HCO_3^- is not directly reabsorbed by the renal tubules; instead, it must first be converted to H_2CO_3, with the H^+ secreted into the tubular lumen in exchange for the Na^+ that is transported from the lumen. The HCO_3^- is reabsorbed indirectly by conversion to CO_2 within the tubular lumen, and most of the H^+ is reabsorbed after its conversion to water within the lumen. HCO_3^- reabsorption is an active process but is not accomplished in the conventional manner via an active pump for HCO_3^- either at the luminal or basolateral membranes. Rather, **HCO_3^- reabsorption involves the tubular secretion of H^+.**

A. **Proximal reabsorption.** Since the glomerular filtration rate (GFR) is about 180 L/day and the plasma $[HCO_3^-]$ is about 24 mEq/L (24 mmol/L), the daily filtered load of HCO_3^- is 4320 mEq (i.e., 180 L/day × 24 mEq/L). Almost all of this filtered HCO_3^- is reabsorbed.

1. Between 80% and 85% of the filtered load of HCO_3^- is reabsorbed proximally.
   a. The secretion of H^+ by the proximal tubule and the thick segment of the ascending limb of the loop of Henle is mediated primarily by the luminal $Na^+ = H^+$ antiporter, which accounts for two-thirds of the total H^+ secretion by the nephron.

    b. The Na^+-H^+ countertransporter is a secondary active transport system, because the energy for H^+ secretion is derived from the lumen-to-cell Na^+ concentration gradient and not directly from the hydrolysis of ATP.

    c. The net result is that for every H^+ secreted into the lumen, a HCO_3^- enters the blood in the peritubular capillaries.

2. Other characteristics of proximal tubular function

    a. Ammonium (NH_4^+) can substitute for H^+ on the Na^+-H^+-exchanger and hence provide a mechanism for NH_4^+ secretion.

    b. The proximal tubule is the major nephron site for the production and secretion of NH_4^+.

    c. The amount of NH_4^+ added to the luminal fluid is equal to the amount of NH_4^+ excreted in the final urine.

    d. Every H^+ secreted into the lumen leaves a HCO_3^- within the tubular cell that is passively transported into the systemic circulation via the $3HCO_3^-$-$1Na^+$ symporter located in the basolateral membrane. Most (90%) of the HCO_3^- transport across the basolateral membrane occurs via this cotransporter.

    e. The proximal tubule is the major site for the intraluminal generation of titratable acid.

3. Characteristics of the Na^+-H^+ antiporter

    a. The main determinant of proximal Na^+ and water reabsorption

    b. Promotes HCO_3^- reabsorption via the secretion of H^+

    c. Promotes active Cl^- reabsorption by operating in parallel with the Cl^--formate exchanger

    d. Provides the concentration gradient for passive Cl^- reabsorption (paracellular) by promoting preferential HCO_3^- and water reabsorption.

4. The presence of carbonic anhydrase on the microvilli of the luminal border (brush border) of the proximal tubules catalyzes the rapid extracellular dehydration of H_2CO_3 to form CO_2 and water.[*]

5. CO_2 diffuses back into the proximal tubular cell, where it is rehydrated by intracellular carbonic anhydrase into H_2CO_3. The HCO_3^- formed by the dissociation of H_2CO_3 is passively reabsorbed into the peritubular blood along with Na^+, which is actively transported into the peritubular blood. The H^+ formed by the dissociation of H_2CO_3 serves as a source for another H^+ to be secreted.

6. It is important to note that the Na^+ delivered to the peritubular capillaries comes from the filtrate in the lumen, but the HCO_3^- transported into the capillaries is synthesized within the proximal tubular cell.

7. Any secreted H^+ that combines with HCO_3^- in the lumen to bring about HCO_3^- reabsorption DOES NOT contribute to the urinary excretion of acid. Thus, most of the secreted H^+ is used to accomplish HCO_3^- reabsorption and not H^+ excretion (Figures 37-1 and 37-2).

8. Referring to this process as HCO_3^- reabsorption, then, seems inaccurate, since the HCO_3^- that appears in the peritubular capillaries is not the same HCO_3^- that was filtered. Moreover, most of the H^+ that was secreted into the lumen is not excreted in the urine but is incorporated into water and reabsorbed.

9. There is no absolute maximal tubular transport capacity for HCO_3^-, since the reabsorptive capacity for HCO_3^- varies directly with the fractional reabsorption of Na^+.

B. | **Reabsorption from the distal and collecting tubules**

1. The remaining 10%–15% of the filtered HCO_3 is reabsorbed in the distal tubule (thick segment of the ascending limb of the loop of Henle) and the collecting tubules (type A intercalated cells).

---

[*]Intracellular carbonic anhydrase is found throughout the renal tubule, including the distal convoluted tubule and collecting duct. In the proximal convoluted tubule, carbonic anhydrase also is located on the luminal cell membranes.

2. H^+ secretion by the distal nephron occurs primarily via the H^+-ATPase (i.e., $3H^+$-AT-Pase uniporter) pump in the luminal membrane of the type A intercalated cell. Aldosterone enhances the activity of this pump.

3. HCO_3^- returns to the circulation across the basolateral membrane of the collecting duct (type A intercalated cell) via a $Cl^- HCO_3^-$ exchanger.

4. Other characteristics of the cortical collecting duct (CCD)
   a. The capacity to reabsorb HCO_3^- via H^+ secretion by the H^+-ATPase uniporter in the luminal border of the A cells (intercalated cells).
   b. The capacity to secrete HCO_3^- via the electroneutral Cl^--HCO_3^- antiporter in the luminal membrane of the B cells (intercalated cells).

C. **Addition of new HCO_3^-.** In addition to the renal conservation of HCO_3^-, the kidneys **add** newly synthesized HCO_3^- to the plasma so that the quantity of HCO_3^- in the renal vein exceeds the amount that entered the kidneys.

1. The addition of new HCO_3^- to the plasma does not involve the HCO_3^- reabsorbed into the tubule but the HCO_3^- **generated** within the tubular cell via the hydration of CO_2 and dissociation of H_2CO_3. This process is similar to the scheme for the reabsorption of filtered HCO_3^-; however, **the HCO_3^- that is generated within the tubular cell does not represent filtered HCO_3^-.**

2. The renal contribution of new HCO_3^- is accompanied by the excretion of an equivalent amount of acid in the urine in the form of titratable acid, NH_4^+, or both.

3. The amount of new HCO_3^- formed per day (approximately 70–100 mEq) is much less than the quantity of filtered HCO_3^- reabsorbed per day (more than 4320 mEq).

4. When a secreted H^+ combines with a **nonbicarbonate** buffer in the lumen, it is excreted.

5. It is essential to appreciate that the loss of filtered HCO_3^- in the urine is equivalent to the addition of H^+ to the body, since both are derived from the dissociation of H_2CO_3.

6. Also essential to understand is that the excretion of H^+ is quantitatively equivalent to the addition of new HCO_3^- to the body.

IV. EXCRETION OF TITRATABLE ACID (Figure 37–3; Table 37–1)

A. **Filtration of HPO_4^{2-}.** Titratable acid denotes that portion of H^+ bound to filtered buffers and equals the amount of alkali, in the form of sodium hydroxide (NaOH), required to titrate urine back to the normal pH of blood (i.e., the number of milliequivalents of H^+ added to the tubular fluid that combined with phosphate or organic buffers).

1. Titratable acid is largely attributed to the conversion of HPO_4^{2-} to $H_2PO_4^-$. Additional buffer species that may contribute to titratable acid are creatinine, uric acid, β-hydroxybutyrate, and SO_4^{2-}.

2. Titratable acid is a poor measure of the total amount of H^+ secreted by the tubules, since most of the acid produced by this secretion is H_2CO_3, which disappears from the urine as CO_2. However, the H^+ that is trapped by anions of noncarbonic acids remains in the final urine in the form of titratable acid.

3. Titratable acid is a measure of the content of weak acids. It is not a measure of the H^+ that combines with ammonia (NH_3) to yield NH_4^+, because the pK' of the NH_3/NH_4^+ buffer system is high (9.2).

4. The proximal tubule is the major nephron site where titratable acid is formed. Additional titratable acid is generated along the collecting duct by a H^+-ATPase pump.

B. **Excretion of $H_2PO_4^-$.** The exchange of H^+ for Na^+ converts dibasic sodium phosphate ($Na_2HPO_4^{2-}$) in the glomerular filtrate into dihydrogen phosphate (NaH_2PO_4), which is ex-

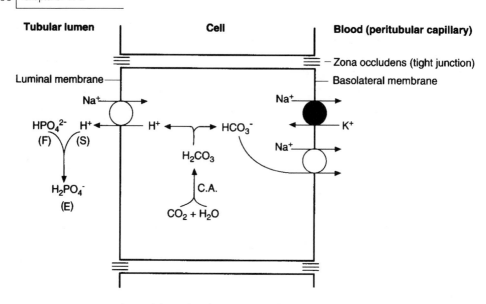

FIGURE 37-3. Formation of titratable acid in the proximal tubule. Note that a "new" HCO_3^- is returned to the peritubular capillary for every H^+ that is secreted and excreted. *C.A.* = carbonic anhydrase; ● = Na^+-K^+-adenosine triphosphatase (ATPase) pump; ○ = protein carrier; *F* = filtered; *S* = secreted; E = excreted.

TABLE 37-1. Urinary Acid Excretion in Health and Disease (in mEq H^+/day)

Urinary Acid	Normal Excretion	Excretion in Diabetic Ketoacidosis
Titratable acid	10–30	75–250
Ammonium	30–50	300–500
Total	40–80	375–750

creted in the urine as titratable acid. The H^+ secreted into the tubules, therefore, can react with filtered HPO_4^{2-} rather than the filtered HCO_3^-.

1. Besides HCO_3^-, HPO_4^{2-} represents a major filtered conjugate base.* Furthermore, the $HPO_4^{2-}/H_2PO_4^-$ buffer pair provides an excellent buffer system because it has a pK' of 6.8.

2. The **blood** $HPO_4^{2-}/H_2PO_4^-$ molar ratio is 4:1. The H^+ secretory system converts much of the HPO_4^{2-} to $H_2PO_4^-$ in the tubular fluid, resulting in a urinary $HPO_4^{2-}/H_2PO_4^-$ molar ratio of 1:4. The acidification of the phosphate buffer system occurs significantly in the proximal tubule, and much of the H^+ generated by the formation of H_2SO_4 and H_3PO_4 during protein and phospholipid metabolism is excreted in this way.

3. H^+ secreted into the lumen that reacts with HCO_3^- is not excreted, whereas H^+ secreted into the lumen that reacts with a nonbicarbonate buffer remains in the tubular fluid and is excreted.

4. Urinary phosphate is the major anion contributing to urine acid excretion.

5. Virtually all of the filtered phosphate is reabsorbed by the Na^+-phosphate symporter of the proximal tubular brush border.

*Since about 75% of the filtered HPO_4^{2-} is reabsorbed, only about 25% of the filtered HPO_4^{2-} is available for buffering.

C. Role of aldosterone in H$^+$ excretion. Aldosterone exerts its major renal effect on the collecting duct (type A intercalated cells and principal cells).

1. Aldosterone plays an important role in regulating collecting duct HCO$_3^-$ reabsorption via its stimulatory effect on H$^+$ secretion.

2. Aldosterone stimulates H$^+$ secretion directly on the tubular cell.

3. Aldosterone stimulates H$^+$ secretion indirectly by increasing Na$^+$ reabsorption.

V. **EXCRETION OF AMMONIUM (NH$_4^+$)** [Figures 37–4 A and C; see Table 37–1]. Unlike phosphate, NH$_3$ enters the tubular lumen not by filtration but by tubular synthesis and secretion, which normally are confined to the distal and collecting tubules.

A. Secretion of NH$_3$. NH$_3$ is synthesized mainly by the deamidation and deamination of glutamine in the presence of glutaminase. Most of the **NH$_4^+$** excreted in the urine is produced in the **proximal** tubular cells from amino acids, primarily glutamine.

1. The NH$_4^+$ that are formed are actively secreted into the lumen and are excreted in the final urine at a rate equal to their secretion rate.

2. With regard to proximal NH$_4^+$ secretion, it must be emphasized that the traditional view that states that NH$_3^+$ combines with the H$^+$ derived from the dissociation of H$_2$CO$_3$ is incorrect. Instead, the H$^+$ produced in the metabolism of glutamine results in the formation of NH$_4^+$ within the proximal tubular cell (see Figure 37–4).

3. The mechanism of distal nephron NH$_4^+$ excretion is different from that in the proximal tubule (see Figures 33–1; 37–4).

B. Formation of NH$_4^+$. The NH$_3^+$/NH$_4^+$ system has a very high pK′ (about 9.2), which means that, at the usual urine pH, almost all the nonpolar NH$_3^+$ that enters the distal tubular lumen immediately combines with H$^+$ to form NH$_4^+$, which is nondiffusible because it is lipid-insoluble. The renal excretion of NH$_4^+$ causes the net addition of HCO$_3^-$ to the plasma.

1. The important physiologic characteristic of the NH$_3^+$/NH$_4^+$ buffer pair is that, as H$^+$ is combined with intraluminal buffer (NH$_3^+$), H$^+$ is excreted in the urine as NH$_4^+$, a substance that does not cause the pH of urine to fall.

2. Under most conditions, the excretion of NH$_4^+$ is quantitatively more important to the acid-base balance of the body than is the excretion of titratable acid. The normal kidney excretes almost twice as much acid combined with NH$_3^+$ (30–50 mEq/day) as titratable acid (10–30 mEq/day) [see Table 37–1].
   a. In chronic severe metabolic acidosis, NH$_3^+$ serves as the major urinary buffer, and NH$_4^+$ excretion can increase from a normal value of 30 mEq/day to 500 mEq/day. However, in chronic acidosis, the excretion of H$_2$PO$_4^-$ may increase by only 20–40 mEq/day.
   b. In diabetic ketoacidosis, the excretion of titratable acid may reach 75–250 mEq/day, whereas the excretion of acid combined with NH$_3^+$ may reach amounts of 300–500 mEq/day. However, the ratio of NH$_4^+$ to titratable acid remains within the normal range of 1 to 2.5.

C. Excretion of H$^+$. The sum of titratable acid and urinary NH$_4^+$ excretion represents the net gain of HCO$_3^-$ for the body fluids.

1. The net amount of fixed acid excreted (in mEq/day) equals the sum of titratable acid and NH$_4^+$ minus the urinary [HCO$_3^-$].

2. Normally, the urine is free of HCO$_3^-$, because all the HCO$_3^-$ remaining in the distal and collecting tubules has combined with secreted H$^+$ and reabsorbed.

3. Aldosterone enhances NH$_3^+$ production via an effect on cellular metabolism.

4. Net acid excretion (NAE) is mathematically expressed as the sum of the excretion rates of titratable acidity (TA) and ammonium (NH$_4^+$) minus the excretion rate of HCO$_3^-$ as:

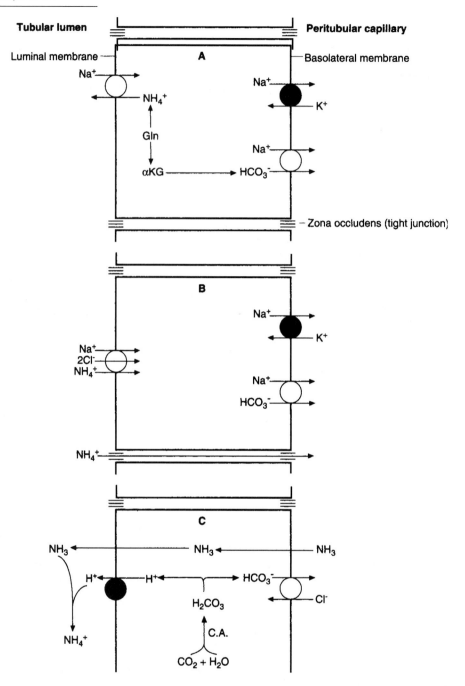

FIGURE 37-4. Mechanism of NH_4^+ transport in the proximal tubule (*A*), the thick ascending limb of the loop of Henle (*B*), and the type A intercalated cells of the collecting duct (*C*). In *A*, glutamine (*Gln*) is taken up by the cells and metabolized into NH_4^+ and α-ketoglutarate (*αKG*). In *B*, NH_4^+ is transported by the Na^+-$2Cl^-$-NH_4^+ symporter and by paracellular transport. In *C*, NH_3 diffuses from the interstitial fluid into the lumen, where it combines with secreted H^+ to form NH_4^+. Note that a "new" HCO_3^- is returned to the peritubular capillary for every H^+ that is secreted and excreted as an NH_4^+. *C.A.* = carbonic anhydrase; ● = H^+- or Na^+-K^+-adenosine triphosphatase (ATPase) pump; ○ = protein carrier.

$$NAE = [(U_{TA} \cdot \dot{V}) + (U_{NH_4^+} \cdot \dot{V})] - (U_{HCO_3^-} \cdot \dot{V})$$

where TA = titratable acid, U = urinary concentration, and $\dot{V}$ = urine flow rate.

VI. BOOKKEEPING OF H⁺ BALANCE AND THE RELATION TO HCO₃⁻ BALANCE: A SUMMARY WITH NORMAL VALUES

A. Filtered load of HCO₃⁻ ($\dot{F}_{HCO_3^-}$)

$$\dot{F}_{HCO_3^-} = GFR \times [HCO_3^-]$$
$$= 180 \text{ L/day} \times 24 \text{ mEq/L}$$
$$= 4320 \text{ mEq/day}$$

where GFR = glomerular filtration rate.

There is no filtered load for H⁺ (<0.1 mEq/day), but the reabsorption of 4320 mEq of HCO₃⁻ requires the **secretion** of 4320 mEq of H⁺!

B. Rate of excretion of H⁺, also termed net acid excretion (NAE), is the sum of the excretion rates ($\dot{E}$) of titratable acid (TA) and ammonium (NH₄⁺) minus the excretion rate of HCO₃⁻. Remember that the excretion rate of H⁺ is about 1 mEq/day per kilogram of body weight.

$$NAE = (\dot{E}_{TA} + \dot{E}_{NH_4^+}) - \dot{E}_{HCO_3^-}$$
$$NAE = [(U_{TA} \cdot \dot{V}) + (U_{NH_4^+} \cdot \dot{V})] - (U_{HCO_3^-} \cdot \dot{V})$$
$$= (20 \text{ mEq/day} + 40 \text{ mEq/day}) - 0 \text{ mEq/day}$$
$$= 60 \text{ mEq/day} = \text{generated or "new" } HCO_3^-$$

Note that the excretion of H⁺ and renal generation of "new" HCO₃⁻ added to the plasma are quantitatively equivalent statements.

C. Secretion rate ($\dot{S}$) of H⁺

$$\dot{S}_{H^+} = \dot{F}_{HCO_3^-} + \dot{E}_{H^+}$$
$$= \dot{F}_{HCO_3^-} + NAE$$
$$= 4320 \text{ mEq/day} + 60 \text{ mEq/day}$$
$$= 4380 \text{ mEq/day}$$

Since the reabsorption of HCO₃⁻ is dependent on the secretion of H⁺, then the secretion of H⁺ is equal to the filtered load of HCO₃⁻ plus the excretion rate of H⁺ (i.e., NAE).

D. Reabsorption rate ($\dot{R}$) of H⁺

$$\dot{R}_{H^+} = \dot{R}_{HCO_3^-} = \dot{F}_{HCO_3^-} - \dot{E}_{HCO_3}$$
$$= 4320 \text{ mEq/day} - 0 \text{ mEq/day}$$
$$= 4320 \text{ mEq/day}$$

Remember that the reabsorption of one HCO₃⁻ requires the secretion of one H⁺. Also, most of the secreted H⁺ is reabsorbed and not excreted.

E. Total HCO₃⁻ added to plasma (T_{HCO3^-})

$$T_{HCO_3^-} = \dot{R}_{HCO_3^-} + NAE$$
$$= 4320 \text{ mEq/day} + 60 \text{ mEq/day}$$
$$= 4380 \text{ mEq/day}$$

NAE is equivalent to "new" HCO₃⁻ generated and added to the blood.

Exercises

1. How does the kidney regulate HCO_3^- concentration?
2. What is titratable acidity?
3. What is urinary ammonium?

DISCUSSION

1. The kidney regulates $[HCO_3^-]$ by two very different processes.
   a. Reabsorption of virtually all of the filtered HCO_3^- mainly by the proximal tubule where H^+ is secreted by the Na^+-H^+ exchanger. The secreted H^+ combines with the filtered HCO_3^- to form H_2CO_3 which is quickly converted to CO_2 and H_2O by luminal carbonic anhydrase. The CO_2 and H_2O are rapidly and passively reabsorbed and reconverted by intracellular carbonic anhydrase to H_2CO_3 which dissociates into H^+ and HCO_3^-. The HCO_3^- is returned to the systemic circulation primarily by a Na^+-$3HCO_3^-$ cotransporter, and the H^+ is transported into the tubular lumen. This is a high-capacity system because a large amount of HCO_3^- is filtered each day and must be reabsorbed:

   180 L/day $\times$ 24 mEq/L = 4320 mEq/day of HCO_3^- which must be reabsorbed!

   This process does not add net HCO_3^- to the extracellular fluid nor secrete net H^+ into the urine. It does nothing to change the acid-base status of the body because the total H^+ content does not change. This process only keeps HCO_3^- from being lost in the urine and prevents metabolic acidosis from developing.
   b. Renal excretion of H^+
   The second way the kidney controls $[HCO_3^-]$ is by eliminating enough H^+ equal to the amount of fixed (noncarbonic) acid produced each day. Remember that the removal of one H^+ is equivalent to the gain of one HCO_3^-. The removal of H^+ from the body by the kidney results in the generation of "new" HCO_3^- to replace the 40–80 mEq/day of HCO_3^-,which was used to buffer the daily production of fixed acid. The kidney does this by two mechanisms:
   (1) The combination of secreted H^+ with the urinary buffer HPO_4^{2-} to form $H_2PO_4^-$ (titratable acidity).
   (2) The formation of urinary NH_4^+, which has two possible origins. Ammonium can be formed in the proximal tubule from glutamine and secreted as NH_4^+ by the substitution for H^+ on the Na^+-H^+ exchanger or by the formation of NH_4^+ in the collecting duct lumen by the combination of secreted H^+ with secreted NH_3. Ammonium excretion is quantitatively more important than the secretion of H^+ in the generation of HCO_3^-.

2. Titratable acidity is the amount of alkali (NaOH) that must be added to a 24-hour urine collection to bring the urine pH to that of arterial blood (7.4). The normal value is 10–30 mEq/day, but it can increase to several hundred milliequivalent if the excretion of urinary weak acids is increased (i.e., ketoacidosis). The bulk of titratable acid is composed of monobasic phosphate ($H_2PO_4^-$) but also includes creatinine, uric acid, and ketoacids.

3. There are two sources of NH_4^+ found in the tubular fluid. In the proximal tubule, NH_4^+ is formed intracellularly from the metabolism of glutamine and secreted as NH_4^+. In the collecting duct, the nonpolar, lipid-soluble NH_3 diffuses (secretion) into the lumen, where it can combine with secreted H^+ to form NH_4^+. In normal subjects 30–50 mEq of H^+ are excreted daily as NH_4^+, but this amount can be increased many times in response to metabolic acidosis. Ammonification is the major renal adaptive response to increased acid loads in metabolic acidosis.

Chapter 38

Primary and Secondary Acid-Base Abnormalities

I. DEFINITIONS AND BASIC CONCEPTS (Tables 38–1, 38–2, 38–3, and 38–4)

A. Acidosis and alkalosis

1. **Acidosis** or **acidemia** is an abnormal clinical condition or process caused by the bodily accumulation of acid (or the loss of base) sufficient to decrease pH below 7.36 or to increase the [H$^+$] above 43.6 nEq/L of blood in the absence of compensatory (secondary) changes.

2. **Alkalosis** or **alkalemia** is an abnormal condition or process caused by the accumulation of base (or the loss of acid) sufficient to raise pH above 7.44 or to decrease the [H$^+$] below 36.3 nEq/L of blood in the absence of compensatory changes.

B. Respiratory and metabolic

1. The adjective **respiratory** denotes that the primary abnormality involves impairment in alveolar ventilation, which results in an abnormally high or low [total CO_2] of the extracellular fluid (ECF).* Table 38–2 lists normal reference values for pH, P_{CO_2}, and [$HCO_3{}^-$]. Note that [H$^+$] is measured in nanoequivalents per liter (nEq/L) and [$HCO_3{}^-$] is measured in milliequivalents per liter (mEq/L).
   a. **Respiratory acidosis** refers to a condition of abnormally high arterial CO_2 tension (P_{CO_2}), which is termed **hypercapnia** (hypercarbia).
   b. **Respiratory alkalosis** refers to a condition of abnormally low arterial CO_2 tension, which is called **hypocapnia** (hypocarbia).

2. The adjective **metabolic** denotes that the primary abnormality involves an abnormal gain or loss of noncarbonic acid by the ECF, which affects [$HCO_3{}^-$].
   a. **Metabolic acidosis** refers to a disturbance that leads to the accumulation of noncarbonic acid in the ECF or to the loss of $HCO_3{}^-$ from the ECF.
   b. **Metabolic alkalosis** refers to an imbalance characterized by a loss of noncarbonic acid or a gain of $HCO_3{}^-$ by the ECF.

C. Primary and secondary factors

1. The factor in the [$HCO_3{}^-$]/S · P_{CO_2} ratio (i.e., [$HCO_3{}^-$] or P_{CO_2}) that undergoes the greater degree of displacement (i.e., the larger proportional change) indicates the **primary abnormality** (see Tables 38–3 and 38–4).
   a. If the [$HCO_3{}^-$]/S · P_{CO_2} ratio becomes less than 20:1, by either decreasing the numerator or increasing the denominator, pH falls ($\uparrow$ [H$^+$]), and acidosis occurs.
   b. If the [$HCO_3{}^-$]/S · P_{CO_2} ratio becomes more than 20:1, by either increasing the numerator or decreasing the denominator, pH rises ($\downarrow$ [H$^+$]), and alkalosis occurs.

2. A **secondary response** in the alternate variable, which occurs in the same direction as the primary abnormality, counteracts the effect of the primary abnormality on the [$HCO_3{}^-$]/S · P_{CO_2} ratio. The secondary change represents **compensation** and acts to minimize the pH alteration produced by the primary disorder.

D. Simple and mixed acid-base disturbances

1. **Simple acid-base imbalances** are caused by one primary factor.

2. **Mixed acid-base imbalances** are caused by more than the primary factor.

---

*[Total CO_2] refers to the dissolved CO_2 (S · P_{CO_2}) plus the [$HCO_3{}^-$].

TABLE 38-1. Definitions of Acid-Base Terms

Acidemia	Serum pH < 7.36
Alkalemia	Serum pH > 7.44
Acidosis	A primary pathophysiologic process that increases the $[H^+]$ and decreases the serum pH
Alkalosis	A primary pathophysiologic process that decreases the $[H^+]$ and increases the serum pH
Metabolic acidosis	A primary process that causes $[HCO_3^-]$ to fall
Metabolic alkalosis	A primary process that causes $[HCO_3^-]$ to rise
Respiratory acidosis	A primary process that causes the PCO_2 to rise
Respiratory alkalosis	A primary process that causes the PCO_2 to fall
Mixed disorder	A condition in which more than one primary acid-base process is occurring
Compensation	A physiologic response to an acidosis or alkalosis that partially returns the pH toward normal

$[H^+]$ = hydrogen ion concentration.
$[HCO_3^-]$ = bicarbonate concentration; PCO_2 = partial pressure of carbon dioxide.

TABLE 38-2. Normal Serum Values for pH, $[H^+]$, $[HCO_3^-]$, and PCO_2

Normal serum pH	7.36–7.44
Normal serum $[H^+]$	40 nEq/L
Normal serum $[HCO_3^-]$	24 mEq/L
Normal serum PCO_2	40 mm Hg

$[H^+]$ = hydrogen ion concentration; $[HCO_3^-]$ = bicarbonate concentration; nEq/L = nanoequivalents per liter; mEq/L = milliequivalents per liter; mm Hg = millimeters of mercury; PCO_2 = partial pressure of carbon dioxide.

TABLE 38-3. Characteristics of the Uncompensated Acid-Base Abnormalities

Acid-Base Abnormality	Primary Disturbance	Effect on:			Compensatory Response
		$[HCO_3^-]/S \cdot PCO_2$	$[H^+]$	pH	
Acidosis					
Respiratory	↑ PCO_2	< 20	↑	↓	↑ $[HCO_3^-]$
Metabolic	↓ $[HCO_3^-]$	< 20	↑	↓	↓ PCO_2
Alkalosis					
Respiratory	↓ PCO_2	> 20	↓	↑	↓ $[HCO_3^-]$
Metabolic	↑ $[HCO_3^-]$	> 20	↓	↑	↑ PCO_2

Note—These conditions are simple disturbances (i.e., they represent the effects of one primary etiologic factor) and thus are termed uncompensated or pure acid-base abnormalities. The compensatory response always occurs in the same direction as the primary disturbance.

TABLE 38-4. Primary and Secondary* Changes in the CO_2/HCO_3^- System

	Acidosis		Alkalosis	
Respiratory	$\dfrac{[HCO_3^-] \;\uparrow}{S \cdot P_{CO_2}}$	< 20:1	$\dfrac{[HCO_3^-] \;\downarrow}{S \cdot P_{CO_2}}$	> 20:1
	$[total\ CO_2]^\dagger \uparrow$		$[total\ CO_2] \downarrow$	
Metabolic	$\dfrac{[HCO_3^-]}{S \cdot P_{CO_2} \;\downarrow}$	< 20:1	$\dfrac{[HCO_3^-]}{S \cdot P_{CO_2} \;\uparrow}$	> 20:1
	$[total\ CO_2]$		$[total\ CO_2]$	

Note—*Dashed arrows* denote direction of compensatory responses. *Thin solid arrows* show changes in [total CO_2] during respiratory imbalances. *Wide arrows* depict direction of change of primary acid-base imbalance and direction of change in [total CO_2]. (Adapted from Christensen HN: *Diagnostic Biochemistry.* New York, Oxford University Press, 1959, p 106.)

*A compensatory (secondary) response in the alternate variable occurs in the same direction and counteracts the effect of the primary disturbance by returning the $[HCO_3^-]$/$S \cdot P_{CO_2}$ ratio toward normal (20:1).

†[Total CO_2] does not always increase in alkalosis or decrease in acidosis. Dissolved CO_2 contributes little to the [total CO_2]. [Total CO_2] provides little information about pulmonary function.

    a. Mixed-type disturbances are not uncommon. Sometimes a primary abnormality of one type is superimposed on a primary abnormality of another type.
        (1) A patient with respiratory acidosis from pulmonary emphysema may develop metabolic acidosis from uncontrolled diabetes or metabolic alkalosis from large doses of corticosteroids used in the treatment of an attack of status asthmaticus.
        (2) A patient with a metabolic acid-base disturbance, in turn, may develop a respiratory acid-base abnormality.
    b. The changes in the variables may be difficult to interpret in mixed acid-base disturbances, because manifestations of one primary abnormality may be either cancelled out or augmented by those of the other primary abnormality. Therefore, **a normal pH may not necessarily mean a normal compensation in mixed acid-base imbalances.**

E. **Plasma $[HCO_3^-]$, CO_2 tension, and $[total\ CO_2]$.** For an adequate analysis of any acid-base disorder, it is necessary to measure pH, CO_2 tension, and the total CO_2 content of blood.

    1. **An acid-base disorder cannot be diagnosed with certainty from the plasma $[HCO_3^-]$ alone.** Although a reduction in the plasma $[HCO_3^-]$ may be due to metabolic acidosis, it also can indicate a renal compensation for respiratory alkalosis. Similarly, an elevated $[HCO_3^-]$ can result from a metabolic alkalosis or the secondary response to respiratory acidosis. Since the aim of therapy is to bring about acid-base balance and not to normalize $[HCO_3^-]$, it is necessary to measure the pH (i.e., $[H^+]$) when acid-base imbalance is suspected.

    2. **Low CO_2 tension** may be due to respiratory alkalosis or a respiratory compensation to metabolic acidosis. Similarly, a **high CO_2 tension** may be caused by respiratory acidosis or a respiratory compensatory response to metabolic alkalosis.

    3. **[Total CO_2]** does not always increase in alkalosis or decrease in acidosis (Figure 38–1; see Table 38–2). About 90% of the [total CO_2] of plasma is contributed by $[HCO_3^-]$, and 5% is contributed by dissolved CO_2 and H_2CO_3. Therefore, dissolved CO_2 contributes little to the [total CO_2]. The [total CO_2] gives little information about the functional status of the lungs.

    4. The physician accepts [total CO_2] and $[HCO_3^-]$ as essentially interchangeable terms. The [total CO_2] normally exceeds the $[HCO_3^-]$ by 1.2 mmol. Most laboratories measure the [total CO_2] and not the $[HCO_3^-]$.

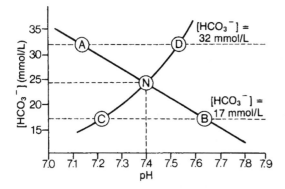

FIGURE 38-1. A pH-[HCO$_3^-$] Davenportgram illustrating that acidosis (*points A and C*) and alkalosis (*points B and D*) cannot be differentiated solely on the basis of [HCO$_3^-$] or [total CO$_2$]. The *[HCO$_3^-$]* pertains to plasma. A = respiratory acidosis; B = respiratory alkalosis; C = metabolic acidosis; D = metabolic alkalosis; and N = normal point. The slope of *line ANB* is a measure of the nonbicarbonate buffer capacity of whole blood. (After Davenport HW: *The ABC of Acid-Base Chemistry*, 5th edition. Chicago, University of Chicago Press, 1969, p 65.)

II. CLINICAL EXPRESSIONS FOR EVALUATION OF ACID-BASE STATUS

A. **Base excess (BE)** [Figure 38–2; Table 38–5]

1. **Definition.** BE refers to the change in the concentration of buffer base [BB] from its normal value, or the **observed [BB] minus the normal [BB]** in mEq/L of whole blood. The range of normality for BE is −2 to +2 mEq/L in arterial whole blood.[†]

   a. The [BB] in normal whole blood is 48 mEq/L, which is arbitrarily set to 0, and deviations (i.e., ±BE) are measured from this reference point.

   b. The normal [BB] of 48 mEq/L equals the sum of all the conjugate bases in 1 L of arterial whole blood. These bases and their concentrations are:
   - **(1)** [HCO$_3^-$] = 24 mEq/L
   - **(2)** [Protein$^-$] = 15 mEq/L
   - **(3)** [Hb$^-$/HbO$_2^-$] = 9 mEq/L

2. **Clinical application.** BE refers principally to the [HCO$_3^-$] but also to other bases in the blood (mainly plasma protein and hemoglobin). However, the [HCO$_3^-$] or [total CO$_2$] is used in acid-base problems as the indicator of BE.

   a. Because [HCO$_3^-$] and BE are influenced only by metabolic processes, there are only two acid-base conditions associated with abnormalities in [HCO$_3^-$] and BE.

   (1) **Metabolic acidosis.** When a metabolic process leads to the accumulation of noncarbonic acid in the body or the loss of HCO$_3^-$, the [HCO$_3^-$] falls, and the BE value becomes negative. Metabolic acidosis is associated with a BE below −5 mEq/L.

   (2) **Metabolic alkalosis.** When a metabolic process causes a loss of acid or an accumulation of HCO$_3^-$, the [HCO$_3^-$] rises above normal, and the BE value becomes positive. Metabolic alkalosis is associated with a BE above +5 mEq/L.

   b. The BE value serves only as a rough guide for alkalosis and acidosis therapy.

B. **Anion gap**

1. **Definition**

   a. The ionic profile (ionogram) of normal serum is depicted in Figure 38–3. The **law of electroneutrality** states that the number of positive charges in any solution must equal the number of negative charges. If every ion present in serum were measured, the concentration of cations would equal the concentration of anions if these concentrations were expressed in mEq/L. Routine serum electrolyte determinations measure essentially all cations but only a fraction of the anions. **This apparent disparity between the total cation concentration and the total anion concentration is termed the *anion gap.*** It is a virtual measurement and does not represent any specific ionic constituent.

   b. The anion gap, which has a normal value of 12 ± 4 mEq/L, reflects the concentra-

---

[†]Because BE is a negative or positive value, the term "base deficit" is avoided.

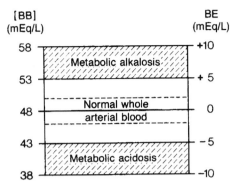

FIGURE 38-2. Diagram illustrating the relationship between base excess *[BE]* and the acid-base status of normal whole arterial blood. BE is the base concentration (in mEq/L), as measured by the titration with strong acid to pH 7.4, at CO_2 tension of 40 mm Hg, and at 37°C. For negative values of BE, the titration must be carried out with strong base. BE measures the change in the concentration of the buffer base (*[BB]*) from its normal value, which is 48 mEq/L in normal whole arterial blood. [BB] is the sum of the buffer anions of blood or plasma. When observed [BB] is less than normal [BB], BE is a negative value; when observed [BB] is greater than normal [BB], BE is a positive value; and when observed [BB] equals normal [BB], BE equals zero. (After Winters RW, et al: *Acid-Base Physiology in Medicine.* Westlake, Ohio, London Co, 1967, p 45.)

tions of those anions actually present but routinely undetermined (i.e., other than $[Cl^-]$ and $[HCO_3^-]$), such as:

(1) Polyanionic plasma proteins (primarily albumin)
(2) Inorganic phosphates
(3) Sulfate
(4) Ions of organic acids (e.g., lactic, β-hydroxybutyric, and acetoacetic acids)

  c. When the anion gap is increased, unmeasured anions fill this gap. (Most of these anions usually are the products of metabolic processes that generate H^+.)

2. Determination of anion gap (Figure 38–4)
  a. The anion gap (AG) equals 16 mEq/L of anions other than HCO_3^- and Cl^- when determined by the following equation:

$$AG = ([Na^+] + [K^+]) - ([HCO_3^-] + [Cl^-])$$

$$= (142\ mEq/L + 5\ mEq/L) - (25\ mEq/L + 105\ mEq/L)$$

$$= 145\ mEq/L - 130\ mEq/L$$

$$= 15\ mEq/L$$

  b. Often the anion gap is calculated with Na^+ as the major cation, because K^+ has a relatively minor quantitative contribution. The equation then becomes:

TABLE 38-5. Base Excess and Metabolic Acid-Base Abnormalities

$[HCO_3^-]$	Base Excess	Metabolic Abnormality	Characteristics
↑	+	Metabolic alkalosis	Noncarbonic acid is lost; HCO_3^- is gained
↓	−	Metabolic acidosis	Noncarbonic acid is gained; HCO_3^- is lost

Adapted from Broughton JO: *Understanding Blood Gases.* Madison, Wisconsin, Ohio Medical Products, form no. 456, 1979, p 8.

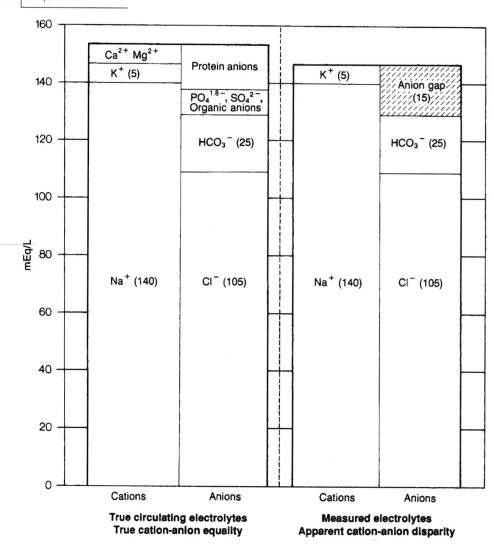

FIGURE 38-3. Ionogram for normal plasma concentrations of anions and cations in mEq/L shows that circulating cations always counterbalance anions, thereby maintaining electroneutrality (*left*). Routine electrolyte analyses measure only a portion of circulating anions, and an apparent cation-anion disparity exists (*right*). This difference, in mEq/L, is termed the anion gap. *Parentheses* indicate concentrations in mEq/L. (Reprinted from Narins RG, et al: Lactic acidosis and elevated anion gap (I). *Hosp Pract* 15:125–136, 1980. Original drawing by Albert Miller.)

$$AG = ([Na^+] - ([HCO_3^-] + [Cl^-])$$
$$= (142 \text{ mEq/L} - (25 \text{ mEq/L} + 105 \text{ mEq/L})$$
$$= 142 \text{ mEq/L} - 130 \text{ mEq/L}$$
$$= 12 \text{ mEq/L}$$

    c. The plasma proteins contribute a significant amount of negative charges and thus anionic equivalence (15 mEq/L). The plasma proteins account, almost stoichiometrically, for the difference between the $[Na^+]$ and the sum of $[HCO_3^-]$ and $[Cl^-]$.

3. Clinical application

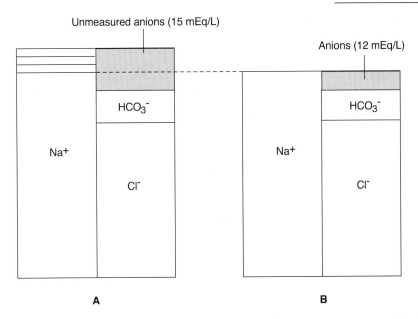

FIGURE 38-4. (*A*) Normal ionogram showing the major cation (Na^+) and the minor cations (K^+, Ca^{2+}, and Mg^{2+}). The major anions are Cl^- and HCO_3^-, but not the minor anions are albumin, phosphate, sulfate, and organic acids such as lactate and acetoacetate. (*B*) Simplified ionogram showing Na^+ as the only cation and making the anion column only as tall as the Na^+ column. The height of the columns indicates relative ion concentration in mEq/L.

a. **Acidification with acids other than HCl**
   (1) Organic acids increase the anion gap. In this case, the lost (neutralized) HCO_3^- is *not* replaced by the routinely unmeasured anions of noncarbonic acids such as lactic acid and the ketoacids. Thus, the anion gap is increased by all metabolic acidoses except the **hyperchloremic acidoses.** With the accumulation of acid, there is rapid extracellular buffering by HCO_3^-. If the acid is HCl, then

$$HCl + NaHCO_3 \rightleftharpoons NaCl + H_2CO_3$$

   The net effect is the milliequivalent-for-milliequivalent replacement of extracellular HCO_3^- by Cl^-. Since the sum of $[Cl^-]$ and $[HCO_3^-]$ remains constant, the anion gap is unchanged in hyperchloremic acidosis.
   (2) It is apparent that the decrease in plasma $[HCO_3^-]$ equals the increase in the anion gap (see Figure 38–3). The presence of an increased anion gap usually indicates an excess of H^+ derived from noncarbonic acid. Whatever the size of the anion gap, **it is the retention of H+—not the particular anion—that is responsible for the acidosis.**
   (a) An increased anion gap due to excess H^+ derived from noncarbonic acid occurs in **metabolic acidosis;** this also may result from a compensatory increase in lactic acid production in response to respiratory alkalosis via activation of the phosphofructokinase step in glycolysis.
   (b) In **respiratory acidosis,** the anion gap is not increased, because excess H^+ is derived from the H_2CO_3 pool, not the noncarbonic acid pool.
b. **Conditions that increase the anion gap** include diabetic and alcoholic ketoacidosis, intoxicant and lactic acidoses, and renal failure.
c. **Conditions that cause metabolic acidosis without an increase in the anion gap** are associated with a high serum $[Cl^-]$ and include diarrhea; pancreatic drainage; ureterosigmoidostomy; ileal loop conduit; treatment with acetazolamide, ammonium chloride, or arginine-HCl; renal tubular acidosis; and, rarely, intravenous hyperalimentation.

d. An elevation in anion gap is also a common finding in metabolic alkalosis owing to the increase in negative charges per albumin molecule, since the pH is farther away from the isoelectric point for albumin of approximately 5.4.

C. Osmolar gap

1. **Definition.** Osmolar gap refers to the disparity between the measured serum (plasma) osmolality and the calculated serum osmolality.

2. **Clinical application.** Osmolar gap measurement provides a reasonably good screening procedure for toxins. Other causes of metabolic acidosis do not affect the osmolar gap, since the metabolic acid simply replaces the HCO_3^- with another anion and HCO_3^- is lost as CO_2.

   a. Serum osmolality is estimated by dividing blood urea nitrogen (BUN) and glucose concentrations (in mg/L) by their molecular weights,[‡] thereby converting them to milliosmoles (mOsm)/L. Doubling the serum $[Na^+]$ (in mEq/L) provides an estimate of the serum ion concentration. With a BUN of 14 mg/dl, plasma glucose of 90 mg/dl, and a plasma $[Na^+]$ of 142 mEq/L, serum (plasma) osmolality (P_{osm}) is estimated as

$$P_{osm} = 2[Na^+] + [BUN\ (mg/L)/28] + [glucose\ (mg/L)/180]$$

$$= 2\ (142) + 140/28 + 900/180$$

$$= 286 + 5 + 5 = 296\ mOsm/kg$$

   b. Circulating intoxicants increase measured serum osmolality without altering serum $[Na^+]$. Therefore, the measured serum osmolality exceeds the calculated serum osmolality, and the difference closely reflects the osmolar concentration of the circulating toxins.

III. ANALYSIS OF ACID-BASE DISORDERS

A. The acid-base algorithm

1. **Example:** pH = 7.35; $[HCO_3^-]$ = 16 mEq/L; PCO_2 = 30 mm Hg. The acid-base disorder in the example can be determined by the three-step approach shown in the algorithm (Figure 38–5).

2. **Examination of the pH**
   a. The disorder can be classified as an acidosis (pH < 7.4).
   b. The disorder can be classified as an alkalosis (pH > 7.4). The example of 7.35 indicates an acidosis.

3. **Determination of metabolic versus respiratory imbalance.** Now the $[HCO_3^-]$ and PCO_2 must be examined.
   a. An acidosis could result from a decrease in $[HCO_3^-]$ (metabolic) or an increase in PCO_2 (respiratory). In the example, the $[HCO_3^-]$ is reduced (16 mEq/L), as is the PCO_2 (30 mm Hg). The disorder in the example must be a metabolic acidosis; it cannot be a respiratory acidosis because the PCO_2 is reduced.
   b. An alkalosis could be the result of an increase in $[HCO_3^-]$ (metabolic) or a decrease in PCO_2 (respiratory). In the example, there is a decline in PCO_2 but the patient has an acidosis (pH = 7.35).

4. **Analysis of the compensatory response**
   a. Metabolic disorders result in compensatory changes in ventilation and thus in PCO_2.
      (1) In compensated metabolic acidosis, the PCO_2 is decreased (as in the example).

[‡]The molecular weight of urea (60) is not used because it is BUN that is measured, and urea contains two nitrogen atoms (2 · 14 = 28).

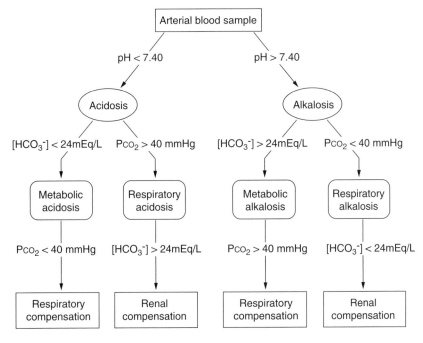

FIGURE 38-5. Algorithm for differentiating simple acid-base imbalances.

    (2) With compensated metabolic alkalosis, the PCO_2 is elevated.
  b. **Respiratory disorders** result in compensatory changes in renal acid excretion and thus in the plasma $[HCO_3^-]$.
    (1) With respiratory acidosis, complete compensation elevates the $[HCO_3^-]$.
    (2) With respiratory alkalosis, complete compensation reduces the $[HCO_3^-]$. In the example, the $[HCO_3^-]$ is reduced; however, the patient is acidotic and not alkalotic.

B. Mixed acid-base disorders

  1. If the compensatory response is not appropriate, a mixed acid-base imbalance should be suspected.
  2. Given the example: $[HCO_3^-] = 20$ mEq/L and $PCO_2 = 55$ mm Hg.
    a. According to the Henderson equation,

$$[H^+] = 24 \frac{PCO_2}{[HCO_3^-]}$$

$$= 24 \frac{55}{20}$$

$$= 66 \text{ nEq/L}$$

$$pH = 9 - \log [H^+]$$

$$= 9 - 1.82$$

$$= 7.18$$

    b. The three-step approach indicates that the disturbance is an acidosis that has a metabolic component ($[HCO_3^-] < 24$ mEq/L) and a respiratory component ($PCO_2 > 40$ mm Hg). Thus, this disorder is mixed. Thus, this disorder is a mixed metabolic acidosis and a respiratory acidosis.
      (1) The compensatory response for a metabolic acidosis is a fall in PCO_2 that is not observed.

(2) The compensation for a respiratory acidosis is an elevation in $[HCO_3^-]$ that is also not observed.

C. Clinical algorithm for the evaluation of acid-base disorders

1. Check the validity of the blood pH using the Henderson equation.

   a. $[H^+] = 24 \dfrac{PCO_2}{[HCO_3^-]}$

   b. Then determine the pH: $pH = 9 - \log [H^+]$

2. Identify the primary acid-base disorder (see Figure 38–5).

3. Calculate the anion gap (AG):
   a. $AG = [Na^+] - ([HCO_3^-] + [Cl^-])$
   b. There are four major causes of high anion gap metabolic acidosis:
   (1) Renal failure
   (2) Lactic acidosis (lactacidosis)
   (3) Ketoacidosis (starvation, diabetic ketoacidosis, and chronic alcoholism)
   (4) Toxins (ingestion of methyl alcohol, ethylene glycol, paraldehyde, and salicylate poisoning)

4. Identify the cause of the primary acid-base imbalance.

5. Observe whether or not there is a compensatory response.

6. Determine the therapeutic regimen to correct the disturbance.

IV. GRAPHIC EVALUATION OF ACID-BASE STATUS: pH-[HCO$_3^-$] DIAGRAM (Figures 38–6; 38–7)

A. Value of diagram. When acid-base data obtained from blood are plotted on the pH-$[HCO_3^-]$ diagram, the physician has a tool that can be used to:

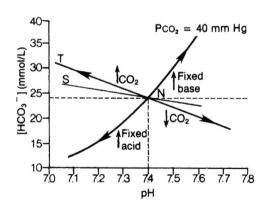

FIGURE 38-6. The pH-$[HCO_3^-]$ diagram showing the buffer curves of separated plasma (*S*) and true oxygenated plasma (*T*). *Point N* denotes the intercept for a normal plasma $[HCO_3^-]$ of 24 mmol/L and a normal pH of 7.4. The slope of the normal in vitro buffer line of true plasma is a function of the hemoglobin content of blood. *Lines S* and *T* are called nonbicarbonate buffer curves, and the steepness of the slopes of these lines is a quantitative assessment of the amount of nonbicarbonate buffer present in the system. These same two lines represent CO_2-titration curves. The steeper the buffer line, the smaller the pH change resulting from a given increase or decrease in CO_2 tension (PCO_2). Vertical arrows indicate increases and decreases in CO_2 tension, fixed acid, or fixed base. (Adapted from Davenport HW: *The ABC of Acid-Base Chemistry,* 5th ed. Chicago, University of Chicago Press, 1969, p 48.)

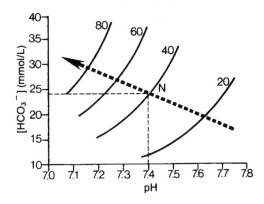

FIGURE 38-7. The pH-[HCO_3^-] diagram with arterial CO_2 tension (P_{CO_2}) isobars for 20, 40, 60, and 80 mm Hg. Each arterial P_{CO_2} isobar is the titration curve of a HCO_3^--H_2CO_3 solution with arterial P_{CO_2} held constant. *Point N* denotes the intercept for a normal plasma [HCO_3^-] of 24 mmol/L and a normal pH of 7.4. The *dashed arrow* represents the buffer line. (After Davenport HW: *The ABC of Acid-Base Chemistry*, 5th ed. Chicago, University of Chicago Press, 1969, p 45.)

1. Diagnose the primary cause of an acid-base abnormality

2. Determine the degree of compensatory response of the kidneys and of the lungs by monitoring the [HCO_3^-] and CO_2 tension, respectively

3. Estimate the concentration of noncarbonic and carbonic acids in the ECF

4. Aid in the choice of therapy to correct an acid-base imbalance

5. Measure the nonbicarbonate buffer power of whole blood by the slope of the buffer line

6. Indicate not only the total buffer activity but also the distribution of the buffering activity between the bicarbonate and nonbicarbonate buffer systems

B. **Construction of diagram: effects of H⁺ and CO_2 on pH.** The basis for plotting pH and [HCO_3^-] on cartesian coordinates is best understood from a consideration of the CO_2/HCO_3^- buffer system:

$$CO_2 + H_2O \rightleftharpoons H_2CO_3 \rightleftharpoons H^+ + HCO_3^-$$

1. **Effect of fixed acid or base on pH**
    a. **Addition of H⁺ at a constant CO_2 tension**
        (1) When H⁺ ions, in the form of fixed (noncarbonic) acid, are added to the CO_2/HCO_3^- system, most of them combine with HCO_3^- to form H_2CO_3, which dehydrates to form CO_2 and water. Thus, the series of reactions in the equation is driven to the left.
        (2) The decrease in [HCO_3^-] closely approximates the amount of H⁺ added only if the solution has no other nonbicarbonate buffer substances. Otherwise, the amount of acid added would be greater than the decrease in [HCO_3^-].
    b. **Addition of base at a constant CO_2 tension**
        (1) When a base is added to the system depicted in the equation, some of the base combines with H⁺, causing more H_2CO_3 to dissociate into H⁺ and HCO_3^-. Here the series of reactions proceeds to the right.
        (2) The increase in [HCO_3^-] determines the amount of base added.
    c. **Principles** (see Figure 38–6)
        (1) When fixed acid or base is added under the conditions described, there is an inverse relationship between [H⁺] and [HCO_3^-], and the primary acid-base disturbance is metabolic. Thus, when fixed acid or base is added, the [H⁺] and [HCO_3^-] change in opposite directions.
        (2) Or, if the direction of change in [HCO_3^-] is the same as that for pH, the primary acid-base abnormality is metabolic.

2. **Effect of CO_2 on pH**
    a. **Addition of CO_2 (see Figure 38–7)**
        (1) An increase in arterial CO_2 tension titrates the blood (and ECF) in the acid direction. This is clear from the equation in III B, which shows that an increase in CO_2

tension causes more CO_2 to hydrate to form H_2CO_3; the H_2CO_3 in turn dissociates into H^+ and HCO_3^-, moving the reactions to the right.

(2) In the CO_2/HCO_3^- system, every molecule of CO_2 that hydrates and dissociates forms one H^+ and one HCO_3^-; therefore, the changes in $[H^+]$ and $[HCO_3^-]$ are exactly equal.

(3) The final $[H^+]$ depends not only on the change in CO_2 tension but also on the buffers in the system. For every H_2CO_3 molecule that has its H^+ taken up by a buffer ion, one HCO_3^- appears in the solution. For example, the reaction with hemoglobin is:

$$H_2CO_3 + Hb^- \rightleftharpoons HHb + HCO_3^-$$

(4) If CO_2 is added to whole blood (which contains many buffer systems), the H^+ rather than remaining in solution, are mostly bound to protein buffers (Pr^-) as:

$$CO_2 + H_2O \rightleftharpoons H_2CO_3 \rightleftharpoons HCO_3^- + H^+$$
$$+$$
$$Pr^-$$
$$\downarrow\uparrow$$
$$H \cdot Pr$$

Therefore, **the CO_2/HCO_3^- system alone is not effective in buffering the changes in pH that are induced by the addition of CO_2.**

b. Removal of CO_2

(1) When CO_2 is removed from the CO_2/HCO_3^- system, fewer CO_2 molecules are available for combination with water to form HCO_3^-.

(2) Thus, not only is CO_2 decreased, but $[H^+]$ and $[HCO_3^-]$ also are decreased and the reactions shift to the left.

c. Principles. The concentration of acid added to a buffer solution by a change in CO_2 tension is equal to the change in $[HCO_3^-]$.§

(1) If CO_2 is added or removed, the $[H^+]$ and $[HCO_3^-]$ change in the same direction, and the primary acid-base disturbance is respiratory.

(2) Or, if the direction of change in $[HCO_3^-]$ is opposite to that for pH, the primary acid-base disturbance is respiratory.

(3) As CO_2 tension is increased or decreased, the values for pH and $[HCO_3^-]$ form coordinates that define a nearly straight line termed the buffer line or the CO_2 titration curve (see Figure 37–7).

d. Summary

(1) When H^+ is added or removed, the $[H^+]$ and $[HCO_3^-]$ change in opposite directions and the acid-base imbalance is metabolic in origin.

(2) When CO_2 is added or removed, the $[H^+]$ and $[HCO_3^-]$ change in the same direction, and the acid-base imbalance is respiratory in origin.

C. **Properties of CO_2 tension (P_{CO_2}) isobars**

1. At constant $[HCO_3^-]$, CO_2 tension is proportional to $[H^+]$. This property can be illustrated using the following form of the Henderson equation to solve for P_{CO_2} (see Chapter 34 V):

$$[H^+] = 24 \frac{P_{CO_2}}{[HCO_3^-]}$$

$$P_{CO_2} = \frac{[H^+]\,[HCO_3^-]}{24}$$

---

§In humans, the serum $[HCO_3^-]$ is 24×10^{-3} Eq/L (24×10^{-3} mol/L), whereas the serum $[H^+]$ is 40×10^{-9} Eq/L (40×10^{-9} mol/L). Therefore, the $[HCO_3^-]$ is 6×10^5 greater than $[H^+]$, and any shift (left or right) in equilibrium has a much greater proportionate effect on $[H^+]$ than on $[HCO_3^-]$.

2. At constant pH (i.e., along any vertical line in Figures 38–6 and 38–7), CO_2 tension is proportional to $[HCO_3^-]$.

V. INTERPRETATION OF ACID-BASE ABNORMALITIES USING THE pH-[HCO$_3^-$] DIAGRAM

(Figure 38–8). Acid-base imbalances are determined graphically with reference to the intercept of the P_{CO_2} isobar of 40 mm Hg and the normal buffer line. The intercept of these two curves marks the point of normality (*N*), which is associated with a pH of 7.4 (the *abscissa*) and a $[HCO_3^-]$ of 24 mmol/L (the *ordinate*). *Point N* **is the triple intercept that defines the pH, $[HCO_3^-]$, and CO_2 tension of true arterial plasma of a normal individual.**

A. **Points to the left** of *point N* (*points A, C, E,* and *F*) indicate acidosis. **Points to the right** of *Point N* (*points B, D, G,* and *H*) indicate alkalosis.

1. *Line NA* represents the direction of an individual's response to an increase in P_{CO_2}. Points to the left of the normal P_{CO_2} isobar (*points A, E,* and *F*) indicate **respiratory acidosis.**
   a. *Point A* denotes a condition of uncompensated respiratory acidosis, which is characterized by a low pH, high $[HCO_3^-]$, and high CO_2 tension.
   b. *Point E* denotes respiratory acidosis (↑ P_{CO_2}) with metabolic acidosis (↓ $[HCO_3^-]$).
   c. *Point F* denotes respiratory acidosis (↑ P_{CO_2}) with metabolic alkalosis (↑ $[HCO_3^-]$).

2. *Line NB* represents the direction of an individual's response to a decrease in CO_2 tension. Points to the right of the normal P_{CO_2} isobar (*points B, G,* and *H*) indicate **respiratory alkalosis.**
   a. *Point B* denotes a condition of uncompensated respiratory alkalosis, which is characterized by high pH, low $[HCO_3^-]$, and low CO_2 tension.
   b. *Point G* denotes respiratory alkalosis (↓ P_{CO_2}) with metabolic acidosis (↓ $[HCO_3^-]$).
   c. *Point H* denotes respiratory alkalosis (↓ P_{CO_2}) with metabolic alkalosis (↑ $[HCO_3^-]$).

B. **Points below** the normal buffer line (*points C, E,* and *G*) indicate conditions with a component of metabolic acidosis (↓ $[HCO_3^-]$). **Points above** the normal buffer lines (*points D, F,* and *H*) indicate conditions with a component of metabolic alkalosis (↑ $[HCO_3^-]$).

1. *Line NC* represents the direction of the development of metabolic acidosis in an individual; the $[HCO_3^-]$ of this individual moves down the normal P_{CO_2} isobar.
   a. *Point C* denotes a condition of uncompensated metabolic acidosis, which is characterized by low pH, low $[HCO_3^-]$, and normal CO_2 tension.
   b. *Point E* denotes metabolic acidosis (↓ $[HCO_3^-]$) with respiratory acidosis (↑ P_{CO_2}).
   c. *Point G* denotes metabolic acidosis (↓ $[HCO_3^-]$) with respiratory alkalosis (↓ P_{CO_2}).

FIGURE 38-8. Pathways of acid-base imbalance. The *[HCO$_3^-$]* pertains to plasma. *Line ANB* represents the normal blood buffer line, and *line CND* represents the normal CO_2 tension (*P_{CO_2}*) *isobar (40 mm Hg).* N = normal point; A = respiratory acidosis (uncompensated); B = respiratory alkalosis (uncompensated); C = metabolic acidosis (uncompensated); D = metabolic alkalosis (uncompensated); E = respiratory acidosis + metabolic acidosis; F = respiratory acidosis + metabolic alkalosis; G = respiratory alkalosis + metabolic acidosis; and H = respiratory alkalosis + metabolic alkalosis. (After Davenport HW: *The ABC of Acid-Base Chemistry,* 5th ed. Chicago, University of Chicago Press, 1969, p 65.)

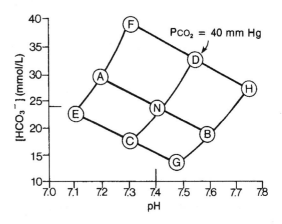

2. *Line ND* represents the direction of the development of metabolic alkalosis in an individual; the [HCO_3^-] of this individual moves up the normal PCO_2 isobar.
   a. *Point D* denotes a condition of uncompensated metabolic alkalosis, which is characterized by high pH, high [HCO_3^-], and normal CO_2 tension.
   b. *Point F* denotes metabolic alkalosis (↑ [HCO_3^-]) with respiratory acidosis (↑ PCO_2).
   c. *Point H* denotes metabolic alkalosis (↑ [HCO_3^-]) with respiratory alkalosis (↓ PCO_2).

C. **Mixed acid-base disturbances,** in which the primary state of acidosis or alkalosis has an additional abnormality with respect to CO_2 tension and [HCO_3^-], are denoted by *points E, F, G,* and *H.*

Case 1

A 22-year-old man with insulin-dependent diabetes mellitus was admitted to the hospital with fever and abdominal pain. His temperature was 102.6°F, his blood pressure was 130/84 and his pulse rate was 86 beats/min. His diabetes was controlled with human recombinant DNA insulin, 15 units in the morning and 10 units at night. A chest x-ray showed a left lobe pneumonia.

Laboratory data

Serum chemistries	Arterial blood gases
[Na^+]: 132 mEq/L	pH: 7.32
[K^+]: 5.2 mEq/L	PCO_2: 20 mm Hg
[Cl^-]: 100 mEq/l	PO_2: 95 mm Hg
[HCO_3^-]: 10 mEq/L	Hemoglobin saturation: 95%
[Glucose]: 600 mg/dl	
BUN: 60 mg/dl	
[Creatinine]: 2.0 mg/dl	
Serum ketones: mildly positive	

1. What steps are taken in the evaluation of this acid-base disorder?

2. What is the diagnosis?

DISCUSSION

The first step is to verify that the pH is correct. This can be quickly and easily done with the Henderson equation, which determines the [H^+] as:

$$[H^+] = 24 \cdot \frac{PCO_2}{[HCO_3^-]}$$

$$= 24 \cdot \frac{20}{10} = 48 \text{ nmol/L}$$

Calculation of pH with the Henderson-Hasselbalch equation is:

$$pH = 9 - \log [H^+]$$

$$= 9 - \log 48$$

$$= 9 - 1.68$$

$$= 7.32 \text{ (normal range: 7.36–7.44)}$$

The arterial blood gases and the pH measurements are correct, and the patient is diagnosed as having acidosis because the pH is less than 7.36.

The second step is to determine the primary acid-base imbalance by examining the serum [HCO_3^-] and the PCO_2. Acidosis could result from a decrease in [HCO_3^-] (metabolic) or an increase in PCO_2 (respiratory). This patient has metabolic acidosis. If the hyperventilation that the patient manifested was the primary cause of the acid-base disturbance, the arterial blood pH would have indicated alkalosis with a pH of more than 7.36. Thus, at this point, the patient has metabolic acidosis with respiratory alkalosis.

The third step is to determine the anion gap (AG).

$$AG = [Na^+] - ([HCO_3^-] + [Cl^-])$$

$$= 132 - (10 + 100)$$

$$= 132 - 110$$

$$= 22 \text{ mEq/L (normal is } 12 \pm 2 \text{ mEq/L)}$$

The increase in the anion gap represents those acid anions (e.g., lactate, ketoacid anions, sulfate, and phosphate) associated with an equimolar reduction in $[HCO_3^-]$. Note that the addition of acid produced a fall in $[HCO_3^-]$, whereas the $[Cl^-]$ remained relatively stable. In patients with an anion gap acidosis, the reciprocity between the anion gap and the $[HCO_3^-]$ decline should always be identified. If this reciprocal relationship is not seen, a complicating acid-base disturbance may coexist.

3. *How would the cause of the elevated anion gap be determined in this patient?*

DISCUSSION

There are four major causes of high anion gap metabolic acidosis: renal failure, lactic acidosis, ketoacidosis (e.g., starvation, diabetes, chronic alcoholism), and toxins (e.g., methyl alcohol, ethylene glycol, paraldehyde, salicylate poisoning). In this patient, the history and physical did not reveal toxin ingestion or alcoholism. The absence of hypoxia (95% hemoglobin saturation with O_2; PO_2 of 95 mm Hg) rules out lactic acidosis. The detection of ketones in the blood and a history of insulin-dependent diabetes mellitus indicates that ketoacidosis caused the increased anion gap.

4. *What was the cause of ketoacidosis in a diabetic controlled with exogenous insulin?*

DISCUSSION

The fundamental cause of diabetic ketoacidosis is a relative or absolute deficiency of insulin. The **major causes of insulin deficiency** are:

a. **Infections** may cause patients to develop anorexia or reduce food intake. Because of the anorexia or fear of developing insulin-induced hypoglycemia, they may stop taking insulin entirely. Nausea and vomiting are common complaints in diabetic patients, occurring during acute ketoacidosis. Frequently, these patients have symptoms of anorexia, early satiety, and postprandial abdominal fullness due to gastroparesis. These symptoms can limit oral nutrition. In patients with severe hyperglycemia, failure to take insulin for 1 or 2 days, particularly when the patient does not eat, may rapidly lead to ketoacidosis. The well-trained patient with diabetes often takes additional insulin during an obvious infectious process. In this patient, pneumonia, which was confirmed by chest x-ray, was the precipitating factor for ketoacidosis. The pneumonia was also the cause of the fever in this patient.

b. **Surgical emergency, trauma, myocardial infarction, and severe emotional stress** represent frequent precipitating causes of uncontrolled diabetes. Abdominal pain in association with ketoacidosis is often misdiagnosed as an acute surgical emergency; however, the abdominal pain in this patient is secondary to the diabetic ketoacidosis.

c. **Chronic, severe overinsulinization** with repeated hypoglycemic reactions may lead to hepatic glycogen depletion and severe ketosis that is disproportionate to the extent of glucosuria and hyperglycemia.

> **d. Associated endocrine disorders** (e.g., acromegaly, Cushing's syndrome, thyrotoxicosis, pheochromocytoma) can antagonize the metabolic effects of insulin.
>
> **e.** In patients with latent or subclinical diabetes, acute deficiency may be produced by **overeating,** particularly carbohydrates.

5. *Describe the pathogenesis of the hyperglycemia, hyperosmolality, shifts of body fluids, and hypovolemia that develop in diabetic ketoacidosis.*

DISCUSSION

The relative or absolute lack of insulin impairs glucose utilization by most tissues (excluding brain tissue), and insulin deficiency combined with excessive glucagon increases hepatic production of glucose from noncarbohydrate sources (i.e., gluconeogenesis is stimulated). Both processes—underutilization of glucose and excessive glucose production—cause progressive hyperglycemia. It is the increased filtered load of glucose, which is due to hyperglycemia, that exceeds the renal reabsorptive capacity and causes glucosuria.

With the relative or absolute lack of insulin, the insulin-sensitive cells (muscle, adipose) are relatively impermeable to glucose; thus, the increasing hyperglycemia progressively raises the osmolality of the extracellular fluid (ECF). In this patient, the osmolar concentration is calculated as:

$$C_{osm} = 2\ [Na^+] + \frac{BUN\ (in\ mg/dl)}{2.8} + \frac{Blood\ glucose\ (in\ mg/dl)}{18}$$

$$= 2\ (132) + \frac{60}{2.8} + \frac{600}{18}$$

$$= 264 + 21 + 33$$

$$= 318\ mOsm/kg\ H_2O$$

As the osmolality of the ECF increases, water diffuses from the intracellular fluid to the ECF, thereby reestablishing transcellular osmotic equivalence and leading to the dilution of the remaining solute, the most abundant of which are the sodium salts. This process progressively dehydrates cells while expanding the ECF. The expansion is transient because of the resulting osmotic diuresis caused by the glucosuria and obligatory salt loss.

During the osmotic diuresis, urinary water losses are disproportionately greater than electrolyte loss, which contributes further to the progressive rise in serum osmolality. Thus, the water loss in patients with diabetic acidosis represents the most serious form of hyperosmotic dehydration and leads to extreme intracellular depletion of water. The water losses through the skin, lungs, and gastrointestinal tract are aggravated by the limited ability of the patient to replace water because of anorexia, vomiting, or coma. This depletion of body fluids leads to contraction of the vascular volume, hypotension, and often shock. The depletion of vascular volume and increased blood viscosity leads to a reduction in renal blood flow and glomerular filtration rate (GFR), which further impairs renal compensatory mechanisms (acid excretion). This results in a more rapidly developing and severe acidosis.

6. *How does protein catabolism contribute to hyperglycemia in insulin-dependent diabetics?*

DISCUSSION

Insulin deficiency (and excess glucagon) increases protein catabolism, which leads to nitrogen loss and increased circulating levels of amino acids, which are gluconeogenic substances and can exacerbate hyperglycemia. The increased endogenous production of urea secondary to tissue breakdown causes an increase in blood urea nitrogen (BUN) due to a decrease in GFR. It also causes a marked increase in renal urea excretion, which contributes a further osmotic effect in addition to that of glucosuria. The destruction of tissue protein is associated with the liberation of intracellular potassium, phosphate, and magnesium, which are lost by urinary excretion as diabetic acidosis proceeds.

7. What does the presence of ketoacids indicate?

DISCUSSION

The generation and maintenance of ketoacid production involve three tissues: adipose tissues, liver, and extrahepatic tissue (muscle, brain). Insulin deficiency and glucagon cause uncontrolled lipolysis, which increases plasma concentrations of both glycerol and free fatty acids (FFA). Glycerol also serves as a gluconeogenic substrate potentiating the hyperglycemia. The ability of liver to rapidly metabolize FFA limits the plasma concentration of these substances and prevents a significant fall in pH. The increased delivery of FFA to the liver increases ketone body production (ketogenesis), which soon leads to increased blood levels of ketone bodies (ketonemia). The liver, unlike other peripheral tissues, is unable to metabolize the ketoacids it synthesizes. Acetoacetate and β-hydroxybutyrate are taken up from the circulation by such tissues as muscle and kidney and are oxidized to CO_2 and H_2O. However, a deficiency of insulin increases fat mobilization and stimulates hepatic ketogenesis. The increased concentration of ketones spills over into the urine (ketonuria). The excretion of ketoacid anions exacerbates the electrolyte (Na^+ and K^+) depletion.

8. What is the best treatment for this patient who has diabetic ketoacidosis?

DISCUSSION

Ketoacidosis may safely, simply, and effectively be treated with cumulative doses of regular insulin under 100 units. Low doses of insulin have been shown to inhibit hepatic glucose production and stimulate peripheral utilization of glucose. This not only effectively reverses hyperglycemia, but it also reverses the ketosis, thereby negating the notion that ketosis or acidemia induces insulin resistance.

The addition of ketoacids to the ECF causes a loss of HCO_3^-, fall in systemic pH, and a compensatory decrease in PCO_2. With therapy, β-hydroxybutyrate and acetoacetate are metabolized to HCO_3^-, thereby improving the ketoacidosis. Thus, it has been argued that since insulin therapy reverses the biochemical abnormalities (including the HCO_3^- deficit) $NaHCO_3$ therapy is not only unnecessary but may be detrimental. It remains necessary to establish volume repletion with normal (0.9%) saline followed by supplements of K^+ and HPO_4^{2-} to allow for the increased uptake of these two ions by insulin treatment as well as their loss in the urine with improvement in GFR.

Chapter 39

Compensatory Mechanisms for Primary Acid-Base Abnormalities

I. TERMINOLOGY

A. **Compensation** is the secondary physiologic process occurring in response to a primary acid-base disturbance by which the deviation of blood pH is ameliorated. Thus, abnormal pH is returned toward normal by **altering the component that is not primarily affected.**

   1. The terms secondary and compensatory may be used to describe a change in the composition of the blood or to describe a process.

   2. The terms secondary and compensatory may be used to describe a process, but they should not be used to describe acidosis or alkalosis, because confusion arises when referring to compensatory responses as "secondary" or "compensatory" acidoses or alkaloses.

B. **Correction** denotes the therapeutic course of action that is directed toward counteracting or altering the factor that is primarily affected. Correction involves the amelioration of the primary underlying abnormality in [H^+], [HCO_3^-], or CO_2 tension. In correction, as in compensation, the pH is returned toward normal.

C. Concept underlying definition of compensation (Table 38–3 and Table 39–1)

   1. In a **metabolic acidosis or alkalosis,** the primary change occurs in the [HCO_3^-] and the adaptive response (compensation) adjusts the ventilation, resulting in a change in P_{CO_2} **in the same direction** as the change in [HCO_3^-]. This response is called **respiratory compensation** for the metabolic process.

   2. In a **respiratory acidosis or alkalosis,** the primary change occurs in the P_{CO_2} and the adaptive response adjusts the reabsorption (reclamation) and generation of [HCO_3^-], resulting in a change in [HCO_3^-] **in the same direction** as the change in P_{CO_2}. This response is termed **metabolic compensation** for the respiratory process.

   3. **Compensation** is a **response** to a **primary pathophysiologic process,** and only the pathophysiologic processes causing a primary change in the [HCO_3^-] or P_{CO_2} should be termed "acidoses" or "alkaloses."

   4. **Examples** with caveats:
      a. The respiratory compensation for a simple metabolic acidosis is hyperventilation, and therefore it is confusing to refer to this compensatory process as a "secondary respiratory alkalosis." Such confusing terms can mislead one to evaluate this simple disorder as a "mixed metabolic acidosis and respiratory alkalosis," which it is not.
      b. Compensation does not mean that the pH will be normalized or even near normalized. Compensation rarely returns pH to a near-normal value. If it did, it would remove the stimulus for the compensation.

II. BASIC MECHANISMS OF COMPENSATORY RESPONSES

A. **Buffers of the extracellular fluid (ECF)** represent the body's first defense mechanism for neutralizing noncarbonic acid. H^+ is transferred across tissue cell membranes in a direction that normalizes blood pH.

B. A deviation in plasma pH acts on the respiratory center to change alveolar ventilation, which, in turn, alters the alveolar CO_2 tension and arterial CO_2 tension to counteract the change in plasma pH. This is called **respiratory compensation** of a primary noncarbonic acid excess or deficit; respiratory compensation usually is not complete (i.e., does not restore pH to normal).

C. **Carbonate ion is released from bone,** which is the predominant source of alkali for neutralizing excess noncarbonic acid added to the ECF.

D. Renal excretion of noncarbonic acid or base increases to eliminate an excess of noncarbonic acid or base or to compensate for the pH changes due to an abnormal arterial CO_2 tension. This is called **renal compensation** of a primary hyper- or hypocapnia.

E. The responses to respiratory acidosis and alkalosis differ from responses to metabolic acid-base disorders in that there is virtually no extracellular buffering of H_2CO_3 in respiratory acidosis because HCO_3^- is not an effective buffer for H_2CO_3.

III. PRINCIPLES OF RESPIRATORY AND RENAL COMPENSATORY RESPONSES

A. **General considerations**

1. Physiologic compensation for major acid-base abnormalities rarely is complete. Therefore, the singular concern of clinical diagnosis is to differentiate the primary cause of the imbalance from the secondary (compensatory) response.

2. Most data indicate that the pH ($[H^+]$) is the most important factor in determining the bodily response to acid-base imbalances. (In both acid and base disturbances, the abnormal pH is returned toward normal.) However, in spite of its critical biologic significance, **a change in pH does not provide all the information needed for quantitative assessment and thus for planning therapy.**
   a. The key determinants of the cause and compensation of acid-base abnormalities are CO_2 tension and $[HCO_3^-]$, not pH.
   b. The most important factor in determining the efficacy of the bodily responses to deviations from the normal acid-base status is pH or $[H^+]$.

B. **Respiratory and renal processes** (see Tables 38–1; 38–2 and Table 39–1)

1. Both respiratory and renal compensatory responses tend to restore the abnormal $[HCO_3^-]/S \cdot P_{CO_2}$ ratio toward its normal value of 20:1.
   a. Primary acid-base disturbances of **metabolic origin** lead to secondary adjustment of the CO_2 tension by changes in the rate of alveolar ventilation.
   b. Primary acid-base disturbances of **respiratory origin** lead to secondary changes in blood $[HCO_3^-]$ by appropriate adjustment of the rate of H^+ secretion/excretion from the renal tubular cell into the tubular lumen.

2. These two processes interact to control the $[H^+]$ of the ECF, and this integration is clearly understood using the mathematical relationship of the Henderson equation (see Chapter 34 V).

$$[H^+] = 24 \frac{P_{CO_2}}{[HCO_3^-]}$$

From this equation, it is apparent that:
   a. An increase in the $[H^+]$, regardless of cause, can be reduced toward normal by a decrease in CO_2 tension, an increase in plasma $[HCO_3^-]$, or by both changes.
   b. A decrease in the $[H^+]$, regardless of cause, can be increased toward normal by an increase in CO_2 tension, a decrease in plasma $[HCO_3^-]$, or by both changes.

TABLE 39-1. Formulas Needed to Evaluate Most Arterial Blood Gases*

Condition Evaluated	Equation
General relationship among pH, [HCO$_3$$^-$], and P$_{CO_2}$	pH α [HCO$_3$$^-$]/P$_{CO_2}$
Anion gap (AG)	AG = [Na$^+$]−([HCO$_3$$^-$]+[Cl$^-$])
Metabolic acidosis	P$_{CO_2}$ = 1.5 [HCO$_3$$^-$] + 8($\pm$2) (P$_{CO_2}$ decreases)
Metabolic alkalosis	P$_{CO_2}$ = 0.9 [HCO$_3$$^-$] + 16 (P$_{CO_2}$ increases)

Respiratory acidosis	For every increment of P$_{CO_2}$ by 10 mm Hg
	Acute: pH decreases by 0.08
	    [HCO$_3$$^-$] increases by 1 mEq/L
	Chronic: pH decreases by 0.03
	    [HCO$_3$$^-$] increases by 4 mEq/L

Respiratory alkalosis	For every decrement of P$_{CO_2}$ by 10 mm Hg
	Acute: pH increases by 0.08
	    [HCO$_3$$^-$] decreases by 2 mEq/L
	Chronic: pH increases by 0.03
	    [HCO$_3$$^-$] decreases by 5 mEq/L

*Full compensation requires 12–24 hours, depending on the acid-base disorder. The formulas for the **metabolic** processes assume that compensation has already been achieved (> 12 hours of acidosis or alkalosis). Most metabolic acidosis or alkalosis develops slowly allowing time for the compensatory processes to develop before the patient presents with symptoms. During the intermediate phase (12–24 hours), the actual values in the table fall between the values predicted for the acute and chronic responses.

IV. ETIOLOGY OF ACID-BASE DISORDERS AND THEIR COMPENSATORY RESPONSES

A. **Metabolic acidosis** is a disorder characterized by a low arterial pH ($\uparrow$ [H$^+$]) or a reduced plasma [HCO$_3$$^-$].

1. **Causes** of metabolic acidosis include:
   a. Gain of noncarbonic (fixed) acid by the ECF, such as excess quantities of the ketoacids (β-hydroxybutyric acid and acetoacetic acid) or lactic acid or the ingestion of alcohol, salicylates, or NH$_4$Cl
   b. Loss of HCO$_3$$^-$ and other conjugate bases, as occurs with severe diarrhea and fistulas (which cause loss of bowel fluids containing HCO$_3$$^-$)
   c. Salicylate toxicity (late effect)

2. **Compensation** for metabolic acidosis includes:
   a. Extracellular buffering primarily by HCO$_3$$^-$
   b. Intracellular buffering primarily by proteins and phosphates
   c. Respiratory compensation by an increase in alveolar ventilation resulting in a decline in the CO$_2$ tension
   d. Renal compensation by an increase in H$^+$ excretion and an increase in HCO$_3$$^-$ reabsorption

B. **Metabolic alkalosis** is a disorder characterized by an elevated arterial pH ($\downarrow$ [H$^+$]) or an increased plasma [HCO$_3$$^-$].

1. **Causes** of metabolic alkalosis include:
   a. Decreased production of noncarbonic acid or a loss of noncarbonic acid via the kidneys or the gastrointestinal system (vomiting)
   b. Excess HCO$_3$$^-$ or other conjugate base by ingestion or infusion
   c. Excessive renal reabsorption of HCO$_3$$^-$
   d. Overtreatment with HCO$_3$$^-$ or lactate

2. Compensation for metabolic alkalosis includes:
   a. Respiratory compensation by hypoventilation resulting in an increase in plasma P_{CO_2}
   b. Renal compensation by an increase in HCO_3^- excretion

C. **Respiratory acidosis** is a disorder characterized by a reduced arterial pH ($\uparrow$ [H^+]), an elevated CO_2 tension (hypercapnia), and a variable increase in the plasma [HCO_3^-].

1. Causes
   a. The common denominator in respiratory acidosis is a reduction in alveolar ventilation.
   b. The most common causes are chronic obstructive pulmonary disease and the overuse of respiratory depressant drugs.

2. Compensation for respiratory alkalosis includes:
   a. Increased renal reabsorption of HCO_3^-
   b. Increased renal H^+ secretion and excretion

D. **Respiratory alkalosis** is a disorder characterized by an elevated arterial pH ($\downarrow$ [H^+]), a low CO_2 tension (hypocapnia), and a variable decrease in the plasma [HCO_3^-].

1. Causes of respiratory alkalosis include:
   a. Hyperventilation (hyperpnea)
   b. Anxiety and hysteria
   c. Salicylate overdosage (early effect)

2. Compensation for respiratory alkalosis includes:
   a. Decreased urinary H^+ excretion
   b. Increased urinary HCO_3^- excretion

V. PATHWAYS FOR COMPENSATION OF PRIMARY ACID-BASE DISTURBANCES: THE pH-[HCO_3^-] RELATIONSHIP (Figure 39–1)

A. **Respiratory acidosis** (*point A*). The system at fault in this condition is the respiratory system, and compensation occurs through metabolic processes.

1. The kidneys excrete more acid and reabsorb more HCO_3^-, returning the [HCO_3^-]/S · P_{CO_2} ratio toward 20:1 and, therefore, returning pH toward normal (*point A_1*).

2. If the CO_2 tension is elevated but the pH is normal, the kidneys had time to retain HCO_3^- to compensate for the elevated CO_2 tension and the process is not acute; that is, the condition has existed at least a few days to give the kidneys time to compensate (*point A_2*).

3. Usually, the body does not fully compensate for respiratory acidosis.

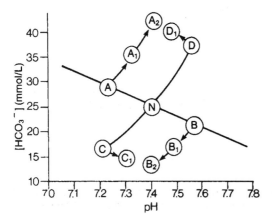

FIGURE 39-1. Effects of renal and respiratory compensation on the pH and plasma [HCO_3^-]. N = normal point; A = respiratory acidosis; A_1 = respiratory acidosis with partial renal compensation; A_2 = respiratory acidosis with complete renal compensation; B = respiratory alkalosis; B_1 = respiratory alkalosis with partial renal compensation; B_2 = respiratory alkalosis with complete renal compensation; C = metabolic acidosis; C_1 = metabolic acidosis with partial respiratory compensation; D = metabolic alkalosis; and D_1 = metabolic alkalosis with partial renal compensation. (After Davenport HW: *The ABC of Acid-Base Chemistry*, 5th ed. Chicago, University of Chicago, Press, 1969, p 65.)

B. **Respiratory alkalosis** (*point B*). In this condition, the acid-base abnormality again is respiratory, and compensation again occurs through metabolic means.

  1. The kidneys compensate by excreting HCO_3^-, thus returning the $[HCO_3^-]/S \cdot P_{CO_2}$ ratio toward 20:1; this compensation takes 2–3 days (*point B$_1$*).

  2. Of the four acid-base abnormalities, only in respiratory alkalosis is the body able to compensate fully; the $[HCO_3^-]/S \cdot P_{CO_2}$ ratio and pH therefore return entirely to normal (*point B$_2$*).

C. **Metabolic acidosis** (*point C*). In this condition, the major abnormality is low $[HCO_3^-]$ or negative base excess (BE), and the compensation is a respiratory process.

  1. By hyperventilation, the CO_2 tension is lowered so that the $[HCO_3^-]/S \cdot P_{CO_2}$ ratio is returned toward 20:1 (*point C$_1$*).

  2. Since the compensatory system is the lungs, compensation can occur rapidly. If the metabolic acidosis is severe, however, the lungs may not be able to expel sufficient CO_2 to compensate fully.

D. **Metabolic alkalosis** (*point D*). In this condition, the major abnormality is a high $[HCO_3^-]$, and the compensation is a respiratory mechanism.

  1. By hypoventilation, the CO_2 tension is elevated so that the $[HCO_3^-]/S \cdot P_{CO_2}$ ratio is increased toward normal (*point D$_1$*).

  2. The body usually cannot compensate fully for metabolic alkalosis.

VI. SUMMARY: CHARACTERISTICS OF UNCOMPENSATED ACID-BASE DISTURBANCES AND THEIR COMPENSATORY RESPONSES (see Table 38–3 and Table 39–1)

A. **Metabolic acidosis**

  1. An uncompensated metabolic acidosis is characterized by a low pH, a low CO_2 content, and a normal CO_2 tension.

  2. When a metabolic acidosis is compensated by a respiratory alkalosis, the pH tends to return toward normal, but the CO_2 content and tension decrease.

B. **Metabolic alkalosis**

  1. An uncompensated metabolic alkalosis is characterized by high pH, a high CO_2 content, and a normal CO_2 tension.

  2. When a metabolic alkalosis is compensated by a respiratory acidosis, the pH tends to return toward normal, but the CO_2 content and tension increase.

C. **Respiratory acidosis**

  1. An uncompensated respiratory acidosis is characterized by a low pH, a high CO_2 content, and a high CO_2 tension.

  2. When a respiratory acidosis is compensated by a metabolic alkalosis, the pH tends to return toward normal, but the CO_2 content increases; the CO_2 tension remains unchanged.

D. **Respiratory alkalosis**

  1. An uncompensated respiratory alkalosis is characterized by a high pH, a low CO_2 content, and a low CO_2 tension.

  2. When a respiratory alkalosis is compensated by a metabolic acidosis, the pH tends to become normal but the CO_2 content decreases; the CO_2 tension remains unchanged.

Exercise

Why do simple acid-base disturbances sometimes look mixed?

DISCUSSION

To emphasize the careful analysis of a compensatory response, consider the patient with a blood gas value that falsely suggests a mixed disturbance. Consider the patient with a history and physical examination that are inconsistent with diabetic ketoacidosis and with a blood gas that reveals a $[HCO_3^-]$ of 12 mEq/L and a PCO_2 of 33 mm Hg. (According to the Henderson equation, these data correspond to a $[H^+]$ of:

$$[H^+] = 24 \ \frac{PCO_2}{[HCO_3^-]} = 24 \ \frac{33}{12} = 66 \ nEq/L$$

and a pH of:

$$pH = 9 - \log [H^+]$$
$$= 9 - 1.82 = 7.18$$

According to Table 39–1, the expected PCO_2 is 26 mm Hg. Does the patient's PCO_2 (33 mm Hg) suggest an impaired compensatory response? There are a number of possibilities.

1. The low level of compensation may simply mean that there was insufficient time for compensation to become fully manifested. Maximal respiratory compensation usually develops within 12–24 hours after onset of the primary disorder. Maximal renal compensation requires 2–4 days. Thus, during the first day of a metabolic disturbance and during the first 2 or 3 days of a respiratory imbalance, the observed undercompensation may be normal.

2. Normal compensatory values apply to the middle 95% of patients, and 5% of patients with an intact compensatory response will be just outside the normal range.

3. It is possible that the patient has a deficiency in the compensatory response, leading to true under- or overcompensation. Hence, if the patient exhibited an early metabolic acidosis, either (a) there was not sufficient time for compensation (uncompensated metabolic acidosis) or (b) if there was sufficient time for compensation, the patient may have a mixed disturbance in acid-base status (metabolic acidosis with respiratory acidosis), in which case there are two coexisting primary disorders—not a primary and a coexisting secondary disorder.

Lastly, if we conclude that this patient has a mixed disorder, it would be possible that the metabolic and respiratory acidoses are present to the same degree. In this case, there would be a decline in pH without a change in $[HCO_3^-]$ and PCO_2. Since the $[HCO_3^-]$ changed (decreased) by 50% while the PCO_2 changed (increased) by about 18%, it is likely that this patient had a metabolic acidosis with a delayed or impaired respiratory compensatory response.

PART VI.   ACID–BASE PHYSIOLOGY

STUDY QUESTIONS

1. To maintain normal H^+ balance, total daily excretion of H^+ should equal the daily

(A) fixed acid production plus fixed acid ingestion
(B) HCO_3^- excretion
(C) HCO_3^- filtered load
(D) titratable acid excretion
(E) ammonium excretion

2. CO_2, which is not an acid, can lead to an increase in the $[H^+]$ of body fluids through the formation of

(A) HCO_3^-
(B) H_2CO_3
(C) lactic acid
(D) acetic acid
(E) phosphoric acid

Questions 3–6

A 25-year-old man suffers from severe diarrhea for about 1.5 hours and reports to the emergency room, where several tests are performed.

3. Based on his history, this patient's arterial pH would be expected to be approximately

(A) 7.32
(B) 7.40
(C) 7.42
(D) 7.45
(E) 7.50

4. The pH of this patient's cerebrospinal fluid would be expected to be approximately

(A) 7.12
(B) 7.22
(C) 7.30
(D) 7.32
(E) 7.40

5. During the compensatory response to his acid-base disorder, this patient's arterial CO_2 tension would most likely be

(A) 32 mm Hg
(B) 40 mm Hg
(C) 46 mm Hg
(D) 50 mm Hg
(E) 60 mm Hg

6. Following the compensatory response, a urinalysis of this patient would most likely indicate

(A) high pH
(B) decreased HCO_3^- excretion
(C) decreased titratable acid excretion
(D) increased Na^+ excretion

7. Titratable acid excretion is a major mechanism for renal excretion of noncarbonic acid. Titratable acid is

(A) mainly in the form of NH_4^+
(B) mainly in the form of monosodium phosphate ($NaHPO_4$)
(C) excreted in higher daily amounts than NH_4^+
(D) formed in the liver
(E) mainly formed in the lumen of the collecting duct

8. An hysterical 35-year-old woman is admitted to the hospital, and the following blood data are collected: $[HCO_3^-] = 22.2$ mmol/L, $PCO_2 = 30$ mm Hg, and $PO_2 = 98$ mm Hg. From these data, the blood $[H^+]$ of this patient would be expected to be

(A) 17.4 nmol/L
(B) 22.5 nmol/L
(C) 28.1 nmol/L
(D) 32.4 nmol/L
(E) 36.7 nmol/L

Questions 9–12

For each acid-base disorder listed below, select the appropriate pair of $[HCO_3^-]$ and CO_2 tension values.

	$[HCO_3^-]$ (mmol/L)	PCO_2 (mm Hg)
(A)	34	65
(B)	10	25
(C)	20	20
(D)	40	45

9. Metabolic acidosis

10. Metabolic alkalosis

11. Respiratory acidosis

12. Respiratory alkalosis

13. Most of the body's total daily acid production is derived from

(A) protein catabolism
(B) triglyceride catabolism
(C) phospholipid catabolism
(D) oxidative metabolism

14. Which one of the following statements about noncarbonic acids is NOT true?

(A) They are called fixed acids.
(B) They are classified as nonvolatile acids.
(C) They are excreted by the kidneys.
(D) They are buffered by both HCO_3^- and non-HCO_3^- buffers.
(E) They are primarily derived from the metabolism of fats.

15. Which one of the following conditions can be a potential consequence of HCO_3^- administration?

(A) Stimulation of pulmonary ventilation
(B) Aggravation of lactic acidosis if present
(C) Inhibition of glycolysis
(D) Decreased affinity of hemoglobin for oxygen
(E) Increased pH of the cerebrospinal fluid

16. A buffer pair (HA/A$^-$) has a pK of 6.4. At a blood pH of 7.4, the concentration of HA is

(A) one-hundredth that of A$^-$
(B) one-tenth that of A$^-$
(C) equal to that of A$^-$
(D) 10 times that of A$^-$
(E) 100 times that of A$^-$

17. Which one of the following statements referring to the renal regulation of $[H^+]$ is true?

(A) The kidneys excrete volatile acid.
(B) The kidneys excrete acid mainly in the form of free H^+.
(C) The kidneys excrete noncarbonic acid.
(D) The kidneys respond to metabolic acidosis mainly by increased excretion of titratable acid.
(E) The kidneys can excrete urine at a pH less than 4.

18. The following blood data are collected from a 27-year-old patient: pH = 7.50, $[HCO_3^-] = 38$ mmol/L, $PO_2 = 80$ mm Hg. Given these findings, what is the expected CO_2 tension (PCO_2) for this patient?

(A) 30 mm Hg
(B) 40 mm Hg
(C) 50 mm Hg
(D) 60 mm Hg
(E) 70 mm Hg

19. Acid-base disturbances associated with an elevated arterial CO_2 content include which one of the following conditions?

(A) Diabetic ketoacidosis
(B) Respiratory alkalosis
(C) Metabolic acidosis
(D) Metabolic alkalosis

20. A 32-year-old woman is admitted to the hospital with suspected partially compensated respiratory acidosis. Which of the following sets of laboratory data would confirm this suspicion?

	[HCO$_3^2$] (mEq/L)	PCO$_2$ (mm Hg)	pH
(A)	17	19	7.9
(B)	31	80	7.22
(C)	9.	30	7.14
(D)	24	45	7.5
(E)	20	25	7.5

21. A semicomatose 19-year-old woman is brought to the emergency room with dry skin, hyperventilation, hypotension, and a rapid pulse rate. The following blood data are obtained:

pH = 7.14
[Na$^+$] = 140 mEq/L
[K$^+$] = 4.5 mEq/L
[Cl$^-$] = 82 mEq/L
[HCO$_3^-$] = 11 mEq/L
PCO$_2$ = 30 mm Hg
[glucose] = 180 mg/dl
From the latter history and laboratory data, the most likely diagnosis is

(A) metabolic alkalosis
(B) metabolic acidosis
(C) respiratory alkalosis
(D) respiratory acidosis
(E) decreased anion gap

22. In metabolic acidosis, the fall in arterial pH is associated with which of the following arterial blood conditions?

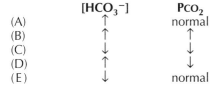

	[HCO$_3^-$]	PCO$_2$
(A)	↑	normal
(B)	↑	↑
(C)	↓	↓
(D)	↑	↓
(E)	↓	normal

23. The following arterial blood data are obtained from a hospitalized 55-year-old man:

[Na$^+$] = 140 mEq/L
[HCO$_3^-$] = 15 mEq/L
[Cl$^-$] = 113 mEq/L
pH = 7.2
From these data, which of the following statements about this patient is true?

(A) The patient has an elevated anion gap
(B) The patient has respiratory acidosis
(C) The [H$^+$] of this patient is higher than 100 nmol/L
(D) The arterial CO$_2$ tension of this patient is approximately normal
(E) The pH of this patient's cerebrospinal fluid (CSF) is decreased markedly

Questions 24–27

For each acid-base disorder listed below, select the appropriate pair of [HCO$_3^-$] and CO$_2$ tension values.

	[HCO$_3^-$] (mmol/L)	PCO$_2$ (mm Hg)
(A)	34	65
(B)	10	25
(C)	20	20
(D)	40	45

24. Metabolic acidosis

25. Metabolic alkalosis

26. Respiratory acidosis

27. Respiratory alkalosis

28. The following blood data are collected from a 58-year-old man: [H$^+$ = 49 nEq/L, PCO$_2$ = 30 mm Hg, and PO$_2$ = 95 mm Hg. From these data, this patient's blood pH would be expected to be

(A) 4.23
(B) 7.31
(C) 8.24
(D) 3.56
(E) 6.17

29. The addition of new bicarbonate to the blood by the kidneys is accomplished by the

(A) intraluminal buffering of protons by HCO_3^- ion
(B) secretion of protons
(C) buffering of protons by HPO_4^{2-}
(D) reabsorption of HCO_3^-
(E) excretion of free H^+ ions in the urine

30. Bone contains about 80% of the total carbon dioxide (CO_2) in the body. The major fraction of the CO_2 is in the form of

(A) carbonate
(B) carbonic acid
(C) bicarbonate
(D) carbon dioxide
(E) carbaminohemoglobin

31. The secretion of H^+ in the proximal tubule is primarily associated with

(A) excretion of K^+
(B) excretion of H^+
(C) reabsorption of HCO_3^-
(D) reabsorption of Ca^{2+}
(E) reabsorption of HPO_4^{7-}

32. A delirious 5-year-old boy is brought to the emergency room. His parents report that he was in good health until 2 hours earlier, when his mental state suddenly began to deteriorate. They suspect he may have swallowed a bottle of aspirin, because they discovered an empty bottle before leaving for the hospital. Laboratory evaluation reveals the following arterial blood data: $[H^+]$ = 18 nmol/L, $[HCO_3^-]$ = 13 mmol/L, P_{CO_2} = 10 mm Hg. This patient's history and blood data are most likely associated with

(A) respiratory alkalosis with partial renal compensation
(B) metabolic alkalosis with partial respiratory compensation
(C) a reduced $[HCO_3^-]$/dissolved CO_2 ratio
(D) a greater than normal CO_2 content

Questions 33–38

For each patient described below, select the set of arterial blood values that coincides with that patient's acid-base condition.

Patient	pH	[HCO$_3^-$] (mEq/L)	[P$_{CO_2}$] (mm Hg)	P$_{O_2}$ (mm Hg)
(A)	7.2	20	50	62
(B)	7.3	33	60	45
(C)	7.3	16	30	105
(D)	7.5	30	38	95
(E)	7.6	20	20	120

33. Patient with chronic respiratory acidosis and partial renal compensation

34. Patient with metabolic acidosis and partial respiratory compensation

35. Patient with uncompensated metabolic alkalosis

36. Patient with respiratory alkalosis and partial renal compensation

37. Patient with highest dissolved CO_2

38. Patient with highest CO_2 content

39. Respiratory alkalosis is characterized by which of the following arterial blood conditions?

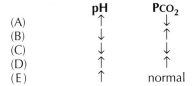

	pH	P_{CO_2}
(A)	↑	↓
(B)	↓	↑
(C)	↓	↓
(D)	↑	↑
(E)	↑	normal

Questions 40–43

Points A-D on the pH-$[HCO_3^-]$ diagram below indicate states of acid-base imbalance; point N indicates a normal acid-base state. Match each of the following conditions with the appropriate lettered point on the diagram.

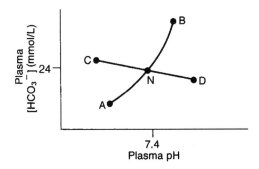

40. Hypocapnia

41. Hypercapnia

42. Ketoacidosis

43. $NaHCO_3$ ingestion

44. The following data were obtained from an arterial blood sample drawn from a hospitalized patient: pH = 7.55, P_{CO_2} = 25 mm Hg, and $[HCO_3^-]$ = 22.5 mEq/L. These findings indicate that the ratio of $[HCO_3^-]$ to dissolved CO_2 is

(A) 5:1
(B) 10:1
(C) 20:1
(D) 30:1
(E) greater than 30:1

45. Patient X has an arterial P_{CO_2} of 30 mm Hg and a plasma HCO_3^- concentration of 22 mM/L. What is the patient's H^+ concentration?

(A) 18 nmol/L; pH = 7.75
(B) 28 nmol/L; pH = 7.56
(C) 33 nmol/L; pH = 7.49
(D) 40 nmol/L; pH = 7.40
(E) 48 nmol/L; pH = 7.32

46. The secretion of H^+ by the proximal tubule occurs primarily by

(A) simple diffusion
(B) facilitated diffusion
(C) secondary active transport
(D) primary active transport
(E) cotransport with Na^+

47. An anxious 27-year-old man is examined in the emergency room, after which the following arterial blood data are obtained:

Blood Chemistry
[Na] = 140 mEq/L
[K^+] = 4 mEq/L
[HCO_3^-] = 19 mEq/L
[Cl^-] = 109 mEq/L

Blood Gas
pH = 7.6
PCO_2 = 20 mm Hg
Po_2 = 98 mm Hg

From these data, the most likely diagnosis is

(A) hypoxia
(B) metabolic alkalosis
(C) metabolic acidosis with respiratory compensation
(D) obstructive lung disease
(E) respiratory alkalosis

48. Which of the following sets of values is indicative of compensated metabolic alkalosis?

	[HCO_3^-] (mEq/L)	PCO_2 (mm Hg)	pH
(A)	20	25	7.50
(B)	40	46	7.56
(C)	17	30	7.30
(D)	34	10	7.70
(E)	17	19	7.90

49. A semicomatose 63-year-old male cigarette smoker presents with labored breathing, chronic coughing, and drowsiness. He has had a "smoker's cough" for 15 years. Physical examination reveals wheezing and slowing of forced expiration as well as cyanosis and bilateral leg edema. Initial laboratory data include the following:

hemoglobin concentration = 18.5 mg/dl
serum pH = 7.32
PCO_2 = 68 mm Hg
Po_2 = 33 mm Hg

From the above findings on history, physical examination, and laboratory testing, the most likely diagnosis is

(A) metabolic acidosis
(B) metabolic alkalosis
(C) respiratory acidosis
(D) respiratory alkalosis

Questions 50–51

The blood pressure falls during a surgical procedure on an anesthetized animal. The arterial blood becomes cyanotic despite the maintenance of normal ventilation. The arterial pH is 7.25, and the arterial CO_2 tension is 40 mm Hg.

50. The acid-base status of the animal is most likely to be

(A) metabolic acidosis with respiratory compensation
(B) respiratory acidosis with metabolic compensation
(C) metabolic acidosis
(D) respiratory acidosis
(E) respiratory alkalosis with renal compensation

51. To increase pH toward normal, in which direction would the ventilation rate be changed and what would be the corresponding change in arterial CO_2 tension?

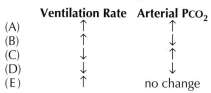

	Ventilation Rate	Arterial PCO_2
(A)	↑	↑
(B)	↑	↓
(C)	↓	↑
(D)	↓	↓
(E)	↑	no change

52. The following arterial blood data are collected from a 42-year-old female patient: [H^+] = 49 nEq/L, PCO_2 = 30 mm Hg, PO_2 = 95 mm Hg. Given these findings, what is the expected arterial bicarbonate concentration [HCO_3^-] for this patient?

(A) 13.2 mEq/L
(B) 14.7 mEq/L
(C) 15.8 mEq/L
(D) 16.5 mEq/L
(E) 17.1 mEq/L

53. Compared with normal, the urinary excretion of acid in metabolic acidosis is best characterized by which of the following patterns?

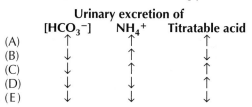

	Urinary excretion of		
	[HCO_3^-]	NH_4^+	Titratable acid
(A)	↑	↑	↑
(B)	↓	↑	↓
(C)	↓	↑	↑
(D)	↓	↓	↑
(E)	↓	↓	↓

Questions 54–58

For each patient described below, select the set of arterial blood values that coincides with that patient's acid-base condition.

Patient	pH	P_{CO_2} (mm Hg)	$[HCO_3^-]$ (mmol/L)
(A)	7.00	70	16
(B)	7.10	27	8
(C)	7.34	70	39
(D)	7.50	48	36
(E)	7.56	26	23

54. Patient with metabolic alkalosis and appropriate respiratory compensation

55. Patient with metabolic acidosis and respiratory acidosis

56. Patient with the highest CO_2 content

57. Patient with the highest $[H^+]$

58. Patient with the highest $[HCO_3^-]/S \cdot P_{CO_2}$ ratio

59. Which of the following statements about the pH of cerebrospinal fluid (CSF) is FALSE?

(A) It is the same as plasma pH during normal acid-base conditions.
(B) It decreases during metabolic alkalosis.
(C) It increases during metabolic acidosis.
(D) It increases during hyperventilation.
(E) It changes in the opposite direction as plasma pH during metabolic acidosis.

60. Which one of the following statements referring to H^+ secretion by the type A intercalated cells of the collecting duct is NOT true?

(A) H^+ can combine with NH_4^+
(B) H^+ can combine with HCO_3^-
(C) H^+ can combine with HPO_4^{2-}
(D) H^+ can remain as free H^+
(E) H^+ is secreted by the H^+-ATPase pump

ANSWERS AND EXPLANATIONS

1. The answer is A [Chapter 32 II A, B 2, Table 32–3; Chapter 37 I B 1, IV, and V C 4]. Total daily production of H^+ from the catabolism of proteins and phospholipids plus any additional fixed acid that is ingested must be matched by the sum of excretion of H^+ as titratable acid plus NH_4^+ to maintain acid-base balance.

2. The answer is B [Chapter 32 I A, III C; Chapter 34 IV B 1 c]. Carbon dioxide (CO_2) is a hydrogen ion (H^+) generator. It is evident that the total reservoir of carbonic acid (H_2CO_3) [i.e., both dissolved CO_2 and H_2CO_3 termed the total "carbonic acid pool"] should be considered the acid component of the HCO_3^- buffer system, and HCO_3^- should be considered the conjugate base. The HCO_3^-/CO_2 buffer system is the most important extracellular fluid (ECF) buffer pair. CO_2, which is not an acid, increases the acidity of a solution through the formation and dissociation of H_2CO_3. Students are often confused by the following series of reactions:

$$CO_2 + H_2O \rightarrow H_2CO_3 \rightarrow H^+ + HCO_3^-$$

because both H^+ and HCO_3^- are formed simultaneously, and there should be no change in pH. However, the HCO_3^- concentration is several orders of magnitude (6×10^5) greater than the H^+ concentration and is correspondingly less affected by any change in the concentration of CO_2 or H_2CO_3.

3–6. The answers are: 3-A, 4-E, 5-A, 6-B [Chapter 34 III B; Chapter 39 IV A; V C; VI A; Figures 34–1, 38–6, 38–8]. The fluid in the small and large intestine is relatively high in HCO_3^-. Therefore, severe diarrhea is a cause of metabolic acidosis, which is the likely diagnosis in this patient. Only one of the given arterial pH values—7.32—is consistent with acidosis.

Increased arterial [H^+] stimulates ventilation, lowering the CO_2 tension of the blood and CSF, resulting in blood acidosis and CSF alkalosis. Thus, in metabolic acid-base alterations, the pH of the blood and CSF change in opposite directions, whereas in respiratory

acid-base abnormalities the pH of the blood and CSF change in the same direction. Since the normal pH of CSF is 7.32, the pH would increase in metabolic acidosis. The only given pH value indicating a CSF alkalosis is 7.40.

Metabolic acidosis is compensated by hyperventilation, which reduces the CO_2 tension and thereby attenuates the reduction in pH. This hyperventilatory response to metabolic acidosis is due to direct stimulation of the medullary respiratory center and of the peripheral chemoreceptors in the carotid and aortic bodies. Only one of the given CO_2 tension values—32 mm Hg—is associated with hypocarbia.

In the absence of therapy with $NaHCO_3$, the renal compensation for a metabolic acidosis requires an increased HCO_3^- reabsorption together with an increased H^+ secretion and excretion. This adaptive response is accomplished by an increased NH_4^+ excretion with a limited ability to enhance titratable acidity via $H_2PO_4^-$ excretion. Thus, the urine will exhibit a low pH.

7. The answer is B [Chapter 37 IV; VI B; Figure 37–3, Table 37–1]. Titratable acid includes the H'' from the fixed (noncarbonic) acids, such as uric acid and ketoacids. It also includes creatinine, but the bulk of the titratable acid comprises monovalent phosphate ($H_2PO_4^-$). Phosphate is not excreted in higher amounts than is NH_4^+, but it is a major component of net acid excretion. Monobasic phosphate is formed mainly in the lumen of the proximal tubule.

8. The answer is D [Chapter 34 V B 2; Chapter 38 III B 2; C 1]. From the data given, this patient's arterial [H^+] is determined to be 32.4 nmol/L. The Henderson equation is used in this case, which is:

$$[H^+] = 24 \frac{P_{CO_2}}{[HCO_3^-]}$$

It is necessary to keep in mind that the units for these factors are: [H^+] (nmol/L, [HCO_3^-] (mmol/L), and P_{CO_2} (mm Hg).

Substituting,

$$[H^+] = 24 \frac{30}{22.2}$$

$$= 32.4 \text{ nmol/L}$$

This patient has a partially compensated respiratory alkalosis. Note that her arterial $[H^+]$ and $[HCO_3^-]$ exhibit a parallel decrease.

9–12. The answers are 9-B, 10-D, 11-A, 12-C [Chapter 38 I B, C; V A, B; Tables 38–3, 38–4; Figure 38–5]. In analyzing these four acid-base disorders, it is necessary to consider both the primary abnormality (i.e., the variable that undergoes the greater degree of change) and the compensatory response (i.e., the alternate variable, which undergoes a lesser degree of change in the same direction).

In metabolic acidosis, there is a primary decrease in $[HCO_3^-]$ and a compensatory decrease in CO_2 tension. Only one pair of values (*B*) shows this pattern. In metabolic alkalosis, there is a primary increase in $[HCO_3^-]$ and a compensatory increase in CO_2 tension. Only one pair of values (*D*) shows this pattern. In respiratory acidosis, there is a primary increase in CO_2 tension and a compensatory increase in $[HCO_3^-]$. Only one pair of values (*A*) shows this pattern. In respiratory alkalosis, there is a primary decrease in CO_2 tension and a compensatory decrease in $[HCO_3^-]$. Only one pair of values (*C*) shows this pattern.

13. The answer is D [Chapter 32 I A; III D]. Most of the body's daily CO_2 production occurs from chemical reactions of the tricarboxylic acid cycle. From this metabolic activity, humans produce about 13,000 mmol of CO_2 daily, or, in acid-base terms, about 13,000 mEq of H^+ per day. The mammalian body produces large amounts of acids from two major sources. The volatile acid H_2CO_3 is produced from CO_2, the end product of oxidative metabolism. A variety of nonvolatile acids (e.g., H_2SO_4, H_3PO_4) are produced from dietary substances.

14. The answer is E [Chapter 32, IV; Table 32–3]. Noncarbonic acids include all acids other than H_2CO_3, such as lactic, acetoacetic, β-hydroxybutyric, hydrochloric, and sulfuric acids. Some noncarbonic acids (lactic, acetoacetic, and β-hydroxybutyric acids) can be converted to CO_2 and eliminated by ventilation (the fate of "volatile" acids). However, when present in large amounts, these acids are eliminated by the kidney (the fate of "nonvolatile" acids). Sulfuric, hydrochloric, and phosphoric acids cannot be catabolized to CO_2 and H_2O and, thus, must be eliminated by renal excretion. Noncarbonic acids can be buffered by both HCO_3^- and non-HCO_3^- buffer systems. Fixed acid is another name for nonvolatile acid. Metabolites of amino acids constitute the major portion of nonvolatile acids.

15. The answer is B [Chapter 32 IV B 5 a; Chapter 36 III A 2 a; Chapter 38 IV B 1 b; Chapter 39 IV B 1, V D]. Pulmonary ventilation is suppressed in response to an increased HCO_3^- concentration. Acidosis inhibits, whereas alkalosis stimulates it; consequently, alkalosis results in elevated plasma lactate levels. Thus, the use of alkali therapy in the treatment of lactic acidosis is controversial because the rising pH with this treatment tends to further increase hyperlactatemia. Bicarbonate ion causes the O_2^- association/dissociation curve to shift to the left, causing a higher affinity of hemoglobin for oxygen. The suppression of ventilatory drive by HCO_3^- leads to an increase in P_{CO_2}. The diffusion of CO_2 across the blood-brain barrier would lead to a decline in the pH of the cerebrospinal fluid.

16. The answer is B [Chapter 34 IV B 1]. Using the Henderson-Hasselbalch equation to calculate the ratio of HA/A^-:

$$pH = pK + \log A^-/HA$$

$$7.4 = 6.4 + \log A^-/HA$$

$$\log A^-/HA = 1.0$$

$$A^-/HA = \text{antilog } 1 = 10$$

$$\text{Therefore } HA/A^- = 1/10 = 0.1$$

17. The answer is C [Chapter 32 IV; Chapter 37 I A, B 1 b; V C]. The kidneys excrete fixed (noncarbonic, or nonvolatile) acid in the forms of titratable acid and ammonium. In the setting of high acid loads (metabolic acidosis), the major increase in acid excretion is mainly in the form of NH_4^+. The lungs, on the other hand, are responsible for the elimination of carbonic (volatile) acid. The minimal urine pH is about 4.4.

18. The answer is C [Chapter 34 IV C 2 b; V B 2; Chapter 38 IV C 1]. From the data given, this patient's arterial CO_2 tension (PCO_2) is determined to be 50 mm Hg (normal = 40 mm Hg). The Henderson equation is used to estimate PCO_2, but $[H^+]$ must be determined first using the Henderson-Hasselbalch equation. Given a pH of 7.5, $[H^+]$ is calculated as:

$$[H^+] = \text{antilog } (9 - pH)$$

$$= \text{antilog } (9 - 7.5)$$

$$= \text{antilog } 1.5 = 31.6 \text{ nmol/L}$$

Substituting to solve for PCO_2,

$$PCO_2 = \frac{[H^+]\,[HCO_3^-]}{24}$$

$$= \frac{(31.6 \text{ nmol/L})\,(38 \text{ mmol/L})}{24}$$

$$= 50 \text{ mm Hg}$$

This patient's increased bicarbonate concentration ($[HCO_3^-]$) indicates a metabolic alkalosis. The elevated bicarbonate levels suppress respiratory drive, leading to compensatory elevation of CO_2 tension. Note that unit analysis cannot be used in this equation.

19. The answer is D [Chapter 38 I E 3; Table 38–4]. The total CO_2 content is mainly a function of HCO_3^- and dissolved CO_2. Therefore, CO_2 content is elevated in metabolic alkalosis and respiratory acidosis. Conversely, CO_2 content declines with decreases in $[HCO_3^-]$ and $[CO_2]$, conditions that are associated with metabolic acidosis and respiratory alkalosis, respectively. Note that $[CO_2]$ denotes the concentration of dissolved CO_2 and is calculated as:

$$[CO_2] = S \cdot PCO_2$$

$$= 0.03 \cdot 40 \text{ mm Hg}$$

$$= 1.2 \text{ mmol/L (normal)}$$

20. The answer is B [Chapter 38 I B 1 a; IV B 2 a; Chapter 39 V A; Tables 38–3, 38–4; Figures 38–5, 38–8, 39–1]. In respiratory acidosis, there is a primary increase in plasma CO_2 tension (PCO_2). The renal compensation for respiratory acidosis is increased HCO_3^- reabsorption, which increases the plasma $[HCO_3^-]$. With partial compensation, the pH would not return to normal. Only one set of data (*B*) indicates hypercapnia with a decrease in pH. Note that the pH and the $[HCO_3^-]/S \cdot PCO_2$ ratio are below normal in this patient, which is consistent with acidosis.

21. The answer is B [Chapter 38 I B 2 a, IV B 1 a; Chapter 39 V C; Tables 38–3, 38–4; Figures 38–5, 38–8, 39–1]. The decreases in arterial pH, $[HCO_3^-]$, and CO_2 tension are consistent with metabolic acidosis. There also is a decreased $[HCO_3^-]/S \cdot PCO_2$ ratio (i.e., 12.2) and a widened anion gap (i.e., 47 mEq/L). The primary disturbance is the marked reduction in $[HCO_3^-]$, and the compensatory response in hyperventilation (as indicated by the hypocapnia). That the $[HCO_3^-]$ decreases and the $[H^+]$ increases is evidence of metabolic acid-base imbalance. The hyperglycemia and dehydration (as evidenced by dry skin) support a diagnosis of diabetes mellitus.

22. The answer is C [Chapter 38 I B 2 a, IV B 1 a; Chapter 39 V C; Tables 38–3, 38–4; Figures 38–5, 38–8, 39–1]. Metabolic acidosis is an acid-base disturbance characterized by a decreased arterial pH (or increased $[H^+]$), a decreased plasma $[HCO_3^-]$, and a compensatory hyperventilation resulting in a decreased arterial CO_2 tension.

23. The answer is D [Chapter 34 V; Chapter 38 II B 2]. From the data given, this patient's arterial CO_2 tension is determined to be 38 mmol/L, which is close to normal (40 mmol/L). The Henderson equation is used to calculate

CO_2 tension. The equation typically is expressed as:

$$[H^+] = 24 \frac{P_{CO_2}}{[HCO_3^-]}$$

Note that when $[HCO_3^-]$ is low, as in this patient, a change in CO_2 tension will have a greater effect on $[H^+]$ than when $[HCO_3^-]$ is normal or high.

$$P_{CO_2} = \frac{[H^+] [NCO_3^-]}{24}$$

First, the $[H^+]$ is calculated from the pH value as:

$$[H^+] = \text{antilog} (9 - pH)$$

$$= \text{antilog} (9 - 7.22)$$

$$= \text{antilog} (1.78)$$

$$= 60 \text{ nmol/L}$$

Then, CO_2 tension can be determined as:

$$P_{CO_2} = \frac{[H^+] [HCO_3^-]}{24}$$

$$= \frac{(60) (15)}{24} = 38 \text{ mm Hg}$$

Thus, the CO_2 tension of this patient is within normal limits, and therefore respiratory compensation has not occurred. The acid-base disturbance of this patient is attributable to a hyperchloremic metabolic acidosis.

To determine CO_2 tension, the Henderson equation is rearranged as:

$$AG = [Na^+] - [HCO_3^- + Cl^-]$$

$$= 140 \text{ mEq/L} - (15 \text{ mEq/L} + 113 \text{ mEq/L})$$

$$= 140 \text{ mEq/L} - 128 \text{ mEq/L} = 12 \text{ mEq/L}$$

Notice that, in this type of acidosis, the anion gap (AG) is normal. The pH of the cerebrospinal fluid (CSF) in metabolic acidosis usually is elevated because of the compensatory hyperventilatory response to the metabolic acidosis. In this patient, there is no evidence of significant hyperventilation, and therefore the pH of the CSF would not increase significantly. The axiom to remember is that metabolic acid-base alterations evoke opposite changes in the pH of the CSF and blood, whereas respiratory acid-base disturbances bring about parallel changes in the pH of CSF and blood.

24–27. The answers are: 24-B, 25-D, 26-A, 27-C [Chapter 38 I B, III A 3; Chapter 39 I C; Tables 38–3 and 38–4; Figure 38–5]. In analyzing these four acid-base disorders, it is necessary to consider both the primary abnormality (i.e., the variable that undergoes the greater degree of change) and the compensatory response (i.e., the alternate variable, which undergoes a lesser degree of change in the same direction).

In metabolic acidosis, there is a primary decrease in $[HCO_3^-]$ and a compensatory decrease in CO_2 tension. Only one pair of values (B) shows this pattern. In metabolic alkalosis, there is a primary increase in $[HCO_3^-]$ and a compensatory increase in CO_2 tension. Only one pair of values (D) shows this pattern. In respiratory acidosis, there is a primary increase in CO_2 tension and a compensatory increase in $[HCO_3^-]$. Only one pair of values (A) shows this pattern. In respiratory alkalosis, there is a primary decrease in CO_2 tension and a compensatory decrease in $[HCO_3^-]$. Only one pair of values (C) shows this pattern.

28. The answer is B [Chapter 34, IV C 1; V B 2]. From the data given, this patient's blood pH is determined to be 7.31. To determine the arterial pH, it is first necessary to calculate the arterial $[HCO_3^-]$ using the Henderson equation:

$$[HCO_3^-] = 24 \frac{P_{CO_2}}{[H^+]}$$

$$= 24 \frac{30}{49}$$

$$= 14.7 \text{ mmol/L}$$

Then, applying the Henderson-Hasselbalch equation, the arterial pH is determined as

$$pH = pK = + \log \frac{[HCO_3^-]}{S \cdot P_{CO_2}}$$

$$= 6.1 + \log \frac{14.7 \text{ mmol/L}}{0.9 \text{ mmol/L}}$$

$$= 6.1 + \log 16.3$$

$$= 6.1 + 1.21$$

$$= 7.31$$

This patient has a partially compensated metabolic acidosis. It is important to note that the $[HCO_3^-]/S \cdot PCO_2$ ratio is equal to 16.3, which indicates a significant respiratory response (hyperventilation) to the metabolic problem. Thus, this metabolic acidosis is alleviated by a response that involves the respiratory system.

29. The answer is C [Chapter 37 I B 1 b, III C, IV B; Table 37–1; Figure 37–3]. Most of the H^+ that is secreted (more than 4000 mEq per day) is buffered by luminal HCO_3^- and reabsorbed. Only the H^+ that combines with luminal nonbicarbonate buffers (HPO_4^{2-} or NH_3)' is excreted and thereby adds new HCO_3^- to the body. The catabolism of glutamine is also associated with the secretion and subsequent excretion of NH_4^+, thereby contributing to the formation of new HCO_3^-. Thus, the combination of H^+ with a buffer other than HCO_3^- accomplishes not only HCO_3^- conservation but also the addition of a new HCO_3^- that raises the HCO_3^- concentration of blood. The reabsorption of HCO_3^- must be contrasted to the generation of new HCO_3^-. The excreted H^+ ion in urine is largely (99%) in the form of H^+ bound to buffers and can be assessed by measuring urinary acidity and ammonium. Urine pH by itself fails to provide any information about H^+ bound to buffers.

30. The answer is A [Chapter 35 I A 2 b (1) (2)]. Total CO_2 includes all of the substances shown in answers A through E. However, the largest fraction (about two-thirds) of the total CO_2 is in the form of carbonates combined with Na, Ca^2 and other cations in bone crystals. The remaining one-third consists of HCO_3^- found in the hydration shell of the hydroxyapatite crystal. The total bone carbonate is about 50 times the amount of HCO_3^- found in the ICF and ECF together.

31. The answer is C [Chapter 27 III A, J 1; Chapter 37 III A; Figures 27–3, 37–1, 37–2]. In the proximal tubule, most of the H^+ is actively secreted into the tubular lumen via the Na^+-H^+ antiporter. Most of this H^+ combines with HCO_3^- in the tubular fluid to form CO_2 and water. The CO_2 diffuses into the proximal tubular cells, where H_2CO_3 is resynthesized

and dissociated into H^+ and HCO_3^-. The HCO_3^- exits the cells through the basolateral border via the $3HCO_3^--1Na^+$ symporter. Carbonic anhydrase is located on the luminal surface of the cells as well as inside the cells and facilitates the dehydration (lumen) and hydration (intracellular) of carbonic acid. The urinary buffer existing in the highest amount is HCO_3^-.

32. The answer is A [Chapter 38 I B 1, IV B 2 b; Chapter 39 V B; Tables 38–3 and 38–4; Figures 38–5, 39–1]. The variable that shows the greatest degree of change in this patient is arterial CO_2 tension (PCO_2), which is decreased by 75% compared with a 46% decrease in $[HCO_3^-]$. These findings are consistent with respiratory alkalosis, which, in this case, is due to hyperventilation brought on by early salicylate toxicity. The resultant hypocapnia reduces tubular H^+ secretion, so the HCO_3^- reabsorption is attenuated, causing a compensatory loss of urinary HCO_3^-. The arterial pH of this patient can be calculated using the Henderson-Hasselbalch equation as:

$$pH = pK + \log \frac{[HCO_3^-]}{S \cdot PCO_2}$$

$$= 6.1 + \log \frac{13 \text{ mmol/L}}{0.3 \text{ mmol/L}}$$

$$= 6.1 + \log 43.3$$

$$= 6.1 + 1.6$$

$$= 7.7$$

Note that the increased ratio of $[HCO_3^-]/S \cdot PCO_2$ is consistent with alkalotic states. This condition must be differentiated from metabolic alkalosis, which is associated with increases in arterial $[HCO_3^-]$, CO_2 tension, and pH.

33–38. The answers are: 33-B, 34-C, 35-D, 36-E, 37-B, 38-B [Chapter 34 IV B 2, 3; Chapter 38 1 E 3; IV A-B; Chapter 39 IV-VI; Figures 38–5; 38–7; 38–8]. *Patient B* has respiratory acidosis with partial renal compensation. Respiratory acidosis is caused by increased CO_2 tension, which reduces the $[HCO_3^-]/S \cdot PCO_2$ ratio and thus the pH. Whenever CO_2 tension rises, $[HCO_3^-]$ also must increase somewhat because of the dissociation of H_2CO_3 formed by the hydration of CO_2. The kidney responds by conserving $[HCO_3^-]$ via increased H^+ secretion, with acid excreted as $H_2PO_4^-$ and NH_4^-.

Patient C has metabolic acidosis with partial respiratory compensation. Metabolic acidosis means a primary decrease in $[HCO_3^-]$, which decreases the $[HCO_3^-]/S \cdot 1\ P_{CO_2}$ ratio and thus the pH. The $[HCO_3^-]$ may be lowered by the addition of H^+ or by the loss of HCO_3^-. Respiratory compensation occurs by increased ventilation via the action of H^+ in the peripheral and central chemoreceptors.

Patient D has uncompensated metabolic alkalosis. In this condition, the increase in $[HCO_3^-]$ causes an increase in the $[HCO_3^-]/S \cdot P_{CO_2}$ ratio and thus the pH. Respiratory compensation occurs by a reduction in alveolar ventilation, which tends to raise CO_2 tension (not evident in *patient D*).

Patient E has respiratory alkalosis with partial renal compensation. Respiratory alkalosis is caused by a decrease in CO_2 tension, which increases the $[HCO_3^-]/S \cdot P_{CO_2}$ ratio and thus the pH. Renal compensation occurs by increased HCO_3^- excretion.

Patient B has both the highest amount of dissolved CO_2 and the highest total CO_2 content. Dissolved CO_2 is determined by multiplying the CO_2 tension (in mm Hg) by the CO_2 tension solubility constant, S, as

$$\text{dissolved } CO_2 = S \cdot P_{CO_2}$$

$$= 0.03 \cdot 60$$

$$= 1.8 \text{ mmol/L}$$

Total CO_2 content is the sum of $[HCO_3^-]$ and dissolved CO_2. It is calculated in *patient B* as total CO_2 content

$$= [HCO_3^-] + S \cdot P_{CO_2}$$

$$= 33 + 0.03 \cdot 60$$

$$= 33 + 1.8$$

$$= 34.8 \text{ mmol/L}$$

39. The answer is A [Chapter 38 I B 1 b, IV B 2 b; Tables 38–3, 38–4; Figures 38–5, 38–8]. Respiratory alkalosis is an acid-base disturbance characterized by an increased arterial pH (or decreased $[H^+]$), a decreased CO_2 ten-

sion (hypocapnia), and a variable reduction in arterial $[HCO_3^-]$ due to renal compensation.

40–43. The answers are: 40-D, 41-C, 42-A, 43-B [Chapter 38 I B 1–2; Chapter 39 IV A–D]. In analyzing these four uncompensated acid-base disturbances, it is important to consider the CO_2 tension and $[HCO_3^-]$ rather than the pH, because CO_2 tension and $[HCO_3^-]$ are the key determinants of the cause of, and compensation for, these disturbances.

Point D represents a patient with increased PH ($\downarrow [H^+]$) brought about by respiratory alkalosis. This condition is characterized by a primary decrease in CO_2 tension (hypocapnia) and a variable secondary decrease in plasma $[HCO_3^-]$. Metabolic acidosis also is characterized by declines in these two variables, but the pH is decreased ($\uparrow [H^+]$) as well. Respiratory alkalosis is defined as alveolar ventilation greater than the existing need of the body to eliminate CO_2. This excess in alveolar ventilation, called hyperventilation, results in a reduced arterial CO_2 tension. Hyperpnea is the general term used to describe any increase in ventilatory effort. With respiratory alkalosis, there is a decline in the [total CO_2].

Point C represents a patient with decreased pH ($\uparrow [H^+]$) caused by respiratory acidosis. This clinical disorder is characterized by a primary increase in CO_2 tension (hypercapnia) and a variable secondary increase in plasma $[HCO_3^-]$. The common denominator in respiratory acidosis is hypoventilation, which is defined as alveolar ventilation insufficient to excrete CO_2 rapidly enough to meet the existing needs of the body. With respiratory acidosis, there is a relatively small increment in the [total CO_2], because the major fraction of the CO_2 content is composed of HCO_3^-.

Point A represents a patient with diabetes mellitus, which is the most common cause of ketoacidosis. This overproduction of ketoacids is caused by a deficiency of insulin, which leads to: (1) increased lipolysis and an increased delivery of free fatty acids to the liver and (2) the preferential conversion of free fatty acids to ketoacids rather than to triglycerides. Thus, metabolic acidosis is characterized by a low arterial pH ($\uparrow H^+$]), a reduced $[HCO_3^-]$, and a compensatory hyperventilation resulting in hypocapnia. The renal compensatory response for respiratory alkalosis also diminishes the plasma $[HCO_3^-]$, but the pH in that disorder is elevated ($\downarrow$ H$^+$]). Overproduction of ketoacids causes acidosis by two mechanisms: (1) a decrease in plasma [HCO$_3^-$] with an increase in the anion gap and (2) overloading of the renal capacity to excrete H$^+$ resulting in a loss of Na$^+$ and a failure to recover NaHCO$_3$. In metabolic acidosis, there is a decline in the [total CO$_2$]. Furthermore, ketoacidosis, like lactic acidosis, differs from other forms of metabolic acidosis in that the anion associated with H$^+$ can be metabolized back to HCO$_3^-$, as β-hydroxybutyrate$^-$ + O$_2$ $\rightarrow$ CO$_2$ + H$_2$O + HCO$_3^-$.

β-Hydroxybutyrate represents about 75% of the circulating ketoacids in diabetic ketoacidosis. It can be seen from the latter chemical equation that the metabolism of the β-hydroxybutyrate anion results in the regeneration of the HCO$_3^-$ that was neutralized in buffering the H$^+$. Since the HCO$_3^-$ is replaced by an anion that is metabolized back to HCO$_3^-$, there is no actual loss of HCO$_3^-$ from the body in ketoacidosis (or lactic acidosis). Insulin administration decreases the accumulation of β-hydroxybutyric acid and allows the metabolism of the acid ions back to HCO$_3^-$.

Point B represents a patient with metabolic alkalosis. Excessive ingestion of NaHCO$_3$ can result in metabolic alkalosis and an increase of pH ($\downarrow$ [H$^+$]). Metabolic alkalosis is characterized by an increase in the plasma [HCO$_3^-$] and a compensatory increase in the CO$_2$ tension produced by a decline in alveolar ventilation. Since elevation of plasma [HCO$_3^-$] can be due to the renal compensation for chronic respiratory acidosis, the diagnosis of metabolic alkalosis cannot be made without measuring the pH. Metabolic alkalosis is associated with a large increase in the [total CO$_2$].

44. The answer is D [Chapter 34, IV B; Chapter 38 I C; Tables 38–3 and 38–4; Figure 38–5]. In alkalotic states, the [HCO$_3^-$]/S · P$_{CO_2}$ ratio exceeds the normal 20:1, due to either an increase in [HCO$_3^-$] (metabolic alkalosis) or a decrease in CO$_2$ tension (respiratory alkalosis). The normal ratio of 20:1 is derived as:

$$\frac{[HCO_3^-]}{S \cdot P_{CO_2}} = \frac{24 \text{ mmol/L}}{0.03 \cdot 40 \text{ mm Hg}}$$

$$= \frac{24 \text{ mmol/L}}{1.2 \text{ mmolL}} = \frac{20}{1}$$

In this alkalotic patient, the [HCO$_3^-$]/S · P$_{CO_2}$

is 30:1. This ratio can be determined by substituting the patient's blood data into the above equation, as:

$$\frac{[HCO_3^-]}{S \cdot P_{CO_2}} = \frac{22.5 \text{ mmol/L}}{0.03 \cdot 25 \text{ mm Hg}}$$

$$= \frac{22.5 \text{ mmol/L}}{0.75 \text{ mmol/L}} = \frac{30}{1}$$

45. The answer is A [Chapter 34 IV C 2 b, V B 2]. The total daily production of fixed acid from the catabolism of proteins and phospholipids together with an additional acid via ingestion must be matched by the excretion of H$^+$, which is equal to the sum of titratable acid and NH$_4^+$ to maintain acid-base balance.

46. The answer is C [Chapter 27 III J; Chapter 37 III; Figures 27–3, 37–1, and 37–2]. Two-thirds of the total H$^+$ secretion occurs via the Na$^+$–H$^+$ antiporter and takes place mainly by the proximal tubule. This countertransporter is a secondary active transport system whereby the active secretion of H$^+$ is energized by the lumen to cell Na$^+$ concentration gradient. Of course, this secretory carrier depends on metabolic energy (ATP) insofar as the Na$^+$ electrochemical gradient is maintained by the Na$^+$–K$^+$-ATPase pump.

47. The answer is E [Chapter 38 I B 1 b; IV a, B 2 a, V A 2; Chater 39 IV D, V B; Tables 38–3 and 38–4; Figures 38–5, 39–1]. The most likely diagnosis is respiratory alkalosis resulting from anxiety-induced hyperventilation. The key determinants of the cause and compensation of the acid-base disorder are the arterial CO$_2$ tension and [HCO$_3^-$]. The greater reduction in CO$_2$ tension than in [HCO$_3^-$] indicates that the primary disturbance is respiratory alkalosis. That both the arterial [HCO$_3^-$] and [H$^+$] change in the same direction further supports the diagnosis of a respiratory acid-base imbalance. Both obstructive and restrictive lung diseases are common causes of respiratory acidosis.

48. The answer is B [Chapter 38 I, III A, IV B 1, V B 2; Tables 38–3 and 38–4; Figure 38–5, 38–8]. The hallmarks of metabolic alkalosis are elevated [HCO_3^-], which is the primary event, and elevated CO_2 tension, which is the compensatory event. Also, the [H^+] decreases and the [HCO_3^-] increases. The only other patient set of values showing an increased [HCO_3^-]–set D–does not exhibit an increase in CO_2 tension.

49. The answer is C [Chapter 34 IV C; V B; Chapter 38 I, III A, IV B 2, V A I; Tables 38–3, 38–4; Figures 38–5, 38–8]. This patient has an acidosis caused by CO_2 retention (i.e., respiratory acidosis). The condition is partially compensated by renal retention of HCO_3^-. The [HCO_3^-] can be determined using either the Henderson-Hasselbalch equation or the Henderson equation.

Using the Henderson-Hasselbalch equation, the [HCO_3^-] is determined as

$$pH = pK' + \log \frac{[HCO_3^-]}{S \cdot P_{CO_2}}$$

$$7.32 = 6.1 + \log \frac{[HCO_3^-]}{0.03 \cdot 68 \text{ mm Hg}}$$

$$7.32 = 6.1 + \log [HCO_3^-] - \log 2.04$$

$$\log [HCO_3^-] = 7.32 - 6.1 + 0.31$$

$$= 1.53$$

antilog 1.53 = 33.9 mmol/L

Using the Henderson equation, the [HCO_3^-] is determined as

$$[HCO_3^-] = 24 \frac{P_{CO_2} \text{ (mm Hg)}}{[H^+] \text{ (nmol/L)}}$$

$$= 24 \frac{68 \text{ mm Hg}}{47.9 \text{ nmol/L}}$$

$$= 34.1 \text{ mmol/L}$$

The patient's hypoxemia could be due to a pulmonary diffusion barrier. The cyanosis is caused by a greater than normal concentration of reduced hemoglobin (greater than 5 g/dl of arterial blood in the deoxy state). The leg edema could be due to the increased retention of HCO_3^- and Na^+, resulting in an increase in plasma volume. The hypoxemia causes polycythemia and constriction of vascular smooth muscle of the pulmonary circulation, leading to pulmonary hypertension, elevated right atrial pressure, and increased capillary pressure. The increase in capillary pressure causes fluid movement into the interstitial space and, ultimately, edema.

50–51. The answers are: 50-C, 51-B [Chapter 38 IV B 1; Chapter 39 IV A1–2]. The acid-base abnormality is metabolic acidosis without respiratory compensation. Since the respiratory response to metabolic acidosis is hyperpnea, hypocapnia would be expected, but is not observed in this case. Moreover, the imbalance cannot be attributed to respiratory acidosis, which would be characterized by an elevated arterial CO_2 tension. It is apparent that a mechanical respirator maintained the animal's CO_2 tension at a constant level.

The pH of arterial blood is a function of two variables: [HCO_3^-] and CO_2 tension. A compensatory response occurs in the alternate variable and in the same direction as the primary abnormality. In this case, the decline in [HCO_3^-] (i.e., metabolic acidosis) would be associated with a parallel decline in CO_2 tension, the alternate variable. To bring this about, there would be a hyperventilatory response and a resultant decline in CO_2 tension.

52. The answer is B [Chapter 34, V B]. From the data given, this patient's arterial bicarbonate concentration ([HCO_3^-]) is determined to be 14.7 mmol/L (mEq/L). Arterial [HCO_3^-] is easily estimated using the Henderson equation, which is stated as:

$$[HCO_3^-] = 24 \frac{P_{CO_2}}{[H^+]}$$

where [HCO_3^-] is expressed in mmol/L, [H^+] in nmol/L, and P_{CO_2} in mm Hg. Substituting,

$$[HCO_3^-] = 24 \frac{30}{49}$$

$$= 14.7 \text{ mmol/L}$$

The acid-base disturbance in this case is an almost completely compensated metabolic acidosis (pH 7.32).

53. The answer is C [Chapter 37 IV, V, VI B]. The kidney responds to an increased acid load by augmenting renal ammonia (NH_3) production and, consequently, ammonium (NH_4^+) excretion. There is a smaller increase in the excretion of titratable acid (primarily in the form of $H_2PO_4^-$. Thus, the decreased pH and decreased HCO_3^- excretion and increased H^+ excretion (in the form of NH_4^+ and $H_2PO_4^-$) are consistent with metabolic acidosis.

54–58. The answers are: 54-D, 55-B, 56-C, 57-A, 58-E [Chapter 34 IV C 2; V B 2; Chapter 38 I C, I E 3; IV B; V; Chapter 39 IV, V; Figure 38–8]. *Patient D* has a metabolic alkalosis with partial respiratory compensation. Metabolic alkalosis can result from ingestion of alkaline substances (e.g., antacids) or from loss of acid (as occurs in vomiting). The total CO_2 content also is increased in metabolic alkalosis. The compensation for this condition is hypoventilation or excretion of an alkaline urine. Note that *patient D* shows partial compensation, as evidenced by the increased CO_2 tension. The $[HCO_3^-]/S \cdot P_{CO_2}$ ratio and pH are increased.

Patient B has a metabolic acidosis with partial respiratory compensation. Metabolic acidosis can result from increased fixed (noncarbonic) acid production (as occurs in diabetic ketoacidosis), increased acid retention (as occurs in renal failure with subsequent accumulation of $H_2PO_4^-$), or loss of base (as occurs in diarrhea). The total CO_2 content also is decreased in metabolic acidosis. The compensation for this condition is hyperventilation or excretion of an acid urine. Note that *patient B* shows partial compensation, as evidenced by the decrease in CO_2 tension. The $[HCO_3^-]/S \cdot P_{CO_2}$ ratio and pH are decreased.

Patient C has the highest plasma CO_2 content (i.e., $[HCO_3^-] + S \cdot P_{CO_2}$). This patient has respiratory acidosis, a condition caused by CO_2 retention resulting from hypoventilation, which may be due to pulmonary disease. The compensation for this condition is an increase in both HCO_3^- reabsorption and in H^+ excretion in the form of $H_2PO_4^-$ and NH_4^+. Note that *patient C* shows nearly complete compensation, as evidenced by the increased $[HCO_3^-]$ and return of PH toward normal. The $[HCO_3^-]/S \cdot P_{CO_2}$ ratio is only slightly decreased (i.e., 18:1 versus the normal 20:1).

Patient A has the lowest pH and thus the highest $[H^+]$. This patient has metabolic acidosis without compensation. $[H^+]$ can be calculated as

$$[H^+] = \text{antilog}\, (9 - pH)$$
$$= \text{antilog}\, (9 - 7)$$
$$= \text{antilog}\, 2$$
$$= 100 \text{ nmol/L}$$

or estimated as

$$[H^+] = 24\, \frac{P_{CO_2}}{[HCO_3^-]}$$
$$= 24\, \frac{70}{16}$$
$$= 24\, (4.38)$$
$$= 105 \text{ nmol/L}$$

Patient E has the highest $[HCO_3^-]/S \cdot P_{CO_2}$ ratio (i.e., 29.5:1). This patient has respiratory alkalosis, a condition caused by loss of CO_2 due to anxiety or hysteria leading to hyperventilation. The compensation for respiratory alkalosis is excretion of an alkaline urine. This patient shows partial renal compensation, as evidenced by the slight decline $[HCO_3^-]$. *Patient E* has a slightly lower than normal CO_2 content.

59. The answer is A [Chapter 34, III B; Table 34–3; Figure 34–1]. The $[HCO_3^-]$ of cerebrospinal fluid (CSF) and arterial blood are similar (approximately 24 mmol/L); however, the arterial pH (7.4) is higher than the pH of CSF (approximately 7.32), because the CO_2 tension of CSF is approximately 48 mm Hg compared with 40 mm Hg in arterial blood. Acute metabolic alkalosis depresses ventilation, increasing the CO_2 tension of the blood and CSF; this results in CSF acidosis and blood alkalosis. Thus, in metabolic acid-base disturbances, the $[H^+]$ of CSF and blood changes in opposite directions, and in respiratory acid-base disturbances, the $[H^+]$ of CSF and blood changes in the same direction.

60. The answer is A [Chapter 37 III B 1, 2; Figure 37–2]. H^+ is secreted into the lumen of the collecting duct primarily by the electrogenic H^+-ATPase pump. This H^+ can combine with any of the available urinary buffers such as

NH_3, HPO_4^{-2}, and HCO_3^-. It cannot combine with NH_4^+ because it is an acid, not a buffer. A very small amount (trivial) of H^+ can remain as free H^+. The amount of H^+ bound to buffers depends on the amount of buffer present, the pK of the buffer, and the amount of H^+ secreted. It is important to appreciate that of all the urinary buffers only NH_3 is secreted into the lumen. The other buffers (HCO_3^-, HPO_4^{2-}) enter the nephron by glomerular filtration.

PART VII

GASTROINTESTINAL PHYSIOLOGY

Michael B. Wang

Chapter 40

Structure and Function of the Gastrointestinal (GI) Tract

I. **STRUCTURE.** The digestive system is composed of a long muscular tube—the gastrointestinal (GI) tract, or alimentary canal—and a set of accessory organs (Figure 40–1).

A. The **GI tract** consists of the oral cavity, pharynx, esophagus, stomach, small intestine, large intestine, rectum, and anal canal.

B. The **accessory organs** include the tongue, teeth, salivary glands, pancreas, liver, and gallbladder.

C. The **lining of the GI tract** is composed of:

1. **Two muscular layers (the circular muscle and the longitudinal muscle)**, which are responsible for propelling food along the GI tract

2. A **mucosal layer,** which contains the epithelial cells responsible for the absorption of nutrients and the secretion of mucus and enzymes

D. **Neuronal control** of the GI tract is provided by **extrinsic and intrinsic (enteric) neurons.**

1. **Extrinsic nervous control comes from the parasympathetic and sympathetic nervous systems**.
   a. **Parasympathetic innervation**
      (1) Parasympathetic nerve fibers come from
         (a) The **vagus nerve,** which innervates the striated muscle of the esophagus, the stomach, the small intestine, and the ascending colon
         (b) The **pelvic nerve,** which innervates the lower portion of the colon and the striated muscle of the external anal canal
      (2) **Parasympathetic nerve activity**
         (a) **Increases GI motility and secretion**
         (b) **Decreases the activity of sphincters**
   b. **Sympathetic innervation**
      (1) **Sympathetic fibers** reach all levels of the GI tract from the celiac, mesenteric and hypogastric ganglia.
      (2) **Sympathetic nerve activity**
         (a) **Increases sphincter tone**
         (b) **Reduces blood flow to the GI tract**

2. The intrinsic nervous system is composed of the **myenteric and submucosal plexuses**.
   a. The extrinsic nerve fibers synapse on neurons within the intrinsic nervous system.
   b. Intrinsic nervous system activity can act independently of the extrinsic nervous system.

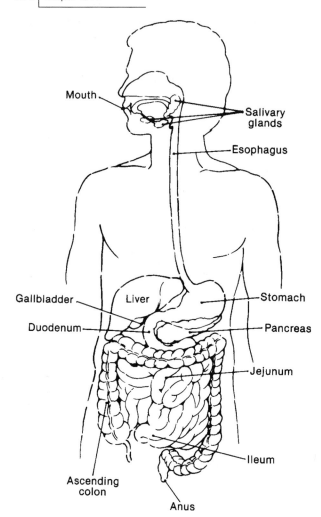

FIGURE 40-1. The gastrointestinal (GI) tract.

3. Sensory fibers. A large portion of the neurons within the extrinsic and intrinsic nervous systems are mechanical and chemical sensory fibers that provide the central nervous system with information about the activity of the GI tract and initiate reflexes that control the motility and secretion of the gut.

II. **FUNCTION.** The digestive system is responsible for breaking down food and supplying the body with water, nutrients, and electrolytes needed to sustain life. Before food can be used by the body, it must be ingested, digested, and absorbed—processes that involve coordinated movement of muscle and secretion of various substances.

A. Ingestion involves:

1. Placing food into the mouth

2. Chewing the food into smaller pieces (mastication)

3. Moistening the food with salivary secretions

4. Swallowing the food (deglutition)

B. **Digestion.** During digestion, food is broken down into small particles by the grinding action of the GI tract and then degraded by digestive enzymes into usable nutrients.

1. **Starches** are degraded by amylases into monosaccharides.

2. **Proteins** are degraded by a variety of enzymes (e.g., pepsin, trypsin) into dipeptides and amino acids.

3. **Fats** are degraded by lipases and esterases into monoglycerides and free fatty acids.

C. **Absorption.** During absorption, nutrients, water, and electrolytes are transported from the GI tract (principally from the small intestine) to the circulation.

Case Study

A 25-year-old man visits his doctor complaining of recurrent diarrhea. He says his stools are frothy, bulky, and smell "awful." He has lost about 25 pounds over the last month. A test for blood in his stool is negative, but he is anemic and bruises easily. He says he feels weak all the time and his muscles frequently go into spasms (tetany). He spent the last 6 months studying in the tropics. He is diagnosed with tropical sprue.

   1. *Why has he lost weight?*

DISCUSSION

Tropical sprue is a generalized malabsorption disorder of unknown origin that affects individuals who have traveled in the tropics. Failure to absorb nutrients causes the weight loss. The disease is self-limiting, and patients usually recover in several months. Treatment with antibiotics can speed recovery.

   2. *Why are his stools frothy, bulky, and malodorous?*

DISCUSSION

Bacterial metabolism of unabsorbed carbohydrates and fats produces the frothy, malodorous stools characteristic of malabsorption syndromes.

   3. *Why is he anemic?*

DISCUSSION

Failure to absorb iron and vitamin B_{12} leads to anemia. Both of these substances (and folate) may have to be replaced as part of the treatment of severe cases of tropical sprue.

   4. *Why does he bruise easily?*

DISCUSSION

Bruising results from failure to absorb vitamin K, and the loss of proteins leads to hypoprothrombinemia.

   5. *Why is he weak?*

DISCUSSION

His weakness is caused by anemia and, perhaps, the hypokalemia connected with the dehydration associated with his diarrhea.

6. *What causes his tetany?*

DISCUSSION

Tetany results from hyperexcitable nerves and muscle, a condition caused by decreased serum calcium levels. Serum calcium levels fall because calcium is not being absorbed.

Chapter 41

Ingestion of Food

I. **CHEWING.** After food is placed into the mouth, it is cut and ground into smaller pieces by chewing (mastication).

A. **The chewing reflex.** Although chewing is a voluntary act, it is coordinated by reflex centers in the brain stem that facilitate the opening and closing of the jaw.

1. When the mouth opens, stretch receptors in the jaw muscles initiate a reflex contraction of the masseter, medial pterygoid, and temporalis muscles, causing the mouth to close.

2. When the mouth closes, food comes into contact with buccal receptors, eliciting a reflex contraction of the digastric and lateral pterygoid muscles, causing the mouth to open.

3. When the jaw drops, the stretch reflex causes the entire cycle to be repeated.

4. The tongue contributes to the grinding process by positioning the food between the upper and lower teeth.

B. **Function of chewing**

1. Chewing **breaks food into smaller pieces,** which:
   a. Makes it easier for the food to be swallowed
   b. Breaks off the indigestible cellulose coatings of fruits and vegetables
   c. Increases the surface area of the food particles, making it easier for them to be digested by the digestive enzymes

2. Chewing **mixes the food with salivary gland secretions,** which:
   a. Initiates the process of starch digestion by salivary amylase
   b. Initiates the process of lipid digestion by lingual lipase
   c. Lubricates and softens the bolus of food, making it easier to swallow

3. Chewing **brings food into contact with taste receptors** and **releases odors** that stimulate the olfactory receptors. The sensations generated by these receptors increase the pleasure of eating and initiate gastric secretions.

II. **LUBRICATION OF FOOD BY SALIVA**

A. **Salivary glands**

1. The **parotid glands,** located near the angle of the jaw, are the largest glands. They secrete a watery fluid.

2. The **submandibular** and **sublingual glands** secrete a fluid that contains a higher concentration of proteins and so is more viscous.

3. Smaller glands are located throughout the oral cavity. Those in the tongue secrete lingual lipase.

B. **Composition of saliva.** The salivary glands secrete a relatively high volume of fluid (0.5–1 L/day) containing electrolytes and proteins.

1. **Formation of saliva.** Saliva is secreted into the salivary ducts by acinar cells that line the beginning of the salivary duct.
   a. Salivary flow rates and enzymatic secretions are increased by parasympathetic nervous system activity.

    b. The initial electrolyte composition of saliva is similar to plasma.

  2. Modification of saliva. The ductal cells that line the tubular portions of the salivary ducts change the composition of saliva. Ductal cells reabsorb Na^+ and Cl^- and secrete K^+ and HCO_3^-.

    higher

    Lower

    a. At high flow rates, there is less time for reabsorption and secretion, and, therefore, saliva contains ~~lower~~ concentrations of Na^+ and Cl^- and ~~higher~~ concentrations of K^+.

    b. At low flow rates there is more time for reabsorption and secretion and, therefore, saliva contains ~~higher~~ */lower* concentrations of Na^+ and Cl^- and ~~lower~~ *higher* concentrations of K^+.

    c. HCO_3^- **concentration increases when salivary flow increases because** HCO_3^- **secretion is increased when salivary glands are stimulated by the parasympathetic nervous system.**

  4. Proteins. Two types of proteins are found in saliva.

    a. The **enzymes** α-amylase (ptyalin) and lingual lipase begin the process of starch and fat digestion.

    b. Mucin is a glycoprotein that lubricates the food.

C. | **Control of salivary secretion**

  1. Salivary secretion is controlled entirely by **autonomic nervous system (ANS) reflexes.**

    a. Parasympathetic nerve stimulation causes the salivary gland cells to secrete a large volume of watery fluid that is high in electrolytes but low in proteins.

    b. Sympathetic nerve stimulation causes the salivary glands to secrete a small volume of fluid that contains a high concentration of mucus.

  2. Salivary reflexes are elicited by the thought, aroma, or taste of food or by the presence of food within the alimentary canal.

  3. Salivary gland metabolism and growth are both stimulated by increased ANS activity.

D. | **Functions of saliva.** Salivary secretions perform a number of important functions.

  1. Protection. Salivary secretions protect the mouth by:

    a. Cooling hot foods

    b. Diluting any hydrochloric acid (HCl) or bile regurgitated into the mouth

    c. Washing food away from the teeth and destroying harmful bacteria within the mouth

  2. Digestion. Salivary secretions begin the process of starch and fat digestion.

    a. α-**Amylase** can digest most of the ingested starches into disaccharides before they reach the small intestine. α-Amylase is ultimately inactivated by the low pH of the stomach.

    b. Lingual lipase begins to break down ingested fats while they are in the mouth, stomach, and upper portions of the small intestine.

  3. Lubrication. Salivary secretions lubricate the food, making swallowing easier, and moisten the mouth, facilitating speech.

III. SWALLOWING (DEGLUTITION)

A. | **Phases of swallowing**

  1. Oral (voluntary) phase. During the voluntary phase, the tongue forms a bolus of food and forces it into the oropharynx by pushing up and back against the hard palate.

  2. Pharyngeal phase

    a. The pharyngeal phase is coordinated by a swallowing center in the medulla and lower pons. It is initiated by sensory fibers that detect the presence of food within the oropharynx.

      (1) The nasopharynx is closed by the soft palate, preventing regurgitation of food into the nasal cavities.

      (2) The palatopharyngeal folds are pulled medially, forming a passageway for the food to move into the pharynx.

      (3) The glottis and vocal cords are closed and the epiglottis swings down over the larynx, guiding the food toward the esophagus and away from the airways.

      (4) The bolus of food is pushed into the esophagus by the peristaltic contractions of the pharynx and the opening of the upper esophageal sphincter.

  b. Respiration is inhibited for the duration of the pharyngeal phase of swallowing (1–2 seconds).

3. Esophageal phase. After reaching the esophagus, food is propelled into the stomach by primary, which is part of the swallowing reflex. The strength of peristaltic contractions is proportional to the size of the bolus entering the esophagus.

  a. Esophageal structure. The esophagus is about 20–25 cm in length and is isolated from the oral cavity by the **upper esophageal sphincter (UES)** and from the stomach by the **lower esophageal sphincter (LES).**

      (1) The **UES** is a true anatomical sphincter formed by the cricopharyngeal muscle. The UES is a **striated muscle** and is completely under the control of the vagal fibers that innervate the esophagus. UES tone is maintained by the continual firing of the vagal fibers originating from the **nucleus ambiguus.** The neurotransmitter released by these fibers is **acetylcholine (ACh).**

      (2) The **upper third of the esophagus,** like the UES, is striated muscle that is under the control of vagal fibers emerging from the nucleus ambiguus.

      (3) The **lower two thirds of the esophagus** is composed of **smooth muscle.** Its activity is regulated by vagal fibers originating within the **dorsal motor nucleus.** These fibers innervate intrinsic neurons within the muscle layers of the esophagus that release an inhibitory neurotransmitter (either **vasoactive intestinal peptide [VIP] or nitric oxide [NO]).**

      (4) The distal 2 cm of the esophagus forms the **LES.** Although the LES is not a separately identifiable muscle, its contractile characteristics are quite different from the rest of the esophageal smooth muscle. During quiescent (nonperistaltic) periods, tonic activity of the vagal fibers innervating the esophagus causes the smooth muscle of the LES to contract. In contrast, the remainder of the smooth muscle within the esophagus is flaccid when not undergoing peristaltic contractions.

  b. Types of esophageal peristalsis. There are two types of esophageal peristalsis, primary and secondary.

      (1) Primary esophageal peristalsis is initiated by swallowing. It begins when food passes into the esophagus from the pharyngeal cavity.

         (a) As soon as the food enters the esophagus, the UES contracts to prevent regurgitation of food into the mouth, and the LES relaxes so that food can pass from the esophagus into the stomach.

         (b) The peristaltic wave travels rather slowly (3–4 cm/sec), taking about 8 seconds to push the food from mouth to stomach. The force of gravity causes liquids to pass through the esophagus at a much faster rate.

         (c) After food enters the stomach, the LES contracts to prevent regurgitation of food into the esophagus.

         (d) If swallowing is not accompanied by the passing of food into the esophagus, the ensuing peristaltic wave will be very weak or may not occur at all.

      (2) Secondary peristalsis is initiated by the presence of food within the esophagus. Any material remaining in the esophagus stimulates mechanical or irritant receptors.

         (a) After primary peristalsis is completed, any food remaining in the esophagus stretches mechanical receptors, initiating another peristaltic wave.

         (b) Secondary peristaltic waves continue until all of the swallowed food is removed from the esophagus.

  c. Coordination of esophageal peristalsis

      (1) Primary esophageal peristalsis is coordinated by vagal fibers emerging from the swallowing center within the medulla that are activated as part of the swallowing reflex. **Vagotomy,** which eliminates the efferent fibers emerging from the swallowing center, would prevent the initiation of primary esophageal peristalsis.

(2) **Secondary esophageal peristalsis is coordinated by the intrinsic nervous system** of the esophagus. Afferent fibers innervate stretch receptors within the wall of the esophagus and thereby activate the appropriate fibers in the intrinsic nervous system. Because intrinsic rather than vagal nerves are involved, **vagotomy** would have little or no effect on secondary esophageal peristalsis.

B. Disorders of swallowing

1. **Esophageal reflux** may occur if the intragastric pressure rises high enough to force the LES open, if the LES is unable to maintain its normal tone, or if the LES is forced through the diaphragm and into the thoracic cavity (i.e., hiatal hernia).

   a. During pregnancy, the growing fetus may push the top of the stomach into the thorax. The low intrathoracic pressure (compared to the higher intra-abdominal pressure) causes the LES to expand, allowing reflux to occur.

   b. Reflux of stomach acid causes esophageal pain (heartburn) and may lead to irritation of the esophagus or bronchioles (due to aspiration).

2. **Achalasia** is a neuromuscular disorder of the lower two thirds of the esophagus that leads to absence of peristalsis and failure of the LES to relax. Food accumulates above this sphincter, taking hours to enter the stomach and dilating the esophagus.

Case 1

A 65-year-old man comes to his physician complaining of recurrent heartburn. He also says that he is having difficulty "getting his food down," that the food "seems to be sticking to his throat," and that, on many occasions, small amounts of food are regurgitated. At first, the problem occurred only when he ate quickly but now it occurs all the time, even when he is only drinking. He is diagnosed with achalasia.

1. What causes his heartburn (pyrosis)?

DISCUSSION

Pain localized to the chest may be associated with ischemic heart disease, with gastroesophageal reflux, or with spasms of the esophagus.

2. What produces the symptom of dysphagia (a feeling that passage of food through the esophagus is being obstructed)?

DISCUSSION

Dysphagia can be caused by narrowing of the lower esophageal sphincter or by damage to the neurons or muscles responsible for normal esophageal peristalsis.

3. Why did the problem occur with solids before liquids?

DISCUSSION

Under normal circumstances, the LES can dilate to a diameter of 3 to 4 cm. If the LES is constricted, large food particles will not be able to pass into the stomach. Further constriction will limit all solid food, and eventually even liquids will have a hard time entering the stomach.

4. What physiological treatments are available?

DISCUSSION

Achalasia is a motor disorder of the esophagus in which the LES fails to relax during swallowing. It is typically caused by damage to enteric interneurons that release VIP or NO. Treatment consists of mechanically enlarging the LES so that contractions do not entirely close the opening, surgically removing all or part of the LES, or preventing contractions with drugs such as nifedipine, a calcium channel blocker that relaxes smooth muscle, or botulinum toxin, which prevents the release of ACh from excitatory interneurons. Achalasia also can occur secondarily to reflux disease or a blockage of the LES by a tumor.

Case 2

A 35-year-old woman comes to the emergency room complaining of severe chest pains. An electrocardiogram (EKG) and enzyme study rule out cardiac disease. She is then evaluated for gastroesophageal reflux disease using a barium swallow, esophageal endoscopy, and the Bernstein test, in which 0.1 N HCl is infused into the esophagus.

> *1. What is gastroesophageal reflux?*

DISCUSSION

Gastroesophageal reflux may occur when (1) emptying of the stomach does not occur normally (e.g., because of pyloric sphincter disease); (2) when the gastric contents are pushed up against the esophagus (e.g., when the patient is lying down); or (3) when the LES fails to contract between swallows. If the acid erodes the esophageal protective layer, the presence of acid (or bile) in the refluxed fluid may cause pain.

> *2. How do the barium swallow, esophageal endoscopy, and the Bernstein test help in the diagnosis of esophageal reflux disease?*

DISCUSSION

A barium swallow is used to monitor the movement of fluid following ingestion radiographically. In severe reflux disease, regurgitation can be observed. Esophageal endoscopy permits the direct visualization of the esophagus lining. If the esophageal lining has been eroded, infusion of HCl will cause pain. Patients without esophagitis do not experience pain when HCl is infused in the Bernstein test.

> *3. What physiological treatments are available?*

DISCUSSION

Treatment is designed to (1) prevent regurgitation (e.g., by reducing weight or propping up head and chest with pillows when sleeping); (2) increase gastric emptying (by avoiding fatty foods that delay gastric emptying or giving drugs, such as cisapride, that increase gastric emptying); or (3) reduce acid production with H_2 blockers.

CHAPTER 42

Stomach

I. ANATOMY (Figure 42–1)

A. Functional components

1. The three functional parts of the stomach are the **fundus, corpus** (body), and **antrum.** Gastric contents are isolated from other parts of the gastrointestinal (GI) tract by the lower esophageal sphincter (LES) proximally and by the pylorus (pyloric sphincter) distally.

2. The antrum and pylorus are anatomically continuous and respond to nervous control as a unit.

B. Musculature

1. As elsewhere in the gut, each muscle layer in the stomach forms a functional syncytium and, therefore, acts as a unit. In the fundus, where the layers are relatively thin, the strength of contraction is weak; in the antrum, where the muscle layers are thick, the strength of contraction is greater.

2. The stomach and duodenum (the uppermost part of the small intestine) are divided by a thickened muscle layer called the pyloric sphincter.

C. **Innervation**

1. **Intrinsic.** The interconnected **myenteric (Auerbach's) plexus** and **submucosal (Meissner's) plexus** within the stomach wall comprise the intrinsic innervation of the stomach, as they do innervation elsewhere in the gut. They are **directly responsible for peristalsis** and other contractions. Because this system is continuous between the stomach and duodenum (see Figure 42–3), peristalsis in the antrum influences the duodenal bulb.

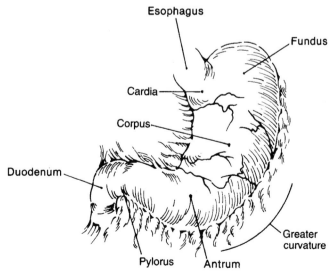

FIGURE 42-1. The stomach.

    a. The **myenteric plexus** is located between the layers of the circular and longitudinal muscles of the stomach.

    b. The **submucosal plexus** is located between the layers of the circular muscle and mucosa on the luminal surface of the stomach.

2. Extrinsic. Autonomic innervation is dual—both **sympathetic,** via the celiac plexus, and **parasympathetic,** via the vagus nerve. Sympathetic innervation inhibits motility, and parasympathetic innervation stimulates motility. Together, the two systems modify the coordinated motor activity that arises independently in the intrinsic nervous system.

II. MOTILITY.

Complex patterns of motility move food through the stomach, where it can be broken down further by gastric secretions and then propelled into the small intestine. Only small amounts of food are digested or absorbed in the stomach.

A. Function.

Gastric motility serves three basic functions.

1. Storage. When food enters the stomach, the orad region—primarily the fundus— enlarges to accommodate the food.

2. Mixing. The presence of food in the caudad stomach—primarily the corpus and antrum—increases the contractile activity of the stomach.

    a. The enhanced contractile activity (a combination of **peristalsis** and **retropulsion**) mixes the food with stomach acid and enzymes, breaking it into smaller and smaller pieces.

    b. When the food is mixed into a pasty consistency, it is called **chyme.**

3. Emptying. When the chyme is broken down into small enough particles, it is propelled through the pyloric sphincter into the intestine.

B. Storage is accomplished by receptive relaxation and accommodation.

When food enters the stomach, the contractile activity of the fundus is inhibited, enabling the stomach to easily accommodate 1 to 2 L of food.

1. Receptive relaxation is initiated as part of the peristaltic process, causing swallowing and esophageal motility.

2. Accommodation is initiated in response to a bolus of food entering the stomach. Stretch receptors in the orad stomach detect the presence of food and initiate a vagovagal reflex producing receptive relaxation.

3. The **inhibitory neurotransmitter** responsible for receptive relaxation and accommodation is either VIP or NO.

4. Effects of vagotomy. Sectioning the vagus nerve prevents or greatly diminishes receptive relaxation and accommodation, because vagal reflexes produce both processes.

C. Peristalsis.

Peristaltic contractions are initiated near the fundal-corpus border and proceed caudally, producing a peristaltic wave that propels the food toward the pylorus.

1. Mechanics of peristalsis. Peristaltic contractions are produced by periodic changes in membrane potential, called **slow waves,** or the **basic electrical rhythm (BER)** [Figure 42–2]. These waves are responsible for the rhythm and force of gastric contractions.

    a. Gastric slow waves are initiated by pacemaker cells within the wall of the stomach.

    b. Slow waves consist of an **upstroke** and **plateau** phase and occur at a rate of approximately three to four waves per minute.

    c. The **velocity** of the waves is 1 cm/sec when they sweep over the corpus and increases to 3–4 cm/sec in the antrum.

    d. Although the electrophysiological basis for the slow waves is not entirely known, it is assumed that the upstroke is due to the flow of Na^+ and Ca^2 into the cell and that the plateau is dependent primarily on the flow of Ca^{2+} into the cell.

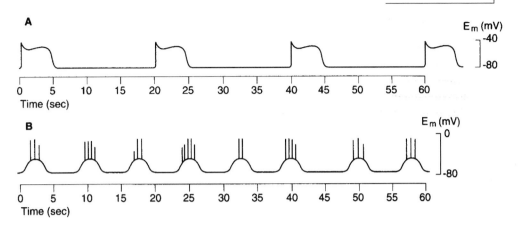

FIGURE 42–2. Basic electrical rhythm (BER), or slow waves, as recorded from smooth muscle cells of (*A*) the stomach and (*B*) the middle of the intestine. The slow waves of the stomach are 5–7 seconds in duration and occur at a rate of 3–5 waves/min; the slow waves of the intestine are more frequent (12 waves/min in the duodenum and 8 waves/min in the ileum) and have spikes superimposed on their plateaus. Ca^{2+} entering the smooth muscle cell during the slow wave produces mechanical activity. In the stomach, acetylcholine (ACh) increases contractile activity by increasing the amplitude and duration of the plateau phase of the slow wave. In the intestine, ACh increases the strength of contraction by increasing the frequency of spikes appearing on top of the slow wave.

2. **Force of peristalsis.** The force of peristaltic contractions is regulated by gastrin and acetylcholine (ACh). These hormones:
   a. **Increase the size of the slow wave plateau potential,** which increases the amount of Ca^{2+} entering the cell from the extracellular fluid (ECF)
   b. **Activate second messengers** that release Ca^{2+} from the sarcoplasmic reticulum (SR)

D. **Retropulsion.** Retropulsion is the back-and-forth movement of the chyme caused by the forceful propulsion of food against the closed pyloric sphincter (Figure 42–3).

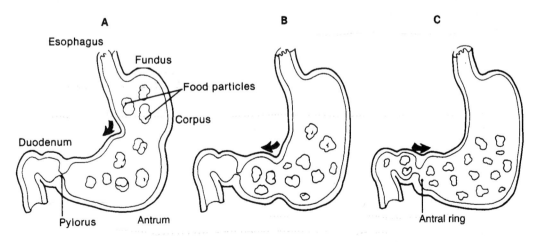

FIGURE 42–3. Peristaltic contractions begin in the midstomach (*A*) and proceed caudally, pushing the food toward the pylorus (*B*). When the food reaches the pylorus (where pieces of food that are small enough flow into the duodenum), a mass contraction of the terminal antrum pushes the food back toward the corpus through a narrow antral ring (*C*). The backward movement of the food is called retropulsion.

1. The wave of peristaltic contraction reaches the pyloric sphincter before the chyme does. Thus, when the chyme reaches the sphincter, it is pushed back into the body of the stomach.

2. The forward and backward movement of the chyme (caused by peristalsis and retropulsion) breaks the chyme into smaller and smaller pieces and mixes it with the gastric secretions present within the stomach.

E. **Gastric emptying** occurs when the chyme is decomposed into small enough pieces (typically less than 1 mm³)to fit through the pyloric sphincter.

1. Each time the chyme is pushed against the pyloric sphincter, a small amount (2–7 ml) may escape into the duodenum.

2. The amount of chyme passing through the pylorus depends on the size of the particles. If the particles are too large, none of the chyme will enter the duodenum.

3. Therefore, the rate of gastric emptying of solids depends on the rate at which the chyme is broken down into small particles.

4. Liquids empty much faster than solids. The rate at which liquids empty is proportional to pressure within the orad stomach, which increases slowly during the digestive period.

F. **Regulation of gastric emptying**

1. **Local reflexes**
   a. **Excitatory reflexes,** initiated by expansion of the antrum, are responsible for increasing gastric motility. Although these reflexes do not require the vagus nerve, vagotomy decreases the magnitude and coordination of stomach contractions.
   b. **Inhibitory reflexes.** A variety of stimuli act on the duodenum to initiate **enterogastric reflexes** that slow the rate of gastric emptying.
      (1) **Purpose.** Enterogastric reflexes prevent the flow of chyme from exceeding the ability of the intestine to handle it.
      (2) **Causes.** High osmolarity, low pH, fat and protein digestion products, low osmolality, the caloric content of food, and distention of the duodenal wall all elicit an enterogastric reflex.

2. **Hormones** released from the stomach and intestine also influence gastric motility.
   a. **Excitatory effects. Gastrin,** released into the circulation in response to antral distention or food breakdown products, enhances gastric contractions.
   b. **Inhibitory effects.** A variety of intestinal hormones, collectively called **enterogastrones,** inhibit gastric contractions. **Cholecystokinin (CCK)** and **secretin** are two known enterogastrones. The identity and mode of action of other enterogastrones remain to be discovered.
      (1) **CCK** is released from the duodenum in response to fat or protein digestion products. CCK probably acts by blocking the excitatory effects of gastrin on gastric smooth muscle (see Chapter 43 IV C 3).
      (2) **Secretin** is released from the duodenum in response to the presence of acid. Secretin most likely has a direct inhibitory effect on smooth muscle (see Chapter 43 IV C 3).

3. **Migrating motor complex (MMC).** During the interdigestive period, any food left in the stomach is removed by the MMC.
   a. The MMC is a peristaltic wave that begins within the esophagus and travels through the entire GI tract (see Chapter 43 III B 3).
   b. The peristaltic wave occurs every 60–90 minutes during the interdigestive period.
   c. The hormone **motilin** which is released from endocrine cells within the epithelium of the small intestine, increases the strength of the MMC.

G. **Vomiting** (or **emesis**) is the forceful expulsion of the food from the stomach and intestine.

1. **Initiation.** Vomiting may be initiated by direct activation of the **vomiting center** in the

medulla or by activation of the **chemoreceptor**
the brain stem.

a. The **vomiting center** may be activated direct
injury or increases in intracranial pressure. V
rectly, it causes **projectile vomiting** a rapid
nausea.

b. The **chemoreceptor trigger zone** may be acti
within the GI tract or by circulating emetic ag
sulfate. Vomiting caused by activation of the
nied by nausea.

2. Mechanical sequence of vomiting

    a. Vomiting begins with a deep inspiration follov

    b. Next, a pressure wave originating in the intest
ach.

    c. Finally, an increase in abdominal pressure forc.. ... chyme into the esophagus and
out of the mouth.

    d. Retching may precede vomiting. Retching involves all of the involuntary motions of
vomiting but without the production of vomitus. The chyme is not ejected because
the abdominal and thoracic pressures are not sufficient to overcome the resistance of
the upper esophageal sphincter (UES).

III. GASTRIC SECRETION

A. General considerations

1. Function. Gastric secretions aid in the breakdown of food into small particles and continue the process of digestion begun by salivary enzymes. About 2 L/day of gastric secretions are produced.

2. Phases of gastric secretion

    a. The cephalic phase of gastric secretion is initiated by the thought, sight, taste, or smell of food. It is dependent on the integrity of the vagal fibers innervating the stomach.

      (1) Secretion of hydrochloric acid (HCl) from parietal cells, gastrin from G cells, and pepsinogen from peptic (chief) cells is stimulated by vagal efferent fibers.

      (2) Almost half of the gastric secretions released during a meal occur as a result of cephalically induced vagal stimulation.

    b. The gastric phase of secretion is initiated by the entry of food into the stomach. Food entering the stomach buffers acid, raises pH, and allows other stimuli (e.g., vagal fibers, gastrin) to release acid.

      (1) Distention of the corpus, acting through local and vagovagal reflexes, results in an increase in HCl secretion.

      (2) Distention of the antrum initiates vagally mediated and local reflexes that result in gastrin release from antral G cells. Gastrin release is inhibited at low pH (<3).

      (3) Low pH activates local reflexes, which enhance pepsinogen secretion.

      (4) Although the rate of gastric secretion during the gastric phase is less than during the cephalic phase, it continues for a longer time. Thus, the two phases contribute about the same amount of secretion.

    c. The intestinal phase of secretion begins as the chyme begins to empty from the stomach into the duodenum. Overall, little gastric secretion occurs during the intestinal phase.

3. Gastric secretory cells are located on the surface of the stomach and in glands that are buried within the mucosa.

    a. Oxyntic glands are located in the fundus and corpus of the stomach. They contain three types of secretory cells. *intrinsic factor*

      (1) The parietal (oxyntic) cells secrete **HCl.** These cells are also responsible for the

of **intrinsic factor,** which is necessary for the absorption of vitamin B_{12} [in the] ileum of the small intestine (see III E; Chapter 43 VII E 3).

[chie]f **(chief) cells** secrete **pepsinogen,** the precursor for the proteolytic enzyme [p]epsin.

Mucous cells secrete mucus.

Pyloric glands are located in the antrum and pyloric regions of the stomach. They contain **G cells** and some mucous cells. **G cells** are responsible for the release of the hormone **gastrin.** (stimulates HCl release from parietal cells)

- **(1)** There are two forms of gastrin, G-17 (little gastrin, a 17-amino-acid peptide) and G-34 (big gastrin, a 34-amino-acid peptide). Although G-17 is more potent than G-34, the larger gastrin is found in higher concentrations within the circulation.
- **(2)** Gastrin is released from the basolateral surface of the G cells, enters the circulation, and travels to the orad stomach, where it stimulates parietal-cell HCl secretion.

B. HCl secretion

1. Functions of HCl
- **a.** HCl participates in the breakdown of protein.
- **b.** It provides an optimal pH for the action of pepsin.
- **c.** It hinders the growth of pathogenic bacteria.

2. Mechanism of HCl secretion (Figure 42–4)
- **a.** HCl is secreted into the parietal cell **canaliculi** by a three-step process.
  - **(1)** The active transport process is begun by the transport of K^+ and Cl^- into the canaliculi. Cl^- is transported either by a pump or through a channel. The flow of Cl^- creates a negative potential inside the canaliculi, causing K^+ to flow passively into the canaliculi.
  - **(2)** H^+ is then exchanged for K^+ by the **H^+–K^+-ATPase pump.**
  - **(3)** Water enters the canaliculi down the osmotic gradient created by the movement of HCl into the canaliculi.
- **b.** The H^+ entering the canaliculi is supplied by the dissociation of carbonic acid (H_2CO_3 into H^+ and bicarbonate (HCO_3^-) within the parietal cell.
  - **(1)** H_2CO_3 is formed from the reaction:

$$CO_2 + H_2O \rightarrow H_2CO_3 \rightarrow H^+ + HCO_3^-$$

  to HCl   back to blood in exchange
                              for Cl⁻

  - **(2)** The formation of H_2CO_3 from CO_2 is catalyzed by the enzyme **carbonic anhydrase.** Acetazolamide, a carbonic anhydrase inhibitor, blocks the formation of HCl by the parietal cell.
  - **(3)** The HCO_3^- diffuses back into the plasma (creating the alkaline tide associated with gastric secretion) in exchange for Cl^-, thus providing Cl^- for the initial step in the secretory process [see III B 2 a (1)].
- **c.** Most of the HCl that is secreted into the stomach is neutralized and reabsorbed within the small intestine. However, if the gastric contents are lost before they enter the small intestine (e.g., by vomiting), a severe alkalosis may ensue.
- **d.** The active transport processes involved in the generation of HCl require a large amount of adenosine triphosphate (ATP). The ATP is generated by mitochondria found in very high concentration (40% of cell volume) within the parietal cell.
- **e.** The pH of the parietal cell secretion can be as low as 0.8 (i.e., a H^+ concentration of approximately 150 mmol, or almost 4 million times as great as the H^+ concentration of plasma).
- **f.** The **H^+–K^+-ATPase** pump can be irreversibly inhibited by the drug **omeprazole,** which is now used for the treatment of duodenal and gastric ulcers.

3. Substances affecting HCl secretion
- **a. Stimulation of HCl secretion.** ACh, histamine, and gastrin act directly on the parietal cell to stimulate HCl secretion (Figure 42–5). In addition, ACh and gastrin may directly stimulate the mast cell to secrete histamine.
  - **(1)** ACh, a neurotransmitter, is released from nerve cells innervating the parietal cell.

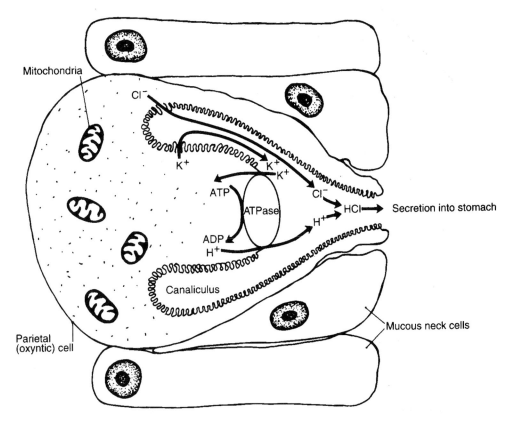

FIGURE 42–4. Hydrochloric acid (HCl) being formed by the parietal cell. Cl⁻ and K⁺ are secreted into canaliculi by separate transporters, which may be channels or carriers. H⁺ is exchanged for K⁺ by an ATPase active transport system, allowing HCl to be secreted into the stomach. Numerous mitochondria provide energy for the active transport process. (Adapted from Guyton AC: *Textbook of Medical Physiology,* 8th edition. Philadelphia, WB Saunders, 1991, p 64.)

      (2) Histamine is released from mast cells located within the corpus.
         (a) Histamine can stimulate HCl secretion directly or can potentiate the secretion produced by ACh or gastrin.
         (b) Histamine is classified as a **paracrine agent** because it diffuses from its release site to the parietal cells (rather than traveling within the circulation, as does a hormone).
         (c) The commonly used anti-ulcer drugs (i.e., cimetidine and ranitidine) are histamine antagonists that block the H₂ receptor on the parietal cell.
      (3) Gastrin is released from G cells in the distal stomach (see III A 3 b). Gastrin is classified as a hormone because it travels to its target cell through the circulation. A variety of substances affect gastrin secretion (see III C).
   b. Inhibition of HCl secretion. Somatostatin inhibits HCl secretion by parietal cells and gastrin secretion by G cells. Somatostatin is released from interneurons within the enteric nervous system.

  4. Regulation of gastric acid (HCl) secretion
    a. Stimulation during the cephalic phase. The vagus nerve stimulates the release of ACh and inhibits the release of somatostatin from interneurons within the enteric nervous system, thus enhancing the secretion of HCl (see Figure 42–5).

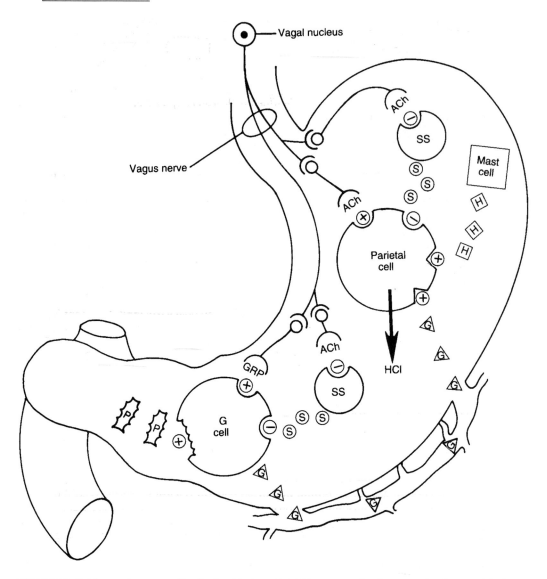

FIGURE 42–5. Many substances affect hydrochloric acid (*HCl*) secretion by the parietal cell. Acetylcholine (*ACh*) from the vagus nerve, histamine (*H*) from mast cells, and gastrin (*G*) from G cells all stimulate the parietal cell directly to secrete HCl. The release of gastrin into the circulation, in turn, is stimulated by gastrin-releasing peptide (*GRP*) and protein digestion products (*P*). Somatostatin (*S*), released from somatostatin cells (*SS*), inhibits the release of both gastrin and HCl. Thus, the stimulation of vagal fibers, which causes the release of ACh and GRP but inhibits the release of somatostatin, has an amplified positive effect on parietal-cell HCl secretion. + = stimulation; − = inhibition. (Adapted from Johnson LR [ed]: *Gastrointestinal Physiology*, 3rd edition. St. Louis, CV Mosby, 1985, p 72.)

    b. Stimulation during the gastric phase. The amount of ingested protein is the most im-
    portant determinant of acid secretion during the gastric phase.
        (1) Protein is a good buffer and thus keeps the pH of the stomach at an optimal level
           for acid secretion.
        (2) Amino acids and peptides directly stimulate parietal cells to secrete acid.

(3) Alcohol and caffeine also cause the release of HCl and gastrin.

c. **Inhibition during the gastric phase.** The most potent inhibitor of HCl secretion during the gastric phase is the presence of acid in the stomach. If the pH of the stomach falls below 2, acid secretion stops. Acid secretion is inhibited by two mechanisms.

   (1) A low pH directly inhibits HCl and gastrin secretion.

   (2) Lowering the pH also releases somatostatin, which inhibits the secretion of gastrin by the G cells and HCl by the parietal cells (see Figure 42–5).

d. **Stimulation during the intestinal phase.** The presence of protein digestion products within the duodenum causes an increase in HCl secretion.

   (1) Although G cells have been identified within the duodenum, gastrin is not thought to cause the increase in acid secretion.

   (2) An as yet unidentified hormone, called **entero-oxyntin,** is postulated to be responsible for the increase in acid secretion.

   (3) Amino acids circulating in the blood after being absorbed from the intestine may also stimulate HCl secretion.

e. **Inhibition during the intestinal phase.** Acid secretion is inhibited when food enters the duodenum. Because the major effect of food entering the duodenum is inhibition of acid secretion, loss of the proximal intestine increases gastric secretion (and motility).

   (1) H^+, fatty acids, and increased osmolarity stimulate the release of enterogastrones from the duodenum.

   (2) The most important of the enterogastrones may be **gastric inhibitory peptide (GIP),** which inhibits both gastrin release and parietal cell secretion of HCl. GIP is thought to act by stimulating the release of somatostatin, which, in turn, inhibits the parietal and G cells. GIP is also involved in the release of insulin.

C. Gastrin secretion

1. **Functions of gastrin**
   a. Gastrin stimulates HCl secretion.
   b. It increases gastric and intestinal motility.
   c. It increases pancreatic secretions.
   d. It is necessary for the proper growth of GI mucosa.

2. **Substances affecting gastrin secretion**
   a. **Stimulation of gastrin secretion.** Bombesin [gastrin-releasing peptide (GRP)] most likely is the neurotransmitter responsible for stimulating G cells to secrete gastrin. The vagus nerve increases the release of GRP during the cephalic phase (see Figure 42–5).
   b. **Inhibition of gastrin secretion.** Somatostatin inhibits gastrin secretion. The vagus nerve inhibits the release of somatostatin during the cephalic phase.

3. **Regulation of gastrin secretion**
   a. In general, gastrin secretion is regulated by the same mechanisms that regulate HCl secretion (i.e., vagal stimulation, pH, enterogastrones).
   b. In addition, several foods and food breakdown products (**secretagogues**) directly stimulate the release of gastrin. These include protein digestion products, alcohol, and coffee (both caffeinated and decaffeinated).

D. Pepsinogen secretion from Chief Cells

1. **Function of pepsinogen. Pepsin,** the active form of pepsinogen, is a proteolytic enzyme that begins the process of protein digestion (see Chapter 43 VII B 2 a).

2. **Regulation of pepsinogen secretion.** Pepsinogen is released from the chief cells of the oxyntic glands during all three phases of digestion.
   a. **Cephalic phase.** During the cephalic phase of digestion, vagally stimulated cholinergic neurons within the enteric nervous system directly stimulate chief cells to release pepsinogen.
   b. **Gastric phase.** During the gastric phase of digestion, low pH activates local reflexes that enhance pepsinogen secretion. The low pH of the stomach also is responsible for

converting pepsinogen into pepsin. Again, ACh is the transmitter that stimulates the chief cells.

c. **Intestinal phase.** Secretin enhances pepsinogen release. Thus, the presence of H^+ within the duodenum during the intestinal phase of digestion may contribute to pepsinogen secretion.

E. | Intrinsic factor from parietal cells

1. **Definition.** Intrinsic factor is a glycoprotein secreted by the parietal cells of the gastric mucosa, chiefly by those in the fundus.

2. **Function.** Intrinsic factor is required for the **absorption of vitamin B_{12}.**
   a. Intrinsic factor forms a complex with vitamin B_{12}.
   b. The intrinsic factor—B_{12} complex is carried to the terminal ileum, where the vitamin is absorbed (see Chapter 43 VII E 3).

IV. GASTRIC MUCOSAL BARRIER.
The gastric mucosal barrier protects the gastric lining cells from damage by intraluminal HCl, or **autodigestion.**

A. | Autodigestion is prevented by

1. **Mucus, which contains HCO_3^-** and, therefore, neutralizes much of the acid before it reaches the cellular lining of the stomach

2. **A high blood flow** that rapidly carries away any acid that penetrates the cellular lining

3. The **high turnover rate** of the gastric mucosa. Approximately 5×10^5 mucosal cells are shed each minute, replacing the entire mucosa in 1–3 days. Any damaged cells are quickly replaced.

4. **Prostaglandins** which are responsible for maintaining the gastric mucosal barrier.

B. | The **rate of repair** of mucosal injury depends on the extent of injury and varies from as little as 48 hours for restricted desquamation to up to 3–5 months if damage has left only the deepest portions of the gastric pits intact.

C. | **Ulcer therapy.**
Ulcer repair is aided by drugs that neutralize gastric acid (e.g., nonprescription antacids) or prevent acid release, such as proton pump inhibitors (see III B 2 f) and H_2 blockers [see III B 3 a (2) (c)] and by antibiotics against *Helicobacter pylori,* which is a major cause of gastric and duodenal ulcers.

V. GASTRIC DIGESTION AND ABSORPTION

A. | Digestion

1. **Carbohydrate digestion** in the stomach depends on the action of salivary amylase, which remains active until halted by the low pH in the stomach.

2. **Protein digestion.** About 10% of ingested protein is broken down completely in the stomach. Gastric pepsin facilitates later digestion of protein by breaking apart meat particles.

3. **Fat digestion** is minimal due to the restriction of gastric lipase activity to triglycerides containing short-chain (<10 carbons) fatty acids. Acid and pepsin break emulsions so that fats coalesce into droplets, which float and empty last.

B. | Absorption

1. **Nutrients.** Very little absorption of nutrients takes place in the stomach. The only substances absorbed to any appreciable extent are highly lipid-soluble substances (e.g., the un-ionized triglycerides of acetic, propionic, and butyric acids). Aspirin at gastric pH is

un-ionized and fat soluble; after absorption, it ionizes intracellularly, damaging mucosal cells and ultimately producing bleeding. Ethanol is absorbed rapidly in proportion to its concentration.

2. **Water** moves in both directions across the mucosa. It does not, however, follow osmotic gradients. Water-soluble substances, including Na^+, K^+, glucose, and amino acids, are absorbed in insignificant amounts.

Case 1

A 45-year-old man schedules an appointment with his physician because he is always tired. During the visit he complains of constant stomach distress. A blood test reveals pernicious anemia. A serum gastrin test and stomach biopsy are then ordered. He is diagnosed with gastritis of the orad stomach.

> 1. How does inflammation of the orad stomach cause pernicious anemia?

DISCUSSION

Pernicious anemia is caused by insufficient vitamin B_{12} (cobalamin) absorption resulting from diminished intrinsic factor secretion. Gastritis reduces secretion by destroying the parietal cells.

> 2. What will his serum gastrin levels reveal?

DISCUSSION

Destroying parietal cells results in less acid secretion, which causes the stomach fluids to have a higher pH. Gastrin secretion is regulated by pH—the lower the pH, the less gastin is secreted; the higher the pH, the more gastrin is secreted. In gastritis, the high pH of the luminal contents results in a serum gastrin level higher than normal.

> 3. What treatment is necessary?

DISCUSSION

The pernicious anemia must be treated with parenteral administration of vitamin B_{12}. If the inflammatory process producing the gastritis (e.g., *H. pylori*) can be identified, it can be treated. Most often, chronic gastritis confined to the orad stomach is an autoimmunological process for which there is no general treatment.

Case 2

A 23-year-old woman calls her physician because of a constant gnawing pain in the upper part of her abdomen. The pain is worse between meals, and she often wakes up with severe pain. The physician recommends that she try taking antacids before each meal and before going to bed and schedules an office visit later in the week. The antacids relieve most of the pain. In the office, her physician does a test for occult blood, which turns out to be positive. She is diagnosed with duodenal ulcer and given a proton-pump inhibitor and an antibiotic against *H. pylori*. Her symptoms completely disappear within a few weeks.

> **1.** What causes a duodenal ulcer?

DISCUSSION

Duodenal ulcers, like gastric ulcers, are mucosal lesions produced by HCl acid and pepsin. The presence of the bacterium *Helicobacter pylori* promotes ulcer formation, presumably by weakening the protective mechanisms that normally prevent ulcers from forming. Almost all patients with duodenal ulcers (and most patients with gastric ulcers) are infected with *H. pylori,* but not everyone with *H. pylori* has ulcers. Although patients with duodenal ulcers may have excessive acid production, not all patients do. However, the stomach contents empty more rapidly in patients with duodenal ulcers, and the duodenal mucosal cells secrete less HCO_3^- than in normal patients when acid enters the duodenum.

2. *Why is her pain worse between meals and at night?*

DISCUSSION

Food is a major buffer of stomach acid. After meals, and particularly at night, food is absent from the stomach. As a result, the pH of the stomach can decrease to 1 or 1.5. The high concentration of acid erodes the mucosa and causes pain.

3. *How do antacids work?*

DISCUSSION

Antacids, such as HCO_3^- Mg $(OH)_2$ and $Al(OH)_3$, work by buffering stomach acids. They are destroyed when they neutralize the acid and, therefore, must be taken often to be effective. Aluminum tends to cause constipation and magnesium tends to cause diarrhea, so the two antacids often are mixed in commercial preparations.

4. *What does a positive test for occult blood indicate?*

DISCUSSION

The term *occult blood* refers to small amounts of blood found in the stool. The presence of blood in the stools may be detected using Hemoccult test paper. The test paper contains guaiac resin, which turns blue when mixed with hydrogen peroxide and hemoglobin. The test can be performed on a stool sample obtained during a rectal examination or by the patient after defecation. Often the only symptom that patients with ulcer disease (or other GI lesions) have is fatigue that results from the constant loss of small amounts of blood. Sometimes a positive test for occult blood indicates a GI disorder before any symptoms develop.

5. *Why is the drug therapy so effective?*

Proton pump inhibitors completely block the formation of gastric acid and, therefore, immediately relieve the pain associated with duodenal ulcers. Elimination of the *H. pylori* infestation of the stomach and intestine almost always prevents recurrence of the ulcers.

CHAPTER 43

Small Intestine

I. **OVERVIEW.** The small intestine is the major site of *digestion* and *absorption* of carbohydrates, proteins, and fats in the gastrointestinal (GI) tract. The action and secretions of several *accessory organs* (see II B) are essential to the digestive and absorptive functions of the small intestine. Nutrients and fluids that are not absorbed in the small intestine are passed on to the colon.

II. **ANATOMY**

A. **Small intestine**

1. The small intestine has three parts: the **duodenum,** the **jejunum,** and the **ileum** (see Figure 40–1).

2. Although the small intestine is approximately 5 m long, it has an **absorptive area** of over 250 M^2.
   a. Its large surface area is created by numerous folds of the intestinal mucosa (**valvulae conniventes**); by densely packed **villi,** which line the entire mucosal surface; and by **microvilli,** which protrude from the surface of the intestinal cells.
      (1) The epithelial cells from which the microvilli protrude are called **enterocytes.**
      (2) The microvilli (about 1 μm long and 0.1 μm in diameter) give the intestinal mucosa its characteristic *brush border* appearance.
   b. The **blood supply** of the villus is ideally organized to collect the nutrients after they are absorbed across the brush border membrane.
      (1) Each villus is supplied by an arteriole, which gives rise to a capillary tuft at the tip of the villus. The capillaries coalesce into venules, which drain into the portal vein. The portal vein carries the absorbed nutrients to the liver.
      (2) Branches of the lymphatics, called **lacteals,** also extend to the tip of the villus. These vessels carry absorbed fats to the thoracic duct from which they enter the general circulation.

B. The **accessory organs** involved in intestinal digestion and absorption are the **pancreas,** the **liver,** and the **gallbladder.**

1. The **pancreas** secretes various substances that aid in intestinal digestion, including HCO$_3$−, which neutralizes the acidic content of chyme entering the small intestine.

2. The **liver** secretes bile, which is necessary for fat digestion and nutrient absorption.
   a. Bile travels from the liver through **bile ducts** to reach the duodenum of the small intestine.
   b. The **sphincter of Oddi,** located at the distal end of the duodenum, forms the opening that connects the small intestine to the **common bile duct.**
      (1) This sphincter controls the flow of bile into the small intestine (see V A 4, V E 2 a).
      (2) When the sphincter is closed, bile cannot enter the small intestine and must be stored in the gallbladder.
   c. The **portal circulation** carries bile that has been absorbed from the terminal ileum back to the liver (see V C; Figure 43–1).

3. The **gallbladder** stores bile during the interdigestive period.

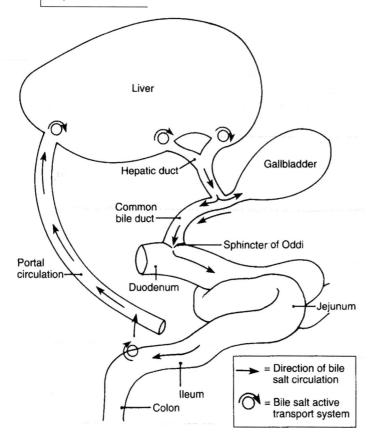

FIGURE 43–1. The enterohepatic circulation. Bile acids are absorbed from the terminal ileum by a Na^+-dependent active transport system and then rapidly sequestered by hepatocytes in the liver and returned to the gallbladder or duodenum. Each day, about 20% of the bile acid pool escapes the enterohepatic circulation (thus becoming lost to excretion) and must be resynthesized by the liver.

In the figure: Liver, Gallbladder, Hepatic duct, Common bile duct, Sphincter of Oddi, Portal circulation, Duodenum, Jejunum, Ileum, Colon.

Legend:
- → = Direction of bile salt circulation
- ↻ = Bile salt active transport system

III. MOTILITY

A. Contractile activity

1. **Function.** Contractile activity of the smooth muscles lining the small intestine serves two major functions:
   a. Mixing the chyme with the digestive juices and bile to facilitate digestion and absorption
   b. Propelling the chyme from the duodenum to the colon

2. Transit time. It usually takes about 2–4 hours for the chyme to move from one end of the small intestine to the other.

B. Types of movements

1. **Segmentation is** the most common type of intestinal contraction.
   a. During segmentation, about 2 cm of the intestinal wall contracts, forcing the chyme back toward the stomach (oradly) and toward the colon (aboradly).
   b. When the muscle relaxes, the chyme returns to the area from which it was displaced.
   c. This back-and-forth movement enables the chyme to become thoroughly mixed with the digestive juices and to make contact with the absorptive surface of the intestinal mucosa.
   d. Segmentation contractions occur about 12 times/min in the duodenum and 8 times/min in the ileum. The contractions last for 5–6 seconds.
   e. Segmentation occurs throughout the digestive period.

2. **Peristaltic contractions** also occur in the small intestine.

    a. Although peristaltic contractions occasionally propel food along the entire length of the intestine, they rarely involve more than a short segment of the intestine.

    b. Peristalsis is not considered an important component of intestinal transit.

3. The **migrating motor complex (MMC;** see Chapter 42 II F 3) spreads over the intestine during the interdigestive period.

    a. The MMCs sweep out the chyme remaining in the small intestine during the interdigestive period.

    b. MMCs occur every 60–90 minutes and last for about 10 minutes.

C. **Propulsion of chyme.** During the digestive period, the higher frequency of segmentation in the proximal intestine (duodenum) than in the distal intestine (ileum) propels the chyme slowly toward the colon.

    1. When the chyme is pushed distally, it is less likely to be forced back by a segmentation contraction.

    2. In contrast, when the chyme is pushed towards the stomach, it is quickly pushed toward the colon again by a segmentation contraction in the more proximal region of the small intestine.

D. **Control of intestinal motility.** The frequency and strength of segmentation contractions in the intestine are controlled by the **slow waves** (see Figure 42–2).

    1. **Generation.** Segmentation contractions can occur only if the slow waves produce **spikes,** or **action potentials.** Spikes appear on the slow waves when the membrane potential is sufficiently depolarized.

    2. **Frequency**

        a. The frequency of segmentation contractions is directly related to the frequency of the slow waves.

        b. Slow wave frequency is controlled by **pacemaker cells** within the wall of the intestine and is not influenced by neural activity or circulating hormones.

    3. **Strength**

        a. The strength of a segmentation contraction is proportional to the frequency of the spikes generated by the slow wave. The amplitude of the slow wave controls the frequency of the slow waves. Therefore, the greater the slow wave amplitude, the greater the frequency of spikes generated and the greater the strength of the contraction.

        b. Slow wave amplitude is controlled by the hormones released during digestion.

            (1) Gastrin, cholecystokinin (CCK), motilin, and insulin increase the slow wave amplitude.

            (2) Secretin and glucagon reduce the slow wave amplitude.

IV. PANCREATIC SECRETIONS

A. **Pancreatic cell types and their functions.** The pancreas contains endocrine, exocrine, and ductal cells.

    1. The **endocrine cells,** arranged in small islets within the pancreas, secrete **insulin, glucagon, somatostatin,** and **pancreatic polypeptide** directly into the circulation.

    2. The **exocrine cells** are organized into acini that produce four types of digestive enzymes: **peptidases, lipases, amylases,** and **nucleases,** which are responsible for digesting proteins, fats, carbohydrates, and nucleic acids, respectively. In their absence, malabsorption syndromes develop.

    3. Each day, the **ductal cells** secrete about 2–2.5 liters of pancreatic juice containing a high concentration of **bicarbonate (HCO_3^-).** The HCO_3^- neutralizes gastric acid and regulates the pH of the upper intestine. Failure to neutralize the chyme as it enters the intestine will result in duodenal ulcers.

B. | **Composition of pancreatic secretions**

1. The ductal cells of the pancreatic ducts secrete a fluid that is high in HCO_3^- typically about 100 mEq/L) and low in Cl^- (about 50 mEq/L).
   a. The high concentration of $HCO3_3^-$ and low concentration of Cl^- is produced by a HCO_3^-–Clk^- exchanger on the apical membrane of the ductal cells.
      (1) The ductal cells originally secrete fluid containing an electrolyte composition similar to plasma.
      (2) Cl^- is secreted into the pancreatic ducts by the CFTR (cystic fibrosis transport regulator).
      (3) HCO_3^- is transported into the pancreatic ducts in exchange for Cl^-.
      (4) H^+ is actively transported out of the cell across the basal membrane by a Na^+-H^+ exchanger.
      (5) Acinar cells, which are primarily responsible for secreting pancreatic enzymes, secrete a fluid that is mostly NaCl.
   d. The concentration of HCO_3^- increases when pancreatic flow rates increase.
      (1) At low flow rates, equal volumes of pancreatic juice come from ductal and acinar cells.
      (2) At high flow rates, the proportion of the pancreatic juice secreted by the ductal cells, which have a high HCO_3^- concentration increases.

2. **Enzymes.** The pancreas secretes three major types of pancreatic enzymes: **amylases, lipases,** and **proteases.**
   a. **Pancreatic α-amylase** is secreted in its active form. It hydrolyzes glycogen, starch, and most other complex carbohydrates, except cellulose, to form disaccharides.
   b. **Pancreatic lipases** (lipase, cholesterol lipase, and phospholipase) (see VII C 1 a) are secreted in their active forms. The enzymes that hydrolyze water-insoluble esters require bile salts to work. Water-soluble esters can be hydrolyzed without the action of bile salts.
   c. **Pancreatic proteases (trypsin** and **the chymotrypsins)** are secreted in their inactive zymogen form (trypsinogen and the chymotrypsinogens, respectively) (see VII B 2 b).
      (1) Trypsinogen is converted to trypsin by enterokinase (also called enteropeptidase) or by trypsin itself (autocatalysis).
      (2) The chymotrypsinogens are converted to their active form by trypsin.
   d. **Trypsin inhibitor** is secreted by the same cells and at the same time as the pancreatic proenzymes. Trypsin inhibitor protects the pancreas from autodigestion.

C. | **Control of pancreatic secretion.** Like gastric secretion, pancreatic secretion is divided into the following three phases:

1. **Cephalic phase.** The thought, sight, smell, or taste of food produces the cephalic phase of pancreatic secretion. Both acinar and ductal cell secretions are enhanced by vagal stimulation.
   a. Enzyme secretion by the acinar cells is stimulated directly by vagal fibers that release acetylcholine (ACh) or by cholinergic interneurons that are stimulated by the vagal preganglionic fibers.
   b. Although the vagus nerve can also cause HCO_3^- secretion by ductal cells, its ability to stimulate HCO_3^- secretion is not nearly as great as its ability to stimulate the release of enzymes.

2. **Gastric phase.** Pancreatic secretion is enhanced during the gastric phase by distention and food breakdown products.
   a. **Distention** of the antrum and corpus initiates a vagovagal reflex resulting in a low volume of pancreatic secretion containing both HCO_3^- and enzymes. ACh is the transmitter.
   b. **Food breakdown products** (primarily amino acids and peptides) can stimulate pan-

creatic secretions because of their ability to cause the G cells of the antrum to release gastrin. Gastrin produces a low-volume, high-enzyme pancreatic secretion.

3. **Intestinal phase.** The major stimulants for pancreatic secretion are the hormones cholecystokinin (CCK) and secretin. They are released from endocrine cells in the duodenum and jejunum during the intestinal phase of pancreatic secretion.
   a. **CCK,** in addition to its effect on the gallbladder (see V E 2 a), is a potent stimulant of pancreatic enzyme secretion. It is secreted by I cells within the duodenum.
      (1) Like gastrin, CCK is found in two physiologically active forms, an octapeptide called CCK-8 and a 33-chain polypeptide, CCK-33.
      (2) The actions of CCK are potentiated by secretin. By itself, secretin has no effect on enzyme secretion.
   b. **Secretin** was the first hormone ever discovered. Its primary effect is to increase HCO_3^- secretion by the pancreas. It is secreted by S cells within the duodenum.
      (1) The actions of secretin are potentiated by CCK. By itself, CCK has no effect on HCO_3^- secretion.
      (2) Because they are potentiators of each other's action, small concentrations of CCK and secretin together can produce significant amounts of pancreatic HCO_3^- and enzyme secretions, while either one alone would have little or no effect.
   c. **Control of CCK and secretin release.** CKK and secretin are secreted from endocrine cells in response to the entrance of chyme into the small intestine.
      (1) **Amino acids** (primarily **phenylalanine**), **fatty acids,** and **monoglycerides** are the major stimuli for CCK secretion.
      (2) **Low pH** (<4.5), caused by the presence of gastric acid (HCl) in the intestine, is a potent stimulus for the release of secretin.
   d. A vagovagal reflex, which greatly potentiates the effects of secretin and CCK, is activated during the intestinal phase of digestion.
   e. ACh potentiates the effects of both CCK and secretion. Thus, vagal stimulation is much more potent in stimulating pancreatic secretions when CCK and secretin are present in the plasma.

V. BILIARY SECRETIONS

A. General features of bile

1. **Function.** Bile is required for the digestion and absorption of fats and for the excretion of water-insoluble substances such as cholesterol and bilirubin.

2. **Formation.** Bile is formed by liver epithelial cells, called **hepatocytes,** and by epithelial cells lining the bile ducts, called **ductal cells.** Between 250 and 1100 ml of bile are secreted daily.

3. **Storage.** Although it is secreted continuously, bile is stored in the gallbladder during the interdigestive period.

4. **Release.** Bile is released into the duodenum during the digestive period only after chyme has triggered the release of CCK, which then produces contraction of the gallbladder and relaxation of the sphincter of Oddi.

B. Composition of bile

1. **Bile acids**
   a. **Primary bile acids** (**trihydroxycholic acid** and **dihydroxychenodeoxycholic acid**) are synthesized from cholesterol and converted into bile salts by the hepatocytes as follows.
      (1) Cholesterol is absorbed through microvilli lining the serosal (antiluminal) border of the hepatic epithelial cells.
      (2) The bile acids are conjugated with either taurine or glycine to form bile salts.

(3) The bile salts are actively secreted into a canaliculus on the lateral (luminal) surface of the hepatocyte, from which they then drain into the bile duct.

(4) Because bile salts are not lipid soluble, they remain within the intestine until reaching the ileum, where they are actively absorbed (see VII C 2).

b. Secondary bile acids are formed by deconjugation and dehydroxylation of the primary bile salts by intestinal bacteria, forming **deoxycholic acid** and **lithocholic acid.**

2. Bile pigments

a. Bilirubin and **biliverdin,** the two principal bile pigments, are metabolites of hemoglobin formed in the liver and conjugated as glucuronides for excretion. They are responsible for the golden yellow color of bile.

b. Intestinal bacteria metabolize bilirubin further to **urobilin,** which is responsible for the brown color of stool.

c. If bilirubin is not secreted by the liver, it builds up in the blood and tissues, producing **jaundice**.

3. Phospholipids (primarily **lecithins**) are, after bile salts, the most abundant organic compound in bile.

a. Although the phospholipids are normally insoluble in water, they are solubilized by the bile salt micelles.

b. The **micelles** are able to solubilize other lipids more effectively when they are composed of bile salts and phospholipids than when they are composed of bile salts alone.

4. Cholesterol, although present in only small amounts, is an important component of bile.

a. Cholesterol is essentially insoluble in water and thus must be solubilized by bile salt micelles before it can be secreted in the bile (see VII C 2).

b. Biliary secretion of cholesterol is important because it is one of the few ways in which cholesterol stores can be regulated.

5. Electrolytes. The electrolyte composition of bile is similar to that of pancreatic juice and plasma (see IV B 1).

C. **Enterohepatic circulation** is the recirculation of bile salts from the liver to the small intestine and back again. This circulation is necessary because of the limited pool of bile salts available to help break down and absorb fat (see Figure 43–1).

1. Path of circulation. Bile salts travel from the liver to the duodenum via the common bile duct. When the bile salts reach the terminal ileum, they are reabsorbed into the portal circulation. The liver then extracts them from the portal blood and secretes them once again into the bile.

a. Bile salts are reabsorbed only in the terminal ileum. No reabsorption of bile salts occurs in the duodenum or jejunum.

b. From 90%–95% of the bile salts that enter the small intestine are actively reabsorbed from the lower ileum back into the portal circulation.

c. The remaining bile salts are excreted into the feces.

2. Circulating pool. The total circulating pool of bile salts (consisting of primary and secondary bile acids) is approximately 3.6 g. Because 4–8 g of bile salts are required to digest and absorb a meal (more if the meal is high in fat), the total pool of salts must circulate twice during the digestion of each meal. Consequently, the bile salts usually circulate 6–8 times daily.

3. Bile salt synthesis and replacement. The rate of bile salt synthesis is determined by the rate of return to the liver. The usual rate is 0.2–0.4 g/day, which replaces normal fecal losses. The maximal rate is 3–6 g/day. If fecal losses exceed this rate, the total pool size decreases.

4. Clinical implications. Because bile salts are required for proper digestion and absorption of fats, any condition that disrupts the enterohepatic circulation (e.g., ileal resection or small intestinal diseases such as sprue or Crohn's disease) leads to a decreased bile acid pool and malabsorption of fat and fat-soluble vitamins. The clinical manifestations of such conditions are steatorrhea and nutritional deficiency. An increase in fecal losses of bile salts results in watery diarrhea, because bile salts inhibit water and Na^+ absorption in the colon.

D. **Control of biliary secretion.** The volume of biliary secretion and the amount of bile in that secretion are regulated separately.

1. **The bile-independent fraction of biliary secretion** refers to the amount of **fluid,** composed of electrolytes and water, that is secreted each day by the liver. Although this fluid, by definition, is secreted with the bile, its secretion is controlled separately from bile secretion.

   a. Secretion of this fluid is controlled by the hormone **secretin.**
   b. The fluid resembles the secretion of the pancreatic ductal cells in the following ways (see IV B 1, IV C):
   (1) The fluid is secreted by ductal cells.
   (2) Its secretion is controlled by secretin.
   (3) It has a high concentration of HCO_3^-.

2. **The bile-dependent fraction of biliary secretion** refers to the quantity of **bile salts** secreted by the liver.

   a. The amount of bile salts secreted is directly related to the amount of bile reabsorbed by the hepatocytes (i.e., the more bile reabsorbed from the portal circulation, the more bile secreted by the liver).
   (1) The total amount of bile is relatively constant. Because the liver has limited synthetic capacity, there is a limit to the amount of bile that can be secreted.
   (2) Substances that enhance bile secretion are called **choleretics.** Bile salts and bile acids are the major choleretics.
   b. Unlike the bile-independent secretion, the **synthesis and secretion of bile** by the liver is not under any direct hormonal or nervous control. However, CCK increases bile flow indirectly by increasing the release of bile from the gallbladder (see V E 2 a).

E. **Gallbladder**

1. **Functions.** The gallbladder stores and concentrates the bile during the interdigestive period and empties its contents into the duodenum during digestion.

   a. **Storage.** During the interdigestive period, the bile secreted by the liver is collected in the gallbladder. The gallbladder typically stores 20–50 ml of bile.
   (1) The bile is highly **concentrated** within the gallbladder by the reabsorption of water.
   (2) Water is reabsorbed by the osmotic gradient produced by the active reabsorption of Na^+ and HCO_3^-.
   b. **Contraction.** During digestion, the gallbladder contracts, emptying its contents into the duodenum.

2. **Control**

   a. **CCK is the major stimulus** for gallbladder contraction and sphincter of Oddi relaxation. When chyme enters the small intestine, **fat and protein digestion products** directly stimulate the secretion of CCK [see IV C 3 c (1)].
   b. **Vagal stimulation** of the gallbladder also causes gallbladder contraction and sphincter of Oddi relaxation. Vagal stimulation occurs directly during the cephalic phase of digestion and indirectly via a vagovagal reflex during the gastric phase of digestion.

3. **Effects of cholecystectomy.** Bile, not the gallbladder, is essential to digestion. After removal of the gallbladder, bile empties slowly but continuously into the intestine, allowing digestion of fats sufficient to maintain good health and nutrition. Only high-fat meals need to be avoided.

4. **Gallstones** form in an estimated 10%–30% of the population, although only a fraction, perhaps 20% of these, ever produce symptoms. In Western societies, about 85% of gall-

stones are composed chiefly of cholesterol; the remainder are pigment stones, composed chiefly of calcium bilirubinate.

    a. Cholesterol and lecithin, both of which are insoluble in water, are kept in solution in bile through the formation of micelles (see VII C 2 a). When the proportions of lecithin, cholesterol, and bile salts are altered, cholesterol crystallizes, leading to stone formation. Cholesterol stones are radiolucent.

    b. Calcium bilirubinate stones can form when infection of the biliary tree leads to bacterial deconjugation of conjugated bilirubin. Unconjugated bilirubin, which is insoluble in bile, then precipitates to begin the stone-forming process. Calcium bilirubinate stones are radiopaque.

VI. INTESTINAL SECRETIONS

A. **Mucus** most likely serves a protective role, preventing HCl and chyme from damaging the intestinal wall. Mucus is secreted by:

    1. Brunner's glands, which are located within the duodenum

    2. Goblet cells located along the length of the intestinal epithelium and in the intestinal crypts, called the crypts of Lieberkühn

B. **Enzymes** capable of breaking down small peptides and disaccharides are associated with the microvilli of the epithelial cells lining the intestine. Although these enzymes are not secreted into the intestine, they are able to digest small peptides and disaccharides during the absorptive process.

C. **Water and electrolytes** are secreted by all the epithelial cells of the intestine.

    1. The watery secretion provides a solvent into which the products of digestion are dissolved.

    2. If excessive amounts of fluid are produced (as happens when the enterotoxin responsible for cholera stimulates massive fluid secretion), potentially life-threatening watery diarrhea can result.

VII. DIGESTION AND ABSORPTION

A. **Carbohydrates.** The **three major carbohydrates** in the human diet are the disaccharides—**sucrose** (cane sugar) and **lactose** (milk sugar)—as well as the polysaccharide starches (which may be in either the straight-chain form, **amylose,** or the branched-chain form, **amylopectin**). **Cellulose,** another plant polysaccharide, is present in the diet in large amounts, but no enzymes in the human digestive tract can digest it, so it is excreted unused. Dietary intake of carbohydrates is 250–800 g/day, which represents 50%–60% of the diet.

    1. Digestion. Carbohydrates must be digested into monosaccharides before being absorbed from the GI tract.

        a. Although starch digestion, by **salivary α-amylase,** begins in the mouth, almost all carbohydrate digestion occurs within the small intestine.

        b. Pancreatic α-amylase digests carbohydrates into a variety of oligosaccharides.

        c. The oligosaccharides are digested into monosaccharides by brush border enzymes such as **maltase, lactase,** and **sucrase.**

        d. The end products of carbohydrates are **fructose, glucose,** and **galactose.**

    2. Mechanisms of absorption

        a. Glucose and **galactose** are absorbed by a common **Na⁺-dependent active transport system.**

            (1) The carrier has two binding sites for Na⁺ and one to which either one molecule of glucose or galactose can bind.

    (2) Because two Na$^+$ are transported down their electrochemical gradient, a large amount of energy is available for transport; thus, almost all of the glucose and galactose present in the intestine can be absorbed.

  b. **Fructose is absorbed by facilitated transport.** Fructose absorption occurs readily because most of the fructose is rapidly converted into glucose and lactic acid within the intestinal epithelial cells, thus maintaining a high concentration gradient for diffusion.

  c. After being absorbed into the enterocytes, the monosaccharides are transported across the basolateral membrane by facilitated diffusion. They then diffuse from the intestinal interstitium into the capillaries of the villus.

  d. Absorption of monosaccharides is not regulated. The intestine can absorb over 5 kg of sucrose each day.

  e. Failure to absorb carbohydrates results in diarrhea and intestinal gas.

    (1) The unabsorbed carbohydrates act as osmotic particles and draw excessive fluids into the intestine, resulting in diarrhea.

    (2) The flora of the intestine and colon metabolize the unabsorbed carbohydrates, producing a variety of gases [hydrogen (H_2), methane (CH_4), and CO_2], as well as a variety of intestinal irritants.

    (3) **Lactose intolerance** is the most common cause of carbohydrate malabsorption. It results from the inability of the goblet cells to produce lactase.

      (a) Avoidance of milk or milk products prevents the symptoms from developing.

      (b) Lactose intolerance in adults, where it is most common, is not usually a problem. However, in infants, the diarrhea-produced dehydration can be life-threatening.

B. **Proteins.** The daily dietary protein requirement for adults is 0.5–0.7 g/kg of body weight. For children 1–3 years old, it is 4 g/kg.

1. **Sources.** The protein that is found in the intestines comes from two sources.

  a. **Endogenous proteins,** totaling 30–40 g/day, are secretory proteins as well as the protein components of desquamated cells.

  b. **Exogenous proteins** are dietary proteins, which total at least 75–100 g daily in the average American diet.

2. **Digestion.** Proteins must be digested into small polypeptides and amino acids before being absorbed.

  a. About 10%–15% of the protein entering the GI tract is digested by **gastric pepsin** secreted by chief cells. Protein digestion within the stomach is important primarily because the protein digestion products act as secretagogues, stimulating the secretion of proteases by the pancreas.

  b. **Pancreatic proteases** play a major role in protein digestion. The proteases, such as trypsin, are secreted in an inactive form and must be converted into an active form within the intestine (see IV B 2 c).

    (1) **Enterokinase,** an enzyme secreted by the epithelial cells of the duodenum and jejunum, converts the inactive trypsinogen into trypsin.

    (2) Trypsin then autocatalyzes the conversion of trypsinogen to trypsin as well as activating the other proteases.

  c. **Peptidases,** secreted by the intestinal epithelial cells, continue the digestive process begun by the pancreatic proteases, eventually converting the ingested proteins to small polypeptides and amino acids.

3. **Mechanisms of absorption**

  a. A variety of **Na$^+$-dependent active transport systems** have been identified for the transport of tripeptides, dipeptides, and amino acids. Polypeptides with more than three peptides are poorly absorbed.

    (1) Separate transporters are present for the absorption of basic, acidic, and neutral amino acids. At least two different polypeptide transporters exist.

    (2) Tripeptides and **d**ipeptides are absorbed in greater quantities than amino acids.

  b. Once inside the enterocytes, intercellular peptidases digest some of the polypeptides to amino acids.

    c. Amino acids and the remaining polypeptides are transported across the basolateral membrane of the enterocytes by facilitated or simple diffusion. They then enter the capillaries of the villus by simple diffusion.

    d. Almost all of the ingested protein is absorbed by the intestine. Any protein that appears in the stool derives from the bacteria within the colon or from cellular debris.

    e. **Malabsorption** of amino acids due to lack of adequate transporters (e.g., the malabsorption of neutral amino acids that occurs in **Hartnup disease**) is relatively rare. Inadequate absorption of proteins due to lack of trypsin is a common consequence of pancreatic diseases.

C. **Fats. Daily dietary fat intake** varies widely, from 25–160 g.

  1. **Digestion.** Although the serous glands of the tongue secrete lingual lipase, very little, if any, lipid digestion occurs in the mouth or stomach. Unlike carbohydrates and proteins, lipids are absorbed from the GI tract by **passive diffusion.** However, before the lipids can be absorbed, they must first be made soluble in water. **Bile salts** are required for the solubilization of lipids.

    a. **Pancreatic lipases.** The pancreas secretes three different lipases (see IV B 2 b).

      (1) **Pancreatic lipase** is a fairly specific lipase that cleaves fatty acids from the 1 and 1′ positions of triglycerides, leaving a 2-monoglyceride.

      (2) **Cholesterol esterase** cleaves the fatty acid from cholesterol esters, leaving free cholesterol.

      (3) **Phospholipase A$_2$** cleaves the fatty acids from phospholipids such as phosphatidylcholine.

    b. **Emulsification of lipids.** Lipids must be broken down into small droplets (less than 1 μm in diameter) or **emulsified** into fat globules by bile acids and lecithin (a component of bile) before being digested.

    c. Fat digestion by the pancreatic lipases occurs very rapidly after emulsification because of the large surface-to-volume ratio of the small globules.

  2. **Mechanism of absorption**

    a. **Micelle formation.** The emulsified products of lipid digestion (e.g., monoglycerides, cholesterol) must form **micelles** with bile salts before they can be absorbed.

      (1) **Micelles** are small (about 5 nm in diameter) spherical aggregates containing some 20–30 molecules of lipids and bile salts.

      (2) The **bile salts** are on the outside of the micelle. The 2-monoglycerides and lysophosphatides have their hydrophobic chains facing the interior of the micelle and their polar ends facing the surrounding water phase. The cholesterol and fat-soluble vitamins are located within the fat-soluble interior of the micelle.

    b. **Absorption of lipids and bile salts from micelles**

      (1) The micelles move along the microvilli surface, allowing their lipids to diffuse across the microvilli membrane and into the enterocytes.

      (2) Lipids, cholesterol, and the fat-soluble vitamins are removed rapidly from the micelles once the micelles make contact with the microvilli.

      (3) The rate-limiting step in lipid absorption is the migration of the micelles from the intestinal chyme to the microvilli surface.

      (4) The bile salts, freed of their associated lipids, are absorbed in the terminal ileum by a Na$^+$-dependent active transport process.

      (5) Normally, all of the ingested lipid is absorbed. Fat present in the stool is derived from the intestinal flora.

    c. **Formation of chylomicrons by enterocytes**

      (1) Once inside the enterocytes, the digested lipids enter the **smooth endoplasmic reticulum** (ER), where they are reconstituted.

        (a) 2-Monoglycerides are combined with fatty acids to produce triglycerides.

        (b) Lysophosphatides are combined with fatty acids to form phospholipids.

        (c) Cholesterol is re-esterified.

      (2) The re-formed lipids coalesce into **chylomicrons** (small lipid droplets about 1 nm in diameter) within the smooth ER.

(3) The chylomicrons are transported out of the cell by exocytosis. β-lipoprotein, which is synthesized by the enterocytes, covers the surface of the chylomicrons. In the absence of β-lipoprotein, exocytosis will not occur, and the enterocytes become engorged with lipids.

d. Transport of lipids into circulation
  (1) After exiting the cell, the chylomicrons merge into larger droplets that vary in size from 50–500 nm, depending on the amount of lipids being absorbed.
  (2) The large lipid droplets then diffuse into the lacteals, from which they enter the lymphatic circulation.
  (3) Almost all digested lipids are totally reabsorbed by the time the chyme reaches the midjejunum, with most of the absorption occurring in the duodenum.

e. Lipid malabsorption is much more common than carbohydrate or protein malabsorption. It usually results from one of the following two conditions:
  (1) The pancreas does not secrete sufficient quantities of lipase.
  (2) The liver does not secrete sufficient quantities of bile.

D. | Water and electrolytes

1. Water
  a. The small intestine, in addition to absorbing most of the dietary Na^+ and water, must also absorb the 7–8 L of water and 20–30 g of Na^+ that are contained in salivary, gastric, biliary, and pancreatic secretions. Failure to reabsorb water from the intestine can lead to rapid dehydration and circulatory collapse.
  b. Water undergoes **passive, isosmotic reabsorption** in the small intestine.
    (1) Active reabsorption of electrolytes and nutrients creates an osmotic gradient favoring the reabsorption of water.
    (2) Because osmotic equilibrium is rapidly achieved, the fluid in the intestine is always isotonic to plasma.
  c. In the duodenum, the osmotic pressure created by the entering chyme causes water to flow into the intestine.
  d. In the jejunum and ileum, the reabsorption of sodium chloride (NaCl) creates an osmotic gradient favoring the reabsorption of water.

2. NaCl
  a. Na^+ reabsorption is a two-step process.
    (1) First, Na^+ and Cl^- are transported from the lumen into the enterocyte.
    (2) Then, they are transported across the basolateral membrane into the intestinal interstitium.
  b. Na^+ enters the enterocyte in three ways.
    (1) About 30% is transported into the cell by a Na^+-glucose, Na^+-amino acid, or Na^+-(di- or tri-) peptide cotransport system.
    (2) About 30% is transported into the cell by a neutral Na^+ Cl^- cotransport system.
    (3) The remainder enters the cell passively down an electrochemical gradient.
  c. Once inside the enterocyte, Na^+ is transported across the basolateral membrane by a Na^+-K^+-ATPase active transport system.
  d. For the most part, Cl^- flows passively through the enterocyte down the electrochemical gradient established by the active transport of Na^+.

E. | Vitamins and minerals

1. Fat-soluble vitamins (A, D, E, and **K)** become part of the micelles formed by bile salts and are absorbed along with other lipids in the proximal intestine.

2. Water-soluble vitamins (C, and the **B vitamins biotin, folic acid, nicotinic acid, B_6 [pyridoxine], B_2 [riboflavin],** and **B_1 [thiamine]**) are absorbed by facilitated transport or a Na^+-dependent active transport system in the proximal small intestine.

3. Vitamin B_{12} absorption is more complex than that of other vitamins.
  a. In the stomach, vitamin B_{12} is bound to an **R protein,** which is a specific binding protein.

b. The gastric parietal cells secrete another vitamin B_{12}-binding protein called **intrinsic factor.** However, the affinity of intrinsic factor for vitamin B_{12} is less than that of R protein, so most of the B_{12} is bound to R protein in the stomach.

c. In the intestine, pancreatic proteases cleave vitamin B_{12} from the R protein, allowing it to bind to intrinsic factor.

d. The intrinsic factor–B_{12} complex binds to a receptor on ileal enterocytes.

    (1) Absorption of the vitamin B_{12} from the intrinsic factor-B_{12} complex can occur only after the complex binds to the receptor.

    (2) In the absence of intrinsic factor, minimal amounts of vitamin B_{12} can be absorbed by diffusion. Thus, if large amounts of the vitamin are ingested, enough B_{12} can be absorbed to prevent **pernicious anemia.**

4. Ca^{2+} absorption within the small intestine is regulated to maintain Ca^{2+} balance. Normally, about 25%–80% of the daily intake of Ca^{2+} 1000 mg) is absorbed.

a. Ca^{2+} absorption occurs via a membrane-bound carrier that is activated by **vitamin D.**

    (1) Vitamin D_3 is converted to **25-hydroxyvitamin D_3** by the liver.

    (2) The kidney converts the **25-hydroxyvitamin D_3** to **1,25-dihydroxyvitamin D_3** by a process that is regulated by parathyroid hormone.

    (3) 1,25-dihydroxyvitamin D_3 then enters the enterocyte where it induces the formation of a Ca^{2+} carrier that inserts on the luminal surface of the enterocyte.

b. Ca^{2+} is transported out of the cell by a Ca^{2+}-ATPase active transport system and by a $Na+$- Ca^{+2+} exchange system.

5. Iron absorption is necessary to maintain normal iron balance. However, very little (0.75 mg for men and 1.5 mg for women) of the 15–25 mg of iron ingested each day is actually absorbed.

a. Iron is absorbed primarily within the **duodenum** and **jejunum.**

b. Iron can be absorbed either as **heme** (derived from meat) or as a **free ion.**

c. The ferrous ion (Fe^{2+}) is absorbed more efficiently than the **ferric ion (Fe^{3+})**

d. Ascorbic acid (vitamin C) promotes iron absorption by reducing Fe^{3+} to Fe^{2+} and by preventing iron from forming insoluble complexes within the chyme.

e. Stomach acid tends to break insoluble iron complexes apart and thus facilitates iron absorption.

f. Four separate steps are involved in the transport of iron from the intestine to the plasma.

    (1) First, the iron is transported across the apical membrane of the enterocyte by a specific iron carrier system.

    (2) Second, the iron binds to **apoferritin,** an iron-binding protein, to form **ferritin.**

    (3) In order to leave the enterocyte, the iron must dissociate from ferritin and bind to an intracellular carrier protein that shuttles it to the basolateral membrane, where it is transported out of the cell.

    (4) Upon entering the intestinal interstitium, the iron is transported to the plasma by **transferrin,** a β-globulin.

g. The **amount of iron absorbed** depends on the amount of intracellular and extracellular transport protein (transferrin) compared to the amount of ferritin.

    (1) If a large amount of transferrin is available, iron can be transported rapidly from the enterocyte to the plasma.

    (2) If little transferrin is available, most of the iron remains trapped in the enterocyte and is eventually excreted when the cells are desquamated.

    (3) When iron stores are depleted, such as after a hemorrhage, transferrin synthesis increases.

Case 1

A 35 year old woman visits her physician because of severe, unremitting abdominal pains. She reports failing nauseated and weak and states that she has lost weight over the last

several months and that her stools are bulky. **Physical examination reveals a mild fever and tachycardia. She is found to have a high blood glucose level and an abnormal glucose tolerance test. A tentative diagnosis of chronic pancreatitis is confirmed by an X-ray of the pancreas which shows extensive calcification.**

1. Why has she lost weight? Why does she have bulky stools?

DISCUSSION

Chronic pancreatitis is most often caused by excessive alcohol ingestion but may result from gallstones or severe malnutrition. In many cases the cause is not known.

Pancreatitis interferes with the endocrine and exocrine functions of the pancreas. The inability to excrete sufficient amounts of digestive enzymes prevents the breakdown and consequently, the absorption of food. The excretion of large quantities of fluid (diarrhea) undigested fats (called steatorrhea) results in a large volume (as much as 2 to 3 liters per day) of bulky, oily stools.

2. Why is she weak? Why is she tachycardic?

DISCUSSION

The tachycardia (rapid heart rate) could result indirectly from the cardiovascular response to volume depletion or directly from the effect of temperature on the pacemaker cells of the heart.

3. Why does she have a high blood sugar and an abnormal glucose tolerance test?

DISCUSSION

The high blood sugar and abnormal glucose tolerance test are signs of diabetes which are most likely caused by damage to the pancreatic β-cells.

Case 2

A severely dehydrated young child is brought to the emergency room by her parents. She has had diarrhea and has been vomiting for the last 24 hours. She is tachycardiac, hypotensive and lethargic. Her parents report that they were at the county fair the day before she became sick. A tentative diagnosis of cholera is made and confirmed by identifying the bacteria *Vibrio cholerae* in the stool. An isotonic oral rehydrating solution containing Na$^+$ (90 mM), K$^+$ (20 mM), and glucose (110 mM) is given.

1. How does V. cholerae cause diarrhea?

DISCUSSION

The cholera toxin binds to the surface of the intestinal epithelial cells. An activated subunit of the toxin enters the cell where it transfers ADP-ribose to the G$_s$-protein, causing continuously activation of adenylyl cyclase. The consequent accumulation of cAMP causes increased Cl$^-$ secretion and decreased Na$^+$ reabsorption. The accumulation of NaCl causes the osmotic flow of water into the intestine, producing high volumes of watery diarrhea.

2. Why does the rehydrating solution contain glucose?

DISCUSSION

The toxin affects only the ion transporting mechanisms of the intestine. The Na^+-glucose co-transporters still function to reabsorb Na^+, glucose and water. By providing excess glucose, these transporters can reabsorb adequate quantities of fluid until the cholera toxin is removed from the GI tract (typically 2 or 3 days).

3. Why does the rehydrating solution contain so much K^+?

DISCUSSION

The colon secretes K^+. The amount of K^+ lost from the body increases during periods of diarrhea. When the diarrhea is severe, as it in cholera, the lost K^+ must be replaced.

CHAPTER 44

Large Intestine

I. **OVERVIEW.** The **colon,** or large intestine (Figure 44–1), absorbs some of the nutrients and most of the fluids passed into it from the small intestine. Under normal circumstances, all but 50–100 ml of the 1500 ml received from the small intestine is absorbed. Any nutrients or fluids that cannot be absorbed are passed into the feces.

II. **MOTILITY**

A. **Function.** The **contractile activity** of the large intestine serves two functions.

  1. It enhances the efficiency of water and electrolyte absorption.

  2. It promotes the excretion of the fecal material remaining in the colon.

B. **Types of movements**

  1. **Haustral shuttling** *similar to segmentation s.m. intestine*

    a. Bands of muscle divide the large intestine into sac-like segments called **haustrations.** Although the haustrations are present when the colon is empty, the entry of food into the colon causes an increase in colonic contractile activity.

    b. The dynamic formation and disappearance of haustrations squeeze the chyme, moving it back and forth along the colon in a manner similar to that described for the segmentation contractions in the small intestine (see Chapter 43 III A 1).

  2. **Peristalsis,** here, as elsewhere in the gut, is a progressive contractile wave preceded by a wave of relaxation. Peristaltic-like segmentation contractions move the chyme very slowly (5 cm/hr) along the colon. It can take up to 48 hours for chyme to traverse the colon.

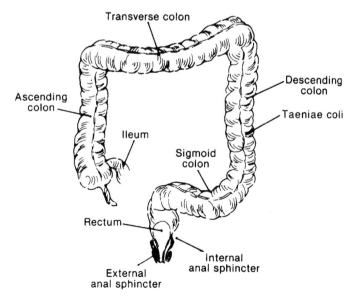

FIGURE 44–1. The large intestine.

3. Mass movements. Occasionally (three to four times daily) the chyme is swept rapidly along the colon by a peristaltic wave called a mass movement. The mass movement forces fecal material into the rectum.

4. The **frequency** of contractions is greater in the rectum than in the sigmoid colon, causing retrograde movement of fecal material. Because of this orad movement of fecal material, the rectum usually is empty, and material placed into it, such as a suppository, will be pushed up into the colon.

5. The overall effect of the **neural input to the colon is inhibitory.** Thus, elimination of the enteric nervous system, as occurs in **Hirschsprung's disease,** leads to a large increase in colonic tone.

C. Defecation

1. Fecal material entering the rectum is evacuated by defecation, during which:
  a. The smooth muscles of the distal colon and rectum contract, propelling the fecal material into the anal canal
  b. The **internal and external anal sphincters** both relax
  c. The abdominal and diaphragmatic muscles contract, increasing the intra-abdominal pressure and forcing the feces through the anal canal

2. Defecation involves both voluntary and reflex activity.
  a. When fecal material expands the rectum, a **rectosphincteric reflex** relaxes the internal anal sphincter, contracts the external anal sphincter, and generates the urge to defecate.
  b. Voluntary control mechanisms then either maintain contraction of the external anal sphincter (which is composed of skeletal muscle innervated by the pudendal nerves) to prevent defecation or allow it to relax so that defecation can occur.
  c. If defecation does not occur, the internal anal sphincter closes, and the rectum relaxes to accommodate the fecal material within it.
  d. Individuals lacking α-motoneuronal control over the external anal canal will defecate whenever the rectum is filled with fecal material.

III. ABSORPTION, SECRETION, AND GAS PRODUCTION

A. Water.
The colon is unable to absorb more than 2–3 L/day. Thus, if most of the 8–10 L entering the intestine (either as ingested water or as gastric, pancreatic, or biliary secretions) is not absorbed in the small intestine, severe diarrhea can occur.

B. Na^+ and Cl^-.
The colon absorbs most of the Na^+ and Cl^- that escapes absorption in the small intestine.

C. K^+,
on the other hand, is secreted by the colon. Its concentration typically rises from its ileal concentration of 9 mEq/L to 75 mEq/L by the time the fluid reaches the end of the large intestine.

D. Aldosterone.
Although the small intestine has no way to regulate absorption of Na^+ or K^+, the hormone aldosterone controls these processes in the colon. **Aldosterone** enables the colon to absorb all of the Na^+ in the fecal fluid. However, in doing so, it causes significant amounts of K^+ to be lost from the body.

E. Intestinal gas

1. There are three sources of gas in the gastrointestinal (GI) tract.
  a. **Swallowed air,** including air released from food and carbonated beverages, enters the stomach, from which it is removed by eructation or passed into the intestines with chyme.

b. Gas is formed by **bacterial action** in the ileum and large intestine.
c. Some gases diffuse into the GI tract from the **bloodstream.**

2. Gas in the colon differs in volume and source from gas in the small intestine.
   a. Small intestine. The small amount of gas present usually is the result of swallowed air. This gas most likely will be passed on to the colon.
   b. Colon
      (1) Colonic gas, or flatus, is produced in large volumes—up to 7–10 L/day.
      (2) The gas is produced chiefly through the breakdown of undigested nutrients that reach the colon.
      (3) The main components of flatus are CO_2, CH_4, H_2, and nitrogen gas (N_2). Because all of these gases except N_2 diffuse readily through the intestinal mucosa, the volume of flatus expelled is reduced to about 600 ml/day.

Case

A 10-year-old boy is brought to the pediatrician because of abdominal pain, bloating, and an inability to defecate. No feces are present within the rectum. A barium enema shows a markedly constricted sigmoid colon and a large expansion of the more proximal colon. A biopsy reveals the absence of enteric neurons in the distal colon. A diagnosis of Hirschsprung's disease (aganglionic megacolon) is made.

1. What is constipation?

DISCUSSION

Constipation is a clinical condition in which bowel movements are infrequent (less than three per week) or incomplete. It is often accompanied by difficult or painful defecation, a feeling of bloating or abdominal pain.

2. Why does the absence of enteric neurons produce intense constriction of the bowel?

DISCUSSION

The major neurotransmitters released by enteric neurons are VIP and NO. Therefore, the overall effect on the spontaneously active enteric nervous system is inhibition of gastrointestinal smooth muscle. Destruction of the enteric nervous system leads to increased contractile activity of GI smooth muscle. In Hirschsprung's disease the lesion typically occurs in the distal colon and rectum, leading to an obstructed colon. Aganglionic megacolon is a congenital disease which is usually discovered in infancy. However, in some cases the obstruction is less severe and symptoms do not appear until adolescence.

STUDY QUESTIONS

1. Which of the following secretions is most dependent on vagal stimulation?

(A) Saliva
(B) Hydrochloric acid (HCl)
(C) Pepsin
(D) Pancreatic juice
(E) Bile

2. The major stimulus for primary peristalsis in the esophagus is

(A) presence of food in the esophagus
(B) swallowing
(C) regurgitation of food from the stomach
(D) closing of the upper esophageal sphincter (UES)
(E) opening of the lower esophageal sphincter (LES)

3. Which of the following will inhibit stomach contractions?

(A) Acetylcholine (ACh)
(B) Motilin
(C) Gastrin
(D) Secretin
(E) Histamine

4. Gastric acid secretion increases when food enters the stomach because

(A) protein digestion products directly stimulate the parietal cells to release hydrochloric acid (HCl)
(B) food raises the pH of the stomach, allowing more acid to be released
(C) both
(D) neither

5. Gastric parietal cells secrete

(A) gastrin
(B) motilin
(C) cholecystokinin (CCK)
(D) intrinsic factor
(E) secretin

6. Which of the following can occur without brain stem coordination?

(A) Chewing
(B) Swallowing
(C) Primary esophageal peristalsis
(D) Vomiting
(E) Gastric emptying

7. The major stimulus for gastric acid (HCl) secretion during the cephalic phase is

(A) histamine
(B) gastrin
(C) secretin
(D) somatostatin
(E) acetylcholine (ACh)

8. The major stimulus for the release of secretin is

(A) protein digestion products
(B) histamine
(C) somatostatin
(D) hydrochloric acid (HCl)
(E) cholecystokinin (CCK)

9. Fats are transported from intestinal cells to blood plasma primarily in the form of

(A) micelles
(B) chylomicrons
(C) triglycerides
(D) fatty acids
(E) monoglycerides

10. Acetylcholine (ACh) is required for the contraction of

(A) the lower esophageal sphincter (LES)
(B) the upper esophageal sphincter (UES)
(C) both the LES and UES
(D) the antrum

11. The major stimulus for receptive relaxation of the stomach is

(A) food in the stomach
(B) food in the intestine
(C) secretin
(D) cholecystokinin (CCK)
(E) motilin

12. The motility pattern primarily responsible for the propulsion of chyme along the small intestine is

(A) the migrating motor complex (MMC)
(B) peristaltic waves
(C) myogenic contractions
(D) haustrations
(E) segmentation

13. Gastric acid (HCl) secretion is inhibited by

(A) somatostatin
(B) entero-oxyntin
(C) high pH
(D) amino acids
(E) acetylcholine (ACh)

14. The major factor controlling the secretion of bile salts from the liver is the amount of

(A) secretin released during a meal
(B) fat entering the small intestine
(C) bile acids produced by the liver
(D) bile reabsorbed from the intestine
(E) cholecystokinin (CCK) released during a meal

15. Micelle formation is necessary for absorption of

(A) bile salts
(B) iron
(C) cholesterol
(D) alcohol
(E) B vitamins

16. Secondary bile acids are formed

(A) in the liver from cholesterol
(B) by the conjugation of bile acids with taurine or glycine
(C) both
(D) neither

17. Na^+-dependent transport is responsible for the absorption of all of the following EXCEPT

(A) vitamin E
(B) amino acids
(C) glucose
(D) bile salts

18. Intestinal motility is increased by all of the following EXCEPT

(A) cholecystokinin (CCK)
(B) secretin
(C) gastrin
(D) insulin
(E) motilin

19. All of the following stimulate cholecystokinin (CCK) secretion EXCEPT

(A) amino acids
(B) fatty acids
(C) hydrochloric acid (HCl)
(D) bile acids

20. All of the following effects are caused by secretin EXCEPT

(A) stimulation of pancreatic bicarbonate (HCO_3^-) secretion
(B) enhancement of bile acid secretion
(C) potentiation of pancreatic enzyme secretion by cholecystokinin (CCK)
(D) inhibition of gastric muscle contraction

21. A Na^{+-}-dependent active transport system is necessary for the intestinal absorption of all of the following EXCEPT

(A) dipeptides
(B) bile salts
(C) fructose
(D) vitamin C
(E) glucose

22. Which stimulus is most important for the regulation of gastric acid (HCl) secretion?

(A) Secretin
(B) Histamine
(C) Cholecystokinin (CCK)
(D) Bombesin
(E) Motilin

23. Which stimulus is most important for the regulation of gastrin secretion?

(A) Secretin
(B) Histamine
(C) Cholecystokinin (CCK)
(D) Bombesin
(E) Motilin

24. Which stimulus is most important for the regulation of pancreatic enzyme secretion?

(A) Secretin
(B) Histamine
(C) Cholecystokinin (CCK)
(D) Bombesin
(E) Motilin

25. Which stimulus is most important for the regulation of gallbladder emptying?

(A) Secretin
(B) Histamine
(C) Cholecystokinin (CCK)
(D) Bombesin
(E) Motilin

26. Which stimulus is most important for the regulation of emptying of the intestine during the inter-digestive period?

(A) Secretin
(B) Histamine
(C) Cholecystokinin (CCK)
(D) Bombesin
(E) Motilin

27. Where does the absorption of bile acids occur?

(A) Fundus of the stomach
(B) Antrum of the stomach
(C) Duodenum of the intestine
(D) Ileum of the intestine
(E) Colon

28. Where does the secretion of gastrin occur?

(A) Fundus of the stomach
(B) Antrum of the stomach
(C) Duodenum of the intestine
(D) Ileum of the intestine
(E) Colon

29. Where does the secretion of intrinsic factor occur?

(A) Fundus of the stomach
(B) Antrum of the stomach
(C) Duodenum of the intestine
(D) Ileum of the intestine
(E) Colon

30. Where does the secretion of K^+ occur?

(A) Fundus of the stomach
(B) Antrum of the stomach
(C) Duodenum of the intestine
(D) Ileum of the intestine
(E) Colon

31. Where does the absorption of iron occur?

(A) Fundus of the stomach
(B) Antrum of the stomach
(C) Duodenum of the intestine
(D) Ileum of the intestine
(E) Colon

ANSWERS AND EXPLANATIONS

1. The answer is A [Chapter 42 II C 1; Chapter 42 III B 2–3, D 2 a–b; Chapter 43 IV C, V D 2]. Salivary flow is entirely dependent on the autonomic nervous system (ANS). Vagal stimulation produces a large volume of watery fluid, while sympathetic stimulation causes the secretion of proteins (mucus and some enzymes). Secretion of hydrochloric acid (HCl), pepsin, pancreatic juice, and bile is influenced by vagal stimulation but can occur without it.

2. The answer is B [Chapter 42 III A 3 b (1)]. Primary esophageal peristalsis is part of the swallowing response and occurs whether or not food enters the esophagus. The intensity of the peristalsis, however, increases if food is present. If the esophagus is not emptied by primary peristalsis, the presence of food in the esophagus will initiate another peristaltic reflex, called secondary peristalsis.

3. The answer is D [Chapter 42 II F 2 b (2)]. Secretin has a direct inhibitory effect on the smooth muscle fibers forming the stomach wall. Acetylcholine (ACh) and motilin, and possibly gastrin, increase the force of stomach contractions. Histamine has no direct effect on stomach contractions.

4. The answer is C [Chapter 43 III B 3 b]. Gastric acid secretion is increased directly by protein digestion products and inhibited when the pH of the stomach is reduced. The buffering action of food promotes gastric acid secretion by keeping the pH from falling too low.

5. The answer is D [Chapter 42 III A 3 a (1)]. Parietal cells, located in the oxyntic glands of the orad stomach (fundus and corpus), secrete hydrochloric acid (HCl) and intrinsic factor. Gastrin is secreted by G cells located in the pyloric glands of the distal stomach (antrum). Secretin and cholecystokinin (CCK) are secreted by endocrine cells in the proximal intestine. Motilin is secreted from endocrine cells within the epithelium of the small intestine.

6. The answer is E [Chapter 42 II E, F 1 a]. Gastric emptying of solids occurs when the contractile activity of the stomach reduces the size of the particles within the food sufficiently for them to pass through the pyloric sphincter.

Stomach contractions are elicited by reflexes initiated by antral distention and by gastrin. Although the strength of the contractions is reduced by vagotomy, contractions can still occur. Chewing, swallowing, primary (but not secondary) peristalsis, and vomiting all are coordinated by specific regions of the brain stem.

7. The answer is E [Chapter 42 III B 4]. During the cephalic phase of gastric acid (HCl) secretion, the sight, smell, or thought of food activates cholinergic [acetylcholine (ACh)-releasing] vagal fibers, which stimulate the release of HCl from antral parietal cells.

8. The answer is D [Chapter 43 IV C 3 c (2)]. Secretin and cholecystokinin (CCK) are hormones released from endocrine cells located in the proximal intestine. Although the release of both hormones is stimulated by the presence of chyme in the small intestine, it is the low pH resulting from hydrochloric acid (HCl) in the chyme that is the major stimulus for the release of secretin. Protein digestion products (e.g., amino acids, particularly phenylalanine) stimulate both secretin and CCK secretion, but are the major stimuli for CCK secretion. CCK potentiates the effects of secretin but does not affect its release. Somatostatin and histamine have no effect on CCK or secretin secretion.

9. The answer is B [Chapter 43 VII C 2 c]. Chylomicrons are small lipid droplets within the enterocytes that are reconstituted from the lipid digestion products formed in the intestine. The chylomicrons are transported from the enterocytes by exocytosis by the intestinal fluid surrounding the intestine. The chylomicrons are then absorbed into the intestinal lacteals, from which they enter the circulation.

10. The answer is B [Chapter 41 III A 3 a (1)]. The upper esophageal sphincter (UES) is composed of striated muscle and is stimulated by cholinergic [acetylcholine (ACh)-releasing] vagal fibers. The lower esophageal sphincter (LES) is composed of smooth muscle, which normally is maintained in a contracted state by a myogenic process. ACh regulates the force of peristaltic contractions in the antrum but is not required to stimulate them.

11. The answer is A [Chapter 42 II B 2]. When food distends the orad stomach (fundus and corpus), it produces a vagovagal reflex by which noncholinergic, nonadrenergic fibers relax the stomach. About 2 L of food can be accommodated in the stomach when receptive relaxation is at its maximum.

12. The answer is E [Chapter 43 III B 1]. Although the major functions of segmentation are the mixing of chyme with digestive juices and exposing the products of digestion to the intestinal wall, segmentation is also responsible for pushing the chyme along the intestine. Propulsion occurs because the frequency of segmentation is higher in the more proximal intestine than it is in the distal intestine. Thus, it is more likely for the chyme to move toward the colon than it is to move toward the stomach. Peristaltic waves move chyme along the intestine, but these are not frequent enough to propel the food into the colon. The migrating motor complex (MMC) empties the intestine of the small amount of chyme remaining in the intestine during the interdigestive period.

13. The answer is A [Chapter 42 III B 3 b]. Gastric acid (HCl) secretion is inhibited by low pH in the stomach and by somatostatin released from interneurons within the enteric nervous system. Acetylcholine (ACh), the hormone known as entero-oxyntin, and amino acids all stimulate gastric acid secretion.

14. The answer is D [Chapter 43 V D 2 a]. The amount of bile synthesized each day is not sufficient to absorb all of the fat digested. However, because the bile salts are absorbed by the intestine and returned to the liver, they can be used over and over again. The amount of bile secreted each day is thus proportional to the amount absorbed from the intestine.

15. The answer is C [Chapter 43 VII C 2 a, b (2)]. Micelles are necessary for absorption of dietary lipids such as cholesterol. Bile salts, iron, and B vitamins are absorbed by membrane-bound active transport systems. Alcohol is both water- and fat-soluble and so can diffuse directly across the membranes.

16. The answer is D [Chapter 43 V B 1]. Secondary bile acids are formed in the intestine by the deconjugation and dehydroxylation of primary bile acids. Primary bile acids are synthesized from cholesterol in the liver and then conjugated with taurine or glycine to form primary bile salts.

17. The answer is A [Chapter 43 VII A 2 a, B 3 a, C 2 b (4), E 1]. Amino acids and glucose are absorbed in the proximal intestine by Na^+-dependent active transport systems. Bile salts are reabsorbed by a Na^+-dependent active transport system located within the terminal ileum. Vitamin E is a fat-soluble vitamin and is absorbed by passive diffusion along with other lipids in the proximal intestine.

18. The answer is B [Chapter 43 III D 3 b]. Secretin decreases intestinal and gastric contractile force. Cholecystokinin (CCK), gastrin, insulin, and motilin all increase intestinal contractions.

19. The answer is D [Chapter 43 IV C 3 c]. Amino acids, particularly phenylalanine, fatty acids, and monoglycerides all directly stimulate the release of cholecystokinin (CCK) from intestinal endocrine cells. Hydrochloric acid (HCl), which lowers the pH of chyme entering the intestine, also causes CCK secretion. Bile acids do not influence CCK secretion.

20. The answer is B [Chapter 42 II F 2 b; Chapter 43 IV C 3 b, V D 1 a]. Although secretin regulates the volume of biliary secretion, it neither enhances nor inhibits the secretion of bile salts. Secretin's major effect is to stimulate bicarbonate (HCO_3^- secretion by the pancreas and the liver. In addition, it potentiates the effect of cholecystokinin (CCK) on pancreatic enzyme secretion. Secretin also diminishes gastric emptying, probably by directly reducing gastric smooth muscle contractility.

21. The answer is C [Chapter 43 VII A 2 a-b, B 3 a, C 2 b (4), E 2]. Unlike glucose, which depends on a Na^+-dependent active transport system for absorption, fructose is absorbed by facilitated diffusion. Active transport for fructose is not required because the intracellular fructose concentration is maintained at a low value by intracellular enzymes that rapidly convert fructose to glucose and lactose. Bile salts, vitamin C, and dipeptides all rely on Na^+-dependent active transport systems to be absorbed.

22–26. The answers are: 22-B, 23-D, 24-C, 25-C, 26-E [Chapter 42 II F 3 c, III B 3 a, C 2 a; Chapter 43 IV C 3 a, V E 2 a]. Gastric acid (HCl) secretion is stimulated by acetylcholine (ACh), histamine, and gastrin. It is inhibited by somatostatin.

Gastrin secretion is stimulated by bombesin [also called gastrin-releasing peptide (GRP)] and inhibited by somatostatin.

Cholecystokinin (CCK) and secretin both stimulate the pancreas. CCK, however, is responsible for the secretion of pancreatic enzymes. CCK is also responsible for stimulating the gallbladder to contract.

Motilin, a hormone released from the small intestine, increases the strength of the migrating motor complex (MMC) and may be responsible for initiating it. The MMC, which occurs every 60–90 minutes during the inter-digestive period, starts in the stomach and sweeps along the entire gastrointestinal (GI) tract. It is thought to be responsible for emptying the small intestine of any chyme remaining after the completion of a meal.

27–31. The answers are: 27-D, 28-B, 29-A, 30-E, 31-C [Chapter 42 III A 3 a (1), b; Chapter 43 VII C 2 b (4), E 5, a; Chapter 44 III C]. Bile acids are absorbed in the terminal ileum by a Na^+-dependent cotransport process.

Gastrin is secreted by G cells contained in the pyloric glands of the distal stomach (antrum and pylorus).

Intrinsic factor, necessary for the absorption of vitamin B_{12}, is secreted by parietal cells located in the proximal stomach (fundus).

The colon secretes K^+ into the chyme. About 10% of the daily K^+ load is excreted by the colon; the remainder is excreted by the kidney.

Iron is absorbed primarily within the duodenum and jejunum.

PART VIII
ENDOCRINE PHYSIOLOGY

John Bullock

Chapter 45

Physical and Chemical Characteristics of Hormones

I. **DEFINITION.** In the classic definition, hormones are secretory products of the ductless glands, which are released in catalytic amounts into the bloodstream and transported to specific target cells (or organs), where they elicit physiologic, morphologic, and biochemical responses. In reality, the requirement that hormones be secreted into the bloodstream is too restrictive, because they also can act locally (Figure 45-1A). For example:

A. **Paracrine hormones** can be conveyed over short distances by diffusion through the intersti-

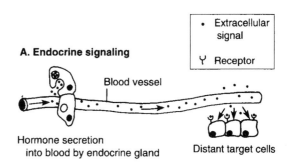

A. Endocrine signaling

Blood vessel

Hormone secretion
into blood by endocrine gland

Distant target cells

• Extracellular signal

Y Receptor

B. Paracrine signaling

Secretory cell

Adjacent target cell

C. Autocrine signaling

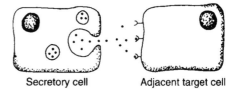

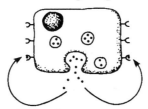

Target sites on same cell

FIGURE 45-1. The three methods of hormone information transfer. Cell-to-cell signaling can occur over long distances via hormone secretion into the bloodstream (*A*) or over short distances via hormone diffusion through the interstitium (*B*). A hormone also may act directly on the cell that produces it (*C*). [Adapted from Darnell J, Lodish H, Baltimore D (eds): *Molecular Cell Biology,* 2nd edition. New York, WH Freeman, 1990, p 710.]

tial space to act on neighboring cells as regulatory substances; therefore, they have a site of action close to their site of secretion (see Figure 45-1B).

B. **Neurocrine communication** (endocrine signaling) involves the release of chemical messengers from nerve terminals (see Figure 45-1C). Neurocrine substances may reach their target cells via one of three routes.

1. The **neurotransmitter can be released directly** into the intercellular space, cross the synaptic junction, and inhibit or activate the postsynaptic cell.
   a. Neurocrine substances are inactivated by degrading enzymes and by reuptake of the substances by neurons.
   b. Examples of neurocrine substances secreted by this route are acetylcholine (ACh) and norepinephrine.

2. A **neural signal can be transferred via a gap junction,** which is a membrane specialization between nerve cells; between nerve terminals and endocrine cells; and between endocrine cells. Gap junctions allow the movement of small molecules and electric signals from one cell to another, creating a functional **syncytium.**

3. The third potential route is identical to the classic neurosecretory mechanism, which involves the **release of a peptide or neurohormone from a neurosecretory neuron** into the blood followed by the interaction of this neuron hormone with specific receptors on distant target cells (see Chapter 46 III, IV). Examples of such neurocrine substances are oxytocin and antidiuretic hormone (ADH). The effector sites of neurohormones are not always endocrine cells.

C. **Autocrine hormones** regulate the activity of the same cells that produce them (see Figure 45-1C). **Autocoid** is a term used to designate a compound that is synthesized at, or close to, its site of action. This contrasts with circulating hormones, which act on tissues distant from their site of synthesis. Prostaglandins are autocoids.

II. HORMONE-SECRETING TISSUES. Virtually all organs in the body exhibit endocrine function.

A. The most studied endocrine organs and examples of the hormones they produce are listed in Table 45-1.

B. Other organs with endocrine function and the hormones they produce are:

1. Heart: atrial natriuretic peptide (ANP)

2. Kidney: 1,25-dihydroxycholecalciferol (calcitriol)

3. Liver: 25-hydroxycholecalciferol (calcidiol), somatomedin [insulin-like growth factor I (IGF-I)]

4. Pineal gland: melatonin

5. Skin: calciferol (vitamin D_3)

6. Gastrointestinal (GI) tract: gastrin, cholecystokinin (CCK), secretin, vasoactive intestinal peptide (VIP)

III. FUNCTIONS. Hormones regulate existing fundamental bodily processes but do not initiate cellular reactions de novo. In contrast to vitamins, hormones serve no nutritive role in responsive tissues and are not incorporated as a structural moiety into another molecule.

A. **Regulation of biochemical reactions.** As regulators, hormones stimulate or inhibit the rate and magnitude of biochemical reactions by their control of enzymes and, thereby, cause morphologic, biochemical, and functional changes in target tissues. Although they are not

TABLE 45-1. Principal Endocrine Organs and Hormones They Produce

Organ	Examples of Hormones
Pituitary gland	Tropic hormones (e.g., adrenocorticotropic hormone, growth hormone, prolactin)
Hypothalamus	Hypophysiotropic hormones [e.g., releasing hormones (e.g., thyrotropin releasing hormone], antidiuretic hormone, oxytocin
Thyroid gland	Thyroxine, 3,5,3'-triiodothyronine, calcitonin
Adrenal glands	Mineralocorticoids (e.g., aldosterone), glucocorticoids (e.g., cortisol), catecholamines (e.g., epinephrine, norepinephrine)
Parathyroid glands	Parathyroid hormone
Gonads	Testosterone, estradiol, progesterone
Pancreatic islets	Insulin, glucagon, somatostatin

used as energy sources in biochemical reactions, hormones modulate energy-producing processes and regulate the circulating levels of energy-yielding substrates (e.g., glucose, fatty acids).

B. **Regulation of bodily processes.** Hormones regulate growth, maturation, differentiation, regeneration, reproduction, pigmentation, behavior, metabolism, and chemical homeostasis. For example, the steroid and thyroid hormones primarily act to regulate the rate of transcription of specific genes to alter the synthesis of specific proteins. Slower processes (e.g., growth, reproduction, metabolism) require longer periods of continual hormone stimulation in contrast to rapid coordination of the body (e.g., reflex contraction of a somatic muscle), which is regulated by the nervous system.

IV. PHYSICAL CHARACTERISTICS

A. **Chemical composition.** The three major classes of hormones are: steroids, proteins and polypeptides, and amino acid derivatives (i.e., catecholamines and thyroid hormones). No polysaccharides or nucleic acids are known to function as hormones.

B. **Plasma concentration.** Hormones usually are secreted into the circulation in extremely low concentrations.

1. Peptide hormone concentration is between 10^{-12} mol/L and 10^{-10} mol/L.

2. Epinephrine and norepinephrine concentrations are 2×10^{-10} mol/L and 13×10^{-10} mol/L, respectively.

3. Steroid and thyroid hormone concentrations are 10^{-9} mol/L and 10^{-6} mol/L, respectively.

C. **Latent period.** The time interval between the application of a stimulus and a response is known as the latent period. The time between a neural stimulus and the contraction of a muscle may be only 8 msec, in contrast to the latent period associated with hormones, which can be as long as seconds, minutes, hours, or days.

1. Following the administration of **oxytocin,** milk ejection occurs in a few seconds.

2. The metabolic response to **thyroxine** can take as long as 3 days.

D. **Postsecretory modification.** Such changes occur by the proteolytic cleavage of peptide hormones or by enzymatic conversion of steroids and thyroid hormones at sites beyond the site of secretion. This peripheral conversion to more active hormonal forms occurs in the liver, kidney, fat, or bloodstream, as well as in the target tissues themselves.

E. **Circulating forms.** The binding of serum proteins (e.g., globulin) to hormones protects the hormones against clearance by the kidneys, slows the rate of degradation by the liver, and provides a circulating reserve of hormones. Only unbound hormones pass through capillaries to produce their effects or to be degraded.

F. **Hormone receptors.** Unique molecular groups in or on target cells interact with hormones to initiate a characteristic response. The specificity of a hormone depends on the formation of a strong noncovalent bond with its receptor (Figure 45-2; see Chapter 46 I). The major factor that determines the response to a hormone is the cellular receptor and the postreceptor machinery coupled to it.

1. **Mechanisms**
    a. The interaction of a ligand (i.e., hormone or agonist) with its receptor is the first step in the transduction of the hormonal signals from outside of the cell to the inside, where it can modulate function.
    b. The receptors play two roles in the signal transduction process.
        (1) They bind the extracellular signaling molecule (hormone, or ligand, or agonist) at the cell surface with both high affinity and specificity.
        (2) They relay the information in this ligand-binding event to sites within the cell, leading to modification of cellular metabolism and/or growth.
    c. The signal produced by hormone binding is transduced intracellularly via multiple effector pathways that include cAMP, cGMP, arachidonic acid, diacylglycerol (DAG), inositol triphosphate (IP_3), Ca^{2+}, and other ions. They are produced by enzymes (e.g., adenylyl and guanylyl cyclases, phospholipases A and C) and ion channels. In many cases, the hormone-receptor complexes do not interface directly with these effectors, but rather act via an intermediate modulating signal transducer such as guanine nucleotide-binding regulatory proteins (G proteins).

2. **Classification.** There are four common classes of membrane receptors (see Figure 45-2).
    a. **G protein–coupled receptors** (e.g., pituitary tropic hormones, glucagon, epinephrine, norepinephrine, parathyroid hormone, prostaglandins)
    b. **Ligand-gated ion channels,** which include neurotransmitters such as acetylcholine (ACh), γ-aminobutyric acid (GABA), and glycine
    c. **Receptor kinases** such as membrane receptors that contain effector (enzyme) activity [(e.g., tyrosine or serine kinase as an intrinsic part of the structure (receptors for insulin and growth factors)]
    d. **Receptor-linked kinases** that have no intrinsic enzyme activity [e.g., growth hormone, prolactin, cytokines (interleukins)]

3. **Receptor location**
    a. Receptors for steroid hormones and iodothyronines (thyroid hormone): primarily localized within the nucleus (internal receptors)
    b. Receptors for peptide and polypeptide hormones, catecholamines, and prostaglandins (integral membrane proteins): interspersed within the phospholipid bilayer of the plasma membranes of target cells (external receptors)

4. **Spare receptors.** A maximum physiologic response of a target cell is observed even when the concentration of a hormone is lower than that required to occupy all of the receptors on that cell. Therefore, most of the receptors (~ 97%) are referred to as spare (reserve) receptors.

5. **Changes in receptor number** (down-regulation, up-regulation)
    a. Hormone-sensitive cells respond to high concentrations of certain hormones by reducing the number of cell surface receptors, thus decreasing sensitivity to the hormone. For example, elevated ambient insulin concentrations cause a loss or inactivation of insulin receptors in liver cells, fat cells, and white blood cells (WBCs).
    b. Catecholamines exert their effects via plasma membrane receptors, and thyroid hormones have receptors in the target cell nucleus. Excess thyroid hormone leads to an

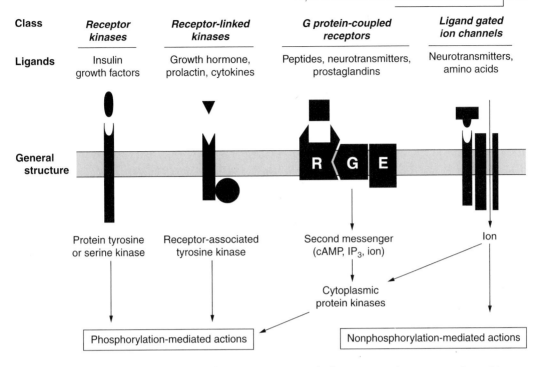

Class	Receptor kinases	Receptor-linked kinases	G protein-coupled receptors	Ligand gated ion channels
Ligands	Insulin growth factors	Growth hormone, prolactin, cytokines	Peptides, neurotransmitters, prostaglandins	Neurotransmitters, amino acids
General structure		R G E		
	Protein tyrosine or serine kinase	Receptor-associated tyrosine kinase	Second messenger (cAMP, IP$_3$, ion)	Ion
			Cytoplasmic protein kinases	
	Phosphorylation-mediated actions		Nonphosphorylation-mediated actions	

FIGURE 45-2. Four major classes of membrane receptors exist for hormones and neurotransmitters. Many growth factors, including insulin, bind to cell-surface receptors that act as protein tyrosine kinases stimulating the phosphorylation of proteins on tyrosine residues. Growth hormone, prolactin, and many cytokines act on receptors that associate with cytoplasmic tyrosine kinases. A third class of agonists binds to receptors (R) that are coupled to separate effector (E) molecules by G proteins (G). Effectors may be enzymes that produce second messengers that, in turn, can activate distinct protein (generally serine/threonine) kinases. The fourth major class of receptors includes ligand gated ion channels. Some of these are self-contained, as illustrated on the right. In others, the receptor and the ion channel are coupled by G proteins, as shown in the center. (Modified from Kahn CR, Smith RJ, and Chin WW: Mechanism of action of hormones that act at the cell surface. In *Williams Textbook of Endocrinology,* 9th edition. Edited by Wilson JD, Foster DW, Kronenberg HM, and Larsen PR. Philadelphia, WB Saunders, 1998, p 100.)

increased number of catecholamine receptors in the myocardium of experimental animals. This may explain the catecholamine-like effects noted in hyperthyroid patients who produce normal amounts of catecholamines.

    (1) Hyperthyroid patients have tachycardia and palpitations, effects observed with excessive catecholamines (pheochromocytoma). These cardiac symptoms can be ameliorated by the administration of a β-blocker such as propranolol.

    (2) The increase in cardiac β-adrenergic receptors in hyperthyroidism makes the heart more responsive to catecholamines.

  c. Angiotensin II decreases the number of its receptors on adrenocortical cells and increases the number of its receptors in vascular smooth muscle.

6. Receptor density

  a. Approximately 10^4 to 10^5 receptors exist on the surface of a polypeptide hormone target cell.

  b. Approximately 3×10^3 to 10^4 intracellular receptors exist per steroid target cell.

7. Receptor responses (Figure 45-3)

  a. Maximal hormonal responses may occur when less than 100% of receptors are occupied.

  b. When only the number of receptor sites per cell is reduced, there is a proportional reduction in the concentration of hormone-receptor complex and in biological response (for each hormone concentration), with a shift in the dose-response curve to the right.

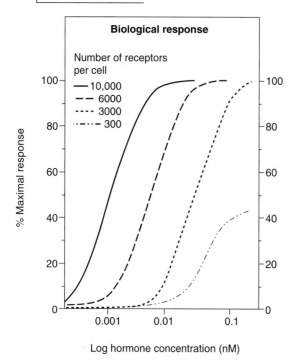

FIGURE 45-3. In a system with many spare receptors, a 50% fall in receptor number produces a small rightward shift in the dose-response curve for hormone action with no change in maximal response. A decrease in maximal response occurs only when receptor concentration falls to a very low level (a 97% decrease in this example). Note that a maximal response occurs when fewer than 100% (10,000 receptors per cell) are occupied. This does not mean that some receptors are inactive. Rather, all receptors are active, but occupancy of only a small fraction is sufficient to produce the final bioeffect.

 c. In some cases, a maximal hormonal response occurs with as few as 50 to 100 receptors occupied, even though the cell has tens or hundreds of thousands of receptors for a particular hormone.

 d. It is important to appreciate that all receptors are active, and the occupancy of only a small fraction is sufficient to produce a biological effect.

G. **Half-life.** Most hormones are metabolized rapidly after secretion. In general, peptide hormones are short-lived in the circulation, whereas steroids and thyroid hormone have a significantly longer half-life because they are bound to plasma proteins.

H. **Degradation.** The interaction of hormones with their target cells is followed by intracellular degradation.

 1. Degradation of protein hormones and amines occurs after binding to membrane receptors and internalization of the hormone-receptor complex.

 2. Degradation of steroids and thyroid hormones occurs after binding of the hormone-receptor complex to the chromatin.

I. **Inactivation and excretion.** Only a small fraction of the circulating hormone is removed by most target tissues. Hormone inactivation occurs in the liver and kidney.

 1. Hormone degradation uses many enzymatic mechanisms such as hydrolysis, oxidation, hydroxylation, methylation, decarboxylation, sulfation, and glucuronidation.

 2. Only a small fraction (< 1%) of any hormone is excreted intact in the urine or feces.

V. CHEMISTRY (Table 45-2)

A. **Proteins and polypeptides.** These substances, which are generally water-soluble, circulate unbound in plasma.

TABLE 45-2. Characteristics of the Principal Classes of Hormones

Characteristic	Peptides	Steroids and Calcitriol*	Amines	
			Catecholamines	Thyroid Hormone
Solubility				
In aqueous solvents (hydrophilic)	Excellent	Limited†	Good	Limited
In nonaqueous solvents (lipophilic)	Poor	Excellent	Limited	Good
Biosynthetic pathway	Single peptide, prohormone, or preprohormone	Multiple enzymes	Multiple enzymes	Multiple enzymes
Postsecretory modifications	Very rare‡	Common	None	Common
Storage of preformed hormone	Often substantial	Minimal	Substantial	Substantial
Degradation products	Irreversibly inactive	Sometimes retain or regain activity	Inactive	Inactive
Plasma binding proteins	Very rare	Yes	Limited	Yes
Half-life	Short (minutes)	Long (hours)	Very short (seconds)	Very long (hours to days)
Receptors	Cell surface	Nucleus	Cell surface	Nucleus
Site of action	Plasma membrane	Nucleus	Plasma membrane	Nucleus
Mechanism of action	Stimulates production of second messenger	Stimulates production of specific mRNAs	Stimulates production of second messenger	Stimulates production of specific mRNAs

*Calcitriol = 1,25-dihydroxyvitamin D_3.
†Stored as cholesterol esters in lipid droplets.
‡Although most translational processing is presecretory (i.e., it occurs within the cell), in some instances, postsecretory modifications occur (i.e., additional proteolytic modifications take place outside of the cell).

1. Structure
  a. The peptide and protein hormones vary greatly in size. For example, **thyrotropin-releasing hormone (TRH)** is a tripeptide, whereas **human chorionic gonadotropin (hCG)** consists of 243 amino acid residues.
  b. The molecular weights of the pituitary tropic hormones, which consist of about 200 amino acid residues, vary from 23,000 to 25,000 daltons. (The average molecular weight of an amino acid residue is 120; thus, multiplying the number of residues by 120 is a good estimate of the molecular weight of a peptide or protein.)

2. Synthesis. Many of the protein-type hormones are synthesized on the rough endoplasmic reticulum as **prohormones** or **preprohormones.** These precursor hormones undergo posttranslational cleavage by an endopeptidase within the Golgi complex prior to secretion of the biologically active hormone.
  a. Growth hormone (GH) and **prolactin** are synthesized as prohormones.
  b. Proopiomelanocortin (POMC), synthesized in the pituitary and hypothalamus, is a prohormone complex that contains peptide hormone moieties including adrenocorticotropic hormone (ACTH; corticotropin), melanotropin, lipotropin, and endorphins.
  c. Insulin and **parathyroid hormone (PTH)** are synthesized as preprohormones, which are hydrolyzed to prohormones and then further hydrolyzed to the hormone that is secreted.

3. Storage and secretion. Protein and polypeptide hormones are secreted by endocrine organs derived from ectoderm (pituitary gland*; tuberoinfundibular, supraoptic, and paraventricular nuclei) as well as organs derived from endoderm (pancreatic islets of Langerhans, thyroid gland, parathyroid glands). The primordial cells that give rise to the parafollicular cells (C cells) of the thyroid gland are derived from neural crest precursors.
  a. Protein and polypeptide hormones are stored exclusively in subcellular membrane-bound secretory granules within the cytoplasm of endocrine cells.
  b. These hormones are released into the blood by exocytosis, which involves fusion of the secretory granule and cell membrane followed by extrusion of the granular contents into the bloodstream (i.e., exocytosis).

4. Half-life of various peptide/protein hormones
  a. ADH and oxytocin: < 1 minute
  b. Insulin: 7 minutes
  c. Prolactin: 12 minutes
  d. ACTH: 15–25 minutes
  e. Luteinizing hormone (LH): 15–45 minutes
  f. Follicle-stimulating hormone (FSH): 180 minutes
  g. GH: 6–20 minutes

B. **Amino acid derivatives.** Catecholamines, which are water-soluble, and thyroid hormones, which are lipid-soluble, circulate in the plasma bound mainly to binding globulins.

1. Structure
  a. Catecholamines are derived from the amino acid tyrosine. Thyroid hormones are derived from two iodinated tyrosine residues. Hormones derived from tyrosine also are called **phenolic derivatives.**
  b. Catecholamines and thyroid hormones both retain the aliphatic α-amino group. Introduction of a second hydroxyl group in the ortho position on the benzene ring is characteristic of the catecholamines, whereas iodination of the benzene ring distinguishes the thyroid hormones.
  c. Thyroid hormones are the only substances in the body that contain iodine.

2. Synthesis. Epinephrine and norepinephrine are synthesized in the chromaffin cells,

---

*The anterior and posterior lobes of the pituitary gland are derivatives of buccal ectoderm and neural ectoderm, respectively.

which are modified postganglionic neurons (see Chapter 50 I B–D). Thyroid hormones are synthesized in thyroid follicular cells (see Chapter 53 I, IV).

3. **Storage and secretion.** The amine hormones are secreted by endocrine tissues derived from the neural crest (adrenal medulla) and from endoderm (thyroid gland).
   a. Catecholamines are stored in secretory granules. Secretion occurs when the membrane of the chromaffin granules fuses with the plasma membrane, causing the granular contents to be extruded into the circulation.
   b. Thyroid gland secretions are called **iodothyronines**—compounds resulting from the coupling of two iodinated tyrosine molecules. Thyroid hormones are stored outside follicular cells in the form of **thyroglobulin,** a glycoprotein precursor found in the lumen of the cells. The 5 mg of thyroid hormone stored in the normal thyroid gland is sufficient to last about 2 months. Following endocytosis and proteolysis of thyroglobulin, thyroid hormone is secreted into the bloodstream by simple diffusion.
   c. **Calcitriol** (1,25-dihydroxyvitamin D_3) is stored as a precursor in the form of 7-dehydrocholesterol or cholecalciferol (vitamin D_3) in the skin.

4. **Circulation and half-life**
   a. Epinephrine and norepinephrine exist in plasma either in the free form or in conjugation with sulfate or glucuronide. Most circulating epinephrine is bound to blood proteins (mainly albumin); norepinephrine does not bind to blood proteins to any appreciable degree.
   b. Most thyroid hormones are bound to thyroxine-binding globulin.
   c. The half-life of various amine hormones is as follows:
      (1) Epinephrine: 10 seconds
      (2) Norepinephrine: 15 seconds
      (3) Triiodothyronine: 1 day
      (4) Thyroxine: 7 days

C. **Steroid hormones.** These lipid-soluble substances circulate in the plasma bound to carrier proteins called **steroid-binding globulins.**

1. **Structure.** Steroids are a group of biologically active substances, including androgens, estrogens, progesterone, glucocorticoids, and mineralocorticoids. 25-Hydroxyvitamin D_3 and 1,25-dihydroxyvitamin D_3 are modified steroids called **secosteroids.**
   a. Steroids consist of three cyclohexyl rings and one cyclopentyl ring combined into a single structure. They are derived from the cyclopentanoperhydrophenanthrene nucleus consisting of a fully hydrogenated phenanthrene (rings A, B, and C), to which is attached a hydrogenated cyclopentane ring (ring D). This fully saturated, four-ring structure consisting of 17 carbon atoms is the hypothetical parent compound, gonane or sterane.
   b. The secosteroids, which are vitamin hormones, lack a B ring and, therefore, consist of two cyclohexyl rings (rings A and C) and one cyclopentyl ring (ring D).

2. **Synthesis and secretion.** Steroids are synthesized and secreted by the endocrine organs derived from mesoderm (adrenal cortex, testis, ovary). The placenta also synthesizes and secretes steroids.
   a. Steroids are derived from cholesterol. The first, and rate-limiting, step in steroid synthesis is conversion of cholesterol to pregnenolone. Depending on the product, hydroxylations of the steroid nucleus may occur at carbons 11, 17, 18, or 21.
   b. There is little storage of steroids. Instead, steroid-producing cells store esterified cholesterol in the form of lipid droplets, which serve as precursors. Steroids are released in the circulation by simple diffusion. Cholesterol can be obtained from three sources.
      (1) Preformed cholesterol transported in association with low-density lipoproteins (LDLs), which are internalized and hydrolyzed within lysosomes that release cholesterol for steroid biosynthesis
      (2) Cholesterol synthesized anew from two-carbon units (acetyl coenzyme A) [acetyl-CoA]

(3) Cholesterol liberated from cholesterol esters stored within lipid droplets

c. Cell surface receptors for some ligands such as LDL are also integral membrane proteins and function to translocate the ligand (e.g., ACTH, LH) to intracellular sites where the ligands act to alter cellular function.

3. Half-life of various steroid hormones
   a. Aldosterone: 30 minutes
   b. Cortisol: 90–100 minutes
   c. 1,25-Dihydroxyvitamin D_3: 15 hours
   d. 25-Hydroxyvitamin D_3: 15 days

Case

A 30-year-old athletic woman is diagnosed with an insulinoma on the basis of laboratory results that reveal hyperinsulinemia and hypoglycemia. However, she exhibits few symptoms of hypoglycemia despite the adenoma, even during her daily 3-minute runs for aerobic exercise.

1. In general, what symptoms are associated with hypoglycemia?

DISCUSSION

Hypoglycemia elicits a prompt and marked increase in adrenomedullary catecholamine secretion and sympathetic nerve stimulation. Thus, symptoms of hypoglycemia can include neurogenic manifestations such as sweating, palpitations, weakness, and confusion, as well as neuroglycopenic symptoms such as confusion, drowsiness, dizziness, and blurred vision. Neuroglycopenic symptoms predominate.

2. What conditions are characteristic of insulinoma?

DISCUSSION

The most consistent abnormality with insulinoma is failure of a normal decrease in insulin secretion as the plasma glucose concentration declines in the postabsorptive state. This results in relative hyperinsulinemia (i.e., plasma insulin levels that are inappropriately high for the ambient glucose concentration). This reduced effectiveness (insulin resistance) could be caused by:

   1. Decreased levels of circulating insulin antagonists [growth hormone (GH), cortisol, glucagon, and epinephrine]

   2. Anti-insulin antibodies

   3. Anti-insulin receptor antibodies

   4. Insulin receptor defects (decreased number, binding affinity, or sensitivity)

   5. Postreceptor defects (defective signal transduction mechanism or cellular response mechanism)

   6. Enzyme (hepatic) defects in glucose production by glycogenolysis or gluconeogenesis

   The most important causes of insulin resistance are tissue defects (conditions 4, 5, and 6). The hypoglycemia indicates that the rate of glucose efflux from the circulation exceeds that of glucose influx into the circulation. This can result from excessive glucose efflux (excessive glucose utilization or renal excretion of glucose) or deficient glucose influx (deficient endogenous glucose production in the absence of exogenous delivery, or both). Chronic hyperinsulinemia would be expected to decrease the number of insulin receptors (down-regulation) or the binding affinity of these receptors for insulin. With chronic hypoglycemia and the adrenergic response, lipolysis is activated by the counterregulatory hormones, and more fatty acids and glycerol are released. Therefore, patients with insulinoma usually have sufficiently high levels of the alternate fuels to prevent hypoglycemia from excessive oxidation of glucose.

3. What accounts for the relative absence of symptoms?

DISCUSSION

It is important to appreciate that despite the insulinoma, this woman does not have low circulating levels of fatty acids, an expected insulin effect. This lack of effect of insulin on triacylglycerol metabolism could be due to:

1. Adaptation to chronic hyperinsulism (e.g., down-regulation of insulin receptors in adipocytes)

2. Chronically high levels of epinephrine, which stimulates lipolysis

3. Chronic hypoglycemia, which limits the availability of glucose and also the formation of glycerophosphate which is necessary for lipogenesis

As a result of such mechanisms, fatty acids may be more readily available to her than to a normal athlete. Furthermore, the oxidation of fatty acids to regenerate muscle adenosine triphosphate (ATP) could be a glucose-sparing mechanism.

Chapter 46

Hormonal Control Systems

I. **HOMEOSTASIS AND STEADY STATE.** A major function of the endocrine system is to maintain the homeostasis of the internal environment. This condition of relative constancy in the concentration of dissolved substances, in temperature, and in pH is a basic requirement for the normal function of cells.

A. The concept of **homeostasis** as a constancy of physiologic variables must be modified, because many regulated organismic processes are not constant but conform to a persistent endogenous or exogenous **rhythm.** For example, humans demonstrate a **circadian pattern** in the levels of plasma 17-hydroxycorticosteroids. Such 24-hour cycles are not solely a response to fluctuating environmental stimuli but also are a result of internal endogenous oscillators whose phases are influenced by environmental stimuli.

1. In humans, certain corticosteroids (e.g., cortisol) have a rhythmic pattern of secretion, with secretory rates highest early in the morning and lowest late at night. Accordingly, plasma cortisol concentration is at a peak between 6 A.M. and 8 A.M. and at a nadir between midnight and 2 A.M. (Figure 46-1).
   a. This circadian rhythm persists but shifts to correspond with a change in sleeping habit (e.g., during illness, night work, changes in longitude, and total bed rest or confinement).
   b. For this reason, treatment of patients with exogenous corticosteroids is on an alternate-day dosage regimen, whereby the entire dose is given in the morning of every other day. This dosage schedule simulates the normal adrenocortical secretory rhythm.
2. The rhythmic pattern of corticosteroid secretion occurs in isolated adrenal glands and even in single adrenocortical cells.

B. The term **steady state** indicates that a function or a system is unvarying with time, but that the system is not in true equilibrium. The system is said to be in a **dynamic equilibrium,** because matter and energy flow into the system at a rate equal to that at which matter and energy flow out of the system.

II. **HYPOTHALAMIC–HYPOPHYSIAL AXES AND FEEDBACK CONTROL.** The hypothalamus has **neural control** over hormone secretion by the posterior lobe of the pituitary gland. The secretory activity of the anterior lobe is controlled by **hypothalamic hormones,**

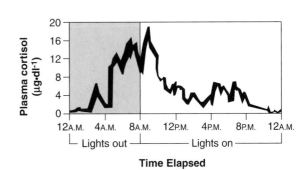

FIGURE 46-1. Pulsatile and diurnal nature of cortisol secretion.

which are secreted into the **hypothalamic–hypophysial portal system** (the hypophysial portal system). Only those hypothalamic hormones that regulate the anterior pituitary are hypophysiotropic hormones.

A. **Hypophysial portal system** (Figure 46-2). The median eminence has a poorly developed blood–brain barrier, and there is relatively little arterial blood perfusing the cells of the anterior lobe. The blood supply of the anterior lobe is derived from branches of the internal carotid arteries (mainly the superior hypophysial artery).

1. The posterior lobe derives its blood from a capillary plexus emanating from the inferior hypophysial artery. This capillary plexus drains into the dural sinus. The neural tissue of the upper infundibular stem (neural stalk) and of the median eminence is supplied largely by branches of the superior hypophysial artery. The median eminence is the specialized area of the hypothalamus located beneath the inferior portion of the third ventricle. It is a storage and release center for hypophysiotropic hormones.

2. The **primary capillary plexus,** which emanates from the superior hypophysial artery, forms a set of long portal veins that carry blood downward into the anterior lobe.

3. The portal veins, which give rise to the **secondary capillary plexus,** constitute about 90% of the blood supply to the cells of the anterior lobe. The secondary capillary plexus drains into the dural sinus.

4. The anterior lobe receives its remaining blood from the short portal veins, which originate in the capillary plexus of the inferior hypophysial artery at the base of the infundibular stem.

5. The capillary beds of the portal system consist of fenestrated capillaries and represent openings in the blood–brain barrier.

B. **Feedback control** is an important mechanism regulating hormone synthesis and secretion (Figure 46-3).

1. **Hypothalamic–pituitary–target gland model.** The paradigm for feedback control is the interaction of the pituitary gland with target endocrine tissues (thyroid gland, adrenal cortex, gonads). Unbound circulating hormones produced by target endocrine organs in-

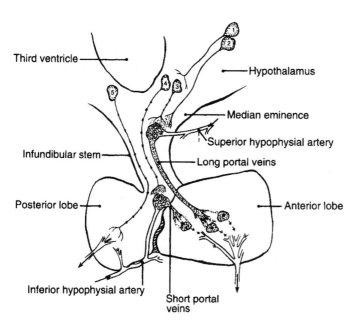

FIGURE 46-2. Anatomic relationship of the hypothalamus and pituitary gland, showing the hypophysial portal system and neurons involved in control of the pituitary gland. Neuron five (5) represents the peptidergic neurons of the supraopticohypophysial and paraventriculohypophysial tracts. Neurons four (4) and three (3) are the peptidergic neurons of the tuberohypophysial tract. Neuron one (1) and neuron two (2) are monoaminergic neurons. (Adapted from Gay VL: The hypothalamus: physiology and clinical use of releasing factors. *Fertil Steril* 23:51, 1972.)

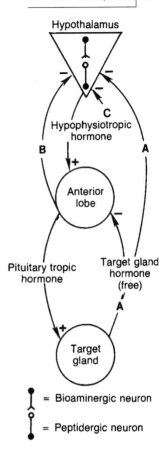

FIGURE 46-3. The three levels of feedback mechanisms for controlling hormone secretion: long-loop feedback (*A*), short-loop feedback (*B*), and ultrashort-loop feedback (*C*). Plus signs indicate stimulation, and minus signs indicate negative feedback.

hibit the hypothalamic–pituitary system, causing a decrease in the secretion of pituitary tropic hormones, which, in turn, control the secretion by the endocrine target glands. Virtually all hormone secretions are controlled by some type of feedback control.

2. **Negative feedback control** occurs on three levels.
   a. **Long-loop feedback.** Peripheral gland hormones and substrates arising from tissue metabolism can exert long-loop feedback control on both the hypothalamus and the anterior lobe of the pituitary gland. Long-loop feedback, which usually is negative but occasionally can be positive, is particularly important in the control of thyroid, adrenocortical, and gonadal secretions.
   b. **Short-loop feedback.** Negative feedback also can be exerted by the anterior pituitary tropic hormones on the synthesis or release of the hypothalamic releasing or inhibiting hormones, which collectively are called **hypophysiotropic hormones.**
   c. **Ultrashort-loop feedback.** Evidence suggests that the hypophysiotropic hormones may inhibit their own synthesis and secretion via a control system referred to as ultrashort-loop feedback.

III. **NEUROSECRETORY NEURONS** (see Figure 46-2). Neural control of the pituitary gland is exerted through neurohumoral secretions that arise from specialized neurosecretory neurons (peptidergic neurons) and are carried by the bloodstream to a target site.

A. **Structure and function**

   1. Neurosecretory neurons are glandular, unmyelinated secretory cells with two functions.

    a. They act as typical neurons, in that they conduct action potentials.

    b. They also function as endocrine glands, in that they synthesize and release neurohormones either directly into the general circulation (as in the case of the neurosecretory neurons of the pars nervosa) or into a portal system (as in the case of the hypophysiotropic neurons, which release their neurohormones into the primary plexus of the hypophysial portal system).

  2. A neurosecretory cell system consists of axons that do not innervate tissues but terminate directly on or near blood vessels. This differentiates these cells from typical neurons, which release neurotransmitters at localized synaptic regions. The functional complex of a neurosecretory neuron together with a blood vessel (hemocoele) is called a **neurohemal organ.**

B. **Classification.** Neurosecretory neurons in humans are restricted to the hypothalamus, where they occur as two distinct populations of cells that secrete neurohormones (Tables 46-1 and 46-2).

  1. The **magnocellular neurosecretory system** refers to the neurosecretory neurons of the supraoptic and paraventricular nuclei, which together form the supraopticohypophysial tract. Magnocellular neurons synthesize and secrete the neurohormones antidiuretic hormone (ADH) and oxytocin.

  2. The **parvicellular** (also called parvocellular) **neurosecretory system** refers to the neurosecretory neurons of the tuberoinfundibular tract. These neurons of the medial basal hypothalamus have axons that terminate directly on the capillaries of the portal vessels in the median eminence, and they form a final common pathway for neuroendocrine function (see Table 46-1).

    a. The parvicellular neurosecretory neurons mainly are peptidergic. However, an important exception is the dopaminergic neurosecretory neurons that form and secrete **prolactin-inhibiting factor (PIF).**

    b. The secretory products of the parvicellular neurosecretory neurons are called hypophysiotropic hormones (releasing/inhibiting hormones).

    c. Blood concentrations of hypophysiotropic hormones in portal blood are 10 to 20 times higher than in peripheral blood.

TABLE 46-1. Neuroendocrine Transducer Systems

Neuroendocrine System	Hormone
Magnocellular neurosecretory neurons	
Posterior lobe	
Supraoptic	Antidiuretic hormone (ADH)
Paraventricular	Oxytocin
Parvicellular neurosecretory neurons	
Median eminence	Hypophysiotropic hormones
Preganglionic fibers	
Adrenal medulla	Epinephrine*
Postganglionic fibers	
Pineal gland	Melatonin†
Juxtaglomerular apparatus	Renin†

After Martin JB, et al: Neuroendocrine transducers and neurosecretion. In *Clinical Endocrinology*. Philadelphia, FA Davis, 1977, p 4.
*Acetylcholine (ACh) is the neurotransmitter preceding epinephrine release.
†Norepinephrine precedes the release of both melatonin and renin.

TABLE 46-2. Characteristic Features of the Neurosecretory Control Systems

Feature	Parvicellular System	Magnocellular System
Neural input	Norepinephrine, dopamine, serotonin	Acetylcholine
Nuclei	Arcuate nucleus	Supraoptic and paraventricular nuclei
Tract	Tuberoinfundibular	Supraopticohypophysial
Terminus	Median eminence, upper infundibular stem	Pars nervosa (infundibular process)
Neurohormones	Neuropeptides (hypophysiotropic hormones), polypeptides	Neuropeptides (arginine-ADH, oxytocin), nonapeptides
Type of endocrine neuron	Peptidergic	Peptidergic
Stimuli	Monoamines	Acetylcholine
Vascular elements	Hypophysial portal system	Capillary bed (systemic)

C. **Neural control.** Neural information is transmitted to the parvicellular and magnocellular neurosecretory cells by **monoaminergic neurons.** Most of the cell bodies of the monoaminergic neurons are located in the mesencephalon and lower brain stem.

1. The monoaminergic neurons that innervate the parvicellular neurons produce and secrete biogenic amines, which modulate the hypothalamic release of the hypophysiotropic hormones.

2. The function of the magnocellular neurosecretory neurons is controlled by cholinergic and noradrenergic neurotransmitters.
   a. Acetylcholine (ACh) stimulates the release of ADH and oxytocin.
   b. Norepinephrine inhibits the secretion of ADH and oxytocin.

3. Because the secretion of the parvicellular and magnocellular peptidergic neurons is regulated by biogenic amines, the neurosecretory neurons can correctly be viewed as **neuroeffector** cells.

IV. **NEUROENDOCRINE TRANSDUCERS.** These endocrine glands convert neural signals into hormonal signals. Neural control of endocrine tissues occurs in three ways (Figures 46-4 and 46-5).

A. **Direct innervation of autonomic secretomotor neurons**

1. **Pancreatic islets of Langerhans**
   a. The islets of Langerhans have a postganglionic parasympathetic innervation. Increased vagal activity to the beta cells stimulates insulin release only during periods of elevated blood sugar.
   b. The islets of Langerhans also have a postganglionic sympathetic innervation. When the sympathetic nerves to the beta cells are stimulated or when norepinephrine or epinephrine is infused, the predominant effect is inhibition of insulin secretion.

2. **Pineal gland.** This endocrine structure of the diencephalon is classified as a periventricular organ because it borders on the third ventricle.
   a. The pinealocytes are innervated by the postganglionic (adrenergic) sympathetic fibers, which originate in the superior cervical ganglia of the sympathetic chain.
   b. When the neurotransmitter norepinephrine is released by the autonomic fibers, it stimulates the synthesis and release of melatonin and other indoleamine hormones.
   c. The pineal gland, like other periventricular organs (e.g., the median eminence), has a poorly developed blood–brain barrier.

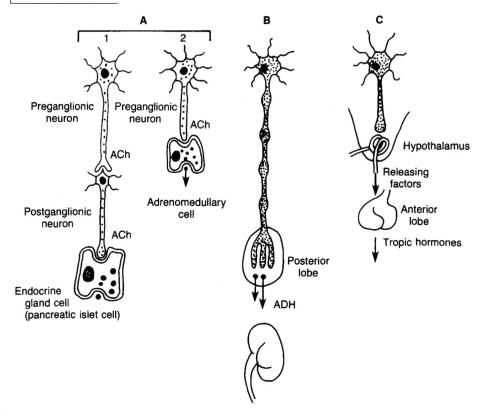

FIGURE 46-4. The three types of neuroendocrine transducers. (*A*) Secretomotor neurons control endocrine glands by direct innervation via autonomic fibers; the adrenal medulla is the only autonomic neuroeffector that is innervated by preganglionic neurons. *A1* = the autonomic nervous system (ANS); *A2* = the sympathoadrenomedullary axis; *ACh* = acetylcholine. (*B*) Magnocellular neurosecretory neurons control the posterior lobe of the pituitary gland, and (*C*) parvicellular neurosecretory neurons control the anterior lobe. (Reprinted from Martin JB, et al: Neuroendocrine transducers and neurosecretion. In *Neuroendocrinology.* Philadelphia, FA Davis, 1977, p 5.)

3. **Juxtaglomerular cells.** These granular cells of the juxtaglomerular apparatus (JGA) receive a postganglionic input, which, when stimulated, leads to the release of the proteolytic enzyme renin. According to the neuroendocrine transduction concept, renin can be classified as a hormone.

4. **Adrenal medulla.** This endocrine structure is composed of chromaffin cells and is innervated by preganglionic (cholinergic) sympathetic fibers, which, when stimulated, cause the release of the adrenomedullary hormones epinephrine and norepinephrine. The prior release of ACh at the synapses causes the secretion of these catecholamines.

B. **Magnocellular neurosecretory regulation of the posterior lobe** (see Table 46-2, Figure 46-4, and Figure 46-5)

1. Depolarization of the magnocellular neurosecretory cells by ACh released at synapses on the cell bodies of these neurons causes the release of ADH and oxytocin. The axons of these neurons terminate directly on the blood vessels of the posterior lobe, but they do not innervate the vessels.

2. The neural input to the cell bodies of the magnocellular neurons is cholinergic, and the hormonal output consists of peptide hormones.

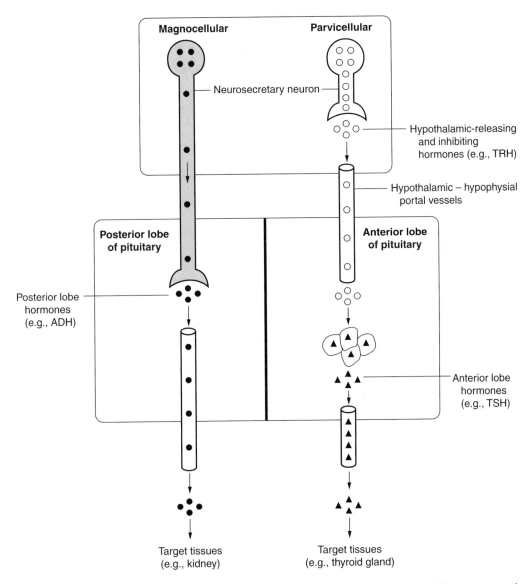

FIGURE 46-5. Schematic figure showing the relationship between the hypothalamus and the posterior and anterior lobes of the pituitary gland. Filled circles are posterior pituitary hormones; open circles are hypothalamic hormones; triangles are anterior pituitary hormones. ADH = antidiuretic hormone; TRH = thyrotropin-releasing hormone; TSH = thyroid-stimulating hormone. (Modified from Costanzo, LS: *Physiology*, Philadelphia: WB Saunders, 1998, p 348.)

C. **Parvicellular neurosecretory regulation of the anterior lobe** (see Table 46-2 and Figure 46-5)

   1. The anterior lobe lacks a direct nerve supply, but the pituitary gland does possess an innervation. The neurons in the anterior lobe are exclusively postganglionic sympathetic, which are **vasomotor fibers** and not secretomotor fibers.

   a. The hypothalamic regulation of the anterior lobe is achieved through the tuberohypophysial neurons of the medial basal hypothalamus. These peptidergic neurons synthesize and secrete specific hypophysiotropic hormones, which enter the hypophysial portal system and stimulate or inhibit the secretion of anterior pituitary hormones.

    b. The arcuate nucleus (nucleus infundibularis) is the main site of origin of the fine un-myelinated axons of the tuberoinfundibular pathway; however, tuberohypophysial neurons exist throughout the hypophysiotropic area, including the ventromedial nuclei and the periventricular and preoptic areas. The arcuate nucleus serves as the final neural link in the neurovascular connection between the hypothalamus and the anterior lobe.

  2. The intermediate lobe of the adenohypophysis in humans is considered to be a vestigial tissue because it is poorly developed.

    a. β-melanocyte-stimulating hormone (β-MSH) has been isolated from the human pituitary, but β-MSH activity in human plasma originates mainly from the corticotropes in the pars distalis.

    b. The melanotropins are synthesized by proteolytic cleavage of proopiomelanocortin (POMC).

Case

A 4-year-old girl is brought to the physician's office by her concerned mother. The mother has noted that the girl is beginning to undergo breast enlargement and has experienced some vaginal bleeding.

    1. What is the diagnosis?

DISCUSSION

The girl is experiencing premature thelarche and some signs of premature menarche. The diagnosis is sexual precocity, which has been defined as the development of secondary sex characteristics beginning before the age of 8 years in girls and 9 1/2 years in boys. The majority of cases in girls involve premature activation of the hypothalamic–pituitary–ovarian axis.

    2. What management is most appropriate?

DISCUSSION

The treatment goal must be the reduction of sex steroid (estrogen) levels. By constant exposure to gonadotropin-releasing hormone (GnRH) or potent agonistic (naforelin) analogues of GnRH, inhibition of the pituitary–ovarian axis occurs. The underlying mechanism in this setting is the down-regulation of GnRH receptors located on the anterior pituitary, resulting in the suppression of luteinizing hormone (LH) and follicle-stimulating hormone (FSH) secretion. In turn, the decline in gonadotropin levels secondarily reduces ovarian function.

  In addition, this therapy is effective in the treatment of a variety of endocrinopathies, including endometriosis, androgen excess, hirsutism, menstrual cycle–related disorders, and prostatic carcinoma. Furthermore, with the inhibition of ovulation by GnRH analogues, a new avenue of approach to contraception can be explored.

  Pulsatile administration of GnRH is necessary to effect normal cyclic gonadotropin release. In patients with "hypothalamic amenorrhea" (hypothalamic hypogonadism) who do not have normal pulsatile GnRH input to the pituitary, the use of a programmed pulsatile pump containing GnRH can restore ovulation and pregnancy can be achieved. It is imperative to appreciate that the mode of hormone administration (constant versus cyclic) can change the therapeutic goal.

Chapter 47

Pituitary Gland (The Hypophysis)

I. EMBRYOLOGY. The pituitary gland is in close anatomic relation to the hypothalamus. This relationship has both embryologic and functional significance.

A. The anterior lobe of the pituitary gland, the **adenohypophysis,** is derived from the primitive gut by an upward extension (Rathke's pouch) of the epithelium of the primitive mouth cavity (stomodeum). The adenohypophysis is a derivative of buccal oral ectoderm.

B. The neural or posterior lobe, the **neurohypophysis,** develops as a downward evagination of the neural tube at the base of the hypothalamus (infundibulum) and, therefore, represents a true extension of the brain. Neuroregulation of this structure is achieved by direct neural connections. The neurohypophysis is a derivative of neural ectoderm.

II. MORPHOLOGY

A. **Gross anatomy** (see Figure 46-2)

   1. General structure
   a. The pituitary gland lies in a bony walled cavity, the **sella turcica,** in the sphenoid bone at the base of the skull.
   b. The **dura mater** completely lines the sella turcica and nearly surrounds the gland.
   c. The **pituitary (hypophysial) stalk** and its blood vessels reach the main body of the gland through the diaphragma sellae. The pituitary stalk consists of the infundibular stem and the adenohypophysial tissue that is contiguous with the infundibular stem.

   2. Adenohypophysial structure. The anterior lobe has three components.
   a. The **pars distalis** represents the bulk of the anterior lobe in humans and receives most of its blood supply from the superior (anterior) hypophysial artery, which gives rise to the hypophysial portal system. The pars distalis is the source of the pituitary tropic hormones.
   b. The **pars intermedia** lies between the pars distalis and the neural lobe and is a vestigial structure in humans. It is relatively avascular and is considered almost nonexistent in humans.
   c. The **pars tuberalis** is an elongated collection of secretory cells, which superficially envelops the infundibular stem and extends upward as far as the basal hypothalamus. It is the most vascular portion of the anterior lobe but it is not a site for hormone synthesis.

   3. Neurohypophysial structure
   a. **Components**
      (1) The **median eminence,** located beneath the third ventricle, is a small, high vascular protrusion of the dome-shaped base of the hypothalamus, which is designated grossly as the tuber cinereum. The floor of the third ventricle is designated the infundibulum because it resembles a funnel.
      (2) The **infundibular stem** (neural stalk) of the posterior lobe arises in the median eminence.
      (3) The **pars nervosa** retains its neural connection with the ventral diencephalon.
   b. **Dominant features** of the posterior lobe are the **neurosecretory neurons** that form the **magnocellular neurosecretory system.** These unmyelinated nerve tracts arise from the supraoptic and paraventricular nuclei within the ventral diencephalon and de-

scend through the infundibulum and neural stalk to terminate in the posterior lobe. The posterior lobe and median eminence are storage and secretory sites for hormones and, therefore, the posterior lobe is not correctly termed an endocrine gland.

B. **Histology**

1. **Cells.** Two major types of cells are found in equal numbers in the anterior lobe.
   a. **Chromophils** (granular secretory cells) exist in two forms.
      (1) **Acidophils** (eosinophils) account for about 80% of the chromophils and are the cellular source of prolactin and growth hormone (GH). The somatotrophs (acidophils) are the most abundant cell type in the pituitary gland.
      (2) **Basophils** comprise about 20% of the chromophils and are the source of thyroid-stimulating hormone (TSH), adrenocorticotropic hormone (ACTH), luteinizing hormone (LH), follicle-stimulating hormone (FSH), and β-lipotropic hormone (β-LPH).
   b. **Chromophobes** (agranular cells) are not precursors of the chromophils and are now known to have an active secretory function. Most of these cells likely are degranulated secretory cells.

2. **Neurons** in the anterior lobe are almost exclusively postganglionic sympathetic fibers that innervate blood vessels.

3. **Nerve fibers** of the neurohypophysial system terminate mostly in the pars nervosa. Interspersed between these neurosecretory fibers are numerous glial cells called **pituicytes,** whose function, other than structural support, remains unknown.

C. **Vascular supply** (see also Chapter 46 II A and Figure 46-2). A basic tenet of the neurovascular hypothesis is that the concentration of the hypophysiotropic hormones is greater in hypophysial portal blood than at any other site in the vasculature.

1. In humans, the capillaries at the base of the hypothalamus are formed directly from branches of the superior hypophysial arteries, which arise from the internal carotid arteries. There are few vascular anastomoses between the hypothalamic artery and the superior hypophysial artery. The crucial regulatory connection between the hypothalamus and the anterior lobe is via the hypophysial portal vessels.

2. The intermediate lobe is not perfused directly by the hypophysial portal system but it contains bioaminergic secretomotor fibers originating in the hypothalamus.

3. The blood supply to the posterior lobe is largely separate from that of the anterior lobe. The blood supply to the median eminence is greater than that to the entire pituitary gland.

III. **HORMONES OF THE POSTERIOR LOBE: ANTIDIURETIC HORMONE (ADH) AND OXYTOCIN** (see Table 46-1). The physiologic aspects of ADH are described in Chapter 29. The physiologic aspects of oxytocin are described below.

A. **Synthesis and storage**

1. Like ADH, oxytocin is a nonapeptide* that is synthesized within the cell bodies of the peptidergic neurons of the magnocellular neurosecretory system.

2. This polypeptide is synthesized in the paraventricular and supraoptic nuclei of the hypothalamus and, like ADH, is stored in the posterior lobe of the pituitary gland.

B. **Stimuli for release.** Stimulation of cholinergic nerve fibers results in oxytocin secretion (Figure 47-1A).

1. Stimulation of the tactile receptors in the areolar region of the female breast during suckling activates somesthetic neural pathways, which transmit neural signals to the hypo-

---

*If the two cysteine residues are counted together as a single cystine residue, ADH and oxytocin are correctly classified as octapeptides.

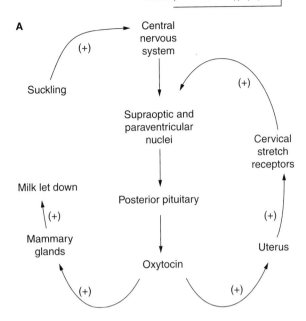

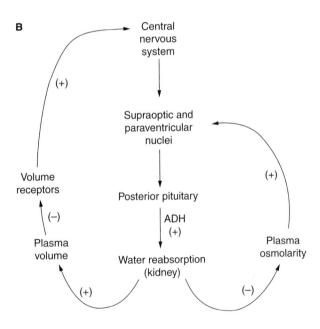

FIGURE 47-1. (*A*) Regulation of oxytocin secretion showing a positive feedback arrangement. Oxytocin stimulates the uterus to contract, causing the cervix to stretch. Increased cervical stretch is sensed by neurons in the cervix and transmitted to the hypothalamus, which signals more oxytocin secretion. Oxytocin secreted in response to suckling forms an open-loop feedback system in which positive input is interrupted when the infant is satisfied and stops suckling. (*B*) Regulation of vasopressin secretion. Increased blood osmolality and decreased blood volume are sensed in the brain or thorax, respectively; these conditions increase vasopressin secretion. Vasopressin, acting principally on the kidney, produces changes that restore osmolality and volume, thereby shutting down further secretion in a negative feedback system.

thalamus. This leads to the reflex secretion of oxytocin into the bloodstream and to milk release following a latent period of 30–60 seconds. This reflex is called the **milk let-down** or **milk ejection reflex.**

  a. Oxytocin causes milk release in lactating women by contraction of the myoepithelial cells, which cover the stromal surface of the epithelium of the alveoli, ducts, and cisternae of the mammary gland.

  b. Oxytocin secretion can be conditioned so that the physical stimulation of the nipple no longer is required. Thus, lactating women can experience milk release in response to the sight and sound of a baby.

   c. While oxytocin aids in the process, its presence is not absolutely required for successful nursing in humans.

   2. Genital tract stimulation such as that which occurs during coitus and parturition may also cause an oxytocin secretory response.

   3. Men may also produce oxytocin, and release occurs during genital tract stimulation. The role of this neurohypophysial hormone in men is unknown.

C. **Inhibition of release**

   1. Emotional stress and psychic factors such as fright may inhibit milk let-down.

   2. Excitation of adrenergic fibers to the hypothalamus inhibits peptide release. Activation of the sympathetic neurons with the concomitant release of norepinephrine and epinephrine inhibits oxytocin secretion.

   3. Ethanol inhibits endogenous oxytocin release, resulting in reduced myometrial contractility.

   4. Enkephalins also inhibit oxytocin release.

D. **Physiologic effects**

   1. Oxytocin stimulates contraction of the smooth muscle (myoepithelium) of the lactating mammary gland (milk ejection).

   2. It also stimulates contraction of the smooth muscle of the uterus (myometrium).
   a. The sensitivity of the myometrium to exogenous oxytocin during pregnancy increases as pregnancy advances.
   b. Oxytocin plays a role in labor and has been shown to be a useful therapeutic agent in the induction of labor.

IV. **HORMONES OF THE ANTERIOR LOBE.** The principal hormones of the anterior lobe of the pituitary gland can be classified conceptually into two groups: hormones that stimulate other endocrine glands to secrete hormones and hormones that have a direct effect on nonendocrine target tissues. Only the latter group is described here, using GH and prolactin as examples.

A. **Growth hormone (GH)** also is known as human growth hormone (HGH), somatotropic hormone (STH), and somatotropin.

   1. **Synthesis, chemistry, and general characteristics**
   a. GH represents approximately 4%–10% of the wet weight of the pituitary gland, equivalent to 5–15 mg. A single, unbranched polypeptide chain, it contains 191 amino acid residues.
   b. GH is synthesized by the acidophils of the anterior lobe of the human pituitary gland and is stored in very large amounts in the pituitary.
   c. Humans exhibit a **species specificity** for GH, and only human and monkey GH preparations have biologic activity in humans. Researchers have synthesized GH in bacteria using recombinant DNA techniques.
   d. Like all other pituitary hormones, GH is secreted episodically at 2-hour intervals. The large diurnal fluctuations represent integrations of many small secretory episodes. A regular nocturnal peak in GH secretion occurs 1–2 hours after the onset of deep sleep, which correlates with stage 3 or stage 4 slow-wave sleep.
   e. The plasma GH concentration in the growing child is not significantly higher than that in the adult whose growth has ceased.
   f. About half of the plasma GH is bound to a GH-binding protein.

   2. **Control of secretion.** The release of GH is primarily under the control of two hypophysiotropic hormones (Figure 47-2; Table 47-1).
   a. **Stimuli for release.** Somatotropin-releasing hormone (SRH), which has been identified as a 44-amino acid peptide, is the releasing hormone for GH. However, several pharmacologic, physiologic, and psychic agents are known to stimulate GH release.

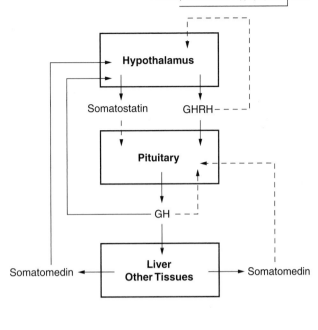

FIGURE 47-2. Regulation of growth hormone (GH) secretion. The hypothalamic peptide (GHRH) stimulates GH release, while the hypothalamic peptide somatostatin inhibits it. Negative feedback occurs via the peripheral mediators of GH action: somatomedins, also known as insulin-like growth factors (IGFs). Negative feedback occurs both via somatomedin inhibition of GHRH action and by somatomedin stimulation of somatostatin release. GH inhibits its own secretion by short-loop feedback and stimulates somatostatin secretion. In addition, GHRH inhibits its own release via ultra–short-loop feedback.

TABLE 47-1. Regulation of Somatotropin (Growth Hormone) Secretion

Stimulation	Inhibition
Growth hormone–releasing hormone	Somatostatin (octreotide)
Hypoglycemia* (insulin)	Hyperglycemia
Falling free fatty acids	Rising free fatty acids
Rising amino acids (arginine, leucine)	Somatomedins (via somatostatin stimulation)
Fasting, starvation	
Stages 3 and 4 sleep	Growth hormone
Stress	Cortisol
Exercise	Pregnancy
Glucagon	
Estrogens, androgens	Obesity
Dopamine,† acetylcholine, serotonin	Senescence
α-Adrenergic agonists	β-adrenergic agonists
Bromocriptine‡	
Antidiuretic hormone	

*This effect depends on intracellular glycopenia, because administration of 2-deoxyglucose, a competitive inhibitor of glucose, causes intracellular glucose deficiency and stimulates growth hormone secretion in spite of its hyperglycemic effect.

†Dopamine often inhibits growth hormone secretion in acromegaly.

‡Bromocriptine tends to stimulate growth hormone secretion in normal subjects. It suppresses secretion of insulin, glucagon, and thyroid-stimulating hormone.

(1) Monoaminergic and serotoninergic pathways are mediators of GH release; thus, α-adrenergic, dopaminergic, and serotoninergic agonists as well as β-adrenergic antagonists all stimulate GH release in humans.

(2) Bromocriptine (a dopamine agonist), enkephalins, endorphins (β-endorphin), and opiates stimulate GH secretion.

(3) Insulin-induced hypoglycemia is a potent stimulus of GH secretion, as are pharmacologic doses of glucagon and vasopressin.

(4) Physiologic stimuli include hypoglycemia, increased plasma concentrations of amino acids (arginine, leucine, lysine, tryptophan, and 5-hydroxytryptophan), and decreased free fatty acid concentrations. In addition, estrogens stimulate GH synthesis and secretion.

(5) Moderate-to-vigorous exercise; emotional stress; and stress resulting from fever, surgery, anesthesia, trauma, pyrogen administration, and repeated venipuncture stimulate GH secretion. Fasting or starvation leads to elevated GH secretion after 2 or 3 days.

b. Inhibitors of secretion. GH secretion is regulated by three feedback loops.

(1) GH-releasing hormone (GHRH) inhibits its own release via an ultra-short feedback loop.

(2) Somatomedin inhibits GHRH secretion and stimulates somatostatin secretion which, in turn, inhibits GH secretion.

(3) GH can inhibit its own secretion via a short-feedback loop mechanism that operates between the anterior lobe and the median eminence. Somatotropin-inhibiting hormone (SIH; somatostatin) inhibits the synthesis and release of GH and TSH.

    (a) Somatostatin is a tetradecapeptide (14 amino acid residues) that has been chemically synthesized.

    (b) Somatostatin is a product of the parvicellular neurosecretory neurons that terminate in the median eminence and produce hypophysiotropic hormones. It also is found in other parts of the brain, in the gastrointestinal (GI) tract, and in the delta cells of the pancreatic islets.

    (c) In addition to inhibiting GH secretion, somatostatin blocks the secretion of insulin, glucagon, and gastrin and inhibits the intestinal absorption of glucose. These effects produce a state of hypoglycemia.

(4) The secretion of GH in response to the aforementioned stimuli often is blunted in obese individuals.

(5) Glucocorticoids decrease GH secretion, but their predominant effect is the interference with the metabolic actions of GH.

(6) A decline in GH secretion is observed in late pregnancy, despite the presence of high estrogen levels.

    (a) Impaired glucose tolerance is common, and clinical diabetes occurs frequently, despite the above-normal insulin secretion in response to a glucose load during pregnancy.

    (b) Pregnancy regularly antagonizes the action of insulin and increases the pancreatic secretory capacity of both normal and diabetic individuals.

    (c) The development of gestational diabetes probably occurs because of a greater degree of insulin antagonism caused by normal plasma concentrations of human placental lactogen (HPL).

3. Physiologic and metabolic effects (Figures 47-3 and 47-4)

a. Stimulation of growth of bone, cartilage, and connective tissue

(1) The effects of GH on skeletal growth are mediated by a family of polypeptides called **somatomedins** [also termed insulin-like growth factors (IGFs)], which are synthesized mainly in the liver. (Thyroid hormone and insulin also are necessary for normal osteogenesis.) The growth-promoting effects of GH are largely attributed to the somatomedins.

    (a) IGF-I, a peptide of 70 amino acid residues, circulates in a bound form in plasma with a binding protein (IGFBP-3).

    (b) The measurement of IGF-I or the GH-dependent protein (IGFBP-3) are reliable indices of overall GH secretion.

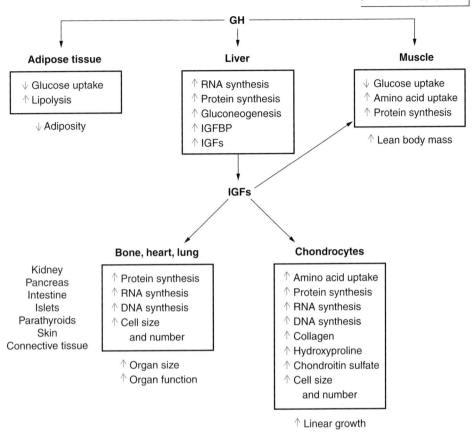

FIGURE 47-3. Biological actions of growth hormone (GH). The effects on linear growth, organ size, and lean body mass are mediated by insulin-like growth factors (IGFs) [somatomedins] produced in the liver. IGFBP = insulin-like growth factor–binding protein. Adapted with permission from Berne RM, Levy MN: *Physiology,* 4e. Mosby, Philadelphia, 1998, p. 895.

    (2) Somatomedin may be produced in nonhepatic tissue as well; somatomedin activity has been found in the serum, kidney, and muscle tissue.
        (a) Receptors for somatomedin exist in chondrocytes, hepatocytes, adipocytes, and muscle cells.
        (b) Somatomedin has insulin-like effects on tissues, including lipogenesis in adipose tissue, increased glucose oxidation in fat, and increased glucose and amino acid transport by muscle.
    (3) GH, through somatomedin, stimulates proliferation of chondrocytes and the appearance of osteoblasts. The increase in the thickness of the epiphysial (cartilaginous) end-plate accounts for the increase in linear skeletal growth.
    (4) After epiphysial fusion, bone length can no longer be increased by GH, but bone thickening can occur through periosteal growth. It is this growth that accounts for the changes seen in hypersomatotropism (acromegaly).
    (5) These reactions are the biochemical correlates of protein synthesis in general body growth and also account for the hyperplasia and hypertrophy associated with increased tissue mass.
  b. Protein metabolism
    (1) GH has predominantly anabolic effects on skeletal and cardiac muscle, where it stimulates the synthesis of protein, RNA, and DNA.
    (2) GH reduces circulating levels of amino acids and urea (i.e., it promotes nitrogen retention), which accounts for the term **positive nitrogen balance.** Urinary urea concentration also is decreased.

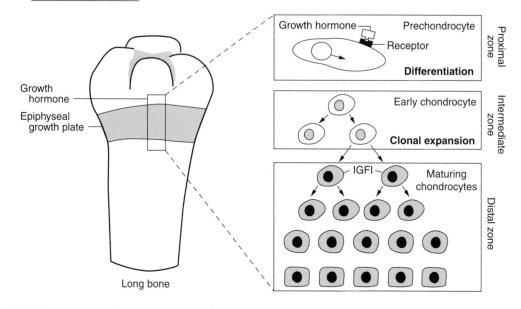

FIGURE 47-4. Metabolic actions of growth hormone (GH). GH acts directly at the epiphyseal (cartilagenous or growth) plate to stimulate linear growth and stimulates differentiation of prechondrocytes into early chondrocytes. Insulin-like growth factor-I (IGF I) stimulates clonal expansion and maturation of chondrocytes.

      (3) GH promotes amino acid transport and incorporation into proteins.

      (4) GH does not enhance muscle mass or strength in young, GH-sufficient adults, although it was a popular illicit drug among athletes at one time. However, it has been associated with an increase in exercise capacity.

  c. Fat metabolism

      (1) GH has an overall catabolic effect on adipose tissue. It stimulates the mobilization of fatty acids from adipose tissue, leading to a decreased triglyceride content of fatty tissue and increased plasma levels of free fatty acids, glycerol, and ketoacids.

      (2) GH increases hepatic oxidation of fatty acids to the ketone bodies, acetoacetate and β-hydroxybutyrate. The muscle takes up all of the products of lipolysis* and converts them to acetyl coenzyme A (acetyl-CoA).

      (3) Glucose cannot be made from fat because the end-product of fat metabolism (catabolism) is acetyl-CoA.

  d. Carbohydrate metabolism. GH is a diabetogenic hormone. Because of its anti-insulin effect, GH has a tendency to cause hyperglycemia.

      (1) GH can produce an insulin-resistant diabetes mellitus primarily because of its lipolytic effect but also because of a decrease in glucose transport.

         (a) Free fatty acids can antagonize the effect of insulin to promote glucose uptake by skeletal muscle and adipose tissue.

         (b) Free fatty acids can stimulate gluconeogenesis. Under conditions of caloric restriction (or starvation), amino acids from muscle protein, lactate–pyruvate from muscle glycogen, and glycerol from adipose tissue serve as gluconeogenic substrates (see Figure 48-5).

            i. The increased free fatty acids inhibit glucose utilization (glycolysis), and this decline in glucose transport (uptake) decreases lipogenesis. This requires glucose for the formation of glycerophosphate from the reduction of dihydroxyacetone phosphate (DHAP) because fat cells lack the glycerokinase enzyme.

*Fatty acids, glycerol, acetoacetate, and β-hydroxybutyrate.

      ii. The increase in free fatty acid levels contribute to the GH-induced **insulin resistance.**

    (c) Excess acetyl-CoA production favors gluconeogenesis, because pyruvate carboxylase requires acetyl-CoA to form oxaloacetate from pyruvate. Oxaloacetate is the rate-limiting factor in gluconeogenesis.

    (d) Acetyl-CoA inhibits glycolysis by inhibition of pyruvate kinase.

    (e) Free fatty acids stimulate hepatic glucose synthesis mainly via the stimulation of fructose biphosphatase. At the same time, pyruvate kinase and phosphofructokinase both are inhibited by free fatty acids, which block glycolysis and favor gluconeogenesis. Citrate also blocks glycolysis at the phosphofructokinase step.

  (2) The indirect inhibition of glycolysis by GH diverts glucose into muscle glycogen, inhibits glucose transport, and decreases glycogen breakdown. This maintenance of muscle glycogen is called the glycostatic effect of GH (i.e., GH spares carbohydrate). In diabetics, GH stimulates hepatic glucose production derived either from glycogenolysis or gluconeogenesis.

  (3) When glycogen storage is saturated, glucose-6-phosphate inhibits phosphorylation of glucose by hexokinase leading, in turn, to the inhibition of glucose uptake.

  (4) GH induces an elevation in basal plasma insulin levels (insulinotropic effect).

  (5) Because of its anti-insulin effect, GH inhibits glucose transport in adipose tissue. Because adipose tissue requires glucose for triglyceride synthesis, GH antagonizes insulin-stimulated lipogenesis.

  e. Mineral metabolism. GH promotes renal reabsorption of Ca^{2+}, phosphate, and Na^+.

4. Endocrinopathies

  a. Disorders associated with increased GH

    (1) Growth retardation can occur when GH levels are increased and somatomedin levels are depressed (e.g., in kwashiorkor). (In the African pygmy, who is resistant to the action of GH, both GH and somatomedin levels are normal. A decrease in GH receptors causes the growth retardation.)

    (2) Overproduction of GH during adolescence results in **giantism,** which is characterized by excessive growth of the long bones. Patients may grow to heights of as much as 8 feet.

    (3) Excessive GH secretion during adulthood, after the epiphysial (growth) plates of long bones have fused, causes growth in those areas where cartilage persists. This leads to **acromegaly,** a condition characterized by coarse facial features, underbite (prognathism),* prominent brow, enlarged hands and feet, and soft tissue hypertrophy (e.g., cardiomegaly, hepatosplenomegaly, and renomegaly).

  b. Disorders associated with decreased GH

    (1) Decreased GH secretion in immature persons leads to stunted growth, or **dwarfism,** which is accompanied by sexual immaturity, hypothyroidism, and adrenal insufficiency.

    (2) GH deficiency may be part of an overall lack of anterior pituitary hormones (**panhypopituitarism**) or from an isolated genetic deficiency. Selective GH deficiency is rare in adults. Clinical manifestations may include impaired hair growth and a tendency toward fasting hypoglycemia.

  c. Treatment

    (1) The treatment of choice for hypersomatotropism is selective surgical extirpation of the pituitary adenoma without damage to other pituitary functions. Bromocriptine is effective in suppressing, but not normalizing, GH levels in most acromegalic patients. This substance tends to stimulate GH secretion in normal individuals. The somatostatin analogue octreotide is very effective in the treatment of long-term acromegaly.

    (2) Disorders associated with GH deficiency can be treated with human GH.

---

*Mandibular prognathism characterizes acromegaly and maxillary prognathism characterizes hyposomatotropism.

B. **Prolactin.** This hormone also is known as lactogenic hormone, mammotropic hormone, and galactopoietic hormone. The only clearly established role for prolactin is the initiation and maintenance of lactation.

1. **Synthesis, chemistry, and general characteristics**
   a. Prolactin is synthesized in the pituitary acidophils.
   b. Human prolactin is a single peptide chain containing 198 amino acid residues.
   c. It does not regulate the function of a secondary endocrine gland in humans.

2. **Control of secretion.** Two hypothalamic neurosecretory substances have been implicated in prolactin secretion.
   a. **Stimuli for release.** Prolactin-releasing factor (PRF) is the putative releasing hormone for prolactin. PRF has not been identified or chemically synthesized; however, one of these releasing factors is thyrotropin-releasing hormone (TRH), which also causes the release of TSH.
      (1) Prolactin secretion increases about 1 hour after the onset of sleep, and this increase continues throughout the sleep period. The nocturnal peak occurs later than that for GH.
      (2) Prolactin secretion is enhanced by exercise and by stresses such as surgery under general anesthesia, myocardial infarction, and repeated venipuncture.
      (3) Plasma prolactin levels begin to increase by the eighth week of pregnancy and usually reach peak concentrations by the 38th week.
      (4) Nursing and breast stimulation are known to stimulate prolactin release. Oxytocin has been shown to act directly on lactotrophs to stimulate prolactin release, which suggests a physiologic role for oxytocin as a prolactin-releasing factor. This role is most evident around the time of ovulation when estrogen levels are also high. Estrogens are potent stimulators of prolactin secretion that act directly at the level of the pituitary.
      (5) Serum prolactin levels are elevated in those patients with primary hypothyroidism who are believed to have high TRH levels in the hypophysial portal circulation.
      (6) Dopamine antagonists (phenothiazine and tranquilizers), adrenergic blockers, and serotonin agonists stimulate prolactin secretion.
      (7) Pituitary stalk section and lesions that interfere with the portal circulation to the pituitary gland also cause prolactin release.
   b. **Inhibitors of release.** Normally, the control of prolactin secretion is under constant inhibition via prolactin-inhibiting factor (PIF).
      (1) Dopamine, the most important PIF physiologically, is secreted into the hypophysial portal vessels.
      (2) Serotonin antagonists and dopamine agonists (bromocriptine) block the secretion of prolactin. Bromocriptine administered during the postpartum period reduces prolactin secretion to nonlactating levels and terminates lactation.

3. **Physiologic effects**
   a. Because prolactin does not have an important role in maintaining the secretory function of the corpus luteum, it is not a gonadotropic hormone in women.
   b. Prolactin plays an important role in the development of the mammary glands and in milk synthesis.
      (1) During pregnancy, the mammary duct gives rise to lobules of alveoli, which are the secretory structures of this tissue. This differentiation requires prolactin, estrogens, and progestogens. In this way, prolactin acts at the breast to block lactation. Once the lobuloalveolar system is developed, the role of prolactin and corticosteroids in milk production, although essential, becomes minimal. GH and thyroid hormone enhance milk secretion.
      (2) Immediately following pregnancy, prolactin stimulates galactosyltransferase activity, leading to the synthesis of lactose.
      (3) In women, high serum levels of prolactin are associated with suppressed LH secretion and anovulation, which account for an absence of menses (amenorrhea) during postpartum lactation.

    (a) With continued nursing, FSH levels rise, but LH levels remain low.

    (b) In the early postpartum period, both the FSH and LH levels are low, presumably because of suppression of gonadotropin-releasing hormone (GnRH).

4. Endocrinopathy. Hyperprolactinemia, although not a rare condition, frequently is undiagnosed because galactorrhea occurs in only about 30% of cases.

    a. Signs and symptoms. In women, elevated serum prolactin manifests as infertility and amenorrhea. In men, hyperprolactinemia is a cause of impotence and decreased libido.

    b. Treatment. Therapy for prolactin hypersecretion includes administration of bromocriptine, a dopamine agonist that lowers prolactin levels and usually restores normal gonadal function. A potent long-acting dopamine agonist [cabergoline (Dostinex)] has been shown to be more effective in reducing prolactin than bromocriptine (Parlodel).

Case Study

A 48-year-old man seeks medical attention because his friends have remarked about changes in his appearance. His shoe size has increased from a 9C to an 11EEE over the past 5 years, and his dental plate has had to be remade three times in 6 years.

    On physical examination, he exhibits coarse physical features. His tongue is enlarged, and the interdental spaces are increased. An eye test shows a loss of both temporal visual fields. His hands and feet are enlarged, with spade-like fingers. Hepatomegaly is also evident. Laboratory studies show a fasting blood glucose of 150 mg/dl and a fasting growth hormone (GH) level of 60 ng/ml (normal, < 2.5 ng/ml), which does not decrease after a 75-g oral glucose load. The blood level of insulin-like growth factor-1 (IGF-1) is 690 ng/ml (normal, 24–153 ng/ml). Magnetic resonance imaging (MRI) reveals a large pituitary mass.

    1. Why did the physician measure the GH level?

DISCUSSION

This man's features and his history of changes in appearance and shoe size strongly suggest an excess of GH. A tumor of pituitary somatotrophs usually causes this condition, which is known as acromegaly.

    2. What other peptide is certainly elevated in the patient's plasma? What is the source of this peptide?

DISCUSSION

GH stimulates the synthesis of a peptide mediator called somatomedin or insulin-like growth factor-1 (IGF-1). This is produced in the liver and in many other tissues that contain GH target cells. Plasma somatomedin levels are high in patients with GH-secreting tumors.

    3. What has caused the changes in the patient's facial features, tongue, hands, feet, and liver?

DISCUSSION

GH, via somatomedin, stimulates proliferation of chondrocytes, osteoblasts, and connective tissue cells, causing excess linear growth in children. As a result, giantism occurs and stimulates appositional (periosteal) bone growth in adults, whose bone growth centers are already closed. This causes widening of digits, thickened vertebrae, ribs, skull bones, and mandible, with resultant alteration in facial features and position of the teeth. In addition, stimulation of visceral parenchymal cell growth occurs, which causes enlargement of organs such as the liver and kidneys (organomegaly). Growth of soft tissues increases lean body mass.

> **4.** *What is the normal effect of glucose administration on the plasma GH level? Why did no change occur in this patient?*

DISCUSSION

Glucose normally suppresses GH release to levels less than 2 ng/ml. When GH is secreted autonomously by an acidophilic tumor (as in this case), there is usually no response to glucose administration.

> **5.** *Why is the fasting plasma glucose level elevated, and what change in the plasma insulin level would you expect to find?*

DISCUSSION

GH is an insulin antagonist that inhibits insulin-stimulated glucose uptake by muscle cells as well as the insulin effects on the liver. Thus the fasting plasma glucose level rises. In response to the high glucose levels, plasma insulin levels will also be elevated. Excessive secretion of GH can lead to insulin-resistant diabetes mellitus. In addition, GH directly stimulates growth of pancreatic islet beta cells. GH is also a gluconeogenic hormone.

Chapter 48

Adrenal Gland: Medulla

I. EMBRYOLOGY

A. The neural crest gives rise to neuroblasts, which eventually give rise to the autonomic post-ganglionic neurons, the adrenal medulla, and the spinal ganglia.

B. The adrenal medulla consists of chromaffin cells (pheochromocytes), which are neuroecto-dermal derivatives and the functional analogues of the sympathetic postganglionic fibers of the autonomic nervous system (ANS).

C. In early fetal life, the adrenal medulla contains only norepinephrine.

II. MORPHOLOGY

A. **Gross anatomy**

1. The adrenal medulla represents essentially an enlarged and specialized sympathetic ganglion and is called a **neuroendocrine transducer** because a neural signal to this organ evokes hormonal secretion.

2. The adrenal medulla is the only autonomic neuroeffector organ without a two-neuron motor innervation. It is innervated by long sympathetic preganglionic, cholinergic neurons that form synaptic connections with the chromaffin cells.

3. Small clumps of chromaffin cells also can be found outside the adrenal medulla, along the aorta and the chain of sympathetic ganglia.

B. **Histology**

1. **Cells.** There are two types of adrenomedullary chromaffin cells. Individual cells contain either **norepinephrine** or **epinephrine,** which is stored largely in subcellular particles called chromaffin granules. These granules are osmiophilic, electron-dense, membrane-bound secretory vesicles.
   a. Approximately 80% of the chromaffin granules in the human adrenal medulla synthe-size epinephrine (adrenaline). The remaining 20% synthesize norepinephrine (nora-drenaline).
   b. The chromaffin granules contain catecholamines, protein, lipids, and adenine nu-cleotides [mainly adenosine triphosphate (ATP)].
      (1) One of the proteins localized in the particulate fraction is the enzyme, dopamine-β-hydroxylase.
      (2) Soluble acidic proteins found in the granules are called **chromagranins.**
   c. Secretion, in which the total contents of the granule are released by exocytosis, takes place through fenestrated capillaries, which overcome diffusion barriers.

2. **Neurons**
   a. The preganglionic sympathetic fibers that innervate the adrenal medulla traverse the splanchnic nerve, which contains myelinated (type B) secretomotor fibers emanating mainly from lower thoracic segments (T5 and T9) of the ipsilateral intermediolateral gray column of the spinal cord.
   b. The chromaffin cells do not have axons; therefore, they are functional analogues of the postganglionic neurons.

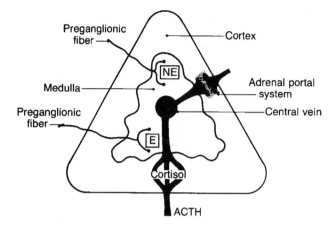

FIGURE 48-1. The adrenal portal vascular system constitutes a functional connection between the cortex and medulla and has a high cortisol concentration. NE = norepinephrine; E = epinephrine; ACTH = adrenocorticotropic hormone. (Adapted from Pohorecky LA, Wurtman RJ: Adrenocortical control of epinephrine synthesis. *Pharmacol Rev* 23(1):1–35, 1971.)

C. **Vascular supply** (Figure 48-1)

1. **Arterial blood** to the adrenal gland reaches the outer capsule from branches of the renal and phrenic arteries, with a less important arterial input directly from the aorta. The adrenal medulla is perfused by blood vessels in two ways.

    a. A type of **portal circulation** exists in the adrenal gland where the cortex and medulla are in juxtaposition. From the capillary plexus on the outer adrenal capsule most of the blood enters venous sinuses, which drain into and supply the medullary tissue. Thus, most of the blood perfusing the adrenal medulla is derived from the portal system and is, therefore, partly deoxygenated.

    b. There also exists a direct arterial blood supply to the medulla via the **medullary arteries,** which traverse the cortex.

2. **Venous blood** drains via a single central vein, composed almost entirely of bundles of longitudinal smooth muscle fibers, which pass along the longitudinal axis of the gland.

III. ADRENOMEDULLARY HORMONES: PHENOLIC DERIVATIVES

A. The adrenal medulla synthesizes and secretes biogenic amines. These dihydroxylated phenolic amines, or **catecholamines,** are epinephrine and norepinephrine. Most of the met-enkephalin in the circulation also originates in the adrenal medulla. Enkephalins are pentapeptides that function as neurotransmitters or neuromodulators, which normally are localized in neuronal processes and terminals.

1. **Epinephrine** is produced almost exclusively in the adrenal medulla, with smaller amounts synthesized in the brain. Essentially all circulating epinephrine is derived from the adrenal medulla.

2. **Norepinephrine** is widely distributed in neural tissues, including the adrenal medulla, sympathetic postganglionic fibers, and central nervous system (CNS). In the brain, the concentration of norepinephrine is the highest in the hypothalamus. The norepinephrine content of a tissue reflects the density of its sympathetic innervation. Norepinephrine has been demonstrated in almost all tissues except the placenta, which is devoid of nerve fibers.

B. Humans who have undergone bilateral adrenalectomies excrete practically no epinephrine in the urine. However, urinary levels of norepinephrine remain within normal limits, indicating that the norepinephrine originates from extra-adrenal sources (i.e., the terminals of the postganglionic sympathetic fibers and the brain).

IV. CONTROL OF CATECHOLAMINE SYNTHESIS (Figure 48-2)

A. The biosynthetic pathway originates with L-tyrosine, which is derived from the diet or from the hepatic hydroxylation of L-phenylalanine by phenylalanine hydroxylase. Tyrosine is hydroxylated in the cytoplasm by tyrosine hydroxylase to L-dopa (3,4-dihydroxyphenylalanine). The process requires tetrahydrobiopterin as a cofactor. Tyrosine hydroxylase is the rate-limiting enzyme in the overall biosynthesis of epinephrine.

B. Dopa is converted in the cytosol to **dopamine** (3,4-dihydroxyphenylethylamine) by a nonspecific aromatic L-amino acid decarboxylase (dopa decarboxylase), which requires pyridoxal phosphate as a cofactor.

C. Dopamine enters the chromaffin granule, where it is converted to L-norepinephrine by dopamine-β-hydroxylase, which exists exclusively in the granule. Ascorbate serves as the hydrogen donor. This enzyme is located in the granulated vesicles of sympathetic nerve endings and the chromaffin granules of the adrenomedullary chromaffin cells.

1. Norepinephrine is the end product in approximately 20% of chromaffin cells.

2. In about 80% of chromaffin cells, norepinephrine diffuses back into the chromaffin cytoplasm. There, it is N-methylated by phenylethanolamine-N-methyltansferase (PNMT) using S-adenosylmethionine as a methyl donor. The resulting L-epinephrine must enter the chromaffin granule after its conversion in the cytosol by PNMT.
   a. PNMT is selectively localized in the adrenal medulla, the only site where it exists in significant concentrations.
   b. PNMT activity is induced by very high local concentrations of glucocorticoids (cortisol), which are found only in the adrenal portal blood draining the adrenal cortex.

V. CONTROL OF CATECHOLAMINE SECRETION

A. **General considerations**

1. **Acetylcholine (ACh)** provides the major physiologic stimulus for the secretion of the adrenomedullary hormones. In addition, angiotensin II, histamine, and bradykinin stimulate catecholamine secretion.
   a. Catecholamine release is stimulated by ACh from the preganglionic sympathetic nerve endings innervating the chromaffin cells.
   b. The final common effector pathway activating the adrenal medulla is the cholinergic preganglionic fibers in the greater splanchnic nerve.
   c. ACh causes the depolarization of the chromaffin cells followed by the release of cate-

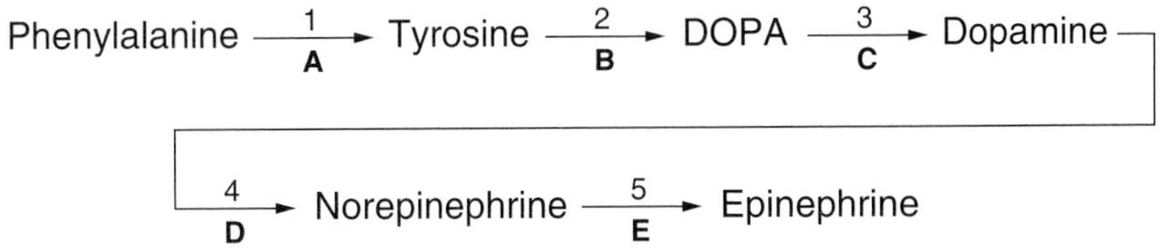

FIGURE 48-2. Biosynthesis of adrenomedullary catecholamines. 1 = phenylalanine hydroxylase (cytosol); 2 = tyrosine hydroxylase (cytosol); 3 = dopa decarboxylase (cytosol); 4 = dopamine-β-hydroxylase (granule); 5 = phenylethanolamine-N-methyltransferase (cytosol); A = tetrahydrobiopterin → dihydrobiopterin, molecular O_2; B = tetrahydrobiopterin → dihydrobiopterin, molecular O_2; C = pyridoxal phosphate, molecular O_2; D = ascorbate → dehydroascorbate, molecular O_2; E = S-adenosyl methionine (SAM) → S-adenosyl homocysteine, molecular O_2.

cholamines by **exocytosis.** Ca^{2+} influx secondary to membrane depolarization is the central event in **stimulus-secretion coupling.**

2. **Cortisol and adrenocorticotropic hormone (ACTH).** Because catecholamine synthesis is dependent on cortisol, the functional integrity of the adrenal medulla indirectly depends on a functional pituitary gland for ACTH secretion and a functional median eminence for corticotropin-releasing hormone (CRH) secretion. CRH is a hypophysiotropic hormone produced by the parvicellular nuclei of the ventral diencephalon.

B. **Physiologic and psychological stimuli for release.** The adrenal medulla constitutes the neuroeffector of the sympathoadrenomedullary axis that is activated during states of emergency. This response to stress is called the **fight-or-flight reaction.** Among the conditions in which the sympathetic nervous system is activated are fear, anxiety, pain, trauma, hemorrhage and fluid loss, asphyxia and hypoxia, changes in blood pH, extreme cold or heat, severe exercise, hypoglycemia, and hypotension. During hypoglycemia, the adrenal medulla is activated selectively. In humans, epinephrine and norepinephrine appear to be released independently by specific stimuli.

1. Anger and active aggressive states or situations are associated with increased norepinephrine secretion.

2. States of anxiety are associated with increased epinephrine secretion. In addition, epinephrine release is increased by tense but passive emotional displays or threatening situations of an unpredictable nature.

3. Angiotensin II potentiates the release of catecholamines.

4. Plasma concentrations of epinephrine vary according to physiologic or pathologic state as follows:
   (a) Basal level: 25–50 pg/ml (6×10^{-10} mol/L)
   (b) Hypoglycemia: 230 pg/ml
   (c) Diabetic ketoacidosis: 500 pg/ml
   (d) Severe hypoglycemia: 1500 pg/ml

C. **Regulation of adrenergic receptors.** A reciprocal relationship exists between catecholamine concentration and the number and function of adrenergic receptors.

1. A sustained decrease in catecholamine secretion is associated with an increased number of adrenergic receptors in target cells and an increased responsiveness to catecholamines. Conversely, a chronic increase in catecholamine secretion is associated with a decreased number of adrenergic receptors in target cells and a decreased responsiveness to catecholamines (down-regulation).

2. This relationship may account for the phenomenon of **denervation hypersensitivity,** which is observed in sympathetic neuroeffectors following autonomic fiber denervation.

VI. METABOLISM AND INACTIVATION OF CIRCULATING CATECHOLAMINES

A. **General considerations.** The plasma half-life of epinephrine and norepinephrine is 10 seconds and 15 seconds, respectively. The biologic effects of circulating catecholamines are terminated rapidly by both nonenzymatic and enzymatic mechanisms.

1. **Neuronal uptake.** Sympathetic nerve endings have the capacity to take up amines actively from the circulation. This active uptake of circulating catecholamines leads to nonenzymatic inactivation by intraneuronal storage and to enzymatic inactivation by a mitochondrial enzyme called **monoamine oxidase (MAO).** Neuronal uptake ("reuptake") is the major route of norepinephrine removal from synaptic clefts. Then, cytosolic catecholamines can be either retransported into storage vesicles or deaminated by MAO.

2. **Extraneuronal uptake.** The formation of catecholamine metabolites locally in innervated

tissues and systemically in the liver, kidney, lung, and gut implies catecholamine uptake by a variety of cells.

3. **Inactivation.** Circulating epinephrine and norepinephrine are metabolized predominantly in the liver and kidney.

B. **Metabolic pathways for catecholamine inactivation** (Figure 48-3)

1. **MAO** is found in very high concentrations in the mitochondria of the liver, kidney, stomach, and intestine. MAO catalyzes the oxidative deamination of a number of biogenic amines, including the intraneuronal and circulating catecholamines.
   a. The combined actions of MAO and **aldehyde oxidase** on epinephrine and norepinephrine produce 3,4-dihydroxymandelic acid by oxidative deamination.
   b. The combined actions of MAO and aldehyde oxidase on the O-methylated metabolites of epinephrine and norepinephrine (metanephrine and normetanephrine, respectively) produce 3-methoxy-4-hydroxymandelic acid [vanillylmandelic acid (VMA)] by oxidative deamination.

2. **Catechol-O-methyltransferase (COMT)** is found in the soluble fraction of tissue homogenates with the highest levels in liver and kidney. COMT is considered mainly as an extraneuronal enzyme, but it is also found in postsynaptic membranes. COMT metabolizes circulating catecholamines in the kidney and liver and metabolizes locally released norepinephrine in the effector tissue.
   a. COMT, which requires S-adenosylmethionine as a methyl donor, produces normetanephrine from norepinephrine, metanephrine from epinephrine, and VMA from 3,4-dihydroxymandelic acid by 3-O-methylation.
   b. Of the available tests, increased urinary metanephrines have the highest diagnostic sensitivity and specificity for pheochromocytoma.

C. **Significance of catecholamine metabolites**

1. Only 2%–3% of the catecholamines are excreted directly into the urine, mostly in conjugation with sulfuric or glucuronic acid. Most of the catecholamines produced daily are excreted as the deaminated metabolites, VMA and 3-methoxy-4-hydroxyphenylglycol (MOPG). Only a small fraction is excreted unchanged or as metanephrines.

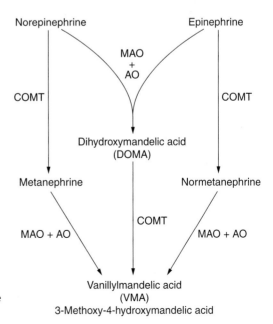

FIGURE 48-3. Metabolism of norepinephrine and epinephrine by catechol-O-methyltransferase (COMT), monoamine oxidase (MAO), and aldehyde oxidase (AO).

2. Under normal circumstances, epinephrine accounts for a very small proportion of urinary VMA and MOPG. Because the majority is derived from norepinephrine, urinary VMA and MOPG reflect the activity of the nerve terminals of the sympathetic nervous system rather than that of the adrenal medulla.

3. The excretion of unchanged epinephrine or plasma epinephrine provides a better index of the physiologic activity of the sympathoadrenomedullary system than does the excretion of catecholamine metabolites, because the latter reflects, to a considerable extent, norepinephrine that is metabolized within nerve endings and the brain and never released at adrenergic synapses in the active form.

VII. PHYSIOLOGIC ACTIONS OF CATECHOLAMINES (Tables 48-1 and 48-2; Figure 48-4). The effects of adrenomedullary stimulation and sympathetic nerve stimulation gen-

TABLE 48-1. Some Physiologic Effects of Catecholamines and Types of Adrenergic Receptors

Effector Organ	Receptor Type	Response
Eye		
Radial muscle	α	Contraction (mydriasis)
Ciliary muscle	β	Relaxation for far vision
Heart*		
Sinoatrial node	β	Increase in heart rate (increase in rate of diastolic depolarization and decrease in duration of phase 4 of sinoatrial nodal action potential)
Atrioventricular node	β	Increase in conduction velocity and shortening of functional refractory period
Atria	β	Increase in contractility
Ventricles	β	Increase in contractility and irritability
Blood Vessels*	α	Constriction (arterioles and veins)
	β	Dilation
Bronchial muscle	β	Relaxation (bronchodilation)
Gastrointestinal tract		
Stomach	β	Decrease in motility
Intestine	α, β	Decrease in motility
Sphincters	α	Contraction
Urinary bladder		
Detrusor muscle	β	Relaxation
Trigone and sphincter	α	Contraction
Skin		
Pilomotor muscles	α	Piloerection
Sweat glands	α	Selective stimulation (adrenergic sweating)*
Uterus	α	Contraction
	β	Relaxation
Liver	α	Glycogenolysis
Muscle	β	Glycogenolysis
Pancreatic islets	α	Inhibition of insulin secretion
	β	Stimulation of insulin secretion
Kidney (afferent arterioles)	β	Renin secretion

Adapted from Morgan HE: Function of the adrenal glands. In *Best and Taylor's Physiological Basis of Medical Practice,* 10th edition. Edited by Brobeck JR. Baltimore, Williams & Wilkins, 1979.
*See Table 48-2 and Figure 48-4.

TABLE 48-2. Cardiovascular Effects of Catecholamines in Humans*

Cardiovascular Function	Epinephrine	Norepinephrine	Isoproterenol
Systolic blood pressure	+ +	+ + +	0 +
Diastolic blood pressure	−	+ +	− −
Mean blood pressure	+ 0 −	+ +	− −
Total peripheral resistance	− −	+ + +	− − −
Heart rate (chronotropic effect)	+	−	+ +
Stroke output (inotropic effect)	+ +	+	+ +
Cardiac output	+ + +	− 0	+ + +

0 = no effect; + = increased; − = decreased. The number of symbols indicates the approximate magnitude of the response.

*Administration in therapeutic doses of 0.1–0.4 μg/kg/min IV or 0.5–1.0 mg SC.

[Adapted with permission form Craig CR, Stitzel RE (eds.): *Modern Pharmacology,* 2nd edition. Boston, Little, Brown, 1986, p 161.]

erally are similar. However, in some tissues, epinephrine and norepinephrine produce different effects owing to the existence of two types of adrenergic receptors, **alpha** (α) and **beta** (β) receptors, which have different sensitivities for the various catecholamines and, therefore, produce different responses. **Epinephrine** is the single most active endogenous amine on both α and β receptors.

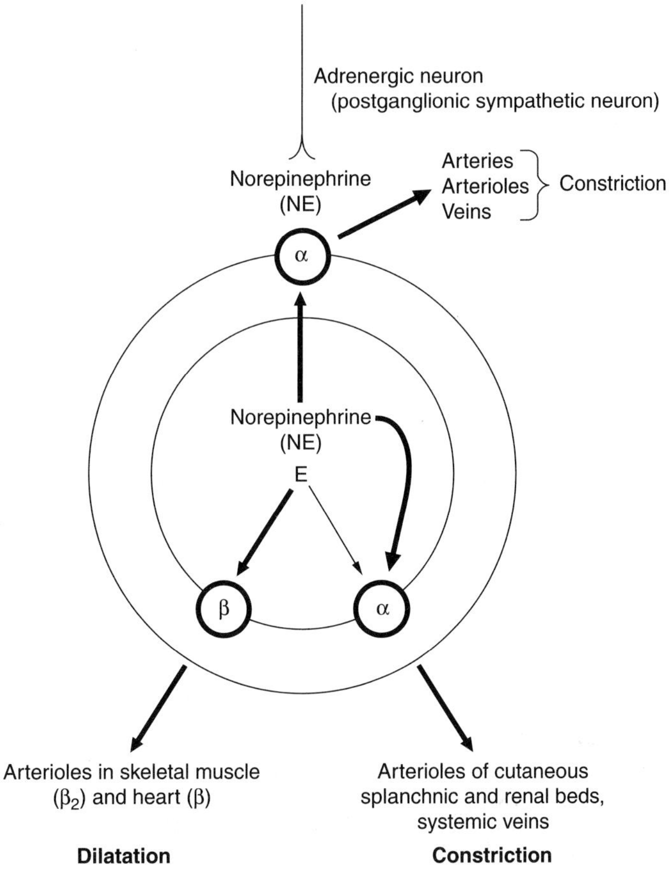

FIGURE 48-4. Effects of catecholamines on blood vessels. Norepinephrine released from sympathetic nerves causes constriction throughout the vascular tree by activation of α-adrenergic receptors. Circulating epinephrine can activate α- and β-adrenergic receptors of the vascular smooth muscle cells. The latter is of particular importance in skeletal muscle and the heart, where the β-adrenergic inhibitory effect of the catecholamine predominates. In other resistance vessels and veins epinephrine causes mainly α-adrenergic activation. E = epinephrine; NE = norepinephrine.

A. The **α-adrenergic receptors** are sensitive to both epinephrine and norepinephrine. These receptors are associated with most of the excitatory functions of the body and have at least one major inhibitory function (i.e., inhibition of intestinal motility).

B. The **β-adrenergic receptors** respond to epinephrine and, in general, are relatively insensitive to norepinephrine. These receptors are associated with most of the inhibitory functions of the body and have one important excitatory function (i.e., excitation of the myocardium).

VIII. **BIOCHEMICAL EFFECTS OF CATECHOLAMINES** (Figure 48-5). Norepinephrine has little direct effect on carbohydrate metabolism; however, both norepinephrine and epinephrine can inhibit glucose-induced secretion of insulin from the beta cells of the pancreatic islets of Langerhans. Hence, epinephrine is a diabetogenic hormone.

A. **Carbohydrate metabolism.** Because hepatic stores of glycogen are limited (about 100 g) and decrease only transiently after epinephrine activation, lactate derived from muscle glycogen (300 g) is the major precursor for hepatic **gluconeogenesis,** the process that sustains hepatic glucose formation and secretion. Gluconeogenesis mainly accounts for the hyperglycemic action of epinephrine in normal physiologic states. In pathologic states (e.g., pheochromocytoma), the diabetogenic action of catecholamines is caused by the inhibition of insulin secretion and the gluconeogenic effect of these hormones (usually norepinephrine), which are secreted in excessive amounts. Because propranolol attenuates hyperlactacidemia and hyperglycemia, this implies that epinephrine-induced glycogenolysis in muscle and in the liver is mediated by the β and α receptors, respectively (see Table 48-1).

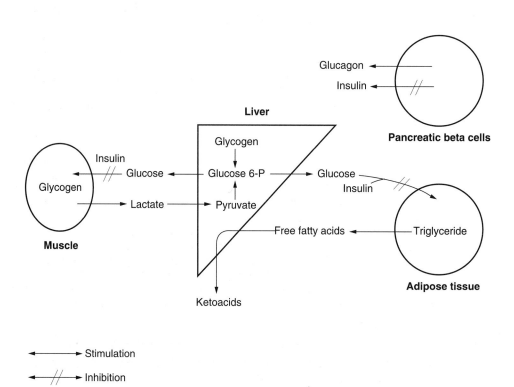

FIGURE 48-5. Metabolic actions of epinephrine. Epinephrine stimulates gluconeogenesis and inhibits glucose utilization. In addition, it stimulates lipolysis and ketogenesis, and inhibits insulin secretion. The net effect is hyperglycemia, together with elevated plasma free fatty acids and ketoacids. Epinephrine increases insulin resistance.

1. **Glycogenolysis in the liver**
   a. Epinephrine stimulates glycogenolysis in the liver via the Ca^{2+}-activated glycogen phosphorylase and the inhibition of glycogen synthetase. Glucose-6-phosphatase, found mainly in the liver and in lesser amounts in the kidney, forms free glucose, which increases blood glucose.
   b. Because glucagon stimulates and insulin suppresses hepatic glycogenolysis, the effects of epinephrine on insulin secretion (suppression) and glucagon secretion (stimulation) reinforce the breakdown of glycogen and the increase in hepatic glucose secretion.
   c. Epinephrine also increases the hepatic production of glucose from lactate, amino acids, and glycerol, all of which are gluconeogenic substances.

2. **Glycogenolysis in muscle**
   a. Epinephrine stimulates glycogenolysis in muscle by a β-adrenergic receptor mechanism involving the stimulation of adenylyl cyclase and cyclic adenosine 3′,5′-monophosphate (cAMP)–induced stimulation of glycogen phosphorylase. Concomitantly, glycogen synthetase activity is reduced.
   b. Muscle lacks glucose-6-phosphatase, and epinephrine-induced glycogenolysis in muscle **does not directly increase blood glucose.** The glucose-6-phosphate is metabolized to lactate or pyruvate, which is converted to glucose by the liver.
   c. The ultimate physiologic effect of epinephrine-stimulated glycogenolysis in muscle is increased hepatic glucose secretion (hyperglycemia) via the hepatic conversion of muscle lactate to glucose.

3. **Hyperglycemic effects of epinephrine** on the liver are important only in conjunction with the effects of epinephrine on glucagon and insulin secretion together with its glycogenolytic effect on muscle in acute emergency situations. Epinephrine in physiologic concentrations does not have a direct glycogenolytic effect in the liver.
   a. Much higher amounts of epinephrine than glucagon are required to cause hyperglycemia. However, epinephrine has a more pronounced hyperglycemic effect than glucagon for the following important reasons.
      (1) Epinephrine inhibits insulin secretion, while glucagon stimulates insulin secretion; therefore, the hyperglycemic effect of glucagon is attenuated by insulin.
      (2) Epinephrine stimulates glycogenolysis in muscle, thereby providing lactate for hepatic gluconeogenesis.
      (3) Epinephrine stimulates glucagon secretion, which amplifies the hyperglycemic effect of epinephrine.
      (4) Epinephrine stimulates ACTH secretion, which then stimulates cortisol secretion. Cortisol also is a potent gluconeogenic hormone via the hepatic conversion of alanine to glucose.
      (5) Circulating catecholamines inhibit muscle glucose uptake, which is in contrast to the effect of glucagon (gluconeogenesis).
   b. Epinephrine indirectly inhibits insulin-mediated facilitated diffusion of glucose by muscle and adipose tissue via its blockade of insulin secretion.
   c. Catecholamines also directly inhibit glucose uptake by the suppression of glucose transporter proteins in the cell membranes of skeletal and cardiac muscle cells and adipocytes. The GLUT-4 transporter, which is found exclusively in cardiac and skeletal muscle and in adipose tissue, is specifically responsible for the glucose utilization stimulated by insulin.

B. **Fat metabolism.** In humans, the major site of lipogenesis from glucose is the liver.

1. A man of average size has fat stores that contain about 15 kg of triglyceride, some of which can be metabolized to free fatty acids.

2. Epinephrine stimulates lipolysis by activating triglyceride lipase, which is called the intracellular **hormone-sensitive lipase.** The activation of this enzyme is via the β-adrenergic receptor (i.e., cAMP).

3. Mobilization of free fatty acids from stores in adipose tissue supplies a substrate for keto-

genesis in the liver. Acetoacetate and β-hydroxybutyrate are transported from the liver to the peripheral tissues, where they are quantitatively important as energy sources.

   a. Cardiac muscle and the renal cortex use fatty acids and acetoacetate in preference to glucose, whereas resting skeletal muscle uses fatty acids as the major source of energy.

   b. During extreme conditions such as starvation and diabetes, the brain adapts to the use of ketoacids. Ketoacids also are oxidized by skeletal muscle during starvation.

C. **Gluconeogenesis** refers to the formation of glucose from noncarbohydrate sources. Gluconeogenesis occurs in the liver and the kidney.

   1. Gluconeogenic substances include pyruvate, lactate, glycerol, odd-chain fatty acids, and amino acids. However, the major source of endogenous glucose production is protein, with a small fraction available from the glycerol contained in fat. All of the constituent amino acids in protein tissue, with the exceptions of leucine and lysine, can be converted to glucose.

   2. The conversion of even-chain fatty acids is not possible in the mammalian liver because of the absence of the enzymes necessary for the de novo synthesis of the four-carbon dicarboxylic acids from acetyl coenzyme A (acetyl-CoA).

IX. ENDOCRINOPATHIES

A. **Hyposecretion** of catecholamines, as occurs during tuberculosis and malignant destruction of the adrenal glands or following adrenalectomy, probably produces no symptoms or other clinical features.

   1. Catecholamine production from the sympathetic nerve endings appears to satisfy the normal biologic requirements, because the adrenal medulla is not necessary for life.

   2. The functional integrity of the adrenal medulla can be determined experimentally by the administration of 2-deoxy-D-glucose. This nonmetabolizable carbohydrate induces intracellular glycopenia and extracellular hyperglycemia.

   3. Spontaneous deficiency of epinephrine is unknown as a disease state, and adrenalectomized patients do not require epinephrine replacement therapy.

B. **Hypersecretion** of catecholamines from chromaffin cell tumors (pheochromocytomas) produces demonstrable clinical features. Secretion from tumors occurs by simple diffusion.

   1. Pheochromocytoma patients have sustained or paroxysmal hypertension. Unlike patients with essential hypertension, pheochromocytoma patients exhibit orthostatic hypotension.

   2. The hypersecretion of catecholamines is associated with severe headache, sweating (cold or **adrenergic sweating**), palpitations, chest pain, extreme anxiety with a sense of impending death, pallor of the skin caused by vasoconstriction, and blurred vision.

   3. Most pheochromocytomas contain predominantly norepinephrine, and most affected patients secrete predominantly norepinephrine into the bloodstream. Evidence of epinephrine hypersecretion increases the likelihood that the tumor origin is in the adrenal medulla. However, an extra-adrenal site should not be excluded.

   a. If epinephrine is secreted primarily, the heart rate is increased.

   b. If norepinephrine is the predominant hormone, the pulse rate decreases reflexly in response to marked hypertension.

   4. Urinary excretion of catecholamines, metanephrines, and VMA are increased.

C. **Treatment** requires surgical removal of the tumor. Ninety percent of pheochromocytomas are benign.

Case Study

A 32-year-old male electrician experiences frequent episodes of headache, hyperhidrosis (sweating), and heart palpitations that usually occur with work that involves sudden movements or changes in body position. He describes these paroxysms as "attacks" with a sudden onset that last from minutes to hours and then subside gradually. The episodes have occurred two or three times per week over a 3-month period. The man also reports that during these "attacks" he experiences anxiety, apprehension, tremulousness, pain in the chest, weakness, and a sense of impending doom that made him feel "washed out." He ascribed them to "nerves" because he recently separated from his wife.

> 1. *What is the relationship between changes in body position and the episodes of sweating, palpitations, and anxiety?*

DISCUSSION

The man has the symptoms of a pheochromocytoma. Changes in body position provoke the classic triad of paroxysmal symptoms—episodic palpitations, diaphoresis, and headache—by displacing the abdominal contents. Actions such as lifting, straining, bending, or strenuous exertions of any kind that press on the tumor and release catecholamines result in the symptoms. About 90% of pheochromocytomas are solitary, unilateral, encapsulated adrenomedullary tumors, which are not innervated, unlike normal adrenal medullary chromaffin cells. Thus, catecholamines are released by simple diffusion into the bloodstream and not by exocytosis.

Physical examination reveals a blood pressure of 185/125 mm Hg seated and 145/112 mm Hg standing, and a heart rate of 96 beats/min seated and 108 beats/min standing. The man receives a prescription for clonidine to control his blood pressure and a tricyclic antidepressant to calm his "nerves." The physician refers him to a hypertension clinic for further evaluation.
A magnetic resonance imaging (MRI) scan reveals a mass in the left adrenal area. The following laboratory results are obtained on a 24-hour urine collection: metanephrines, 3.2 mg (normal, < 1.3 mg); norepinephrine, 918 μg (normal, < 80 μg); epinephrine, 7.2 μg (normal, < 20 μg); dopamine, 205 μg (normal, < 400 μg); and VMA, 17.6 mg (normal, < 9 mg). A 2-hour postprandial oral glucose tolerance test yields a result of 400 mg/dl (normal, < 140 mg/dl).

> 2. *How are pheochromocytomas and hypertension associated?*

DISCUSSION

Pheochromocytomas remain an important cause of correctable hypertension. Hypertension (usually severe and refractory to antihypertensive medications) is the cardinal sign of pheochromocytoma. In most cases, the diagnosis is suspected because a patient has a hypertensive crisis, an anxiety attack, or difficult-to-control hypertension. Anxiety states may be confused with pheochromocytoma, but mental stress or psychological tension does not usually provoke a crisis, although anxiety may accompany the attack.
The syndrome of **h**ypertension, **h**eadache, **h**yperhidrosis, **h**eart palpitations, and **h**yperglycemia (the 5 Hs) is highly predictive of pheochromocytoma. Indeed, the man's 2-hr postprandial blood glucose (400 mg/dl) is indicative of severely impaired glucose tolerance, which is caused by the inhibition of insulin secretion by catecholamines acting via the α-adrenergic receptor on the pancreatic islets (beta cells). In short, catecholamines are diabetogenic hormones.

> 3. *Would you expect clonidine and a tricyclic antidepressant to be effective?*

DISCUSSION

Certain prescribed drugs, including tricyclic antidepressants, antidopaminergic agents, and naloxone, may precipitate a hypertensive crisis in the presence of pheochromocytoma. β-Blockade that is not preceded by adequate α-blockade may also precipitate a hypertensive crisis. This effect is the result of α-receptor activation with enhanced vasoconstriction due to blockade of β-receptors that promote vasodilation.

The antihypertensive drug clonidine, a centrally acting presynaptic α_2-agonist, inhibits central sympathetic outflow. It should not have been administered to this patient, who also was taking a tricyclic antidepressant, because these drugs block its hypotensive effect. In this patient, clonidine decreases his blood pressure despite high circulating levels of catecholamines. Such a finding indicates that the physiologic release of norepinephrine from axon terminals of sympathetic postganglionic neurons is more significant than the levels of circulating catecholamines.

Other features in the history may suggest pheochromocytoma; for example, patients showing an increase in blood pressure after receiving certain antihypertensive drugs, especially β-adrenergic antagonists and guanethidine.

    4. How would you prepare this patient for surgery to remove the pheochromocytoma?

DISCUSSION

At least 90% of pheochromocytomas are benign and can be totally excised. However, adrenergic blockade is required preoperatively to control blood pressure and prevent intra-operative hypertensive crises. After adequate α-adrenergic blockade is achieved, β-adrenergic blockade may be initiated. β-adrenergic blockade alone may evoke a more severe hypertension due to unopposed α-adrenergic stimulation.

The drug of choice is phenoxybenzamine, an irreversible, long-acting, noncompetitive α-antagonist. This agent also permits expansion of blood volume, which is usually decreased as a result of excessive vasoconstriction. Metyrosine (α-methylparatyrosine), which inhibits the synthesis of catecholamines by blocking tyrosine hydroxylase, is used in those patients who have persistent catecholamine-producing tumors that cannot be treated with combined α- and β-adrenergic blockade (phenoxybenzamine and propranolol, respectively).

    5. What could underlie the man's orthostatic hypotension?

DISCUSSION

Orthostatic hypotension is frequently observed in pheochromocytoma, as it is in this patient. Attributed to plasma volume contraction (hypovolemia), it also likely reflects catecholamine desensitization and dysautonomia. A significant postural decline in blood pressure should suggest pheochromocytoma.

Chapter 49

Adrenal Gland: Cortex

I. **ADRENAL CORTEX: STRUCTURE AND FUNCTION.** This section describes the physiologic and biochemical aspects of **glucocorticoids,** the most important of which is **cortisol** (also known as **hydrocortisone**).

A. **Embryology.** Morphologically and physiologically, the fetal adrenal gland differs strikingly from that of the adult. However, through all stages of life, the function of the adrenal cortex is dependent on adrenocorticotropic hormone (ACTH).

1. The adrenal cortex is a mesodermal derivative. It is axiomatic that all endocrine glands derived from mesoderm synthesize and secrete steroid hormones.

2. The outer **neocortex,** which is the progenitor of the adult cortex, comprises about 15% of the total volume of this organ, and the inner **fetal zone** (inner zone or **fetal cortex**) constitutes about 85%.

3. The adrenal gland is larger at birth than it is during adulthood because the fetal zone undergoes rapid involution during the first few months of extrauterine life and completely disappears by 3–12 months postpartum.

4. Near term, the fetal cortices of the fetal adrenal glands secrete 100–200 mg of steroids daily in the form of sulfoconjugates, the principal one of which is the biologically weak androgen, **dehydroepiandrosterone (DHEA) sulfate.** This 17-ketosteroid is an androgen containing 19 carbon atoms.

B. **Morphology of the adult adrenal cortex**

1. **Gross anatomy**
   a. The adrenal glands are paired structures situated above the kidneys.
   b. Normally, each gland weighs about 5 g, of which the cortex constitutes approximately 80%.

2. **Histology and function.** The adrenal cortex consists of three distinct layers or **zones** of cells.
   a. The outermost layer, the **zona glomerulosa,** is the site of **aldosterone** and **corticosterone** synthesis. Aldosterone is the principal mineralocorticoid of the human adrenal cortex.
   b. The wider, middle zone is the **zona fasciculata,** and the innermost layer is the **zona reticularis.** The two inner zones of the adrenal cortex should be considered a functional unit, where mainly **cortisol** (and some corticosterone) and **DHEA** are synthesized.

C. **Adrenocortical hormones: corticosteroids** (Tables 49-1 and 49-2)

1. **Secretion**
   a. The human adrenal cortex secretes two glucocorticoids (cortisol and corticosterone*), one mineralocorticoid (aldosterone), biosynthetic precursors of three end products (progesterone, 11-deoxycorticosterone, and 11-deoxycortisol), and androgenic substances (DHEA and its sulfate ester).
   b. The normal human adrenal cortex does not secrete physiologically effective amounts of testosterone or estradiol.

---

*At physiologic concentrations, corticosterone has glucocorticoid activity.

TABLE 49-1. Average 8:00 A.M. Plasma Concentration and Secretion Rate of Corticosteroids in Adults

Corticosteroid	Plasma Concentration (μg/dl)	Secretion Rate (mg/day)
Cortisol	13	15
Corticosterone	1	3
11-Deoxycortisol	0.16	0.40
Deoxycorticosterone	0.07	0.20
Aldosterone	0.009	0.15
18-Hydroxycorticosterone	0.009	0.10
Dehydroepiandrosterone (DHEA)	0.5	15
DHEA sulfate	115	15

Adapted with permission from Genuth SM: The adrenal glands. In *Physiology, 3rd ed.* Edited by Berne RM, Levy MN. St. Louis, CV Mosby, 1993, p 958.

2. Transport

a. Under physiologic circumstances, about 90% of the plasma cortisol is bound to **cortisol-binding globulin** (CBG; transcortin), which is an α-globulin. [In addition to binding cortisol, transcortin has a high binding affinity for progesterone, deoxycorticosterone (DOC), corticosterone, and some synthetic analogues.] About 6% of the plasma cortisol is bound to plasma **albumin,** and about 4% is **unbound** and represents the physiologically active steroid.

b. The 90% of the plasma cortisol bound to plasma protein represents the metabolically inactive pool, which serves as a reservoir for free hormone.

c. Most (80%) of the cholesterol precursor for adrenal steroid synthesis is provided by plasma lipoproteins [low-density lipoproteins (LPLs)] by a specific membrane receptor-mediated pathway.

3. Biosynthesis of adrenal steroids: enzymes (Table 49-3). Five oxidative CYP (formerly P450) enzymes act at various ring carbons of cholesterol (Figure 49-1).

a. CYP11A1 (side-chain cleavage enzyme) cleaves the side chain between carbons 20 and 22 of cholesterol.

b. CYP11B1 (11β-hydroxylase) catalyzes β-hydroxylation at C-11.

c. CYP17 (17α-hydroxylase) catalyzes the hydroxylation of C-17.

d. CYP21A2 (21-hydroxylase) catalyzes the hydroxylation at C-21.

e. 3β-hydroxysteroid dehydrogenase (3β-HSD) catalyzes the conversion of:

(1) Pregnenolone to progesterone

TABLE 49-2. Blood Production Rates of Adrenal Androgens

Androgenic Steroid	Plasma Concentration (μg/dl)	Blood Production Rate (mg/day)
Testosterone		
Men	0.8	7.0
Women*	0.034	0.34
Androstenedione		
Men	0.06	1.4
Women	0.14	3.4

Reprinted from Mulrow PJ: The adrenals. In *Physiology and Biophysics.* Edited by Ruch TC, Patton HD. Philadelphia, WB Saunders, 1973, p 229.
*In women, about 50% of the blood testosterone is derived from androstenedione.

TABLE 49-3. Nomenclature and Location of Steroidogenic Enzymes*

Trivial Name	Past	Current	Location	Inhibitors
Aromatase	P450$_{arom}$	CYP19	ER (m)	—
Cholesterol side-chain cleavage enzyme; desmolase	P450$_{SCC}$	CYP11A1	M	Aminoglutethimide, ketoconazole, etomidate
3β-hydroxysteroid dehydrogenase	3β-HSD	3β-HSD	ER (m)	Cyanoketone
17α-hydroxylase/ 17,20-lyase	P450$_{C17}$	CYP17	ER (m)	—
17β-hydroxysteroid dehydrogenase	17β-HSD	17β-HSD	Cytosol, ER (m)	—
21-hydroxylase	P450$_{C21}$	CYP21A2	ER (m)	—
11β-hydroxylase	P450$_{C11}$	CYP11B1	M	Metyrapone, ketoconazole, etomidate
Aldosterone synthase; corticosterone 18-methylcorticosterone oxidase/lyase	P450$_{C11AS}$	CYP11B2	M	—

E = endoplasmic reticulum; m = microsome; M = mitochondrion.

*Other inhibitors of steroidogenic enzymes include mitotane. Mifepristone (RU486) does not inhibit biosynthesis of steroids but competitively inhibits peripheral actions of glucocorticoids and progestagens. Mifepristone is an effective abortifacient and has been used to treat hypercorticosolism and meningioma.

> **(2)** 17α-hydroxypregnenolone to 17α-hydroxyprogesterone
> **(3)** DHEA to androstenedione
> **f.** CYP11B2 converts corticosterone to aldosterone.

4. Corticosteroidogenesis (Figure 49-2)
   a. Uptake of cholesterol. Free cholesterol is the preferred precursor of the corticosteroids, although the adrenal cortex can form cholesterol from acetyl coenzyme A (acetyl-CoA). Most stored adrenal cholesterol is esterified with fatty acids; it is the cholesterol ester content that is reduced following ACTH stimulation of the fasciculata–reticularis complex.
   b. Side-chain cleavage of cholesterol. The rate-limiting step in corticosteroidogenesis is the mitochondrial conversion of cholesterol to pregnenolone by 20,22-desmolase.

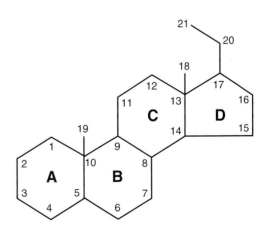

FIGURE 49-1. Basic steroid ring structure. The four rings are identified by letters, and individual carbon atoms comprising the steroid ring are numbered. Substituent groups in derivative steroid molecules are designated by the number of the carbon atom to which they are attached. Double bonds in the ring structure are identified by the carbon atom with the lower number.

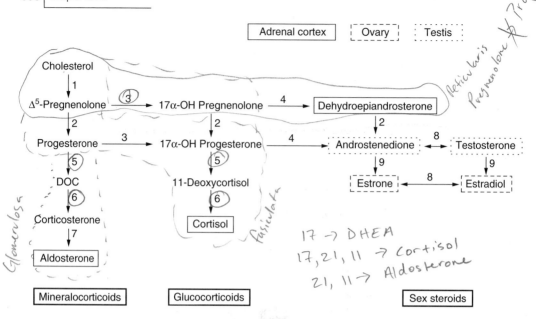

FIGURE 49-2. Summary of steroidogenesis in the adrenal cortex, testis, and ovary. Notice that there is no interconversion between mineralocorticoids and glucocorticoids. 18-hydroxycorticosterone is a by-product rather than an intermediate and, therefore, it is not shown. *1* = 20,22 desmolase; *2* = 3 β-hydroxysteroid dehydrogenase + Δ 5-isomerase; *3* = 17 α-hydroxylase; *4* = 17,20 desmolase; *5* = 21-hydroxylase; *6* = 11 β-hydroxylase; *7* = aldosterone synthase; *8* = 17-hydroxysteroid dehydrogenase; *9* = aromatase.

    c. Pregnenolone: the common precursor of all steroid hormones. Conversion of pregnenolone to progesterone requires two enzymes—3β-hydroxysteroid dehydrogenase and Δ⁵-isomerase.

    d. Hydroxylation. These reactions follow sequentially after the formation of pregnenolone and progesterone and require $NADPH_2$, molecular O_2, and a cytochrome P450 oxygen donor system.

        (1) The hydroxylation reactions in the biosynthesis of aldosterone occur sequentially at the C-21, C-11, and C-18 positions.

        (2) The hydroxylation reactions in the biosynthesis of cortisol occur sequentially at the C-17, C-21, and C-11 positions.

    e. Sex steroid pathways. Both pregnenolone and progesterone are substrates for the microsomal enzyme, 17α-hydroxylase, which is found not only in the adrenal cortex but also in the testis and ovary.

        (1) Pregnenolone is converted to 17α-hydroxypregnenolone, which can either continue along the Δ⁵-pathway to the synthesis of androgens or enter the glucocorticoid pathway.

        (2) Progesterone is converted to 17α-hydroxyprogesterone, which can either proceed along the Δ⁴-pathway to the synthesis of androgens or enter the mineralocorticoid pathway.

        (3) The zona glomerulosa, which lacks 17α-hydroxylase, does not have the capacity to synthesize 17α-hydroxyprogesterone. For this reason, the zona glomerulosa cannot synthesize cortisol.

            (a) The conversion of pregnenolone to DHEA is in the Δ⁵-pathway.

            (b) The conversion of progesterone to androstenedione is in the Δ⁴-pathway.

    f. Glucocorticoid/mineralocorticoid pathways. Both progesterone and 17α-hydroxyprogesterone are substrates for the microsomal enzyme, 21-hydroxylase.

        (1) Progesterone is converted to 11-deoxycorticosterone, which is in the mineralocorticoid pathway. 11-deoxycorticosterone is synthesized in the inner zone of the adrenal cortex (zona fasciculata).

(2) 17α-Hydroxyprogesterone is converted to 11-deoxycortisol, which is in the glucocorticoid pathway.

(3) 11-Deoxycorticosterone and 11-deoxycortisol are not precursors for the synthesis of each other.

g. **Diverging pathways.** Both 11-deoxycorticosterone and 11-deoxycortisol are acted on by mitochondrial 11β-hydroxylase.

(1) 11-Deoxycorticosterone forms corticosterone in the mineralocorticoid pathway.

(2) 11-Deoxycortisol is converted to cortisol, the principal glucocorticoid of the human adrenal cortex.

(3) Corticosterone differs from cortisol only in that the former substance lacks a 17α-hydroxyl group. Although this structural difference is small, it accounts for a very large difference in the biologic activity of these two hormones.

h. **Aldosterone synthesis.** Some of the corticosterone serves as the substrate for another mitochondrial enzyme, 18-hydroxylase.

(1) This reaction leads to the formation of 18-hydroxycorticosterone.

(2) 18-Hydroxycorticosterone is converted to aldosterone by the mitochondrial enzyme, 18-hydroxysteroid dehydrogenase, which is found only in the zona glomerulosa.

i. **Synthesis and secretion of sex steroids**

(1) Androgens. The adrenal cortex secretes four androgenic hormones: androstenedione, testosterone, DHEA, and DHEA sulfate. Quantitatively, the most important sex steroids produced by the human adrenal cortex are DHEA and DHEA sulfate. Except for testosterone, adrenocortical androgens are relatively weak and serve as precursors for hepatic conversion to testosterone.

(a) DHEA is derived from 17α-hydroxypregnenolone by the action of 17,20-desmolase.

(b) DHEA is mainly conjugated with sulfuric acid and, as such, is bound to plasma protein. While in this bound form, DHEA is not readily excreted but circulates in higher concentrations than any other adrenal steroid.

(c) DHEA is the principal precursor of urinary 17-ketosteroids; however, the most abundant urinary 17-ketosteroids are androsterone and etiocholanolone.

(d) DHEA and DHEA sulfate have androgenic activity by virtue of their peripheral conversion to testosterone. DHEA sulfate is active as a minor precursor of other 19-carbon steroids formed in the gonads and placenta, which are sites of sulfatase activity.

(i) Normal excretion rates for 17-ketosteroids are 5–14 mg/day in women and 8–20 mg/day in men.

(ii) Normally, adrenocortical precursors represent the bulk of the urinary 17-ketosteroid pool, with a smaller contribution from the gonads.

(iii) The main androgen secreted by premenopausal women is androstenedione, about 60% of which is of adrenocortical origin.

(2) Estrogens. The human adrenal cortex can synthesize minute amounts of estrogen. The adrenal cortex makes its major contribution to the body's estrogen (estrone) pool indirectly by supplying androstenedione together with DHEA and its sulfate as substrates for conversion to estrogens by subcutaneous fat, hair follicles, mammary adipose tissue, and other tissues.

5. Metabolism of corticosteroids

a. **General considerations**

(1) Corticosteroid inactivation occurs by:

(a) Enzymatic reduction of the Δ^{4-5} double bond in the A-ring to form **dihydrocortisol**

(b) Enzymatic reduction of the ketonic oxygen substituent at the C-3 position to form **tetrahydrocortisol**

(c) Conjugation with glucuronic acid to form a water-soluble metabolite that is readily excreted by the kidney

(2) The major urinary metabolite of cortisol is **tetrahydrocortisol glucuronide.**

b. **Hepatic conversion.** The liver is the major extra-adrenal site of corticosteroid metabolism.

    (1) Cortisol can be enzymatically converted to cortisone by 11β-hydroxysteroid dehydrogenase and excreted as **tetrahydrocortisone glucuronide.**

    (2) The ketonic oxygen substituent on the C-20 position of cortisol and other steroids can be enzymatically converted to a hydroxyl group. These steroids can be subjected to A-ring reduction, conjugated, and excreted as glucuronides.

        (a) Cortisol is converted to **cortol glucuronide.**

        (b) Cortisone is converted to **cortolone glucuronide.**

        (c) Progesterone forms **pregnanediol glucuronide.**

        (d) 17α-Hydroxyprogesterone forms **pregnanetriol glucuronide.**

    (3) Steroids that contain a 17α-hydroxyl group are ketogenic. Cortisol can be enzymatically converted to a 17-ketosteroid by 17,20-desmolase. About 5% of cortisol appears in the urine as a 17-ketosteroid.

    (4) Aldosterone also can undergo A-ring reduction and conjugation to form **tetrahydroaldosterone glucuronide.**

  c. Conversion in other extra-adrenal tissues. Muscle, skin, fibroblasts, intestine, and lymphocytes also can carry out oxidation–reduction reactions at the C-3, C-11, C-17, and C-20 positions of the corticosteroid molecule.

D. **Control of adrenocortical function** (see Figure 46-3). Physiologic control of the rate of cortisol secretion occurs via a double negative feedback loop, a mechanism that is characteristic of most neuroendocrine control systems.

  1. Regulation of ACTH secretion

    a. The parvicellular peptidergic neurons of the hypothalamus release **corticotropin-releasing hormone** (CRH), which stimulates the secretion of ACTH from the anterior lobe of the pituitary gland via the hypophysial portal system. CRH is a polypeptide consisting of 41 amino acid residues.

    b. Neurotransmitters secreted by the monoaminergic neurons that innervate the peptidergic neurons regulate CRH secretion from the tuberoinfundibular neurons.

        (1) Cholinergic neurons stimulate hypothalamic secretion of CRH. Serotonin also is a stimulatory signal to CRH neurons.

        (2) Adrenergic neuron activity inhibits release of CRH. Another known inhibitor of CRH secretion is **γ-aminobutyric acid (GABA).**

    c. Hypothalamic CRH and vasopressin [antidiuretic hormone (ADH)], which are colocated in the peptidergic neurons terminating in the median eminence, stimulate secretion of corticotropin.

        (1) Thus, cortisol has a negative feedback effect on both CRH and ADH, which are cosecreted into the portal system.

        (2) Adrenal insufficiency removes this negative feedback effect, leading to elevations in both plasma ACTH (corticotropin) and ADH.

        (3) The deleterious effect of cortisol deficiency (water intoxication) is largely related to increased release of ADH, as evidenced by the ability of an ADH antagonist to reverse this defect in water excretion.

  2. Precursors of ACTH: chemistry (Figure 49-3). Endorphins are structural derivatives of β-lipotropic hormone (β-LPH). The lipotropin-related peptides (β-LPH and β-endorphin) and ACTH share a common glycoprotein precursor molecule (molecular weight: about 31,000 daltons), proopiomelanocortin (POMC), which is synthesized in the corticotropes of the pars distalis of the pituitary gland.

    a. POMC is activated by proteolytic cleavage to yield 10 individual peptides that have been **classified into four groups:**

        (1) ACTH and corticotropin-like intermediate lobe peptide (CLIP)

        (2) Lipotropic hormones (lipotropins), represented by β- and γ-LPH

        (3) Melanocyte-stimulating hormones (MSHs), represented by α-, β-, and γ-MSH

        (4) Opioid peptides or endorphins, represented by α-, β-, and γ-endorphins

    b. POMC consists of **three major chemical moieties.**

        (1) The N-terminal fragment (16 K) is cleaved to form γ-MSH.

        (2) ACTH consists of the fragment containing amino acid residues 1–39.

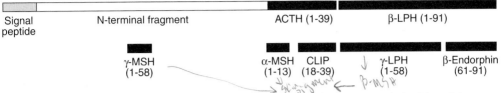

FIGURE 49-3. Diagram of the structure of the POMC molecule and the hormones derived from it by proteolysis. The precursor POMC protein contains a leader sequence (signal peptide) followed by a fragment that contains the sequence of α-MSH (amino acids 51–62), the ACTH molecule (1–39) that contains the sequences for α-MSH (ACTH 1–13) and CLIP (ACTH 18–39), and the β-lipotropin (1–91) molecule that contains the sequences of γ-MSH (1–58) and β-endorphin (61–91). The latter also includes the sequence for met-enkephalin (first five amino acids of β-endorphin). ACTH = adrenocorticotropic hormone; CLIP = corticotropin-like intermediate lobe peptide; MSH = melanocyte-stimulating hormone; POMC = proopiomelanocortin. [Reproduced from Griffen JE, Ojeda SR (eds): *Textbook of Endocrine Physiology,* 3rd edition. New York, Oxford University Press, 1996, p 112.]

      (a) ACTH is cleaved to produce α-MSH, which consists of the fragment containing amino acid residues 1–13. In humans, α-MSH normally is not synthesized in significant quantities.
      (b) ACTH also is cleaved into CLIP, which consists of the fragment containing amino acid residues 18–39.
   (3) β-LPH consists of the fragment containing amino acid residues 1–91. β-LPH is the precursor of the endogenous opioids, γ-LPH and β-endorphin.
      (a) γ-LPH consists of the β-LPH fragment containing amino acid residues 1–58.
         (i)   In nonhuman species, γ-LPH is converted by proteolytic cleavage to β-MSH, which is the fragment containing amino acid residues 41–58.
         (ii) In humans, β-MSH and α-MSH are not formed in significant quantities, because the intermediate lobe is vestigial in adult humans. β-MSH does not exist as such in normal human plasma.
      (b) β-Endorphin consists of the β-LPH fragment containing amino acid residues 61–91.
         (i)   β-Endorphin is cleaved into γ-endorphin, which is the fragment containing amino acid residues 61–77.
         (ii) γ-Endorphin forms α-endorphin, which is the fragment containing amino acid residues 61–76.

3. Precursors of ACTH: distribution. The endogenous opioids (endorphins) do not cross the blood–brain barrier.
  a. POMC is synthesized in the anterior and intermediate lobes of the pituitary gland, in the hypothalamus and other areas of the brain, and in several peripheral tissues including the placenta, gastrointestinal (GI) tract, and lung.
    (1) In the human **pituitary gland,** POMC exists principally in the anterior lobe where it is synthesized by basophils. POMC is the precursor of ACTH and β-LPH, which are secreted together from the basophils [see Chapter 47 II B 1 a (2)].
      (a) ACTH and β-LPH occur within the same pituitary cell and possibly within the same secretory granule.
      (b) The intermediate lobe does not produce ACTH and β-LPH as final secretory products.
    (2) In the **brain,** the concentrations of ACTH and β-LPH are much lower than in the anterior lobe, and all neural cells or fibers that contain ACTH also contain β-LPH. The highest extrapituitary concentrations of ACTH, α-MSH, β-LPH, γ-LPH, and β-endorphin exist in the hypothalamus followed by the limbic system.
  b. β-Endorphin
    (1) β-Endorphin is the principal opioid peptide in the **pituitary gland,** and it exists in the highest concentration in the intermediate lobe of experimental animals. In the human pituitary, β-endorphin generally is confined to the cells of the anterior

lobe. In response to acute stress, the pituitary gland secretes ACTH and β-endorphin concomitantly.

(2) **Other sites.** β-Endorphin has been found in the human pancreas, placenta, semen, as well as elsewhere in the male reproductive tract, and it also exists in the plasma and cerebrospinal fluid (CSF).

4. Negative feedback action of corticosteroids

a. Of the endogenous corticosteroids, only cortisol has ACTH-suppressing activity. The synthetic glucocorticoid, **dexamethasone,** is a potent inhibitor of ACTH secretion and, therefore, of endogenous glucocorticoid secretion.

b. The negative feedback of cortisol is exerted at the level of the pituitary gland and the ventral diencephalon.

(1) If free cortisol levels are supraphysiologic, ACTH secretion is suppressed and the adrenal cortex ceases its excretory activity and undergoes **disuse atrophy.**

(2) Conversely, if plasma free cortisol levels are subnormal, the anterior lobe is released from inhibition by cortisol, ACTH secretion rises, and the adrenal cortex secretes more cortisol and becomes hypertrophic.

5. Hypophysial–adrenocortical rhythm. Normally, blood ACTH levels are higher in the morning than in the evening. This accounts for the diurnal rhythms in cortisol secretion, plasma cortisol concentration, and 17-hydroxycorticosteroid excretion (see Figure 46-1).

6. Hypophysial–adrenocortical response to stress. The normal hypothalamic–hypophysial–adrenocortical control system can be overridden by a variety of challenges, which collectively are referred to as **stress.**

a. Among the stresses shown to induce increased activity are severe trauma, pyrogens, hypoglycemia, histamine injection, electroconvulsive shock, acute anxiety, burns, hemorrhage, exercise, infections, chemical intoxication, pain, surgery, psychological stress, and cold exposure.

b. In stress conditions, ACTH secretion is stimulated despite the fact that systemic levels of cortisol are much higher than those required to inhibit ACTH secretion completely in unstressed conditions.

E. **Physiologic effects of glucocorticoids** (Figure 49-4). Of the naturally occurring steroids, only cortisol, cortisone, corticosterone, and 11-dehydrocorticosterone have appreciable glucocorticoid activity. Full recovery from hypothalamic–hypophysial–adrenocortical suppression may require as long as 1 year following cessation of all steroid therapy.

1. Anti-inflammatory effects. Glucocorticoids inhibit inflammatory and allergic reactions in several ways.

a. They stabilize lysosomal membranes, thereby inhibiting the release of proteolytic enzymes.

b. They decrease capillary permeability, thereby inhibiting diapedesis of leukocytes.

c. Glucocorticoids reduce the number of circulating lymphocytes, monocytes, eosinophils, and basophils.

(1) The decreased number of these formed elements in blood is caused primarily by a redistribution of the cells from the vascular compartment into the lymphoid tissue (e.g., spleen, lymph nodes, bone marrow). Cellular lysis is not a major mechanism for decreasing the number of these cells in the human circulation.

(2) The decrease in circulating basophils accounts for the fall in blood histamine levels and the abrogation of the allergic response.

(a) The migration of inflammatory cells from capillaries is decreased.

(b) Glucocorticoids lessen the formation of edema and, thereby, reduce the swelling of inflammatory tissue.

(3) Glucocorticoids cause an increase in the number of circulating neutrophils owing to the accelerated release from bone marrow and a reduced migration from the circulation. Steroids also inhibit the ability of neutrophils to marginate to the vessel wall.

d. Glucocorticoids cause involution of the lymph nodes, thymus, and spleen, which leads to decreased antibody production.

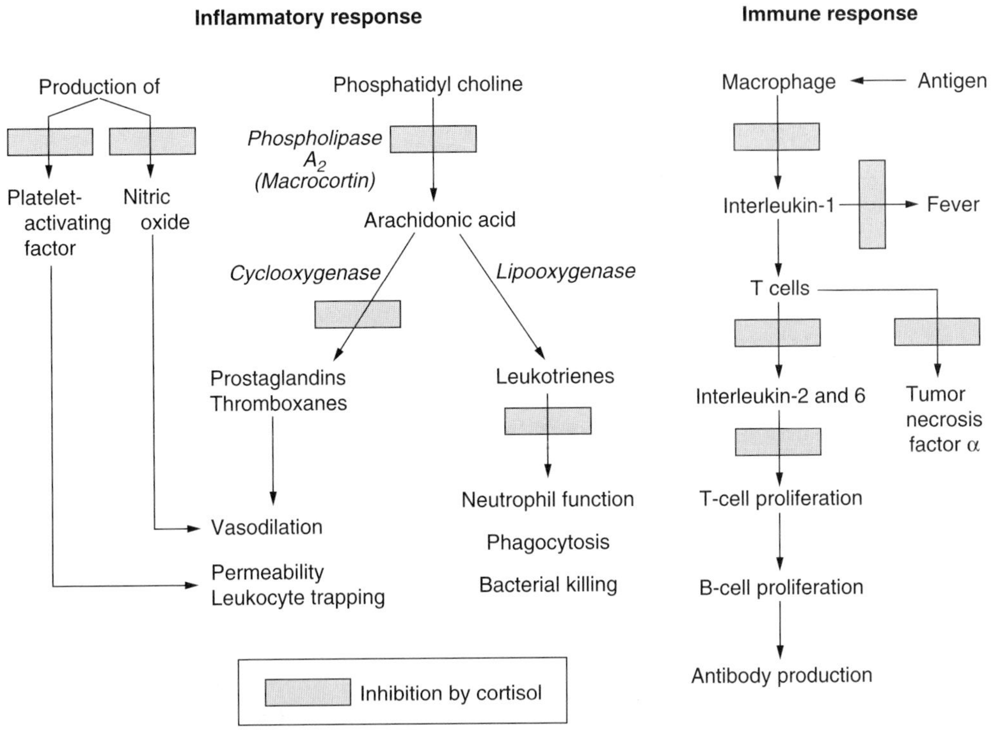

Inflammatory response   **Immune response**

Inhibition by cortisol

FIGURE 49-4. Cortisol inhibition in inflammation and immune system responses: mechanisms involved. Inhibition of the enzymes phospholipase and cyclooxygenase and the synthesis of nitric oxide and platelet-activating factor impairs the vascular component of inflammation, inhibition of leukotriene actions impairs neutrophil phagocytosis and bactericidal abilities, and inhibition of antigen presentation and macrophage cytokine release impairs proliferation and cytokine release of T-cells. Ultimately, B-cell function is reduced so that both cellular and humoral immunity are decreased. [Reproduced from Berne RM, Levy MN (eds): *Physiology,* 4th edition. Philadelphia, Mosby, 1998, p 947.]

    (1) This lymphocytopenic effect aids in the prevention or reduction of the immune response by organ transplant recipients.
    (2) Because recipients pretreated with large doses of glucocorticoids are susceptible to intercurrent infections, antibiotics are a necessary adjunct to the steroid therapy.
    (3) Antibody production is not suppressed in humans at conventional steroid doses; however, chronic administration of high doses of glucocorticoids leads to an impairment of host-defense mechanisms.
  e. Glucocorticoids lead to an increase in the total blood count because of the increased numbers of neutrophils, erythrocytes, and platelets. The increase in circulating erythrocytes (polycythemia) results from the stimulation of hematopoiesis. The total white blood cell (WBC) count does not decrease because of mobilization of neutrophils.

 2. Anti-immunity effects (see Figure 49-4)
  a. A decrease in basophils, eosinophils, and thymus-derived lymphocytes (T cells) occurs.
  b. Decreased production and release of cytokines suppresses cell-mediated immunity.
    (1) The decline in interleukin-1 (IL-1) caused by macrophages leads to a fall in T lymphocytes.
    (2) The fall in IL-2 by T lymphocytes leads to a decline in T cells.
  c. Decreased proliferation of B lymphocytes leads to a fall in immunoglobulin (antibody) production, which causes suppression of humoral-mediated immunity.
  d. Involution of lymph nodes and thymus occurs.

3. **Antiallergenic effects**
   a. Glucocorticoids are antiallergenic because they protect against the release of secretory products of granulocytes, mast cells, and macrophages, which have vesicles containing serotonin, histamine, and hydrolases that contribute to the inflammatory response. These substances (mediators) inhibit cellular degranulation, inhibit histamine synthesis, and stabilize the lysosomal membranes.
   b. These mediators and lysosomal enzymes are released in response to arachidonate metabolites, cell injury, reaction with antibodies, and phagocytosis.

4. **Renal effects**
   a. Glucocorticoids restore the glomerular filtration rate (GFR) and renal plasma flow to normal levels following adrenalectomy. Mineralocorticoids do not have these effects.
   b. Glucocorticoids facilitate free-water excretion (clearance) and uric acid excretion. They are necessary for the rapid excretion of a water load.

5. **Gastric effects.** Cortisol increases gastric flow and gastric acid secretion, while it decreases gastric mucosal cell proliferation. The latter two effects lead to peptic ulceration following chronic cortisol treatment.

6. **Psychoneural effects.** Individuals who have been receiving chronic high-dose therapy with glucocorticoids may become initially euphoric and then psychotic, paranoid, and depressed. High cortisol levels can cause insomnia, mood changes, reduced memory function, depression, irritability, and lower seizure threshold.

7. **Antigrowth effects**
   a. Large doses of cortisol have been shown to antagonize the effect of active vitamin D metabolites on the absorption of Ca^{2+} from the gut, to inhibit mitosis of fibroblasts, and to cause degradation of collagen. All of these effects lead to osteoporosis, which is a reduction in bone mass per unit volume with a normal ratio of mineral-to-organic matrix.
   b. The breakdown of collagen leads to an increase in urinary hydroxyproline excretion, and high cortisol levels decrease intestinal absorption of Ca^{2+} by antagonizing the action of $1,25(OH)_2D_3$.
   c. Glucocorticoids inhibit the anabolic actions of growth hormone (GH) and insulin-like growth factor-1 (IGF-1), particularly in bone.
   d. Chronic supraphysiologic doses of glucocorticoids suppress GH secretion and inhibit somatic growth.
   e. Glucocorticoids delay wound healing because of the reduction of fibroblast proliferation. Connective tissue is reduced in quantity and strength.
   f. Although glucocorticoids increase the ability of muscle to perform work, large doses lead to muscle atrophy and muscular weakness.

8. **Vascular effect.** Cortisol in pharmacologic doses enhances the vasopressor effect of norepinephrine. In the absence of cortisol, the vasopressor action of catecholamines is diminished, and hypotension ensues. Thus, corticosteroids have a role in the maintenance of normal arterial systemic blood pressure and volume through their support of vascular responsiveness to vasoactive substances. [Cortisol enhances catecholamine synthesis via its activation of the epinephrine-forming enzyme, phenolethanolamine-N-methyltransferase (PNMT).]

9. **Stress adaptation.** Glucocorticoids allow mammals to adapt to various stresses (trauma, cold, illness, starvation) in order to maintain homeostasis.
   a. Resistance to stress is not increased by the administration of glucocorticoids.
   b. Stress is associated with the activation of the hypothalamic–hypophysial–adrenal axis.

F. | **Metabolic effects of glucocorticoids** (Figure 49-5 and Table 49-4)

1. **Carbohydrate metabolism.** Cortisol is a carbohydrate-sparing hormone and, therefore, exerts an anti-insulin effect, which leads to hyperglycemia and insulin resistance.
   a. Glucocorticoids maintain blood glucose and the glycogen content of the liver by pro-

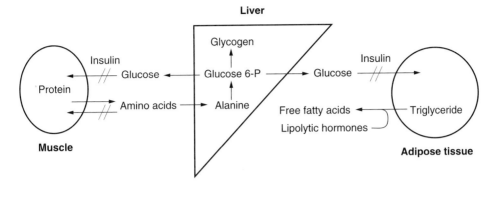

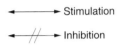 Stimulation

Inhibition

FIGURE 49-5. Metabolic actions for cortisol. Cortisol enhances gluconeogenesis, glycogenesis, proteolysis (muscle), and lipolysis. The net effect is hyperglycemia, together with hyperproteinemia, and elevated plasma free fatty acids. Cortisol promotes hepatic glycogen formation and hepatic protein synthesis. The net effect of cortisol is an increase in body fat. The most important overall action of cortisol is to promote the conversion of protein (gluconeogenesis). This effect leads to hyperaminoacidemia together with the storage and release of glucose (liver) and fatty acids (adipose tissue).

moting the conversion of amino acids to carbohydrates and the storage of carbohydrate as hepatic glycogen.

b. Cortisol is hyperglycemic principally because of its gluconeogenic activity, which is related to its protein catabolic effect on extrahepatic tissues, especially muscle.

   (1) The proteolytic effect of glucocorticoids results in the mobilization of amino acids from muscle and in an increase in plasma amino acid concentration.

   (2) Alanine is quantitatively the major gluconeogenic amino acid precursor in the liver. Like acetyl-CoA, alanine inhibits pyruvate kinase activity.

TABLE 49-4. Enzyme Activities Increased by Cortisol

Provide Carbon Precursors	Convert Pyruvate to Glycogen	Release Glucose	Synthesize Fat
Alanine transaminase	Pyruvate carboxylase	Glucose-6-phosphatase	Lipoprotein lipase
Tyrosine transaminase	Phosphoenolpyruvate carboxykinase Phosphoglyceraldehyde dehydrogenase		Glucose-6-phosphate dehydrogenase
Tryptophan pyrrolase	Aldolase		
Threonine dehydrase	Fructose 1,6-biphosphatase		
Serine dehydrase	6-Phosphofructo-2-kinase/ fructose 2,6-biphosphatase Phosphohexoisomerase Glycogen synthase		

    c. Cortisol also exerts an anti-insulin effect by blocking glucose transport in muscle and adipose tissue. This effect accounts for the phenomenon of glucose intolerance or an eventual "steroid diabetes"; thus, it is a diabetogenic hormone.

    d. Glucocorticoids augment the activity of key gluconeogenic enzymes by the induction of de novo hepatic enzyme synthesis.

        (1) The gluconeogenic pathway has three steps that differ from those in the glycolytic pathways as a result of their thermodynamic irreversibility. These enzymes and their substrates are as follows.

            (a) Glucose-6-phosphate → glucose (glucose-6-phosphatase)

            (b) Fructose 1,6-bisphosphate → fructose-6-phosphate (fructose 1,6-bisphosphatase)

            (c) Conversion of pyruvate to phosphoenolpyruvate requires two steps:

                (i) Pyruvate → oxaloacetate (pyruvate carboxylase)

                (ii) Oxaloacetate → phosphoenolpyruvate (phosphoenolpyruvate carboxykinase)

        (2) Glucocorticoids are associated with activation of glycogen synthetase by glucose-6-phosphate and of pyruvate carboxylase by acetyl-CoA. They also are associated with indirect inhibition of glycolysis by free fatty acids, resulting in increased glucogenesis and glycogenesis.

    e. Cortisol also indirectly inhibits the activities of glycolytic enzymes, which accounts for its anti-insulin effect. Enzymes that are blocked by the effect of glucocorticoids include glucokinase, phosphofructokinase, and pyruvate kinase.

    f. Glucocorticoids mobilize fatty acids from adipose tissue to the liver, where metabolism of free fatty acids may lead to products that inhibit glycolytic enzymes and favor gluconeogenesis.

        (1) The glycerol released from the fat cell with the fatty acids also serves as a secondary substrate for gluconeogenesis.

        (2) The cortisol-inhibited glycolysis in peripheral tissue probably is indirectly blocked via the inhibition of the key glycolytic enzyme, phosphofructokinase, by the elevated concentration of plasma free fatty acids.

    g. Glucocorticoids are associated with compensatory hyperinsulinemia following hyperglycemia.

2. Protein metabolism. The most important gluconeogenic substrates are amino acids derived from proteolysis in skeletal muscle.

    a. Cortisol enhances the release of amino acids from proteins in skeletal muscle and other extrahepatic tissues, including the protein matrix of bone.

        (1) The amino acids released, especially the glucogenic amino acid **alanine,** are transported to the liver and converted to glucose.

        (2) Increased glucose production by cortisol via gluconeogenesis is associated with increased urea production via the conversion of amino nitrogen to urea. This effect accounts for the increased urinary nitrogen excretion.

        (3) The proteolysis in skeletal muscle brings about a negative nitrogen balance.

    b. The amino acids taken up by the liver are used not only to form glucose or glycogen but also to build new protein. This protein anabolic effect at the level of the liver is an important exception to the overall protein catabolic effect of cortisol.

    c. Equally important is the ability of glucocorticoids to inhibit the de novo synthesis of protein, probably at the translational level. This is called an **antianabolic effect** of cortisol.

3. Fat metabolism. Glucocorticoids are lipolytic hormones. Their lipolytic effect is in part from the potentiation of the lipolytic actions of other hormones such as GH, catecholamines, glucagon, and thyroid hormone.

    a. Glucocorticoids favor the mobilization of fatty acids from adipose tissue to the liver, where the metabolism of fatty acids inhibits glycolytic enzymes and promotes gluconeogenesis. As a result of increased fatty acid oxidation, glucocorticoids may lead to ketosis, especially in the context of diabetes mellitus.

        (1) The major site of stimulation is the gluconeogenic enzyme, fructose 1,6-bisphosphatase, which is activated by fatty acids.

(2) At the same time, pyruvate kinase and phosphofructokinase are inhibited by fatty acids. Thus, glycolysis is inhibited while gluconeogenesis proceeds.

b. Glucocorticoids also indirectly stimulate lipolysis by blocking peripheral glucose uptake and utilization. They inhibit re-esterification of fatty acids within adipocytes by inhibiting the use of glucose. In addition, cortisol stimulates the differentiation of adipose cells from preadipocytes to adipocytes.

c. Fatty acid synthesis is inhibited in the liver by cortisol, an effect not observed in adipose tissue. The overall effect of glucocorticoids on fat is to induce a redistribution of fat together with an increase in total body fat (i.e., truncal obesity). The increase in body weight is not a result of a growth effect caused by the accretion of protein. (Recall that cortisol is an antigrowth hormone.)

    (1) There is characteristic centripetal distribution of fat (i.e., an accumulation of fat in the central axis of the body) with wasting of the extremities.

        (a) The deposition of fat in the facies is called "moonface."

        (b) The deposition of fat in the suprascapular region is referred to as "buffalo hump" or "dowager's hump."

        (c) Excessive fat distribution leads to a pendulous abdomen.

    (2) Glucocorticoid-induced obesity reflects increased food intake rather than a change in the rate of lipid metabolism.

d. Chronic excessive amounts of cortisol lead to hyperlipidemia and hypercholesterolemia. Glucocorticoids increase appetite and, thereby, play a role in obesity.

e. The obesity of hypercortisolism may be due to a defective leptin receptor. Leptin is a protein hormone produced and secreted exclusively by adipose tissue in proportion to its mass.

    (1) In experimental animals (mice), leptin decreases food intake, and absence of leptin produces obesity.

    (2) In humans, leptin is reduced following weight reduction and fasting. Leptin levels are increased in obesity.

    (3) Most human obesity is associated with leptin resistance rather than leptin deficiency.

    (4) Glucocorticoids increase leptin synthesis in adipocytes, and insulin also stimulates leptin synthesis.

f. The lipogenesis observed in hypercortisolism is, in part, related to increased lipoprotein lipase activity in adipocytes and also to elevated glucose-6-phosphate dehydrogenase activity. The increased activity of this dehydrogenase leads to elevated generation of $NADPH_2$, a necessary cofactor for fat synthesis.

II. ENDOCRINOPATHIES OF THE ADRENAL CORTEX (Figures 49-6 and and 49-7; see Figure 49-2)

A. Hypofunctional lesions

1. Primary adrenal insufficiency: deficiency of three adrenal hormones—cortisol, aldosterone, and DHEA

a. Clinical problems due mainly to aldosterone deficiency include anorexia, weakness, weight loss, vomiting, hyperpigmentation, hyponatremia (natriuresis), hyperkalemia, hypotension, metabolic acidosis, increased plasma ADH, hyposmotic dehydration, and elevated plasma ACTH.

b. The decline in plasma ketosteroids leads to the loss of pubic hair, reduced muscle mass, and loss of libido in women and reduced libido in men. Amenorrhea may also occur.

c. Hypoglycemia is the result of increased peripheral glucose utilization associated with increased sensitivity to insulin, with impaired gluconeogenesis, hepatic glucose production, and glycogen synthesis.

d. Vomiting and abdominal pain often are prodromal to an adrenal crisis.

2. Secondary adrenal insufficiency: deficiency of two adrenal hormones—cortisol and DHEA

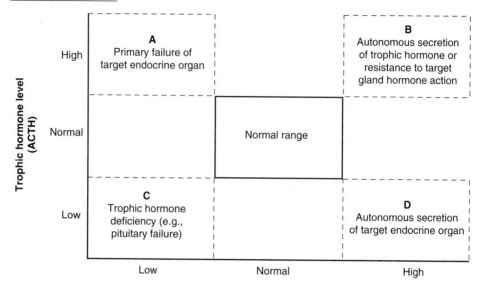

FIGURE 49-6. Paradigm for assessment of endocrine status. Most hormone systems are under some regulatory feedback control. For example, thyroid hormone and TSH; testosterone or progesterone and LH; plasma $[Ca^{2+}]$ and PTH; angiotensin II or plasma $[K^+]$ and aldosterone; estradiol or inhibin and FSH. In each of the above "pairs," the first substance is on the abscissa and the second substance is on the ordinate. A = primary adrenal insufficiency or congenital adrenal hyperplasia; B = secondary hypercortisolism due to a pituitary neoplasm or ectopic ACTH syndrome; C = secondary adrenal insufficiency due to a hypothalamic or hypophysial lesion; D = primary hypercortisolism due to an adrenal neoplasm. ACTH = adrenocorticotropic hormone; FSH = follicle-stimulating hormone; LH = luteinizing hormone; PTH = parathyroid hormone; TSH = thyroid-stimulating hormone. [Reproduced from Griffen JE, Ojeda SR (eds): *Textbook of Endocrine Physiology,* 3rd edition. New York, Oxford University Press, 1996, p 94.]

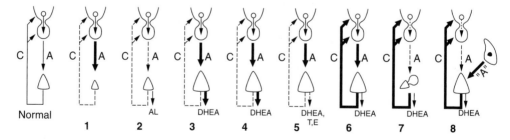

FIGURE 49-7. Diseases of endocrine regulation in the hypothalamic–hypophysial–adrenocortical axis in various endocrinopathies. In **hypocortisolism,** *1* = primary adrenal insufficiency (deficiency of AL, C, DHEA) and *2* = secondary adrenal insufficiency (deficiency of C, DHEA, normal AL). In **hypocortisolism** [adrenogenital syndrome (congenital adrenal hyperplasia)—enzyme deficiencies], *3* = 21-hydroxylase (CYP21A2): deficiencies of C, DOC, and AL, with increased DHEA; *4* = 11β-hydroxylase (CYP11B1)—deficiencies of C and AL with increased DHEA and DOC; and *5* = 17α-hydroxylase (CYP17)—deficiencies of C, DHEA, T, and E, with increased DOC. In **hypercortisolism (Cushing's syndrome),** *6* = ACTH-dependence (secondary hypercortisolism (Cushing's disease, pituitary neoplasm)—excess C; *7* = ACTH-independence [primary hypercortisolism (adrenal neoplasm)]—excess C and DHEA. *7 and 8* = ACTH-dependence [ectopic ACTH syndrome (ectopic neoplasm—excess C, A = adrenocorticotropic hormone (ACTH); C = cortisol; DHEA = dehydroepiandrosterone (adrenal); AL = aldosterone; DOC = deoxycorticosterone (adrenal); T = testosterone (testis); and E = estradiol (ovary).

    a. Most symptoms are associated with cortisol deficiency (e.g., hypoglycemia). Clinical signs are similar to those of primary insufficiency (see II A 1 a). However, dehydration, hyperpigmentation, and hyperkalemia do not occur, and hypotension is less prominent.

    b. Affected patients can regulate Na^+, K^+, and H^+ balance because normal renin–angiotensin–aldosterone function is maintained and hypovolemia is rare. However, hyponatremia can occur due to elevated ADH levels.

    c. 17-Ketosteroids are absent or low and may cause loss of libido in women and result in azoospermia because of panhypopituitarism.

B. Hyperfunctional lesions: Cushing's syndrome

  1. Hypercortisolism with the loss of the circadian (diurnal) secretory rhythm of cortisol is the hallmark of Cushing's syndrome. However, the pulsatile pattern of hormone secretion persists.

    a. ACTH-dependent hypercortisolism (elevated ACTH): autonomous ACTH secretion

      (1) Cushing's disease (secondary hypercortisolism) characterized by elevated ACTH and cortisol together with bilateral adrenal hyperplasia due to a pituitary neoplasm

      (2) Ectopic ACTH syndrome (tertiary hypercortisolism) characterized by elevated ACTH and cortisol with bilateral adrenocortical hyperplasia due to a nonendocrine tumor (e.g., bronchogenic carcinoma)

    b. ACTH-independent hypercortisolism (low ACTH)

      (1) Cushing's syndrome caused by primary adrenocorticalism (elevated cortisol)

      (2) Atrophic adrenal gland ipsilateral to the adrenal neoplasm and outside the neoplasm

      (3) Atrophic adrenal gland contralateral to the adrenal neoplasm

  2. Major clinical manifestations include the following:

    a. Increased cortisol secretory rate

    b. Hypertension due to Na^+ retention

    c. Insulin resistance (hyperglycemia due to gluconeogenesis and hyperinsulinemia)

    d. Increased plasma levels of DHEA and urinary excretion of 17-ketosteroids

      (1) Women: oligomenorrhea or amenorrhea, hirsutism, decreased libido

      (2) Men: decreased libido, impotency

    e. Osteopenia (osteoporosis) [reversible]

    f. Weight gain (centripetal obesity)

    g. Muscle wasting and weakness

    h. Mental lability: depression, irritability, insomnia, psychosis, manic depression

    i. Glucose intolerance (hyperglycemia) and hyperinsulinemia

  3. Cushing's syndrome can be caused by partially autonomous pituitary tumors or by autonomous adrenal or ectopic tumors.

C. Enzyme deficiencies: congenital adrenal hyperplasia (CAH). This condition is also known as adrenogenital (AG) syndrome.

  1. Major biochemical lesions: 21-, 11-, and 17-hydroxylase deficiencies—CYP21A2, CYP11B1, and CYP17, respectively.

    a. Hypocortisolism, elevated ACTH, and adrenocortical hyperplasia are the hallmarks of all AG syndromes.

    b. The adrenal fasciculata (cortisol-producing zone) and glomerulosa (aldosterone-producing zone) are hypofunctional, but the reticularis overproduces androgen (DHEA).

    c. A continuum of physical manifestations exist due to the spectrum of severity of enzyme deficiency.

  2. CAH due to a CYP21A2 deficiency

    a. Two forms of 21-hydroxylase deficiency are recognized in neonates, namely, a simple "virilizing" form and a "salt wasting" form.

    b. Hyperandrogenism, which is caused by the loss of negative feedback regulation of ACTH by cortisol, is a key feature.

(1) The weak androgen DHEA that is present in high amounts in CAH is partly metabolized to testosterone outside the adrenal gland.

(2) DHEA may also be aromatized to estrone, which is converted to estradiol. This is primarily responsible for the termination of linear bone growth.

(3) The excess androgen accelerates both linear growth and epiphysial closure, so that despite the early accelerated growth velocity, bone age advances rapidly, and adult height is diminished.

c. Electrolyte (Na^+) and fluid losses cause hyponatremia, hyperkalemia, acidosis, dehydration, hypoglycemia, vascular collapse, hypotension and increased plasma renin activity, and cardiac arrest.

d. In boys, this enzyme deficiency appears in early infancy as sexual precocity but usually they have a normal sexual development. Some untreated men may be fertile, but others have a reversible azoospermia.

e. In girls, this enzyme deficiency appears as virilization (masculinization) with clitoral hypertrophy, hirsutism, and sexual ambiguity (female pseudohermaphroditism) [i.e., male phenotype]. In untreated adult women, reproductive function is impaired because of irregular menses.

f. Internal genital morphogenesis is concordant with gonadal sex in females and males.

g. Patients with salt-wasting require long-term therapy with both mineralocorticoids and glucocorticoids.

h. It is important to appreciate that patients with a CYP21A2 deficiency are functionally similar to patients with primary adrenal insufficiency, except that the latter have atrophic adrenal cortices.

3. **CAH due to a CYP11B1 deficiency**

a. The elevated production of DOC induces Na^+ and water retention with induction of hypertension, which is a hallmark of CYP11B1 deficiency. Affected patients also tend to present with hypoglycemia due to hypocortisolemia.

b. The volume expansion and hypertension suppress aldosterone secretion and plasma renin activity.

c. The mineralocorticoid excess (DOC) also causes hypokalemia.

d. Decreased cortisol production results in elevated ACTH secretion, which impairs conversion of 11-deoxycortisol (a nonbioactive glucocorticoid) to cortisol and of deoxycorticosterone (DOC, a weak mineralocorticoid*) to corticosterone in the zona fasciculata, resulting in the accumulation of these steroid precursors.

e. The increased flow of substrate proximal to the deficient enzyme also results in excess androgen (DHEA) secretion, which contributes to increased urinary level of 17-ketosteroids.

f. The excess androgens masculinize the external genitalia of the female fetus and neonate, leading to genital ambiguity (female pseudohermaphroditism).

g. Postnatally, untreated males and females exhibit progressive virilization, rapid somatic growth, and skeletal maturation, which lead to early puberty in boys and hyperandrogenism in girls. In young adulthood men experience acne, and women present with hirsutism and menstrual irregularities.

h. Treatment involves exogenous glucocorticoids.

4. **CAH due to a CYP17 deficiency**

a. A defect in the CYP17 enzyme occurs in both the adrenal cortex and gonads (testis and ovary) and results in impaired synthesis of 17α-hydroxyprogesterone and thus of cortisol, androgens, and estrogens.

b. Decreased cortisol synthesis causes increased secretion of corticotropin which, in turn, results in excessive secretion of 17-deoxysteroids by the adrenal cortex, including the mineralocorticoid DOC, corticosterone, and 18-hydroxycorticosterone, all of which do not depend on 17α-hydroxylase.

c. Plasma levels of progesterone are also increased.

---

*When DOC is produced in large quantities, it can cause hypertension.

d. Excess DOC secretion leads to hypertension, hypokalemic alkalosis, and suppression of plasma renin activity. Secondarily, suppressed aldosterone synthesis and secretion is observed.

e. Corticosterone, a weak glucocorticoid, is elevated and prevents the symptoms of glucocorticoid deficiency.

f. Testosterone, estradiol, and DHEA production, which depends on 17α-hydroxylase, are also low.

   (1) The impaired gonadal steroidogenesis explains the elevated follicle-stimulating hormone (FSH) and luteinizing hormone (LH) [hypergonadotropic hypogonadism].

   (2) The reduction in testicular and ovarian sex steroid synthesis underlies the appearance of the female phenotype.

   (3) Females have normal internal and external genital tracts, but the hypogonadism at puberty results in sexual infantilism.

   (4) Hypogonadism in the male results in male pseudohermaphroditism with incomplete internal genital ducts and/or external genitalia that are incompletely masculinized (sexual infantilism). There may be sexual ambiguity.

   (5) The hypogonadal male with a CYP17 deficiency is characterized by the absence of Müllerian duct derivatives and Wolffian duct derivatives are hypoplastic.

g. Treatment requires glucocorticoid together with sex steroids.

D. **Hyperfunctional lesions: primary aldosteronism** (Conn's syndrome)—aldosterone-producing adenoma (APA) [see Chapter 30]

1. Aldosterone, the principal mineralocorticoid, is synthesized in the zona glomerulosa by the action of aldosterone synthase (CYP11B2), which converts corticosterone to aldosterone.

2. Aldosterone secretion is regulated primarily by the renin–angiotensin system and by the concentration of K^+ but is also affected by the circadian secretion of ACTH.

   a. Aldosterone modulates the transepithelial transport of Na^+ and K^+, and plasma acid–base balance. Recall that Na^+ is a major determinant in the regulation of extracellular fluid (ECF) volume.

   b. DOC is synthesized in the zona fasciculata and is under the control of ACTH.

3. Benign APAs are autonomous but typically exhibit a diurnal pattern of aldosterone secretion, with a peak in the early morning and a nadir in the late afternoon or evening. This pattern suggests that aldosterone synthesis is under the control of ACTH.

   a. In patients with APA, aldosterone secretion does not increase normally in response to assumption of an upright posture, due to marked suppression of the renin–angiotensin system.

   b. Tumors of APA patients are insensitive to angiotensin II.

4. Aldosterone also elevates K^+ secretion by the collecting ducts (principal cells).

   a. This results in hypokalemia, which impairs insulin secretion and results in glucose intolerance or overt diabetes.

   b. Some patients may experience frontal headaches, muscular weakness or flaccid paralysis caused by hypokalemia, or polyuria and nocturia resulting from the hypokalemia-induced renal concentrating defect.

   c. Patients rarely exhibit edema owing to Na^+ "escape," in which the Na^+-retaining effects of chronic aldosteronism are lost, possibly mediated by a compensatory increase in atrial natriuretic peptide (ANP) secretion.

Case Study

A 48-year-old woman goes to the local emergency department because of an abrupt onset of lower back pain. Radiographic examination shows a compression fracture of the third lumbar vertebra along with evidence of osteoporosis in the spine. Further history reveals a 50-pound

weight gain over the preceding 3 years, muscle weakness, and a tendency to bruise easily. She also complains of increasing emotional lability, including bouts of euphoria and depression. Sleep is also disturbed. Her previously regular menses are now only occurring every 4 to 6 months.

Physical examination shows an obese woman, with excess adipose tissue largely in the face, above the clavicles, and about the trunk. The extremities are thin and exhibit muscle atrophy. The skin is thin, with bruises that cannot be accounted for by trauma. Large purple marks are evident over the abdomen. Excess hair growth is present on the upper lip and skin. Neurologic examination shows weakness of proximal muscle groups but normal deep tendon reflexes. Blood pressure is 164/102 mm Hg, and heart rate is 76 beats/min.

Laboratory findings show a fasting plasma glucose of 180 mg/dl. Serum electrolytes show a slight increase in bicarbonate and a slight decrease in potassium.

1. *What is the most likely endocrine cause of this clinical picture?*

DISCUSSION

The constellation of signs and symptoms is a classic picture of excess endogenous cortisol, or of exogenously administered glucocorticoid (Cushing's syndrome).

2. *How does this hormonal disturbance produce the patient's symptoms and signs?*

DISCUSSION

Cortisol creates an antianabolic (i.e., catabolic) metabolic state. The muscle mass shows increased proteolysis with a resulting decrease in the size and number of muscle fibers. As a result, weakness and atrophy are present. In bone, collagen synthesis is inhibited and the rate of bone resorption is increased, which leads to osteopenia and to fractures. Calcium absorption from the gastrointestinal (GI) tract is diminished because of inhibition of the action of 1,25-(OH)$_2$ vitamin D$_3$. This adds to the difficulty in maintaining bone mass. Inhibition of collagen synthesis in skin and blood vessel walls leads to thinning of these tissues and to fragility of capillaries; this also causes bruising and purple bands (striae) in the skin. Appetite is stimulated centrally by cortisol, but the excess of ingested calories is selectively deposited in certain depots for reasons currently unexplained. Cortisol decreases rapid eye movement (REM) sleep and increases the amount of time awake.

All of these effects stem from the binding of cortisol to its nuclear glucocorticoid receptor. This modulates the transcription of numerous genes.

3. *Why is the fasting plasma glucose level elevated? Would you expect the plasma insulin level to change?*

DISCUSSION

Cortisol inhibits the insulin-stimulated uptake of glucose by muscle and augments gluconeogenesis in the liver and is an insulin antagonist. These effects combine to raise fasting plasma glucose. Plasma insulin increases in response to the rise in plasma glucose.

4. *What accounts for the hypertension and slight abnormalities in the plasma levels of bicarbonate and potassium?*

DISCUSSION

Cortisol also binds to the mineralocorticoid receptor and an excess of cortisol can therefore mimic aldosterone actions on the kidney to produce sodium retention, edema, hypertension, hypokalemia, and metabolic alkalosis.

5. What other hormones are likely to be present in excess in this patient?

DISCUSSION

If hypersecretion of cortisol is caused by a pituitary lesion, plasma **adrenocorticotropic hormone (ACTH)** will be elevated or at least inappropriately normal in the face of elevated cortisol levels. This resetting of the normal relationship between cortisol and ACTH can be demonstrated by administering an appropriate dose of a synthetic glucocorticoid such as dexamethasone. In a normal individual, this markedly decreases both plasma ACTH and plasma cortisol levels, but in an individual with a hyperfunctional pituitary, plasma ACTH and cortisol decrease little, if any. However, if a very large dose of dexamethasone is given, even the abnormal corticotrophs will be shut off, and plasma ACTH and cortisol will decrease significantly.

Abnormal expression of the ACTH precursor gene by a nonendocrine tumor will be manifest by a very high plasma level of ACTH, with no suppression when dexamethasone is given. In addition, such high levels of ACTH may cause hyperpigmentation of the skin because of the melanocyte-stimulating hormone (MSH) sequence within ACTH.

It is imperative to point out that this patient's plasma ACTH level was low—evidenced by the absence of hyperpigmentation of her skin. The low plasma ACTH concentration was caused by elevated cortisol secretion from an adrenal neoplasm. The elevated cortisol was responsible for the negative feedback inhibition of ACTH secretion. The concluding statement is that Cushing's syndrome is always characterized by hypercortisolism; however, ACTH levels can be high (pituitary or ectopic neoplasm) or low (adrenocortical neoplasm).

The loss of regular menses and the increasing facial hair suggest an excess of adrenal androgen secretion. Plasma levels of **dehydroepiandrosterone (DHEA)** and **androstenedione** will likely be elevated. These weak androgens may then be converted to the potent androgen, testosterone, in peripheral tissues.

Physicians eventually determine that the primary locus of this woman's disease is the gland from which the hormonal disturbance originated. She undergoes surgical removal of the gland. Postoperatively, she experiences satisfactory weight loss and the return of a normal emotional state. However, she also develops generalized weakness, lethargy, and loss of appetite. Her blood pressure falls to 98/62 mm Hg.

6. What is now wrong with the patient? How has this condition developed?

DISCUSSION

The original cause of this patient's hypercortisolism was an adrenal adenoma; therefore, her plasma ACTH level was very low because of negative feedback. As a result, the remaining adrenal cortical tissue was atrophic and nonfunctioning.

Immediately after removal of the adrenal adenoma, the plasma cortisol falls to low levels, which produce the postoperative symptoms and low blood pressure. This situation can persist for many months until, first, her adrenocorticotrophs recover from prolonged suppression and, second, her remaining adrenal cortical cells increase in size and number and recover their ability to secrete normal amounts of cortisol.

Chapter 50
The Testis

I. EMBRYOLOGY

A. Normal sex differentiation in the embryo

1. There are three sequential processes:
   a. Chromosomal (genotypic) sex is established at **fertilization.**
   b. **Chromosomal sex** causes the indifferent gonad to develop into an ovary or testis.
   c. **Gonadal sex** determines phenotypic sex. **Phenotypic sex** refers to the internal genital tracts, the urethras, and the external genitalia.

2. Both male and female embryos develop bipotential and neutral sex anlagen during the first 6 weeks of gestation, at which time sexual dimorphism is apparent (Tables 50-1 and 50-2 and Figure 50-1).
   a. The **bipotential gonad** (also known as the primordial, primitive, indifferent, or ambisexual gonad) consists of a medulla, a cortex, and primordial germ cells.
      (1) The bipotential gonadal anlagen, which gives rise to either the testes or ovaries, can be identified in human embryos by 30 days after fertilization.
      (2) These germ cells are embedded in a layer of cortical epithelium surrounding a core of medullary mesenchymal tissue.
      (3) At 6 weeks, the seminiferous tubules begin to form from the medulla.
      (4) The cortical region (from which the female gonad develops) undergoes regression.
   b. **Primordia of internal genitalia**
      (1) A paired set of wolffian (male) ducts
      (2) A paired set of müllerian (female) ducts
   c. **Neutral external genitalia.** In contrast to the internal genitalia, the external genitalia in both sexes develop from common anlagen, which are the urogenital sinus, the genital sinus, the genital tubercle, the genital swelling, and the genital (urethral) folds.

B. Testicular differentiation (Figure 50-2)

1. The earliest sign of male development occurs at approximately 6 weeks, at which time the bipotential gonad begins to differentiate as a testis. This process is referred to as **testis differentiation.**
   a. In the absence of testis determination, ovarian determination takes place several weeks after the time of testis determination.
   b. The gene product that triggers testis determination is termed **testis-determining factor (TDF).**
   c. The Y chromosome encodes the gene for TDF.
   d. A candidate for the TDF gene was isolated from the sex-determining locus on the Y chromosome and is termed **sex-determining region Y gene,** or **SRY gene.**
   e. The TDF gene product causes Sertoli cell differentiation and all subsequent events reflect Sertoli cell activity.

2. The earliest correlate of male differentiation is the appearance of large numbers of Sertoli cells at about 6 to 7 weeks and the subsequent organization of seminiferous tubules containing Sertoli cells and primordial germ cells.
   a. Germ cells (gonocytes and spermatogonia) undergo mitotic division within the testicular cords.
   b. Selective destruction of germ cells occurs before they reach the gonad and, therefore, they do not play a role in the initiation of testis differentiation.
   c. Meiosis does not occur before puberty in the male, but it does in the female.

TABLE 50-1. Six Parameters of Sexual Dimorphism

Parameter	Determining Factors	
	Male Development	**Female Development**
Genetic sex	Heterogametic (XY)	Homogametic (XX)
Gonadal sex	Y-linked testis-determining factor (TDF)	Oocytes
Genital ducts	Testosterone; anti-müllerian hormone	Innate tendency
External genitalia	*Dihydrotestosterone	Innate tendency
Gender role	Psychosocial factors	Psychosexual factors
Puberty	Testosterone	Estradiol

*Dihydrotestosterone can substitute for testosterone in the virilization of the embryonic wolffian ducts; however, the converse is not true.

TABLE 50-2. Sexual Anlagen and Their Derivatives

Anlage	Male Derivatives	Female Derivatives
Medulla of primordial gonad	Testis	—
Cortex of primordial gonad	—	Ovary
Wolffian duct	Epididymis, vas deferens, seminal vesicles	—
Müllerian duct	—	Oviducts (fallopian tubes), uterus, upper vagina
Urogenital sinus	Prostate, prostatic urethra	Urethra, lower vagina
*Urethral folds	Penile urethra, shaft of the penis	Labia minora
†Genital swellings	Scrotum	Labia majora
Genital tubercle	Glans penis	Clitoris

*The genital folds elongate and fuse to form the shaft of the penis.
†The fusion of the urethral fold converts the genital swellings into the scrotum (male) or the labia majora (female).

  3. Leydig (interstitial) cells appear at 8 weeks (i.e., about 1 week after the appearance of Sertoli cells).
     a. The Leydig cells are equipped with membrane receptors for human chorionic gonadotropin (HCG) and luteinizing hormone (LH) and synthesize and secrete testosterone.
        (1) At 8–9 weeks of fetal life, the Leydig cells secrete testosterone in response to chorionic gonadotropin secreted by the placenta.
        (2) While HCG is the major fetal gonadotropin, pituitary gonadotropins become more significant in later gestation and influence phallic growth and testicular descent.
        (3) Fetal pituitary gonadotropin secretion is regulated by hypothalamic gonadotropin-releasing hormone (GnRH).
        (4) Testosterone in the male fetus suppresses gonadotropin release by negative feedback.
     b. By 14 weeks the Leydig cells make up more than half the volume of the testis.
     c. At the end of the fourth month, the number of fetal Leydig cells decreases and only a few remain at term.

INDIFFERENT STAGE

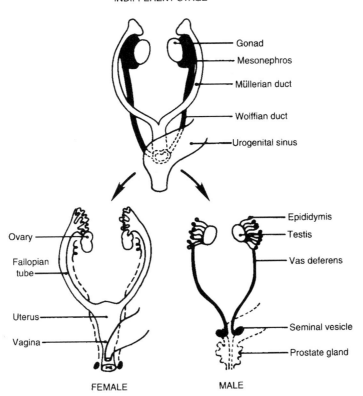

FIGURE 50-1. Sex differentiation of the gonad and the internal genitalia. Up to 6 weeks gestation, the gonad is a bipotential structure (*indifferent stage*), and the urogenital tract in both sexes consists of two pairs of genital ducts (i.e., the wolffian and müllerian ducts) and a mesonephros, all of which terminate in the urogenital sinus. In the female, the gonad develops into an ovary and the müllerian ducts become organized into the fallopian tubes, uterus, and upper vagina, while the wolffian ducts remain vestigial. In the male, a testis develops and the wolffian ducts differentiate into the epididymis, vas deferens, and seminal vesicle, while the müllerian ducts regress. (Reprinted from Wilson JD: Embryology of the genital tract. In *Campbell's Urology,* 4th ed. Edited by Harrison JH, et al. Philadelphia, WB Saunders, 1977, p 1473.)

4. The final stage of testis differentiation is descent through the inguinal canal to reach the scrotum at about 34 to 35 weeks of gestation.

5. By puberty, the testes usually have developed sufficiently to perform the functions of spermatogenesis and steroidogenesis. Generally, puberty begins between the ages of 12 and 14 years. In the United States, 95% of normal boys show signs of puberty by the age of 16 years.

C. **Ovarian differentiation** (see Tables 50-1 and 50-2 and Figure 50-1; see also Chapter 51)

1. The ovary can be identified histologically by about day 70.

2. The female gonad develops from the cortical region of the primitive gonad.

3. In the absence of testis determination, ovarian determination takes place.

4. In general, differentiation of the ovary occurs several weeks after the time of testis determination.
   a. Granulosa cells appear, and as they surround the germ cells, they commit them to oocyte formation.

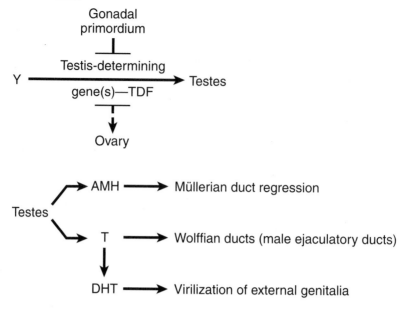

FIGURE 50-2. Testis determination and hormones involved in male sex differentiation. Testis-determining factor (TDF) triggers testis determination. T = testosterone; DHT = dihydrotestosterone; AMH = antimüllerian hormone, or müllerian-inhibiting factor.

    b. Hilar cells form later in development.

  5. In the absence of antimüllerian hormone, the female ducts (müllerian ducts) proliferate and form the oviducts, uterus, and upper two thirds of the vagina.
    a. The development of the female external genitalia is independent of ovarian influence.
    b. The female internal genitalia are functionally committed to become female as early as 8 weeks.

  6. In the absence of androgen, the wolffian ducts degenerate and the external genitalia maintain the neutral, female form.

D. Hormonal regulation of male development (see Table 50-1; Figures 50-2 and 50-3)

  1. The two principal components of male phenotypic development, wolffian duct differentiation and virilization of the urogenital sinus and external genitalia, are under control of testosterone and dihydrotestosterone.

  2. Virilization of the male embryo is mediated by three hormones.
    a. Antimüllerian hormone (AMH) is a peptide hormone produced by the Sertoli cells.
      (1) AMH appears at around 7 weeks of gestation, at the time of Sertoli cell differentiation.
      (2) AMH causes regression of the müllerian ducts and thus prevents development of the uterus, oviducts, and upper vagina.
      (3) Müllerian duct regression is induced by the local paracrine action of AMH secreted by the Sertoli cells of the ipsilateral testis.
    b. Testosterone from the Leydig cells of the fetal testis mediates virilization of the wolffian ducts.
      (1) The wolffian ducts differentiate into the vas efferens, epididymis, vas deferens, ejaculatory ducts, and the seminal vesicles.
      (2) This effect of testosterone is a local paracrine effect from the ipsilateral testis.
      (3) In other target tissues (prostate and external genitalia), testosterone must be converted to dihydrotestosterone before there is an androgenic effect.

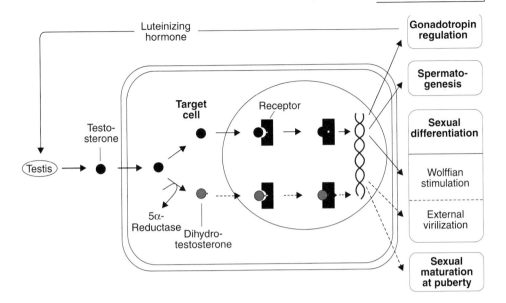

FIGURE 50-3. Normal androgen physiology. The major actions of androgens are shown in the right panel. Testosterone is shown to either bind to the androgen receptor in the nucleus of the target cell directly or following conversion to dihydrotestosterone (DHT). Testosterone and DHT bind to the same nuclear receptor resulting in the formation of a hormone-receptor complex, which interacts with the chromatin. Some actions of androgens are mediated by testosterone (*solid arrows*) or by dihydrotestosterone (*dashed arrows*). From Wilson JD, Foster DW, Kronenberg HM, et al: *Williams Textbook of Endoc*rinology, 9th ed. Philadelphia, WB Saunders, 1998, p 828.

   c. Dihydrotestosterone (DHT) is formed at its site of action from testosterone and causes masculinization of the prostate and external male genitalia.

     (1) The urogenital sinus and external genitalia contain active 5α-reductase, which converts testosterone to dihydrotestosterone, which masculinizes these structures.

     (2) DHT is therefore necessary for the virilization of the following structures:

       (a) Urogenital sinus, which gives rise to the prostate and prostatic urethra

       (b) The genital folds, which elongate and fuse to form the shaft of the penis

       (c) The genital swellings, which fuse to form the scrotum

       (d) The genital tubercle, which becomes the glans penis

     (3) DHT and testosterone combine with the same nuclear receptor; however, DHT is the most potent natural androgen.

II. MORPHOLOGY

A. Gross anatomy

   1. The testes normally are situated in the scrotum, where they are maintained at a temperature that is 2°C lower than normal body temperature. The lower temperature is necessary for normal spermatogenesis.

   2. The seminiferous tubules have an aggregate length of approximately 250 meters and constitute about 90% of the testicular volume.

B. Functional histology. The testis consists of two functional regions:

   1. Interstitial cell compartment. Leydig cells are located between the seminiferous tubules and produce androgenic steroids. This nontubular tissue comprises about 10% of the testicular volume.

   a. Leydig cells are numerous at birth but virtually disappear within the first 6 months of postnatal life.

   b. The reappearance of Leydig cells marks the onset of puberty.

   c. At puberty, the fibroblast-like cells of the testis serve as stem cells that differentiate into Leydig cells.

2. Seminiferous tubular compartment (Figure 50-4). The basic cellular components of the tubules are the germinal cells and the nongerminal (Sertoli) cells.

   a. The spermatogonia and Sertoli cells lie on the basal lamina. The developing germinal cells (spermatocytes) are found between the Sertoli cells.

   b. Specialized tight junctions between the Sertoli cells form a blood–testis barrier and divide the tubule into the outer, or basal, compartment and an inner, or adluminal, compartment.

3. Spermatogonia serve as a pool of undifferentiated nonmotile stem cells in the outer compartment.

   a. The majority of the spermatogonia undergo continuous mitotic division to provide additional stem cells.

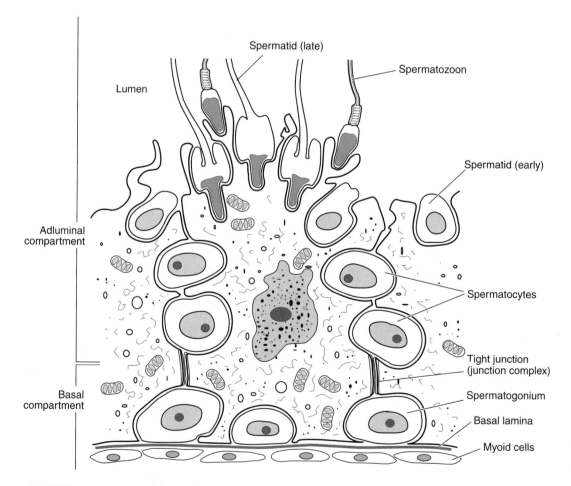

FIGURE 50-4. Diagram of the seminiferous tubule showing the Sertoli cell cytoplasm and developing spermatocytes. Note that both the spermatogonial and Sertoli cells lie on the basal lamina (basal membrane). (Adapted from Wilson JD, Foster DW, Kronenberg HM, Larsen PR: Williams Textbook of Endocrinology, 9th ed. Philadelphia, WB Saunders, 1998, p 822.)

b. A minority of the spermatogonia undergo further differentiation by meiosis, a process unique to the germinal epithelium.

c. Each spermatogonial cell undergoing differentiation gives rise to 16 primary spermatocytes, each of which then enters meiosis and gives rise to 4 spermatids and ultimately 4 spermatozoa. Thus, 64 spermatozoa can develop from each spermatogonium.

d. Spermatogenesis requires about 70 days in man, and the transport of sperm cells through the epididymis to the ejaculatory duct requires an additional 12–21 days.

e. Both testes of the young adult male form 123 ($\pm$ 18) million sperm daily during the reproductive years.

f. There are four phases of spermatogenesis (Figure 50-5):

   (1) Primary spermatocytes, formed during mitotic division of spermatogonia contain 23 **chromosomal pairs** identical to those in the spermatogonia and are, therefore, diploid cells.

   (2) The euploid primary spermatocytes under two meiotic (reduction) divisions. The first meiotic (haploid) division reduces the number of chromosomes by half, by forming secondary spermatocytes each containing 23 **chromosome pairs** (23 maternal and 23 paternal chromosomes).

   (3) Each secondary spermatocyte then undergoes a second meiotic division, giving rise to two spermatids, each of which contains 23 **single chromosomes.** Thus, four haploid spermatids are formed from the original primary spermatocyte.

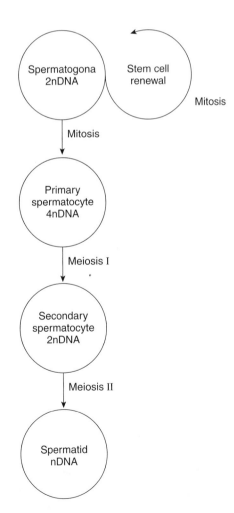

FIGURE 50-5. Representation of stem cell (spermatogonium) renewal pathway and differentiation pathway of the germinal cells. n = haploid; 2n = diploid; 4n = tetraploid.

(4) The spermatids differentiate into mature spermatozoa, a process called **spermio-genesis,** which is characterized by the absence of cell division.

g. Spermatogenesis requires LH and FSH.

(1) FSH (gametogenic hormone) stimulates spermatogenesis by:

(a) Stimulating mitosis of Sertoli cells, increasing their number during puberty

(b) Promoting maturation of Sertoli cells

(c) Binding to surface receptors on Sertoli cells and spermatogonia

(2) LH influences spermatogenesis indirectly by stimulating testosterone synthesis in the Leydig cells.

4. Sertoli cells are nonmotile and, in the mature testis, nonproliferating tubular cells that lie on the basal lamina.

a. Structural features. The Sertoli cells extend through the entire thickness of the germinal epithelium from the basement membrane to the lumen. The tight junctions between the bases of the Sertoli cells serve two functions (see Figure 50-4).

(1) They divide the seminiferous tubular epithelium into two functional pools: a basal compartment containing the spermatogonia and an adluminal compartment containing the spermatogonia and spermatids.

(2) They form an effective permeability barrier within the seminiferous epithelium, which is defined in man as the blood–testis barrier that limits the transport of many substances from the blood to the seminiferous tubular lumen. This barrier maintains germ cells in an immunologically privileged location, because mature sperm cells are very immunogenic when introduced into the systemic circulation.

b. Functions

(1) Secretion of antimüllerian hormone, the glycoprotein that causes regression of the müllerian ductal system

(2) Maintenance of the blood–testis barrier

(3) Regulation of germ cell maturation

(4) Provision of mechanical support for maturing gametes

(5) Phagocytosis of residual bodies of spermatid cytoplasm. Thus, the residual bodies are not cast off into the lumen but are retained within the epithelium throughout the spermiation process.

(6) Secretion of a watery, solute-rich (K^+ and HCO_3^-) fluid into the seminiferous lumen. These cells actively pump ions into the intercellular spaces to create a standing osmotic gradient that moves water from the Sertoli cell base to the free surface of the lumen. This fluid movement provides a driving force for conveying sperm from the testis to the epididymis, where most of this isosmotic fluid is reabsorbed.

(7) Conversion of androgenic precursors to estradiol

(8) Production of specific proteins, viz, androgen-binding protein (ABP) for secretion into the seminiferous tubule lumen. ABP maintains a high local testosterone concentration in the seminiferous tubules.

(9) Synthesis of inhibin, which regulates FSH secretion by negative feedback at the level of the pituitary.

(10) In the fetus, Sertoli cells secrete a meiosis-inhibiting factor, which suppresses germ cell proliferation and differentiation beyond the primitive spermatogenial stage.

III. HORMONES OF THE TESTIS: STEROIDS (Table 50-3)

A. Secretion and transport

1. Testosterone is the major hormone produced by the Leydig cells of the testis. Like all naturally occurring androgens, testosterone consists of 19 carbon atoms.

a. Testosterone is not stored in the testis. Cholesterol esters, the major precursor for testosterone biosynthesis, are stored in the lipid droplets in the Leydig cells.

b. A normal man secretes 4–9 mg of testosterone daily. More than 97% of secreted testosterone is bound to plasma proteins; 68% is bound to albumin, and 30% is bound to testosterone-binding globulin (also called sex hor-

TABLE 50-3. Major Gonadal Steroids in Adult Men

Steroid	Plasma Concentration (ng/dl)	Relative Androgenic Activity
Testosterone	650	100
Dihydrotestosterone	45	250–300
Androstenedione	120	10–20

mone–binding globulin, because it binds estradiol as well). A very small percentage of the plasma testosterone is unbound.

2. **Androstenedione** also is secreted by the testis at a rate of about 2.5 mg/day and is an important steroid precursor for blood estrogens in men.
   a. Many non-endocrine tissues (e.g., brain, skin, fat, liver, placenta, and gonads) have the enzyme CYP19 (cytochrome P450 aromatase), which converts testosterone to estradiol and androstenedione to estrone by peripheral conversion.
   b. Major portions of blood estradiol and estrone in normal men are derived from blood testosterone and androstenedione, respectively.
   c. In addition, the Sertoli and Leydig cells of the testis secrete small amounts of estradiol.

3. **Dihydrotestosterone** (DHT) is synthesized by the testis, probably because of the action of **5α-reductase** from the Sertoli cells on testosterone secreted by the Leydig cells.
   a. Only 20% of plasma dihydrotestosterone is synthesized in the testis. Most of the DHT is derived from the peripheral conversion of testosterone, which serves as a prohormone in the skin and male reproductive tract (prostate gland and seminal vesicles).
   b. DHT has more than twice the biologic activity of testosterone.

B. **Testicular steroidogenesis: the Leydig cell** (see Figure 49-2 and Table 49-3)
   1. Luteinizing hormone (LH) activates 20,22-desmolase (CYPIIAI) and, therefore, is the pituitary gonadotropin that regulates testosterone synthesis by the Leydig cells.
   2. The key step in steroidogenesis is the conversion of cholesterol to pregnenolone.
   3. The CYPIIAI enzyme is the rate-limiting enzyme for steroid synthesis in all steroid-producing tissues.
   4. In the developing male fetus, the stimulus for testosterone synthesis is HCG, which is the placental hormone secreted in highest amounts during the first trimester of pregnancy.
   5. Androgen biosynthesis in the human testis proceeds preferentially via the Δ^5 pathway from pregnenolone to dehydroepiandrosterone (DHEA) before entering the Δ^4 pathway as androstenedione and testosterone.
   6. Five enzymatic processes are involved in the conversion of cholesterol to testosterone.
      a. Side chain cleavage of cholesterol by 20,22-desmolase (CYPIIAI) to form pregnenolone
      b. Conversion of pregnenolone to 17α-hydroxypregnenolone via 17α-hydroxylase (CYP17)
      c. Conversion of 17α-hydroxypregnenolone to DHEA via 17,20-lyase (CYP17). **Enzyme CYP17 has both 17-hydroxylase and 17,20-lyase activities.**
      d. Conversion of DHEA to androstenedione via 3β-hydroxysteroid dehydrogenase (3β-HSD11)
      e. Reduction of androstenedione to testosterone via 17-hydroxysteroid dehydrogenase (CYP17 HSD)
   7. Some pregnenolone may be converted via 3β-HSDII to progesterone, which can be hy-

droxylated at the C-17 position (CYP17) prior to its conversion to androstenedione along the Δ^4 pathway.

8. Androstenedione is the common final precursor in the synthesis of testosterone.

9. The 17-ketosteroids (e.g., androstenedione) are, in effect, pro-androgens, since their peripheral conversion to the 17β-hydroxysteroids, testosterone and DHT, is required for biological activity (Figure 50-6).

C. **Metabolism**

1. **Dihydrotestosterone formation.** Testosterone can serve as a prohormone and be metabolized by 5α-reductase to the more active androgen, dihydrotestosterone. The activity of 5α-reductase is high in the skin, prostate gland, seminal vesicles, epididymis, and liver. This enzyme also is present in testicular tissue.

  a. Androgen target tissues are thought to be the principal sites of dihydrotestosterone formation. The nuclear membrane and microsomes of androgen-sensitive tissues are the physiologically important sites for conversion of testosterone to dihydrotestosterone. Therefore, dihydrotestosterone not only is secreted by the testis into the circulation but also is synthesized mainly from testosterone that has entered the cells of androgen-dependent tissues.

  b. The formation of dihydrotestosterone is an irreversible reduction reaction; therefore, dihydrotestosterone cannot serve as a proestrogen.

  c. The anlagen of the prostate gland and external genitalia can form dihydrotestosterone prior to the onset of virilization. Dihydrotestosterone is formed from testosterone prior to the secretion of significant amounts of testosterone from the testis. The wolffian duct derivatives can form dihydrotestosterone after the onset of androgen secretion and after differentiation of the male genital system is far advanced.

  d. Dihydrotestosterone can be metabolized further to 17-ketosteroids and polar derivatives found in the urine.

2. **Estradiol and estrone formation.** Testosterone and androstenedione can be converted to estradiol and estrone, respectively, by the action of aromatase. Thus, the estrogens in the male are derived from direct secretion by the testis and from peripheral conversion of circulating androstenedione and testosterone.

  a. Aromatization of circulating androgens is the major pathway for estrogen formation in the male.

  b. Aromatases are membrane-bound enzymes found in the brain, skin, liver, mammary tissues, and most significantly, the adipose tissue.

3. **17-Ketosteroid formation.** Testosterone can be metabolized to less active metabolites that are conjugated in the liver and excreted into the urine as 17-ketosteroids.

  a. **Androsterone** and **etiocholanolone** are the major urinary metabolites of testosterone. **Testosterone glucuronide** and **5α-androstanediol glucuronides** are among the other androgenic metabolites measured in urine.

    (1) Testosterone glucuronide originates mainly in the liver from testosterone, androstenedione, and dihydrotestosterone. The measurement of plasma testosterone is the mainstay for assessing Leydig cell function.

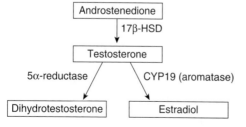

FIGURE 50-6. Conversion of the 17-ketosteroid androstenedione to testosterone via 17β-hydroxysteroid dehydrogenase and the conversion of testosterone to active metabolites in peripheral tissues (i.e., adipose tissue, liver, and target organs).

(2) 5α-Androstanediol glucuronides arise from the testosterone metabolites in both the liver and the skin. Because an increased 5α-reductase activity in the skin and other extrahepatic tissues is produced by increased androgen secretion, the measurement of urinary 5α-androstanediol glucuronides has been recommended as an index of clinical androgenicity.

b. The **excretory rate** for urinary 17-ketosteroids in normal men is 15–20 mg/day.

(1) Of this amount, 20%–40% are of testicular origin. The remainder are adrenocortical secretions, the major one of which is **dehydroepiandrosterone (DHEA).**

(2) Because the urinary 17-ketosteroid pool reflects mainly adrenocortical activity, a measurement of the 17-ketosteroid secretion is not a good index of testicular function.

IV. HORMONAL CONTROL OF TESTICULAR FUNCTION (Figures 50-7 and 50-8; see also Figure 46-3)

A. **Hypothalamic-hypophysial-seminiferous tubular axis:** Follicle-stimulating hormone (FSH)

1. The action of **FSH** appears to be on the Sertoli cell and not on spermatogonia themselves; however, the germinal epithelium is the primary site of **action** of FSH.

2. LH and FSH are required for spermatogenesis. Because the effects of LH are mediated by testosterone, testosterone and FSH are two hormones that act directly on Sertoli cells to promote gametogenesis and secretion of regulatory proteins.

a. Exogenous testosterone alone does not promote spermatogenesis in men lacking Leydig cells. Spermatogenesis requires that a high concentration of testosterone be produced locally by LH action on Leydig cells.

b. Sertoli cells synthesize **androgen-binding protein** by an FSH-dependent process. This protein binds testosterone and dihydrotestosterone, which provide a local androgenic pool to support spermatogenesis.

c. Sertoli cells also synthesize **inhibin** in response to FSH secretion. This protein inhibits FSH secretion by direct negative feedback on the pituitary gland. Inhibin is not known to suppress secretion of FSH-releasing hormone (GnRH), a decapeptide produced by the parvicellular peptidergic neurons. The selective rise in plasma FSH levels in individuals with damaged seminiferous tubules is from a reduced secretion of inhibin.

3. Normal spermatogenesis occurs in men with a 5α-reductase deficiency. Dihydrotestosterone is not required for normal sperm development.

4. Plasma physiologic levels of androgens have little effect on the inhibition of FSH secretion.

5. FSH indirectly affects testosterone synthesis by increasing the number of LH receptors on the Leydig cell.

6. Testosterone administration has little effect on FSH secretion, and very large doses are required to suppress FSH in the male.

B. **Hypothalamic-hypophysial-Leydig cell axis:** Luteinizing hormone (see Figures 46-3, 50-7, and 50-8)

1. **Gonadotropin-releasing hormone** (GnRH) is a decapeptide synthesized in the cell bodies of the parvicellular neurosecretory neurons in the hypothalamus and secreted into the hypophysioportal blood.

a. GnRH secretion is pulsatile and, in adult men, occurs at a frequency of 8 to 14 pulses per day.

b. The release of GnRH is controlled by peptidergic neurons whose axons are highly concentrated in the arcuate nucleus and the median eminence.

c. The secretion of LH has been shown to be concordant with the frequency of a hypothalamic "pulse generator."

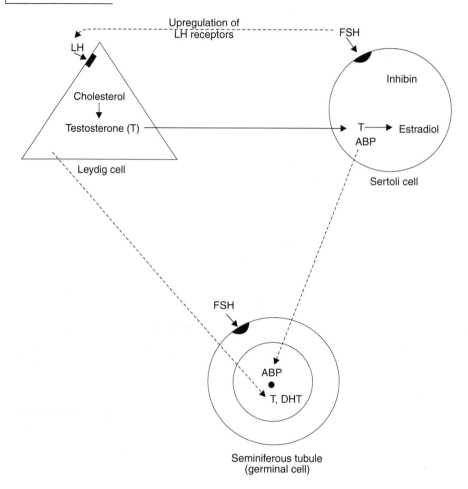

FIGURE 50-7. The triad model of the testis: Leydig cell, Sertoli cell, and germinal cell. Neither FSH nor LH appears to act directly on germ cells but affect germinal cell function by acting on the Sertoli cell and Leydig cell, respectively. LH binds to surface receptors on the Leydig cell and FSH binds to surface receptors on the Sertoli cell. However, the primary site of **action** of FSH is the epithelium of the seminiferous tubule (gametogenesis). Androgen receptors are present in Sertoli cells and Leydig cells but not in germinal epithelium. Androgen-binding protein (ABP) requires FSH and testosterone; therefore, androgen affects germinal cell function. FSH plays an indirect role in steroidogenesis by increasing the number of LH receptors on the Leydig cell. DHT = dihydrotestosterone.

2. The pituitary responds to GnRH with a synchronous secretion of LH and FSH, which stimulate steroidogenesis and gametogenesis, respectively.
   a. The LH receptors are located on the plasma membrane of the Leydig cell.
   b. The FSH receptors are found on the surface of the Sertoli cell.

3. The rate of testosterone synthesis and secretion by Leydig cells is stimulated primarily by LH. The secretion of testosterone, in turn, inhibits LH secretion. It is unbound testosterone that suppresses LH secretion. The major target of negative feedback is the hypothalamus.

4. Both testosterone and estradiol can inhibit LH secretion; however, since dihydrotestosterone can also suppress LH, androgen conversion to estrogen is not a prerequisite for this inhibitory action on the hypothalamus and pituitary gland.

5. Some neurosecretory neurons of the hypothalamus secrete a releasing hormone into the hypophysial portal system, which then conveys it to the anterior lobe of the pituitary gland.

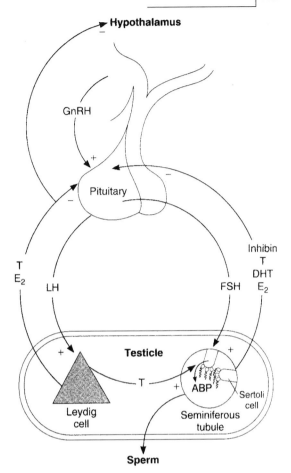

FIGURE 50-8. Hypothalamic-pituitary-testicular axis. Secretion of testosterone by the testis (Leydig cell) is stimulated by LH, whereas the maturation and growth of the tubule cells are stimulated by FSH. The secretion of testosterone in turn inhibits the secretion of LH; however, it is likely that the major target of negative feedback is the hypothalamus. A peptide secretion of the testis, inhibin, which is secreted by the tubular epithelium (Sertoli cell) exerts a direct inhibitory effect on FSH secretion. Testosterone negative feedback is exerted on neurons that project to the LHRH (GnRH) neurons and not on the LHRH peptidergic neurons themselves. $GnRH$ = gonadotropin-releasing hormone; LH = luteinizing hormone; FSH = follicle-stimulating hormone; T = testosterone; DHT = dihydrotestosterone; ABP = androgen-binding protein; E_2 = estradiol; + = positive influence; − = negative influence.

    a. GnRH stimulates the pituitary basophils.
    b. GnRH also is called LH-releasing hormone (LHRH) and FSHRH because it elicits the secretion of both LH and FSH.

  6. Testosterone and estradiol independently control LH secretion by negative feedback at two separate sites: the hypothalamus (GnRH) and the pituitary (LH).
    a. Testosterone negative feedback is exerted mainly on the opiatergic neurons that project to the LHRH neurons.
    b. Testosterone plays a minor role in the inhibition of LH secretion at the level of the pituitary.
    c. The negative feedback effects of estradiol are at both the hypothalamic and pituitary levels.
    d. In contrast to testosterone, estradiol exerts a significant direct inhibitory effect on LH secretion at the pituitary level.
    e. Inhibition of LHRH also occurs because of estradiol that is formed by local hypothalamic conversion of testosterone.

V. PHYSIOLOGIC EFFECTS OF ANDROGENS (Tables 50-4, 50-5, and 50-6)

A. **Reproductive function.** Androgens are essential for the control of spermatogenesis, the maintenance of the secondary sex characteristics, and the functional competence of the accessory sex organs.

TABLE 50-4. Major Actions of Androgenic Hormones

Life Stage	Testosterone	Dihydrotestosterone
Fetal period	Development of epididymis, vas deferens, and seminal vesicles	Development of penis, penile urethra, scrotum, and prostate gland
Puberty	Growth of penis, seminal vesicles, musculature, skeleton, and larynx	Growth of scrotum, prostate gland, pubic hair, and sebaceous glands
Adulthood	Spermatogenesis	Prostatic secretions

Reprinted from Genuth SM: The reproductive glands. In *Physiology,* 2nd ed. Edited by Berne RM, Levy MN. St. Louis, CV Mosby, 1988, p 999.

TABLE 50-5. Actions of Androgen

In utero
  External genitalia development (dihydrotestosterone)
  Wolffian duct development (testosterone)
Prepubertal
  Male behavioral effects
Pubertal
  External genitalia
    Penis and scrotum increase in size and become pigmented
    Rugal folds appear in scrotal skin
  Hair growth
    Mustache and beard develop; scalp line undergoes recession
    Pubic hair develops
    Axillary, body hair appears
  Linear growth
    Pubertal growth spurt
    Androgens interact with growth hormone to increase somatomedin C (IGF1) levels
  Accessory sex organs
    Prostate and seminal vesicles enlarge, and secretion begins
  Voice
    The pitch is lowered because of enlargement of larynx and thickening of vocal cords
  Psyche
    More aggressive attitudes are manifest
    Sexual potential develops
  Muscle mass
    Muscle bulk and strength increase
    Positive nitrogen balance
Adult
  Hair growth
    Androgenic patterns are maintained
    Male baldness may be initiated
  Psyche
    Behavioral attitudes and sexual potency are maintained
  Bone
    Bone loss and osteoporosis are prevented
  Spermatogenesis
    Interaction with FSH to modulate Sertoli cell function and stimulate spermatogenesis
  Hematopoiesis
    Erythropoietin-stimulated
    Direct marrow effect on erythropoiesis

TABLE 50-6. Physiologic and Biochemical Effects of Androgens

Testosterone	Dihydrotesterone
Stimulates differentiation of the wolffian ducts into the epididymis, vas deferens, and the seminal vesicles	Stimulates differentiation of the genital tubercle, genital swellings, genital folds, and urogenital sinus into penis, scrotum, penile urethra, and prostate, respectively, in the fetus
Causes enlargement of the larynx and thickening of the vocal cords resulting in a deeper voice	During puberty, promotes growth of the scrotum and prostate and stimulates prostatic secretions
Is the major local hormone required for initiation and maintenance of spermatogenesis. Stimulates pubertal growth spurt and terminates linear bone growth by acceleration of epiphyseal closure	Stimulates the hair follicles and produces the male pattern of hair growth characterized by beard growth, diamond-shaped pubic escutcheon, relatively large amounts of body hair, and the recession of the temporal hairline (which in some men culminates in baldness)
Causes enlargement of the penis and seminal vesicles (with or without dihydrotestosterone)	Increases production of sebum by the sebaceous glands with consequent development of acne, especially during puberty
Causes enlargement of the muscle mass (especially shoulder and pectoral muscles) at puberty	
Causes nitrogen retention (positive nitrogen balance) accounting for protein anabolism	
Androgen suppression of LHRH and LH by negative feedback is largely a function of testosterone	
Increases circulating levels of low-density lipoprotein (LDL) cholesterol and decreases plasma high-density lipoprotein (HDL) cholesterol	
Favors accumulation of upper body, abdominal, and visceral fat	
Stimulates erythropoiesis	
Stimulates renal Na^+ reabsorption	
Initiation of sexual drive (libido) and erectile function (potency)	

1. The accessory sex organs consist of excretory ducts and glands that transmit spermatozoa and that secrete seminal fluid necessary for the survival and motility of spermatozoa after ejaculation. The major accessory sex organs are the prostate gland and seminal vesicles.

2. The secondary sex characteristics are the physiologic characteristics of masculinity (e.g., growth of facial hair, recession of hair at the temples, enlargement of the larynx, thickening of the vocal cords).

3. Seminal plasma, the fluid in which spermatozoa normally are ejaculated, originates almost entirely from the prostate gland and seminal vesicles.
    a. The volume of the human ejaculate (semen) is 2–5 ml, most of which is contributed by the seminal vesicles.
        (1) The prostate gland is the origin of citric acid, acid phosphatase, zinc, and spermine.
        (2) The seminal vesicles are the source of prostaglandins, fructose, ascorbic acid, and phosphorylcholine. Metabolism of fructose provides energy for sperm motility.

    b. Sperm represents less than 10% of the ejaculate volume. The ejaculate contains about 120 million spermatozoa per ml of semen, for a total of approximately 400 million sperm cells.

B. **Biologic effects** (see Table 50-6). Androgens stimulate cell division as well as tissue growth and maturation and are classified as protein anabolic hormones. (This anabolic effect in muscle is referred to as the **myotropic effect** of androgens.) Only testosterone and dihydrotestosterone have significant biologic activity. The 17-ketosteroids, androstenedione, DHEA, and etiocholanolone, are weak androgens but important metabolites of testosterone.

    1. In the adolescent, androgens produce linear growth, muscular development, and retention of nitrogen, potassium, and phosphorus. Testosterone also accelerates epiphysial fusion of the long bones. The skeletal development during puberty, particularly of the shoulder girdle, is pronounced. Dihydrotestosterone is the active androgen in all adult tissues containing 5α-reductase, **with the notable exception of muscle.**

    2. Testosterone stimulates differentiation of the wolffian duct system into the epididymis, vas deferens, and seminal vesicles; dihydrotestosterone stimulates organogenesis of the urogenital sinus and tubercle into the prostate gland, penis, urethra, and scrotum.

    3. Androgens produce a low-pitched voice; stimulate growth of chest, axillary, and facial hair; and cause temporal hair recession.

    4. Androgens are responsible for libido and potentia.

    5. Testosterone is a requisite for normal spermatogenesis.

    6. Regulation of gonadotropin secretion

VI. THE NEGATIVE FEEDBACK PARADIGM: INTERPRETATIONS OF ALTERATIONS IN TROPIC AND TARGET HORMONE PAIRS (Table 50-7 and Figure 50-9)

A. Almost all hormone systems are under some regulatory feedback control; measuring both members of a hormone pair (e.g., testosterone and LH) provides information that is not apparent from individual measurements.

    1. This relationship can be applied to pituitary tropic hormones and the hormones secreted by their target glands.

    2. This same relationship can also apply to ionized Ca^{2+} and parathyroid hormone; glucose and insulin; plasma osmolality and antidiuretic hormone; and Na^+ and aldosterone.

TABLE 50-7. Interpretations of Alterations in Tropic and Target Gland Hormones Based on Negative Feedback Control Systems

Condition	Sex Steroids	LH	FSH
Removal of gonads	↓	↑	↑
Postmenopausal women	↓	↑	↑
Administration of testosterone (or methyl testosterone)	↑	↓	(↓)
Administration of inhibin	—	—	↓
Constant infusion of GnRH	↓	↓	↓

LH = luteinizing hormone; FSH = follicle-stimulating hormone; GnRH = gonadotropin-releasing hormone.

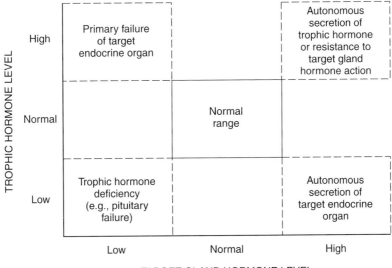

FIGURE 50-9. Paradigm depicting interpretations of alterations in tropic and target gland hormone pairs (e.g., testosterone and LH). It can also be used for hormones and substances that are regulated by that hormone (e.g., Ca^{2+} and parathyroid hormone, Na^+ and aldosterone, and glucose and insulin). The independent variable is on the abscissa and the dependent variable is on the ordinate. From Griffin JE, Ojeda SR (eds): *Textbook of Endocrinology,* 3rd ed. New York, Oxford University Press, 1996, p 94.

B. The measurement of the hormone pair permits the assessment of the effects of a hormone on its regulatory control mechanism.

   1. In the context of the pituitary and its target endocrine glands, finding low levels of both members of the hormone pair indicates the major lesion to be a tropic hormone deficiency.

   2. High levels of target hormone coupled with low levels of tropic hormone indicate autonomous secretion of the target endocrine organ or treatment with exogenous hormones.

   3. Elevated levels of both members of a hormone pair can suggest several forms of hormonal imbalance.

   a. Autonomous secretion of a tropic hormone can arise at the normal (endocrine) site or at an ectopic (non-endocrine) site.

   b. Combined elevations in tropic and target hormone can result from resistance to the action of the target endocrine gland hormone.

   c. The cause of the elevation of both members of a hormone pair can often be determined from the clinical findings.

   (1) Autonomous hypersecretion of the tropic hormone results in clinical evidence of target gland hormone excess.

   (2) Target hormone resistance is usually associated with target gland hormone deficiency.

Case

An 18-year-old woman consulted a physician because of her failure to initiate menses (menarche). She had experienced normal breast development at age 12 years, but no pubic or axillary hair had ever appeared. Her height is 5 ft 6 in; weight, 120 lb, blood pressure, 110/70 mmHg; and pulse, 60 beats/min. She swims competitively but denies steroid use. She also trains daily by swimming laps for 2 hours. The general physical examination was normal and confirmed

the presence of well-developed breasts. The external genitalia were those of a normal female. The vagina, however, ended in a blind pouch and no cervix was seen. Neither ovaries nor a uterus was palpable. Within the inguinal areas, a 1.5-cm mass was felt on each side. Use Figures 50-C1 and 50-C2, Tables 50-C1 and 50-C2, and the following discussion to assist in the diagnosis of this patient.

DISCUSSION

The complete form of testicular feminization has been recognized for years. Patients are phenotypic women who come to medical attention because of inguinal hernias (infants) or because of primary amenorrhea (adolescents). The phenotype is of a normal woman except axillary and pubic hair are diminished. Breast development and distribution of body fat are feminine; the external genitalia are unambiguously female; and the clitoris is normal. The vagina is short and blind-ending; the uterus and oviducts are absent; testes are located in the abdomen, the inguinal canal, or labia majora. Spermatogenesis is absent.

> **1.** From these findings, what do you suggest for a diagnosis?

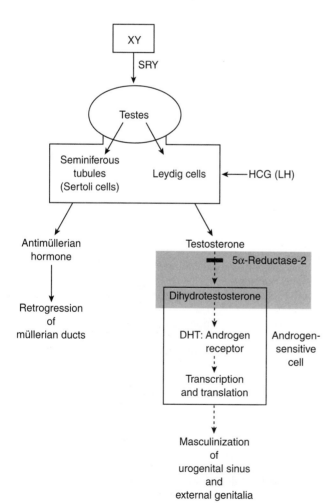

FIGURE 50-C1. A diagrammatic scheme of male pseudohermaphroditism caused by complete or partial androgen resistance illustrating defects in the androgen receptor that result in absent or reduced binding of androgens or impaired function of the ligand-bound receptor.

TABLE 50-C1. Clinical Features of Complete Androgen Resistance

Karyotype:	46,XY
Inheritance:	X-linked recessive
Genitalia:	Female with blind vaginal pouch
Wolffian duct derivatives:	Usually absent; less commonly, rudimentary or hypoplastic
Müllerian duct derivatives:	Absent or vestigial
Gonads:	Testes
Habitus:	Scant or absent pubic and axillary hair; breast development and female habitus at puberty; primary amenorrhea ("hairless woman")
Hormone and metabolic profile:	Increased plasma LH and testosterone concentration; increased estradiol (for men); FSH levels often normal or slightly increased Resistance to androgenic and metabolic effects of testosterone
Androgen receptor studies:	Genetic heterogeneity; mutations can lead to low or undetectable amount of normal receptor (receptor-negative), unstable receptor (thermolabile, partial receptor deficiency), or the receptor-positive form

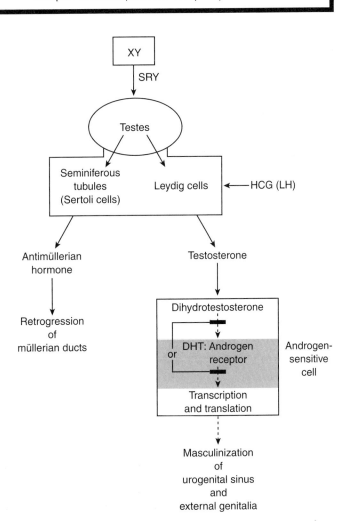

FIGURE 50-C2. A diagrammatic scheme of male pseudohermaphroditism resulting from 5α-reductase deficiency.

TABLE 50-C2. Clinical Features of 5α-Reductase-2 Deficiency

Karyotype:	46,XY
Inheritance:	Autosomal recessive
Genitalia:	Usually ambiguous with small, hypospadiac phallus; blind vaginal pouch
Wolffian duct derivatives:	Normal
Müllerian duct derivatives:	Absent
Gonads:	Normal testes
Habitus:	Partial virilization at puberty without gynecomastia; decreased facial and body hair, no temporal hair recession; prostate not palpable
Hormone profile:	Decreased ratio of 5α/5β C_{21}- and C_{19}-steroids in urine; increased plasma testosterone/dihydrotestosterone (T/DHT) ratio before and after HCG stimulation; modest increase in plasma LH and decreased conversion of T to DHT in vivo

DISCUSSION

This individual could have an XX karyotype. The blind ending to the vagina and absence of the uterus could be explained by failure of embryologic development of the müllerian ducts bilaterally. This, however, would not explain the presence of apparent gonads in the inguinal canals, nor would it explain the absence of sexual hair, which implies deficient androgenic stimulation.

This phenotypic female patient is an example of male pseudohermaphroditism where the gonads are exclusively testes but the genital ducts or genitalia or both are incompletely masculinized. Two major forms of this condition have been identified: end-organ resistance to androgenic hormones (testicular feminization syndrome) and errors in testosterone metabolism by peripheral tissues (5α-reductase deficiency). This patient presents with unambiguous female external genitalia; a blind vaginal pouch; absent müllerian structures (uterus, oviducts); testes located in the inguinal canal; and usually absent wolffian derivatives. At adolescence, female secondary sexual characteristics developed and include normal breasts and female body habitus but no menses. Pubic and axillary hair is sparse or absent, as in this patient.

If this patient had 5α-reductase deficiency, the wolffian derivatives would be normal with ambiguous external genitalia. At puberty there would be virilization without gynecomastia and the prostate would not be palpable. This patient also has normal testes.

    2. *Does she exhibit primary or secondary amenorrhea?*

DISCUSSION

The patient exhibits primary amenorrhea because the patient has never experienced menses.

    3. *Could this individual have an XY sex chromosome karyotype? If so, what diagnoses might explain her condition? What would be inconsistent with each of these possibilities?*

DISCUSSION

This individual certainly could have an XY chromosome karyotype. If she were XY, the completely female external genitalia suggest an absence of androgenic activity, because androgens are required to masculinize the external genitalia in a normal male. The lack of sexual hair confirms the absence of androgenic activity. The lack of androgen could also be accounted for by a defect in the synthesis of testosterone, by deficient production of dihydrotestosterone from testosterone because of deficiency of the enzyme 5α-reductase, or by the lack of an androgen receptor.

Defects in testosterone synthesis are usually partial and do not produce absolute androgen deficiency. Therefore, wolffian duct development occurs, and external genitalia are ambiguous rather than completely feminine. A lack of testosterone would also not account for the breast development, because the breasts are estrogen dependent and androgens are a necessary precursor to estrogen synthesis. Dihydrotestosterone is required for in utero masculinization of the external genitalia (though not for wolffian duct development). Hence, dihydrotestosterone deficiency could account for the feminine pattern. However, during puberty, testosterone itself, without conversion to dihydrotestosterone, can stimulate growth of the penis, but this obviously did not occur in the patient.

Dihydrotestosterone deficiency would also not induce marked breast development, because normal testosterone levels would still balance normal estrogen levels and inhibit breast development in an XY individual. **Absence of the androgen receptor would explain all of the patient's findings.** Without tissue receptors, testosterone could not promote wolffian duct development, and dihydrotestosterone could not masculinize the external genitalia. The growth of sexual hair could not be stimulated. Lack of androgen receptor in the breast tissue would also allow unopposed estrogen action and therefore normal or even excessive breast development.

    4. What are the inguinal masses likely to look like histologically?

DISCUSSION

The inguinal masses in the XY individual would be testes, because differentiation of the indifferent gonads into testes requires the Y chromosome. The spermatogenic apparatus would be poorly developed, however, because of the lack of essential local testosterone action on Sertoli cells and possibly on the germ cells themselves. The Leydig cells would be hyperplastic, reflecting high rates of testosterone production. This would compensate for resistance to the testosterone action caused by androgen receptor deficiency.

    5. For this karyotype, what are the patient's plasma levels of estradiol, testosterone, LH, and FSH likely to be?

DISCUSSION

For this XY individual, the plasma LH level would be elevated because of loss of negative feedback by testosterone on the pituitary gonadotrophs, which would also lack the androgen receptor. The high LH levels would stimulate increased secretion of testosterone by the hyperplastic Leydig cells. In turn, high testosterone levels would lead to overproduction of estradiol by the testes and also by peripheral conversion. The plasma level of FSH would be normal because of normal production of inhibin by the Sertoli cells.

If this were an XX individual with failure of müllerian duct development, the levels of testosterone, estradiol, LH, and FSH in the plasma would all be normal.

In an XO individual, plasma estradiol would be low because granulosa cell function is absent. Plasma testosterone might also be low because of a lack of theca cell function. Plasma LH would be high because of a lack of negative feedback by estradiol. Plasma FSH would be high because of a lack of inhibin production caused by absence of granulosa cells.

    6. Comment on the development of her internal genitalia.

DISCUSSION

The müllerian duct derivatives are absent because of the Sertoli cell secretion of AMH and the wolffian duct derivatives are absent or vestigial due to androgen (testosterone) resistance.

    7. Do you think this patient has a prostate gland?

DISCUSSION

The primary defect is a deficient number of androgen receptors for dihydrotestosterone and testosterone. Therefore, the prostate is hypoplastic and not palpable.

> **8.** *Why could you rule out a congenital isolated GnRH deficiency?*

DISCUSSION

GnRH deficiency is ruled out because of a number of a hormonally-dependent responses. Müllerian duct regression requires a functional testis in terms of Sertoli cell function and therefore, FSH section. Testosterone production and secretion requires LH secretion, which regulates Leydig cell function. The hallmark of androgen resistance is an elevated plasma LH and testosterone in the absence of virilization. Breast development requires estradiol formation from aromatization of testosterone. Deficiency of GnRH is ruled out by the presence of breast development.

> **9.** *Would a 17-hydroxylase deficiency be consistent with the findings in this patient?*

DISCUSSION

No. An adrenogenital syndrome due to a 17-hydroxylase deficiency is associated with retardation of sexual development in both males and females.

> **10.** *Is this patient an example of male or female pseudohermaphroditism?*

DISCUSSION

This patient is an example of male pseudohermaphroditism because the gonads are exclusively testes but the genital ducts and external genitalia are incompletely masculinized. This karyotypic male is phenotypically female.

> **11.** *Do you think that this patient had a 5α-reductase deficiency?* Explain your answer.

DISCUSSION

No. With a 5α-reductase deficiency, there is partial virilization at puberty without gynecomastia. Also, there would be normal wolffian duct differentiation in this enzyme deficiency (see Table 50-C2).

> **12.** *Predict the response to exogenous testosterone administration.*

DISCUSSION

This patient would not be responsive to exogenous testosterone treatment. It would not be indicated to inform the patient directly that genetic sex and phenotypic sex do not coincide. It would probably be prudent to remove the testes before puberty or soon after it begins, and to follow this with estrogen therapy to promote the development of female secondary sexual characteristics. This 46,XY patient who was raised as a female should not be a candidate for gender reassignment. Following the above therapeutic measures, it is very probably that this woman could marry and have a normal sexual life. Of course, she could not have children.

Chapter 51
Ovary and Placenta

I. **OVARY**

A. **Embryology**

1. **Internal genitalia** (see Figure 50-1). The primordia of both male and female genital ducts, which are derived from the mesonephros, are present in the fetus at 7 weeks gestation. The paired **müllerian ducts** form parallel to the paired **wolffian ducts.** In the female fetus, the upper ends of the müllerian ducts are the anlagen of the fallopian tubes (oviducts), whereas the lower ends join to form the uterus, cervix, and upper end of the vagina.

   a. The uterus and fallopian tubes, which develop from the müllerian ducts, do not require the presence of an ovary.

   b. In the absence of a fetal testis, müllerian duct–inhibiting factor (antimüllerian hormone) and testosterone are not secreted by the fetal Sertoli cells and Leydig cells, respectively. Moreover, dihydrotestosterone is not formed from testosterone. Without the presence of these three hormones, at 10–11 weeks gestation, the müllerian ducts begin to differentiate and the wolffian ducts undergo regression.

   c. This process of female genital duct development is completed at 18–20 weeks gestation.

2. **External genitalia**

   a. The external genitalia of both sexes begin to differentiate at 9–10 weeks gestation. In the female, this process proceeds without any known hormonal influence.

   b. The external genitalia and urethra in both sexes develop from common anlagen, which are the urogenital sinus and the genital tubercle, genital folds, and genital swelling.

      (1) The urogenital sinus gives rise to the lower portion of the vagina and to the urethra.

      (2) The genital tubercle is the origin of the clitoris.

      (3) The genital swelling is the primordium of the labia majora.

      (4) The genital folds develop into the labia minora.

3. **Ovary.** In the absence of the H-Y antigen, the gonadal primordium develops into an ovary, provided that germ cells are present. Ovarian development occurs several weeks later than does testicular differentiation.

   a. At 8 weeks, when the testicular secretion of testosterone begins and before the ovarian differentiation is completed, the fetal "ovary" has the capacity to synthesize **estradiol.**

      (1) It is unlikely that the fetal ovary contributes significantly to the circulating estrogens in the fetus. The fetus is exposed to estrogen (**estriol**) of placental origin. The site of estradiol synthesis by the primordial ovary is not known.

      (2) The ovary has no role in sex differentiation of the female genital tract.

   b. Also at about 8 weeks gestation, the cortex of the primitive gonad undergoes active mitosis, and epithelial cells infiltrate the gonad as a syncytium of tubules and cords. Primordial germ cells are carried along with this inward migration.

      (1) Proliferation of the cortex ceases at about 6 months.

      (2) The **rete ovarii** secretes a meiosis-inducing factor.

      (3) The germ cells begin to proliferate to form **oogonia.** This mitotic process is maximal between 8 and 20 weeks, after which it diminishes, ceases, and never is resumed.

   c. Unlike the fetal testis, the fetal ovary begins gametogenesis. **Oogenesis,** the formation of primary oocytes from oogonia, begins at 15 weeks and reaches a peak between 20 and 28 weeks gestation (Figure 51-1).

      (1) The oogonium is unique in that it is the only female cell in which both X chromosomes are active.

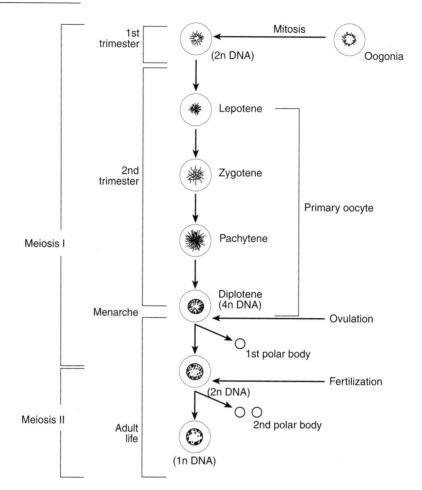

FIGURE 51-1. The life cycle of the oocyte. During the first trimester of fetal life, the oogonium undergoes mitosis. The first meiotic division (meiosis I) begins during the second trimester but is arrested at the diplotene stage (4n DNA). After menarche, at the time of ovulation, meiosis I resumes in the oocyte with the extrusion of the first polar body (2n DNA). Meiosis II is initiated at the time of fertilization and is completed with the extrusion of the second polar body (1n DNA) immediately following conception. Fusion with the male pronucleus restores the nuclear content to 2n DNA. One X chromosome is inactivated in the female early in development and can be visualized as an A chromatin or Barr body in the inner surface of the nuclear membrane of somatic cells. Note that when mitotic division ceases and the cells enter meiosis, they are then termed oocytes.

      (2) The **primary oocytes** enter a prolonged prophase (diplotene stage) of the first meiotic division and remain in this state until ovulation occurs over a period from 12 to 50 years later.
          (a) Before ovulation, the first polar body is extruded, thus completing the first meiotic division.
          (b) The haploid secondary oocyte immediately begins a second meiotic division but remains in metaphase and does not extrude the second polar body until the ovum is penetrated by a sperm.
      (3) The **diploid primary oocytes** become enveloped by a single layer of flat granulosa cells and in this form are called **primordial follicles.** The formation of primordial follicles reaches a peak between 20 and 25 weeks.
      (4) The primordial follicle is the morphologic marker of fetal ovarian development.
   d. Also between 20 and 25 weeks, the gonad has acquired the morphologic appearance

of an ovary. During this period, the plasma concentration of pituitary FSH reaches a peak and the first **primary follicles** appear [see I B 1 b].

B. **Ovarian follicles: Folliculogenesis** (Figure 51-2)

1. There are two major classes of follicles: **nongrowing** and **growing.**
    a. **Nongrowing follicles**
       (1) The primordial follicles represent a pool of nongrowing follicles.
       (2) The primordial follicles are formed in the fetal ovary between the sixth and ninth months of gestation.
       (3) Since the primary oocytes in the follicle have entered meiotic prophase, all oocytes that are capable of participating in reproduction during a woman's life are formed at birth.
    b. **Growing follicles,** which are recruited from the primordial follicles, can be divided into five classes: primary, secondary, tertiary, graafian, and atretic.
       (1) The first three stages of growth can occur in the absence of the pituitary.
       (2) A recruited primordial follicle can differentiate into the primary, secondary, and early tertiary in the absence of the pituitary; therefore, the differentiation of the preantral follicle does not require FSH.
       (3) When a growing follicle reaches the early tertiary stage, its continued development depends on FSH.

2. **Preantral follicles**
    a. **Primordial follicles** represent a pool of **nongrowing** follicles from which all dominant preovulatory follicles are selected.
       (1) Each primordial follicle is composed of an outer single layer of granulosa cells and a small immature oocyte arrested in the dictyotene stage of meiosis.
       (2) Both the granulosa and the oocyte are enveloped in a thin membrane called the basal lamina.
       (3) These follicles (oocyte and granulosa cells) lack a direct blood supply.
       (4) The primordial follicle is the fundamental reproductive unit of the ovary.
       (5) The number of primordial follicles (and thus oocytes) decreases from several million at birth to several hundred thousand at menarche.
    b. **Primary follicles** form when the flattened epithelial cells become cuboidal inside the basal lamina and undergo mitotic division to form a multilayered stratum granulosum.
       (1) The oocyte enlarges and forms a band of mucoid substance called the zona pellucida.
       (2) The zona pellucida separates the granulosa cells from the oocyte.
    c. **Secondary follicles** are formed by further proliferation of granulosa cells and by the final phase of oocyte growth.
       (1) Stromal cells outside the basal lamina differentiate into a concentric connective tissue layer which gives rise to the follicular theca.
          (a) The portion of the theca contiguous to basal lamina forms the theca interna.
          (b) The thecal cells that merge with the surrounding stroma are designated theca externa.
       (2) The secondary follicle acquires an independent blood supply consisting of arterioles that do not penetrate the basal lamina.
    d. **Tertiary follicles** are characterized by further hypertrophy of the theca and the early process of antrum formation called cavitation.
       (1) The antrum is a fluid-filled space and contains estrogen.
       (2) The theca interna is transformed into theca interstitial cells which will become steroidogenic cells which synthesize and secrete androgens (androstenedione) in response to gonadotropins (FSH and LH).
       (3) The oocyte and the granulosa remain avascular.

3. **Antral (graafian) follicles** (see Figure 51-2)
    a. In response to gonadotropins (FSH and LH), the follicle increases in size to form a graafian follicle.
       (1) If a tertiary follicle is selected to ovulate it may grow 75-fold, increasing from 0.4 mm to 30 mm in diameter.

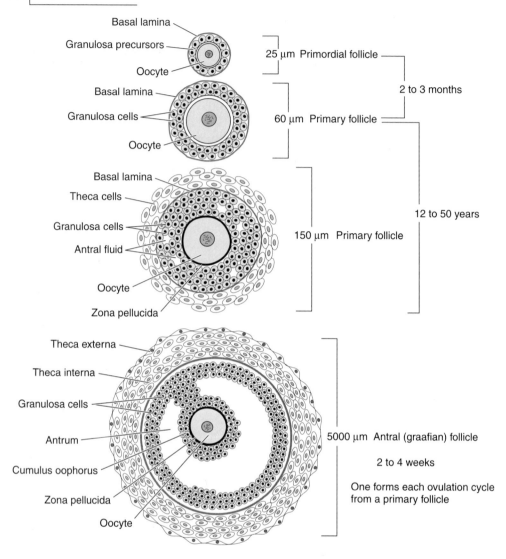

FIGURE 51-2. Schematic representation of the development of an ovarian follicle (not to scale). (Redrawn from Berne RM, Levy MN: *Physiology.* St. Louis, Mosby, 1983, pp 1069–1115, with permission. From Griffen JE, Ojeda SR, editors: *Textbook of Endocrinology,* 3rd ed. New York, Oxford University Press, p 176.)

        (2) The growth of the graafian follicle is accomplished by granulosa and theca prolif-
eration and follicular fluid accumulation in the antrum.
    b. The average time for the development of a primary follicle to the point of ovulation is
10 to 14 days.
  4. Atretic follicles
    a. Once a primordial follicle is recruited to initiate growth, it either develops into a
dominant preovulatory follicle or it degenerates by a process termed **atresia.**
    b. The atresia of follicles is due to apoptosis.

C. **The corpus luteum**

  1. The extrusion of the mature oocyte (secondary) from the ovary is caused by an LH surge
at midcycle in response to an elevation in plasma estradiol concentration [150 picograms
per ml (pg/ml)].

a. The **onset** of the LH surge occurs 34 to 36 hours before ovulation.

b. The **peak** of the LH surge occurs 12 to 24 hours before ovulation.

c. At midcycle of the menstrual cycle LH initiates the resumption of meiosis and the secondary oocyte reaches the second meiotic metaphase following the extrusion of the first polar body just prior to ovulation. Ovulation occurs 16 to 20 hours after the peak of the LH surge.

d. Meiosis is again arrested, and is completed with the release of the second polar body immediately following fertilization.

2. After ovulation the basement membrane separating the granulosa from the theca breaks down and blood vessels invade the granulosa cells.

3. The cells of the corpus luteum are derived from both the follicle and the theca.

a. The granulosa cells become the granulosa-lutein cells (large cells).

b. The theca cells are transformed into the theca-lutein cells (small cells).

D. **Oogenesis** (see Figures 51-1 and 51-2)

1. **Fetal oogenesis.** The period of oogonial proliferation results in a peak population of about 6–7 million germ cells in the two ovaries at 5 months gestation. Included in this group of cells are oogonia, oocytes in various stages of prophase, and degenerating germ cells. This total number of germ cells decreases to 2 million at term. The number of primordial follicles present in the ovary at birth rapidly diminishes thereafter.

2. **Postnatal oogenesis.** By 6 months postpartum, all of the oogonia have been converted to primary oocytes. By the onset of puberty, the number of primary oocytes has decreased to about 400,000.

3. **Prepubertal oogenesis.** Between birth and puberty, the primary oocyte is surrounded by the zona pellucida and six to nine layers of granulosa cells. These follicles are in varying stages of development.

4. **Pubertal oogenesis.** In contrast to the male who produces spermatogonia and primary spermatocytes continuously throughout life, the female cannot form oogonia beyond 28 weeks gestation and must function with a declining pool of oocytes.

a. Meiosis in the female results in the formation of one viable oocyte. In contrast, each primary spermatogoniurn in the male ultimately gives rise to 64 spermatozoa.

b. Oogenesis in the female begins in utero in response to meiosis-stimulating factor, whereas in the male, spermatogenesis is arrested at the spermatogonial stage in response to meiosis-inhibiting factor.

c. Just prior to ovulation, the first polar body is extruded from the primary oocyte, which completes the first meiotic division, and forms a secondary oocyte.

(1) This haploid cell immediately begins the second meiotic division but remains in metaphase.

(2) Extrusion of the second polar body (**polocyte**) does not occur until the mature ovum (ootid) is fertilized by a sperm cell. Fertilization normally occurs in the ampulla of the fallopian tube.

E. **Morphology**

1. **Gross anatomy**

a. The ovaries are ovoid glands with a combined weight of 10–20 g during the reproductive years.

b. The ovaries are anchored to the **broad ligament** by the **mesovarium.**

2. **Functional histology of the ovary and uterus**

a. **Ovary**

(1) **Structural divisions** include the **cortex** (which is lined by the germinal epithelium and contains all of the oocytes), the **inner medulla,** and the **hilus** (i.e., the point where the ovary attaches to the mesentery).

(2) **Functional subunits** include the **follicle** and **oocyte** (each consisting of **theca cells** and **granulosa cells**) and the **corpus luteum.**

(3) Gametogenesis in the female denotes **folliculogenesis,** which leads to the formation of a mature ovum.
   (a) During the preovulatory phase, the functional unit of the ovary is the follicle.
   (b) During the postovulatory phase, the functional unit of the ovary is the corpus luteum.
(4) Steroidogenesis in the ovary is the synthesis and secretion of **estradiol** and **progesterone.** Although steroidogenesis occurs in three morphologic units (i.e., the follicle, corpus luteum, and stroma), only the follicle and corpus luteum are major steroid-producing units.
   (a) Theca (interna) cells produce androstenedione and testosterone, which diffuse into the granulosa cells.
   (b) Granulosa cells synthesize estradiol and estrone from androgenic precursors produced by the theca cells.

b. Uterus
   (1) Layers. The uterus consists of two major tissue layers.
      (a) The outer layer, the **myometrium,** is a thick layer of smooth muscle.
      (b) The inner layer of the uterus is the **endometrium.** At the height of its development, during the luteal phase, the endometrium is approximately 5 mm thick. On the basis of blood supply, the endometrium can be divided into two major layers.
         (i) The **stratum basale** (stratum basalis) is the abluminal (deeper) layer of the endometrium. This layer functions as the regenerative layer in the growth and differentiation of endometrial tissue that is sloughed during menses.
         (ii) The **stratum functionale** (stratum functionalis) is the adluminal (superficial) layer of the endometrium, which is shed during menses.
   (2) Endometrial blood supply
      (a) The stratum basale receives its vascular supply from the **basal (straight) arterioles,** which arise from the uterine radial arteries.
      (b) The stratum functionale is perfused by the **spiral (coiled) arterioles,** which also emanate from the radial arteries.
      (c) Thus, the arcuate arteries give off radial arteries, and the radial arteries bifurcate to form the basal and coiled arteries.

F. **Hormones of the ovary: steroids.** Ovarian hormones include two phenolic steroids—**estradiol** (C-18) and **estrone** (C-18)—and the progestogen, **progesterone** (C-21).

1. Secretion and transport (Tables 51-1 and 51-2)
   a. Estrogens. Over 70% of circulating estrogens are bound to sex steroid-binding globulin, and 25% are bound to plasma albumin.
      (1) Estradiol is the principal and biologically most active estrogen secreted by the ovary. Ovarian estradiol accounts for more than 90% of the circulating estradiol.
      (2) Estrone, a weak ovarian estrogen, also is formed by the peripheral conversion of **androstenedione.**
         (a) In premenopausal women, most of the circulating estrone is derived from estradiol by conversion via 17-hydroxysteroid dehydrogenase (17β-HSD).
         (b) In postmenopausal women, estrone is the dominant plasma estrogen and is derived via the prohormone pathway. Specifically, estrone is derived from the conversion of adrenocortical androstenedione in peripheral tissues (mainly liver). In obese women, there is a significant peripheral conversion of androstenedione to estrone by adipose tissue. This extraovarian synthesis of estrogen is implicated in the higher incidence of endometrial carcinoma in obese women.
      (3) Estriol, the weakest of all the naturally occurring estrogens, is synthesized by the placenta and the liver but not the ovary. In nongravid women, estriol is formed in the liver as a conversion product of estradiol and estrone.
   b. Progesterone is not bound to sex hormone-binding globulin. The progesterone is bound primarily to CBG (transcortin) and albumin.

2. Ovarian steroidogenesis (Figure 51-3; see also Figure 49-2). The two pathways for biosynthesis of ovarian steroids have in common the conversion of cholesterol to pregnenolone, a reaction stimulated by LH and FSH via 20,22-desmolase.

TABLE 51-1. Types of Steroids and their Systemic Concentrations and Rates of Synthesis in Women

Steroid	Plasma Concentration (ng/dl)	Production Rate (μg/day)
Estrogens (C-18)		
Estradiol		
Early follicular phase	6	80
Late follicular phase	50	700
Middle luteal phase	20	300
Estrone (C-18)		
Early follicular phase	5	100
Late follicular phase	20	500
Middle luteal phase	10	250
Progestogens (C-21)		
17-Hydroxyprogesterone		
Early follicular phase	30	600
Late follicular phase	200	4000
Middle luteal phase	200	4000
Progesterone (C-21)		
Follicular phase	100	2000
Luteal phase	1000	25,000
Testosterone (C-19)	40	250
Dihydrotestosterone (C-19)	20	50
Androstenedione (C-19)	150	3000
Dehydroepiandrosterone (C-19)	500	8000

Reprinted from Lipsett MB: Steroid hormones. In *Reproductive Endrocrinology: Physiology, Pathophysiology and Management.* Edited by Yen SSC, Jaffe RB. Philadelphia, WB Saunders, 1978, p 84.

TABLE 51-2. Serum FSH and LH Concentrations During the Life Cycle of the Normal Female*

Stage of Life	FSH[†]	LH[†]
Prepubertal period (5–11 years)	4.5	3.9
Puberty (11–13 years)	6.8	8.2
Reproductive period		
Follicular phase	8.3	12.8
Midcycle	19.3	83.5
Luteal phase	6.9	11.6
Postmenopausal period	96.0	66.0

Adapted from Ontjes DA, Walton J, Ney RL: The anterior pituitary gland. In *Metabolic Control of Disease,* 8th edition. Edited by Bondy PK, Rosenberg LE. Philadelphia, WB Saunders, 1980, p 1192.

*Mean values without standard deviations.

[†]Concentrations expressed in milli-International units.

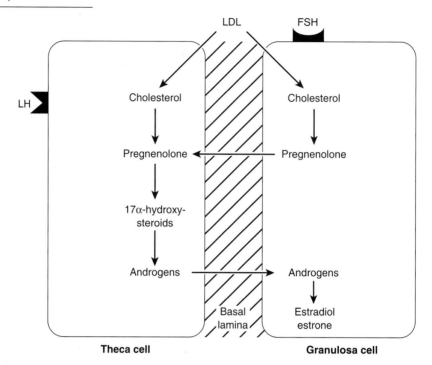

FIGURE 51-3. The two cell-two gonadotropin ovarian model. The theca* and granulosa cells cooperate in the synthesis of estrogen. The theca cells produce mainly androgens in response to LH; the granulosa cells respond to FSH by producing pregnenolone from plasma cholesterol, and by aromatizing androgens to estrogens. *LDL* = low-density lipoproteins. (From Goodman HM: *Basic Medical Endocrinology,* 2nd edition. New York, Raven Press, 1994, p 281.)

    a. One pathway proceeds by way of the Δ^5-pathway, which involves the synthesis of 17α-hydroxypregnenolone and DHEA via 17α-hydroxylase and 17,20-lyase, respectively.

    b. CYP17 is an enzyme that catalyzes both the hydroxylation of the C-17 of progesterone or pregnenolone (17α-hydroxylase) **and** the cleavage of the 2-carbon side chain at C-17 (17,20-lyase**).

        (1) DHEA,[†] a 17-ketosteroid, is converted to another androgenic 17-ketosteroid, androstenedione,[†] by 3β-hydroxysteroid dehydrogenase[††] and Δ^5-reductase.

        (2) Androstenedione can be reduced by 17-hydroxysteroid dehydrogenase to testosterone, which is a reversible reaction.

        (3) Testosterone is a precursor of estradiol via an aromatase (CYP19) reaction.

    c. The other pathway proceeds via the conversion of pregnenolone to progesterone by 3β-hydroxysteroid dehydrogenase and Δ^5-isomerase. Progesterone is the initial compound in the Δ^4-pathway.

        (1) Progesterone is converted to 17α-hydroxyprogesterone by 17α-hydroxylase (CYP17).

        (2) 17α-Hydroxyprogesterone is another precursor for androstenedione via another 17,20-lyase** step.

        (3) Androstenedione and testosterone are interconvertible with the enzyme 17-hydroxysteroid dehydrogenase (17β-HSD).

        (4) Androstenedione and testosterone are converted to estrone and estradiol, respectively, by the action of aromatase (CYP19). These two 18-carbon steroids (estrogens) also are interconvertible with 17-hydroxysteroid dehydrogenase (17β-HSD).

*For the remainder of this chapter, the term **theca** denotes **theca interna.**
**Also 17,20-desmolase.
[†]These 17-ketosteroids are steroids that consist of 19 carbon atoms.
[††]Also 3 β-HSD.

3. **Metabolism of ovarian steroids.** The liver is the major site of steroid metabolism.
   a. **Catabolism of progestogens**
      (1) Progesterone is converted to **pregnanediol.**
      (2) 17α-Hydroxyprogesterone is catabolized to **pregnanetriol.**
   b. **Catabolism of estrogens**
      (1) Large quantities of both estradiol and estrone are hydroxylated (primarily in the liver) at the C-16 position to form **estriol.**
      (2) Another major catabolic route for estrogens is hydroxylation at the C-2 and C-4 positions, which yields the **catecholestrogens.**
   c. **Estrogens are excreted** in the urine in the form of soluble conjugates.
      (1) Estriol, catecholestradiol, and catecholestrone are excreted primarily as glucuronidates.
      (2) Estrone is excreted primarily as a sulfate conjugate.

G. Ovarian function

1. **Menstruation**
   a. **Menarche** refers to the onset of menstruation, which normally occurs between the ages of 12 and 14 years. Prior to menarche, minimal amounts of estrogen are produced by the peripheral conversion of androgens.
   b. **Menstrual cycle**
      (1) **Duration.** Although a duration of 25–30 days is considered typical, a cycle length of 28 days is the exception rather than the rule in adult women. In early adolescence, the cycle is characterized by irregular menses and anovulation.
      (2) **Temporal reference points** (Figure 51-4). The menstrual cycle conventionally begins with the first day of menstruation, when the endometrial lining is shed along with blood and uterine secretions. Days of the menstrual cycle are measured using two different reference points.
         (a) One system designates the first day of menses as **day 1** and the last day of the cycle as **day 28.**
         (b) The other system designates the day of the LH peak (ovulation) as **day 0,** with preovulatory days indicated with a **minus sign** and postovulatory days indicated with a **plus sign.**
2. **Menopause** refers to the cessation of menses, which typically occurs at about the age of 50 years. Menopause is a result of primary hypogonadism (i.e., cessation of ovarian steroid secretion) and is associated with an increased gonadotropin (predominantly FSH) secretion (see Table 51-2).

H. Ovarian (menstrual) cycle (see Figure 51-4)

1. The menstrual cycle is divided into two major periods: the **follicular phase** (days 1 through 14) and the **luteal phase** (days 15 through 28).

2. **The preovulatory phase**
   a. The follicular phase begins with the onset of menstruation and ends with ovulation.
   b. The follicular phase is also referred to as the preovulatory, proliferative, or **estrogenic phase.**
   c. The follicular phase is dominated by estradiol, which is the estrogen secreted by the developing follicle in response to FSH secretion from the pars distalis of the adenohypophysis.
   d. The follicular phase is marked by follicular growth and maturation and by endometrial proliferation. This phase generally lasts 8–9 days but can be quite variable (10–16 days). During this phase, the stratum basalis regenerates a stratum functionalis, and, by the end of this phase, one follicle (rarely more) has reached the final stage of growth.
      (1) A **primary follicle** begins as an oocyte surrounded by a single layer of cuboidal epithelial cells called granulosa cells. The primary follicle becomes multilaminar by the mitosis of the granulosa cells, which occurs with maturation.
      (2) Upon cavitation of the granulosa, an **antrum** is formed, which is filled with **liquor**

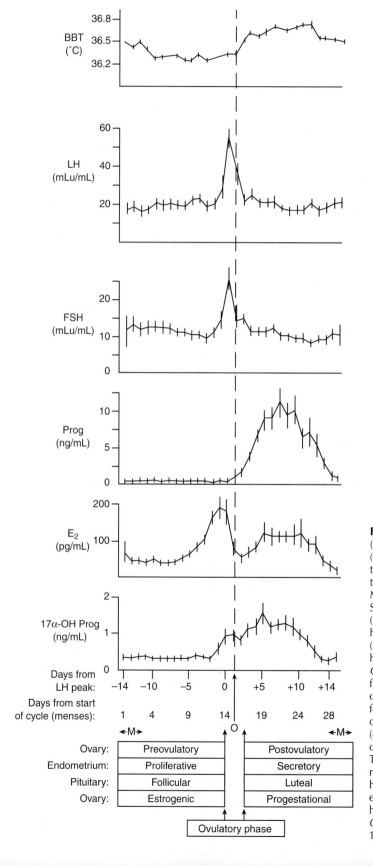

FIGURE 51-4. Hormonal (ovarian and pituitary), uterine (endometrial), and basal body temperature (*BBT*) correlates of the normal menstrual cycle. Mean plasma concentrations (± SEM) of luteinizing hormone (*LH*), follicle-stimulating hormone (*FSH*), progesterone (*Prog*), estradiol (*E₂*) and 17α-hydroxyprogesterone (*17α-OHProg*) are shown as a function of time. Ovulation occurs early on day 15 (day +1) following the LH surge, which occurs at midcycle on day 14 (day 0). *M* = menses, *O* = ovulation. (Adapted from Thorneycroft IA, et al: The relation of serum 17-hydroxyprogesterone and estradiol 17-β levels during the human menstrual cycle. *Am J Obstet Gynecol* 111:947–951, 1971.)

folliculi secreted by the granulosa cells. The developing follicle now is called the **secondary follicle** (vesicular follicle or, more commonly, graafian follicle).
  - **(a)** The granulosa cells secrete a protective shell, the **zona pellucida,** which surrounds the oocyte.
  - **(b)** The stroma gives rise to a bilaminar **theca,** which surrounds the granulosa cells but is separated from them by a basal lamina (**lamina propria**).
    - **(i)** The **theca interna** is a well-vascularized layer consisting of steroid-secreting cells that lie on the basal lamina. The blood vessels do not penetrate this membrane and, therefore, the granulosa cells are avascular until after ovulation.
    - **(ii)** The **theca externa** is peripheral to the theca and is composed mainly of fibrous connective tissue. It is less vascular than the theca interna.
  - **(3)** Just prior to ovulation, the primary oocyte of the secondary follicle completes the first meiotic division, which began prior to birth, and forms a secondary oocyte with a haploid nucleus and the first polar body. The second meiotic division takes place in the ampulla of the oviduct and occurs only if fertilization occurs.

3. **Ovulation.** The secondary oocyte is released from the graafian follicle by a process called **ovulation,** which usually occurs early on **day 15** of the average cycle. (In reference to the LH peak, this midcycle event occurs on **day 1,** that is, one day following the LH surge.) After ovulation, the egg lives for about 20 hours following ovulation unless conception takes place.
  - **a.** LH initiates the process of luteinization of the theca and the granulosa cells and enhances progesterone secretion.
  - **b.** The **onset** of the LH surge is a relatively precise indicator of ovulation; it occurs 34 to 36 hours before the release of the ovum from the follicle.
  - **c.** The **peak** of LH secretion occurs 12 to 24 hours prior to ovulation. Thus ovulation occurs **early** on day 15.
  - **d.** Immediately before the LH peak, estradiol levels in the plasma fall.
  - **e.** The ovulatory peak of FSH is thought to be stimulated by progesterone; FSH increases the granulosa cell LH receptors.

4. **Postovulatory phase.** The next 13–14 days constitute the postovulatory phase, during which the endometrium is prepared for the possible implantation of the fertilized ovum, which is a blastocyst when it arrives in the uterine cavity. This phase is relatively constant in duration. As a result, the day of ovulation can be estimated by subtracting 14 days from the total length of the menstrual cycle.
  - **a.** Following ovulation, the remainder of the cycle (progestational or luteal phase) is **dominated by progesterone.**
  - **b.** After ovulation, estradiol levels decrease; there is a shorter, broader, and flatter secondary estradiol rise at midluteal phase and a second decrease at the end of the menstrual cycle.
  - **c.** The circulating levels of LH and FSH during the progestational phase are below those observed during the follicular phase, but they begin to rise again, especially FSH, at the end of the cycle.
  - **d.** If fertilization does not occur, implantation also does not occur because the hormonal maintenance of the endometrial growth and differentiation is withdrawn.
  - **e.** Without conception, ischemia and necrosis of the luminal endometrium result after 14 days, and the ensuing menses marks the beginning of another menstrual cycle.
  - **f.** If conception occurs, the functional lifespan of the corpus luteum is extended, and it continues to secrete estradiol and progesterone at increasing rates during the first 6–8 weeks gestation.

I. Neuroendocrine control of the menstrual cycle: an overview (Figure 51-5)

1. Pituitary function is regulated by the feedback effects of gonadal hormones on the pituitary and the hypothalamus.
  - **a.** All gonadal steroids—estrogens, progestogens, and androgens—bind to pituitary receptors to influence gonadotropin secretion.
  - **b.** Unlike other feedback control systems, estrogens exert both negative and positive feedback effects.

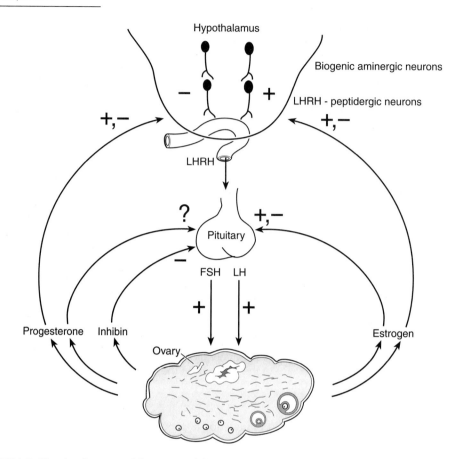

FIGURE 51-5. The development of the ovarian follicle is largely under the control of FSH; ovulation is caused by LH. Depending on the dose, time course, and previous hormonal status, estrogen can either inhibit or stimulate the secretion of LH through both negative and positive feedback controls. Progesterone can also either stimulate or inhibit LHRH secretion, depending on the hormonal status, but its effects at the pituitary level are relatively insignificant. The early preovulatory rise in progesterone augments the ovulatory gonadotropin surge (for FSH) while the later rise of progesterone in the luteal phase is inhibitory. Estrogens also have a variable feedback effect, with short-term administration causing an initial decrease in response to GnRH, longer-term administration causing a positive feedback effect, and chronic administration also causing a negative feedback effect. It is important to appreciate that steroid hormone feedback regulation of the hypothalamus-pituitary-gonadal axis occurs at both the pituitary and hypothalamic levels.

    c. The neurons projecting to the hypothalamus are targets of gonadal steroids.
    d. The inhibitory effects of estradiol on LH and FSH are **primarily** at the level of the pituitary; however, the secretion of FSH is more sensitive to inhibition than is the secretion of LH.
    e. The **positive** feedback action of estradiol occurs at the level of the pituitary when its plasma concentration rises above 150 pg/ml for at least 36 hours.
    f. Rising estradiol levels initiate both LH and FSH surges but a small amount of progesterone prior to ovulation may be necessary.
    g. Progesterone negative feedback acts primarily at the level of the central nervous system.

  2. Control of follicular development and ovulation (see Figures 51-4 and 51-5)
    a. During the follicular phase of the cycle, the LHRH generator operates at a frequency of 1 pulse per hour (circhoral) resulting in the synchronous secretion of LHRH into the pituitary portal circulation.

      (1) This approximate circhoral frequency of GnRH secretion is observed in castrated and postmenopausal subjects and at the midcycle surge in the release of LH in women with normal cycles.

      (2) The LHRH pulse generator is localized in the medial basal hypothalamus and the secretion of LHRH is influenced by neurons whose terminals end on the arcuate nucleus.

      (3) The pulsatile release of LHRH is based on the concordance between pulses of LHRH in pituitary portal blood and LH pulses in the peripheral blood.

   b. In response to gonadotropin secretion, the graafian follicle develops and matures, secreting increasing quantities of estradiol.

      (1) Estradiol exerts its inhibitory effects on both the hypothalamus and the pituitary.

      (2) Inhibition of FSH (and LH) occurs at low levels of estradiol but is more complete at high levels.

      (3) Progesterone at high concentrations inhibits LH (and FSH) primarily at the level of the hypothalamus; at low concentrations, progesterone increases LH release.

      (4) During follicular maturation, plasma estradiol levels exceed a threshold of about 150 to 200 pg/ml for at least 36 hours. The inhibitory (negative feedback) effect of the steroid is suddenly reversed and the pituitary secretes a preovulatory surge of LH and FSH (positive feedback effect of estradiol at the level of the pituitary).

   c. Under the influence of LH, the ruptured graafian follicle luteinizes and the rapidly growing corpus luteum secretes increasing quantities of progesterone.

   d. In the absence of conception, the corpus luteum involutes 14 to 15 days after its formation, and the levels of estradiol and progesterone decline.

   e. FSH receptors are located exclusively on the granulosa cells; LH receptors are located both on the granulosa cells and the theca cells.

   f. FSH is the gametogenic hormone that regulates the growth and maturation of the follicle.

   g. LH is the luteotropic hormone that regulates the function and the lifespan of the corpus luteum.

J. **Ovarian cycle and neuroendocrine control of ovarian function** (Figure 51-6; see also Figures 46-3 and 51-4). The ovarian cycle is associated with the secretion of ovarian steroids (estradiol and progesterone), which, in turn, are regulated by FSH and LH from the pituitary

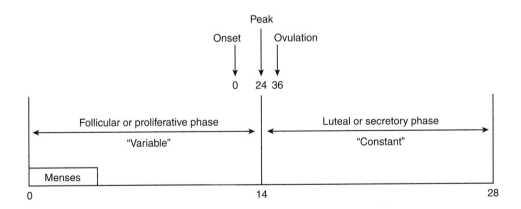

FIGURE 51-6. Relationship of the LH surge and menstrual cycle length. The onset of the LH peak begins about 24 hours before the surge (peak), and ovulation occurs about 36 hours after the onset of the LH peak. Ovulation occurs early on day 15 (day +1) [see I C 1].

gland. A single hypothalamic hormone, GnRH, differentially regulates the secretion of FSH and LH.

1. **Preovulatory phase.** Under the influence of FSH and LH, the primary follicle begins to develop. The combined effects of LH on the theca* cells to produce androgenic pro-estrogens and of FSH on the granulosa cells to aromatize these androgens to estrogens (estradiol) result in a slowly increasing blood estradiol concentration. During the preovulatory phase, the dominant gonadotropic hormone is FSH, and the dominant steroid is estradiol. Therefore, the preovulatory phase of the ovarian cycle also is referred to as the **follicular phase, the estrogenic phase, or the proliferative phase.**

   a. Plasma estradiol concentration reaches a peak about 24 hours prior to the surge in LH secretion, or about 36 hours prior to ovulation. The peak in plasma estradiol concentration occurs on day 13 (day −1).*

      (1) As the plasma estradiol concentration increases, it exerts a negative feedback on the hypothalamic-hypophysial complex, resulting in a gradual decline in FSH. LH levels rise slightly through the follicular phase.

      (2) Inhibin secretion by the granulosa cells also exerts a negative feedback effect on FSH secretion.

   b. The peak in plasma estradiol concentration exerts a positive feedback on the hypothalamic-hypophysial axis, causing a reflex release of GnRH and a concomitant surge in pituitary LH secretion 24 hours later, on day 14 (day 0).

      (1) A lesser increase in plasma FSH secretion occurs on day 14 (day 0).

      (2) Increased plasma estradiol levels inhibit FSH secretion both directly and indirectly at the level of the pituitary gland and ventral diencephalon, respectively.

      (3) The midcycle surge of LH requires estradiol in plasma concentrations of approximately 150 pg/ml for at least 36 hours.

   c. The follicular phase usually lasts 14 days, but any variability in the duration of the menstrual cycle usually is attributable to variability in the length of the follicular phase. It should be noted that the follicular phase begins with the first day of menses, while the proliferative phase of the endometrium begins with the last day of menses.

   d. There is a fall in the plasma estradiol level following the estradiol peak. Note in Figure 51–3 that this fall in plasma estradiol precedes ovulation.

   e. During the preovulatory phase, the plasma progesterone concentration remains very low.

      (1) The bulk of this progesterone is derived from the peripheral conversion of adrenal progestogens; however, large amounts of progesterone exist within the follicular antrum.

      (2) The principal progestin secreted by the granulosa cells during the late follicular phase is 17α-hydroxyprogesterone.

2. **Ovulatory phase.** Ovulation occurs early on day 15 (day +1) in response to the surge of LH secretion that occurred 24 hours earlier.

   a. Ovulation refers to the extrusion of a haploid secondary oocyte into the peritoneal cavity. The oocyte enters the oviduct (fallopian tube) where fertilization occurs.

   b. The rupture of the secondary follicle by the midcycle surge of LH leads to the formation of a new endocrine tissue (i.e., the corpus luteum), which involves proliferation, vascularization, and luteinization of the theca and granulosa cells. LH, therefore, is called the **luteotropic hormone of the menstrual cycle.**

3. **Postovulatory phase.** LH also maintains the functional status of the corpus luteum during the postovulatory phase. The hormone secreted in the greatest amounts by the corpus luteum during this phase is progesterone. For these reasons, the postovulatory phase also is called the **luteal phase** and the **progestational phase, or secretory phase.** The length of the luteal phase is remarkably constant at approximately 14 days. Therefore, the time of ovulation can be estimated by subtracting 14 days from the duration of the menstrual cycle.

   a. The decline in estrogen secretion prior to ovulation and at the time of ovulation removes the positive feedback effect of estradiol on gonadotropin secretion.

---

*Also throughout this chapter, the cycle days are numbered with reference to the onset of menses and with reference to the LH peak (in parentheses).

b. Both FSH and LH levels fall after their midcycle peaks but remain sufficiently high to stimulate the newly formed lutein-theca cells and lutein-granulosa cells to secrete estradiol, estrone, and progesterone.

c. About 6 days after ovulation, on day 21 (day +7), the plasma concentrations of progesterone and 17α-hydroxyprogesterone peak coincidently with the second peak of plasma estradiol concentration. Note in Figure 51-4 that this second peak is lower and broader than the estradiol peak that occurs during the preovulatory phase.

d. The plasma concentrations of progesterone during the entire ovarian cycle are higher than those of estradiol. **The units of concentration for progesterone (ng/ml) are 1000 times greater than for estradiol (pg/ml).**

e. The effect of the raised plasma estradiol and progesterone levels is a negative feedback on FSH and LH, respectively. Progesterone acts as an antiestrogen at this time because it inhibits LH secretion when the second estradiol peak occurs.

f. LH levels continue to decline during the luteal phase, while FSH levels begin to rise progressively during the late luteal phase.

g. The total amount of estradiol secreted during the follicular phase is comparable to that secreted during the luteal phase. This can be appreciated by comparing the areas under the estradiol curve during these two phases, using day 15 (day +1) as the dividing line between the follicular and luteal phases.

h. Unless conception occurs and is followed by implantation of the blastocyst, the corpus luteum undergoes involution following the reduction in gonadotropin secretion.
  (1) The declines in estradiol and progesterone secretion remove the negative feedback effect on the hypothalamic-hypophysial complex.
  (2) The corpus luteum regresses after about 14 days of steroid hormone secretion.

i. Progesterone is associated with a 0.2°C–0.5°C rise in basal body temperature, which occurs immediately following ovulation and which persists during most of the luteal phase (see Figure 51-4).
  (1) The basal body temperature dips during the follicular phase.
  (2) This temperature increment is used clinically as an index of ovulation.
  (3) Progesterone halts endometrial mitosis but causes maturation and differentiation of the endometrium.

K. | **Endometrial cycle**

1. **Hormonal effects on the myometrium.** Estradiol and progesterone are antagonistic with respect to their effects on the myometrium: estrogens promote uterine motility, and progestogens inhibit myometrial contractility.

2. **Hormonal effects on the endometrium.** Estradiol and progesterone are synergistic with respect to their effects on the endometrium during the proliferative and secretory phases.
  a. The **proliferative (preovulatory) phase** of the menstrual cycle refers to the endometrial changes that occur in response to estradiol.
    (1) Estrogens stimulate mitosis of the stratum basale, which regenerates the stratum functionale.
    (2) Estrogens stimulate angiogenesis (neovascularization) in the stratum functionale as well as stimulate the growth of secretory glands. The blood vessels become the spiral arterioles that perfuse the stratum functionale. The glands contain glycogen but are nonsecretory at this time.
    (3) The cervical epithelium secretes a watery mucus in response to estrogen stimulation.
    (4) The proliferative phase involves growth of the endometrium from 0.5 to 5 mm in depth.
  b. The **secretory (postovulatory) phase** is characterized by secretion of large amounts of both progesterone and estradiol by the corpus luteum. The endometrium during this secretory phase is hyperemic and has a "lace curtain" or "Swiss cheese" appearance.
    (1) Progesterone promotes differentiation of the endometrium, including elongation and coiling of the mucous glands (which secrete a thick viscous fluid containing glycogen) and spiraling of the blood vessels.

(2) Unless fertilization occurs, hormone secretion by the hypothalamic-hypophysial complex and ovarian steroid secretion decline on about day 25 (day +11).

   (a) Menses, beginning on day 1 (day −14) of the following cycle, starts with vasoconstriction of the spiral arterioles, which causes ischemia and necrosis. The average duration of menstrual flow is 4 to 6 days.

   (b) The necrotic tissue releases vasodilator substances, causing vasodilation. The necrotic walls of the spiral arterioles rupture, causing hemorrhage and shedding of cells over a period of 4–5 days.

L. **Physiologic effects of ovarian steroids** (Table 51-3)

1. Estrogens have important protein anabolic effects. Estrogens are responsible for the growth and development of the fallopian tubes, uterus, vagina, and external genitalia as well as the maintenance of these organs in adulthood. These steroids also promote cellular proliferation in the mucosal linings of these structures.

   a. Endometrium. Estrogens stimulate the regeneration of the stratum functionalis during the proliferative phase of the endometrial cycle by increasing mitosis.

   (1) The water content and blood flow to the endometrium are increased markedly.

   (2) The spiral arterioles of the stratum functionalis are especially sensitive to estrogens and grow rapidly under their influence.

   b. Myometrium. Estrogens increase the amount of contractile proteins (i.e., actin and myosin) in the myometrium and, thereby, increase spontaneous muscular contractions. Estrogens also sensitize the myometrium to the action of oxytocin, which promotes uterine contractility.

   c. Cervix. Under the influence of estrogens, the uterine cervix secretes an abundance of copious thin, watery mucus during the follicular phase. Progesterone causes the formation of a thick, viscous, cervical mucus during the luteal phase.

   (1) This fluid can be drawn into very long threads when placed between two glass slides. This is a clinical index of estrogen activity called **spinnbarkheit.**

   (2) Cervical mucus also demonstrates the phenomenon of crystallization when it is dried on a glass slide. The characteristic **ferning pattern** is from the accumulation of sodium chloride. This phenomenon also is used diagnostically as an index of endogenous estrogen secretion.

   d. Breast. Estrogens promote the development of the tubular duct system of the mammary gland. Estrogens are synergistic with progesterone in stimulating the growth of the lobuloalveolar portions of this gland.

   e. Bone. Estrogens, like androgens, exert a dual effect on skeletal growth in that they cause an increase in osteoblastic activity, which results in a growth spurt at puberty.

   (1) Estrogens hasten bone maturation and promote the closure of the epiphysial (cartilagenous) plates in the long bones more effectively than does testosterone. Therefore, the female skeleton usually is shorter than the male skeleton.

   (2) Estrogens are responsible for the oval or roundish shape of the female pelvic inlet. This inlet in the male is spade-shaped.

   (3) Estrogens, to a lesser degree than testosterone, promote the deposition of bone matrix by causing Ca^{2+} and HPO_4^{2-} retention. In large amounts, estrogens also promote retention of Na^+ and water.

   f. Liver. Estrogens stimulate the hepatic synthesis of the transport globulins, including thyroxine-binding globulin and transcortin.

   (1) This results in increased plasma concentrations of thyroxine and cortisol but unchanged amounts of free thyroxine.

   (2) Pregnant women often are in a state of mild hyperadrenocorticism because the elevated placental progesterone competes with cortisol for binding sites on transcortin, thus increasing plasma free cortisol.

2. Progesterone

   a. Endometrium. The endometrium, which proliferates under the influence of estrogens, becomes a secretory structure under the influence of progesterone.

   (1) The endometrial glands become elongated and coiled and secrete a glycogen-rich fluid.

   (2) Progesterone accounts for the differentiation of the stratum functionalis.

TABLE 51-3. Physiologic Effects of Estradiol and Progesterone

Estradiol	Progesterone
General —Promotes development of female secondary sexual characteristics	**General** —Serves as a precursor for steroid hormones —Increases basal body temperature
Pituitary-hypothalamus —Inhibits FSH secretion by negative feedback —Sensitizes pituitary to secrete prolactin —Inhibits (high levels) LH secretion by negative feedback —Stimulates midcycle surge of LH (and FSH) by positive feedback on pituitary	**Pituitary-hypothalamus** —Inhibits LH secretion by negative feedback —Stimulates midcycle FSH peak
Vagina —Causes thickening of vaginal mucosa	
Mammary Glands —Promotes development of lactiferous ductal system	**Mammary Glands** —Promotes alveolar growth and development of ductal system
Ovary —FSH increases FSH receptors on granulosa cells; FSH (in presence of estradiol) increases LH receptors on granulosa cells; LH stimulates theca cells —Proliferation and development of granulosa cells	**Ovary** —Stimulates theca cells to secrete androgens —Inhibits further follicular development
Uterus —Promotes uterine growth: hypertrophy of myometrium and hyperplasia of endometrium —Causes thinning of cervical fluid (spinnbarkheit) —Up-regulates estradiol and progesterone receptors —Promotes uterine motility	**Uterus** —Arrests endometrial mitosis —Inhibits myometrial contraction —Induces secretory activity of endometrium —Increases viscosity of cervical fluid —Promotes maturation and differentiation of endometrium —Down-regulates estradiol and progesterone receptors
	Uterus (Pregnancy) —Causes implantation (nidation) of the fertilized ovum (blastocyst) —Causes formation of decidua (decidualization) of maternal endometrium
Kidney —Promotes renal Na$^+$ retention ("ferning" of cervical fluid)	**Kidney** —Antagonizes the action of aldosterone on the kidney
Bone —Enhances bone growth, density, and maturation leading to epiphyseal closure	

FSH=follicle-stimulating hormone; *LH*=luteinizing hormone

  b. **Cervix.** Under the influence of progesterone, the mucus secreted by the cervical glands is reduced in volume and becomes thick and viscid. This consistency of cervical mucus together with the absence of "ferning" provide presumptive evidence that ovulation and luteinization have occurred.
  c. **Myometrium.** Progesterone decreases the frequency and amplitude of myometrial contractions.
  d. **Breast.** This steroid also promotes lobuloalveolar growth in the mammary gland.
  e. **Kidney.** Progesterone promotes renal excretion of Na^+ (anti-aldosterone effect).

II. ENDOCRINE PLACENTA

A. Placenta formation

  1. **Timetable of early placental function** (days measured from ovulation). The gestational period, measured from the time of conception (ovulation) to parturition, is 38 weeks (266 days) [see footnote on page 658].
     a. Pregnancy is considered to last 280 days from the first day of the last menstrual period if menses are regular at 28 days.
     b. The embryologic date (266 days) is 2 weeks shorter than the obstetric date (280 days).
     c. **Day 0:** Fertilization occurs in the distal portion of the oviduct or **ampulla.**
        (1) Fertilization triggers the final stage of the second meiotic division of the oocyte. The second polar body is extruded from the secondary oocyte, and a haploid number of chromosomes are present in the female pronucleus.
        (2) The lifespan of an unfertilized ovum is less than 20 hours following ovulation; sperm cells are viable for about 48 to 72 hours after ejaculation.
     d. **Day +3 or +4:** The morula enters the uterine cavity.
     e. **Day +5 or +6:** The morula forms a cavity, the **blastocoele,** which is transformed into a **blastocyst.**
     f. **Day +7:** The blastocyst is implanted into the endometrium. By the end of 1 week, a primitive uteroplacental circulation begins to develop.
     g. **Day +11:** The human embryo is deeply embedded and enclosed by the endometrium.
     h. **Day +21:** The placenta is fully functional.

  2. **Early placental formation**
     a. At the time of implantation, or **nidation,** the blastocyst consists of two cellular masses (Figure 51-7).
        (1) The inner cell mass, the **embryoblast,** will form the embryo and, eventually, the fetus.
        (2) The outer rim of cells, the **trophoblast,** forms the attachment to the endometrium and gives rise to the fetal membranes.
     b. The endometrium, under the influence of progesterone secreted by the corpus luteum, is transformed into a **decidua,** which is the maternal portion of the placenta that surrounds the conceptus. The decidua is the endometrium of pregnancy.
     c. The decidua basalis constitutes the maternal portion of the placenta and the chorion makes up the fetal portion of the placenta.

  3. **Placental development.** The trophoblast, which is entirely fetal in origin, develops into the placenta. The trophoblast forms two cell layers (see Figure 51-6).
     a. The inner layer forms the **cytotrophoblast,** which is on the fetal side of the blastocyst and is the progenitor of the syncytiotrophoblast.
     b. The outer layer forms the **syncytiotrophoblast.** The mature synctiotrophoblast is derived from the cytotrophoblast.

B. Hormones of the placenta (Figures 51-8, 51-9, 51-10, and 51-11). The fetus, placenta, and mother are interdependent and constitute a functional unit called the **feto-placento-maternal unit.**

  1. The syncytiotrophoblast serves as an endocrine organ secreting human chorionic gonadotropin (HCG); chorionic thyrotropin; chorionic somatomammotropin (HCS), also called human placental lactogenic; progesterone; and estrogens.

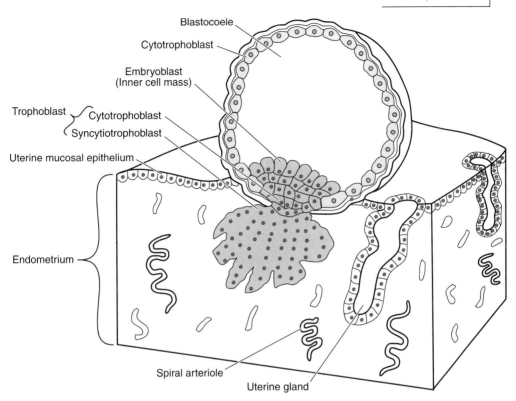

FIGURE 51-7. Structures formed by an implanting conceptus within the uterine endometrium. Note that the blastocyst attaches to the endometrium with the embryonic pole facing the uterine cavity.

2. The pregnant woman at or near term produces 15–20 mg/day of estradiol, 50–100 mg/day of estriol, 250–300 mg/day of progesterone, 1–2 mg/day of aldosterone, and 3–8 mg/day of deoxycorticosterone (DOC). By itself, the placenta is an incomplete steroid-producing organ.

3. **Human chorionic gonadotropin (HCG)** is a polypeptide containing 236 amino acid residues, making it the largest active peptide hormone produced in humans.
   a. **Synthesis and secretion.** The syncytiotrophoblast is the source of HCG, which is secreted soon after fertilization.
   b. **Plasma concentration**
      (1) HCG reaches a plasma peak between 60 and 90 days gestation. This peak is 200 times greater than the LH peak at the height of the ovulatory surge.
      (2) HCG is detectable in maternal blood as early as 6–8 days after conception, which forms the basis for the immunologic pregnancy test.
      (3) HCG measurement in maternal blood is a useful index of the functional status of the trophoblast.

4. **Progesterone** (see Figures 51-8, 51-9, 51-10, and 51-11)
   a. **Synthesis and secretion**
      (1) Placental progesterone is derived mainly from maternal cholesterol (LDL-cholesterol); the fetus does not contribute significantly to placental progesterone formation.
      (2) Progesterone is a requirement for the maintenance of pregnancy including **early pregnancy** (implantation).
      (3) This C-21 steroid is synthesized by the syncytiotrophoblast. Most (85%) of the progesterone formed in the trophoblast is secreted into the maternal compartment.
   b. **Plasma concentration** of placental progesterone rises steadily throughout gestation,

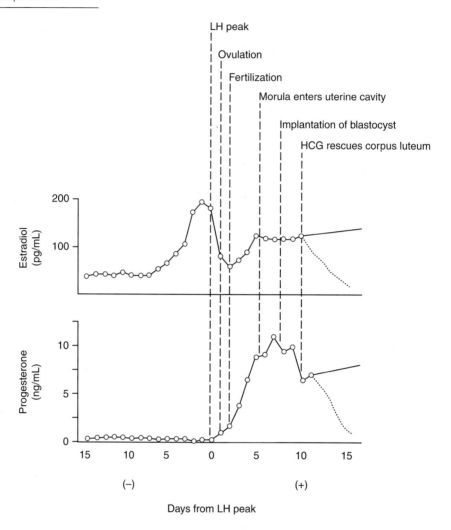

FIGURE 51-8. Relation between events of early pregnancy and steroid hormone concentrations. By the 10th day after the LH peak, there is sufficient HCG to maintain and increase estrogen and progesterone production, which would otherwise decrease (*dotted lines*) at this time. (From Goodman HM: *Basic Medical Endocrinology,* 2nd edition. New York, Raven Press, 1994, p 299.)

reaching a maximal plateau at 36–40 weeks. There is no significant drop in plasma progesterone concentration prior to labor.

   (1) Both 17α-hydroxyprogesterone and progesterone from the corpus luteum reach a peak 3–4 weeks postconception in response to HCG secretion.

   (2) At 6–8 weeks postconception, progesterone reaches a nadir, while 17α-hydroxyprogesterone continues to decline. The 17α-hydroxyprogesterone levels reflect corpus luteal secretion. The secondary rise in plasma progesterone reflects placental (trophoblast) secretion and is referred to as the **luteal-placental shift** (7 weeks postconception). After the eighth week of pregnancy, the syncytiotrophoblast is the most active fetal or maternal endocrine organ.

   (3) An intact materno-placental circulation will produce essentially normal progesterone levels, even in the event of fetal death.

 c. Metabolism. The principal urinary metabolite of progesterone is pregnanediol, which is a marker of placental function.

 d. Conversion to fetal corticoids

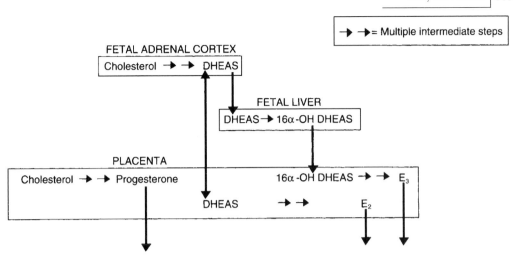

FIGURE 51-9. Pathways of steroid hormone biosynthesis in the feto-placental unit. *DHEAS* = dehydroepiandrosterone sulfate; *16α-OH DHEAS* = 16α-hydroxydehydroepiandrosterone sulfate; E_2 = estradiol; E_3 = estriol. (Adapted from Wilson JD, Foster DW: *Williams Textbook of Endocrinology,* 7th edition. Philadelphia, WB Saunders, 1985, p 423.)

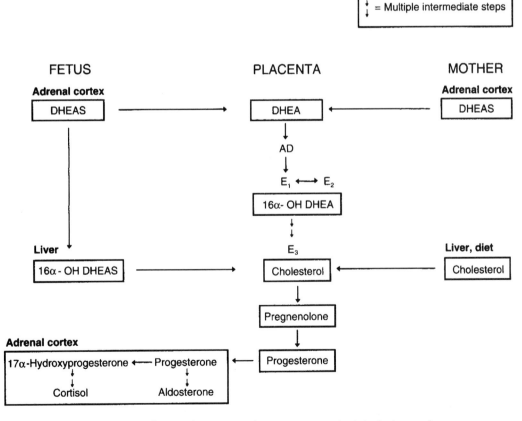

FIGURE 51-10. The primary pathways of estrogen and progesterone synthesis in the human feto-maternoplacental unit. Note that the steroids are produced from both fetal and maternal substrates. *DHEA(S)* = dehydroepiandrosterone (sulfate); *16α-OH DHEA(S)* = 16α-hydroxydehydroepiandrosterone (sulfate); *AD* = androstenedione; E_1 = estrone; E_2 = estradiol; E_3 = estriol.

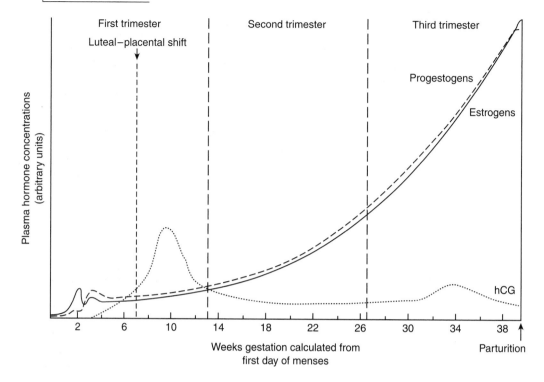

FIGURE 51-11. The patterns of maternal plasma hormone concentrations that occur during pregnancy. *HCG* = human chorionic gonadotropin. (Adapted from Laycock J, Wise P: *Essentials of Endocrinology,* 2nd edition. New York, Oxford University Press, 1983, p 155.)

    (1) The placenta produces pregnenolone from maternal cholesterol, but it lacks the enzymes necessary for androgen synthesis (i.e., 17α-hydroxylase and 17,20-desmolase, CYP17 and 17,20-lyase, respectively).

    (2) Pregnenolone synthesized by the placenta is oxidized to progesterone by 3β-hydroxysteroid dehydrogenase/Δ^5-isomerase (3β-HSD).

    (3) Placental progesterone circulates to the fetal adrenal cortex, where it is hydroxylated at positions C-17, C-21, and C-11 to form aldosterone and cortisol. Thus, in early pregnancy, the fetus requires placental progesterone to synthesize corticoids, because the fetal zone of the adrenal cortex has a relative block in the 3β-hydroxysteroid dehydrogenase/Δ^5-isomerase system.

    (4) Beyond 10 weeks gestation, the fetal adrenal cortex no longer depends on placental progesterone for synthesis of aldosterone and cortisol.

  5. Estrogens (see Figures 51-8, 51-9, 51-10, and 51-11). Quantitatively, estriol is the major estrogen of human pregnancy, with smaller amounts of estradiol and estrone produced.

    a. Synthesis and secretion

      (1) These C-18 steroids are synthesized by the syncytiotrophoblast.

      (2) Estriol is produced primarily from androgenic precursors formed in the fetal zone of the adrenal cortex and the liver. The principal adrenal steroid is **DHEA,** which is a ketosteroid. DHEA is sulfoconjugated (sulfated) by sulfokinase* in the fetal adrenal to **DHEAS.**

        (a) DHEAS is the predominant precursor for estradiol and estrone synthesis after

---

*Fetal sulfokinase conjugates metabolites of pregnenolone, progesterone derivatives, and the androgens (DHEA) found in the high levels of the feto-placental unit.

DHEAS is deconjugated by placental sulfatase. These two estrogens contribute to the estriol pool by conversion in the maternal liver.

(b) DHEAS is converted in the fetal liver to 16α-hydroxydehydroepiandrosterone sulfate by 16α-hydroxylase. This enzyme is not found in the placenta.

b. Plasma concentration. Like progesterone, the plasma estriol concentration rises steadily throughout gestation, reaching a maximal plateau at 36–40 weeks. The secretory curve for estriol parallels that for progesterone and correlates well with the fetal growth curve.

(1) Plasma estriol concentrations reflect the functional status of the feto-placental unit. Falling levels indicate impending fetal death.

(2) Even with fetal death, plasma progesterone levels can remain within normal limits.

(3) Ninety percent of estradiol and estriol formed in the trophoblast is secreted into the maternal compartment.

C. Physiologic effects of placental hormones

1. HCG is classified as an anterior pituitary-like hormone with biologic actions that mimic those of LH (i.e., it can be used to induce ovulation).

a. HCG is a second luteotropic hormone, in that it maintains the function of the corpus luteum until the feto-placental unit is autonomous in terms of hormone synthesis (about 7 weeks postconception).

b. HCG converts the corpus luteum of menstruation into the corpus luteum of pregnancy, thereby extending the functional lifespan of the corpus luteum.

c. HCG stimulates the corpus luteum of early pregnancy to secrete 17α-hydroxyprogesterone and lesser amounts of progesterone, which reach a peak 3–4 weeks postconception. Blood 17α-hydroxyprogesterone level is an excellent indicator of corpus luteal function during early pregnancy, because the placenta lacks significant 17α-hydroxylase activity (CYP17).

d. HCG stimulates the fetal testis to secrete testosterone at a time prior to fetal pituitary LH secretion.

e. HCG may serve as a tropic agent for the fetal zone (inner zone) of the adrenal cortex, which secretes DHEA.

2. Progesterone

a. Progesterone inhibits uterine motility by hyperpolarization of the uterine myometrium.

b. It converts the secretory endometrium of the luteal phase of the menstrual cycle to the decidua during pregnancy. Progesterone maintains the decidua.

c. Synergistic action of progesterone and estrogen is required to induce development of the lubuloalveolar compartment, which prepares the breasts for lactation. Progesterone acts primarily on the lobuloalveolar compartment.

d. Progesterone has an immunosuppressive role in protecting the fetus.

e. Progesterone contributes to the growth and development of the fetus (e.g., by acting as a precursor for corticoid synthesis by the fetal adrenal cortex).

f. Progesterone promotes renal excretion of Na^+, which antagonizes the effects of increased aldosterone levels found in pregnancy.

3. Estrogens. The estrogenic effects of pregnancy are primarily caused by estradiol, the most potent of the estrogens.

a. Estrogens mediate the growth and development of the maternal reproductive organs.

(1) The gravid uterus increases 18-fold (about 1700%) in weight, beginning as a 60 g organ in the nongravid state.

(2) During the gestational period, the uterus lengthens from 7 cm to 30 cm.

(3) Uterine volume at term is 500–1000 times greater than that before pregnancy.

(4) The increase in uterine size during pregnancy occurs by stretching and hypertrophy of the myometrium.

b. Estrogens stimulate hepatic synthesis of thyroxine-binding globulin, steroid hormone-binding globulin, and angiotensinogen as well as stimulating renal renin secretion. The latter two effects lead to increased angiotensin II synthesis.

    c. Estrogens stimulate development of the lactiferous ductal system in the mammary gland.

    d. Just before term, the estrogen-to-progesterone ratio increases and the uterus is dominated by estrogen.

Case

A 27-year-old woman presents requesting ovulation induction for a history of infertility. She had some breast development, as well as axillary and pubic hair development at an age of 11–12 years but has never had spontaneous menses. Evaluation at the age of 20 years showed low gonadotropins. She was treated with hormone replacement therapy until age 25. Amenorrhea persisted after the estrogen and progestin were stopped. She then underwent ovulation induction with clomiphene citrate (50 mg 3 5 days) and exogenous gonadotropins (150 IU Pergonal 3 5 days) without ovulation.

    She denies hirsutism, acne, galactorrhea, headaches, and vasomotor flushes. She does not exercise and denies any history of an eating disorder. There is no family history of amenorrhea. Her husband's semen analysis is normal. Physical examination was unremarkable except for a height of 5 ft and a weight of 99 lb.

    Repeat laboratory evaluation showed: LH , 0.8 mIU/ml (N for basal LH 5 0.8–26 mIU/ml); FSH 3.9 mIU/ml (N for basal FSH 5 1.4–9.6 mIU/ml) and estradiol , 20 pg/ml (N basal estradiol 5 20–60 pg/ml). Thyroid function tests and prolactin were normal.

    1. What is her diagnosis?

DISCUSSION

This patient exhibits hypogonadotropic hypogonadism, characterized by primary amenorrhea, low plasma gonadotropins, and low plasma estradiol. Because pituitary function is otherwise normal, this diagnosis is based on a GnRH deficiency. **Hypothalamic amenorrhea** is a term that describes patients with secondary amenorrhea associated with low urinary gonadotropins in the absence of a pituitary tumor. These patients also appear to have defective hypothalamic GnRH secretion, characterized by a decrease in pituitary LH pulse frequency or amplitude compared to normal. This is a common cause of secondary amenorrhea and is often related to stress, weight loss, severe exercise, and dieting. These latter conditions can result in the slowing of the GnRH pulse generator resulting in low FSH and the attenuation of follicular growth. Estradiol levels will also decline due to the decline in FSH. The development of this case (discussion of question 4) provides evidence for a diagnosis of **hypothalmic hypogonadism.**

    2. What is a normal menstrual cycle length?

DISCUSSION

Normal menstrual cycle length is between 25 and 35 days, although at the extremes of reproductive life (i.e., adolescence and perimenopause), there is a greater variability in cycle length because of an increased incidence of anovulatory cycles. The normal menstrual cycle requires precise integration of hormonal events at the level of the hypothalamus, pituitary, ovary, and uterus (endometrium). Thus, there are four levels of control of the normal cycle that constitute the reproductive "hardware."

    1. The hypothalamus provides the obligatory "software" program for intermittent (pulsatile) gonadotropin-releasing hormone (GnRH) secretion, which is approximately circhoral.

    2. The pituitary must receive the GnRH signal and secrete pulsatile LH and FSH in a response that is concordant with the GnRH pulse. The pituitary responds acutely to estradiol stimulation with positive feedback leading to the LH surge, which is essential for ovulation. It is rare that the pituitary is a cause of the malfunction of the brain-pituitary-ovarian-uterine axis.

3. The ovary processes the gonadotropin signals, follicle stimulating hormone (primary go-nadotropin in the follicular phase) and luteinizing hormone (primary gonadotropin in the luteal phase), which results in the sequential secretion of steroids. The ovary is also responsible for the housing, maintenance, growth, and maturation of the preovulatory follicle and oocyte. Together with the hypothalamus, the ovary serves as the second time-keeper.

4. The endometrium in response to the ovarian steroids creates a uterine environment conducive to the implantation of an embryo (blastocyst). In short, the endometrium creates a nidus for implantation which occurs on or about the 22nd day of a 28-day cycle. The uterus is the least demanding component of this 4-part system in that sequential physiologic estradiol and progesterone priming can result in pregnancy quite easily when properly timed to the intrauterine transfer of a donated embryo.

The follicular phase of the menstrual cycle begins on day-1 of menses and includes folliculogenesis, selection of a dominant follicle, and rising levels of estradiol from this dominant follicle, resulting ultimately in positive feedback and a preovulatory LH surge. The luteal phase begins immediately after ovulation and is characterized by estradiol and progesterone secretion from the corpus luteum (with progesterone resulting in the endometrial secretory changes which are necessary for implantation). This phase ends with menses that results from the removal of hormonal support. The luteal phase is fairly constant in length (12–16 days); therefore, the major variability is in the follicular phase.

3. What is the definition of amenorrhea?

DISCUSSION

Amenorrhea is defined as (1) the absence of menstruation for 3 to 6 months in women with past menses (referred to as secondary amenorrhea) or (2) the absence of menarche by the age of 16 years in girls who have never menstruated (**primary amenorrhea**). Amenorrhea is a normal phenomenon in prepubertal girls, during pregnancy and lactation, and after menopause. The most common cause of secondary amenorrhea is pregnancy followed by hyperprolactinemia.

It should be regarded as pathologic when it is present at any other time during the normal reproductive years unless the woman is chronically using oral contraceptives.

Primary amenorrhea is defined as (1) the absence of menses with no evidence of breast development by the age of 14 years or (2) the absence of menses with breast development by the age of 16 years. **Secondary amenorrhea** is absence of menses for 3–6 months in a patient who previously menstruated. Menstrual disorders can be divided into two main categories: disorders of the uterus or outflow tract and (2) disorders of ovulation.

4. Is she a candidate for ovulation induction? If so, what are chances of conceiving?

DISCUSSION

In spite of her previous ovulation induction history, she remains an excellent candidate for further therapy, because patients with hypogonadotropic hypogonadism have high conception rates with both exogenous gonadotropins and pulsatile GnRH. Pulsatile GnRH appears to be the drug of choice, as pregnancy rates are high and the risk of multiple gestation and ovarian hyperstimulation appears to be lower than with exogenous gonadotropins.

The patient did not respond to clomiphene citrate, which is not surprising, because clomiphene is an antiestrogen and, therefore, is more likely to be effective in patients with circulating endogenous estrogens. Clomiphene interferes with hypothalamic or pituitary estrogen receptor binding and leads to increased levels of serum gonadotropins. If this woman had an elevated prolactin level, ovulation induction could be effected by bromocriptine, a dopamine agonist. This patient was treated with intravenous pulsatile GnRH and successfully conceived (Figure 51-C1). It should be pointed out that the mode of luteinizing hormone-releasing hormone (LHRH) [GnRH] administration (i.e., continuous or pulsatile) is critical. **Continuous** stimulation of the

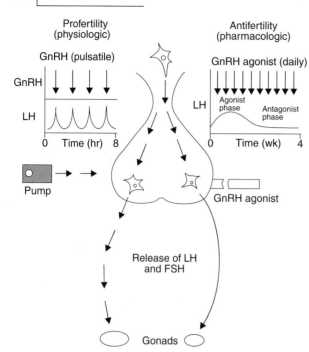

FIGURE 51-C1. Modes of action of GnRH (physiologic) and its analogs (pharmacologic). The physiologic use (*left*) of GnRH requires the pulsatile administration of natural GnRH. Information regarding GnRH secretion has been inferred from the pulsatile secretion of LH in the peripheral circulation. In the pharmacologic use (*right*), GnRH agonists are administered daily or as a depot treatment. They evoke an initial agonist phase of several days to weeks followed by desensitization and a long-term inhibition of gonadotropin secretion that is virtually complete and readily reversible when the GnRH agonist is discontinued. *LH* = luteinizing hormone; *FSH* = follicle-stimulating hormone.

pituitary by GnRH agonists results in the down-regulation of GnRH receptors on the pituitary after an initial stimulation. The plasma levels of FSH and LH become essentially undetectable, resulting in the reversible suppression of the pituitary-gonadal axis and suppression of gonadal (ovarian or testicular) steroid secretion. Such "biochemical castration" has clinical application in the treatment of endometriosis, uterine fibroids, precocious puberty, and prostatic carcinoma.

On the other hand, the restoration of a physiologic pattern of GnRH stimulation by the pulsatile administration of GnRH can restore normal patterns and levels of gonadotropins and sex steroids and induce monotocous ovulation. The pulsatile administration of GnRH agonists is useful in the treatment of women with primary amenorrhea, hypothalamic amenorrhea (the patient in this case), polycystic ovarian disease, and some women with panhypopituitarism. Pulsatile GnRH treatment is also useful in the restoration of fertility in men. The route of pulsatile administration of GnRH agonists is intravenous with the use of a portable pump.

    5. If she did not choose ovulation induction would she need any hormonal intervention?

DISCUSSION

If fertility were not a goal in this patient, estrogen replacement therapy would be recommended, because osteoporosis is a risk in any patient with hypothalamic amenorrhea. Therapy could be accomplished with either oral contraceptives or a menopausal hormone replacement regimen. Contraception in women could also be brought about by the continuous provision of GnRH, which leads to down-regulation of the pituitary GnRH receptors.

Chapter 52

Pancreas

I. ENDOCRINE PANCREAS AND METABOLISM

A. **Histology and function of the islets of Langerhans** (Figure 52–1). The endocrine pancreas consists of **islets of Langerhans,** which form 2% of the pancreatic tissue.

1. Each islet consists of approximately 3000 cells.

2. The human endocrine pancreas consists of approximately one million islets.

3. **Cells.** Four types of cells have been identified.
   a. **Alpha cells** make up about 25% of the islet cells and are the source of glucagon, which consists of 29 amino acid residues.
   b. **Beta cells** constitute about 60% of the islet cells and are associated with insulin synthesis. This polypeptide consists of 51 amino acid residues.
   c. **Delta cells** form about 10% of the islet cells and are the source of somatostatin, which is a tetradecapeptide.
   d. **Pancreatic polypeptide (PP or F)** cells form approximately 5% of the islet cells and synthesize a polypeptide that contains 36 amino acid residues.

4. **Neurotransmitters and epinephrine.** Unmyelinated postganglionic sympathetic and parasympathetic nerve fibers terminate close to the three cell types (alpha, beta, and delta cells) and modulate pancreatic endocrine function via the secretion of neurotransmitters.
   a. **Acetylcholine** secretion causes insulin release only when glucose levels are elevated. Acetylcholine appears to inhibit somatostatin release.
   b. **Norepinephrine** secretion from sympathetic stimulation via activation of the α-receptor leads to inhibition of insulin release. Norepinephrine stimulates somatostatin release.

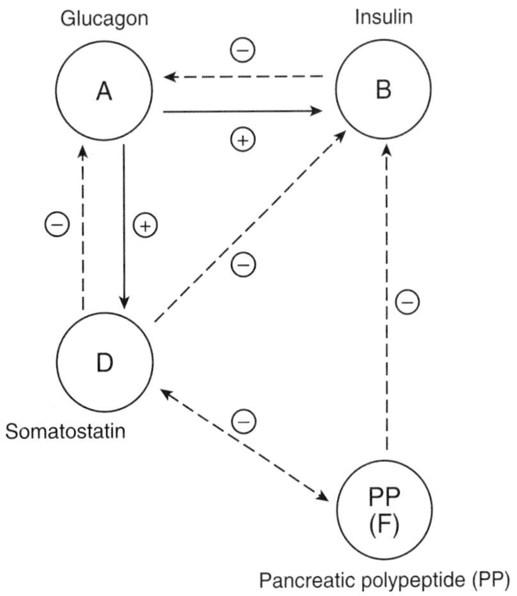

FIGURE 52–1. The paracrine system of the pancreatic islet cells. The pattern of islet cell hormone secretion represents an integrated response by all of the islet cells to humoral, neural, and paracrine regulation. *Plus signs* and *solid arrows* indicate stimulation; *minus signs* and *dashed arrows* denote inhibition. A = alpha cell; B = beta cell; D = delta cell; PP (F) = pancreatic polypeptide cell.

    c. Epinephrine. Despite the dual α- and β-adrenergic receptor system in beta cells, the α-adrenergic action of epinephrine predominates, so that insulin secretion is inhibited. (Insulin release is mediated by a β-adrenergic receptor.) [see Chapter 48 VII, Table 48-1]

  5. Control of secretions. The alpha, beta, and delta cells constitute a functional syncytium, which forms a paracrine control system for the coordinated secretion of pancreatic polypeptides (see Figure 52–1 and Table 52–1).

    a. Insulin inhibits alpha cell secretion (glucagon), thereby increasing peripheral glucose uptake and opposing glucagon-mediated glucose production (gluconeogenesis).

    b. Glucagon stimulates beta cell secretion (insulin) and delta cell secretion (somatostatin) leading to hypoglycemia, which, in turn, increases hepatic glucose production and opposes hepatic glucose storage.

    c. Somatostatin inhibits alpha cell (glucagon) and beta cell (insulin) secretion, producing hypoglycemia and inhibition of intestinal glucose absorption. The lowering of blood glucose levels by somatostatin in diabetic patients probably results from the inhibition of glucagon secretion and reduced intestinal absorption of glucose.

    d. PP inhibits insulin and somatostatin secretion via a direct pancreatic effect.

B. | **Biosynthetic organization of the beta cell**

  1. Human proinsulin is a single-chain polypeptide of 86 amino acid residues, with a molecular weight of approximately 9000 daltons.

    a. Intracellular proteolytic cleavage of proinsulin forms insulin and C-peptide.

    b. The conversion of proinsulin is not fully completed, and about 5% of the secretory product of the beta cell is proinsulin, which has about 5% of the biological activity of insulin.

    c. C-peptide increases glucose uptake into skeletal muscle in both normal subjects and subjects with type 1 diabetes mellitus (DM).

    d. The plasma half-life of proinsulin is 15 minutes.

  2. C-peptide is the connecting peptide remaining after cleavage of proinsulin to insulin. In humans, it consists of 31 amino acid residues.

    a. Beta cell secretory products consist of equimolar amounts of insulin and C-peptide; therefore, circulating C-peptide concentrations reflect beta cell activity.

    b. The normal fasting concentration of C-peptide in peripheral blood is approximately 1.0–3.5 ng/ml.

    c. C-peptide increases glucose uptake into skeletal muscle in both normal subjects and type 1 diabetes mellitus.

    d. The plasma half-life of C-peptide is 30 minutes.

  3. Insulin is stored in the beta cell granules as a crystalline hexamer complex with two atoms of zinc per hexamer. In plasma, insulin is transported as a monomer.

    a. Insulin has a molecular weight of about 6000 daltons and contains 51 amino acid residues.

Table 52-1. Effects of Islet Hormones on the Secretory Activities of Islet Cells: Paracrine Effects Among Various Islet Cells

	Secretory Activity			
Hormone	**Insulin Secretion**	**Glucagon Secretion**	**Somatostatin Secretion**	**Pancreatic Polypeptide Secretion**
Insulin	. . .	Inhibits	. . .	. . .
Glucagon	Stimulates	. . .	Stimulates	. . .
Somatostatin	Inhibits	Inhibits	. . .	Inhibits
Pancreatic polypeptide	Inhibits	. . .	Inhibits	. . .

    b. Insulin secretion requires the presence of extracellular Ca^{2+}. Inside the beta cell, Ca^{2+} binds to a Ca^{2+}-binding protein called **calmodulin.**

    c. The plasma half-life of insulin is 5 minutes.

C. **Control of insulin secretion (Figures 52–1 and 52–2, Tables 52–1 and 52–2)**

  1. Carbohydrates

    a. Monosaccharides that can be metabolized (e.g., hexose, triose) are more potent stimuli of insulin secretion than carbohydrates that cannot be metabolized (e.g., mannose, 2-deoxy-D-glucose).

    b. The principal stimulus for insulin release is glucose. As the blood glucose level rises above 4.5 mmol/L (80 mg/dl), it stimulates the release and synthesis of insulin.

    c. Substances that inhibit glucose metabolism (e.g., 2-deoxy-D-glucose, D-mannoheptulose) interfere with insulin secretion.

    d. The reduction of glucose to sorbitol may contribute to insulin secretion.

    e. Glucose also stimulates somatostatin release.

  2. Gastrointestinal (GI) hormones

    a. The plasma concentration of insulin is higher after oral administration of glucose than after it has been administered intravenously, even though the arterial blood glucose concentration remains lower. This augmented release of insulin following an oral glucose dose is a result of the secretion of GI hormones, including:

      (1) Gastric inhibitory peptide, which appears to be the principal GI potentiator of insulin release

      (2) Gastrin

      (3) Secretin

      (4) Cholecystokinin (CCK)

    b. GI hormones also augment somatostatin release.

  3. Amino acids

    a. Amino acids vary in their ability to stimulate beta cells. Among the essential amino acids, in decreasing order of effectiveness, are arginine, lysine, and phenylalanine.

    b. The stimulation of insulin secretion by oral administration of amino acids exceeds that of intravenously administered amino acids. Protein-stimulated secretion of CCK, gastrin, or both may mediate this effect.

    c. The analogues of leucine and arginine that cannot be metabolized also stimulate insulin secretion.

  4. Fatty acids and ketone bodies are not known to have an important role in the regulation of insulin secretion in humans. The ingestion of medium-chain triglycerides causes a small increment in insulin levels.

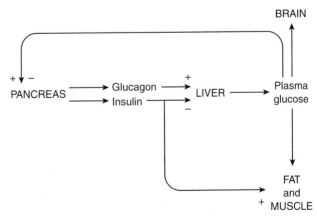

FIGURE 52-2. Plasma glucose has direct effects on the pancreas to increase insulin and decrease glucagon secretion during hyperglycemia, and to increase glucagon and decrease insulin secretion during hypoglycemia. Glucagon stimulates glucose production, and insulin suppresses glucose production from the liver and increases glucose uptake in muscle and fat via the GLUT-4 transporter. Glucose uptake is not insulin-dependent in the brain or liver.

Table 52-2. Agents that Affect Insulin Secretion

Primary Stimuli	Secondary Stimuli	Inhibitors
Physiologic		
Glucose	Glucagon	Somatostatin
Mannose	Secretin	Epinephrine*
Leucine†	Cholecystokinin	Norepinephrine*
Arginine	Gastrin	Starvation
Lysine	Gastric inhibitory peptide	Exercise
Short-chain fatty acids	Acetylcholine*	
Long-chain fatty acids	Prostaglandin E_1 and E_2	
Acetoacetate‡	Obesity	
β-Hydroxybutyrate		
Pharmacological		
N-Acetylglucosamine	Theophylline	Diazoxide
Glyceraldehyde	Caffeine	Mannoheptulose
Dihydroxyacetone	Isobutyl-methylxanthine	2-Deoxyglucose
Glucosamine	Sulfonylureas	Iodoacetate
Inosine	β-adrenergic agonists	α-adrenergic agonists

*Parasympathetic and sympathetic neural input to the pancreatic beta cells stimulate and inhibit insulin secretion, respectively.

†Alanine does not stimulate insulin secretion; however, it is a stimulus for glucagon secretion.

‡Ketoacids cause release of insulin.

5. Islet hormones. Glucagon stimulates insulin secretion and somatostatin inhibits insulin secretion. Somatostatin inhibits gastrin and secretin secretion, glucose absorption, and GI motility.

6. Other hormones
   a. Growth hormone (GH) induces an elevation in basal insulin levels that precedes a change in blood glucose levels, suggesting a direct beta-cytotropic effect.
   b. Hyperinsulinemia also has been observed with exogenous and endogenous increments of corticosteroids, estrogens, progestogens, and parathyroid hormone. Since blood glucose concentrations are not reduced with these hormones, it is inferred that these hormones have an anti-insulin effect.

7. Obesity. Hyperinsulinemia is observed in obese patients. An increase in body weight in the absence of a disproportionate increase in body fat does not affect insulin levels.

8. Ions. Both K^+ and Ca^{2+} are necessary for normal insulin and glucagon responses to glucose. Therefore, hypokalemia leads to glucose intolerance.

9. Cyclic nucleotides. Cyclic adenosine 3′, 5′-monophosphate is a releaser of insulin.

D. **Biochemical actions of insulin** (Figure 52–3, Figure 52–4, Table 52–3, Table 52–4, Table 52–5)

1. Carbohydrate metabolism
   a. Liver
      (1) In general, the liver takes up glucose when the circulating concentration is high and releases it when the blood glucose level is low.
      (2) Glucose transport in hepatocytes depends on an insulin-insensitive isoform of the glucose transporter (GLUT-2), and net uptake or release of glucose depends on whether the concentration of free glucose is higher in the extracellular fluid (ECF) or in the intracellular fluid (ICF).
      (3) The two enzymes that catalyze phosphorylation of glucose to glucose-6-phosphate are hexokinase and glucokinase.

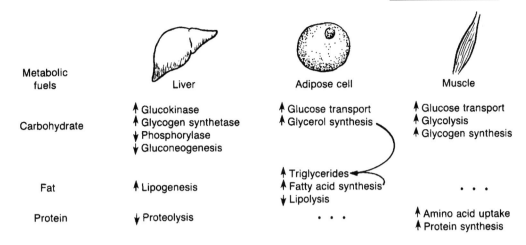

FIGURE 52-3. The major target sites and metabolic actions of insulin. Insulin is primarily involved in the regulation of metabolic processes, the principal manifestation of which is the control of plasma glucose concentration. (Reprinted from Felig P: Pathophysiology of diabetes mellitus. *Med Clin North Am* 55:821–834, 1971.)

(a) **Hexokinase** is saturated at normal plasma glucose concentrations and is not regulated by insulin.

(b) Hexokinase is found in most tissues, has a high affinity (low K_m = 0.1 mM; K_m = Michaelis constant) for glucose and other hexoses, and has a low V_{max} (maximum velocity).

(c) **Glucokinase** is only half-saturated at blood glucose concentrations between 90 and 100 mg/dl (5.0–5.5 mmol/L). Thus, the activity of this enzyme is insulin- and glucose-dependent.

(d) Glucokinase is found only in liver, has a low affinity (high K_m = 10 mM) for

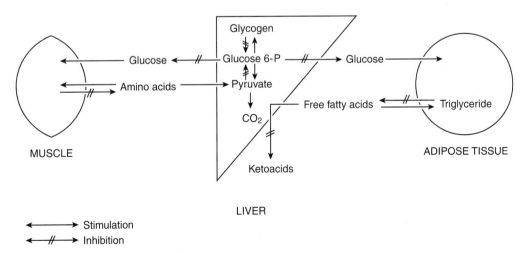

FIGURE 52-4. Metabolic effects of insulin on fat, protein, and carbohydrate. Insulin is protein anabolic and lipogenic. It promotes both the utilization (glycolysis) and storage (glycogenesis) of glucose. The net effect is the decline in the plasma concentrations of glucose, free fatty acids, amino acids, and ketoacids. Note the decline in hepatic fatty acid uptake with a resultant decline in plasma ketoacid levels.

Table 52-3. Insulin-Dependent and Insulin-Independent Tissue Based on Glucose Transport

Dependent	Independent
Muscle (resting)	Nerve
Adipose	Renal epithelium
	Intestinal epithelium
	Erythrocytes
	Liver*

*Very small concentrations of insulin are also required for glucose uptake by exercising skeletal muscle; therefore, the insulin requirement for glucose transport by exercising muscle is reduced but not eliminated.

      glucose only, and has a high V_{max}. It is active when glucose concentrations are relatively high.

(4) Dephosphorylation requires the activity of glucose-6-phosphatase, which is suppressed by insulin.

(5) The phosphorylation of fructose-6-phosphate by phosphofructokinase is enhanced by insulin. A decrease in phosphofructokinase activity favors the reversal of glycolysis.

(6) Insulin diminishes hepatic glucose output by activating glycogen synthetase and

Table 52-4. Biochemical Effects of Insulin on Target Tissues

Effect	Tissue
Rapid effects	
Increased membrane transport of glucose	Muscle, adipose
Increased membrane transport of amino acids	Muscle, adipose, liver
Intermediate effects	
Carbohydrate metabolism	
Increased glycogen synthesis	Muscle, liver
Decreased glycogenolysis	Muscle, liver
Increased glycolysis	Muscle, liver, adipose
Decreased gluconeogenesis	Liver
Lipid metabolism	
Increased lipogenesis	Liver, adipose
Increased esterification	Liver, adipose
Decreased lipolysis	Adipose
Increased cholesterol synthesis	Liver
Decreased ketogenesis	Liver
Increased utilization of dietary lipid	Liver, adipose
Decreased fatty acid oxidation	Liver, adipose
Protein metabolism	
Increased protein synthesis	Liver, muscle, adipose
Decreased proteolysis	Liver, muscle
Long-term effects	
Promotion of cell growth	
Promotion of cell division	
Promotion of DNA synthesis	
Promotion of RNA synthesis	

Table 52-5. Characteristics of the Five Facilitated-Diffusion Glucose Transporters

Transporter	Tissue Distribution	Characteristics
GLUT-1	High concentrations in brain, erythrocytes, and endothelial cells	Responsible for low level of basal glucose uptake to sustain energy generation carried out by all cells
GLUT-2	Kidney, small intestine epithelia, liver, pancreatic beta cells	Low-affinity glucose transporter; has a role in sensing glucose concentrations in islet
GLUT-3	Neurons, placenta	High-affinity glucose transporter
GLUT-4	Skeletal muscle, cardiac muscle, adipocytes	Main insulin-responsive glucose transporter via fusion of intracellular vesicles with the plasma membrane
GLUT-5	Small intestine, sperm, kidney, brain, adipocytes, muscle	Fructose transporter; very low affinity for glucose

The principle mechanism for glucose transport in most mammalian cells is facilitated diffusion, catalyzed by the GLUT family of transporters. On stimulation by insulin, many of the intracellular vesicles containing GLUT-4 transporters fuse with the plasma membrane, thereby increasing the total number of glucose transporters in the plasma membrane. In the absence of insulin, most of the GLUT-4 reverts to the intracellular location, whereas most of the GLUT-1 remains associated with the plasma membrane. Glucose (and galactose) and neutral amino acids enter intestinal and renal epithelia at the brush border by secondary active transporters (cotransporters or symporters) driven by the Na^+ concentration gradient. However, these substances leave cells at the basolateral membrane primarily by facilitated transporters.

by inhibiting gluconeogenesis. The key intermediary reaction in gluconeogenesis is between pyruvate and phosphoenolpyruvate. This reaction requires the enzymes pyruvate carboxylase and phosphoenolpyruvate carboxykinase. The latter enzyme is inhibited in the presence of glucose and insulin.

  b. Fructose-2,6 bisphosphate (F-2,6 P_2): A third messenger (Figure 52–5)
    (1) The phosphorylation state of phosphofructokinase II (PFK II) is controlled by cyclic adenosine monophosphate-dependent protein kinase and insulin-dependent phosphatase.
    (2) F-2,6 P_2, the third messenger, stimulates phosphofructokinase I (PFK I) at catalytic concentrations, and it coordinately inhibits the opposing enzyme, fructose-1,6 bisphosphatase (F-1,6 P_2ase).
      (a) This inhibition has the effect of directing substrate traffic downward to the triose level.
      (b) A decreased F-2,6 P_2 concentration reverses the effect of the third messenger (on the downward flow of substrates through the glycolytic pathway) resulting in the facilitation of upward flow of substrates (i.e., gluconeogenesis).
    (3) Summary. High F-2,6P_2 favors lipogenesis from glucose (downward flow), and low F-2,6 P_2 permits gluconeogenesis from trioses (upward flow).
  c. Muscle. The **insulin-dependent facilitated diffusion mechanism** for glucose is found in skeletal and cardiac muscle (GLUT-4).
    (1) Muscle is the principal site of insulin-stimulated glucose disposal in vivo; less glucose is transported into adipose tissue.
    (2) Glucose transport across muscle cell membranes requires insulin.
    (3) Insulin activates glycogen synthetase, which causes glycogen synthesis, and phosphofructokinase, which causes glucose utilization.
    (4) Glucose uptake in exercising muscle is not dependent on *increased* insulin secretion. In resting muscle, glucose is a relatively unimportant fuel, with the oxidation of fatty acids supplying most of the energy.
  d. Adipose tissue. The **insulin-dependent facilitated diffusion mechanism** for glucose is found also in adipose tissue (GLUT-4).

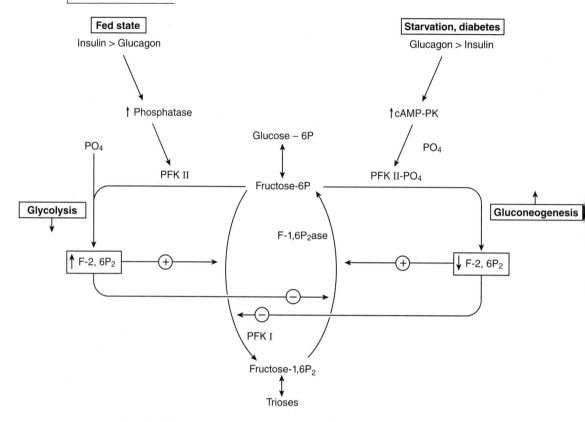

FIGURE 52-5. The role of fructose-2,6 bisphosphate (F-2,6P$_2$) in the regulation of phosphofructokinase I (PFK I) and fructose-1,6 bisphosphatase (F-2,6P$_2$ase). Substrate flow (glycolysis versus gluconeogenesis); regulated by controls exerted on these enzymes. F-2,6 P$_2$ase in the liver cell increases in the fed state, that is, in the presence of glucose, when the molar ration of insulin:glucagon is high. F-2,6 P$_2$ase concentration decreases when the hormone ratio is reversed; that is, in starvation and diabetes. The enzyme phosphofructokinase II (PFK II), which catalyzes the formation of F-2,6P$_2$, is oddly bifunctional; when it is phosphorylated, it functions as a phosphatase and diminishes the concentration of F-2,6P$_2$, but when it is dephosphorylated, it acts as a kinase and increases the production of F-2,6P$_2$ and therefore its concentration. *CAMP-PK* = cyclic adenosine monophosphate-dependent protein kinase; *Fructose-6P* = fructose-6-phosphate; *Glucose-6P* = glucose-6-phosphate.

    (1) Insulin acts primarily to stimulate glucose transport.
    (2) Insulin activates glycogen synthetase and phosphofructokinase.
    (3) The major end products of glucose metabolism in fat cells are fatty acids and α-glycerophosphate. The fat cell depends on glucose as a precursor of α-glycerophosphate, which is important in fat storage because it forms esters with fatty acids to form triglycerides (triacylglycerols).

  2. Fat metabolism. Insulin is a lipogenic and an antilipolytic hormone.
    a. Liver
      (1) When insulin and carbohydrate are available, the human liver is quantitatively a more important site of fat synthesis than is adipose tissue.
      (2) In the absence of insulin, the liver does not actively synthesize fatty acids, but it is capable of esterifying fatty acids with **glycerol,** which is phosphorylated by glycerokinase.
        (a) Glycerol must be phosphorylated before it can be used in the synthesis of fat.
        (b) In the absence of glycolytic breakdown of glucose to α-glycerophosphate, glycerokinase permits the esterification of fatty acids.

(3) In the absence of insulin, there is an increase in fat oxidation and in the production of ketone bodies. Insulin exerts a potent antiketogenic effect.

(4) Insulin promotes the synthesis and release of **lipoprotein lipase,** which is an extracellular enzyme that hydrolyzes both chylomicron and very-low-density lipoprotein (VLDL) triglyceride.

    (a) Lipoprotein lipase catalyzes the hydrolysis of circulating lipoprotein triglyceride to fatty acids and glycerol.

    (b) Lipoprotein lipase is the key enzyme in the removal of lipoprotein triglyceride and thereby is important in the formation of both light and heavy lipoprotein (LDL and HDL).

    (c) Lipoprotein lipase is active at the luminal surface of the capillary endothelial cell, and under normal conditions is completely absent from the circulation.

    (d) The highest lipoprotein lipase activity is found in the heart, but lipoprotein lipase is distributed in adipose tissue, lactating mammary gland (and milk), lung, skeletal muscle, aorta, corpus luteum, brain, and placenta.

  b. Adipose tissue

    (1) Insulin deficiency also decreases the formation of fatty acids in adipose tissue.

    (2) The major effect of insulin-stimulated glucose uptake in human fat cells is to provide α-glycerophosphate for esterification of free fatty acids. The absence of α-glycerophosphate formation from glycolysis during insulin deficiency prevents the esterification of free fatty acids, which are constantly released from triglycerides in the adipocytes.

    (3) The lipolytic effect in the absence of insulin is caused by an increase in the hormone-sensitive lipase known as triglyceride lipase, the activity of which is normally inhibited by insulin.

3. Amino acid and protein metabolism. Insulin is an important protein-anabolic hormone, and it is necessary for the assimilation of a protein meal. The protein-anabolic effect of insulin is not dependent on increased glucose transport.

  a. In diabetic patients, the muscle uptake of amino acids is reduced, and elevated postprandial blood levels are observed.

  b. During severe insulin deficiency, **hyperaminoacidemia** involving branched-chain amino acids (i.e., valine, leucine, and isoleucine) is present.

  c. Insulin increases uptake of most amino acids into muscle and increases the incorporation of amino acids into protein.

  d. Insulin increases body protein stores through four mechanisms:

    (1) Increased tissue uptake of amino acids

    (2) Increased protein synthesis

    (3) Decreased protein catabolism

    (4) Decreased oxidation of amino acids

4. Electrolyte metabolism

  a. Insulin lowers serum K^+ concentration. This hypokalemic action of insulin is caused by stimulation of K^+ uptake by muscle and hepatic tissue.

  b. Diabetic patients have a proclivity toward developing hyperkalemia in the absence of acidosis.

  c. Insulin has an antinatriuretic effect.

5. Membrane polarization

  a. Insulin decreases membrane permeability to both Na^+ and K^+, but it decreases Na^+ permeability to a greater extent, causing hyperpolarization of mammalian muscle.

  b. The membrane hyperpolarization produced by insulin is the cause, not the result, of the net shift of K^+ from the extracellular to the intracellular space.

6. Integration of insulin action: A summary (Figure 52–6)

  a. Insulin is a very effective hypoglycemic hormone for two major reasons.

    (1) It promotes both hepatic and muscle glycogen deposition.

    (2) It enhances glucose utilization (glycolysis).

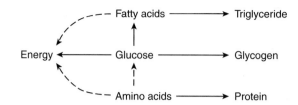

FIGURE 52-6. Insulin exerts integrated and synergistic actions in the promotion of the storage of body fuels. It enhances the storage of fat and protein, and it promotes both the storage and utilization of carbohydrates. *Solid arrows* denote stimulation, and *dashed arrows* indicate inhibition. (Reprinted from Felig P: Disorders of carbohydrate metabolism. In *Metabolic Control and Disease,* 8th edition. Edited by Bondy PK and Rosenberg LE. Philadelphia, WB Saunders, 1980, p 294.)

    b. For glucose transport, the major insulin-independent tissues are brain, erythrocytes, liver, and epithelial cells of the kidney and intestine.

    c. Insulin is the primary anabolic hormone in the body for the following reasons.

        (1) Inhibition of hepatic gluconeogenesis decreases the hepatic requirement for amino acids.

        (2) The protein anabolic effect of insulin reduces the output of amino acids from muscle, thereby decreasing the availability of glucogenic amino acids for gluconeogenesis.

        (3) Glucose uptake by muscle is stimulated, providing an energy source that spares fatty acids, the release of which is inhibited by the antilipolytic action of insulin.

        (4) Fat accumulation is enhanced by increased hepatic lipogenesis.

        (5) The antilipolytic action of insulin (inhibition of hepatic oxidation of fatty acids) is a result of the formation of α-glycerophosphate from glucose in the fat cell.

        (6) The antilipolytic action of insulin at the level of the adipose cell reinforces the insulin-mediated inhibition of hepatic ketogenesis and gluconeogenesis by depriving the liver of precursor substrates for ketogenesis and the energy source (fatty acids) and cofactors (acetyl-CoA) necessary for gluconeogenesis.

E. | **Control of glucagon secretion** (Table 52–6 and Figure 52–7)

    1. Metabolic fuels

Table 52-6. Factors that Regulate Glucagon Secretion

Stimuli	Inhibitors
Hypoglycemia	Hyperglycemia
Low fatty acid levels	High fatty acid levels
Most amino acids	Ketone bodies
Epinephrine	Secretin
Norepinephrine	Somatostatin
Acetylcholine	Serotonin
Dopamine	
Gastrin	
Cholecystokinin	
Gastric inhibitory polypeptide	
Vasoactive intestinal polypeptide	
Exercise	
Starvation	

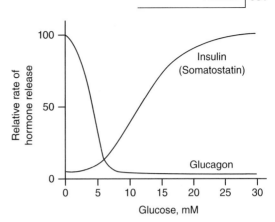

FIGURE 52-7. Dose-response curves for glucose suppression of glucagon secretion and for glucose stimulation of insulin secretion.

    a. Hypoglycemia stimulates glucagon secretion and hyperglycemia inhibits it.
    b. Amino acids (e.g., arginine, alanine) also are stimuli for glucagon release.
    c. Decreasing circulatory levels of fatty acids are associated with glucagon release.

2. GI hormones
    a. CCK, gastrin, secretin, and gastric inhibitory peptide stimulate glucagon secretion.
    b. The potentiation of glucagon secretion by the ingestion of a protein meal is probably mediated via CCK secretion.

3. Fatty acids inhibit glucagon release.

F. **Biochemical actions of glucagon.** The major site of action of glucagon is the liver (Table 52–7 and Figure 52–8). In almost all aspects the actions of glucagon are the exact opposite to those of insulin.

1. Carbohydrate metabolism
    a. Glucagon has a hyperglycemic action, resulting primarily from stimulation of hepatic glycogenolysis.
    b. Glucagon is an important gluconeogenic hormone.
    c. The hyperglycemic action of epinephrine is amplified by its stimulation of glucagon secretion and its inhibition of insulin secretion (see Chapter 48 VIII A 3).

Table 52-7. Effects of Glucagon on Intermediary Metabolism

Effect	Tissue
Carbohydrate metabolism	
Stimulation of glycogenolysis	Liver
Inhibition of glycogen synthesis	Liver
Stimulation of gluconeogenesis	Liver, kidney cortex
Inhibition of glycolysis	Liver
Lipid metabolism	
Stimulation of lipolysis	Adipose
Stimulation of ketogenesis	Liver
Inhibition of triglyceride synthesis	Liver
Protein metabolism	
Stimulation of proteolysis	Liver, muscle

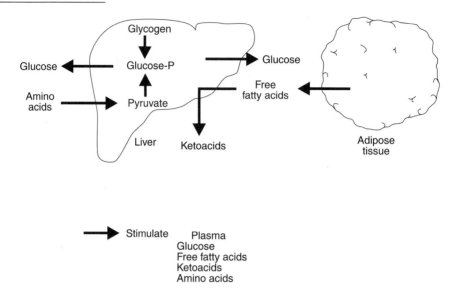

FIGURE 52-8. Effect of glucagon on the overall flow of fuels results in tissue release of glucose, fatty acids, and ketoacids into the circulation and hepatic uptake of amino acids for gluconeogenesis.

    d. Suppression of glucagon secretion by glucose is not essential for normal glucose tolerance as long as insulin is available.

2. Fat metabolism
    a. Glucagon is a lipolytic hormone because of its activation of hormone-sensitive lipase (triglyceride lipase) in adipose tissue by cyclic adenosine monophosphate.
    b. Glucagon causes an elevation in the plasma level of fatty acids and glycerol.
        (1) Glycerol is utilized as a gluconeogenic substrate in the liver.
        (2) The oxidation of fatty acids as an energy substrate accounts for the glucose-sparing effect of glucagon.
        (3) Glucagon is essential for the ketogenesis brought about by the oxidation of fatty acids. In the absence of insulin, glucagon can accelerate ketogenesis, which leads to metabolic acidosis.

3. Protein metabolism
    a. Glucagon has a net proteolytic effect in the liver (negative nitrogen balance).
    b. This peptide is gluconeogenic, an effect that leads to increased amino acid oxidation and urea formation.
    c. In addition to its protein catabolic effect, glucagon has an antianabolic effect—inhibition of protein synthesis.

G. **Control of somatostatin secretion** (Table 52–8). Somatostatin has many important physiologic actions in addition to inhibiting GH (somatotropin) secretion (see Chapter 47 IV A 2 b).

    1. Somatostatin is a decapeptide synthesized in the delta cells of the pancreatic islets.

    2. There is a parallelism between the agents that promote the secretion of somatostatin (see Table 52–8) and those that stimulate the release of insulin (see Table 52–2), because the same metabolites and GI tract hormones promote the secretion of both hormones.

    3. Somatostatin has been isolated from nerve terminals throughout the brain, spinal cord, and peripheral ganglia, where it can function as a peptidergic neurotransmitter.

H. **Physiologic actions of somatostatin** (Table 52–9) Somatostatin inhibits the secretion of both glucagon and insulin and produces a 30%–50% decrease in blood glucose concentration following infusion into volunteers.

Table 52-8. Agents that Affect Somatostatin Secretion

Stimuli
Glucose
Arginine, leucine, amino acid mixtures, cholecystokinin
Gastrin
Gastric inhibitory polypeptide
Secretin
Glucagon
Inhibitors
Epinephrine
Diazoxide

Table 52-9. Biological Activities of Somatostatin

Endocrine—inhibition of secretion of:
Pituitary
Growth hormone
Adrenocorticotropin
Thyrotropin
Pancreatic islets
Insulin
Glucagon
Pancreatic polypeptide
Gastrointestinal tract
Gastrin
Cholecystokinin
Secretin
Vasoactive intestinal peptide
Gastric inhibitory polypeptide
Motilin
Nonendocrine—inhibition or reduction of:
Gastrointestinal tract
Gastric acid secretion
Pancreatic bicarbonate and enzyme release
Gastric motility
Gallbladder contraction
Liver
Splanchnic blood flow

1. Somatostatin elicits a parallel fall in hepatic glucose production.

2. The hypoglycemic effect is mediated by suppression of glucagon secretion, since somatostatin has no direct effect on glucose metabolism.

3. The prevention of ketoacidosis and reduction of hyperglycemia by somatostatin following the withdrawal of insulin from type 1 diabetic subjects has raised the possibility that this hormone might prove useful as an adjunct to insulin treatment in the management of type 1 diabetes.

I. Control of pancreatic polypeptide (PP) secretion (Table 52–10)

1. PP has been located in parts of the GI tract, but the pancreas is the major source of PP.

2. There is a marked hyperplasia of the PP cells (F cells) in type 1 diabetes of long duration.

Table 52-10. Factors which Affect Pancreatic Polypeptide Secretion

Factor	Effect on Secretion
Amino acids (arginine)	Stimulates
Glucose	Inhibits
Somatostatin	Inhibits
Acetylcholine	Stimulates
β-Adrenergic agonists	Stimulates
α-Adrenergic agonists	Inhibits

Table 52-11. Actions of Pancreatic Polypeptide

Endocrine pancreas
 Inhibits insulin secretion
 Inhibits somatostatin secretion

Gastrointestinal tract
 Inhibits pancreatic zymogen secretion
 Inhibits pancreatic bicarbonate secretion
 Decreases gallbladder contractility
 Reduces gastrointestinal motility
 Inhibits gastric acid secretion

3. The secretion of PP appears to be largely under the control of the autonomic nervous system, with the cholinergic stimulation via the vagus providing the major signal for secretion.

4. Blood nutrients and hormones may also play an important role in PP secretion.

5. Obesity has been shown to cause a 50% decline in plasma PP levels.

6. Diabetes (type 1) is associated with an increased plasma concentration of PP.

J. **Physiologic actions of PP** (Table 52–11)

1. PP inhibits the secretion of both insulin and somatostatin without affecting the release of glucagon.

2. PP also affects the exocrine pancreas by inhibiting trypsinogen and bicarbonate-ion secretion.

3. In general, PP slows down the digestive process.

II. PATHOPHYSIOLOGY OF THE ENDOCRINE PANCREAS: DIABETES MELLITUS

A. **Definition:** DM is the relative or absolute deficiency of insulin together with the relative or absolute excess of glucagon.

1. DM is a complex disorder characterized by alterations in carbohydrate, lipid, and protein metabolism resulting from a deficiency of insulin.

2. DM can be differentiated into "insulin-sensitive" and "insulin-insensitive" on the basis of the blood glucose response to insulin administered immediately after an oral load.

3. On average, higher levels of insulin are found in patients with type 2 diabetes, suggesting that insulin resistance contributes to this form of the disease.

B. **Nomenclature.** The terms insulin-dependent DM and non–insulin-dependent DM are no longer used.

1. **Type 1 diabetes** includes patients with severe insulin deficiency.

2. **Type 1A diabetes** refers to immune-mediated diabetes and is characterized by the presence of anti-islet autoantibodies, whether or not a patient currently requires exogenous insulin.

3. **Type 1B diabetes** refers to nonimmune forms of insulin-deficient diabetes.

4. **Type 2 diabetes** involves relative insulin deficiency.

C. **Normal glucose regulation**

1. In normal individuals, insulin secretion is the dominant control system to maintain plasma glucose between 70 and 150 mg/dl.
   a. Normoglycemic control maintains fasting plasma glucose between 70 and 110 mg/dl.
   b. Normal plasma glycated hemoglobin (HbA1c) levels should be equal to or less than 7%.

2. When plasma glucose is low (fasting state), insulin secretion diminishes, hepatic glucose production increases, glucose uptake and utilization by insulin-sensitive tissues such as muscle decrease to a minimum, and insulin-independent glucose utilization is unchanged.

3. When plasma glucose rises postprandially, insulin secretion is elevated, hepatic glucose production decreases, and glucose uptake and utilization by insulin-sensitive tissues increases.

4. In normal individuals, the plasma glucose does not exceed the renal threshold and no glucose is excreted through the kidney.

5. Plasma glucose concentration is the most important determinant of the secretion of the glucoregulatory hormones including insulin, epinephrine, GH, glucagon, and cortisol (Figure 52–9, Table 52–12).
   a. The concentration of plasma glucose is determined by the rate of glucose input from the liver and the rate of removal by the various organs, especially muscle.

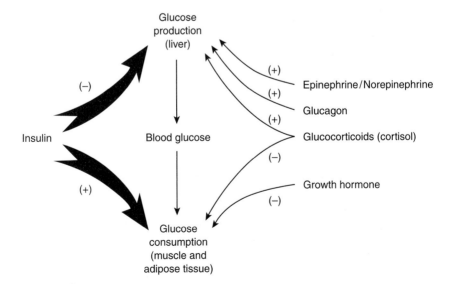

FIGURE 52-9. Interaction of glucoregulatory hormones to maintain the blood glucose concentration. The four counterregulatory hormones (anti-insulin hormones) are shown in the right-hand column. (From Goodman, HM: *Basic medical endocrinology,* 2nd ed. New York, Raven Press, 1994, p 209, Figure 3.)

Table 52–12. Summary of Metabolic Effects of the Glucoregulatory Hormones (Insulin and the Counterregulatory Hormones)

Hormone	Blood Glucose	Glucose Uptake	Glycogenesis	Glycogenolysis	Gluconeogenesis	Glycolysis	Protein	Fat
Somatotropin	↑	↓	↑*	↓*	↑	↓	↑†	↓
Epinephrine	↑	↓	↓	↑	↑	↑	···	↓‡
Cortisol	↑	↓	↑	↓	↑	↓	↓	↑‡**
Glucagon	↑	···	↓	↑	↑	↓	↓	↓‡
Insulin	↓	↑	↑	↑	↓	↑	↑†	↑‡

*Growth hormone and cortisol directly inhibit glucose uptake by muscle; by indirectly inhibiting glycolysis (phosphofructokinase inhibition), these two hormones divert glucose into muscle glycogen and decrease glycogen breakdown.

†Growth hormone and insulin promote protein synthesis and decrease the availability of amino acids for ureogenesis.

‡The four counterregulatory hormones are lipolytic and therefore are ketogenic.

**Cortisol is inherently lipolytic but its net effect is lipogenesis due to hyperphagia.

Note: Of the four counterregulatory hormones, glucagon has essentially one target organ: the liver.

b. Hormones that mobilize fuel and raise plasma glucose concentration in response to hypoglycemia are called counterregulatory (contrainsulin) hormones and include glucagon, epinephrine, cortisol, and somatotropin (Figure 52–10 and Figure 52–11).

c. Thyroid hormone (triiodothyronine) also increases the rate of fuel consumption and the sensitivity of target cells to insulin and the counterregulatory hormones (cortisol and catecholamines).

D. Pathogenesis of hyperglycemia

1. The lack or deficiency of insulin results in an inability to utilize blood glucose for fuel.

2. In diabetes, the body responds as if it were starving even though food is available.

3. The metabolic responses of the untreated insulin-dependent diabetic are essentially the metabolic responses of starvation.

4. Hyperglycemia develops only when there is an absolute or relative deficiency of insulin.

5. Most forms of insulin deficiency occur because of a marked increase in the requirements for insulin (insulin resistance); although insulin secretion becomes higher than normal as a result, it is not high enough to meet physiologic needs (i.e., relative insulin deficiency).

6. The combination of insulin resistance and hyperinsulinemia of type 2 diabetes predisposes patients to develop a high triglyceride and low high-density lipoprotein–cholesterol concentration, high blood pressure, and coronary heart disease.

7. Hyperinsulinemia enhances renal Na^+ retention and increased sympathetic nervous system activity, both of which tend to elevate blood pressure. As many as 50% of patients with essential hypertension appear to be insulin resistant and hyperinsulinemic.

8. Leptin, a polypeptide made by adipose tissue, is one of the physiologic regulators of appetite.
   a. It is secreted into the circulation, binds to a receptor in the hypothalamus, and decreases appetite.
   b. Obese patients, diabetic and nondiabetic, have elevated plasma levels of leptin and are resistant to its effects.

9. Hypertension. Insulin has been shown to (1) promote Na^+ retention by the kidney, (2) increase sympathetic nervous system activity, (3) alter the activity of membrane cation transporters (Na^+-K^+ ATPase and Na^+-H^+ countertransporter) and (4) promote atherogenesis, which decreases arterial compliance.
   a. Hyperglycemia increases osmolarity of the ECF, thus leading to the expansion of the extracellular space.
   b. Renal insufficiency in type 1 and type 2 diabetes contributes to impaired Na^+ and water excretion.

CONTRAINSULIN HORMONES

FIGURE 52-10. Integrated metabolic actions of the counterregulatory hormones in promoting the breakdown and storage of body fuels. *Arrows with a perpendicular mark* denote inhibition of a reaction (compare Figure 52–6). (From Felig, P: Disorders of carbohydrate metabolism. In *Metabolic Control and Disease,* 8th edition. Edited by Bondy PK, Rosenberg LE, Philadelphia, WB Saunders, 1980, p 294.)

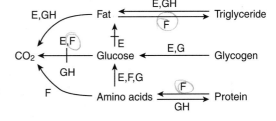

E = Epinephrine   G = Glucagon
F = Adrenal steroids   GH = Growth hormone
   (cortisol)

    c. These factors lead to hypertension with increments in both systolic and diastolic blood pressures.

E. **Classification of DM.** Current classification divides the disease into two major subtypes.

    1. Approximately 10% of all diabetics have type 1 diabetes.

    2. Type 2 diabetics form approximately 90% of the diabetic population.

F. **Salient characteristics of DM** (Table 52–13)

    1. Type 1 diabetes. This form of diabetes is becoming synonymous with autoimmune diabetes.
        a. Insulinopenia and hyperglycemia
        b. Abrupt onset of symptoms
        c. Susceptibility to ketoacidosis
        d. Dependency on exogenous insulin
        e. Metabolic derangements result from the hyperglycemia rather than the intrinsic target tissue defects in insulin action.
        f. The triad of defective insulin secretion, increased glucose production (liver), and decreased glucose clearance (muscle) defines type 1 diabetes.
        g. Increased hepatic glucose production is due to a combination of insulin resistance, hyperglucagonemia, increased free fatty levels, and the increased flow of gluconeogenic substrates to the liver.

    2. Type 2 diabetes
        a. The majority (60%–90%) of these patients exhibit hyperinsulinemia and insulin resistance.
        b. Not ketosis-prone
        c. Not dependent on exogenous insulin, although insulin may be used to treat persistent hyperglycemia that does not respond to diet or oral hypoglycemic agents.
        d. Hepatic glucose production is increased largely because of gluconeogenesis rather than glycogenolysis.
        e. Reduced uptake of glucose by muscle
        f. Conventional wisdom supports the notion that insulin resistance is the primary defect in type 2 diabetes.

Table 52-13. Comparison of Type 1 and Type 2 Diabetes Mellitus

Characteristic	Type 1	Type 2
Concordance rate in monozygotic twins	≤ 50%	95%–100%
HLA association	Yes	No
Circulating islet cell antibodies	Yes (65%–85%)	Absent/low (<10%)
Body weight	Nonobese	Obese (>80%)
Age at onset	Usually <30 years	Usually >40 years
Ketoacidosis	Common	Rare
Circulating insulin levels	Low	Low, normal, or elevated
Inflammatory cells in islets	Present initially	Absent
Islet cell mass	Absent or markedly decreased	Normal or slightly decreased
Insulin response	Sensitive	Resistant (usually not required
Cardinal signs	Polyuria, polydipsia, polyphagia	Overweight (obesity), hyperphagia, and physical inactivity

Case 1

A 21-year-old male medical student experienced increased urination and thirst for 6 weeks, along with a 15-lb weight loss, despite a normal appetite. Fearing that these symptoms meant he had developed diabetes mellitus (DM), he did not seek medical attention promptly. However, when he developed nausea and vomiting for 48 hours, followed by a stuporous state, his college roommate insisted on taking him to the emergency room. There, he was found to be semicoherent, and his oral mucous membranes and skin were dry. Blood pressure was 84/52 and pulse rate was 120 beats/min. He was breathing deeply at a rate of 30 respirations/min. The remainder of the physical examination was within normal limits. A urine sample contained a glucose concentration of 5% and tested strongly positive for acetoacetic acid. Plasma glucose was 800 mg/dl. Sodium was 132 mEq/L, bicarbonate was 5 mEq/L, chloride was 104 mEq/L, and potassium was 5.8 mEq/L. Blood pH was 7.1, PCO_2 was 17 mm Hg, and PO_2 was 95 mm Hg. Blood urea nitrogen was 28 mg/dl, and plasma creatinine was 1.4 mg/dl. On treatment with insulin, intravenous fluids, and potassium, the patient's clinical and biochemical status was restored to normal in 24 hours.

> **1.** *What is the cause of this patient's very high plasma glucose level? Which hormone(s) contribute(s) to the hyperglycemia?*

DISCUSSION

The primary cause of this high plasma glucose level is insulin deficiency resulting from destruction of the beta cells of the pancreatic islets. Secondarily, loss of insulin leads to disinhibition of glucagon secretion from the alpha cells of the islets, and thereby causes glucagon excess. The clinical consequences of insulin deficiency and glucagon excess create a state of stress, which additionally stimulates cortisol secretion, GH secretion, and epinephrine and norepinephrine release. This complete hormonal setting of insulin deficiency arrayed against increases of glucagon, cortisol, GH, and catecholamines generates hyperglycemia.

> **2.** *What are the mechanisms that elevated plasma glucose?*

DISCUSSION

Hepatic glucose production and release are elevated, initially because of exaggerated glycogen breakdown (low insulin, high glucagon, high epinephrine) and subsequently because of increased rates of gluconeogenesis (high glucagon, cortisol, catecholamines, GH, low insulin). The efficiency of glucose uptake by both muscle and adipose tissue is diminished because of impaired glucose transport and intracellular blocks in glucose metabolism (low insulin, high cortisol, high epinephrine). Finally, as dehydration occurs, plasma glucose rises still further because of a reduction in glomerular filtration rate.

> **3.** *Glucose production and release by the liver in part reflect the balance between glycolysis (glucose to pyruvate) and gluconeogenesis (pyruvate to glucose). What control points regulate the rates of bidirectional flow between glucose and pyruvate, and how are these points affected by the relevant hormones?*

DISCUSSION

The bidirectional flow between glucose and phosphoenolpyruvate is determined by the bidirectional flow between fructose-6-phosphate and fructose-1,6-biphosphate. These two phosphates in turn are modulated by the level of fructose-2,6 bisphosphate (F-2,6 P_2). A low ratio of insulin to glucagon decreases the level of F-2,6 P_2 and increases flow toward fructose-6-phosphate and gluconeogenesis by activating fructose-1,6 bisphosphatase (F-1,6 P_2ase) and inhibiting phosphofructokinase. Flow from phosphoenolpyruvate to pyruvate (glycolysis) is determined by the activity of pyruvate kinase, which is diminished by insulin deficiency. Flow from pyruvate to phosphoenolpyruvate (gluconeogenesis) is determined by pyruvate carboxylase and phosphoenolpyruvate carboxykinase, which are increased by high cortisol and glucagon levels and low insulin levels. In brief, the hormonally induced alterations in this patient at key control points favor gluconeogenesis over glycolysis and glucose production over its utilization. (See Figure 52–5.)

F-2,6 P_2, the third messenger, markedly stimulates phosphofructokinase I (PFK I) at catalytic concentrations, and it coordinately inhibits the opposing enzyme, F-1,6 P_2ase. This has the effect of directing substrate traffic downward to the triose level. A decreased F-2,6P_2 concentration has a meaning of its own: by reversing the effect of the third messenger on the downward flow of substrates through the glycolytic pathway, upward flow is facilitated. Thus, high F-2,6P_2 favors glycolysis from glucose, and low F-2,6 P_2 promotes gluconeogenesis from trioses.

> **4.** *What has replaced bicarbonate in the patient's plasma, and by what mechanisms?*

DISCUSSION

Deficiency of insulin plus excess of catecholamines, glucagon, GH, and cortisol generates unrestrained lipolysis of adipose tissue triglycerides. The increased flow of free fatty acids to the liver greatly exceeds that organ's oxidative capacity. Large quantities of four carbon ketoacids are formed (β-hydroxybutyrate and acetoacetate) and released by the liver. These acids have pK values well below 6.1 and require buffering by sodium bicarbonate. This reaction produces the sodium salts of the keto acids and carbonic acid. The latter dehydrates to carbon dioxide and water.

> **5.** *Why is the patient breathing rapidly, and why is the blood pH low* (Figure 52-C1)?

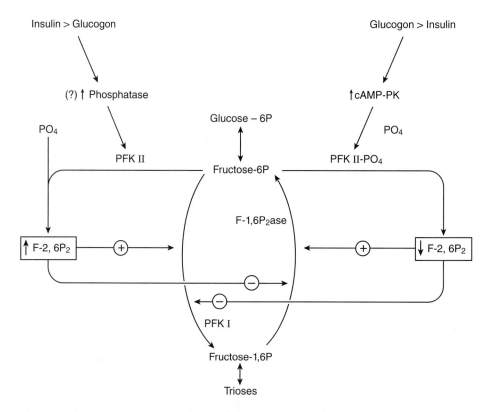

FIGURE 52-C1. The regulation of glycolysis and gluconeogenesis. Fructose 2,6 bisphosphate (F-2, 6-P_2) stimulates glycolysis by activating phosphofructokinase I (PFKI) which converts fructose 6-phosphate to fructose 1,6-bisphosphate and inhibits gluconeogenesis by deactivating fructose-1,6 bisphosphatase, which converts fructose 1,6 bisphosphate to fructose 6-phosphate.

DISCUSSION

Excess production of CO_2 stimulates central chemoreceptors and peripheral chemoreceptors by increasing extracellular hydrogen ion concentrations. This increases the rate of ventilation. However, the resultant fall in the partial pressure of carbon dioxide ($PaCO_2$) produced by this patient's maximum respiratory effort failed to compensate for the marked reduction in plasma bicarbonate. According to the Henderson-Hasselbalch equation, an increase in blood hydrogen ion concentration occurs; that is, a fall in pH.

6. *Why is the blood pressure low and the pulse rate high?*

DISCUSSION

For 6 weeks, high plasma glucose levels created a filtered load of glucose that exceeded the tubular maximum for renal tubular glucose reabsorption. The glucose that escaped reabsorption caused an osmotic diuresis. This, along with the lessened oral intake of water and the gastrointestinal (GI) losses from vomiting, resulted in severe dehydration and hypovolemia that lowered the blood pressure. In turn, decreased baroreceptor firing caused a reflex tachycardia.

7. *What levels of free fatty acids and triglycerides might you expect in plasma?*

DISCUSSION

Plasma free fatty acids will be high because of increased lipolysis. Plasma triglycerides will be high because of increased production of very-low-density lipoprotein (VLDL) from the increased free fatty acid load to the liver. This elevation of triglycerides will be aggravated by decreased clearance of VLDL from plasma because of loss of adipose tissue lipoprotein lipase activity when insulin is deficient.

8. *What levels of amino acids might you expect in plasma?*

DISCUSSION

Plasma branched-chain amino acids will be high because of increased muscle proteolysis in the absence of insulin and because of elevated cortisol levels. The high amino acid flow to the liver sustains accelerated rates of gluconeogenesis.

9. *What other hormone levels would be increased in plasma?*

DISCUSSION

Plasma aldosterone will be high, stimulated by the renin–angiotensin system, which is activated by the patient's hypovolemia. Plasma antidiuretic hormone (ADH) will be high, mostly stimulated by a high plasma osmolality from glucose and secondarily by hypovolemia.

10. *What contributed to this patient's weight loss?*

DISCUSSION

There are three components to the patient's weight loss: (a) extracellular fluid (ECF) losses from osmotic diuresis and vomiting; (b) loss of adipose mass because insulin deficiency leads to increased lipolysis and decreased reesterification of free fatty acids by glycerol phosphate; and (c) loss of lean body mass because insulin deficiency accelerates proteolysis and diminishes protein synthesis. In addition, somatomedin levels fall, further decreasing protein synthesis.

11. *What caused his thirst and increased appetite?*

DISCUSSION

High plasma osmolality plus hypovolemia stimulates thirst. Appetite increases in response to wasting large quantities of calories as glucose in the urine.

12. *What other constituents of the urine would be present in excessive quantities, especially when one considers that he had no food intake for 48 hours?*

DISCUSSION

Urea nitrogen excretion will be elevated, reflecting high rates of amino acid use for gluconeogenesis instead of for protein synthesis. Ammonia excretion will be elevated as a means of buffering excess hydrogen ion generated by the presence of elevated ketoacids in the tubular urine. Potassium, phosphate, and magnesium excretion will be increased because these intracellular electrolytes are released when glycogen and protein stores diminish.

13. *What effect would insulin treatment have on his plasma bicarbonate, pH, potassium, and phosphate levels?*

DISCUSSION

Restoration of insulin will inhibit lipolysis and reduce production of ketoacids. This will result in an increase in plasma bicarbonate and pH. Plasma potassium will fall for several reasons: (a) insulin directly stimulates potassium uptake by cells; (b) as insulin diminishes ketoacid levels and extracellular fluid (ECF) acidosis, potassium will move from ECF to intracellular fluid (ICF) in exchange for hydrogen ion released from intracellular buffers; and (c) as insulin decreases plasma glucose, water will move from extracellular space to the intracellular space, and potassium will be carried along by solvent drag. Plasma phosphate will fall because insulin stimulates cellular uptake of phosphate as glucose transport is increased and phosphorylated glucose intermediates are formed.

14. *Comment on the distribution of water in the intracellular fluid (ICF) and extracellular fluid (ECF).*

DISCUSSION

This patient will exhibit hyperosmotic dehydration, in which there is a reduction in the volumes of the intracellular fluid (ICF) and extracellular fluid (ECF) with increased osmolalities of both major fluid compartments. The movement of water from the ICF to the ECF along an osmotic gradient due to hyperglycemia contributes in large measure to the decrease in Na^+ concentration (hyponatremia).

Chapter 53

Thyroid Gland

I. HISTOLOGY AND FUNCTION

A. **Thyroid components.** The functional unit of the thyroid gland is the **follicle (acinus)** surrounded by a rich capillary plexus.

1. The follicular (acinar) **epithelium** consists of a single layer of cuboidal cells.
   a. The cell height of the follicular epithelium varies with the degree of stimulation of thyroid-stimulating hormone (TSH; Figure 53–1).
   b. The glandular epithelium varies with the degree of stimulation, becoming columnar when active and flat when inactive.
   c. When stimulated, the follicles are depleted of colloid; when unstimulated, the follicles accumulate colloid.

2. The **lumen** of the follicle is filled with a clear amber, proteinaceous fluid called **colloid,** which is the major constituent of the thyroid mass.

3. **Microvilli** extend into the colloid from the apical (adluminal) border, which is the site of the iodination reaction. The initial phase of thyroid hormone secretion (i.e., resorption of the colloid by endocytosis) also occurs in the apical border.

4. The **parafollicular (C) cells,** which secrete **calcitonin,** do not border on the follicular lumen.

B. **Thyroid functions**

1. **Hormone secretion.** The thyroid gland secretes two hormones, which are **iodothyronines** and therefore derivatives of the amino acid **tyrosine.**

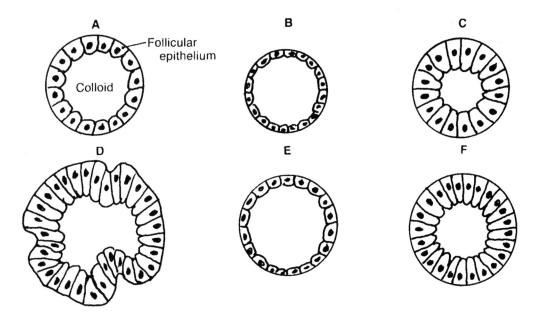

FIGURE 53-1. The thyroid follicle in various functional states. A = normal; B = exogenous thyroid hormone treatment (atrophy); C = iodide deficiency goiter; D = administration of goitrogenic agent; E = iodide administration; and F = thyrotoxicosis (Graves' disease).

  a. The major secretory product of the thyroid gland is **3,5,3′,5′-tetraiodothyronine (thyroxine),** which is abbreviated as T_4 to denote the four iodide atoms. The other thyroid hormone is **3,5,3′-triiodothyronine,** which is abbreviated as T_3. T_3 is secreted in small amounts.

  b. Only these two thyronines have biologic activity.

    (1) The **molar activity** ratio of T_3 to T_4 is 10:1 in most systems.

    (2) The **secretory ratio** of T_4 to T_3 is 10–20:1.

    (3) The **plasma concentration ratio** of free T_4 to free T_3 is 2:1. Most of the T_3 in the plasma is derived from monodeiodination of T_4 by the action of monodeiodinase (5′-deiodinase) found in peripheral tissue. The storage ratio of T_4 to T_3 bound to thyroglobulin is approximately 10:1, and the storage ratio of T_4 to reverse T_3 bound to thyroglobulin is about 30:1.

  c. **Reverse 3,3′,5′-triiodothyronine (rT$_3$)** is a biologically inactive thyronine formed by peripheral conversion catalyzed by 5-deiodinase.

2. Related functions. The thyroid cell performs two parallel functions in the synthesis of thyroid hormone.*

  a. It synthesizes a soluble protein substrate called **thyroglobulin.**

    (1) This glycoprotein is not only the site of formation of T_4 and T_3, but also is the storage form of the two hormones.

    (2) Thyroglobulin also is the storage form of thyroid hormone.

    (3) Each thyroglobulin molecule contains approximately 134 tyrosyl residues, of which only about 25 to 30 are iodinated, and only 6 to 8 form iodothyronines.

    (4) Both T_4 and T_3 are held in peptide linkage with thyroglobulin.

  b. The thyroid cell accumulates inorganic iodide from the plasma against an electrochemical gradient.

II. DISTRIBUTION OF THYROID IODIDE

A. Iodide intake

1. In the United States, the daily dietary iodine intake is between 300 and 1000 μg.

2. The recommended minimum intake is 150 μg per day (about 1 mg per week) to maintain euthyroidism because iodine is added to salt and iodate is added to bread.

3. During pregnancy the recommended intake is 200 μg per day.

4. The minimum intake required to prevent goiter is 75 μg per day.

5. The neonatal iodide requirement is 40 μg per day.

B. Thyroid iodide

1. The thyroid gland contains 5–7 mg of iodide.

  a. Of the total iodide, 95% is in the extracellular space (i.e., stored in the colloid as thyroglobulin). Thus, colloid constitutes part of the transcellular fluid compartment.

    (1) Two thirds of the total iodide content in the colloid is in the form of biologically inactive **iodotyrosines.**

    (2) One third of the colloid iodide content is in the form of biologically active **thyronines** (i.e., T_4 and T_3).

    (3) The molar storage ratio of T_4 to T_3 is 9:1, and the molar storage ratio of iodotyrosines to iodothyronines is 2:1.

  b. The remaining 5% of the total thyroid iodide is in the intracellular space of the follicular epithelium.

2. The thyroid gland contains the body's largest iodide pool.

3. Thyroid hormone is a derivative of phenol.

C. Storage. The storage function is an important aspect of thyroid function.

1. There are approximately 5 to 7 mg (5000 to 7000 μg) of T_4 stored in the thyroid gland.

---

*The term "thyroid hormone" denotes thyroxine (T_4) and triiodothyronine (T_3).

Table 53-1. Percentage of T_3 and T_4 Bound to Thyroid-Binding Proteins in Plasma

Hormone	TBG	TBPA	TBA
T_4	70–75%	15–20%	5–10%
T_3	70–75%	. . .	25–30%

TBA = thyroxine-binding albumin; TBG = thyroxine-binding globulin; TBPA = thyroxine-binding prealbumin.

2. This would be sufficient for approximately 2 to 3 months in the absence of any thyroidal secretion.

III. HORMONE TRANSPORT: EXTRACELLULAR BINDING PROTEINS.
Extracellular binding proteins for thyroid hormone are in the plasma, while the storage form of thyroid hormone (thyroglobulin) is in the follicular lumen (colloid) [Table 53–1].

A. Thyroxine-binding proteins. Virtually all (99.95%) of T_4 is bound to plasma proteins, leaving about 0.05% unbound (free). About 99.5% of T_3 is bound to plasma proteins. This portion of unbound hormones represents the biologically active hormone. Thyroxine is mainly associated with two of the three binding proteins.

  1. Thyroxine-binding globulin (TBG) binds about 75% of the plasma T_4. In normal individuals, one third of the available binding sites on TBG are saturated with T_4.

  2. Thyroxine-binding prealbumin (TBPA) binds about 15%–20% of the circulating T_4. This binding protein is called transthyretin.

  3. About 9% of the T_4 is bound to albumin (TBA).

  4. Under normal conditions only about one third of the available binding sites on TBG are occupied by T_4.

B. Triiodothyronine-binding proteins

  1. Almost all (99.5%) of T_3 is transported bound to TBP.

  2. About one fourth T_3 is bound to albumin, and practically none is bound to thyroxine-binding prealbumin.

  3. About 0.5% of the T_3 is unbound. The lower affinity of T_3 for the plasma binding proteins (and thus the higher concentration of unbound T_3) contributes to the greater biologic activity of T_3.

IV. BIOSYNTHESIS AND RELEASE OF THYROID HORMONE.
The thyroid gland accumulates or "traps" iodide by an active transport mechanism that operates against both a concentration and an electric gradient. The normal thyroid iodide-to-plasma iodide concentration ratio is 25–40:1. This ratio may reach 200:1 in hyperthyroid states.

A. Thyroid hormone biosynthesis: A quantitative overview (Figure 53–2)

  1. T_4 is synthesized solely in the thyroid gland, whereas T_3 is produced by both the thyroid gland and by peripheral conversion of T_4 at extrathyroidal sites.

  2. The total daily thyroidal production rate of T_4 is about 80 μg, all of which is derived from thyroidal secretion.
  a. Approximately 80% of this T_4 (64 μg) is monodeiodinated either at the 5' or at the 5 position to form T_3 or reverse T_3, respectively, in which T_4 is considered a prohormone.
  (1) About 40% of the 80 μg of T_4 secreted daily (32 μg) is peripherally metabolized via 5'-deiodinase to form 80% of the 30 μg of T_3 produced each day (24 μg/day).

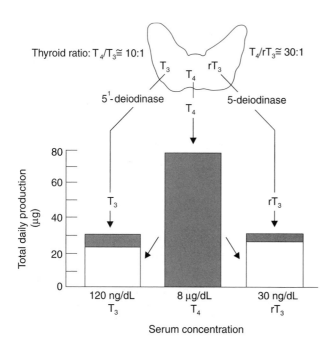

FIGURE 53-2. Sources and daily production rates (in μg) of circulating T_4, T_3, and rT_3 (reverse T_3) in normal adults, showing the distribution into components of direct secretion by the thyroid and peripheral conversion of secreted thyroxine. The T_4/T_3 and T_4/rT_3 ratios shown at the top are those in thyroglobulin. (From Griffin JE and SR Ojeda (eds): *Textbook of Endocrine Physiology*, 3rd ed. New York, Oxford University, 1996, Figure 13–4.)

    (2) The other 40% of the 80 μg of T_4 secreted daily (32 μg) is peripherally converted via 5-deiodinase to form 85% of the 30 μg of rT_3 produced per day (25.5 μg/day).
  b. The remaining 20% of intrathyroidal T_3 production (6 μg) represents direct thyroidal secretion.
  c. The remaining 15% of thyroidal rT_3 production (4.5 μg) represents direct thyroidal secretion.

B. **Synthesis.** All of the biosynthetic steps are stimulated by TSH (Figure 53–3).

  1. **Iodide uptake** (Figure 53–4)
    a. Active iodide uptake occurs at the basal membrane of the thyrocyte by the Na^+-I^- symporter, which is linked to the Na^+-K^+-ATPase pump.
    b. A normal thyroidal iodide uptake is about 150 μg per day.
    c. Iodide diffuses along an electric gradient into the lumen, where the luminal iodide-to-follicular cell iodide concentration ratio is 5:1.
    d. Radioactive iodide uptake by the thyroid gland is a useful therapeutic index of the functional status of the thyroid gland. A 24-hour uptake normally ranges between 10% and 35% of the administered dose.
    e. Iodide-131, a beta emitter, is used in the routine quantitative assessment of radioactive iodine uptake.
    f. The radionuclides technetium-99m and iodine-123 are used in the radionuclide imaging of the thyroid (scintigraphy). Technetium-99m is trapped by the thyroid gland but is not organified.

  2. **Oxidation** of iodide is mediated by thyroid peroxidase (TPO) and forms active iodide, which may be in the form of iodinium ion (I^+), a free radical of iodine called iodate ion (IO_3^-), iodine (I_2) or hypoiodous acid (HOI).
    a. The oxidation of iodide requires hydrogen peroxide (H_2O_2), which is an oxidant (electron acceptor).

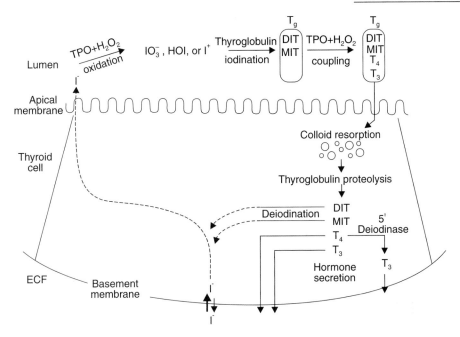

FIGURE 53-3. Steps of thyroid hormone synthesis and secretion. *TPO* = thyroid peroxidase; IO_3^- = iodate; T_g = thyroglobulin; *MIT* = monoiodotyrosine; *DIT* = diodotyrosine; *HOI* = hypoiodous acid; *ECF* = extracellular fluid; T_4 = thyroxine; T_3 = triiodothyronine. I^+, HOI, or IO_3^- are possible forms of active iodide. (From Griffin JE and SR Ojeda (eds): *Textbook of Endocrine Physiology,* 3rd ed. New York, Oxford University, 1996, p 262, Figure 13–2.)

    b. The active iodide is covalently bound (organified) to some of the tyrosyl residues of thyroglobulin.

3. Organification of iodide (iodination of tyrosyl residues of thyroglobulin)
    a. This reaction occurs in exocytotic vesicles fused with the apical membrane, i.e., at the cell–lumen interface.
    b. The substrate for iodination is thyroglobulin.
    c. Iodination also requires TPO.
    d. This process results in mono- or diiodination of about 15 of the 134 tyrosine residues of thyroglobulin to form monoiodotyrosine (MIT) and diiodotyrosine (DIT), respectively.

4. Coupling (condensation) of iodotyrosines occurs and forms biologically active thyronines (T_3 and T_4).
    a. The iodothyronines are formed in exocytotic vesicles at the apical border of the follicular cell and are held in peptide linkage with thyroglobulin (as are the tyrosines).
    b. T_4 synthesis requires the fusion of two DIT molecules, and T_3 synthesis requires the condensation of an MIT molecule with a DIT molecule.
    c. TPO also mediates the coupling reaction; therefore, this reaction is also oxidative.
    d. This reaction also requires H_2O_2 as an oxidant.

5. Secretion begins with the reuptake of thyroglobulin, which is engulfed by pinocytotic extensions of microvilli from the apical (lumical) membrane, forming endocytotic vesicles (colloid droplets; Figure 53–3).

6. The endocytotic vesicles **fuse** with lysosomes to form phagolysosomes, which migrate to the base of the cell and release their hydrolytic enzymes.

7. The **release** of hormones involves the following reactions:
    a. The digestion of thyroglobulin by lysosomal proteases releases all iodinated amino acids (iodotyrosines and iodothyronines).

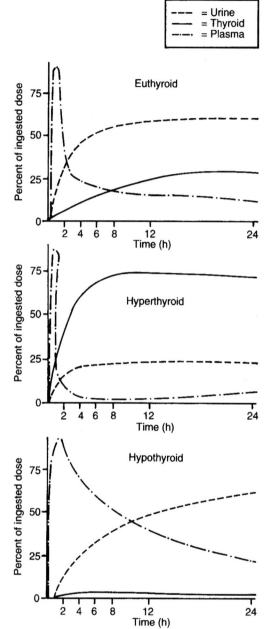

FIGURE 53-4. Twenty-four-hour radioactive iodine uptake by individuals on a relatively low-iodine diet. Percentages are plotted against time after an oral dose of radioactive iodine for plasma, urine, and the thyroid gland. In hyperthyroidism, plasma radioactivity falls rapidly, then rises again as a result of release of labeled T_4 and T_3 from the thyroid gland. (Adapted from Ingbar SH and Woeber KA: *Textbook of Endocrinology,* 4th ed. Edited by Williams RH. Philadelphia, WB Saunders, 1968, p 144.)

  (1) Iodotyrosines are largely prevented from being secreted by the action of an intra-cellular iodotyrosine deiodinase that is specific for iodotyrosines.
  (2) The iodide released from MIT and DIT is available for reutilization and forms the "second iodide" pool, which provides more iodide for new hormone formation than does new iodide uptake.
 b. The T_3 and T_4 diffuse into the extracellular fluid and enter the circulation, where over 99% binds to thyroxine-binding proteins.

V. METABOLISM AND EXCRETION OF THYROID HORMONE

A. T_4 is the iodothyronine found in highest concentration in plasma and is the only one that arises solely by direct secretion from the thyroid gland.

B. Most of the T_3 present in plasma is derived from the peripheral conversion of T_4 by mono-deiodination via 5'-deiodinase.

  1. The extrathyroid deiodination of T_4 accounts for over 80% of the circulating T_3.

  2. The liver, kidney, and pituitary deiodinate T_4 to form T_3.

C. Thyroid hormone is metabolized by deiodination, deamination, and conjugation with glucuronic acid. The conjugate then is secreted via the bile duct into the intestine.

D. In normal individuals, T_4 and T_3 are excreted mainly in the feces, with a small amount appearing in the urine.

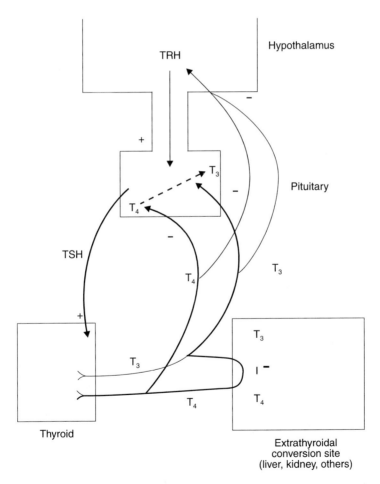

FIGURE 53-5. The hypothalamic-pituitary-thyroid axis. Thyroid-stimulating hormone (TSH) regulates the thyroid glandular synthesis and secretion of T_4 and T_3; T_3 is also produced in many other tissues by deiodination of T_4. TSH secretion is regulated by serum T_4, serum T_3, T_3 produced from T_4 within the pituitary, and thyrotropin-releasing hormone (TRH). T_4 and T_3 probably also regulate TRH secretion. $(-)$ = inhibitory effect; $(+)$ = stimulatory effect. (From Felig P, Baxter JD, and Frohman LA (eds): *Endocrinology and Metabolism*, 3rd ed. New York, McGraw-Hill, 1995, p 445, Figure 10–11.)

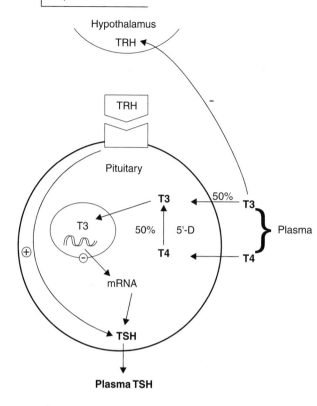

FIGURE 53-6. Regulation of thyrotropin (TSH) from the pituitary thyrotrope. Thyrotropin-releasing hormone (TRH) is under the negative feedback influence by circulating free thyroid hormones, in which TRH mRNA levels are inversely proportional to circulating T_3 levels. The circulating TSH level reflects the net negative influence of thyroid hormone and the positive stimulation of TRH on TSH synthesis and release from the thyrotrope. About 50% of nuclear T_3 arises from local conversion of T_4 by 5′-deiodinase (5′-D) within the thyrotrope and 50% comes directly from the circulation. This contrasts with peripheral tissues, where 80% of the nuclear T_3 is derived from plasma. (From Falk SA (ed): *Thyroid Disease: Endocrinology, Surgery, Nuclear Medicine and Radiotherapy,* 2nd ed. Philadelphia, Lippincott-Raven, 1997, p 38, Figure 5.)

VI. CONTROL OF THYROID FUNCTION (see Figures 53–5 and 53–6)

A. **Hypothalamic-hypophysial-thyroid axis.** TSH secretion is influenced by four factors: thyrotropin-releasing hormone (TRH) secretion from the median eminence, the blood level of unbound T_4, the blood level of unbound T_3 generated by the peripheral conversion of T_4 to T_3, and the peripheral conversion of T_4 to T_3 within the pituitary gland.

1. **TRH** is a tripeptide synthesized by the parvicellular peptidergic neurons in the hypothalamus.
   a. TRH is transported to the median eminence, where it is stored. From there, TRH is released into the hypophysial portal system and is carried to the anterior lobe of the pituitary gland.
   b. TRH stimulates the basophils (**thyrotropes**) to secrete TSH.
   c. TRH secretion is also influenced by thyroid hormone; T_3 decreases TRH secretion by the hypothalamus.

2. **TSH** stimulates the thyroid follicle to secrete thyroid hormone, most of which is bound to plasma protein carriers.
   a. TSH stimulates the series of enzymatic reactions that lead to the synthesis of the iodothyronines.
   b. The circulating TSH level reflects the net effect of the negative feedback of thyroid hormone and the positive stimulation of TRH on TSH synthesis and secretion from the thyrotrophs.
   c. All of the inhibition of TSH secretion can be accounted for by the T_3 produced by the monodeiodination of T_4 in the pituitary by 5′-deiodinase.
   d. The pituitary is under constant stimulation by TRH, but the responsiveness of the pituitary to TRH is regulated by the free thyroid hormone in the blood (T_3 within the pituitary); therefore, thyroid hormone can inhibit the effect of TRH on TSH secretion.

3. Other regulators
   a. Estrogens enhance TSH secretion.
   b. Large doses of iodide inhibit thyroid hormone release and thereby cause decreases in serum T_4 and T_3 concentrations and an increase in TSH secretion.
   c. Somatostatin inhibits TSH secretion and the response to TRH.
   d. Dihydroxyphenylethylamine (dopamine), dope, and bromocriptine decrease the basal secretion of TSH.

B. Thyroid autoregulation

1. Thyroid function also is regulated by an intrinsic control system that maintains the constancy of thyroid hormone stores.
   a. The high concentrations of intrathyroidal **inorganic** iodide lead to the inhibition of thyroid release.
   b. High concentrations of **organic** iodide (thyroid hormone) lead to a decrease in iodide uptake.

2. Both of these effects reduce the fluctuation in thyroid hormone secretion when an acute change occurs in the availability of a requisite substrate (e.g., iodide).

C. Goiter

1. Any enlargement of the thyroid gland is called a **goiter,** and antithyroid substances that cause thyroid enlargement are called **goitrogens.**
   a. Goitrogens are substances that block the synthesis of thyroid hormone.
   b. A goiter does not define the functional state of the thyroid gland.

2. If the goitrogen reduces thyroid hormone synthesis to subnormal levels, TSH secretion is enhanced.

3. Goitrogens lead to the increased synthesis of endogenous TSH, which is responsible for the formation of a hypertropic thyroid gland (goiter).

D. Antithyroid drugs (ATDs)

1. Drugs that inhibit thyroid hormone synthesis
   a. ATDs are used in the treatment of hyperthyroidism.
   b. Since ATDs reduce thyroid hormone levels that lead to elevated TSH secretion, ATDs are called goitrogens.

2. ATDs are grouped into two classes: agents that block iodide transport and those that inhibit the organification of iodide and the coupling of iodotyrosyl residues in thyroglobulin.
   a. Drugs that block iodide uptake
      (1) They include monovalent anions such as pertechnetate (TcO_4^-), perchlorate (ClO_4^-), thiocyanate (SCN^-), and nitrate (NO_3^-).
      (2) These anions are competitive inhibitors of iodide transport.
      (3) SCN^- and ClO_4^- are no longer used because of their toxicity.
      (4) Pertechnetate-99m, a gamma emitter, is a useful radioisotope for thyroid imaging (scintiscanning) because it is transported into the thyroid, but, unlike iodide, it is not organified and therefore diffuses back into the circulation.
   b. ATDs that block organification of iodide and coupling reactions
      (1) This family of drugs includes the thionamides (propylthiouracil, methimazole, and carbimazole), which contain a thiourea moiety in their structure.
      (2) Carbimazole is hydrolyzed to methimazole in vivo.
      (3) In vivo these ATDs inhibit iodination of tyrosine residues on thyroglobulin by interacting with TPO; therefore, they inhibit TPO-mediated oxidation and thyroglobulin iodination.
      (4) Thionamides also inhibit the TPO-mediated coupling reaction.
      (5) In summary, these ATDs serve as TPO substrates, and are themselves iodinated,

shunting oxidized iodide away from the tyrosyl residues, thereby reducing iodotyrosine formation.

(6) Propylthiouracil also inhibits 5'-deiodinase, leading to a reduction in the extrathyroidal synthesis of T_3.

3. Other drugs that affect thyroid function

a. Radiodine I-131 is the most common treatment of thyrotoxicosis (Graves' disease).

b. Lithium carbonate, which is used in the treatment of bipolar depression, inhibits thyroid hormone release and synthesis (organification of iodide) and may cause goiter and hypothyroidism.

c. Excess iodide. In spite of a highly efficient autoregulatory system, excess iodide can in unusual circumstances lead either to the development of a goiter and hypothyroidism or thyrotoxicosis in individuals with a preexisting goiter.

d. Iodine deficiency ranks as the most common cause of thyroid biosynthetic failure worldwide.

(1) This condition is associated with a hypothyroid goiter.

(2) With lesser degrees of iodine deficiency a euthyroid goiter is more likely.

e. Thyrotoxicosis. Thyroid-stimulating antibody causes the hyperthyroidism of Graves' disease.

(1) The antibody to the TSH receptor is known as thyroid-stimulating immunoglobulin (TSI), or TSH-receptor antibody.

(2) This IgG immunoglobulin causes a diffuse hyperthyroid goiter.

(3) TSH levels in hyperthyroidism are depressed.

(4) TSI reacts with the TSH receptor to stimulate both function and growth of the thyroid gland.

VII. PHYSIOLOGIC EFFECTS OF THYROID HORMONE

A. Thyroid hormone receptors in the nuclei of most tissues mediate nearly all of the known physiologic actions of thyroid hormone.

1. T_4 and T_3 exist within cells both free and bound to cytosol, microsomes, mitochondria, and nuclei (chromatin).

2. T_3 constitutes nearly all the nuclear-bound hormone; therefore, T_4 can be considered largely as a prohormone.

3. T_4 has some intrinsic biological activity.

4. The physiologic actions of thyroid hormone are growth, differentiation, calorigenesis, and TSH (and TRH) suppression.

B. Thyroid hormone increases the **basal metabolic rate (BMR)** of most cells in the body. The normal BMR for adult euthyroid males is 35–40 kcal/m^2 body surface/hr. Normal BMR is 6%–10% lower in euthyroid females.

1. Exceptions to this effect occur in the gonads, brain, lymph nodes, thymus, lung, spleen, dermis, and some accessory sex organs.

2. A correlate of the increase in BMR is an increase in the size and the number of mitochondria together with an increase in the enzymes that regulate oxidative phosphorylation.

3. The increase in BMR also is associated with an increase in Na$^+$-K$^+$-ATPase (Na$^+$-K$^+$ pump) activity. The fluxes of Na$^+$ (efflux) and K$^+$ (influx) are estimated to require 10%–30% of the total basal energy consumed by cells.

4. The increase in BMR accounts for the thermogenic calorigenic effect of thyroid hormone.

C. Thyroid hormone is essential for normal **bone growth and maturation** as well as for the maturation of neurologic tissue, especially the brain.

1. In hypothyroidism, there is a marked decrease in the myelination and arborization of neurons in the brain.

2. If hypothyroidism is untreated, mental retardation occurs (cretinism).

D. Thyroid hormone is necessary for normal **lactation.**

VIII. **METABOLIC EFFECTS OF THYROID HORMONE**

A. **Carbohydrate metabolism**

1. In physiologic amounts, thyroid hormone potentiates the action of insulin and promotes glycogenesis and glucose utilization.

2. In pharmacological amounts, thyroid hormone is a hyperglycemic agent.
  a. Thyroid hormone potentiates the glycogenolytic effect of epinephrine, causing glycogen depletion.
  b. Thyroid hormone is gluconeogenic in that it increases the availability of precursors (lactate and glycerol) for glucose production.
  c. In large doses, thyroid hormone accelerates intestinal glucose absorption.
  d. The thermogenic effects of thyroid hormone are accompanied by increased peripheral and splanchnic utilization of glucose.
    (1) The increased need for glucose is balanced by increased hepatic glucose output.
    (2) The increased hepatic glucose production is provided by increased gluconeogenesis and glycogenolysis.
  e. High levels of thyroid hormone lead to glucose intolerance.

B. **Protein metabolism**

1. In physiologic amounts, thyroid hormone has a potent protein anabolic effect.

2. In large doses, thyroid hormone has a protein catabolic effect.

3. Thyroid hormone inhibits synthesis of glycosaminoglycan and fibronectin in fibroblasts.

C. **Fat metabolism**

1. Thyroid hormone stimulates all aspects of lipid metabolism, including synthesis, mobilization, and utilization. On a net basis, the lipolytic effect is greater than the lipogenic effect.

2. The increase in lipolysis provides fatty acids that can be oxidized to generate energy for thermogenesis.

3. There is a general inverse relationship between thyroid hormone levels and plasma lipids.
  a. Elevated thyroid hormone levels are associated with decreases in blood triglycerides, phospholipids, and cholesterol.
  b. High levels of thyroid hormone also are associated with increases in plasma free fatty acids and glycerol.

D. **Vitamin metabolism.** The metabolism of fat-soluble vitamins is affected by thyroid hormone. For example, thyroid hormone is required for the hepatic synthesis of vitamin A from carotene and the conversion of vitamin A to retinene.

1. In hypothyroid states, the serum carotene is elevated, and the skin becomes yellow.

2. This skin condition differs from that observed in jaundice in that the sclera of the eye is not yellow.

IX. **CONTROL OF THYROID HORMONE SECRETION: THE HYPOTHALAMO-PITUITARY-THYROIDAL AXIS** (Table 53–2)

Table 53-2. The Hypothalamo-Pituitary-Thyroidal Axis

	Circulating or Release Rate		
	T$_4$	TSH	TRH
1. Primary hypothyroidism	↓	↑	↑
2. Pituitary hypothyroidism (also called secondary hypothyroidism)	↓	↓	↑
3. Hypothalamic hypothyroidism (also called tertiary hypothyroidism)	↓	↓	↓
4. Graves' disease	↑	↓	↓

TRH = thyroid-releasing hormone; TSH = thyroid-stimulating hormone.

Case 1

A 34-year-old woman has a 3-month history of nervousness, tremor, palpitation, increased sweating, and discomfort with heat. She had lost 15 pounds despite increased food intake. She also noted muscle weakness and easy fatigability with exercise to which she was ordinarily accustomed. She had missed two consecutive menstrual periods. On physical examination, her pulse rate was 110 beats/min at rest and rose to 150 beats/min with 30 seconds of rapid stair climbing. Blood pressure was 150/60 and respiration rate was 20/min. Her skin was warm and moist, her speech was rapid, her gaze had a stare quality, and her movements were hyperkinetic. She exhibited a tremor and very rapid reflexes, and she was unable to rise without assistance from a squatting position. The cardiac impulse was hyperdynamic, and the thyroid gland was diffusely enlarged. Laboratory studies showed a total serum T$_4$ level of 26 μg/dl (normal 5–12 μg/dl), a free T$_4$ of 4.1 ng/dl (normal 0.8 to 2.4 ng/dl), and a serum TSH of 0.01 mIU/ml (normal 0.5 to 5 mIU/ml). A 24-hour uptake of radioactive iodine was 70% (normal 8%–30%). A pregnancy test was negative. The patient was treated with a thiouracil drug. Four weeks later her symptoms had improved, and serum T$_4$ had decreased to 11 μg/dl. However, after 12 weeks of the same dose of the thiouracil drug, serum T$_4$ had decreased further to 4 μg/dl, and she complained of the recurrence of fatigue with lethargy and intolerance to cold. Her weight had increased 20 pounds to a level above her usual healthy weight. Resting pulse was 54 beats/min. The thyroid gland, which had begun to decrease in size with drug treatment, had now grown even larger than before treatment.

> *1. By what mechanisms did an excess of thyroid hormone cause the various symptoms and physical findings this patient exhibited? How did her cardiac output and systemic vascular resistance compare with normal?*

DISCUSSION

Loss of weight despite normal food intake indicates negative caloric balance caused by energy expenditure exceeding energy intake. An excess level of thyroid hormone has increased the patient's basal or resting metabolic rate that is, the rate of oxygen utilization was above normal. In addition, thyroid hormone excess has caused a negative nitrogen balance, with the rate of protein degradation exceeding the rate of protein synthesis, so that lean body mass and bone mass have declined along with adipose tissue. The high basal metabolic rate (BMR) induced by thyroid hormone is accompanied by increased heat production, which causes intolerance to high environmental temperatures and stimulates mechanisms of heat loss, such as sweating and hyperventilation. Nervousness, tremor, rapid reflexes, and tachycardia reflect increased adrenergic nervous system activity. Muscle weakness is caused by a loss of muscle mass that results from enhanced proteolysis. Increased fatigability with exercise is caused by inefficient generation of adenosine triphosphate (ADP) and reduced stores of creatine phosphate. The patient's cardiac output has been increased through thyroid hormone-induced increases in preload, cardiac contractility, and stroke volume. Systemic vascular resistance is decreased; this is attributable to local vasodilation caused by increased rates of tissue metabolism.

2. *What was her serum level of triiodothyronine (T3) likely to be and why? Would this contribute to her clinical state?*

DISCUSSION

The serum T_3 level would be elevated. This is largely attributable to the high serum level of T_4, from which most T_3 is derived by peripheral conversion. To a lesser extent T_3 secretion is increased by the enlarged thyroid gland. T_3 is the active metabolite of T_4, and it binds with 10-fold greater affinity to the nuclear thyroid hormone receptor. Therefore, increased T_3 accounts for most of the patient's clinical signs.

3. *Why was her serum thyroid-stimulating hormone (TSH) so low?*

DISCUSSION

Excess secretion of thyroid hormone almost always results from disease intrinsic to the thyroid gland, and therefore such secretion is autonomous and independent of thyroid-stimulating hormone (TSH) stimulation of the gland. The resultant high serum T_4 and T_3 levels inhibit TSH secretion by blocking the effect of thyroid-releasing hormone (TRH) on the pituitary thyrotrophs. The serum TSH level is therefore low.

4. *Under what circumstances could the serum thyroid-stimulating hormone (TSH) have been elevated?*

DISCUSSION

The serum thyroid-stimulating hormone (TSH) level would be elevated only in the rare cases in which hyperthyroidism was either caused by excessive release of thyroid-releasing hormone (TRH) or by secretion of TSH from a pituitary neoplasm.

5. *What was the significance of her elevated radioactive iodine uptake?*

DISCUSSION

An increased rate of synthesis of T_4 requires increased availability of iodide to the thyroid gland. If the total body pool of iodide stays normal, then a larger than normal percentage of that pool must be taken up by the thyroid gland each day to maintain a high level of thyroid hormone synthesis and release.

6. *What is the mechanism of action of the thiouracil drug?*

DISCUSSION

Thiouracil drugs inhibit the enzyme thyroid peroxidase (TPO), which catalyzes all steps in thyroid hormone synthesis from iodide and tyrosine. This enzyme is not required for iodide transport (uptake). In addition to reducing T_4 synthesis and release, thiouracil drugs inhibit the enzyme 5' monodeiodinase and thereby decrease the peripheral production of T_3 from T_4.

7. *What resulted at 12 weeks of therapy from continual exposure to the maximal dose of the thiouracil drug?*

DISCUSSION

Although the thiouracil drug was initially beneficial, continued suppression of thyroid hormone synthesis produced a state of hypothyroidism. The basal metabolic rate (BMR) decreased below normal, leading to inordinate weight gain. Cold intolerance resulted from subnormal thermogenesis. Bradycardia and lethargy resulted from diminished adrenergic nervous system activity.

> **8.** *What was her serum thyroid-stimulating hormone (TSH) level likely to be at that point and why?*

DISCUSSION

When the patient developed hypothyroidism, the decline in negative feedback caused an elevation in the serum level of thyroid-stimulating hormone (TSH). Low serum T_4 and T_3 levels elicit overstimulation of the pituitary thyrotrophs by thyroid-releasing hormone (TRH).

> **9.** *Why did her thyroid gland reenlarge?*

DISCUSSION

The thyroid gland was initially enlarged because of hyperthyroidism (Graves' disease). The later reenlargement of the thyroid gland during thiouracil therapy reflected the trophic action of excess endogenous thyroid-stimulating hormone (TSH) acting through its thyroid plasma membrane receptor to stimulate DNA, RNA, and protein synthesis.

Chapter 54

The Calcitropic Hormones: Parathyroid Hormone, Calcitonin, and Vitamin D

I. ROLE OF Ca²⁺ IN PHYSIOLOGIC PROCESSES

A. **Hemostasis.** Ca^{2+} is necessary for the activation of clotting enzymes in plasma.

B. Ca^{2+} controls **membrane excitation,** and Ca^{2+} influx occurs during the excitatory process of nerve and muscle.

1. Excitable membranes contain specific Ca^{2+} channels.

2. Ca^{2+} entry does not require an active transport process, because the concentration gradient across the membrane is larger for Ca^{2+} than for any other ion.
   a. Ca^{2+} concentration ($[Ca^+]$) in the intracellular fluid (ICF) is about 10^{-7} mol/L.
   b. $[Ca^{2+}]$ in the extracellular fluid (ECF) is about 10^{-3} mol/L (the actual value is 2.5×10^{-3} mol/L).
   c. The $[Ca^{2+}]$ gradient from outside to inside the cell is on the order of 10,000 to 1!

C. Ca^{2+} is bound to cell surfaces and has a role in the **stabilization of the membrane** and **intercellular adhesion.** Within the cell, Ca^{2+} is stored in the mitochondrial membrane, the endoplasmic reticulum (sarcoplasmic reticulum of muscle cells), and the inner plasma membrane.

D. Ca^{2+} is necessary for **muscle contraction** [excitation-contraction (EC) coupling]. It binds to specific Ca^{2+}-binding proteins, such as calmodulin in nonmuscle cells and troponin C in striated muscle cells.

E. Ca^{2+} is essential in all **excitation-secretion processes,** such as the release of hormone by endocrine cells and the release of other products by exocrine cells. It also is essential for **neurotransmitter release.** Calcium binds to the membrane of the secretory vesicles and promotes fusion with the plasma membrane or stimulates the intracellular microtubule/microfilament system.

F. Ca^{2+} is necessary for the production of **milk** and the formation of **bone** and **teeth.**

G. Ca^{2+} acts as a second messenger in the cytosol. Its effects include changes in cell motility, contraction of muscle cells, increased release of secretory proteins, and activation of a number of regulatory enzymes.

H. Ca^{2+} has an essential role in the mineralization of bone.

II. Ca²⁺ DISTRIBUTION

A. **Skeletal storage.** More than 99% of the total body Ca^{2+} is stored in the skeleton.

1. The skeleton of a 70-kg person contains about 1000 g of Ca^{2+}, compared to about 1 g in the extracellular pool.

2. Bone serves as a third-line defense in acid-base regulation by virtue of its CO_3^{2-}, HCO_3^-, and PO_4^{3-} content.

B. Plasma (Figure 54–1). The plasma concentration of total (ionized and nonionized) Ca^{2+} is about 10 mg/dl, which is equivalent to 2.5 mmol/L, or 5 mEq/L. Ionic Ca^{2+} has a plasma concentration of about 1.2 mM/L, or 2.4 mEq/L.

  1. Ca^{2+} is present in the plasma as:
  a. Ionized or free (45%)
  b. Complexed with HPO_4^{2-}, HCO_3^{-}, or citrate ion (10%).
  c. Bound to protein (primarily to albumin) (45%)

  2. Calcium concentration expressed in mg/dl can be converted to mmol/L (mM) by dividing by 4, and to mEq/L by dividing by 2.

  3. The sum of the ionized and complexed Ca^{2+} constitutes the diffusible fraction (55%) of Ca^{2+}. The protein-bound form constitutes the nondiffusible fraction (45%).

  4. Ionized calcium has a higher solubility in acidic solutions (Figure 54–2).

  5. Parathyroid hormone (PTH), calcitonin, and vitamin D regulate the serum ionized Ca^{2+} concentration.

C. Ca^{2+} **pools.** Total body Ca^{2+} can be conceptualized as two major "pools."

  1. The larger Ca^{2+} pool, which contains 99% of the total Ca^{2+}, consists of stable (mature) bone. This represents the Ca^{2+} "pool" that is not readily exchangeable, and it is not available for rapid mobilization.
  a. The size of this non-readily exchangeable (stable) calcium pool is about 1 kg (1,000,000 mg).
  b. The non-readily exchangeable calcium fixed pool is located within the crystal structure of the mineral phase and is the site of action of parathyroid hormone (PTH).

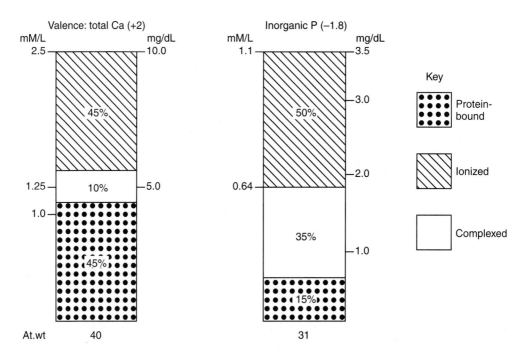

FIGURE 54-1. Distribution of total calcium and inorganic phosphorus in human plasma. The sum of the ionized and complexed fractions constitutes the diffusible fraction and the protein-bound fraction forms the non-diffusible fraction. PTH regulates the ionized fraction of calcium. Approximately 50% of the calcium is in the diffusible form, and about 50% of the calcium is nondiffusible. Approximately 85% of the phosphorus is diffusible and about 15% is nondiffusible.

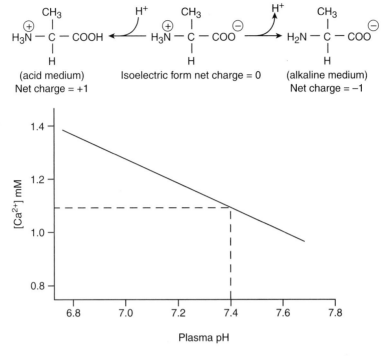

FIGURE 54-2. Plasma ionized calcium concentration as a function of pH. Calcium (ionic) binding to albumin is strongly pH-dependent between pH 7 and 8. An acute increase or decrease in pH will increase or decrease, respectively, the protein-bound fraction of calcium. Thus, in hypocalcemic patients with metabolic acidosis, rapid correction of acidemia with sodium bicarbonate can precipitate tetany, because of increased binding to albumin and, thereby, a decrease in ionized calcium concentration. Respiratory alkalosis caused by hyperventilation also can precipitate tetany in a hypocalcemic patient. In alkaline media, amino acids have a net negative charge, which increases Ca^{2+} binding, whereas in acid media, amino acids have a net positive charge, which decreases Ca^{2+} binding.

    c. The size of the stable phosphorus pool is about 400 g (400,000 mg).

  2. The smaller Ca^{2+} pool, which contains about 1% of the total body Ca^{2+}, consists of labile (young) bone. This Ca^{2+} pool is readily exchangeable because it is in physicochemical equilibrium with the ECF. The pool consists of calcium phosphate salts and provides an immediate reserve for sudden decreases in blood $[Ca^{2+}]$.

    a. This calcium pool represents newly formed bone.

    b. The magnitude of the readily exchangeable calcium pool is approximately 4 g (4000 mg).

    c. One gram of bone crystals is equivalent to a surface area of 100 square meters.

    d. The size of the readily exchangeable phosphorus pool is about 2.2 g (2200 mg).

D. Diet. Balanced diets provide from 800 to 1200 mg of calcium and phosphorus per day.

III. PHOSPHORUS (P) DISTRIBUTION

A. **Skeletal storage.** About 85% of the total body P is stored in the skeleton.

  1. The skeleton contains between 0.5 and 0.8 kg of P, compared to about 0.5 to 0.8 g in the extracellular/intracellular fluid.

  2. Phosphorus is an integral constituent of nucleic acids; phospholipids; complex carbohydrates; glycolytic intermediates; structural, signaling, and enzymatic phosphoproteins; nucleotide cofactors for enzymes and G proteins; and a large number of organic glycolytic intermediates.

B. **Plasma** (see Figure 54–1). The concentration of total (ionized and nonionized P is about 12 mg/dl, of which about 8.5 mg/dl is in the organic form and about 3.5 mg/dl is in the inorganic form.

1. Organic P is composed entirely of phospholipids bound to protein.

2. In clinical settings only the inorganic orthophosphate is routinely measured. About 85% of this inorganic phosphate is ultrafilterable. This inorganic phosphate is found as follows:
   a. Ionized or free P, mainly as HPO_4^{2-} (50% of inorganic P)
   b. Complexed with Na^+, Ca^{2+}, Mg^{2+} (35% of inorganic P)
   c. Bound to protein (15% of inorganic P)

3. Because plasma inorganic phosphate is a mixture of divalent (HPO_4^{2-}) and monovalent ($H_2PO_4^-$) anions, the composite valence of P in plasma is 1.8.* At pH of 7.4 the plasma ratio of $[HPO_4^{2-}]$ to $[H_2PO_4^-]$ is 4:1.

4. Concentrations of phosphorus expressed in mg/dl can be converted to mmol/L by dividing by 3.1, and to mEq/L by dividing by 1.8.

C. **Diet.** Balanced diets provide from 800 to 1500 mg of phosphorus per day.

IV. BONE CHEMISTRY

A. Bone Ca^{2+} is found in the form of **hydroxyapatite crystals.** The empirical chemical formula for this substance is $Ca_{10} (PO_4)_6 (OH)_2$ or $[(Ca_3PO_4)_2]_3 \cdot Ca(OH)_2$. Fluoride ion can replace the OH^- group and form **fluorapatite,** or $[(Ca_3PO_4)_2]_3 \cdot CaF_2$.

1. The calcium:phosphorus ratio in bone is about 1.7:1.

2. A large surface area is provided by the microcrystalline structure of bone. The total bone surface area of the canaliculi and lacunae is 1000 to 5000 m^2!

B. Dry, fat-free bone is two thirds mineral (inorganic) and one third organic matrix.

1. Over 90% of the organic matrix is type 1 collagen and accounts for 95% of the osteoid.

2. The inorganic crystalline structure of bone imparts to it an elastic modulus similar to that of concrete. The compressional strength of bone is greater than that of reinforced concrete.

V. BONE DEVELOPMENT.
Bone is both a tissue and an organ. It consists of cells and an extracellular matrix containing organic and inorganic components. In its early development, bone exists as **osteoid,** an organic, unmineralized matrix surrounding the bone cells that deposited it.

A. **Mesoderm** is the embryonic germ layer that gives rise to cartilage, bone, and muscle.

B. **Neural crest** cells also can differentiate as bone cells, including:

1. Cells that deposit dentin in teeth

2. Cartilage and bone of the head

C. Types of bone

1. Bone is composed of cells and extracellular matrix. Cells account for 2% of the total volume of bone.

---

*80% HPO_4^{2-} and 20% $H_2PO_4^-$. Thus, 0.8×2 plus 0.2×1 is equal to an average valence of 1.8.

2. The extracellular matrix is the predominant component of bone.
   a. One third of the matrix consists of collagen and glycosaminoglycans.
      (1) This organic component is called osteoid.
      (2) A unique feature of the extracellular matrix is that it can be calcified.
   b. Two thirds of the bony matrix is composed of mineral crystals.

3. Bone is subdivided into **cortical** (compact) bone and **trabecular** (cancellous, or spongy) bone.
   a. Compact bone is found in the shafts of long bones and on the surfaces of the pelvis, skull, and other flat bones.
   b. Trabecular bone is found at the ends of long bones, in the vertebrae, and in the internal portions of the pelvis, skull, and other flat bones.

4. About 80–90% of the volume of compact bone is calcified, makes up about 80% of the skeletal mass, and provides biomechanical strength to bone.
   a. The basic unit of cortical bone is called the **osteon.** It consists of concentric layers, or lamellae, of bone arranged around a central channel (haversian canal), which contains the capillary blood supply.
   b. The entire bone is surrounded on its outer surface by the periosteum and is separated from bone marrow by the endosteum.

5. Cancellous (trabecular, or spongy) bone is found in the axial skeleton (skull, ribs, vertebrae, and pelvis) and at the ends of the long bones.
   a. Although only about 20% of the bone mass consists of trabecular bone, its sponge-like organization provides 5 to 8 times as much surface area for metabolic activity as compact bone.
   b. About 15% to 25% of the trabecular bone is calcified, with the remainder being in contact either with a fatty marrow (ends of long bones) or with a hematopoietic marrow (axial skeleton).
   c. The trabeculae are completely surrounded by endosteum.

6. All normal adult bone is lamellar bone, whether it has a compact or a trabecular structure.

VI. **Ca^{2+} REGULATION.** Ca^{2+} regulation involves three tissues—bone, intestine, and kidney; three hormones—PTH, calcitonin, and activated vitamin D_3; and three cell types—osteoblasts, osteocytes, and osteoclasts.

A. **Hormonal control of Ca^{2+} metabolism.** The pituitary gland does not play a major role in regulating the cells that produce PTH, calcitonin, and activated vitamin D_3.

1. **PTH** is a polypeptide that contains 84 amino acid residues. PTH is secreted by the chief cells of the four parathyroid glands.
   a. PTH is the **hypercalcemic hormone** of the body; it exerts its effects on the bone, intestine, and kidney.
   b. PTH regulates only the plasma $[Ca^{2+}]$. An inverse linear relationship exists between plasma $[Ca^{2+}]$ and PTH secretion (Figure 54–3).
      (1) When plasma $[Ca^{2+}]$ falls, PTH secretion increases.
      (2) As plasma $[Ca^{2+}]$ increases, PTH secretion decreases.
      (3) Calcium loads cause inhibition of PTH secretion, inhibition of renal synthesis of $1,25(OH)_2D_3$, decreased intestinal active transport of Ca^{2+}, increased renal excretion of Ca^{2+}, decreased excretion of phosphate, and a decrease in bone resorption.
      (4) Phosphate loads increase PTH secretion, suppress renal synthesis of $1,25(OH)_2D_3$, and inhibit bone resorption.
      (5) An increase in plasma phosphate concentration will directly stimulate PTH secretion and also can indirectly reduce plasma Ca^{2+} concentration, which also enhances PTH secretion.

2. **Calcitonin** is a 32-amino-acid residue polypeptide secreted by the parafollicular (C) cells of the thyroid gland.
   a. Calcitonin is the **hypocalcemic hormone** of the body. It exerts a biologic effect on the bone, intestine, and kidney.

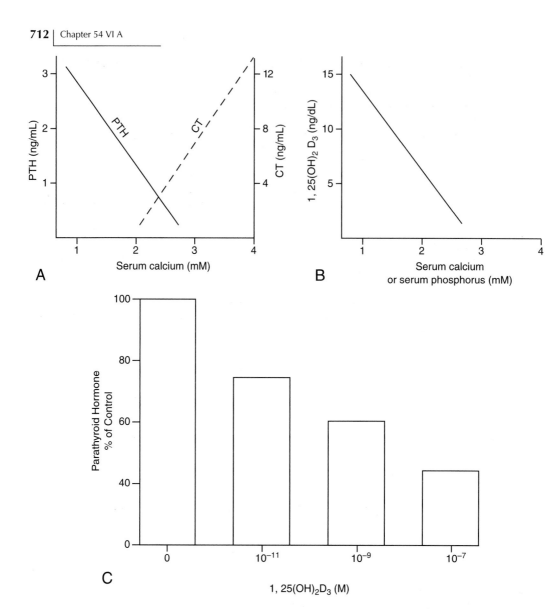

FIGURE 54-3. Relationship between serum calcium concentration and plasma levels of PTH or calcitonin and between serum calcium or phosphorus concentration and plasma $1,25(OH)_2D_3$ Note the parallel relationship between serum calcium concentration and calcitonin. Also note the inverse relationships between serum calcium concentration and PTH (A); serum calcium or serum phosphorus concentration and $1,25(OH)_2D_3$ (B); and between $1,25(OH)_2D_3$ and PTH (C). Parathyroid hormone and calcitriol are the major regulators of Ca^{2+} homeostasis in humans. PTH stimulates the production of calcitriol by activating renal 1 α-hydroxylase, and calcitriol suppresses the synthesis and secretion of PTH (as shown in C). PTH = parathyroid hormone; CT = calcitonin; $1,25(OH)_2D_3$ = calcitriol.

      b. A positive linear relationship exists between plasma $[Ca^{2+}]$ and calcitonin secretion (see Figure 54–3A).
         (1) As plasma $[Ca^{2+}]$ increases, calcitonin secretion increases.
         (2) When plasma $[Ca^{2+}]$ decreases, calcitonin secretion decreases.
      c. Calcitonin release is stimulated by pentagastrin.

    3. Vitamin D_3 (cholecalciferol) is a secosteroid containing 27 carbon atoms, which makes it a steroid hormone. The term "vitamin D" denotes both vitamins D_2 and D_3. In humans, the storage, transport, metabolism, and potency of vitamin D_2 and vitamin D_3 are identical.

  a. The only difference between vitamin D_2 (ergocalciferol) and vitamin D_3 is that D_2 is a 28-carbon secosteroid, because D_2 contains a double bond between C_{22} and C_{23}, and a methyl group on C_{24}.

  b. Vitamin D_2 is a sterol found in yeasts and plants in the form of ergosterol.

  c. Vitamin D_3 is found in fatty fish and cod liver oil.

  d. Vitamin D_3 is both a vitamin when ingested from nutritional sources and a hormone when it is produced in the skin and activated sequentially in the liver and kidney. Therefore, vitamin D_3 is not a true vitamin, unless there is a deficiency of it.

  e. Exposure of the skin to sunlight for 15–20 minutes/day or the irradiation of food has an antirachitic effect.

  f. Intestinal absorption of vitamins D_2 and D_3 occurs principally in the ileum and requires bile salts.

  g. The recommended adequate intake (AI) for vitamin D_3 is between 400 IU (10 μg) per day and 600 IU (15 μg) per day. In the absence of sunlight the AI should be increased by 200 IU per day.

  h. Vitamin D_3 is a second hypercalcemic hormone.

  i. Active metabolites. Only the active metabolites of vitamin D_3 exert biologic activity.

  (1) Calcidiol (25-hydroxyvitamin D_3; 25-hydroxycholecalciferol) is the major blood form of vitamin D_3. This active metabolite is two to five times more effective than vitamin D_3 in preventing rickets.

  (2) Calcitriol (1,25-dihydroxyvitamin D_3; 1,25-dihydroxycholecalciferol) is another active metabolite of vitamin D_3. On a molar basis, it is 100 times more potent than calcidiol.

4. Biosynthesis of active vitamin D_3 (Figure 54–4)

  a. In the epidermis (stratum corneum), the provitamin D_3, 7-dehydrocholesterol, is converted into cholecalciferol (also vitamin D_3) by nonenzymatic photoactivation by solar radiation with energies between 290 and 315 nm (UVB). Ultraviolet B transforms the 4-ring sterol into the 3-ring sterol (secosteroid) called vitamin D_3.

  b. Vitamin D_3 enters the circulation and is bound to the vitamin D_3-binding protein (globulin) and transported to the liver where it is converted to 25-hydroxyvitamin D_3 (also 25OH cholecalciferol, or calcidiol) by hepatic 25-hydroxylase.

  c. Calcidiol is transported to the kidney, where 1α-hydroxylase metabolizes 25OHD$_3$ to 1,25(OH)$_2$D$_3$ [also 1,25(OH)$_2$ cholecalciferol, or calcitriol].

  (1) PTH and hypophosphatemia are the major inducers of this enzyme.

  (2) The target tissues for vitamin D_3 contain a nuclear vitamin D_3 receptor for 1,25(OH)$_2$D$_3$.

  (3) All forms of vitamin D_3 are lipid-soluble.

5. Parathyroid hormone-related protein (PTHrP)

  a. PTHrP mimics PTH as an inducer of bone resorption, renal phosphate excretion (hypophosphatemia), hypercalcemia, and accelerated renal production of 1,25(OH)$_2$D$_3$ in malignancy.

  b. PTHrP and PTH bind to a common receptor; however, each of these hormones also has its own receptor.

  c. PTHrP is the major cause of hypercalcemia in cancer.

B. **Cellular** control of bone metabolism (Figures 54–5 and 54–6)

  1. There are two bone surfaces at which bone is in contact with soft tissue: an external surface (the periosteal surface) and an internal surface (the endosteal surface).

  a. Most of the bone-tissue turnover occurs at bone surfaces, mainly at the endosteal surface where it interfaces with bone marrow.

  b. The osteoblasts and osteoclasts are bone-lining cells that mediate osteogenesis and osteolysis, respectively.

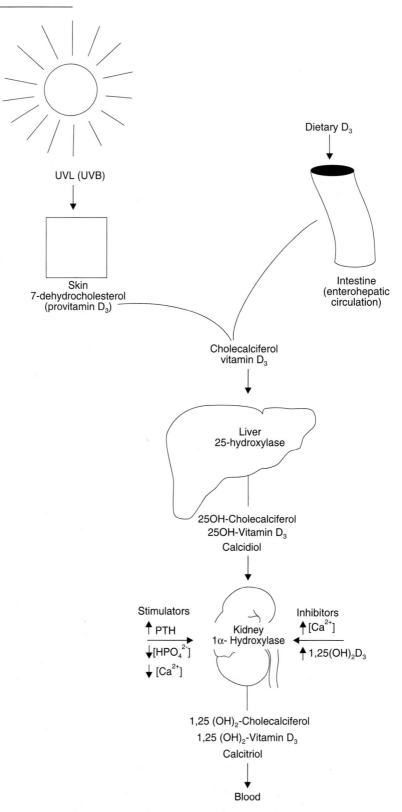

FIGURE 54-4. Biosynthetic activation of vitamin D_3.

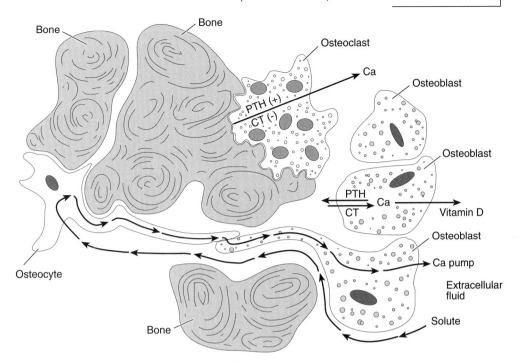

FIGURE 54-5. Relationships among the calcitropic hormones, bone cells, and calcium transport. The shaded areas represent bone crystal. The osteoclast is shown resorbing bone, a process stimulated by parathyroid hormone (PTH) and inhibited by calcitonin (CT). The osteoblasts are shown actively extruding calcium from the bone extracellular fluid (ECF)—between cells and crystals—under the influence of hormones. The canalicular system provides the structure for a functional syncytium between the osteocytes and osteoblasts. (From Greenspan FS, Baxter JD, eds: *Basic and Clinical Endocrinology,* 4th ed. Stamford, CT, Appleton & Lange, 1994, p 230.)

2. **Osteoblasts** are highly differentiated cells that are nonmitotic in their differentiated state. They are the **bone-forming cells** and are located on the bone-forming surface.
   a. Osteoblasts arise from the osteoprogenitor cell.
   b. Osteoblasts are bone-lining cells that synthesize and secrete matrix constituents; that is, collagen and ground substance. The only form of collagen in bone is type 1.
   c. They contain abundant alkaline phosphatase activity, the concentration of which in the serum is used as an index of bone formation.
   d. They have nuclear receptors for PTH, calcitonin, and estrogens.
   e. They are derived from bone marrow mesenchymal stem cells.
   f. Osteocalcin (OC) is another noncollagenous protein secreted by osteoblasts and is accepted as a biochemical marker for osteoblastic activity and hence, bone formation.
      (1) OC is incorporated into the bone matrix.
      (2) During bone resorption, OC is released from the matrix into the circulation, so the serum level has a component of both bone formation and resorption.
      (3) OC is more appropriately a marker for bone turnover rather than a specific marker of osteogenesis.
      (4) OC is the most abundant noncollagenous protein found in bone.
   g. Cells of the osteoblastic lineage are important not only in forming bone but also in initiating resorption.

2. **Osteocytes** are osteoblasts that have become **buried in bone matrix** and are the most numerous of the bone cells in mature bone.
   a. Each cell is surrounded by its own lacuna, but an extensive canalicular system connects osteocytes and surface osteoblasts, forming a functional syncytium, or continuum, by connection of their long cell processes through gap junctions.

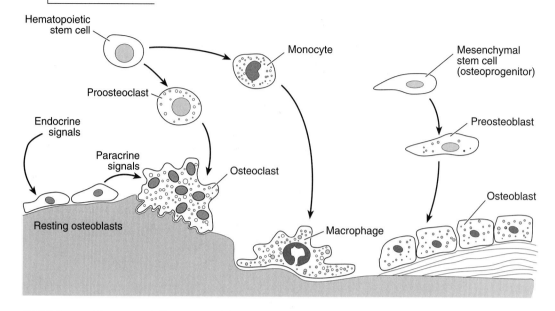

FIGURE 54-6. The process of bone remodeling. Endocrine signals to resting osteoblasts generate local paracrine signals to nearby osteoclasts and osteoclast precursors. The osteoclasts resorb an area of mineralized bone, and local macrophages complete the cleanup of dissolved elements. The process then reverses to formation as osteoblast precursors are recruited to the site and differentiate into active osteoblasts. These lay down new organic matrix and mineralize it. Thus new bone replaces the previously resorbed mature bone. (From Berne RM, Levy MN, eds: *Physiology,* 4th ed. St. Louis, Mosby, 1998, p 853.)

  b. Although historically these cells have been shown to resorb calcified bone, this point recently has been disputed because osteocytes also synthesize new bone matrix at the surface of osteocytic lacunae, which can subsequently become ossified.

 3. Osteoclasts are large, multinucleated (4 to 20 nuclei) cells containing numerous vesicles with lysosomal enzymes. They mediate **bone resorption** at bone surfaces.

  a. These cells contain acid phosphatase.

  b. Osteoclasts are stimulated by PTH and form significant amounts of lactic and hyaluronic acids.

  c. Osteoclasts may cause bone dissolution via an increased local concentration of H^+, which solubilizes bone mineral and increases the activity of enzymes that degrade matrix (collagenase). Urinary hydroxyproline, the major metabolite of collagen, provides an indirect measurement of bone resorption.

  d. The osteoclasts are derived from hematopoietic progenitors in the monocyte/macrophage family. The granulocyte/macrophage-colony-forming units (GM-CFU) are the earliest detectable cells in the osteoclast lineage.

  e. The osteoclast acidifies the extracellular compartment by secreting protons across the ruffled-border membrane by H^+-ATPase uniporters, resulting in bone dissolution.

  f. Osteoclasts contain receptors for calcitonin but not for PTH.

VII. PHYSIOLOGIC ACTIONS OF PTH (Figure 54–7; Table 54–1). Hypocalcemia is the most important stimulus for PTH secretion. Prolonged hypocalcemia can induce proliferation of parathyroid cells together with increased biosynthesis of PTH.

A. Bone

 1. PTH increases mobilization of Ca^{2+} and inorganic phosphate (i.e., osteolysis, or dissolution, or resorption) from the non-readily exchangeable Ca^{2+} pool.

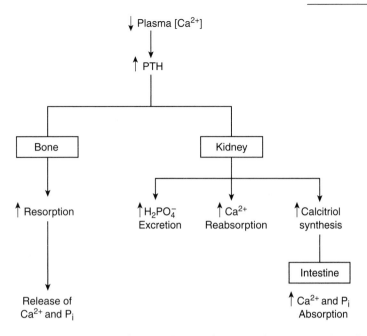

54-7. It is the action of PTH in concert on bone, kidney, and intestine that increases the inflow of Ca^{2+} into the ECF and defends the organism against hypocalcemia. The net effect is hypercalcemia and hypophosphatemia together with hypercalciuria and hyperphosphaturia. P_i = inorganic phosphate.

2. PTH increases osteoclastic cell number and activity, causing release of degradation products of collagen by digestion of osteoid.
   a. With the dissolution of stable bone, hydroxyproline is secreted into the urine.
   b. Urinary hydroxyproline is a marker for collagen metabolism and, thereby, the relative rate of bone resorption (Table 54–2).

3. It is important to note that osteoclasts do not have PTH receptors and that mature osteoclasts cannot respond to PTH.

4. PTH activates osteoclasts by stimulating osteoblasts, which then activate osteoclasts. PTH increases the number of mature osteoclasts by increasing the number of mononuclear, late committed precursors of osteoclasts.

5. Paradoxically, PTH exerts an anabolic action by increasing the formation of trabecular bone.

6. PTH stimulates differentiation of osteoclastic progenitor cells to fuse and form multinucleated osteoclasts.

7. PTH suppresses osteoblast synthesis of collagen and conversion of osteoblastic precursor cells into mature osteoclasts.

8. PTH stimulates release of insulin-like growth factors (IGF I) from osteoblasts.
   a. IGFs enhance bone collagen and matrix synthesis.
   b. IGFs decrease collagenase activity and inhibit bone-collagen degradation.

B. Intestine

1. There is no evidence to support a direct action of PTH on Ca^{2+} and phosphate transport in the intestine.

2. PTH enhances the conversion of $25OHD_3$ to $1,25(OH)_2D_3$, which directly acts on the intestinal enterocytes to increase Ca^{2+} and phosphate absorption.

Table 54-1. Regulation of Calcitropic Hormones: PTH, Calciferol, Calcitonin

Hormone	Stimuli	Inhibitors	Blood		Bone	Intestine		Kidney	
			Ca^{2+}	HPO_4^{2-}		Ca^{2+}	PO_4^{3-}	Ca^{2+}	$H_2PO_4^{-}$
PTH	$\downarrow Ca^{2+} \uparrow P_i$ $\downarrow D_3$	$\uparrow Ca^{2+}, \downarrow P_i$ $\uparrow D_3$	$\uparrow$	$\downarrow$	r	A	A	R	E
Vitamin D_3	$\downarrow Ca^{2+} \downarrow P_i$ $\uparrow PTH \downarrow D_3$	$\uparrow Ca^{2+} \uparrow P_i$ $\downarrow PTH \uparrow D_3$	$\uparrow$	$\uparrow$	r*	A	A	R	R
Calcitonin	$\uparrow Ca^{2+}$	$\downarrow Ca^{2+}$	$\downarrow$	$\downarrow$	$\downarrow$ r	$\downarrow$A	$\downarrow$A	E	E

R = reabsorption; A = absorption; r = resorption; E = excretion; P_i = inorganic phosphate (HPO_4^{2-}); PTH = parathyroid hormone.
Excreted phosphate is in the form $H_2PO_4^{-}$; absorbed phosphate is in the form PO_4^{3-}; and plasma phosphate is mainly in the form HPO_4^{2-}.
*Vitamin D_3 (1,25($OH)_2D_3$) is important for bone mineralization, but there is little direct evidence that it actively participates in this process. Instead 1,25($OH)_2D_3$ promotes the mineralization of osteoid laid down by osteoblasts, by maintaining calcium and phosphorus concentrations within the normal range by the differentiation of bone marrow monocytic stem cells into osteoclasts, which lose their ability to recognize 1,25($OH)_2D_3$.

Table 54-2. Biochemical markers of bone metabolism.

Bone formation
  Osteocalin (OCN) [bone Gla protein]*
  Bone-specific alkaline phosphatase (BSAP)
  Carboxy-terminal extension peptide of type I procollagen
Bone resorption
  Lyslypyridinoline
  Deoxylysylpyridinoline
  N-telopeptide of the cross-links of collagen
  C-telopeptide of the cross-links of collagen
  4-hydroxyproline
  Tartrate-resistant acid phosphatase
  Glycosylated hydroxylysine

---

*Bone Gla (carboxyglutamic acid) protein
Adapted from Favus MJ: *Primer on the Metabolic Diseases and Disorders of Mineral Metabolism,* 4th ed. Philadelphia, Lippincott Williams and Wilkins, 1999, p 129.

C. Kidney: Calcium (Figure 54–8)

1. A typical 70-kg man with a normal glomerular filtration rate (GFR) of 180 L/day filters about 200 mmol of Ca^{2+} per day—about 45% of serum calcium is ultrafilterable (180 L/day × 2.5 mmol/L × 0.45).

2. About 98% of the filtered load is reabsorbed by the nephron. Seventy percent of the filtered load is reabsorbed in the proximal tubule.

3. In the kidney, PTH has three major functions that are essential for the regulation of mineral ion homeostasis:
   a. Reabsorption of Ca^{2+} in the distal nephron
   b. Inhibition of phosphate reabsorption in both the proximal and distal tubules
   c. Stimulation of the synthesis of $1,25OHD_3$ in the proximal tubules

4. In the proximal tubule, PTH decreases Ca^{2+} reabsorption in parallel with a decrease in Na^+ reabsorption.
   a. Although PTH increases net renal Ca^{2+} reabsorption, patients with hyperparathyroidism are hypercalciuric.
   b. Early proximal reabsorption of Ca^{2+} is predominantly paracellular via solvent drag. Ca^{2+} also is transported proximally across the apical membrane along a concentration and an electric gradient. Late proximal Ca^{2+} transport has an active transport component in the basolateral membrane.
      (1) Ca^{2+} enters the cytosol from the lumen down an electrochemical gradient through Ca^{2+} channels.
      (2) Ca^{2+} is transported actively across the basolateral membrane by both a Ca^{2+}-ATPase uniporter and a $3Na^+$-$1Ca^{2+}$ antiporter.

5. PTH-mediated translocation of the Na^+−H^+ antiporter out of the brush border of the proximal epithelial cells leads to the inhibition of proximal HCO_3^- reabsorption, which depends on H^+ secretion. This effect accounts for the metabolic acidosis in hyperparathyroid states.

6. PTH also augments renal gluconeogenesis in the proximal nephron.

7. PTH stimulates the conversion of $25OHD_3$ (calcidiol) to $1,25(OH)_2D_3$ (calcitriol) in the renal proximal tubule, resulting in enhanced Ca^{2+} absorption, bone resorption, and an increase in the filtered load of Ca^{2+}. PTH activates 1α-hydroxylase.

8. About 20% of the filtered load of Ca^{2+} is reabsorbed in the thick ascending limb of the loop of Henle and is regulated by PTH.

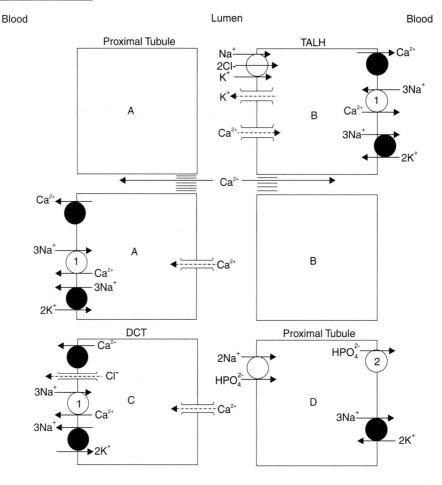

FIGURE 54-8. Calcium transport in the proximal tubule (A); thick ascending limb of the loop of Henle (TALH) (B); and the distal convoluted tubule (DCT) (C). Inorganic phosphate transport in the proximal tubule (D). Solid circles = ATPase pumps; open circles = carrier-mediated secondary active transport (1) or facilitated diffusion (2); and two parallel horizontal lines denote channels (K^+ or Ca^{2+}).

    a. The efflux of K^+ caused by the Na^+-$2Cl^-$-K^+ cotransporter creates a lumen-positive potential that provides a driving force for paracellular Ca^{2+} transport (influx).

    b. Ca^{2+} enters the cytosol via Ca^{2+} channels and is extruded across the basolateral membrane by both a Ca^{2+}-ATPase uniporter and the $3Na^+$-$1Ca^{2+}$ countertransporter.

    c. PTH also stimulates the formation of $1,25(OH)_2D_3$ by stimulating the activity of 1 α-hydroxylase in the proximal tubule.

    d. The vitamin D_3–dependent Ca^{2+}-binding protein calbindin allows large amounts of Ca^{2+} to be translocated intracellularly without altering the $[Ca^{2+}]$.

9. Eight percent of the Ca^{2+} is reabsorbed in the distal convoluted tubule (DCT) and is the major site of regulation of urine Ca^{2+} excretion.

    a. PTH increases Ca^{2+} reabsorption in the DCT by facilitating the opening of luminal channels.

    b. Ca^{2+} enters the cell from the tubular lumen through voltage-sensitive (conductive) Ca^{2+} channels.

    c. PTH increases the Ca^{2+} conductance by increasing the transepithelial potential by increasing Cl^- efflux through conductive channels in the basolateral membrane.

10. Less than 5% of the filtered load for Ca^{2+} is reabsorbed by the collecting duct.

D. Kidney: Phosphorus (see Figure 54–8)

1. An average, healthy 70-kg man with a normal GFR of 180 L/day filters approximately 170 mmol of phosphorus (phosphate) per day, as about 85% of serum inorganic phosphate is ultrafilterable (180 L/day $\times$ 1.1 mmol/L $\times$ 0.85).

2. About 90% of the filtered load is reabsorbed by the nephron.
   a. About 85% of the filtered load for phosphate is reabsorbed proximally against an electrochemical gradient. PTH inhibits phosphate reabsorption in both the proximal tubule and the distal tubule; however, in the presence of PTH, the bulk of proximal phosphorus reabsorption occurs in the initial 25% of this segment.
      (1) Proximal phosphate reabsorption is transcellular (not paracellular).
      (2) Phosphate reabsorption does not occur in the loop of Henle.
      (3) PTH suppresses proximal phosphate reabsorption by decreasing the activity of the $2Na^+\text{-}1HPO_4^{2-}$ electroneutral cotransporter.
   b. Luminal transport of phosphate in the proximal tubule occurs via a $2Na^+\text{-}1HPO_4^{2-}$ symporter.
   c. Transport of phosphate across the basolateral border occurs down a favorable electrochemical gradient via facilitated diffusion.

VIII. **PHYSIOLOGIC ACTIONS OF VITAMIN D$_3$** (Figure 54–9; see also Table 54–1). Activated vitamin D$_3$ is a hydrophilic hormone because it contains three hydroxyl groups; however, it is still very lipid-soluble and acts like a steroid hormone in that it interacts with nuclear receptors in target cells.

A. Bone

1. Vitamin D$_3$ apparently has two kinds of physiologic effects on bone:

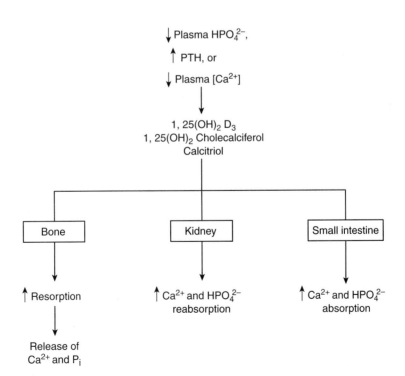

FIGURE 54-9. Major actions of calcitriol on bone, kidney, and intestine that increase Ca^{2+} and P$_i$ in the ECF to promote mineralization of osteoid. In bone, pharmacological doses of 1,25(OH)$_2$D$_3$ mimic the effects of PTH; in physiologic concentrations, it synergizes with PTH.

    a. An antirachitic effect leading to enhanced mineralization
    b. An increase in bone resorption

2. D_3 receptors exist in the nuclei of osteoblasts and osteoprogenitor cells; osteoclasts lack vitamin D_3 receptors. Thus, the activation of osteoclastic progenitors occurs indirectly through the action of calcitriol on osteoblasts.

3. Vitamin D_3 promotes mineralization of osteoid laid down by osteoblasts by maintaining the extracellular Ca^{2+} and phosphorus concentrations within the normal range.
    a. This results in the deposition of calcium hydroxyapatite into the bone matrix.
    b. Increased bone mineralization is also explained by an indirect effect on bone through the intestinal absorption of Ca^{2+} and phosphate.

4. Paradoxically, vitamin D_3 acts directly on bone to promote resorption that mimics the effects of PTH.
    a. Vitamin D_3 induces monocyte-macrophage stem cell progenitors to differentiate and fuse to form osteoclasts.
    b. The activation of the osteoclast by vitamin D_3 is indirect through its action on osteoblasts, which have a spectrum of functions influenced by vitamin D_3, including:
        (1) Proliferation of, and alkaline phosphatase production in, osteoblasts
        (2) Synthesis of osteoblast-derived γ-carboxyglutamic acid protein (osteocalcin)
        (3) Suppression of type I collagen synthesis and promotion of osteocalcin synthesis

5. Calcitriol also binds to D_3 receptors in the parathyroid gland, leading to a diminution in PTH production and release (see Figure 54-3C).

B. Intestine

1. Although Ca^{2+} uptake usually is accompanied by phosphate uptake, the two ions are transported by independent mechanisms, both of which are stimulated by $1,25(OH)_2D_3$.
    a. Vitamin D-sensitive cellular transport of Ca^{2+} through the duodenal enterocyte occurs in three steps:
        (1) Passive uptake of Ca^{2+} through the brush border membrane of intestinal microvilli, which is the rate-limiting step
        (2) Transcellular transport of Ca^{2+} bound to a D_3-induced Ca^{2+}-binding protein called calbindin
        (3) The active extrusion of Ca^{2+} across the basolateral membrane by a D_3-induced Ca^{2+}-ATPase pump

2. Vitamin D_3 stimulates intestinal phosphate uptake via a D_3-stimulated Na^+-coupled phosphate symporter.
    a. Phosphate absorption is mainly passive, with a smaller component of active transport.
    b. Most of the phosphate transport activity is located in the jejunum and ileum; Ca^{2+} absorption occurs principally in the duodenum.

3. Regulation of vitamin D_3 production
    a. PTH and hypophosphatemia directly activate renal 1α-hydroxylase, which catalyzes the conversion of calcidiol to calcitriol.
    b. Hypocalcemia indirectly increases $1,25(OH)_2D_3$ synthesis through its stimulation of PTH secretion (see Figure 54-3C).
    c. Like other steroid hormones, $1,25(OH)_2D_3$ is a negative feedback inhibitor of its own production (see Figure 54-3C).
    d. Calcitriol regulates plasma $[Ca^{2+}]$ also by binding to vitamin D_3 receptors in the parathyroid gland, thereby decreasing the production and secretion of PTH (see Figure 54-3C).
    e. Hypercalcemia indirectly suppresses the activity of the 1 α-hydroxylase through the suppression of PTH secretion, which diminishes the activity of this enzyme, with a resultant reduction in activated vitamin D_3 production.

C. **Kidney**

1. Vitamin D_3 stimulates phosphate reabsorption in the proximal tubule.

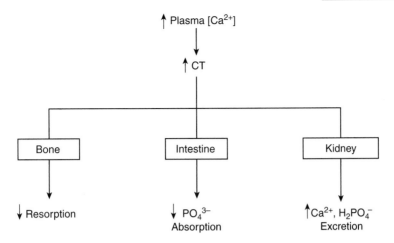

FIGURE 54-10. The hypocalcemic and hypophosphatemic actions of calcitonin on the inhibition of mineral mobilization from the bone; decreased tubular reabsorption and increased excretion of Ca^{2+} and phosphorus ($H_2PO_4^-$); and decreased intestinal absorption of phosphorus (PO_4^{3-}).

  2. Vitamin D_3 promotes distal tubular Ca^{2+} reabsorption via D_3-induced renal calbindins (Ca^{2+}-binding proteins).

  3. Probably the most important effect of $1,25(OH)_2D_3$ on the kidney is the inhibition of 1α-hydroxylase activity, resulting in a decrease in $1,25(OH)_2D_3$ synthesis (see Figure 54-4).

IX. PHYSIOLOGIC ACTIONS OF CALCITONIN (Figure 54–10; see also Table 54–1)

A. Bone

  1. The main biologic effect of CT is to inhibit osteoclastic bone resorption.

  2. When bone turnover is sufficiently high, CT produces hypocalcemia and hypophosphatemia (hypercalciuria and hyperphosphaturia, respectively).

  3. CT does not inhibit bone formation or mineralization.

B. Intestine

  1. CT has no effect on Ca^{2+} absorption but may decrease absorption of phosphorus.

  2. Stimuli for CT secretion include elevated plasma Ca^{2+} concentration and gastrointestinal hormones such as gastrin, pentagastrin, and enteroglucagon.

  3. Somatostatin inhibits CT secretion.

C. Kidney

  1. CT decreases the renal threshold for urinary reabsorption of phosphorus, thus promoting increased urinary phosphorus excretion by the proximal tubule.

  2. CT promotes an increase in the renal fractional excretion of Ca^{2+} at the level of the proximal tubule.

X. ETIOPATHOLOGY OF CALCIUM METABOLISM

A. Osteoporosis

  1. Osteoporosis is the most common metabolic bone disease.

2. It is characterized by a reduction in bone mass with a normal ratio of mineral to organic matrix.

3. The term **osteopenia** is sometimes used to describe reduced bone mass in the absence of symptoms or signs of osteoporosis.

B. **Osteomalacia and rickets**

1. **Osteomalacia** is characterized by an excess of unmineralized bone, which results from the failure of the organic matrix (osteoid) to mineralize normally. Failure to mineralize osteoid seams during normal bone turnover defines osteomalacia, which can occur in both children and adults.

2. **Rickets** is a failure of normal mineralization of the growth plate at the epiphysis of children. It is caused by inadequate mineralization of both osteoid and cartilage at the growing ends of bone in children.

3. Rickets differs from osteomalacia in that it occurs prior to the closure of the epiphyses.

C. **Pathology of the parathyroid-calcium axis** (Table 54–3)

1. Hyperparathyroidism is characterized by an increase in circulating PTH and a decrease in serum phosphate concentration.
  a. Primary hyperparathyroidism. The primary abnormality of the parathyroid glands leads to inappropriate secretion of PTH by a tumor of the parathyroid gland or by ectopic parathyroid tissue. Excess PTH leads to:
    (1) Increased plasma Ca^{2+} and decreased plasma inorganic phosphate concentrations
    (2) Increased urinary excretion of phosphate (phosphaturia), cyclic AMP, and hydroxyproline
    (3) Muscle weakness and fatigability
  b. Secondary hyperparathyroidism. In contrast to primary hyperparathyroidism, the increased secretion of PTH in secondary hyperparathyroidism is an appropriate response to hypocalcemia caused by:
    (1) A vitamin D-deficient diet
    (2) Poor absorption of fat, leading to the concomitant decreased absorption of fat-soluble vitamins (A, D, E, and K)
    (3) Impaired synthesis of $1,25(OH)_2D_3$ due to renal disease
    (4) Increased demand for Ca^{2+}, as during pregnancy and lactation

Table 54-3. Parathyroid Pathologies

Pathology	PTH	$[Ca^{2+}]$	$[P_i]$	Etiology
Primary hyperparathyroidism	↑*	↑	↓	Parathyroid neoplasm (adenoma) Primary parathyroid hyperplasia
Secondary hyperparathyroidism	↑	↓*	↓	Renal disease; vitamin D or Ca^{2+} deficiency; poor fat absorption; cortisol; intestinal malabsorption of vitamin D
Primary hypoparathyroidism	↓*	↓	↑	Thyroid surgery; congenital agenesis or hypoplasia of the parathyroid glands
Secondary hypoparathyroidism	↓	↑*	↑	Vitamin D toxicity
Pseudohypoparathyroidism	↑	↓	↑	Resistance to PTH
Postmenopausal osteoporosis	↓	↑	↑	Menopause; estrogen deficiency
Immobilization osteoporosis	↓	↑	↑	Prolonged immobilization due to spinal cord injury

*represents the initiating factor
P_i = inorganic phosphate; PTH = parathyroid hormone.

(5) The hallmark of vitamin insufficiency and deficiency is low 25-dihydroxyvitamin D_3 in the blood.

2. Hypoparathyroidism is characterized by either low plasma PTH or elevated PTH levels in syndromes associated with resistance to PTH together with an increase in serum phosphate concentration.
   a. **Primary hypoparathyroidism.** The initiating factor is a deficient secretion of PTH by the parathyroid glands caused by:
      (1) A deficiency in the secretion of PTH
      (2) Thyroid surgery with the removal of parathyroid tissue
      (3) The PTH deficiency results in:
         (a) Decreased plasma Ca^{2+} and increased phosphate concentrations
         (b) Hypoparathyroid tetany; i.e., increased neuromuscular excitation such as:
            (i) Percussion of the facial nerve just anterior to the ear lobe resulting in ipsilateral contractions of the facial muscle (Chvostek's sign)
            (ii) Occlusive pressure applied with a blood pressure cuff, resulting in a carpal spasm (Trousseau's sign), appearing as thumb adduction, metacarphophalangeal joint flexion, and interphalangeal joint extension
   b. **Secondary hypoparathyroidism.** In secondary hypoparathyroidism, the initiating factor is the suppression of PTH secretion by increased plasma Ca^{2+} concentration, e.g., by excessive intake of vitamin D, which causes:
      (1) Increased renal Ca^{2+} reabsorption
      (2) Increased intestinal absorption of Ca^{2+}
      (3) Increased resorption of Ca^{2+} from bone
   c. **Pseudohypoparathyroidism.** This disorder is characterized by hypoparathyroidism (i.e., hypocalcemia and hyperphosphatemia), increased secretion of PTH, and target tissue unresponsiveness to the biological actions of PTH.
      (1) The biochemical findings in these patients are identical to those observed in patients with surgical hypoparathyroidism, except that in most patients the plasma PTH is increased, resulting in:
         (a) Decreased bone resorption caused by decreased bone cell responsiveness to PTH
         (b) Increased serum phosphate caused by decreased renal responsiveness to the phosphaturic effect of PTH and decreased synthesis of $1,25(OH)_2D_3$ with decreased intestinal Ca^{2+} absorption
         (c) Increased renal excretion of Ca^{2+} caused again by decreased renal tubular responsiveness to the hypocalciuric effect of PTH
      (2) The PTH-infusion test leading to increased urinary excretion of cAMP remains the most reliable test for pseudohypoparathyroidism.

3. **Postmenopausal osteoporosis.** Because of Ca^{2+} loss from bone, the serum Ca^{2+} level increases following estrogen deficiency.
   a. Because of bone resorption and changes in parathyroid responsiveness to Ca^{2+}, estrogen deficiency also reduces the serum concentration of PTH.
   b. Estrogen deficiency increases serum inorganic phosphate.
   c. There is no reduction in the serum concentration of calcitriol following estrogen deficiency.

4. Immobilization osteoporosis. Prolonged immobilization results in hypercalciuria and hypercalcemia.
   a. This is an example of resorptive (bone-derived) hypercalciuria.
   b. This "disuse osteoporosis" also results in suppression of the PTH1,$25(OH)_2D_3$ axis in that the immunoreactive PTH is markedly reduced.
   c. Serum phosphate levels also are elevated.
   d. Plasma $25OHD_3$ levels remained normal, with depressed levels of plasma $1,25(OH)_2D_3$.

Case 54

A 62-year-old man entered the emergency room with right flank pain. Urinalysis revealed hematuria, and radiographs demonstrated a stone in the right ureter. The stone subsequently was passed spontaneously, and analysis revealed it to be calcium oxalate. Further history disclosed two previous episodes of kidney stones, 10 and 20 years before. Recently, the patient had noted lethargy, polyuria, polydipsia, muscle weakness, and diffuse bone pain. Laboratory studies revealed the following levels: plasma calcium, 12.3 mg/dl (N = 8.4–10.2 mg/dl); phosphate, 1.9 mg/dl (N = 2.7–4.5 mg/dl); creatinine, 1.5 mg/dl (N = 0.8–1.0 mg/dl); and albumin, 5.9 g/dl (N = 1 g/dl). Plasma alkaline phosphatase and urinary hydroxyproline were increased. Urinary calcium excretion was 380 mg/24 hr (N = 250–300 mg/day). After overnight water deprivation, urine osmolality did not exceed 290 mOsm/kg.

1. *Is it certain that this patient has biologically significant hypercalcemia? How would you determine this?*

DISCUSSION

Total plasma calcium consists of a protein-bound portion (approximately 50%) and an ionized portion (approximately 50%). An increase above normal in plasma albumin, as in this patient, could account for a 0.8 mg/dl increase in the total plasma calcium level without increasing the biologically active ionized calcium level. To be certain that the ionized calcium level is increased, it must be measured directly.

2. *What are the most likely hormonal causes of this patient's hypercalcemia?*

DISCUSSION

The most likely hormonal causes are $1,25(OH)_2D_3$ and PTH.

3. *For each hormonal cause, what are the mechanisms by which hypercalcemia is induced?*

DISCUSSION

If excess vitamin D_3 were ingested, the excess would be converted to $25OHD_3$ and then to $1,25(OH)_2D_3$. The latter active metabolite of vitamin D_3 primarily increases calcium absorption from the gut. A second effect is to increase bone resorption. PTH might be secreted in excess by an enlarged neoplastic parathyroid gland. PTH increases reabsorption of calcium from the distal renal tubules; directly stimulates resorption of bone; stimulates renal production of $1,25(OH)_2D_3$ from $25OHD_3$ by activating the 1 α-hydroxylase enzyme; and leads to an increased absorption of calcium from the gut. PTHrp (PTH-related peptide), a larger molecule with an N-terminal amino acid sequence identical to that of PTH, is secreted by a variety of tumors. This molecule mimics all the previously listed actions of PTH by interacting with the PTH receptor.

4. *Which hormonal cause is most likely in view of the low plasma phosphate level?*

DISCUSSION

The low plasma phosphate suggests PTH and PTHrp as the causes of the patient's hypercalcemia. Both molecules increase urinary phosphate excretion by inhibiting reabsorption of phosphate in the proximal renal tubules. This keeps plasma phosphate low. In contrast, $1,25(OH)_2D_3$ increases entry of phosphate into the plasma by stimulating bone resorption; thus, plasma phosphate tends to rise.

5. *What would be the expected effect of hypercalcemia on the plasma levels of the other calcium regulatory hormones?*

DISCUSSION

An excess of $1,25(OH)_2D_3$ would decrease the plasma PTH level by negative feedback from the hypercalcemia and also by direct repression of transcription of the PTH gene. An excess of PTH would increase plasma $1,25(OH)_2D_3$ by stimulating its production, as discussed under question 4. An excess of PTWrp would decrease plasma PTH by negative feedback from the hypercalcemia; $1,25(OH)_2D_3$ would remain normal or increase, depending on the affinity of the renal tubular PTH receptor for PTHrp.

6. *If hyperparathyroidism were present, how would this explain the bone pain and the increase in alkaline phosphatase and urinary hydroxyproline?*

DISCUSSION

Excess PTH stimulates osteoclasts to enlarge, change their shape, and release enzymes that digest bone completely. Pain is associated with weakened bone structure resulting from the accelerated bone reabsorption. The products of collagen breakdown increase hydroxyproline in the urine. Bone formation by osteoblasts is normally coupled to bone resorption; therefore, bone formation also increases, indicated by an elevated plasma alkaline phosphatase.

7. *Why did the patient have polyuria and exhibit inability to concentrate his urine? What would urinary cyclic AMP excretion be if he had hyperthyroidism?*

DISCUSSION

Calcium and sodium share renal tubular reabsorption mechanisms. A high filtered load of calcium decreases sodium reabsorption and causes an osmotic diuresis and polyuria. In addition, high calcium levels inhibit renal responses to ADH. In hyperparathyroidism, urinary cyclic AMP excretion is increased because cyclic AMP is the second messenger for PTH.

8. *When a single, very large parathyroid gland was surgically removed from the patient's neck, the serum calcium fell to 6 mg/dl. What two mechanisms would account for this? In each instance, what would you expect the plasma PTH and plasma phosphate levels to be?*

DISCUSSION

A sharp fall in plasma calcium could result from previous suppression of the uninvolved normal parathyroid glands by hypercalcemia or from their damage during surgery. In this case, plasma PTH would be low and plasma phosphate would be high because of the loss of the inhibitory effect of PTH on renal phosphate reabsorption. Alternatively, the fall in plasma calcium could result from a sudden cessation of excessive rates of bone resorption caused by the high PTH levels. Excessive bone formation could, however, continue until the coupling mechanism restored it to normal. During this period of rebuilding bone, calcium uptake by bone would exceed calcium release from bone, so that plasma calcium would tend to be low. Plasma PTH would be high because of reduced negative feedback. Plasma phosphate would be low because phosphate is also required for bone formation; therefore, its uptake by bone would exceed its release from bone. In addition, the secondarily elevated PTH level would stimulate urinary phosphate excretion.

9. *If the patient hyperventilated when his plasma calcium level was low, what might occur?*

DISCUSSION

Hyperventilation would lead to hypocapnia and respiratory alkalosis. The increase in pH would increase calcium binding to plasma protein, and thereby lower the biologically active ionized fraction of calcium. This can produce neuromuscular irritability with muscle spasms (tetany) and abnormal sensations (paresthesias).

PART VIII. ENDOCRINE PHYSIOLOGY

STUDY QUESTIONS

1. All of the following are biochemical effects of cortisol EXCEPT

(A) hepatic lipogenesis
(B) hepatic gluconeogenesis
(C) muscle proteolysis
(D) hepatic protein anabolism
(E) hepatic glycogenesis

2. Insulin exerts all of the following effects EXCEPT

(A) hyperpolarization of skeletal muscle cells
(B) promotion of lipogenesis
(C) stimulation of glycogen synthase activity
(D) increase in secondary active transport of glucose into muscle cells
(E) increase in glucose transport in adipocytes

3. Which one of the following statements referring to trabecular bone is true?

(A) It constitutes a greater proportion of total bone mass than does cortical bone.
(B) It is found mainly in long bones.
(C) It comprises a greater proportion of total bone surface area than does cortical bone.
(D) It undergoes very little, if any, resorption in adults.
(E) It is surrounded by periosteum.

4. What effect on plasma ion concentrations results from excessive parathyroid hormone (PTH) secretion?

(A) Low plasma inorganic $[HPO_4^{2-}]$
(B) Low plasma $[Ca^{2+}]$
(C) Both
(D) Neither

5. What effect on plasma ion concentrations results from deficient parathyroid hormone (PTH) secretion?

(A) Low plasma inorganic $[HPO_4^{2-}]$
(B) Low plasma $[Ca^{2+}]$
(C) Both
(D) Neither

6. What effect on plasma ion concentrations results from vitamin D intoxication?

(A) Low plasma inorganic $[HPO_4^{2-}]$
(B) Low plasma $[Ca^{2+}]$
(C) Both
(D) Neither

7. Almost all of the active thyroid hormone entering the circulation is in the form of

(A) long-acting thyroid stimulator
(B) thyroglobulin
(C) thyrotropin
(D) thyroxine
(E) triiodothyronine

8. Which of the following is a neurosecretory hormone?

(A) somatotropin
(B) somatostatin
(C) somatomedin
(D) norepinephrine
(E) epinephrine

9. In order to restore fertility in hypophysectomized adult males it is necessary to administer

(A) luteinizing hormone-releasing hormone
(B) gonadotropins
(C) prolactin
(D) gonadotropin-releasing hormone
(E) inhibin

10. Which of the following peptides is synthesized by neurosecretory neurons?

(A) Epinephrine
(B) Norepinephrine
(C) Somatomedin
(D) Somatostatin
(E) Somatotropin

11. Which of the following is a neurosecretory hormone?

(A) Somatostatin
(B) Insulin
(C) Both
(D) Neither

12. An increase in the plasma concentration of a hormone-binding protein would

(A) decrease the response to the hormone
(B) increase the response to the hormone
(C) decrease the concentration of free hormone
(D) increase the concentration of free hormone
(E) decrease the secretion of the hormone from the endocrine tissue

13. All of the following are substrates for monoamine oxidase (MAO) EXCEPT

(A) norepinephrine
(B) vanillylmandelic acid (VMA)
(C) epinephrine
(D) metanephrine
(E) normetanephrine

14. Characteristics of estriol include all of the following EXCEPT

(A) production by the liver
(B) production by the placenta
(C) secretion by theca interna cells of the ovary
(D) quantitatively the major urinary metabolite of the estrogens
(E) the least biologically active of the endogenous estrogens

15. In a normal adult male, treatment with an experimental drug that blocks luteinizing hormone (LH) receptors on the interstitial cells will lead to which one of the following sets of changes in plasma hormone concentrations? ($\uparrow$ = increase; $\downarrow$ = decrease; 0 = no change)

	plasma LH	plasma FSH	plasma testosterone
(A)	$\uparrow$	0	$\downarrow$
(B)	0	$\uparrow$	0
(C)	$\uparrow$	0	$\downarrow$
(D)	$\downarrow$	0	0
(E)	0	$\downarrow$	$\uparrow$

16. A 19-year-old woman has a history of seizure disorder since age 4 and has been controlled by phenobarbital. Hypocalcemia (total serum calcium of 5.4 mg/dl) was first discovered at age 15 years during an evaluation of new-onset bilateral cataracts. There is no family history of hypocalcemia, short stature, or mental retardation. Cvostek and Trousseau signs are positive. Her laboratory data at age 19 are: serum calcium, 6.5 mg/dl (N = 8.4–10.2); ionized calcium, 3.96 mg/dl (N = 4.60–5.24); phosphate, 5.0 mg/dl (N = 2.5–4.4); alkaline phosphatase, 118 IU/dl (N = 53–151); and serum PTH, 138 pg/ml (N < 60); creatinine, 0.9 mg/dl (N = 0.5–1.2); and 25OHD$_3$, 12 ng/ml (N = 10–60). The remainder of the laboratory test results were normal.

What is the differential diagnosis of this patient?

(A) Primary hyperparathyroidism
(B) Vitamin D deficiency
(C) Vitamin D resistance
(D) Pseudohypoparathyroidism
(E) Renal failure

17. Which of the following is a secretory product of the granulosa-lutein cells in nongravid women?

(A) Androstenedione
(B) Pregnenolone
(C) Pregnanediol
(D) Estriol
(E) Estrone

18. The half-life of a hormone in blood is

(A) directly proportional to its rate of secretion
(B) directly proportional to the percentage of the hormone that is bound to its plasma carrier protein
(C) directly proportional to the number of hormone receptors present in the target tissue
(D) inversely proportional to the concentration of its plasma binding protein
(E) inversely proportional to the molecular weight of the hormone

19. The hypophysial portal system

(A) is comprised of one capillary plexus
(B) perfuses the adenohypophysis with venous blood
(C) supplies the pars nervosa with blood
(D) carries pituitary tropic hormones to the pars distalis
(E) receives neurohormones from the secondary capillary plexus

20. Entry of glucose into muscle is

(A) increased by epinephrine
(B) increased by exercise
(C) increased by the transport of free fatty acids into muscle
(D) inversely proportional to plasma glucose concentration
(E) inversely proportional to plasma insulin concentration

21. Which one of the following conditions leads to a diminution in PTH synthesis and secretion?

(A) Increased serum phosphate concentration
(B) Increased plasma $1,25(OH)_2$ vitamin D_3 concentration
(C) Decreased binding of Ca^{2+} to the parathyroid cell membrane receptor
(D) Decreased plasma Ca^{2+} concentration
(E) Increased plasma pH

22. A 49-year-old man visits his family physician because he has had to purchase three pairs of shoes of increasing size within the same year. He also has difficulty speaking because his tongue is enlarged, and he has a severe prominence on his mandible. A laboratory test reveals an elevated plasma growth hormone (GH) concentration. Which of the following tests would confirm the diagnosis of acromegaly?

(A) Oral glucose tolerance test
(B) Injection of insulin
(C) Injection of arginine
(D) Measurement of plasma free fatty acid level
(E) Administration of bromocriptine

23. Administration of exogenous thyroid hormone would likely lead to all of the following EXCEPT

(A) negative feedback inhibition of thyroid-stimulating hormone (TSH) secretion
(B) decreased secretion of triiodothyronine (T_3)
(C) decreased iodide uptake by the thyroid gland
(D) increased O_2 consumption by the brain

24. Hormones that may cause negative nitrogen balance include all of the following EXCEPT

(A) glucagon
(B) thyroid hormone (excess)
(C) cortisol
(D) growth hormone (GH)

Questions 25–32

From the figure select the letter that best depicts the relationship between the plasma concentrations of thyroxine and thyrotropin in the condition outlined in each question. *N* = normal plasma thyroxine and thyroid-stimulating hormone (TSH) levels.

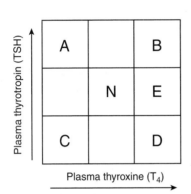

25. The effect of large doses of exogenous triiodothyronine

26. The effect of blocking the intrathyroidal oxidation of iodide

27. The effect of hypophysectomy

28. The effect of hypothalamic disease

29. The effect of primary hyperthyroidism (Graves' disease)

30. The effect of chronic dietary iodide deficiency

31. Generalized resistance to thyroid hormone

32. Hyperthyroidism associated with inappropriate thyroid-stimulating hormone (TSH) secretion

33. Which of the following pairs of structures represents the sites of oxytocin synthesis and secretion, which occurs when a mother nurses her infant?

(A) Median eminence; pars distalis
(B) Adenohypophysis; posterior pituitary
(C) Hypothalamus; pars nervosa
(D) Mammary myoepithelial cells; mammary alveolar cells
(E) Anterior pituitary; posterior pituitary

Questions 34–43

Select the answers from the following graph. Box N represents the normal relationship between plasma [Ca^{2+}] and plasma PTH concentration.

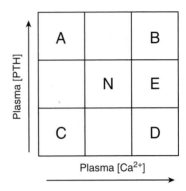

34. Parathyroid adenoma

35. Parathyroidectomy

36. Chronic renal failure

37. Vitamin D$_3$ deficiency

38. Vitamin D$_3$ excess

39. Primary hyperparathyroidism

40. Pseudohypoparathyroidism

41. Osteoporosis (body immobilization)

42. Dietary calcium restriction

43. Increased phosphate loads

44. Oxidation of glucose in muscle is reduced when mobilization of fatty acids is increased because

(A) utilization of fatty acid increases the cellular level of adenosine triphosphate (ATP), which decreases the activity of hexokinase
(B) fatty acids compete with glucose for the oxidized form of nicotinamide adenine dinucleotide (NAD$^+$), which blocks formation of pyruvate
(C) fatty acids compete with glucose for transport across the cell membrane
(D) oxidation of fatty acids increases formation of citrate, which blocks phosphofructokinase
(E) fatty acids inhibit the formation of pyruvate from lactate

45. Epinephrine is a potent hyperglycemic agent because of its ability to do all of the following EXCEPT

(A) stimulate glucagon secretion
(B) stimulate adrenocorticotropic hormone (ACTH) secretion
(C) stimulate hepatic and muscle glycogenolysis
(D) inhibit insulin secretion
(E) inhibit cortisol secretion

46. The effects of insulin include

(A) depolarization of muscle cells
(B) lipolysis
(C) inhibition of glycogen synthase activity
(D) glucose transport into the pancreatic beta cell
(E) increase in secondary active transport of glucose into muscle and fat cells

47. Which one of the following results from the action of parathyroid hormone on the nephron?

(A) Inhibition of 1α-hydroxylase
(B) Stimulation of Ca^{2+} reabsorption in the thick segment of the ascending limb of the loop of Henle
(C) Interaction of PTH with receptors on the luminal membrane of the proximal tubular cells
(D) Stimulation of phosphate reabsorption in the proximal tubule
(E) A fall in the formation of renal calcitriol

48. All of the following statements regarding testosterone are true EXCEPT

(A) it is produced by the fetal testis
(B) it inhibits luteinizing hormone (LH) secretion from the pituitary gland
(C) it is a proestrogen
(D) it is inactivated after conversion to dihydrotestosterone
(E) it accelerates epiphysial closure of the long bones

49. Because hepatic glycogen stores are limited and decrease only temporarily after epinephrine secretion, muscle glycogenolysis is the major mechanism for providing gluconeogenic precursors for hepatic glucogenesis. This gluconeogenic substance derived from muscle is

(A) lactate
(B) acetyl coenzyme A (acetyl-CoA)
(C) glucose
(D) glycerol
(E) alanine

50. Which of the following endocrine organs is larger at birth than in adulthood?

(A) Hypophysis
(B) Thyroid gland
(C) Adrenal gland
(D) Parathyroid glands
(E) Endocrine pancreas

51. An increase in plasma parathyroid hormone (PTH) level would lead to an increase in which of the following?

(A) The number of active osteoblasts
(B) Plasma inorganic phosphate concentration
(C) Renal synthesis of calcitriol
(D) Collagen synthesis
(E) Renal proximal tubular reabsorption of Ca^{2+}

52. Which of the following adrenomedullary enzymes is correctly paired with its substrate?

(A) Phenylethanolamine-N-methyltransferase (PNMT)/epinephrine
(B) Phenylalanine hydroxylase/tyrosine
(C) Dopa decarboxylase/phenylalanine
(D) Dopamine β-hydroxylase/dihydroxyphenylethylamine
(E) Tyrosine hydroxylase/norepinephrine

53. Which of the following adrenergic receptors is linked to relaxation of the detrusor muscle?

(A) Alpha receptor
(B) Beta receptor
(C) Both
(D) Neither

54. All of the following are stimuli for growth hormone (GH) release EXCEPT

(A) bromocriptine
(B) hypoglycemia
(C) stress
(D) obesity
(E) vigorous exercise

Questions 57–60

The following graph shows plasma steroid hormone levels as a function of time during a normal ovarian cycle in a 22-year-old woman. The woman becomes pregnant during this cycle.

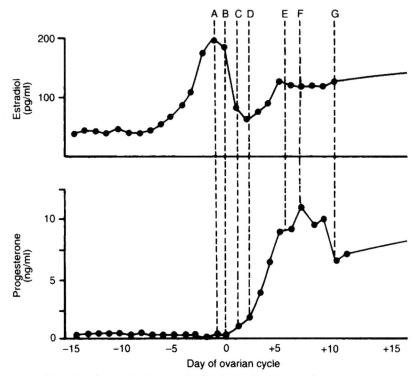

Adapted from Goodman HM: *Basic Medical Endocrinology.* New York, Raven, 1988, p 306.

55. Variation in the length of the menstrual cycle is associated primarily by variation in the

(A) length of the follicular phase
(B) length of menstruation
(C) length of the luteal phase
(D) frequency of sexual intercourse
(E) time between the midcycle FSH surge and ovulation

56. The most biologically active iodothyronine secreted by the thyroid follicles is

(A) triiodothyronine (T_3)
(B) tetraiodothyronine (T_4)
(C) reverse triiodothyronine (rT_3)
(D) thyroglobulin
(E) triiodothyroacetic acid

57. Ovulation is indicated by which of the following lettered points on the graph?

(A) A
(B) B
(C) C
(D) D
(E) E

58. The LH peak is indicated by which of the following lettered points on the graph?

(A) A
(B) B
(C) C
(D) D
(E) E

59. Implantation of the blastocyst corresponds to which of the following points on the graph?

(A) C
(B) D
(C) E
(D) F
(E) G

60. The gradual increases in plasma concentrations of estradiol and progesterone beginning at point G indicate continued steroid secretion by the

(A) placenta
(B) corpus luteum
(C) adrenal cortex
(D) theca interna
(E) ovarian follicle

61. Which one of the following is a metabolic effect of glucagon?

(A) Glycogenesis
(B) Lipogenesis
(C) Glycolysis
(D) Protein anabolism
(E) Gluconeogenesis

62. A 24-year-old woman has regular menstrual cycles of 21–23 days. Ovulation can be expected to occur between cycle days

(A) 7 and 9
(B) 10 and 12
(C) 13 and 15
(D) 16 and 18
(E) 19 and 21

63. Which of the following is a secretory product of the granulosa-lutein cells in nongravid women?

(A) Androstenedione
(B) Pregnenolone
(C) Pregnanediol
(D) Estriol
(E) Estrone

64. Which of the following adrenergic receptors is linked to increased renin secretion?

(A) Alpha receptor
(B) Beta receptor
(C) Both
(D) Neither

65. A 60-year-old woman with rheumatoid arthritis, moderate congestive heart failure, and recent onset of lethargy and fatigue is referred for thyroid evaluation. She has been treated with digoxin, and denies ingestion of foods or drugs containing iodide. Physical exam reveals a pulse rate of 60 beats/min, dry skin, a diffusely enlarged thyroid gland (30 gm), and absent ankle reflexes. Thyroid studies reveal the following (*TSH* = thyroid-stimulating hormone):

	Patient	Normal
T_4:	4.0 μg/dl	4.5–11.5 μg/dl
free T_4:	1.0 ng/dl	0.8–2.4 ng/dl
T_3:	40 ng/dl	70–180 ng/dl
resin T_3 uptake:	28%	25%–35%
TSH:	8 μU/ml	0.5–5 μU/ml

This patient most likely has a diagnosis that is consistent with

(A) primary hypothyroidism
(B) secondary hypothyroidism
(C) a hyperfunctional goiter
(D) excessive ingestion of thyroid extract
(E) thyrotoxicosis

66. Prolactin plays an important role in lactogenesis during lactation. Despite increased prolactin secretion throughout pregnancy, little synthesis of breast milk occurs until after parturition because

(A) plasma cortisol levels are suppressed
(B) secretion of oxytocin does not occur
(C) suckling by the neonate is necessary
(D) there are high plasma levels of estrogen and progesterone
(E) there are high circulating levels of placental lactogen

67. In males, inhibin reduces

(A) libido
(B) testosterone synthesis
(C) spermatogenesis
(D) testosterone secretion
(E) luteinizing hormone-releasing hormone

68. A decrease in cortisol secretion would lead to

(A) increased storage of glycogen in the liver
(B) decreased adrenocorticotropic hormone (ACTH) secretion
(C) decreased adrenomedullary synthesis of epinephrine
(D) increased plasma glucose concentration
(E) increased hepatic protein synthesis

69. True statements about β-endorphin include all of the following EXCEPT

(A) it reacts with the same receptors that bind morphine
(B) it is synthesized by pituitary basophils
(C) it is synthesized from corticotropin
(D) it is a proteolytic cleavage product of proopiomelanocortin (POMC)

70. Activation of the sympathetic nervous system would lead to

(A) increased intestinal motility
(B) increased insulin secretion
(C) relaxation of the pupillary dilator muscle
(D) increased renin secretion
(E) contraction of the ciliary eye muscle

71. The major steroid hormone secreted by the inner zone of the fetal adrenal cortex is

(A) cortisol
(B) dehydroepiandrosterone (DHEA)
(C) progesterone
(D) estriol
(E) corticosterone

72. A 35-year-old woman was planning her pregnancy, but she was diagnosed with hypogonadotropic hypogonadism of hypothalamic origin. Which one of the following would be the therapy of choice to induce ovulation and pregnancy?

(A) Estrogen alone in order to evoke two peaks each month
(B) Progesterone alone in order to evoke a single peak each month
(C) Pulses of GnRH administered every 60 to 90 minutes by a portable intravenous pump
(D) Estrogen and progesterone, taken on a regular monthly schedule to evoke two peaks

73. When is the second meiotic division of the developing ovarian follicle completed?

(A) At puberty
(B) Just prior to ovulation
(C) During the follicular phase of the menstrual cycle
(D) Just after conception
(E) During fetal development

74. A 17-year-old patient with a normal female phenotype is referred to an endocrinology clinic because of sparse pubic and axillary hair and amenorrhea. Chromosomal analysis reveals a male genotype. Further evaluation reveals intra-abdominal testes and circulating testosterone and estrogen concentrations that are characteristic of a normal man. The physician concludes that the patient has testicular feminization syndrome, a genetic end-organ insensitivity to androgen, caused by the absence of androgen receptors. Which of the following findings would be consistent with this syndrome?

(A) Normal wolffian duct development
(B) Normal müllerian duct development
(C) Regression of the internal genitalia
(D) Beard growth following androgen treatment
(E) Normal fertility

75. Which of the following responses is mediated by the β-adrenergic receptor?

(A) Ciliary ocular muscle contraction
(B) Increased intestinal motility
(C) Contraction of the radial eye muscle
(D) Vasoconstriction
(E) Insulin secretion

76. Abnormally high glucocorticoid levels would be associated with an increase in all of the following activities in the **liver** EXCEPT

(A) gluconeogenesis
(B) glycogenesis
(C) glycogenolysis
(D) glucose production
(E) protein synthesis

77. Which of the following adrenergic receptors causes increased insulin secretion?

(A) Alpha receptor
(B) Beta receptor
(C) Both
(D) Neither

78. Glucose transport occurs by insulin-dependent facilitated diffusion in which of the following tissues?

(A) Cardiac muscle
(B) Intestinal epithelium
(C) Renal epithelium
(D) Brain

79. Which of the following catecholamines is elevated in most pheochromocytoma patients?

(A) Epinephrine
(B) Norepinephrine
(C) Both
(D) Neither

80. The cells that contribute most to testicular volume are the

(A) interstitial cells
(B) tubular cells
(C) spermatocytes
(D) connective tissue cells

81. In terms of serum concentration, the major postmenopausal steroid hormone and pituitary tropic hormone are

(A) estradiol and follicle-stimulating hormone (FSH)
(B) estradiol and luteinizing hormone (LH)
(C) estrone and FSH
(D) estrone and LH
(E) estriol and LH

82. Which of the following substances is a substrate for monoamine oxidase (MAO)?

(A) Norepinephrine
(B) Dihydroxymandelic acid
(C) Dihydroxyphenylalanine (DOPA)
(D) Vanillylmandelic acid (VMA)
(E) Tyrosine

83. The primary site of 1,25-dihydroxycholecalciferol formation from its immediate precursor is the

(A) bone
(B) liver
(C) skin
(D) nephron
(E) bloodstream

84. All of the following are biochemical effects of cortisol EXCEPT

(A) hepatic lipogenesis
(B) hepatic gluconeogenesis
(C) muscle proteolysis
(D) hepatic protein anabolism
(E) hepatic glycogenesis

85. Because hepatic glycogen stores are limited and decrease only temporarily after epinephrine secretion, muscle glycogenolysis is the major mechanism for providing gluconeogenic precursors for hepatic glucogenesis. This gluconeogenic substance derived from muscle is

(A) lactate
(B) acetyl coenzyme A (acetyl-coA)
(C) glucose
(D) glycerol
(E) alanine

Questions **86** and **87** refer to the following figure.

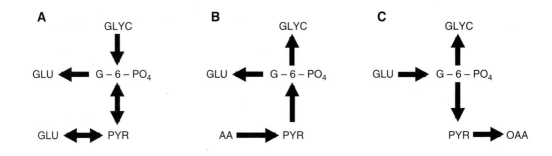

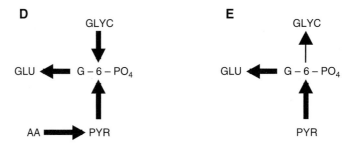

The five panels represent the effect of various hormones on carbohydrate metabolism. *GLYC* = glycogen; *GLU* = glucose; *PYR* = pyruvate; *LAC* = lactate; *AA* = amino acids; *G-6-PO₄* = glucose-6-PO$_4$; and *OAA* = oxaloacetate.

86. Which one of the metabolic pathways refers to the hormone produced by the pancreatic beta cells?

(A) A
(B) B
(C) C
(D) D
(E) E

87. Which one of the metabolic pathways refers to the pancreatic hormone that is elevated in type 1 diabetes mellitus?

(A) A
(B) B
(C) C
(D) D
(E) E

88. Oxytocin is a neurosecretory hormone released from the pars nervosa. Oxytocin secretion promotes all of the following actions EXCEPT

(A) myometrial contraction
(B) lactogenesis
(C) milk ejection
(D) myoepithelial cell contraction

89. Progesterone secretion during the second and third trimesters of pregnancy is a measure of the functional status of the

(A) materno-placental unit
(B) corpus luteum
(C) fetal liver
(D) fetal adrenal gland
(E) maternal ovary

90. Progesterone serves several important functions during pregnancy. All of the following physiologic or biochemical effects require progesterone EXCEPT

(A) stimulation of myometrial contraction
(B) promotion of differentiation and growth of the lactiferous ducts
(C) inhibition of renal Na$^+$ excretion
(D) formation of cortisol by the fetal adrenal cortex in early pregnancy
(E) formation of aldosterone by the fetal adrenal cortex in early pregnancy

91. Which of the following statements that refer to steroid hormones is correct?

(A) They have short circulating half-lives
(B) They are synthesized at a rate similar to their rate of secretion
(C) They are largely bound to plasma albumin
(D) They bind to receptors in the cell membrane of target cells
(E) They are stored in cytoplasmic lipid droplets

92. The physiologic effects of somatotropin are mediated by

(A) receptor-linked tyrosine kinases
(B) somatostatin
(C) a nuclear receptor
(D) insulin
(E) cyclic adenosine monophosphate (AMP)

93. Which of the following endocrine organs is larger at birth than in adulthood?

(A) Hypophysis
(B) Thyroid gland
(C) Adrenal gland
(D) Parathyroid glands
(E) Endocrine pancreas

94. Active vitamin D$_3$ (calcitriol) and parathyroid hormone (PTH) have many similar effects. Which of the following physiologic effects is specific only for calcitriol?

(A) Increased renal phosphate reabsorption
(B) Increased renal Ca^{2+} reabsorption
(C) Increased intestinal Ca^{2+} absorption
(D) Increased plasma [Ca^{2+}]
(E) Decreased plasma [HPO$_4$$^{2-}$]

95. After implantation has occurred, the first missed menstrual period in a healthy female is the result of

(A) degeneration of the corpus luteum
(B) formation of a trophoblast that secretes gonadotropins
(C) formation of a trophoblast that secretes estradiol and progesterone
(D) decreased ovarian synthesis of estradiol and progesterone
(E) placental release of sufficient estradiol and progesterone to prevent menstruation

96. The major steroid hormone secreted by the inner zone of the fetal adrenal cortex is

(A) cortisol
(B) dehydroepiandrosterone (DHEA)
(C) progesterone
(D) estriol
(E) corticosterone

97. Abnormally high glucocorticoid levels would be associated with an increase in all of the following activities in the liver EXCEPT

(A) gluconeogenesis
(B) glycogenesis
(C) glycogenolysis
(D) glucose production
(E) protein synthesis

98. Which of the following catecholamines decreases markedly following bilateral adrenalectomy?

(A) Epinephrine
(B) Norepinephrine
(C) Both
(D) Neither

99. Prostaglandins found in the seminal fluid are secretory products of the

(A) prostate gland
(B) Sertoli cells
(C) seminal vesicles
(D) Leydig cells
(E) epididymis

100. Thyroid peroxidase is required for all of the following steps in thyroid hormone synthesis EXCEPT

(A) iodide uptake
(B) oxidation of iodide
(C) iodination of active iodide
(D) coupling of iodotyrosines
(E) synthesis of iodothyronines

101. Activation of the sympathetic nervous system would lead to all of the following responses EXCEPT

(A) inhibition of peristalsis
(B) contraction of the radial ocular muscle
(C) renin secretion
(D) insulin secretion
(E) vasodilation in skeletal muscle

102. Estriol synthesis during gestation requires all of the following organs EXCEPT the

(A) fetal pituitary gland
(B) fetal liver
(C) neocortex of the fetal adrenal gland
(D) placenta
(E) trophoblast

103. Which of the following is a polypeptide hormone?

(A) Somatostatin
(B) Insulin
(C) Both
(D) Neither

104. All of the following are neuropeptide hormones EXCEPT

(A) antidiuretic hormone (ADH)
(B) β-endorphin
(C) oxytocin
(D) somatomedin
(E) thyrotropin releasing hormone (TRH)

1. The answer is A [Chapter 49 I F 1–3, Figure 49-5]. The overall metabolic effects of cortisol are the release of amino acids from muscle and both the storage and release of glucose and fatty acids. Cortisol inhibits fatty acid synthesis in the liver, and it increases blood glycerol and fatty acid concentrations in concert with other hormones (norepinephrine, epinephrine, glucagon) that increase lipolysis in adipose tissues. Glycerol is an excellent index of lipolysis because, unlike free fatty acids, it is not reused by adipocytes in the resynthesis of triglycerides. Rather, glycerol is used by the liver as a gluconeogenic substrate. Cortisol also promotes synthesis of gluconeogenic enzymes needed to convert the amino acids released from muscle to carbohydrate synthesis in the liver. Glucocorticoids promote proteolysis and inhibit protein synthesis in most tissues except the liver.

2. The answer is D [Chapter 52 I D 1–6, Figures 52-2, 52-3, 52-4, and 52-6; Table 52-4]. Insulin decreases cell membrane permeability to both Na^+ and K^+, but it decreases Na^+ permeability more, causing hyperpolarization of skeletal and cardiac muscle cells and adipocytes but not liver or pancreatic cells. Insulin also promotes lipogenesis, protein anabolism, glycogenesis, and glycolysis. Insulin promotes glucose uptake by muscle adipose tissue and the liver, and it promotes storage and utilization of glucose in all three tissues. Glucose storage by muscle and liver is achieved by formation of glycogen via an increase in glycogen synthase activity. Glucose transport across skeletal and cardiac muscle cells and adipocytes occurs by insulin-dependent facilitated diffusion via the GLUT-4 transporter.

3. The answer is C [Chapter 54 V C 3–5]. Trabecular (cancellous, or spongy) bone is found in the axial skeleton and in the ends of the long bones and makes up about 20% of the skeletal mass. It also has a total surface area that is five to eight times larger than that of compact (cancellous) bone. Because of its much larger surface area, it is remodeled much more actively than cortical bone and contributes more significantly to mineral homeostasis. Trabecular bone is surrounded by endosteum.

4. The answer is A [Chapter 53 VI C, VIII]. Parathyroid hormone (PTH) is the hypercalcemic hormone of the body. The major regulator of PTH synthesis and secretion is serum ionized calcium concentration ([Ca^{2+}]). PTH maintains the normal plasma total calcium concentration at about 5 mEq/L by interacting with the kidney, bone, and intestine. PTH stimulates bone resorption, and it decreases the maximal tubular transport capacity (Tm) for phosphate by decreasing proximal tubular reabsorption of phosphate, resulting in phosphate diuresis. When PTH secretion is high, the fraction of filtered phosphate that is reabsorbed may fall from the normal 80%–95% to 5%–20%. PTH increases the maximal tubular transport capacity for Ca^{2+} by increasing distal tubular reabsorption of Ca^{2+}. Although PTH stimulates renal Ca^{2+} reabsorption, the urinary Ca^{2+} is greater than normal in states of excess PTH because of the increased filtered load of Ca^{2+}.

5. The answer is B [Chapter 53 VI C, VIII]. There is an inverse relationship between the secretion of parathyroid hormone (PTH) and plasma ([Ca^{2+}]): when plasma [Ca^{2+}] falls PTH increases, and when plasma [Ca^{2+}] rises PTH secretion is suppressed. Thus, a decrease in PTH secretion is caused by an increase in plasma [Ca^{2+}]. This increase in Ca^{2+} is associated with a decrease in [HPO_4^{2-}]. Inorganic phosphate has no direct influence on PTH secretion; rather, it is the phosphate-induced decrease in plasma [Ca^{2+}] that stimulates PTH secretion. Conversely, a decrease in plasma inorganic [HPO_4^{2-}] increases plasma [Ca^{2+}] and indirectly inhibits PTH secretion.

6. The answer is D [Chapter 53 VI C, VIII]. Vitamin D_3 toxicity leads to hypercalcemia directly by bone resorption and renal Ca^{2+} absorption and indirectly by mediating PTH-induced intestinal Ca^{2+} reabsorption and indirectly by mediating PTH-induced intestinal Ca^{2+} absorption. This hypercalcemia suppresses PTH secretion, leading to increased plasma [HPO_4^{2-}] and increased renal phosphate reabsorption.

7. The answer is D [Chapter 53 I B]. Almost all of the active thyroid hormone entering the circulation is in the form of thyroxine.

8. The answer is B [Chapter 46 III B 2, C 1 a, Table 46-2; Chapter 47 IV A 2 b]. Of the hormones listed only one, somatostatin, is produced by a neurosecretory neuron. Somatostatin inhibits growth hormone (GH). Somatotropin is produced by the acidophils of the anterior pituitary, the catecholamines by the adrenal medulla, and norepinephrine by the sympathetic postganglionic neurons; somatomedin is of hepatic origin. It is essential to appreciate that the adrenomedullary catecholamines (epinephrine and norepinephrine) are not neurosecretory hormones because they are produced by adrenomedullary chromaffin cells and not by neurosecretory hormones.

9. The answer is B [Chapter 50 II B 3 g]. Both LH (or testosterone) together with FSH are required to restore fertility. LH induces endogenous testosterone secretion and FSH restores normal spermatogenesis. Since this patient has hypogonadotropic hypogonadism due to the extirpation of the pituitary, the hypothalamic hormones (GnRH) lack the pituitary receptors and are, therefore, without effect.

10. The answer is D [Chapter 46 III B 2 a b, Tables 46-1 and 46-2; Chapter 47 IV A 2 b, Figure 47-2]. Somatostatin is a hypophysiotropic hormone produced by the parvicellular neurosecretory neurons that terminate in the median eminence. Somatostatin inhibits secretion of growth hormone (GH; somatotropin), a pituitary tropic hormone. The catecholamines, norepinephrine and epinephrine, are mainly products of the sympathetic postganglionic neurons and the adrenal medulla, respectively. Somatomedin is a hepatic hormone.

11. The answer is A [Chapter 45 V A 1–4, Tables 45-1 and 45-2; Chapter 46 III B 2 a b]. Somatostatin is synthesized in the arcuate nucleus of the tuberoinfundibular neurosecretory neurons that terminate in the median eminence. Somatostatin of hypothalamic origin functions as a neurosecretory hormone. It also is a hypophysiotropic hormone.

12. The answer is A [Chapter 45 IV E, Table 45-2; Chapter 46 II B 1, Figure 46-3]. With an increase in binding protein, the response to either exogenous or endogenous hormone is decreased, because more of the hormone becomes bound, and less is dissociated (free). Also, the total concentration (bound plus free) is increased.

13. The answer is B [Chapter 48 VI B 1, Figure 48-3]. Vanillylmandelic acid (VMA) is the major urinary end product of catecholamine metabolism. Monoamine oxidase (MAO) is a mitochondrial enzyme that catalyzes the oxidative deamination of the catecholamines—dopamine, norepinephrine, and epinephrine. MAO also inactivates the indolamine, serotonin (5-hydroxytryptamine). Substrates for MAO also include normetanephrine and metanephrine.

14. The answer is C [Chapter 51 I F 1 a (3)]. Estriol, the least biologically active natural estrogen, is produced only in the liver and placenta. It is not an ovarian product but represents the predominant urinary end product of estrogen metabolism. In pregnancy, the levels of urinary estriol increase 1000-fold, because estriol is formed by the trophoblast of the placenta. The liver converts estrone and estradiol of ovarian origin into estriol, whereas the trophoblast converts 16α-hydroxydehydroepiandrosterone (16α-OH DHEA) sulfate of fetal adrenal origin into estriol.

15. The answer is A [Chapter 50 IV B 2–6, Figures 50-7, 50-8 and 50-9; Table 50-7]. This experimental drug blocks the effect of LH on the Leydig cell, the major target cell of this gonadotropin. Since testosterone is the major negative feedback inhibitor of LH (and LHRH), the resultant decline in testosterone synthesis and secretion reduces the negative feedback suppression of LH. Therefore, plasma LH levels increase. The major regulation of FSH is via negative feedback by inhibin, a Sertoli cell product. Because this feedback system remains operational, there is no change in FSH levels.

16. The answer is D [Chapter 54 X C 2; Table 54-3]. The differential diagnosis in this clearly hypocalcemic young woman can be divided into hypocalcemia due to absence of or resistance to PTH and hypocalcemia due to non-PTH causes. The most common diagnoses include (1) lack of PTH, (2) resistance to PTH, (3) vitamin D_3 resistance or deficiency, and (4) drug-induced (anticonvulsants). Hypocalcemias may be divided into those causes associated with an appropriate elevation of PTH (secondary hyperparathyroidism), those associated with elevated PTH but no response to the hormone (PTH resistance), and those associated with no elevation of serum PTH (PTH deficiency syndromes).

This patient's elevated serum PTH suggests either vitamin D-mediated causes or the PTH resistance syndromes. Normal serum 25-

hydroxyvitamin D_3 and alkaline phosphatase and elevated serum phosphate exclude vitamin D-deficient or vitamin D-resistant states. Pseudohypoparathyroidism is favored by the elevated serum PTH and elevated phosphate, suggesting that the kidney is unresponsive to even elevated levels of PTH. The normal serum creatinine is indicative of normal renal function. The Chvostek and Trousseau signs are indicative of hypoparathyroid tetany, or increased neuromuscular excitability due to the lowering of the excitability threshold by the low extracellular calcium concentration.

17. The answer is E [Chapter 51 I C 3, E 2 a (4) (b), F 1 a (2), Figure 51-3]. The secretory products of the ovary are estradiol and estrone, which are produced by the granulosa cells of the unruptured follicle and the granulosa-lutein cells of the corpus luteum. Luteinization of the granulosa cells, which depends on LH, involves the appearance of lipid droplets in the cytoplasm. The estrogenic precursors produced by the theca interna (and theca-lutein cells) are androstenedione and testosterone, which are converted by the granulosa (and granulosa-lutein) cells into estrone and estradiol, respectively. The lutein-granulosa cells also produce and secrete progesterone. Thus, androstenedione and pregnenolone are produced, but not secreted, by the ovary. Estriol is not an ovarian product but is synthesized in the liver from estradiol and estrone and in the placenta by the conversion of imported androgens. Pregnanediol is the urinary metabolite of progesterone and is formed in the liver.

18. The answer is B [Chapter 45 IV G, Table 45-2]. Hormones bound to plasma protein-carriers, including mainly the lipid-soluble hormones, have longer half-lives. Furthermore, the half-life is proportional to the binding affinity between the hormone and its protein-carrier. The hormone with one of the highest affinities is thyroxine. Water-soluble (hydrophilic) hormones have much shorter half-lives because they circulate usually as unbound (free) hormone. Notable exceptions are growth hormone and insulin-like growth factor-1 (IGF-1). Also, the larger the aqueous soluble hormones, the longer the half-life. It must be appreciated that larger molecules and plasma protein–bound hormones are not filterable by the glomerulus and this prolongs their circulation time.

19. The answer is B [Chapter 46 II A]. The hypophysial portal system consists of two capillary beds connected by long portal veins. This vascular system provides the major vascular input to the adenohypophysis and delivers the hypophysiotropic hormones released from the media eminence to the pars distalis. The posterior pituitary receives arterial blood via the inferior hypophysial arteries, which are branches of the internal carotid artery. The hypophysial portal system does not receive neurohormones from the secondary plexus. Rather, the secondary plexus delivers neurohormones to the anterior pituitary.

20. The answer is B [Chapter 47 IV A 3 d (1) (a) (b); Chapter 48 VIII A 3 a (5), Figure 48-5; Chapter 52 I D 1 c, Table 52-3]. Muscle is the dominant tissue for insulin-mediated glucose disposal. In addition to its effect on insulin-mediated glucose uptake (GLUT-4), glucose has a mass action effect on glucose transport that is independent of insulin. The raised blood glucose in type 2 diabetes increases the non–insulin-mediated uptake so that, in absolute terms, overall glucose uptake into muscle is no different than in nondiabetic controls. Glucose uptake in exercising muscle is not dependent on increased insulin secretion. In muscle, free fatty acid oxidation spares glucose utilization and, therefore, glucose transport. In the resting state, muscle meets most of its fuel requirements by oxidizing fatty acids. In contrast, during exercise glucose is the major fuel consumed. Insulin increases glucose uptake in muscle and fat by moving GLUT-4 transporters from intracellular vesicles to the plasma membrane. In type 2 diabetes it is possible that the transporter intrinsic activity (not number) of GLUT-4 transporters is reduced with a resultant decline in insulin-dependent glucose transport. High circulating levels of free fatty acids due to elevated levels of cortisol, epinephrine, glucagon, and somatotropin account for the decrease in glucose entry into muscle cells. Exercise improves glucose tolerance, lowers circulating level of insulin, and reduces insulin resistance.

21. The answer is B [Chapter 54 VIII A 5; Figure 54-3C]. Calcitriol decreases the expression of the PTH gene, thereby decreasing the production and secretion of PTH. Increased plasma phosphorus concentration, which leads to a fall in plasma Ca^{2+} concentration, stimulates PTH secretion. A rise in plasma pH leads to a decrease in the plasma concentration of ionized calcium, with a resultant increment in PTH secretion.

22. The answer is A [Chapter 47 IV A 2 b (6) (a), Table 47-1]. A single growth hormone (GH) level cannot be used to rule out acromegaly. The "gold standard" is the demonstration of GH suppression by hyperglycemia during an oral glucose tolerance test. The GH level should decrease to less than 2 ng/ml, but the mean nadir is actually less than 1 ng/ml. The GH response to oral glucose remains the most accurate test for excessive GH secretion. Insulin and arginine are stimulators of GH secretion. The measurement of plasma free fatty acids, which are elevated in acromegalic patients, is nonspecific and therefore not useful.

Dopamine agonists (bromocriptine) and somatostatin analogues (octreotide, lanreotide) are the two classes of drugs that lower GH concentrations in acromegalic patients. One study found whereas clinical improvement occurred in 80%–90% of patients treated with dopamine agonists, less than 20% experienced a reduction in GH or insulin-like growth factor-1 (IGF-1) concentrations to a normal or near-normal level. The somatostatin analogue octreotide suppresses GH more than native somatostatin, thus making it an ideal agent to treat acromegaly. The systemic effects of elevated GH and IGF-1 levels include glucose intolerance, hypertension, sleep apnea, cardiac failure, arthritis, and hyperhidrosis (sweating).

23. The answer is D [Chapter 53 VI A 1 c 2 b –d, Figures 53-5 and 53-6]. Normally, thyroid hormone (T_3 and T_4) is regulated by thyroid-stimulating hormone (TSH), which, in turn, is controlled by thyrotropin releasing hormone (TRH). The circulating levels of T_3 and T_4 also influence TSH release by exerting negative feedback control at the adenohypophysial and, to a lesser extent, hypothalamic levels. TSH influences the structure and function of thyroid follicular cells and regulates all phases of thyroid hormone synthesis, storage, and secretion. Administration of exogenous thyroid hormone leads to disuse atrophy of the thyroid gland via TSH suppression. Thus, iodide trapping and endogenous thyroid hormone secretion are reduced when TSH is suppressed by exogenous thyroid hormone. In most cells of the body, thyroid hormone stimulates the cell membrane enzyme Na^+-K^+-ATPase, thereby increasing O_2 consumption. This effect is not exerted on cells of the brain, lymph nodes, gonads, lungs, spleen, and dermis.

24. The answer is D [Chapter 47 IV A 3 b (2), Figures 47-3; Chapter 49 I F 2 a, Figure 49-5; Chapter 52 I F 3, Table 52-12; Chapter 53 VIII B 2]. Growth hormone (GH), like insulin and normal levels of thyroid hormone, is a potent protein anabolic hormone (i.e., it promotes nitrogen retention and, thus, a positive nitrogen balance). Negative nitrogen balance results when nitrogen losses exceed nitrogen intake, as occurs with deficient dietary protein or in stressful conditions (e.g., tissue trauma, disease states, burns, surgery). Utilization of amino acids in hepatic gluconeogenesis results in negative nitrogen balance. Glucocorticoids (e.g., cortisol) promote muscle proteolysis and inhibit protein synthesis, leading to increased BUN and enhanced nitrogen excretion. Alanine is the predominant amino acid released by muscle. Glucagon is a catabolic hormone for protein in muscle, and it also is an important gluconeogenic hormone. At normal levels, thyroid hormone stimulates protein synthesis. The positive effect of thyroid hormone on body growth is derived largely from stimulation of protein synthesis. In excess amounts, thyroid hormone causes accelerated protein catabolism, leading to increased nitrogen excretion.

25. The answer is C [Chapter 53 VI A 2 b]. High plasma levels of T_3 would also lead to an increase in the intracellular concentration in the pituitary thyrotropes, and thereby decrease their sensitivity to thyrotropin-releasing hormone (TRH). This would result in decreased thyrotopin (TSH) secretion and, subsequently, decreased thyroxine secretion. Of course, the plasma levels of triiodothyronine are elevated because of the exogenous T_3 administration. This high T_3 level would cause thyroid atrophy.

26. The answer is A [Chapter 53 VI D]. If iodide cannot be oxidized to form active iodide, then T_4 and T_3 cannot be synthesized. The low concentration of these hormones will increase the sensitivity of the pituitary thyrotropes to thyroid-releasing hormone (TRH), causing them to secrete more thyroid-stimulating hormone (TSH). In turn, TSH increases thyroidal cell division, resulting in hypertrophy of the thyroid gland (goiter).

27. The answer is C [Chapter 53 VI A 2, Table 53-2]. Hypophysectomy removes the source of thyroid-stimulating hormone (TSH) and without TSH, the secretion of thyroxine becomes minimal. The thyroid gland will also become atrophic.

28. The answer is C [Chapter 53 VI A 1, Table 53-2]. A hypothalamic lesion will reduce the secretion of thyroid-releasing hormone (TRH), leading to attenuation of thyroid-stimulating hormone (TSH) secretion with a resultant decline in thyroxine secretion. Therefore, a hypothalamic lesion will lead to similar qualitative changes in the pituitary-thyroidal axis as those associated with hypophysectomy; however, the changes will be of a lesser magnitude.

29. The answer is D [Chapter 53 VI D 3 e, Table 53-2]. In primary hyperthyroidism, the thyroid hypersecretes T_4 in response to thyroid-stimulating immunoglobulins (TSI) present in the blood. The elevated T_4 increases the intrapituitary concentration of T_3, which, in turn, decreases the sensitivity of the thyrotropes to thyroid-releasing hormone (TRH). This causes thyroid- stimulating hormone (TSH) secretion and plasma TSH to diminish greatly. This T-cell-mediated autoimmunity can be demonstrated against the TSH receptor antigen. These autoantibodies (TSI) behave as thyroid-stimulating hormone, resulting in the formation of a diffuse goiter.

30. The answer is A [Chapter 53 VI D 3 d]. The dietary iodide deficiency results in the reduction of thyroid hormone synthesis and secretion with a resultant reduction in hypothalamic-pituitary negative feedback. This condition is a cause of primary hypothyroidism characterized by reduced thyroid hormone secretion, which causes a hypothyroid goiter due to elevated thyroid-stimulating hormone (TSH) secretion. In long-term iodide deficiency, the $T_4:T_3$ secretion, which is normally 20:1, decreases because the plasma level of T_4 decreases. Since the pituitary thyrotropes depend on plasma T_4 for the intracellular formation of T_3, the thyrotropes become hypersensitive to thyroid-releasing hormone (TRH) and increase their secretion of TSH.

31. The answer is E [Chapter 53 VI A]. Generalized resistance to thyroid hormone defines a condition of reduced inhibition by thyroid hormone of thyroid-stimulating hormone (TSH) secretion in the pituitary (central resistance) and resistance to thyroid hormone action in peripheral tissues (peripheral resistance). The clinical diagnosis of generalized resistance to thyroid hormone is made with the following triad: (1) elevated serum levels of free T_3 and T_4; (2) "inappropriately normal" plasma TSH levels; and (3) peripheral euthyroidism or hypothyroidism.

The figure shows blockages of biological responses to T_4 and T_3 in the pituitary and peripheral tissues, which are characteristic of generalized resistance to thyroid hormone. *Rectangles* denote refractoriness to thyroid hormones. *TSH* = thyroid-stimulating hormone.

32. The answer is B [Chapter 53 VI A]. Thyroid-stimulating hormone (TSH) levels are elevated or inappropriately normal in patients with hyperthyroidism because of TSH-producing tumors. Although such tumors are rare, it is important to be aware of this disorder. Unfortunately, inappropriate treatment for Graves' disease or other forms of hyperthyroidism does occur in patients in whom TSH levels are not initially obtained.

33. The answer is C [Chapter 47 III A]. Like antidiuretic hormone (ADH), oxytocin is secreted from the neurosecretory neuron terminals in the posterior pituitary (pars nervosa), which serves as a storage/release center. The hormones are synthesized in the supraoptic and paraventricular nuclei in the hypothalamus.

34. The answer is B [Chapter 54 VI A, Figure 54-3, X C 1 a, Table 54-3]. The adenoma autonomously secretes large amounts of PTH, which elevates serum Ca^{2+} concentration. The adenoma is not responsive to the usual suppressive effect of elevated Ca^{2+} on PTH secretion. A finding of simultaneous elevation of PTH and serum Ca^{2+} is indicative of primary hyperparathyroidism.

35. The answer is C [Chapter 54 VI A, Figure 54-3, Table 54-3, X C 2 a (2), Table 54-3]. Extirpation of the parathyroid glands removes the source of PTH, and the mechanisms for the maintenance of serum Ca^{2+} are lacking. As a result, serum Ca^{2+} decreases. A finding of simultaneous low serum PTH and Ca^{2+} concentration is indicative of primary hypoparathyroidism.

36. The answer is A [Chapter 54 VI A, Figure 54-3, X C 1 b (3), Table 54-3]. In chronic renal failure, renal phosphate excretion is diminished, resulting in elevated serum phosphorus concentration. In turn, the hyperphosphatemia reduces serum ionized Ca^{2+}. The lower plasma Ca^{2+} elevates PTH; however, PTH is ineffective in raising serum Ca^{2+} that is due to renal failure. The elevated serum phosphate, together with renal damage, decreases the renal synthesis of calcitriol. PTH requires calcitriol to promote bone resorption and intestinal Ca^{2+} and phosphate absorption effectively; therefore, the low serum phosphate is not corrected by the elevated serum PTH.

37. The answer is A [Chapter 54 VI A, Figure 54-3, X C 1 b (1), Table 54-3]. During vitamin D deficiency, intestinal calcium and phosphate absorption are reduced, causing hypocalcemia. The hypocalcemia, in turn, stimulates the parathyroid glands to secrete increased quantities of PTH. PTH acts indirectly on osteoclasts to promote bone resorption and increase Ca^{2+} and phosphate in the blood. PTH also acts on the kidney to promote both tubular Ca^{2+} reabsorption and phosphate excretion. PTH also stimulates renal conversion of $25OHD_3$ to $1,25(OH)_2D_3$, which stimulates the enterocytes to absorb Ca^{2+} and phosphorus via a calcitriol-induced calcium binding protein (calbindin). Calcium absorption occurs principally in the duodenum, and most phosphate transport activity is located in the jejunum and ileum. It is important to appreciate that vitamin D deficiency is a cause of secondary hyperparathyroidism.

38. The answer is D [Chapter 54 VI A, Figure 54-3, X C 2 b, Table 54-3]. Excessive ingestion of vitamin D can cause hypervitaminosis D (D intoxication), which is recognized as hypercalcemia and hyperphosphatemia. As expected, plasma PTH levels are low, resulting in secondary hypoparathyroidism. The hypercalcemia of vitamin D intoxication results from both increased intestinal absorption of Ca^{2+} and the increased resorption of bone.

39. The answer is B [Chapter 54 VI A, Figure 54-3, X C 1 a, Table 54-3]. Primary hyperparathyroidism is a hypercalcemic state due to excessive secretion of PTH. The disease is caused by a benign, solitary adenoma in most cases. Less commonly, primary hyperparathyroidism is due to hyperplasia of all four parathyroid glands. The pathophysiology of primary hyperparathyroidism relates to the loss of normal negative feedback control of PTH by plasma ionized Ca^{2+}. The inappropriately high serum PTH level causes excessive renal Ca^{2+} reabsorption, hypophosphatemia (hyperphosphaturia), and calcitriol synthesis, and increased bone resorption.

40. The answer is A [Chapter 54 VI A, Figure 54-3, X C 2 c, Table 54-3]. This form of hypocalcemia is due to PTH resistance. Thus, these patients are not only hypocalcemic but also hyperphosphatemic. Administration of PTH

to these patients fails to provoke a phosphate diuresis or an increase in serum Ca^{2+}. These patients have elevated plasma PTH levels.

41. The answer is D [Chapter 54 VI A, Figure 54-3, X C 4, Table 54-3]. Weightlessness (as occurs in space flight) and complete, prolonged bed rest due to orthopaedic casting or traction, to spinal cord injury, or to other neurologic disorders regularly leads to accelerated bone resorption and hypercalcemia. The osteoclastic bone resorption, hypercalciuria, and hypercalcemia promptly reverse with the resumption of normal weight-bearing; however, passive range-of-motion exercises are ineffective. Circulating PTH and $1,25(OH)_2D_3$ levels are reduced in this state of hypokinesia.

42. The answer is A [Chapter 54 VI A, Figure 54-3, X C 1 b, Table 54-3]. The pathogenesis of calcium-deficient rickets is similar to that of vitamin D-deficiency rickets in that hypocalcemia causes secondary hyperparathyroidism. PTH increases bone resorption and enhances renal conversion of $25(OH)D_3$ to $1,25(OH)_2D_3$ and increased intestinal Ca^{2+} and phosphorus absorption. Alkaline phosphatase also reflects elevated osteoblastic bone cell activity. These patients have normal $25OHD_3$ levels, demonstrating that they are not necessarily vitamin D deficient, and are hypophosphatemic due to the elevated PTH secretion. Additionally, these patients have increased renal tubular Ca^{2+} reabsorption, decreased renal tubular phosphate reabsorption, low urinary Ca^{2+} excretion, elevated urinary phosphate excretion, and high serum levels of PTH and $1,25(OH)_2D_3$.

43. The answer is A [Chapter 54 VI A, Figure 54-3, X C 1 b, Table 54-3]. The consequences of increased phosphate loads are a decline in serum ionized Ca^{2+}, suppressed renal synthesis of $1,25(OH)_2D_3$, and inhibition of bone resorption. These effects of phosphate are mitigated by the phosphaturic action of PTH. Thus, hypocalcemia can result from hyperphosphatemia. This syndrome can result from delivery of endogenous and exogenous phosphorus loads into the plasma. Settings for increased oral phosphate loading include excessive dietary phosphorus (e.g., milk or phosphoric acid-containing soft drinks), over-aggressive administration of phosphorus supplements (such as neutral phosphate), and colonoscopy preparation (by using oral phosphate-containing laxatives such as Phospho-Soda). Administration of parenteral phosphorus administration (potassium phosphate) to patients with diabetic ketoacidosis, or phosphate-containing parenteral nutrition solutions, particularly in the setting of renal failure, may lead to hypocalcemia.

44. The answer is D [Chapter 47 IV 3 d (1) (a), (e), Figure 47-3; Chapter 49 I F 3 a; Chapter 52 I F 2 b]. Oxidation of free fatty acids inhibits glucose metabolism in muscle because the free fatty acids (and ketones) are oxidized to acetyl coenzyme A (acetyl-CoA). Acetyl-CoA condenses with oxaloacetate to form citrate, a powerful inhibitor of phosphofructokinase, which is the major rate-determining reaction of glycolysis. Growth hormone (GH) and cortisol directly inhibit glucose uptake by muscle and indirectly decrease glucose metabolism in myocytes in two ways: (1) via their lipolytic effect, and (2) via the formation of acetyl-CoA followed by citrate, which inhibits phosphofructokinase.

When glycolysis is inhibited, glucose is diverted into glycogen. In turn, when glycogen storage is saturated, glucose-6-phosphate accumulates and inhibits phosphorylation of glucose by hexokinase, resulting in the inhibition of glucose transport (uptake) by facilitated diffusion. At the same time, pyruvate kinase and phosphofructokinase are both inhibited by free fatty acids, which reduces glycolysis and enhances gluconeogenesis. Acetyl-CoA is also an activator of pyruvate carboxylase, which forms oxaloacetate from pyruvate.

Formation of acetyl-CoA from free fatty acids or ketone bodies is accompanied by conversion of the oxidized form of nicotinamide adenine dinucleotide (NAD^+) to its reduced form, $NADH_2$. The resulting scarcity of NAD^+ limits the oxidation of citrate, which increases in concentration. The scarcity of NAD^+ also limits the conversion of lactate to pyruvate in the liver.

45. The answer is E [Chapter 48 VIII A 3]. Epinephrine is a potent hyperglycemic hormone due mainly to its effects on the liver and pancreas. In the liver, it promotes glycogenolysis and gluconeogenesis, and the glucose-6-phosphate formed by glycogenolysis is hydrolyzed to glucose. Epinephrine-induced glycogenolysis in muscle leads to formation of lactic acid, which is converted to glucose in the liver, further elevating blood glucose. In the pancreas, epinephrine stimulates glucagon secretion and inhibits insulin secretion, both hyperglycemic effects. Epinephrine also stimulates adrenocor-

ticotropic hormone (ACTH) secretion, which, in turn, leads to secretion of cortisol, which is a major hyperglycemic hormone.

46. The answer is D [Chapter 52 D 1 a (6), c, d, 2, 5, Table 52-5]. Glucose enters the beta cell by a specific glucose transporter called GLUT-2 (which also transports glucose into the hepatocyte). Glucose is phosphorylated and metabolized with the generation of adenosine 5'-triphosphate (ATP). The ATP closes the ATP-sensitive K^+ channel, which leads to the depolarization of the B cell membrane and thereby activates a voltage-dependent Ca^{2+} channel. The resultant increase in intracellular Ca^{2+} stimulates insulin secretion. Insulin decreases cell membrane permeability to both Na^+ and K^+, but it decreases Na^+ permeability more, causing hyperpolarization of skeletal and cardiac muscle cells and adipocytes but not of liver or pancreatic cells. Insulin also promotes lipogenesis, protein anabolism, glycogenesis, and glycolysis. Insulin promotes glucose uptake by muscle and adipose tissue but not by the liver, and it promotes storage and utilization of glucose in all three tissues. Glucose storage by muscle and liver is achieved by formation of glycogen via an increase in glycogen synthase activity. Glucose transport across skeletal and cardiac muscle cells and adipocytes occurs by insulin-dependent facilitated diffusion via the GLUT-4 transporter.

47. The answer is B [Chapter 54 VII C 3, 7, D 2 a, Figure 54-8]. PTH stimulates both renal Ca^{2+} reabsorption in the renal distal tubule and the 1α-hydroxylase enzyme. PTH inhibits proximal phosphate and calcium reabsorption which is associated with an increase in urinary phosphate excretion (phosphate diuresis). The receptors for PTH are located on the basolateral membrane of the renal epithelium, not on the luminal (apical) membrane.

48. The answer is C [Chapter 50 I D 2 b, III C 1, IV B 3, V B 1, Tables 50-4 and 50-5]. In skin and target cells of the male reproductive tract, testosterone may be reduced to the more potent androgen, dihydrotestosterone, in a one-way reaction by the enzyme 5α-reductase. Testosterone also is metabolized to estradiol by the action of aromatase in various tissues, including brain, breast, and adipose tissue. During fetal organization, the testis is stimulated by placental human chorionic gonadotropin (HCG) to produce testosterone. The characteristic adolescent "growth spurt" in the male results from an interplay of testosterone and growth hormone (GH), which promote growth of the vertebrae, shoulder girdle, and long bones. This growth is self-limited, as androgens also accelerate epiphysial closure. In adulthood, testosterone is secreted from the testis in response to LH secretion from the pituitary gland; testosterone acts as a negative feedback regulator of LH secretion and, thus, its own secretion.

49. The answer is A [Chapter 48 VIII A, Figure 48-5]. After an overnight fast, about 75% of the hepatic glucose output is derived from glycogen and about 25% from gluconeogenesis. If fasting is prolonged or combined with exercise, the hepatic glycogen stores are depleted much more rapidly, and the percentage contribution from gluconeogenesis increases. The gluconeogenic substrates are lactate, glycerol, and amino acids. The lactate is derived from incomplete oxidation of glucose by the action of epinephrine on muscle, which comprises about 45% of the body mass. Thus, net hepatic glucose synthesis and secretion requires lactate production from muscle glycogenolysis. The major gluconeogenic source of endogenous glucose production by the action of cortisol is alanine, with a smaller fraction available from the glycerol released from triglycerides hydrolyzed in adipose tissue. Acetyl coenzyme A (acetyl-CoA) is not a gluconeogenic substance in mammalian liver. Thus, epinephrine causes hyperglycemia because it stimulates hepatic glycogenolysis and glycolysis together with gluconeogenesis and muscle glycogenolysis while it inhibits insulin secretion.

50. The answer is C [Chapter 49 I A 3]. In the fetus, the adrenal glands are much larger relative to body size than in the adult. In absolute size, they are almost as large at term as the fetal kidneys and are as large as the adult adrenal glands. The fetal zone, or inner zone, of the fetal adrenal cortex undergoes complete involution 4–12 weeks postpartum. The outer zone, or neocortex, undergoes further differentiation into the adult adrenal cortex.

51. The answer is C [Chapter 54 VI A 4, 7, C 3 a b 7]. The major renal effect of parathyroid hormone (PTH) is stimulation of proximal tubular 1α-hydroxylase, an enzyme that converts calcidiol to calcitriol. PTH affects renal Ca^{2+} reabsorption in two ways: it reduces Ca^{2+} reabsorption in the proximal tubule and increases Ca^{2+} reabsorption in the distal tubule. The net effect is an increase in tubular Ca^{2+} reabsorption. This renal effect of PTH can be lessened by the effect of PTH on bone. PTH increases plasma $[Ca^{2+}]$ by promoting bone resorption, which causes an increase in the renal filtered load of Ca^{2+} and, thus, hypercalciuria. Also, PTH inhibits the proximal reabsorption of phosphate, thereby favoring phosphate excretion. PTH acts on bone by dissolving the nonreadily exchangeable calcium phosphate "fixed pool" known as stable bone. PTH activates the osteoclasts—cells that cause osteolysis by their high content of lysosomal enzymes. PTH also stimulates osteocytes, which are bone-bound osteoblasts that mediate osteocytic osteolysis.

52. The answer is D [Chapter 48 V A, Figure 48-2]. The substrate for dopamine β-hydroxylase is dihydroxyphenylethylamine (dopamine), which is converted to norepinephrine within the cytoplasmic granules of the adrenomedullary chromaffin cell or within the vesicle of the postganglionic sympathetic neuron. The other substrates and their enzymes are: epinephrine or norepinephrine/catechol-O-methyltransferase (COMT) or monoamine oxidase (MAO), tyrosine/tyrosine hydroxylase, phenylalanine/phenylalanine hydroxylase, and dihydroxyphenylalanine (dopa)/dopa decarboxylase.

53. The answer is B [Chapter 48 VII A, B, Table 48-1]. The detrusor muscle of the urinary bladder, in contrast to the trigone and sphincter, contains only β-adrenergic receptors, which, when stimulated, evoke relaxation of this smooth muscle. Stimulation of the α-adrenergic receptors of the bladder produces contraction of these smooth muscles. Thus, sympathetic stimulation of the bladder blocks micturition.

54. The answer is D [Chapter 47 IV A 2 a, Table 47-1]. Secretion of growth hormone (GH) in response to various stimuli often is blunted in obesity. Stimuli for GH secretion include norepinephrine, bromocriptine, hypoglycemia, stress, vigorous exercise, insulin, and arginine. The long-term metabolic effects of GH include hyperglycemia owing to gluconeogenesis, glycogenolysis, and lipolysis, all of which explain its anti-insulin effects. GH has a fat catabolic effect, which increases plasma free fatty acid levels. It should be noted that these free fatty acids are not substrates for gluconeogenesis.

55. The answer is A [Chapter 51 I H 2 d, J 1 c, Figure 51-4]. Variability in the length of the follicular phase ranging from 10 to 16 days is the cause for variation in the length of the menstrual cycle. The time between the midcycle FSH and ovulation is quite short (10 to 12 hours).

56. The answer is A [Chapter 53 I B 1 a b, IV A 2 b, Figure 53-2]. Triiodothyronine (T_3) is the most biologically active iodothyronine secreted by the thyroid follicles. In the secretory process, thyroglobulin (the major storage form of thyroid hormone) is degraded to free amino acids, including tetraiodothyronine (T_4), T_3, monoiodotyrosine, and diiodotyrosine. Of these, only T_4 and T_3 are released into the bloodstream, in a ratio of about 20:1. T_3 has three to five times the biologic activity of T_4 and is considered the most biologically active form of thyroid hormone. T_3 also can be formed from T_4 by the action of 5′-deiodinase in peripheral tissues, especially the liver and kidney. The other circulating iodothyronines, such as reverse triiodothyronine (rT_3), tetraiodothyroacetic acid, and triiodothyroacetic acid have much less biologic activity than T_3 and T_4.

57–60. The answers are: 57-C, [Chapter 51 I G 1 b (2) H 3, Figures 51-4 and 51-8] **58-B,** [Chapter 51 H 3, Figures 51-4 and 51-8] **59-D,** [Chapter 51 II A 1 f, Figure 51-8] **60-B** [Chapter 51 II B 4 b (1) (2) 5 b, Figures 51-8 and 51-11, Table 51-1]. In a normal ovarian cycle, the plasma concentration of estradiol peaks (*point A*), triggering a sudden discharge of pituitary gonadotropins [luteinizing hormone (LH) and follicle-stimulating hormone (FSH)] 12–24 hours later. This preovulatory gonadotropin surge (*point B*) is more pronounced for LH than for FSH. Ovulation (*point C*) occurs 16–20 hours after the LH peak and marks the formation of the corpus luteum. LH maintains the functional and morphologic integrity of the corpus luteum for 14 days.

The ovum can be fertilized between 6 and 20 hours following ovulation (*point D*). If fertilization occurs, a morula is formed, which enters the uterine cavity on the third to fourth day postovulation (*point E*). The morula is converted to the blastocyst during the fifth to sixth day postovulation, which is implanted in the endometrial wall of the uterus by the seventh day (*point F*). At *point G*, human chorionic gonadotropin (HCG) rescues the corpus luteum.

The corpus luteum is the principal source of estrogen (estradiol) and progesterone during the first 6–8 weeks gestation. The principal gonadotropic hormone during this period is HCG, which is secreted by the syncytiotrophoblast of the placenta. This anterior pituitary-like hormone has mainly LH activity and is the luteotropic hormone of pregnancy. The trophoblast takes over as the major source of progesterone and estrogen (estriol) secretion by 7 weeks gestation. HCG also stimulates the fetal testis to produce testosterone and the fetal adrenal gland to produce corticoids in early pregnancy.

61. The answer is E [Chapter 52 I F 1–3, Figure 52-8 and Table 52-7]. The metabolic effects of glucagon are the exact opposite to those of insulin. Thus, glucagon is glycogenolytic, gluconeogenic, ketogenic, ureogenic. Equally important, glucagon blocks glycolysis and glucose utilization. The catabolic action on fat (lipolysis) leads to increases in plasma free fatty acids and glycerol. The elevation in ketoacids (ketonuria) results from the partial oxidation of fatty acids. The hyperglycemia results from the promotion of glycogenolysis, gluconeogenesis, and inhibition of glycolysis by glucagon. The hyperaminoacidemia and increased blood urea nitrogen (BUN) are a result of the proteolytic action of glucagon. In summary, glucagon causes a decline in glycogen, fat, and protein stores.

62. The answer is A [Chapter 51 I H 4 a, Figures 51-4 and 51-6]. In this woman with a menstrual cycle of 21–23 days, ovulation would be expected to occur between day 7 and day 9, counting from the first day of menses. The normal menstrual cycle has an average duration of 28 days. The luteal, or postovulatory, phase corresponds to the secretory phase of the endometrium or the progestational phase of the corpus luteum. This phase of the menstrual cycle usually is very constant, lasting about 14 days, while the duration of the follicular phase can be highly variable. Because of the constancy of the postovulatory phase, the time of ovulation can be estimated by subtracting 14 days from the cycle length.

63. The answer is E [Chapter 51 C 3, E 2 a (4) (a), F 1 a (2), and Figure 51-3]. The secretory products of the ovary are estradiol and estrone, which are produced by the granulosa cells of the unruptured follicle and lutein-granulosa cells of the corpus luteum. Luteinization of the granulosa cells, which depends on LH, involves the appearance of lipid droplets in the cytoplasm. The estrogenic precursors produced by the theca interna (and theca-lutein) are androstenedione and testosterone, which are converted by the granulosa (and granulosa-lutein) cells into estrone and estradiol, respectively. The lutein-granulosa cells also produce and secrete progesterone. Thus, androstenedione and pregnenolone are produced, but not secreted, by the ovary. Estriol is not an ovarian product but is synthesized in the liver from estradiol and estrone and in the placenta by the conversion of imported androgens. Pregnanediol is the urinary metabolite of progesterone and formed in the liver.

64. The answer is B [Chapter 30 III B 2 b (1); Chapter 48 VII, Table 48-1]. Renin is synthesized by the juxtaglomerular cells of the afferent arteriole, which receive postganglionic sympathetic innervation. Thus, these autonomic nerves secrete norepinephrine, which stimulates β-adrenergic receptors on the surface of the juxtaglomerular cells.

65. The answer is A [Chapter 53 IV, Figure 53-4, VIII, Table 53-2]. This patient has adult hypothyroidism (myxedema) as evidenced from her lethargic state with fatigue, dry skin, absence of ankle tendon reflexes, and thyroid hormone profile. All forms of hypothyroidism have a relative or absolute reduction of T_4 and T_3 secretion. The plasma thyroid-stimulating hormone (TSH) level is the biologic marker that is more sensitive than the serum T_4 as a test for thyroid dysfunction, because the TSH can detect subclinical disorders, in which serum total T_4 (and T_3) are usually normal. A significant elevation in the serum TSH level is present in all cases of primary hypothyroidism, irrespective of plasma T_4 or T_3 levels. For example, her T_4 level is only slightly below the low normal level and her free T_4 level is within the normal range. Her resin T_3 uptake test is also within the normal range. However, in severe cases of primary hypothyroidism, a significant elevation in plasma TSH will be observed, as this woman's thyroid function tests reveal. It is very rare to see hyperthyroidism due to elevated TSH. The vast majority of patients with thyrotoxicosis (hyperthyroidism) reveal suppressed TSH and elevated TSH-Ab (TSH receptor antibodies). The diagnosis of hypothyroidism due to pituitary or hypothalamic disease is more difficult. The plasma thyroid hormones are low but the TSH levels are not elevated and are usually reduced. The two disorders can be differentiated with exogenous thyroid-releasing hormone (TRH) injection. Hypothyroidism due to pituitary insufficiency is characterized by a low basal TSH and no response to TRH stimulation. Hypothyroidism due to hypothalamic disease is charac-

terized by a delayed and augmented TSH response. It is obvious that her goiter is caused by elevated TSH and that it is hypofunctional. It is imperative to appreciate that a goiter does not determine the thyroidal status in the absence of other findings. Lastly, if she were taking excessive amounts of thyroid extract, she would have suppressed levels of TSH and a much smaller or atrophic thyroid gland. In summary, her elevated TSH in the context of low circulating plasma thyroid hormone is pathognomonic of primary hypothyroidism.

66. The answer is D [Chapter 51 II B 1, Table 51-3; Chapter 47 IV B 2 b (3) (4)]. High circulating levels of estrogen suppress milk production until after parturition. Lactation begins when the maternal breast, primed by long exposure to high levels of prolactin, estrogen, and progesterone, is subjected to sudden withdrawal of these two steroid hormones. Lactation then continues in an environment of relatively high (but declining) prolactin levels and low estrogen and progesterone levels. Suckling provides an essential stimulus for the release of oxytocin and prolactin. Physiologic hyperprolactinemia during pregnancy and lactation is associated with suppression of the hypothalamic-pituitary-ovarian axis. This occurs probably through the prolactin-mediated inhibition of pulsatile secretion of LHRH which, in turn, results in impaired gonadotropin secretion and inhibition of gonadal function. Unlike other pituitary hormones, the primary influence of the hypothalamus on prolactin secretion is inhibitory through the action of the hypophysiotropic hormone called prolactin-inhibiting factor (PIF, or dopamine).

67. The answer is C [Chapter 50 II B 4 b (9), IV A 1, 2 and Figure 50-8]. Inhibin, a peptide hormone produced by the Sertoli cells of the testis, inhibits FSH secretion, not LHRH secretion, leading to a decline in spermatogenesis because FSH is the testicular gametogenic hormone. The negative feedback of inhibin is exerted at the level of the pituitary and suppresses the effect of FSH on its target, the spermatogenic tubules. Inhibin does not affect androgen production by the Leydig cells, which are regulated by LH. Lastly, it is primarily testosterone, not inhibin, that inhibits both LHRH secretion by the hypothalamus and LH secretion by the pituitary.

68. The answer is C [Chapter 48 V A 2]. Because cortisol activates the epinephrine-forming enzyme phenylethanolamine-N-methyltrans-ferase (PNMT), a decrease in cortisol secretion would lead to decreased adrenomedullary synthesis of epinephrine. Another effect of cortisol is to elevate blood glucose through gluconeogenesis and inhibition of peripheral glucose transport and utilization. The proteolytic effect of cortisol in extrahepatic tissues leads to increased transport of amino acids to the liver, where they are used for gluconeogenesis, glycogenesis, and protein synthesis. Hypocortisolism, therefore, would result in decrements in plasma glucose concentration, hepatic glycogen, and hepatic protein. A decline in free blood cortisol levels would also lead to an increase in adrenocorticotropic hormone (ACTH; corticotropin) secretion due to the reduced negative feedback effect of cortisol on the hypothalamic-pituitary complex.

69. The answer is C [Chapter 49 I D 2 b]. The polypeptide known as β-endorphin is formed from β-lipotropin [not from adrenocorticotropic hormone (ACTH)], which is a cleavage product of the prohormone proopiomelanocortin (POMC). POMC and its derivatives are synthesized in the basophils of the pars distalis of the anterior lobe of the pituitary gland. Endorphins, β-lipotropin, and ACTH (corticotropin) also are found in the brain. ACTH can be cleaved to form α-melanocyte-stimulating hormone (α-MSH) and a corticotropin-like peptide called CLIP. β-Endorphin binds with morphine receptors and produces morphine-like responses, such as respiratory depression, analgesia, and miosis.

70. The answer is D [Chapter 48 VII, Table 48-1; Chapter 30 III, Table 30-2]. Activation of the sympathetic nervous system involves stimulation of both α- and β-adrenergic receptors by both norepinephrine and epinephrine. The α-adrenergic response of the pancreatic islet cells is dominant during stimulation; thus, insulin secretion (a response mediated by β-adrenergic receptors) is suppressed. Other responses that are mediated by β-adrenergic receptors include renin secretion, vasodilation, and inhibition of intestinal motility. Vasodilation in skeletal muscle is caused by epinephrine stimulation of β-adrenergic receptors in vascular smooth muscle. Responses mediated by α-adrenergic receptors include inhibition of intestinal motility, contraction of the radial eye muscle (mydriasis), relaxation of the ciliary muscle, and vasoconstriction. Activation of the sympathetic nerves innervating the afferent

and efferent arterioles results in an increase in renin secretion.

71. The answer is B [Chapter 49 I C 1 a, Table 49-1, Figure 49-2]. The chief product of the fetal zone of the adrenal cortex is the weak androgen dehydroepiandrosterone (DHEA), which is secreted as the inactive sulfate ester. DHEA sulfate is converted in the fetal liver to 16α-hydroxydehydroepiandrosterone sulfate, which, on aromatization in the placenta, becomes estriol (estriol is synthesized only by the placenta and adult liver). After the first trimester, the inner zone of the fetal adrenal cortex also can secrete cortisol and aldosterone. Progesterone and corticosterone are synthesized, but not secreted, by the fetal adrenal cortex.

72. The answer is C [Chapter 51 Case 51, discussion of question 4, Figure 51-12]. Because the patient's primary problem resides in the hypothalamus, the pulsatile administration of GnRH (LHRH) will establish a normal pattern of LH and FSH secretion, with the consequent development of a follicle followed by ovulation. Neither estrogen nor progesterone nor any combination of these steroids will allow the follicle to develop. In fact, the combination of these steroids forms the basis for the use of oral contraceptives (i.e., inhibition of FSH and LH). Daily injections of the two gonadotropins will not be efficacious because, without the midcycle secretory spikes of LH and FSH, ovulation will not occur.

73. The answer is D [Chapter 51 I A 3 c (2) (b), Figure 51-1, II A 1 c (1)]. The second meiotic division of the oocyte is not completed until just after fertilization. From the third month of embryonic life, the primary oocytes are arrested in the diplotene phase of the early prophase of meiosis. Completion of this first division occurs just prior to ovulation by the extrusion of the first polar body, resulting in the formation of a secondary oocyte with a haploid number of chromosomes (22 autosomes and 1 sex chromosome). The onset of ovulatory menstrual cycles may lag several months behind menses, which usually occurs between the ages of 12 and 14. The second meiotic division occurs just after conception, yielding a fertilized ovum (zygote) and a second polar body.

74. The answer is C [Chapter 50 I D 1, 2 a–c, Figures 50-2, 50-3 and 50-10, Table 50-8 (see Case 50)]. Patients with testicular feminization have a female phenotype but a male genotype. They have intra-abdominal testes that produce testosterone and estrogen concentrations that are characteristic of normal men, but their tissues are totally unresponsive to androgens because of a lack of androgen receptors and they do not produce sperm. The external genitalia are female because the primordial tissue develops in the female pattern unless stimulated by androgen. The androgen resistance syndromes are disorders in which müllerian duct regression and testosterone synthesis are normal. Male development of the embryo requires müllerian duct inhibiting factor (to prevent the development of female internal genitalia), testosterone (to mediate wolffian duct development), and dihydrotestosterone (to stimulate development of the prostate and male external genitalia). This patient lacks female internal genitalia (because the müllerian duct inhibiting factor exerts its normal action) and lacks male wolffian duct development (because testosterone does not exert its normal stimulatory action). Since both duct systems regress, neither male nor female internal genitalia develop. Secondary sex characteristics, including breast development, appear at puberty in response to the unopposed action of estrogen formed extragonadally from testosterone. This patient has male pseudohermaphroditism, in that the female phenotype in this genetic male is not a result of the presence of both testes and ovaries.

75. The answer is E [Chapter 48 VII, Table 48-1]. Stimulation of either type of receptor in the intestine causes inhibition of peristalsis. Stimulation of β-adrenergic receptors on the pancreatic beta cells evokes insulin secretion.

The ciliary muscle is innervated by both postganglionic sympathetic and postganglionic parasympathetic fibers. Only β-adrenergic, not α-adrenergic, receptors are found in this smooth muscle. β-Adrenergic stimulation causes relaxation of the ciliary muscle, which, in turn, increases the tension on the lens, causing the lens to become thinner and adapted for far vision. The parasympathetic innervation of the ciliary muscle causes it to contract, which, in turn, decreases the tension on the lens, causing the lens to become thick and adapted for near vision (accommodation). Vascular smooth muscle, pancreatic beta cells, and intestinal smooth muscle contain both α- and β-adrenergic receptors. The heart contains only β-adrenergic receptors. The radial eye muscle (pupillary dilator muscle) contains solely α-adrenergic receptors; as the result of sympathetic nerve stimulation, they contract, leading to pupillary dilation (mydriasis).

76. The answer is C [Chapter 49 I F 1 a b d (1) (2), 2 b]. Glucocorticoids are potent hypoglycemic hormones that, at high levels, lead to glucose intolerance. Glucocorticoids stimulate the liver to produce glucose and glycogen owing, in part, to the increased synthesis of key gluconeogenic enzymes. They also promote muscle proteolysis, resulting in the release of amino acids, which (aside from leucine and lysine) are gluconeogenic. The synthesis of hepatic gluconeogenic enzymes accounts for the protein anabolic effect of glucocorticoids in liver. Hepatic glycogenesis occurs via the activation of glycogen synthase by glucocorticoids. The increased hepatic glucose production and secretion involves gluconeogenesis, not glycogen degradation (glycogenolysis).

77. The answer is B [Chapter 48 VII, Table 48-1; Chapter 52 I C, Table 52-2]. Insulin secretion is elicited by stimulation of the β-adrenergic receptor on the surface of the pancreatic beta cell.

78. The answer is A [Chapter 52 I D 1 a (2), c, d 2 (b), Table 52-5]. Glucose is transported by facilitated diffusion in erythrocytes, skeletal and cardiac muscle, and adipocytes. Facilitated diffusion for glucose transport requires a protein-carrier molecule in the cell membrane. The insulin-dependent facilitated diffusion mechanism for glucose is found in skeletal and cardiac muscle and in adipose tissue. Some tissues obtain their glucose requirements by insulin-independent mechanisms; for example, central nervous system (CNS) cells and hepatocytes. In renal and gastrointestinal (GI) epithelium, glucose transport occurs by a secondary active transport system that is not insulin-dependent but is Na$^+$-dependent. Since Na$^+$ and glucose are transported in the same directions, this active transport system is called a symport system.

79. The answer is B [Chapter 48 IX B 3]. Tumors may arise within the sympathoadrenomedullary system. Adrenal chromaffin cell tumors, known as pheochromocytomas, usually arise within the adrenal medulla, are benign, and secrete primarily excessive amounts of norepinephrine. However, pheochromocytoma patients may have signs of both norepinephrine and epinephrine hypersecretion. Most patients have paroxysms of hypertension, tachycardia, sweating, tremor, palpitations, and nervousness. Most lose weight and are hyperglycemic because of the catecholamine-induced inhibition of insulin secretion.

80. The answer is B [Chapter 50 II A 2 B 1]. Ninety percent of the volume of the testis is composed of tubular tissue, with the remaining 10% consisting mainly of nontubular, or interstitial, cells (also called Leydig cells). The seminiferous tubular epithelium contains three cell types: spermatogonia, spermatocytes, and Sertoli cells. Spermatogonia and spermatocytes are germinal cells, and the Sertoli cells are nongerminal cells.

81. The answer is C [Chapter 51 I F 1 a (2) (b), G 1 c, Table 51-2]. In terms of serum concentration, the major postmenopausal steroid and pituitary tropic hormones are estrone and follicle-stimulating hormone (FSH). Menopause, defined as the physiologic cessation of menses, results from a loss in the cyclic ovarian function caused by the failure of the ovary to respond to gonadotropins. The decline in ovarian function causes an increase in pituitary tropic hormones, with a striking increase in plasma FSH concentration relative to the increase in plasma luteinizing hormone (LH) level. Some estrogens continue to be produced in postmenopausal women by the extraovarian conversion of androstenedione of adrenal origin to estrone.

82. The answer is A [Chapter 48 VI B 1, Figure 48-3]. Vanillylmandelic acid (VMA) is the major urinary end product of catecholamine metabolism. Monoamine oxidase (MAO) is a mitochondrial enzyme that catalyzes the oxidative deamination of the catecholamines—dopamine, norepinephrine, and epinephrine. MAO also inactivates the indolamine, serotinin (5-hydroxytryptamine). Substrates for MAO also include normethanephrine and metanephrine. Tyrosine and dihydroxyphenylalanine (DOPA) in the biosynthetic pathway of catecholamines are not MAO substrates.

83. The answer is D [Chapter 54 VI A 4 c, Figure 54-4]. Active vitamin D_3 (1,25-dihydroxycholecalciferol; calcitriol) is formed in the proximal convoluted tubule by conversion (via the action of 1α-hydroxylase) from its immediate precursor, 25-hydroxycholecalciferol (calcidiol). Vitamin D activation begins in the skin, where the previtamin, 7-dehydrocholesterol, is photoactivated by sunlight to lipid-soluble vitamin D_3. Vitamin D_3 then is converted in the liver to calcidiol, the major circulating form of vitamin D_3.

84. The answer is A [Chapter 49 I F 1–3, Figure 49-5]. The overall metabolic effects of cortisol are the release of amino acids from muscle and both the storage and release of glucose and fatty acids. Cortisol inhibits fatty acid synthesis in the liver, and it increases blood glycerol and fatty acid concentrations in concert with other hormones (norepinephrine, epinephrine, glucagon) to increase lipolysis in adipose tissues. Glycerol is an excellent index of lipolysis, because, unlike free fatty acids, it is not reused by adipocytes in the resynthesis of triglycerides. Rather, glycerol is used by the liver as a gluconeogenic substrate. Cortisol also promotes synthesis of gluconeogenic enzymes needed to convert the amino acids released from muscle to carbohydrate synthesis in the liver. Glucocorticoids promote proteolysis and inhibit protein synthesis in most tissues except the liver.

85. The answer is A [Chapter 49 VIII A 2 c, Figure 48-5]. After an overnight fast, about 75% of the hepatic glucose output is derived from glycogen and about 25% from gluconeogenesis. If fasting is prolonged or combined with exercise, the hepatic glycogen stores are depleted much more rapidly and the percentage contribution from gluconeogenesis increases. The gluconeogenic substrates are lactate, glycerol, and amino acids. The lactate is derived from incomplete oxidation of glucose by the action of epinephrine on muscle, which comprises about 45% of the body mass. Thus, net hepatic glucose synthesis and secretion requires lactate production from muscle glycogenolysis. The major gluconeogenic source of endogenous glucose production by the action of cortisol is alanine, with a smaller fraction available from the glycerol released from triglycerides hydrolyzed in adipose tissue. Acetyl coenzyme A (acetyl-coA) is not a gluconeogenic substance in mammalian liver. Thus, epinephrine causes hyperglycemia because it stimulates hepatic glycogenolysis and gluconeogenesis, muscle glycogenolysis, and inhibits insulin secretion.

86. The answer is C [Chapter 52 I D 1, Figures 52-3 and 52-4; Table 52-4]. In carbohydrate metabolism, insulin is glycogenic, glycolytic, and antigluconeogenic. Thus, insulin brings about hypoglycemia by both promoting the polymerization of glucose (glycogenesis) and enhancing glucose utilization (glycolysis). In the figure, there are two glycogenic hormones: cortisol (B) and insulin (C). Cortisol, however, inhibits glucose utilization. There are also two major glycogenic hormones: cortisol (B) and insulin (C). However, cortisol inhibits glucose transport and glycolysis. The other hormone in this series that promotes glycolysis is epinephrine (A), which also promotes glycogenolysis. Hormone D is glucagon, a product of the pancreatic alpha cells; however, glucagon promotes glycogenolysis and inhibits glycolysis. Somatotropin (E) is also hyperglycemia but it inhibits glycolysis without a large effect on glycogen metabolism. Epinephrine (A), cortisol (B), glucagon (D), and somatotropin (E) are all gluconeogenic hormones. These four hormones are anti-insulin hormones and are referred to as the glucose counterregulatory hormones.

87. The answer is D [Chapter 52 I F 1, Figure 52-8, and Table 52-7]. In type 1 diabetes, glucagon (D) is elevated because the inhibitory effect of insulin on glucagon secretion is absent. Glucagon is hyperglycemia because it is glycogenolytic, gluconeogenic, and antiglycolytic. Also, epinephrine increases glucagon secretion in the setting of type 1 diabetes.

88. The answer is B [Chapter 47 III B 1, D, Figure 47-1A]. Prolactin, not oxytocin, causes milk synthesis (lactogenesis); oxytocin evokes milk secretion (ejection). Oxytocin is an octapeptide produced mainly in the paraventricular nucleus of the ventral diencephalon. Because it is synthesized in the magnocellular neurosecretory neurons, oxytocin is classified as a neuropeptide, or neurosecretory hormone. The unmyelinated axons of the paraventricular nucleus contribute to the supraopticohypophysial tract, which terminates in the pars nervosa. The pars nervosa is a release center and not the site of oxytocin synthesis. Oxytocin has two important smooth muscle effects: It causes milk ejection via contraction of the myoepithelial cells of the mammary gland, and it promotes myometrial (uterine) contraction.

89. The answer is A [Chapter 51 II B 4 b (2), Figure 51-11]. The major source of progesterone during the second and third trimesters of pregnancy is the syncytiotrophoblast of the placenta. Maternal cholesterol is the principal source of precursor substrate for the biosynthesis of progesterone. Thus, progesterone levels during pregnancy are an index of the functional status of the materno-placental unit. Plasma progesterone levels during pregnancy are of limited value as an indicator of placental function alone because of the variability of normal levels.

90. The answer is A [Chapter 51 I L 2 a–e, Table 51-3]. By 8 weeks gestation, maternal cholesterol can be converted to progesterone by the placental trophoblast, which becomes the major producer of progesterone. Progesterone is necessary for maintenance of the decidual cells of the endometrium, inhibition of myometrial contraction by the hyperpolarization of uterine smooth muscle cells, and formation of a dense, viscous mucus that seals off the uterine cavity. Progesterone, in synergy with estrogen, promotes the growth and branching of the lobuloalveolar ductal system of the mammary gland. In early pregnancy, placental progesterone serves as a precursor for the synthesis of cortisol and aldosterone by the fetal zone of the adrenal cortex under the stimulation of human chorionic gonadotropin (HCG). Beyond 10 weeks gestation, the outer zone of the fetal adrenal cortex (neocortex) can produce these two corticoids under the stimulation of adrenocorticotropic hormone (ACTH). Progesterone also exhibits a natriuretic effect by antagonizing the action of aldosterone on the renal tubule.

91. The answer is B [Chapter 45 V C 2, 3, Table 45-2]. The synthesis of steroid hormones is normally due to the activation of the synthetic pathway, which increases commensurately with increased secretion. Steroid hormones are largely bound to plasma globulins, which makes them nonfilterable at the glomerulus and accounts for their longer circulating half-lives [e.g., sex hormone–binding globulin and corticosteroid-binding globulin (CBG)]. The lipophilic hormone (steroid) receptors diffuse through the plasma membrane and interact with receptors that are primarily intranuclear. The steroid hormones are stored as prohormones in the form of cholesterol esters in lipid droplets.

92. The answer is A [Chapter 45 IV F 2 d, Figure 45-2]. The major factor determining the tissue response to a hormone is the presence of a cellular receptor for the hormone and the postreceptor machinery to which that receptor is coupled. For peptide hormones the receptors are on the plasma membrane of the target cell. The interaction of the ligand (hormone) with its receptor is the first step in the transduction of the hormonal signals from the outside of the cell to the inside. The membrane receptor for growth hormone (GH) [and prolactin] are glycoproteins, which contain a single transmembrane spanning domain. GH receptors have no intrinsic kinase activity but activate nonreceptor intracellular kinases following hormone binding. Thus, membrane receptors for GH (and prolactin) are classified as receptor-associated tyrosine kinase.

Peptide hormone receptors that contain intrinsic protein tyrosine kinase activity (receptor tyrosine kinases) include insulin and insulin-like growth factor-1 (IGF-1). The largest family of membrane receptors uses an intermediate modulating signal transducer such as G proteins to couple to specific intracellular effector (enzyme) systems (e.g., adenyl cyclase or phosphatidylinositol pathways). Hormones that act through cyclic adenosine monophosphate (cAMP)–mediated mechanisms include glucagon, adrenocorticotropic hormone (ACTH), antidiuretic hormone (ADH) [V_2 receptor], glycoprotein pituitary hormones [luteinizing hormone (LH), follicle-stimulating hormone (FSH), and thyroid-stimulating hormone (TSH)], epinephrine and norepinephrine (β-receptors), and somatostatin. Hormones that do not act through cAMP-mediated mechanisms include epinephrine and norepinephrine (α_1- and α_2-receptors), insulin, ADH (V_1 receptor), GH, and IGF-1. For steroid hormones and iodothyronines (thyroid hormone), the receptors are intracellular (i.e., primarily within the nucleus).

93. The answer is C [Chapter 49 I A 3]. In the fetus, the adrenal glands are much larger relative to body size than in the adult. In absolute size, they are almost as large at term as the fetal kidneys and are as large as the adult adrenal glands. The fetal zone, or inner zone, of the fetal adrenal cortex undergoes complete involution 4–12 weeks postpartum. The outer zone, or neocortex, undergoes further differentiation into the adult adrenal cortex.

94. The answer is A [Chapter 54 VII C 3 b, Figure 54-7, VIII C 1, Figure 54-9, Table 54-1]. Parathyroid hormone (PTH) and active vitamin D_3 (calcitriol) have several similar effects, particularly in Ca^{2+} regulation. However, these two hormones exert different effects on renal phosphate handling: calcitriol promotes phosphate reabsorption, whereas PTH promotes phosphate diuresis. PTH and calcitriol both promote bone resorption, which leads to an increase in serum [Ca^{2+}]. Calcitriol promotes intestinal absorption of Ca^{2+} and phosphate. Although PTH has no direct intestinal effect on Ca^{2+} or phosphate absorption, it does stimulate renal 1α-hydroxylase activity and subse-

quent calcitriol formation; thus, PTH indirectly promotes intestinal absorption of Ca^{2+} and phosphate. In the kidney, PTH promotes distal tubular Ca^{2+} reabsorption, inhibits proximal phosphate reabsorption, and activates proximal 1α-hydroxylase. Calcitriol enhances renal tubular reabsorption of both Ca^{2+} and phosphate. At pharmacologic doses, calcitriol mimics the effects of PTH (i.e., it promotes phosphate excretion).

95. The answer is B [Chapter 51 II C 1 a–c, Figure 51-11]. The trophoblast (syncytiotrophoblast) that is formed secretes human chorionic gonadotropin (HCG) in the first trimester and not estrogen and progesterone for 6 to 8 weeks. It is HCG that is the luteotropic hormone of pregnancy and that stimulates the corpus luteum in early pregnancy, which continues to secrete estradiol and progesterone for 6 to 8 weeks. In time, the placenta will form sufficient estrogen and progesterone to maintain pregnancy, but this will not occur immediately after implantation. No class of steroid other than estrogens and progesterone are formed or secreted by the placenta. The syncytiotrophoblast synthesizes protein hormones in addition to steroids, and after the seventh week of pregnancy (the luteal-placental shift), it is the most active fetal or maternal endocrine organ. HCG is produced about 8 days after ovulation and it "rescues" the corpus luteum from the falling level of pituitary gonadotropins.

96. The answer is B [Chapter 49 I C 1 a, Table 49-1]. The chief product of the fetal zone of the adrenal cortex is the weak androgen dehydroepiandrosterone (DHEA), which is secreted as the inactive sulfate ester. DHEA sulfate is converted in the fetal liver to 16α-hydroxydehydroepiandrosterone sulfate, which, upon aromatization in the placenta, becomes estriol (estriol is synthesized only by the placenta and adult liver). After the first trimester, the inner zone of the fetal adrenal cortex also can secrete cortisol and aldosterone. Progesterone and corticosterone are synthesized, but not secreted, by the fetal adrenal cortex.

97. The answer is C [Chapter 49 I F a b d (1) (2), 2 b]. Glucocorticoids are potent hypoglycemic hormones that, at high levels, lead to glucose intolerance. Glucocorticoids stimulate the liver to produce glucose and glycogen due, in part, to the increased synthesis of key gluconeogenic enzymes. They also promote muscle proteolysis, resulting in the release of amino acids, which (aside from leucine and lysine) are gluconeogenic. The synthesis of hepatic gluconeogenic enzymes accounts for the protein anabolic effect of glucocorticoids in liver. Hepatic glycogenesis occurs via the activation of glycogen synthase by glucocorticoids. The increased hepatic glucose production and secretion involves gluconeogenesis, not glycogen degradation (glycogenolysis).

98. The answer is A [Chapter 48 III B]. The adrenal medulla is a modified sympathetic ganglion consisting of chromaffin cells (pheochromocytes) that are the functional analogs of the postganglionic neurons. About 80% of the adrenomedullary secretion is epinephrine, and 20% is norepinephrine. The plasma concentration ratio of epinephrine to norepinephrine normally is 1:4, the inverse of the secretory ratio. Adrenalectomy causes a precipitous decrement in plasma epinephrine concentration.

99. The answer is C [Chapter 50 V A 3 a (2)]. Prostaglandins found in seminal fluid are secretory products of the seminal vesicles. Chemical analysis of seminal fluid provides an indirect measure of testicular function, because the male accessory sex organs (i.e., the seminal vesicles and prostate gland) are androgen-dependent. The seminal vesicles secrete fructose, prostaglandins, and ascorbate into the seminal plasma; the prostate gland secretes acid phosphatase and citrate into the seminal fluid. Originally, the prostate was believed to be the source of the prostaglandins, and the term has become a misnomer.

100. The answer is A [Chapter 53 IV B 1 a]. The biosynthetic pathway for thyroid hormone has four steps: active uptake of inorganic iodide, oxidation of iodide to active iodide, iodination of the tyrosyl residues on the thyroglobulin molecule, and coupling of iodotyrosines to form iodothyronines. The only step that does not require thyroid peroxidase is the first. Secretion depends on a lysosomal protease.

101. The answer is D [Chapter 48 VII, Table 48-1]. Activation of the sympathetic nervous system involves stimulation of both α- and β-adrenergic receptors by norepinephrine. The α-adrenergic response of the pancreatic islet cells is dominant during stimulation; thus, insulin secretion (a response mediated by β-adrenergic receptors) is suppressed. Other re-

sponses that are mediated by β-adrenergic receptors include renin secretion, vasodilation, and inhibition of intestinal motility. Responses mediated by α-adrenergic receptors include inhibition of intestinal motility, contraction of the radial eye muscle (mydriasis), and vasoconstriction. Vasodilation in skeletal muscle is caused by epinephrine and by stimulation of sympathetic cholinergic nerves.

102. The answer is C [Chapter 51 II B 5 a (2), Figures 51-9 and 51-10]. The neocortex of the fetal adrenal gland does not participate in estriol synthesis during gestation. Estriol is a product of the combined activities of the fetal pituitary gland, the **fetal zone** of the adrenal cortex, the fetal liver, and the syncytiotrophoblast of the placenta. The fetal zone of the adrenal gland is the inner zone that persists only during gestation; the neocortex is the outer zone of the fetal adrenal gland, which is the progenitor of the adult adrenal cortex. In the first trimester, the fetal zone is primarily stimulated by human chorionic gonadotropin (HCG), with adrenocorticotropic hormone (ACTH) [from the fetal pituitary] gaining prominence thereafter. The fetal zone synthesizes dehydroepiandrosterone (DHEA) and its sulfate (DHEAS), which are transported to the placenta after 16α-hydroxylation by the fetal liver. It is 16α-OH DHEAS that is the precursor of placental estriol.

103. The answer is C [Chapter 52 I B 3; G 1; Chapter 29 I B; Chapter 47 III A 1]. Somatostatin and insulin are polypeptides, consisting of 14 and 51 amino acid residues, respectively. Insulin is synthesized in the pancreatic beta cells; somatostatin is synthesized in the pancreatic delta cells as well as many other sites, including the hypothalamus, cerebrum, thymus, thyroid, gastric and intestinal epithelium, skin, heart, and salivary glands. Insulin inhibits glucagon secretion, and somatostatin inhibits secretion of GH, thyroid-stimulating hormone (TSH), insulin, glucagon, pancreatic polypeptide, gut hormones, gastric acid, and pepsin.

104. The answer is D [Chapter 47 IV A 3 a (1) (a)]. The protein anabolic effects of growth hormone (GH) are mediated through a GH-dependent peptide known as somatomedin, which is synthesized in the liver. Important biologic effects of somatomedin include mitogenesis of chondrocytes and bone cells, stimulation of lipogenesis and muscle glycogenesis, and GH-like actions in cartilage (e.g., sulfation of chondroitin). Antidiuretic hormone (ADH) and oxytocin are neuropeptides synthesized mainly in the neurosecretory neurons of the supraoptic and paraventricular nuclei, respectively. Thyrotropin-releasing hormone (TRH) is produced in the neurosecretory neurons of the arcuate nucleus. Endorphins are secretory products of basophils in the adenohypophysis and of brain neurons. Thus, endorphins also can be classified as neuropeptides. Somatomedin is not produced by endocrine neurons called neurosecretory neurons; therefore, it is not a neuropeptide.

COMPREHENSIVE EXAMINATION

QUESTIONS

1. The receptor potential for which sensory system causes the photoreceptors to hyperpolarize when stimulated?

(A) Taste
(B) Olfaction
(C) Audition
(D) Touch
(E) Vision

2. Which of the following decreases the glomerular filtration rate (GFR) and renal blood flow below normal levels?

(A) Glomerulotubular balance
(B) A small increase in efferent arteriolar resistance
(C) Prostaglandin E_2 (PGE_2)
(D) A decrease in afferent arteriolar resistance
(E) A high plasma catecholamine level

3. Which of the following statements applies to aldosterone?

(A) Its secretion is increased by converting enzyme inhibitors
(B) It acts through basolateral membrane receptors to increase luminal membrane sodium channels
(C) It increases Na^+ entry into intercalated cells along the late distal tubule and collecting duct
(D) It increases the amount of Na^+–K^+–ATPase in the principal cells
(E) It decreases the number of K^+ channels on the luminal membrane of the principal cells

4. Extracellular bicarbonate (HCO_3^-) is not an effective buffer for which of the following?

(A) Phosphoric acid
(B) Lactic acid
(C) Sulfuric acid
(D) Carbonic acid
(E) β-hydroxybutyric acid

5. Thyroid hormone is stored primarily in the

(A) plasma
(B) follicular cells
(C) interstitial fluid (ISF)
(D) parafollicular cells
(E) extracellular fluid (ECF)

6. The anti-inflammatory effect of exogenous cortisol is due to

(A) increased capillary membrane permeability
(B) increased formation of leukotrienes
(C) decreased release of pyrogens from granulocytes
(D) activation of macrocortin
(E) increased permeability of lysosomal membranes

7. Which one of the following statements correctly describes a healthy 30-year-old woman with a menstrual cycle of 26 days?

(A) Exogenous estrogen treatment will cause hypertrophy of her ovaries.
(B) Menstruation is caused by the secretion of progesterone from the corpus luteum.
(C) The proliferative phase of the endometrium is caused by the mitogenic action of estradiol secreted by the ovarian follicle.
(D) Plasma estradiol concentration begins to decline prior to ovulation and continues to decrease until menstruation.
(E) The highest plasma level of FSH is associated with the start of menstruation.

Questions 8–9

Lung compliance in a 32-year-old woman is studied. Data collected under control and experimental conditions are listed in the following table.

	Respiratory Rate (breaths/min)	Tidal Volume (ml)	Change in Interpleural Pressure during Inspiration (cm H_2O)
Control	15	600	4
Experimental	25	600	10

8. This patient's lung compliance during control and experimental conditions was

(A) unchanged
(B) 40 ml/breath and 24 ml/breath, respectively
(C) 150 ml/cm H_2O and 60 ml/cm H_2O, respectively
(D) 150 cm H_2O/ml and 60 cm H_2O/ml, respectively

9. This patient can be characterized as having frequency-dependent compliance, which indicates which of the following?

(A) Abnormal surfactant function
(B) Obstructive lung disease
(C) Restrictive lung disease
(D) Pulmonary vascular disease

10. In contrast to motor units that fire later during a movement, motor units that fire at the beginning of a movement

(A) can be tetanized at a lower frequency of stimulation
(B) generate a greater amount of force
(C) have a greater amount of glycogen stored within them
(D) fatigue more rapidly
(E) are innervated by larger alpha motoneurons

11. A 45-year-old man is studied and found to have a respiratory rate of 15 breaths/min, a tidal volume of 0.5 L, and a dead space of 200 ml. The patient is asked to increase his respiratory rate to 30 breaths/min, and his tidal volume is measured at 350 ml. Assuming no change in dead space, which of the following is true regarding alveolar CO_2 tension?

(A) The alveolar CO_2 tension will increase because of the decreased ventilation
(B) The alveolar CO_2 tension will decrease because of the increased ventilation
(C) The alveolar CO_2 tension will not change because it is not affected by respiration
(D) The alveolar CO_2 tension will not change because alveolar ventilation remains constant
(E) The arterial blood pH will decrease because of the increased ventilation

12. A decrease in the osmolality of arterial blood would lead to an increase in urine volume by

(A) increasing the hydrostatic pressure inside the glomerulus
(B) increasing the permeability of the glomerular capillaries to water
(C) inhibiting antidiuretic hormone (ADH) secretion
(D) stimulating the secretion of aldosterone
(E) directly inhibiting the reabsorption of water by the collecting ducts

Questions 13–15

A man undergoes lung volume studies using the helium dilution method. The test begins at the end of a normal expiration. The initial fraction of helium in the spirometer is 0.05, and the helium fraction after equilibration with the lungs is 0.03. The volume of gas in the spirometer is kept constant at 4 L during the procedure by the addition of O_2. According to a spirogram, this patient's vital capacity (VC) is 5 L and his expiratory reserve volume (ERV) is 2 L.

13. What is this patient's functional residual capacity (FRC)?

(A) 1.0 L
(B) 1.7 L
(C) 2.7 L
(D) 3.0 L
(E) 5.0 L

14. What is this patient's residual volume (RV)?

(A) 0.7 L
(B) 1.0 L
(C) 1.7 L
(D) 2.7 L
(E) 3.0 L

15. What is this patient's total lung capacity (TLC)?

(A) 1.7 L
(B) 2.7 L
(C) 3.0 L
(D) 5.0 L
(E) 5.7 L

16. Stimuli for aldosterone secretion include all of the following EXCEPT

(A) angiotensin II
(B) hyperkalemia
(C) hypovolemia
(D) corticotropin
(E) atrial natriuretic peptide (ANP)

17. Alteration in the amount of Ca^{2+} released from the sarcoplasmic reticulum (SR) alters the force of contractions in which of the following muscle type or types?

(A) Cardiac muscle
(B) Skeletal muscle
(C) Smooth and cardiac muscle
(D) Smooth and skeletal muscle
(E) Smooth, cardiac, and skeletal muscle

18. Recruitment of additional muscle fibers alters the force of contractions in which of the following muscle type or types?

(A) Cardiac muscle
(B) Skeletal muscle
(C) Smooth and cardiac muscle
(D) Smooth and skeletal muscle
(E) Smooth, cardiac, and skeletal muscle

19. Amplification of sound stimuli is the function of which component of the auditory system?

(A) Stria vascularis
(B) Scala media
(C) Auditory ossicles
(D) Oval window
(E) Basilar membrane

20. Which of the following factors is responsible for regulation of cerebral blood flow?

(A) Functional hyperemia
(B) Histamine
(C) Hypertension
(D) CO_2 tension (P_{CO_2})
(E) Capillary pressure

21. The actions of atrial natriuretic peptide include an increase in

(A) Na^+ reabsorption in the collecting duct
(B) glomerular filtration rate
(C) extracellular fluid volume
(D) renin secretion
(E) aldosterone secretion

22. According to the concept of glomerulo-tubular balance, which of the following parameters remains constant with an increase in filtered load?

(A) Glomerular filtration rate (GFR)
(B) The absolute amount of Na^+ reabsorption in the proximal tubule
(C) The fractional Na^+ reabsorption in the proximal tubule
(D) The filtered load of Na^+
(E) The excretion rate of Na^+

23. Which of the following results in the greatest increase in renal oxygen consumption?

(A) An increase in oxygen content of the arterial blood
(B) An increase in the renal clearance of inulin
(C) A decrease in the renal clearance of *para*-aminohippuric acid (PAH)
(D) An increase in urine osmolarity
(E) A decrease in urine osmolarity

24. If a substance has a transport maximum, this means

(A) reabsorption is only passive
(B) only a constant fraction of the substance is reabsorbed
(C) reabsorption is not carrier-mediated
(D) below a threshold level, all of the substance is reabsorbed
(E) that it is only secreted into the lumen

25. The nephron segment in which the tubular fluid $[Na^+]$ is greater than that in the medullary interstitium is the

(A) distal convoluted tubule
(B) late proximal tubule
(C) medullary collecting duct
(D) thick ascending limb of the loop of Henle (ALH)
(E) thin ALH

26. During excretion of a maximally concentrated urine, the fluid in the thin ascending limb of the loop of Henle (ALH) has

(A) a lower urea concentration than that found in the fluid within an adjacent descending limb
(B) a lower Na^+ concentration than that in the adjacent interstitial fluid
(C) a lower osmolality than that found in the fluid within an adjacent collecting duct
(D) as osmolality identical to that of the adjacent interstitial fluid (ISF)
(E) a lower osmolality than that found in the afferent arteriolar blood

27. Which of the following substances is the most important for the absorption of Ca^{2+} from the intestine?

(A) Intrinsic factor
(B) Ferritin
(C) Bile salts
(D) Vitamin D
(E) Trypsin

28. Which of the following is an effect of aldosterone?

(A) Increased reabsorption of potassium by the distal nephron
(B) Increased reabsorption of calcium by the proximal tubule
(C) Increased secretion of hydrogen by the proximal tubule
(D) Increased secretion of hydrogen by the intercalated cells of the collecting tubule
(E) Increased reabsorption of sodium by the proximal tubule

29. The major factor determining the long-term extracellular fluid (ECF) volume is

(A) the amount of sodium retained in the ECF
(B) the ECF sodium concentration
(C) the amount of K^+ retained in the ECF
(D) the osmolality of the ECF
(E) antidiuretic hormone (ADH)

30. Which one of the following tends to increase glomerular filtration rate (GFR)?

(A) An increase in glomerular capillary oncotic pressure
(B) Vasoconstriction of the afferent arteriole
(C) An increase in hydraulic pressure in Bowman's capsule
(D) An increase in renal blood flow
(E) Vasodilation of the efferent arteriole

31. Following intravenous infusion of 1 L of 150 mmol/L NaCl, which of the following occurs?

(A) The intracellular fluid (ICF) increases by about 670 ml
(B) The plasma oncotic pressure increases
(C) The interstitial fluid increases by about 750 ml
(D) The hematocrit increases
(E) The extracellular fluid (ECF) increases by 1 L

32. A woman receives an injection of 1 g of mannitol. After equilibration, a plasma sample reveals a mannitol concentration of 0.08 g/L. During the equilibration period, 20% of the mannitol is excreted in the urine. Which of the following statements is correct?

(A) The extracellular fluid (ECF) volume is 1 L
(B) The intracellular fluid (ICF) volume is 1 L
(C) The ECF volume is 10 L
(D) The interstitial fluid volume is 12.5 L
(E) The total body water (TBW) is 40 L

33. Which one of the following transport systems is an example of a primary active transport process?

(A) Na^+–glucose symporter in the proximal tubule
(B) Na^+–alanine cotransporter in renal epithelial cells
(C) Na^+–Ca^{2+} antiporter in the thin ascending loop of Henle
(D) H^+–K^+ exchanger in the collecting tubules
(E) Na^+ conductive channels in the collecting tubule

34. Which of following series correctly lists the substances in the order of lowest to highest clearance?

(A) Na^+, urea, glucose, creatinine, inulin, *para*-aminohippuric acid (PAH)
(B) PAH, inulin, creatinine, glucose, urea, Na^+
(C) Na^+, glucose, urea, inulin, PAH, creatine
(D) Glucose, Na^+, urea, inulin, creatinine, PAH
(E) Na^+, glucose, urea, inulin, creatinine, PAH

35. Most of the body's total daily acid production is derived from

(A) protein catabolism
(B) triglyceride catabolism
(C) phospholipid catabolism
(D) oxidative metabolism
(E) renal bicarbonate excretion

36. Some foodstuffs have an alkalinizing action on body fluids. Which of the following is an example of such an alkalinizing ingested substance?

(A) Sulfur-containing protein
(B) Nucleoprotein
(C) Triglyceride
(D) Phosphoprotein
(E) Fruit juice rich in ascorbate and citrate

37. Extracellular bicarbonate ions do not serve as the effective buffer for

(A) sulfuric acid
(B) phosphoric acid
(C) lactic acid
(D) carbonic acid
(E) β-hydroxybutyric acid

Questions 38–41

Points A–D on the pH–[HCO_3^-] diagram below indicate states of acid-base imbalance; point N indicates a normal acid-base state. Match each of the following conditions with the appropriate lettered point on the diagram.

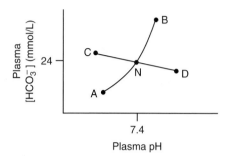

38. Hypocapnia

39. Hypercapnia

40. Ketoacidosis

41. NaHCO$_3$ ingestion

42. A 23-year-old woman with diabetes mellitus is admitted to the hospital. She is dehydrated and hyperpneic. Laboratory examination reveals high urinary concentrations of acetoacetic acid and glucose, blood pH of 7.39, plasma [HCO_3^-] of 19.0 mmol/L, and plasma P_{CO_2} of 33 mm Hg. These data are most suggestive of

(A) metabolic alkalosis with complete renal compensation
(B) metabolic acidosis with complete respiratory compensation
(C) respiratory acidosis with partial renal compensation
(D) respiratory alkalosis with partial renal compensation

43. Which one of the following statements regarding the actions of vitamin D_3 is NOT true?

(A) The renal effect of D_3 on phosphate transport is the same as that for parathyroid hormone.
(B) Osteoblasts have nuclear $1,25(OH)_2$ vitamin D_3 receptors.
(C) It induces the synthesis of calbindin in intestinal enterocytes.
(D) Both bone resorption and mineralization are increased.
(E) It is a hyperphosphatemic hormone.

44. Which of the following is secreted by the zona giomerulosa of the adrenal cortex?

(A) Aldosterone
(B) Antidiuretic hormone (ADH)
(C) Atrial natriuretic peptide (ANP)
(D) Renin
(E) Angiotensin I

45. The shift from curve A to curve B in the hormonal responses (ordinate) to increasing concentration (abscissa) could have been caused by

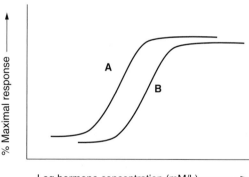

(A) an increase in the number of hormone receptors on the target cells
(B) an increase in the number of target cells
(C) a decrease in the number of target cells
(D) a decrease in the number of hormone receptors on the target cells
(E) a reduction in hormone concentration

46. Hypothalamic hormones

(A) are all neuropeptides
(B) reach the anterior pituitary via axonal connections
(C) cannot cross the blood–brain barrier
(D) include somatotropin
(E) are synthesized in the neurosecretory neurons

47. Growth hormone (GH) synthesis is stimulated by

(A) somatomedin
(B) somatostatin
(C) glucose
(D) arginine
(E) fatty acids

48. Which of the following adrenomedullary enzymes is correctly paired with its substrate?

(A) Phenylethanolamine-N-methyltransferase (PNMT)/epinephrine
(B) Phenylalanine hydroxylase/tyrosine
(C) Dopa decarboxylase/phenylalanine
(D) Dopamine β-hydroxylase/dihydroxyphenylethylamine
(E) Tyrosine hydroxylase/norepinephrine

49. A genetic male (XY) is diagnosed with a 17α-hydroxylase deficiency. Which of the following is correctly associated with this abnormality?

(A) Increased testosterone secretion
(B) Decreased plasma mineralocorticoid
(C) Male phenotype
(D) Male pseudohermaphroditism
(E) Female pseudohermaphroditism

50. Cortisol affects the biosynthesis of epinephrine in the adrenal medulla by

(A) augmenting the conversion of dopamine to epinephrine
(B) activating the epinephrine-forming enzyme
(C) inhibiting the methylation of norepinephrine
(D) activating catechol-O-methyltransferase
(E) increasing the release of acetylcholine (ACh)

51. Antimüllerian hormone causes

(A) wolffian ducts to develop into male internal genitalia
(B) müllerian ducts to develop into female internal genitalia
(C) müllerian ducts to undergo regression, leaving the wolffian ducts to develop
(D) gonadal ridges to develop into testes instead of ovaries
(E) testes to secrete testosterone in early fetal life, causing the wolffian ducts to develop into male external structures

52. The predominant type of biological activity of human menopausal gonadotropin (hMG) is most like that of

(A) progesterone
(B) estradiol
(C) luteinizing hormone
(D) human chorionic gonadotropin
(E) follicle-stimulating hormone

53. Glucagon and epinephrine have several similar effects on carbohydrate metabolism. Which one of the following processes is common to these two hyperglycemic hormones? Both hormones

(A) stimulate insulin secretion
(B) are secreted in response to hypoglycemia
(C) inhibit insulin secretion
(D) inhibit phosphorylase activity
(E) inhibit hepatic gluconeogenesis

54. A 62-year-old woman with asthma presents to the emergency department with a 1-week history of fever, nausea, disorientation, and exacerbation of her asthma. She has a fine tremor, a pulse rate of 160 beats/min with atrial fibrillation, and a temperature of 39°C. A 60-gm diffuse goiter is present. She is delirious, her respiratory status deteriorates, and she requires intubation. Her thyroid function tests are as follows (*TSH* = thyroid-stimulating hormone)

Patient	Normal
T_4: 18.7 μg/dl	4.5–11.5 μg/dl
T_3 resin uptake: 39%	25%–35%
T_3: 650 μg/dl	70–180 μg/dl
TSH: <0.15 μU/ml	0.5–5 μU/ml

These data are most consistent with

(A) primary hypothyroidism
(B) secondary hypothyroidism
(C) exogenous T_3 administration
(D) exogenous T_4 administration
(E) thyrotoxicosis

55. Propylthiouracil administration leads to

(A) a decrease in thyroid mass and an increase plasma T_4
(B) a decrease in both thyroid size and plasma T_4
(C) an increase in both thyroid size and plasma T_4
(D) an increase in thyroid size and a decrease in plasma T_4
(E) no change in thyroid mass and a decrease in plasma T_4

Questions 56–58

The following data were obtained from intracellular recordings of cardiac cells.

	Cell A	Cell B	Cell C
Resting membrane potential (mV)	−50	−60	−80
Capacity for diastolic depolarization	Yes	Yes	No
Intrinsic rate of depolarization (beats/min)	90	45	None

56. Cell A would most likely be found in the

(A) sinoatrial (SA) node
(B) atrial muscle
(C) atrioventricular (AV) node
(D) Purkinje fibers
(E) ventricular muscle

57. Pacemaker activity is exhibited by

(A) cell A
(B) cell B
(C) cell C
(D) cells A and B
(E) cells A, B, and C

58. Cells lacking fast Na^+ current during phase 0 of the cardiac action potential include

(A) cell A
(B) cell B
(C) cell C
(D) cells A and B
(E) cells A, B, and C

59. Which of the following reflexes is most dependent on a vagovagal reflex?

(A) Chewing
(B) Swallowing
(C) Receptive relaxation
(D) Gastric emptying
(E) Intestinal segmentation

60. O_2 delivery to the tissues would be cut in half by a 50% decrease in the normal value of

(A) arterial O_2 tension
(B) minute ventilation
(C) hemoglobin concentration
(D) inspired O_2 tension

61. The bones of the middle ear are primarily responsible for

(A) amplifying the sound waves reaching the ear
(B) detecting the presence of a sound stimulus
(C) locating the source of a sound
(D) discriminating among different frequencies of sound
(E) adapting to a prolonged monotonous sound

62. The hexaxial reference system consists of reference lines generated from

(A) leads V_1–V_6
(B) standard limb leads
(C) augmented limb leads
(D) standard and augmented limb leads
(E) bipolar limb leads

63. Which of the following factors best explains an increase in the filtration fraction?

(A) Increased ureteral pressure
(B) Increased efferent arteriolar resistance
(C) Increased plasma protein concentration
(D) Decreased glomerular capillary hydrostatic pressure
(E) Decreased glomerular filtration area

64. The T wave of the normal electrocardiogram is caused by

(A) atrial depolarization
(B) atrial repolarization
(C) ventricular depolarization
(D) ventricular repolarization

65. A 32-year-old woman is admitted to the hospital with suspected partially compensated respiratory acidosis. Which of the following sets of laboratory data would confirm this suspicion?

	[HCO$_3$$^-$] (mEq/L)	PCO$_2$ (mm Hg)	pH
(A)	17	19	7.9
(B)	31	80	7.22
(C)	9.8	30	7.14
(D)	24	45	7.5
(E)	20	25	7.5

Questions 66–68

A lightly anesthetized man who is breathing spontaneously has a cardiac output of 6 L/min, a heart rate of 75 beats/min, an O_2 consumption of 240 ml/min, and a mixed venous O_2 tension of 40 mm Hg. He is ventilated for 10 minutes at his normal tidal volume but at twice the normal frequency with a gas mixture that is 20% O_2 and 80% N_2. The airway pressure at the end of inspiration is 5 cm H_2O. On cessation of artificial ventilation, the patient does not breathe for 1 minute.

66. The most important factor responsible for the temporary apnea in this patient is reduced activity of the

(A) peripheral chemoreceptors, because of the high O_2 tension
(B) peripheral chemoreceptors, because of the low CO_2 tension
(C) pulmonary stretch receptors that inhibit inspiration
(D) medullary chemoreceptors, because of the low CO_2 tension
(E) medullary chemoreceptors, because of the high O_2 tension

67. During the artificial ventilation, the mixed venous O_2 tension in this patient would be

(A) equal to 40 mm Hg because the metabolic rate was unchanged
(B) greater than 40 mm Hg because the hyperventilation would cause vasoconstriction and less gas exchange with the tissues
(C) greater than 40 mm Hg because of the significant increase in P_{50} of hemoglobin
(D) less than 40 mm Hg because of the hypoxia that would occur from breathing this gas mixture
(E) less than 40 mm Hg because of a decrease in cardiac output

68. During the period of spontanous breathing, this patient had an arteriovenous O_2 difference of

(A) 4 ml/dl
(B) 5 ml/dl
(C) 6 ml/dl
(D) 40 ml/dl
(E) 80 ml/dl

69. Which of the following conditions is most likely to cause acidosis with marked dehydration?

(A) Severe diarrhea
(B) Severe, persistent vomiting
(C) Excessive sweating
(D) Drinking sodium lactate solution
(E) Complete water deprivation for 24 hours

70. Which of the following hormones is correctly paired with its effect on renal electrolyte reabsorption?

(A) Calcitriol/increased HPO_4^{2-} reabsorption
(B) Calcitonin/increased Ca^{2+} reabsorption
(C) Aldosterone/increased K^+ reabsorption
(D) Progesterone/increased Na^+ reabsorption
(E) Calcitonin/increased HPO_4^{2-} reabsorption

71. A red blood cell is placed in a solution. The cell initially shrinks and then returns to its original volume. The red cell's reaction indicates that the solution is

(A) hyperosmotic and hypertonic
(B) hyposmotic and hypertonic
(C) hyperosmotic and isotonic
(D) hyperosmotic and hypotonic
(E) hyposmotic and isotonic

72. Leads V_1 through V_6 measure the electrical activity in the

(A) frontal plane and are bipolar
(B) horizontal plane and are bipolar
(C) frontal plane and are unipolar
(D) frontal plane and are part of a standard 12-lead electrocardiogram (EKG)
(E) horizontal plane and are part of a standard 12-lead EKG

73. Spironolactone, which is an aldosterone antagonist, is injected into the renal artery of a laboratory animal. What are the effects on Na^+ and K^+ excretion, assuming that this drug does not affect the glomerular filtration rate (GFR) or renal blood flow?

	Na^+	K^+
(A)	↑	↑
(B)	↓	↓
(C)	↑	↓
(D)	↓	↑
(E)	↑	unchanged

74. Fatigue-resistant muscle fibers are characterized by high

(A) mitochondria concentrations
(B) myosin-adenosine triphosphatase (ATPase) activity
(C) velocity of shortening
(D) strength-generating capability
(E) glycolytic enzyme concentration

75. Two patients are studied and the following data are collected:

Patient	Respiratory Rate (breaths/min)	Tidal Volume (ml)	Dead Space (ml)
A	20	200	150
B	10	400	150

Which of the following statements about these two patients is true?

(A) The alveolar ventilation is greater in patient A than in patient B
(B) The alveolar ventilation is greater in patient B than in patient A
(C) The alveolar ventilation in both patients is equal
(D) The dead space ventilation in both patients is equal

76. The rate of gastric emptying is controlled primarily by reflexes that occur

(A) during chewing
(B) during swallowing
(C) when chyme enters the stomach
(D) when chyme enters the intestine
(E) during the interdigestive period

77. The regression of the corpus luteum at the end of the postovulatory phase is caused by

(A) a decrease in follicle-stimulating hormone (FSH) secretion
(B) a decrease in luteinizing hormone (LH) secretion
(C) an increase in human chorionic gonadotropin (HCG) secretion
(D) a reduced capacity of the corpus luteum to synthesize steroids
(E) ovarian failure

78. A positive QRS complex in leads aVr and aVF indicates

(A) a normal axis
(B) right axis deviation (RAD)
(C) left axis deviation (LAD)
(D) indeterminate axis
(E) a mean electrical axis (MEA) between 0° and 90°

79. Following the intravenous administration of 1 L of a 150 mmol NaCl solution into a patient with a blood loss, there will be

(A) a decrease in the plasma Na^+ concentration
(B) an increase in the osmolarity of the intracellular fluid (ICF) compartment
(C) an increase in the volume of the ICF compartment
(D) a decrease in the volume of the interstitial fluid (ISF) compartment
(E) a decrease in the colloid oncotic pressure of the plasma

80. When the acetylcholine (ACh) receptors on the pacemaker cells of the heart are activated, there is an increase in the membrane conductance to

(A) K^+
(B) Na^+
(C) Ca^{2+}
(D) Cl^-
(E) K^+ and Na^+

81. Epinephrine inhibits glucose uptake by muscle and adipose tissue. This inhibitory effect is attributed to

(A) glucagon secretion
(B) thyroid hormone secretion
(C) inhibition of insulin secretion
(D) inhibition of growth hormone (GH) secretion
(E) inhibition of cortisol secretion

82. At the end of a normal expiration, a young woman has an interpleural pressure of -5 cm H_2O. Without expiring further, she closes off her nose and mouth and performs a Valsalva maneuver against the closed airway. If the airway pressure is $+20$ cm H_2O during the expiratory maneuver, the interpleural pressure would be

(A) -5 cm H_2O
(B) 5 cm H_2O
(C) 10 cm H_2O
(D) 15 cm H_2O
(E) 20 cm H_2O

Questions 83–85 are based on the figure

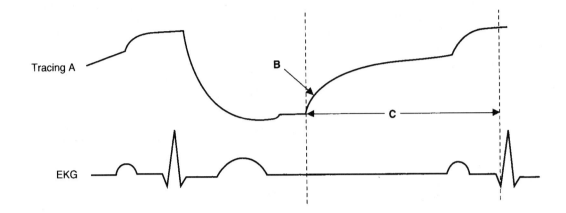

83. Tracing A is a

(A) ventricular pressure pulse
(B) ventricular volume curve
(C) atrial pressure pulse
(D) atrial volume pulse
(E) aortic pressure pulse

84. The point labeled B occurs in what phase of the cardiac cycle?

(A) Atrial contraction
(B) Isovolumic contraction
(C) Rapid ejection
(D) Reduced ejection
(E) Rapid filling

85. The duration of the interval labeled C is decreased by

(A) vagal stimulation
(B) baroreceptor stimulation
(C) arteriolar constriction
(D) an increased heart rate

86. Lesions within the flocculonodular lobe of the cerebellum prevent an individual from

(A) making rapid, alternating movements
(B) moving smoothly when reaching toward a target
(C) keeping the limbs still when resting
(D) grasping an object tightly
(E) maintaining balance when walking

87. Assuming a total body fluid volume of 40 L, 15 L of which are extracellular fluid (ECF) with an osmolarity of 300 mOsm/L, what will be the equilibrium intracellular fluid (ICF) osmolarity if 500 ml of a 0.15 mol/L NaCl solution are infused intravenously?

(A) 164 mOsm/L
(B) 277 mOsm/L
(C) 286 mOsm/L
(D) 300 mOsm/L
(E) 324 mOsm/L

88. A 45-year-old woman with severe vomiting caused by pyloric obstruction would be expected to show

(A) hyperchloremia
(B) an increase in plasma bicarbonate concentration [HCO_3^-]
(C) an increase in alveolar ventilation
(D) acid urine
(E) a decrease in arterial CO_2 tension (Pa_{CO_2})

89. In the formation of HCl by the parietal cells, the transport of H^+ across the parietal cell is coupled with the transport of

(A) K^+
(B) Cl^-
(C) HCO_3^-
(D) H^+
(E) Na^+

90. A newborn genotypic male is found to have an adrenogenital syndrome due to a 17α-hydroxylase defect. Which of the following biochemical reactions in the biosynthesis of gonadal hormones is decelerated in this case of congenital adrenal hyperplasia?

(A) Pregnenolone ← 17α-hydroxypregnenolone
(B) Cholesterol ← pregnenolone
(C) Progesterone ← corticosterone
(D) Deoxycorticosterone ← corticosterone
(E) 17α-Hydroxypregnenolone ← 17α-hydroxyprogesterone

91. Gastric digestion is most important for which of the following substances?

(A) Fats
(B) Carbohydrates
(C) Proteins
(D) Vitamins
(E) Minerals

92. The following blood data are collected from a 27-year-old male patient: pH = 7.50, $[HCO_3^-]$ = 38 mmol/L, Po_2 = 80 mm Hg. Given these findings, what is the expected CO_2 tension (Pco_2) for this patient?

(A) 30 mm Hg
(B) 40 mm Hg
(C) 50 mm Hg
(D) 60 mm Hg
(E) 70 mm Hg

93. The mean electrical axis (MEA) of a ventricular depolarization is −30°. Analysis of the resultant electrocardiogram (EKG) should reveal the largest positive QRS complex in lead

(A) I
(B) II
(C) aVR
(D) AVL
(E) aVF

Questions 94–97

The data below represent the volume of distribution of tritiated water, inulin, and Evans blue dye in a 60-kg man after allowing time for equilibration.

Space	Volume (L)
Tritiated water	35
Inulin	8
Evans blue	3

94. With a hematocrit ratio of 0.40, the man's blood volume is

(A) 2 L
(B) 3 L
(C) 4 L
(D) 5 L
(E) 6 L

95. The interstitial fluid volume is

(A) 3 L
(B) 5 L
(C) 8 L
(D) 11 L
(E) 24 L

96. The extracellullar fluid (ECF) volume is

(A) 2 L
(B) 4 L
(C) 6 L
(D) 8 L
(E) 10 L

97. Assuming that the total body water (TBW) constitutes 70% of the lean body mass (LBM), the amount of body fat in this man is approximately

(A) 5 kg
(B) 10 kg
(C) 15 kg
(D) 20 kg
(E) 25 kg

98. Which of the following is an octapeptide?

(A) Aldosterone
(B) Antidiuretic hormone (ADH)
(C) Atrial natriuretic peptide (ANP)
(D) Renin
(E) Angiotensin I

99. A person with normal vision has a total converging power (without accommodation) of 60 diopters (D). In order to focus an object placed 25 cm from the eye, the converging power of the lens must increase by approximately

(A) 1 D
(B) 2 D
(C) 4 D
(D) 5 D
(E) 10 D

100. The curves below represent the clearances of various substances as a function of their plasma concentrations. Curve E represents the clearance curve for glucose. Following the administration of a substance (phlorizin) that blocks epithelial transport of glucose, the clearance curve for glucose would resemble which of the following curves?

(A) A
(B) B
(C) C
(D) D
(E) E

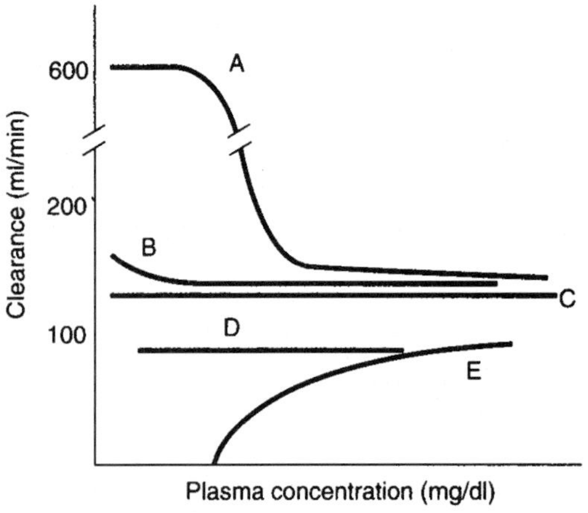

101. Closure of the atrioventricular (AV) valves occurs during which interval of the cardiac cycle?

(A) Atrial contraction
(B) Isovolumic contraction
(C) Rapid ventricular ejection
(D) Reduced ventricular ejection
(E) Isovolumic relaxation

102. A 57-year-old man who is breathing air at sea level has a respiratory exchange ratio of 1. Arterial blood gas analysis of this patient reveals the following: $PO_2 = 85$ mm Hg, $PCO_2 = 30$ mm Hg, and pH = 7.52. This patient's blood data indicate which of the following?

(A) His alveolar-to-arterial O_2 tension difference exceeds 20 mm Hg
(B) His plasma bicarbonate levels are increased
(C) He has been hypoventilating
(D) He has metabolic alkalosis
(E) He has chronic obstructive pulmonary disease (COPD)

Questions 103–104

A female medical student is evaluated for her renal reabsorptive capacity. The following data were obtained 2 hours after the initiation of an inulin infusion.

103. Which of the following is the reabsorption rate of glucose?

	Plasma	**Urine**
Flow rate	—	2 ml/min
Inulin	1.5 mg/ml	90 mg/ml
Glucose	90 mg/dl	0 mg/dl
Concentration of substance X	2 mg/ml	100 mg/ml

(A) Approximately 90 mg/min
(B) Approximately 108 mg/min
(C) Approximately 120 mg/min
(D) Glucose reabsorption must be at its maximum level
(E) The rate of glucose reabsorption cannot be determined from the data presented

104. Assuming that substance X is freely filtered, which of the following statements is correct?

(A) There is net secretion of X
(B) There is net reabsorption of X
(C) There is both reabsorption and secretion of X
(D) The clearance of X could be used to measure the glomerular filtration rate (GFR)
(E) The clearance of X is greater than the clearance of inulin

Questions 105–108

The graph illustrates three curves of glucose filtration, excretion, and reabsorption versus glucose concentration.

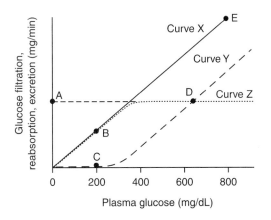

105. At plasma glucose concentrations below 200 mg/dl, curves X and Z are superimposed on each other because

(A) reabsorption and excretion of glucose are equal
(B) all the filtered glucose is reabsorbed
(C) the renal threshold for glucose has been exceeded
(D) glucose reabsorption is saturated
(E) Na^+–glucose cotransport has been inhibited

106. At which of the following points is the excretion rate of glucose equal to the reabsorption rate of glucose?

(A) A
(B) B
(C) C
(D) D
(E) E

107. At which of the following points is the filtered load of glucose equal to the reabsorption rate of glucose?

(A) A
(B) B
(C) C
(D) D
(E) E

108. Curve X represents the excretion curve for

(A) inulin
(B) urea
(C) creatinine
(D) glucose
(E) *para*-aminohippuric acid (PAH)

109. Which of the following statements pertaining to renal Na^+ reabsorption is correct?

(A) In the proximal tubule, it is mainly paracellular
(B) In the proximal tubule, it is mainly transcellular and carrier-mediated
(C) In the thin ascending limb of the loop of Henle (ADH), it requires ATP
(D) In the thick ADH, it is an electrogenic process
(E) In the collecting duct, it takes place mainly across the intercalated cells

110. Starling forces regulate Na^+ and H_2O reabsorption by the proximal tubule. Which of the following changes in Starling forces would increase reabsorption?

(A) Increase in capillary oncotic pressure
(B) Increase in capillary hydrostatic pressure
(C) Decrease in capillary oncotic pressure
(D) Decrease in the permeability of the peritubular capillary to Na^+ and H_2O
(E) Decrease in interstitial pressure

111. Urine concentration would be increased by which of the following?

(A) An increase in plasma antidiuretic hormone (ADH) concentration
(B) A decrease in volume flow through the loop of Henle
(C) A decrease in NaCl reabsorption in the ascending limb of the loop of Henle (ALH)
(D) An increase in volume flow through the vasa recta
(E) Ingestion of 1 L of water

112. An increase in plasma Na^+ concentrations (hypernatremia) with normal blood volumes causes which of the following events?

(A) Release of antidiuretic hormone (ADH) from the posterior pituitary
(B) Release of aldosterone from the adrenal gland
(C) Release of renin from the juxtaglomerular cells
(D) Decrease in renal excretion of Na^+
(E) An increase in free-water reabsorption

113. A drug that blocks the conversion angiotensin I to II is given to a healthy young individual. Plasma levels of the following would be expected to

	Angio-tensin I	Renin	Aldo-sterone	Norepine-phrine
(A)	Increase	Increase	Increase	Increase
(B)	Increase	Increase	Decrease	Decrease
(C)	Decrease	Decrease	Decrease	Decrease
(D)	Decrease	Decrease	Increase	Increase
(E)	Increase	Increase	Decrease	Increase

114. Among the major physiologic actions of PTH is the

(A) increase in intestinal Ca^{2+} absorption
(B) decrease in urinary phosphate excretion
(C) decrease in renal tubular Ca^{2+} reabsorption
(D) inactivation of renal 1α-hydroxylase activity
(E) promotion renal gluconeogenesis

115. Which one of the following conditions causes a decline in the renal synthesis of calcitriol?

(A) Elevated plasma PTH levels
(B) Chronic hepatic failure
(C) Hypocalcemia
(D) Hypophosphatemia
(E) Decreased phosphate loads

116. The highest concentration of urea in the tubule fluid is found in the

(A) thin descending limb of the loop of Henle (DLH)
(B) proximal tubule
(C) medullary collecting duct
(D) distal tubule
(E) thin ascending limb of the loop of Henle (ALH)

117. Which of the following regulates plasma $[Na^+]$?

(A) Aldosterone
(B) Antidiuretic hormone (ADH)
(C) Atrial natriuretic peptide (ANP)
(D) Renin
(E) Angiotensin I

118. Which of the following statements does not apply to hormone receptors?

(A) Increased receptor concentration may result in increased biological action of a fixed concentration of hormone
(B) Many receptors down-regulate in response to high concentrations of their specific hormone
(C) Receptor concentration of one hormone may be regulated by another hormone, which binds to its own receptor
(D) The actions of some hormones do not depend on specific receptors
(E) At the level of the receptor, many peptide hormones produce a maximal biological response when only a small fraction of the total cell-surface receptors are occupied

119. Which of the following structures is classified as an endocrine tissue in humans?

(A) Median eminence
(B) Pars nervosa
(C) Pars distalis
(D) Pars tuberalis
(E) Pars intermedia

120. A pituitary tumor that secretes excessive amounts of growth hormone is likely to cause decreased

(A) plasma concentration of insulin-like growth factor-1 (IGF-1)
(B) uptake of amino acids by muscle
(C) plasma concentration of free fatty acids
(D) tolerance to a glucose load
(E) insulin secretion

121. Which of the following statements applies correctly to the adult human adrenal medulla?

(A) It is innervated solely by preganglionic neurons
(B) It has a parasympathetic innervation
(C) Bilateral adrenalectomy does not affect plasma levels of epinephrine
(D) It secretes mainly norepinephrine
(E) Acetylcholine (ACh) hyperpolarizes the chromaffin cells prior to secretion

122. A 5-year-old boy is referred by the school nurse for clinical testing because of his large size, hoarse voice, increased masculinity, acne, pubic hair, enlarged penis, and hair growth on his upper lip. Physical examination reveals a height of 131 cm (6 standard deviations above the mean), a weight of 31 kg (6 standard deviations above the mean), and a bone age of 12 years. His testes are a normal size for his age. Dehydration is apparent. Laboratory results are:

	Plasma	Urine
$[Na^+]$	110 mEq/L (N = 140)	72 mEq/L
$[K^+]$	9.5 mEq/L (N = 4.5)	15 mEq/L
		17 KS: 4.2 mg/24 hr (N = 0.5)

Which of the following is consistent with these data?

(A) 11β-hydroxylase deficiency
(B) 17α-hydroxylase deficiency
(C) Decreased plasma renin activity
(D) Hypotension
(E) Metabolic alkalosis

123. Chronic injections of supraphysiologic amounts of testosterone in the adult male would be expected to increase

(A) prostatic size
(B) the rate of spermatogenesis
(C) the size and mass of the testes
(D) secretion rate of testosterone by the Leydig cells
(E) secretion rate of inhibin by the Sertoli cells

124. Following a massive hemorrhage during delivery, a 34-year-old woman experiences a failure to lactate and to menstruate. Which of the following is most likely to be associated with this clinical picture?

(A) Elevated prolactin secretion
(B) Excessive urinary Na^+ excretion
(C) Excessive water excretion
(D) Increased sensitivity to insulin
(E) Elevated gonadotropin secretion

125. Which one of the following responses is expected to be present in diabetic ketoacidosis?

(A) Greater than normal amounts of Na^+ and K^+ are lost in the urine
(B) Potassium entry into muscle and fat cells is increased
(C) Alveolar ventilation is below normal
(D) Plasma HCO_3^- concentration is above normal
(E) The urine is alkaline

126. A young woman has puffy skin and a hoarse voice. Her plasma thyrotropin concentration is low but increases markedly in response to thyroid-releasing hormone (TRH) stimulation. She probably has

(A) hyperthyroidism due to a thyroid tumor
(B) hyperthyroidism due to an abnormality in the hypothalamus
(C) hypothyroidism due to a thyroid gland abnormality
(D) hypothyroidism due to a pituitary gland abnormality
(E) hypothyroidism due to a hypothalamic abnormality

127. The secretion of antidiuretic hormone (ADH) would increase in response to which of the following?

(A) Drinking and absorbing 1 L of isotonic NaCl
(B) Weightlessness, as experienced when floating in water
(C) Failure of the right side of the heart
(D) Drinking and absorbing 0.5 L of a 600 mOsm NaCl solution
(E) Drinking and absorbing 1 L of tap water

128. Which of the following inhibits the secretion of aldosterone?

(A) Intravenous infusion of 1 L of isotonic NaCl solution
(B) A fall in plasma osmolality
(C) An increase in plasma potassium concentration
(D) Stimulation of renal nerves
(E) Decrease in sodium delivery to the macula densa

129. In a patient with decreased effective circulating volume (ECV), the resultant increased sympathetic tone results in

(A) suppressed renin secretion
(B) tachycardia
(C) lower peripheral vascular resistance (PVR)
(D) dilated efferent arterioles
(E) stimulated Na^+ reabsorption at the descending limb of the loop of Henle (DLH)

130. Exposure to the sun while working in a hot desert environment for a prolonged time without adequate fluid intake would produce which set of the following changes?

	ICF Volume	ICF Osmolarity	ECF [Na^+]	ECF Osmolarity	Urine Osmolarity
(A)	↓	↓	↑	↑	↑
(B)	↓	↑	↑	↑	↑
(C)	↑	↑	↑	↑	↓
(D)	↓	↑	↓	↑	↑
(E)	↓	↓	↓	↓	↓

131. The following renal function data were obtained for inulin. Urine flow rate: 90 ml/hr

Urine concentration of inulin: 480 mg/ml

Plasma concentration of inulin: 6 mg/ml

Which of the following, in mg/min, is the filtered load for inulin?
(A) 120
(B) 240
(C) 480
(D) 720
(E) 120

132. Which of the following transport pathways is a paracellular transport pathway in the proximal tubule?

(A) Electrogenic Na^+ cotransport with glucose
(B) Bulk flow of Na^+
(C) Electroneutral Na^+–H^+ countertransport
(D) $Na+$ conductive channels
(E) Na^+–K^+–ATPase pump

133. Which of the following statements is most consistent with a filterable substance that is also **actively** reabsorbed from the proximal tubular lumen?

(A) Its renal clearance is lower than that of inulin
(B) Its renal clearance is higher than that of creatinine
(C) The ratio of urinary excretion rate to plasma concentration is the same as that for glucose
(D) The ratio of urinary excretion rate to plasma concentration is greater than that for glucose
(E) Its concentration in the collecting duct is higher than that in plasma

134. β-Adrenergic receptors mediate all of the following responses EXCEPT

(A) ciliary muscle contraction
(B) increased myocardial contractility
(C) vasodilation
(D) insulin secretion
(E) decreased intestinal motility

135. Which one of the following acids is not classified as a nonvolatile acid?

(A) Lactic acid
(B) Acetic acid
(C) Citric acid
(D) Acetoacetic acid
(E) Carbonic acid

136. Which one of the following substances is not an intracellular buffer?

(A) Hemoglobin
(B) Protein
(C) Organic phosphate
(D) Bicarbonate (HCO_3^-)
(E) Carbonate

Questions 137–139

Use the following information obtained for a patient to answer questions 137 through 139:

inulin clearance	170 L/day
plasma [HCO_3^-]	24 mmol/L
urine [HCO_3^-]	0 mmol/L
urine pH	5.8
titratable acid in urine	26 mEq/day
ammonium ion in urine	48 mEq/day

137. Calculate the total amount of secreted H^+ per day in millimoles.

(A) 26
(B) 48
(C) 74
(D) 4154
(E) 4394

138. Calculate the HCO_3^- reabsorption per day in milliequivalents.

(A) 26
(B) 74
(C) 4080
(D) 4250
(E) 4324

139. Determine the amount of new bicarbonate added to the blood per day in milliequivalents.

(A) 26
(B) 48
(C) 74
(D) 4080
(E) 4176

140. In metabolic acidosis, the fall in arterial pH is associated with which of the following arterial blood conditions?

	[HCO_3^-]	P_{CO_2}
(A)	↑	normal
(B)	↑	↑
(C)	↓	↓
(D)	↑	↓
(E)	↓	normal

141. An hysterical, 35-year-old woman is admitted to the hospital, and the following blood data are collected: [HCO_3^-] = 22.2 mmol/L, P_{CO_2} = 30 mm Hg, and P_{O_2} = 98 mm Hg. From these data, the blood [H^+] of this patient would be expected to be

(A) 17.4 nmol/L
(B) 22.5 nmol/L
(C) 28.1 nmol/L
(D) 32.4 nmol/L
(E) 36.7 nmol/L

Questions 142–145

The following data were obtained from an arterial blood sample drawn from a hospitalized patient: pH = 7.55, P_{CO_2} = 25 mm Hg, and $[HCO_3^-]$ = 22.5 mEq/L.

142. This patient's arterial blood findings are consistent with what diagnosis?

(A) Metabolic alkalosis
(B) Respiratory alkalosis
(C) Metabolic acidosis
(D) Respiratory acidosis

143. These findings indicate what ratio of $[HCO_3^-]$ to dissolved CO_2?

(A) 5:1
(B) 10:1
(C) 20:1
(D) 30:1

144. The data indicate that the CO_2 content is approximately

(A) 22 mmol/L
(B) 23 mmol/L
(C) 24 mmol/L
(D) 25 mmol/L
(E) 26 mmol/L

145. The major compensatory response for this patient's acid-base disorder is

(A) hyperventilation
(B) hypoventilation
(C) increased renal HCO_3^- excretion
(D) increased H^+ excretion

146. A 16-year-old boy fractured his right wrist while playing ping pong with a friend. He is short and thin, and his growth rate has been delayed. He developed tetany of his right hand when a blood pressure cuff was applied to his left arm. The following laboratory data were obtained:

plasma total calcium concentration, 6.8 mg/dl (N = 8.5–10.5); serum inorganic phosphate concentration, 1.6 mg/dl (N = 2.5–4.5); excreted Ca^{2+}, 50 mg/day (N = 100–250); excreted phosphate: 625 mg/day (N = 300–600). What is your diagnosis?

(A) Hyperparathyroidism due to a parathyroid tumor
(B) Primary hyperparathyroidism
(C) Primary hypoparathyroidism
(D) Secondary hypoparathyroidism
(E) Vitamin D deficiency

147. Which of the following radiolabeled substances would be helpful in scintigraphic imaging to determine tumor size?

(A) Glucose
(B) Octreotide
(C) Arginine
(D) Insulin
(E) A fatty acid

148. Epinephrine is a potent hyperglycemic hormone because of its ability to inhibit

(A) glucagon secretion
(B) adrenocorticotropic hormone (ACTH) secretion
(C) hepatic glycogenolysis
(D) insulin secretion
(E) cortisol secretion

149. Orchiectomy of the right testis in a 5-week-old 46-XY fetus will lead to

(A) sterility in adulthood
(B) cryptorchidism of the left testis
(C) bilateral failure of wolffian duct growth and differentiation
(D) failure of müllerian duct regression on the right side only
(E) failure to masculinize the external genitalia during gestation

150. Compared to a 25-year-old woman, a 75-year-old woman would be expected to have

(A) lower urinary excretion of estrogen, progesterone, and gonadotropins
(B) lower plasma excretion of estrogen and progesterone, but higher plasma gonadotropins
(C) higher plasma progesterone, but lower plasma estrogen concentrations
(D) lower plasma progesterone, but higher estrogen concentrations
(E) lower plasma estrogen, progesterone with lower plasma gonadotropins

151. History: A 30-year-old woman in her first trimester of pregnancy complains of polyuria, nausea, vomiting, and anorexia. One year ago she weighed 200 lb at a height of 5 feet 4 inches and had a fasting blood glucose of 200 mg/dl. She was treated with caloric restriction and an oral hypoglycemic agent, which resulted in a fasting plasma glucose of 120 mg/dl and postprandial glucose of 180 mg/dl. Three years ago she had a normal pregnancy and delivery with a normal plasma glucose. The diagnosis of her current pregnancy was made 9 weeks ago. Her grandfather and uncle are both diabetics.

The patient weighs 120 pounds with a blood pressure of 130/80 mm Hg, pulse rate of 96/min, respiratory rate of 18/min with a normal body temperature. Except for her pregnancy, her physical exam was unremarkable. Her fasting blood glucose is 115 mg/dl with a 2-hr postprandial glucose of 220 mg/dl. Urinalysis revealed a negative protein, 24-hr glucose excretion was 2 gm, and no ketones in the urine. What is the most likely diagnosis?

(A) Type 1 diabetes and pregnancy
(B) Gestational diabetes only
(C) Type 2 diabetes and pregnancy
(D) Pheochromocytoma
(E) A somatostatin-secreting pancreatic tumor

152. The chronic ingestion of a new compound leads to thyroid gland enlargement and an elevation in plasma thyroxine. What is the most likely action of this compound?

(A) Inhibition of the coupling reactions in the thyroid gland
(B) Stimulation of deiodination of iodotyrosines
(C) Interruption of the negative feedback regulation of thyrotropin
(D) Inhibition of the synthesis of hypothalamic thyrotropin release hormone
(E) Stimulation of the iodide pump

Questions 153–158

The following questions refer to the pressure-volume relationships depicted below. Loop ABEH represents a normal pressure-volume loop.

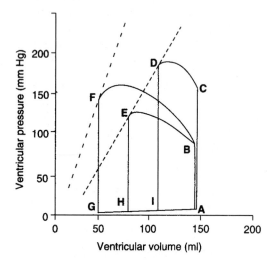

153. Loop ACIDI shows the effect of

(A) increased stroke volume
(B) increased contractility
(C) increased ventricular end-diastolic volume (VEDV)
(D) increased afterload
(E) decreased preload

154. Loop ABFG shows the effect of

(A) increased heart rate
(B) increased contractility
(C) increased ventricular end-diastolic volume (VEDV)
(D) increased afterload
(E) decreased preload

155. In loop ABEH, mitral valve closure occurs

(A) at point A
(B) at point B
(C) at point E
(D) at point H
(E) between points E and H

156. In loop ABEH, ventricular filling occurs during the interval between points

(A) A and B
(B) B and E
(C) E and H
(D) H and A

157. The slope of the line from point G to point A represents

(A) diastolic compliance
(B) systolic compliance
(C) diastolic elastance
(D) systolic elastance

158. The volume of blood in the ventricles at points D, E, or F is referred to as the ventricular

(A) stroke volume
(B) end-diastolic volume (VEDV)
(C) end-systolic volume (VESV)
(D) diastolic reserve volume
(E) residual volume

159. Acetazolamide is administered to a glaucoma patient. Given that this drug inhibits carbonic anhydrase in the renal proximal tubule, which of the following substances will be excreted at a lower rate?

(A) Na^+
(B) H_2O
(C) HCO_3^-
(D) NH_4^+
(E) K^+

160. Reciprocal innervation is most accurately described as

(A) inhibition of flexor muscles during an extension
(B) activation of contralateral extensors during a flexion
(C) reduction of Ia fiber activity during a contraction
(D) simultaneous stimulation of alpha and gamma motoneurons
(E) inhibition of alpha motoneurons during a contraction

161. The graph below shows the diurnal variation in the plasma concentration of which of the following hormones?

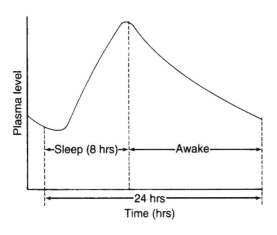

(A) Thyroxine
(B) Insulin
(C) Testosterone
(D) Cortisol
(E) Estradiol

162. During moderate exercise, a patient has a cardiac index of 6.5 L/min/m², a hemoglobin concentration of 12 g/dl, a venous O₂ tension of 30 mm Hg, and a venous O₂ saturation of 50%. Assuming 100% hemoglobin saturation in arterial blood, what is this patient's O₂ consumption?

(A) 150 ml/min/m²
(B) 275 ml/min/m²
(C) 520 ml/min/m²
(D) 790 ml/min/m²
(E) 1030 ml/min/m²

163. The normal sequence of phases of the menstrual cycle is

(A) menses, preovulatory, ovulatory, estrogenic
(B) preovulatory, ovulatory, progestational, menses
(C) ovulatory, progestational, menses, luteal
(D) progestational, menses, follicular, preovulatory
(E) menses, follicular, ovulatory, estrogenic

164. The following arterial blood data are collected from a 42-year-old female patient: [H⁺] = 49 nEq/L, P_{CO_2} = 30 mm Hg, P_{O_2} = 95 mm Hg. Given these findings, what is the expected arterial bicarbonate concentration [HCO₃⁻] for this patient?

(A) 13.2 mEq/L
(B) 14.7 mEq/L
(C) 15.8 mEq/L
(D) 16.5 mEq/L
(E) 17.1 mEq/L

165. If acidosis and hypokalemia result from loss of fluid from the gastrointestinal (GI) tract, the fluid was most likely drained from the

(A) stomach
(B) intestine
(C) gallbladder
(D) pancreas
(E) colon

Questions 166–167

The left ventricular and aortic pressure tracings below were recorded during cardiac catheterization of a 62-year-old patient who complains of chest pain and dizziness on exertion.

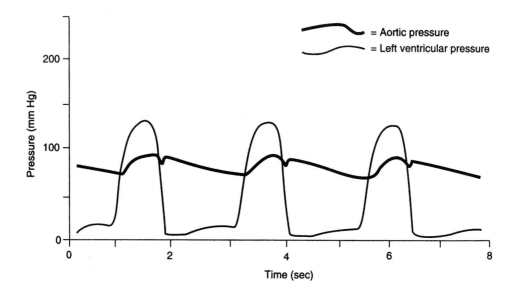

166. The left ventricular and aortic tracings indicate that this patient has

(A) pulmonary valve stenosis
(B) aortic valve stenosis
(C) mitral valve stenosis
(D) aortic valve insufficiency
(E) mitral valve insufficiency

167. Physical examination of this patient would most likely reveal

(A) a systolic murmur
(B) a diastolic murmur
(C) a presystolic murmur
(D) a middiastolic murmur
(E) no first heart sound (S_1)

Questions 168–170

The following arterial blood data are obtained from a patient who is cyanotic at rest: Po_2 = 60 mm Hg, hemoglobin saturation = 85%, Pco_2 = 40 mm Hg, pH = 7.39, and hemoglobin concentration = 18 g/dl. The arterial O_2 tension rises to 295 mm Hg after the patient breathes 100% O_2 at sea level for 20 minutes. Cardiac catheterization reveals normal pressures and an O_2 tension of 40 mm Hg in the right atrium, right ventricle, and pulmonary artery while the patient breathes 100% O_2.

168. The most likely cause of hypoxia in this patient is

(A) a ventilation-perfusion abnormality (physiologic shunt)
(B) a right-to-left anatomic shunt
(C) a left-to-right anatomic shunt
(D) a diffusion defect
(E) hypoventilation

169. The fraction of the cardiac output that represents shunted blood is

(A) 0.2
(B) 0.3
(C) 0.4
(D) 0.5
(E) 0.6

170. The most useful data for locating the site of the shunt would be

(A) O_2 tension in the left ventricle and left atrium
(B) airway resistance
(C) right ventricular and pulmonary arterial pressures
(D) left ventricular pressures
(E) compliance of the lungs

171. A 32-year-old male electrician consults an internist and complains of episodes of palpitations and sweating that occur when he climbs a ladder at work. He feels "washed out" after these attacks, which he ascribes to "nerves." Subsequent examination by the physician leads to a diagnosis of pheochromocytoma. Body fluid analysis of this patient is most likely to reveal a low plasma concentration of

(A) free fatty acids
(B) insulin
(C) fasting glucose
(D) lactate
(E) pyruvate

172. Unloading of muscle spindles can be prevented by

(A) alpha motoneurons
(B) gamma motoneurons
(C) la afferent fibers
(D) lb afferent fibers
(E) C fibers

173. A 32-year-old man can generate an inspiratory pressure of −50 mm Hg intermittently for several minutes. How deep can this man lie underwater while breathing through a tube, if the tube offers no significant resistance to air flow?

(A) 37 mm
(B) 37 cm
(C) 68 mm
(D) 68 cm
(E) 74 cm

174. A 24-year-old diabetic woman was admitted to the hospital in a comatose state and the following data were obtained:

Blood glucose: 40 mg/dl

Plasma C-peptide concentration: within normal limits

Plasma $[K^+]$: 3 mEq/L (N = 4.5 mEq/L)

The tentative diagnosis based on this data is

(A) an adrenomedullary tumor (pheochromocytoma)
(B) an overdose of insulin
(C) an insulinoma
(D) a glucagonoma
(E) a somatostatinoma

175. Which of the following is the correct sequence of events in the tubuloglomerular feedback (TGF) autoregulatory mechanism (DTF = distal tubular flow, MD = macula densa, AR = afferent arteriolar resistance, ER = efferent arteriolar resistance)?

(A) ↓ DTF: MD response: ↑ AR: ↓ GFR
(B) ↑ DTF: MD response: ↑ AR: ↑ GFR
(C) ↑ DTF: MD response: ↑ AR: ↓ GFR
(D) ↓ DTF: MD response: ↑ AR: ↑ GFR
(E) ↓ DTF: MD response: ↓ ER: ↓ GFR

176. Resistance to blood flow through the kidney can be determined by

(A) measuring the clearance of paraaminohippuric acid (PAH)
(B) measuring the hydrostatic pressure difference between the renal artery and renal vein
(C) measuring the renal blood flow
(D) dividing the arteriovenous hydrostatic pressure difference by the renal blood flow
(E) dividing the renal blood flow by the arteriovenous hydrostatic pressure difference

177. The variation in auditory threshold as a function of frequency (the minimum audibility curve) is most related to the properties of the

(A) outer ear
(B) auditory canal
(C) middle ear
(D) tympanic membrane
(E) basilar membrane

Questions 178–179

The following two questions refer to the pressure—volume loop below.

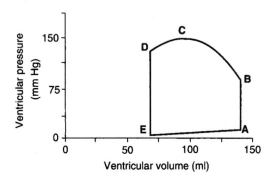

178. Which point on the loop represents the opening of the mitral valve?

(A) Point A
(B) Point B
(C) Point C
(D) Point D
(E) Point E

179. Isovolumic ventricular contraction occurs during the interval between points

(A) A and E
(B) A and B
(C) B and C
(D) C and D
(E) D and E

180. Normally, most of the H^+ is excreted by the kidneys in the form of

(A) HCO_3^-
(B) phosphate ion
(C) NH_4^+
(D) titratable acid
(E) β-hydroxybutyrate ion

181. Following a massive hemorrhage during delivery, a 34-year-old woman experiences a failure to lactate and to menstruate. Which of the following is most likely to be associated with this clinical picture?

(A) Elevated prolactin secretion
(B) Excessive urinary Na^+ excretion
(C) Excessive water excretion
(D) Increased sensitivity to insulin
(E) Elevated gonadotropin secretion

182. Which of the following statements best characterizes the transpulmonary pressure at the base of the lung of a person who is standing?

(A) It is independent of lung volume
(B) It is equal to the transpulmonary pressure at the apex of the lung
(C) It may be negative if the lung is at residual volume (RV)
(D) It causes the basal alveoli to be more dilated than the apical alveoli
(E) It causes the bronchioles at the lung base to be more dilated than those at the apex

Questions 183–186

A patient presents with crushing chest pain, shortness of breath, and marked anxiety. A preliminary diagnosis of acute myocardial infarction is made. Physical examination reveals evidence of pulmonary edema, cardiomegaly, peripheral edema, and pulmonary hypertension. Arterial blood gas analysis, on room air, reveals the following: $P_{CO_2} = 40$ mm Hg, $P_{O_2} = 60$ mm Hg, pH = 7.32, and $[HCO_3^-] = 20$ mEq/L.

183. This patient's blood data are most indicative of

(A) a diffusion abnormality
(B) hypoventilation
(C) a ventilation-perfusion abnormality
(D) left-to-right cardiac shunt

184. The patient is admitted to the CCU, sedated, and given 40% O_2 by respirator, which is set to deliver a tidal volume of 0.6 L at a rate of 16 breaths/min. An inspiratory pressure of 20 mm Hg is required to deliver the tidal volume. If the patient's predicted dead space is 150 ml, then his calculated alveolar ventilation is approximately

(A) 5 L/min
(B) 7 L/min
(C) 9 L/min
(D) 12 L/min
(E) 16 L/min

185. While ventilation continues with 40% O_2, a Swan-Ganz catheter is inserted into the patient's pulmonary artery. A repeat arterial blood analysis reveals a PO_2 of 120 mm Hg, a PCO_2 of 43 mm Hg, and pH of 7.31. These findings indicate that

(A) the pulmonary edema has cleared
(B) gas exchange is completely normal
(C) hemoglobin concentration has increased
(D) the alveolar-to-arterial PO_2 difference is increased

186. This patient's respiratory compliance is

(A) 0.03 L/mm Hg
(B) 0.1 L/mm Hg
(C) 9.0 L/mm Hg
(D) 12.0 mm Hg/L
(E) 26.7 mm Hg/L

187. The greatest amount of fat absorption occurs in the

(A) stomach
(B) duodenum
(C) ileum
(D) colon
(E) rectum

188. The following data were obtained from a 55-year-old man during cardiac catheterization: O_2 consumption = 210 ml/min, O_2 content of right ventricular blood = 11 ml/dl, O_2 content of brachial artery blood = 18 ml/dl, heart rate = 75 beats/min. These data are compatible with which one of the following statements?

(A) The tissues receive 29 ml of O_2/dl of blood
(B) Cardiac output is approximately 1470 ml/min
(C) Pulmonary venous O_2 content is approximately 145 ml/dl of blood
(D) Right ventricular stroke volume averages approximately 40 ml
(E) Cardiac output is extremely high

189. During the process of vitamin B_{12} absorption, almost all of the ingested vitamin B_{12}

(A) binds to intrinsic factor in the stomach
(B) is absorbed in the stomach
(C) both
(D) neither

190. During the first 6–8 weeks of pregnancy, progesterone is secreted mainly by the

(A) maternal adrenal glands
(B) maternal theca interna
(C) corpus luteum
(D) fetal adrenal gland
(E) decidua

Questions 191–193

A 50-year-old man who has smoked two packs of cigarettes a day for 35 years complains of shortness of breath, chronic cough, and production of yellowish, foul-smelling sputum. He has clubbing of his finger nails, and the nail beds and lips are noted to be cyanotic. Arterial blood gas analysis of this patient reveals the following: PO_2 = 55 mm Hg, PCO_2 = 56 mm Hg, HCO_3^- = 35 mEq/L, and pH = 7.4.

191. These blood gas data are most consistent with

(A) acute respiratory failure
(B) inadequate alveolar ventilation
(C) anatomic shunt
(D) anemia
(E) carbon monoxide (CO) poisoning

192. Which of the following pathophysiologic phenomena most likely initiated this patient's syndrome?

(A) Decreased alveolar ventilation followed by increased work of breathing
(B) Bronchial narrowing due to inflammation and edema followed by pulmonary hypertension
(C) Bronchial narrowing due to inflammation and edema followed by increased work of breathing
(D) Hypercapnia followed by pulmonary hypertension
(E) Pulmonary hypertension followed by hypercapnia

193. The acid-base status of this patient's blood is best categorized as

(A) respiratory acidosis, uncompensated
(B) metabolic acidosis, compensated
(C) respiratory acidosis, compensated
(D) lactic acidosis secondary to hypoxia
(E) respiratory alkalosis

Questions 194–197

Questions 194–197 refer to the following diagram, which is an experimental record obtained from an anesthetized dog.

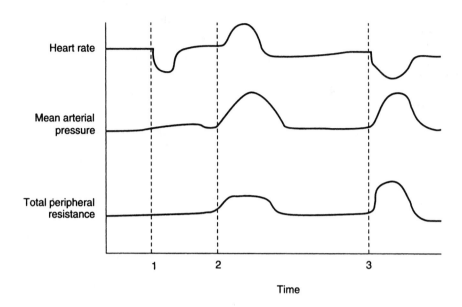

194. The experimental intervention at time 1 most likely represents

(A) electrical stimulation of the lumbar sympathetic nerve roots
(B) electrical stimulation of the superior cervical ganglion (cardiac sympathetic nerves)
(C) administration of a β-adrenergic blocking drug
(D) stimulation of the right vagus nerve
(E) administration of a cholinergic blocking drug

195. The experimental intervention at time 2 most likely represents

(A) electrical stimulation of the sacral sympathetic nerve roots
(B) electrical stimulation of the superior cervical ganglion (cardiac sympathetic nerves)
(C) administration of a sympathetic blocking drug
(D) stimulation of the right vagus nerve
(E) administration of a cholinergic blocking drug

196. A drug was administered at time 3. This drug is most likely classified as a(n)

(A) cholinergic blocking drug (e.g., atropine)
(B) α-adrenergic drug
(C) β-adrenergic drug
(D) β-adrenergic blocking drug
(E) α-adrenergic blocking drug

197. The decrease in heart rate that occurred at time 3 was most likely caused by

(A) the direct effect of the drug on the sino-atrial (SA) node
(B) the direct effect of the drug on the ventricular muscle
(C) the occurrence of ventricular extrasystoles
(D) a reflex effect mediated by the chemoreceptors
(E) a reflex effect mediated by the baroreceptors

198. When the arterial O_2 tension drops from 100 mm Hg to 27 mm Hg with an arterial pH of 7.4 and a CO_2 tension of 40 mm Hg, O_2 content in the blood decreases by about

(A) 10%
(B) 25%
(C) 33%
(D) 50%
(E) 75%

199. Given the following data: glomerular capillary hydrostatic pressure = 47 mm Hg, glomerular capillary colloid oncotic pressure = 28 mm Hg, Bowman's capsule hydrostatic pressure = 10 mm Hg, and Bowman's capsule oncotic pressure = 0 mm Hg, what is the effective filtration pressure (EFP)?

(A) 2 mm Hg
(B) 4 mm Hg
(C) 6 mm Hg
(D) 9 mm Hg
(E) 10 mm Hg

200. Epinephrine-forming enzyme activity is increased directly by

(A) hydrocortisone
(B) acetylcholine
(C) norepinephrine
(D) adrenocorticotropic hormone (ACTH)
(E) 11-deoxycortisol

201. Opening of the aortic valve occurs during which interval of the cardiac cycle?

(A) Atrial contraction
(B) Isovolumic contraction
(C) Rapid ventricular ejection
(D) Reduced ventricular ejection
(E) Isovolumic relaxation

202. Which of the following factors is responsible for increase in microvascular permeability?

(A) Functional hyperemia
(B) Histamine
(C) Hypertension
(D) CO_2 tension (P_{CO_2})
(E) Capillary pressure

203. The following data were obtained in a human subject with a constant glomerular filtration rate (GFR). X, Y, and Z represent three different points on a renal glucose titration curve. Which of the following represents the transport maximum for glucose (mg/min)?

	X	Y	Z
Glucose filtered (mg/min)	100	500	600
Glucose excreted (mg/min)	0	100	200
Glucose reabsorbed (mg/min)	100	400	400

(A) 100
(B) 200
(C) 300
(D) 400
(E) 500

204. Which of the following summarizes the correct sequence of changes following an increase in glomerular capillary pressure?

(A) Increase in glomerular filtration rate (GFR)/decreased NaCl delivery to the macula densa
(B) Increased NaCl concentration in macula densa/vasodilation of efferent arteriole
(C) Increased NaCl delivery to the macula densa/vasoconstriction of the afferent arteriole
(D) Decrease in GFR/dilation of the afferent arteriole by adenosine
(E) Decrease in GFR/increased Na^+ and Cl^- delivery to the macula densa

205. Using the values given below, which of the following is the effective renal blood flow in ml/min?

Plasma [PAH]: 0.2 mg/ml
Urine [PAH]: 48 mg/ml
Urine flow rate: 2.0 ml/min
Hematocrit: 40%
(A) 120
(B) 240
(C) 300
(D) 480
(E) 800

206. In a patient with spasticity, which is the most likely site of injury to the central nervous system (CNS)?

(A) Posterior cerebellum
(B) Vestibular apparatus
(C) Cerebral cortex
(D) Reticular formation
(E) Basal ganglia

207. Which of the following statements about the function of the loop of Henle is correct?

(A) Compared to the transcellular transport of Na^+ by the thick segment, paracellular transport of Na^+ by this same segment is less
(B) Fluid entering the loop of Henle from the proximal tubule is hypotonic to plasma
(C) Fluid leaving the thick ascending limb of the loop of Henle (ALH) is hypertonic to plasma because this segment is water permeable
(D) The major luminal active transport system for Na^+ in the loop of Henle is the $Na^+-2Cl^--K^+$ symporter
(E) The thin descending limb of the loop of Henle (DLH) has a high solute permeability

208. A patient has a urine volume/24 hr of 600 ml, a urine osmolality of 1100 mOsm/kg H_2O, a plasma osmolality of 260 mOsm/kg H_2O, a blood pressure of 120/80 mm Hg, and plasma potassium of 4.1 mM/L. Which of the following could produce these data?

(A) A large increase in antidiuretic hormone (ADH) secretion
(B) A large increase in aldosterone secretion
(C) A large increase in angiotensin II
(D) The total absence of aldosterone
(E) The total absence of ADH

209. Sympathetic nerve stimulation of the renal arterioles (afferent and efferent) causing a marked reduction results in

(A) an increased filtration fraction (FF)
(B) decreased reabsorption of glomerular filtrate
(C) increased glomerular filtration rate (GFR)
(D) increased peritubular capillary pressure
(E) increased glomerular capillary pressure

210. Which of the following actions would produce the greatest increase in the interstitial fluid (ISF) volume?

(A) Sympathetic stimulation
(B) Infusion of 1 L of isotonic saline
(C) Infusion of 1 L of plasma
(D) Infusion of 1 L blood
(E) Infusion of 6% albumin in saline

211. A 70-kg woman receives an intravenous injection of 1 L of isotonic saline. The injection has no effect on capillary hydrostatic pressure. After 15 minutes, which of the following conditions would occur?

(A) Extracellular water would increase by more than 250 ml
(B) Interstitial water would increase by more than 900 ml
(C) Intracellular water would increase by more than 900 ml
(D) Plasma water would be increased by more than 900 ml
(E) Total body water (TBW) would increase by more than 900 ml

212. Facilitated diffusion of a substance

(A) is subject to competition
(B) does not require a carrier-protein
(C) is not saturable
(D) does not exhibit specificity
(E) moves a substance from an area of lower concentration to an area of higher concentration

213. Which of the following statements regarding renal clearance is correct?

(A) Clearance is measured in mg/ml
(B) The clearance of inulin at a plasma concentration of 60 mg/dl is lower than it is at a plasma concentration of 120 mg/dl
(C) Clearance is equivalent to the amount of a substance excreted per unit time
(D) The clearance of *para*-aminohippuric acid (PAH) at a concentration of 80 mg/dl is lower than it is at a plasma concentration of 40 mg/dl
(E) Clearance provides information about the mechanism of renal transport for a substance

214. Epinephrine inhibits glucose uptake by muscle and adipose tissue. This inhibitory effect is attributed to

(A) glucagon secretion
(B) thyroid hormone secretion
(C) inhibition of insulin secretion
(D) inhibition of growth hormone (GH) secretion
(E) inhibition of cortisol secretion

215. More than 90% of the buffering capacity of whole blood is due to

(A) nonbicarbonate buffers in plasma
(B) plasma bicarbonate
(C) nonbicarbonate buffers in the erythrocytes
(D) blood inorganic phosphate
(E) blood inorganic and organic phosphates

216. Carbon dioxide is transported in plasma primarily in the form of

(A) carbaminohemoglobin
(B) bicarbonate ion
(C) carbamates of protein
(D) dissolved CO_2
(E) carbonic acid

217. Which of the following substances causes vasoconstriction?

(A) Adenosine
(B) Angiotensin II
(C) Carbon dioxide
(D) Histamine
(E) Hydrogen ion

218. Respiratory alkalosis is characterized by which of the following arterial blood condition?

	pH	P_{CO_2}
(A)	↑	↓
(B)	↓	↑
(C)	↓	↓
(D)	↑	↑
(E)	↑	normal

219. A woman has hypocalcemia, hyperphosphatemia, and decreased urinary phosphate excretion. Injection of PTH causes hyperphosphaturia. These findings are most consistent with

(A) primary hyperparathyroidism
(B) vitamin D intoxication
(C) vitamin D deficiency
(D) hypoparathyroidism following thyroid surgery
(E) pseudohypoparathyroidism

220. Which of the following hormones is secreted by the posterior pituitary gland?

(A) Follicle-stimulating hormone (FSH)
(B) Luteinizing hormone (LH)
(C) Prolactin
(D) Antidiuretic hormone (ADH)

221. The graph summarizes the relationship between the plasma cortisol concentration (abscissa) and the plasma corticotropin concentration (ordinate). The letter N denotes the normal range of each hormone.

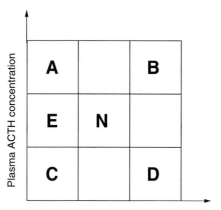

Which of the following letters represents a patient with secondary adrenal insufficiency?

(A) A
(B) B
(C) C
(D) D
(E) E

222. Which steroid hormone is a requirement for the fetal growth and development of both the male internal and external genitalia?

(A) Dihydrotestosterone
(B) Dehydroepiandrosterone (DHEA)
(C) Androstenedione
(D) 17-ketosteroids
(E) Testosterone

223. When is the second meiotic division of the developing ovarian follicle completed?

(A) At puberty
(B) Just prior to ovulation
(C) During the follicular phase of the menstrual cycle
(D) Just after conception
(E) During fetal development

224. Thyroperoxidase (thyroid peroxidase; TPO) functions in

(A) iodination of thyroglobulin
(B) hydrolysis of thyroglobulin
(C) release of thyroxine from thyroglobulin
(D) conversion of T_4 to T_3
(E) iodide transport into the thyrocyte

225. Which of the following factors is responsible for metabolic regulation of blood flow?

(A) Functional hyperemia
(B) Histamine
(C) Hypertension
(D) CO_2 tension (P_{CO_2})
(E) Capillary pressure

226. The substrate for thyroperoxidase in the iodination reaction of thyroid hormone synthesis consists of

(A) free tyrosine residues
(B) thyroxine
(C) tyrosyl residues on thyroglobulin
(D) triiodothyronine
(E) monoiodotyrosine

Questions 227–229

A normal 55-year-old man who lives at an altitude of 11,500 feet is seen for an annual physical examination. Findings on examination include a hemoglobin concentration of 18 g/dl, an arterial O_2 tension of 27 mm Hg, and an arterial pH of 7.40.

227. Based on these findings, this man's arterial O_2 content (ml/dl) would be approximately

(A) 8
(B) 12
(C) 15
(D) 18
(E) 24

228. This man's pulmonary artery pressure is likely to be

(A) normal
(B) lower than normal because of the inhibition of chemoreceptors caused by the low CO_2 tension
(C) higher than normal because of the increased cardiac output
(D) higher than normal because of hypoxic pulmonary vasoconstriction (HPV)

229. The hemoglobin saturation in this man's venous blood is likely to be

(A) normal
(B) less than normal because of the decreased arterial hemoglobin saturation
(C) greater than normal because of the increased cardiac output
(D) greater than normal because of the increased hemoglobin concentration

230. A compound that has a renal clearance 25 times that of creatinine is probably

(A) only filtered at the glomerulus
(B) only secreted by the nephron
(C) both filtered and secreted
(D) synthesized by the nephron and secreted
(E) filtered, secreted, and reabsorbed

231. In renal clearance, the filtered load ($C_x \cdot P_x$) equals the amount excreted ($U_x \cdot \dot{V}$), where P_x is plasma concentration, C_x is plasma clearance, U_x is urine concentration, and $\dot{V}$ is urine flow. If renal plasma flow is 500 ml/min, the filtration fraction is 0.25, P_x is 100 mg/100 ml, U_x is 125 mg/ml, and $\dot{V}$ is 1 ml/min, substance X is

(A) albumin
(B) inulin
(C) *para*-aminohippuric acid (PAH)
(D) actively secreted
(E) totally reabsorbed

232. Relative to the plasma in the efferent arteriole, the fluid in Bowman's capsule has a

(A) higher glucose concentration
(B) higher sodium concentration
(C) higher potassium concentration
(D) lower oncotic pressure
(E) lower sodium concentration

233. All of the following substances are required for thyroxine biosynthesis EXCEPT

(A) active iodide
(B) diiodotyrosine
(C) monoiodotyrosine
(D) thyroglobulin
(E) thyroid peroxidase

234. Rods are able to detect light at much lower intensities than cones for all of the following reasons EXCEPT

(A) the diameter of rods is greater
(B) the rods can more easily detect scattered light within the eye
(C) the number of rods innervating a single ganglion cell is greater
(D) the same light stimulus produces a larger receptor potential in rods
(E) the receptor potential adapts more rapidly in rods

235. Prolactin secretion differs from that of other hormones of the pars distalis because it is

(A) stimulated by dopamine
(B) inhibited by thyrotropin-releasing hormone (TRH)
(C) under tonic inhibition from the hypothalamus
(D) cosecreted with growth hormone (GH)
(E) secreted by the pars intermedia

236. A large dose of insulin is administered intravenously to a normal 34-year-old female patient. This is likely to cause an increase in all of the following EXCEPT

(A) plasma epinephrine concentration
(B) plasma K^+ concentration
(C) adrenocorticotropic hormone (ACTH) secretion
(D) growth hormone (GH) secretion
(E) glucagon secretion

237. The neural crest gives rise to all of the following tissues and cells EXCEPT

(A) Schwann cells
(B) cartilage and bone of the skull
(C) the neural lobe of the pituitary gland
(D) melanocytes
(E) the adrenal medulla

238. A 21-year-old woman presents with hyperpigmentation; blood pressure, 165/105 mm Hg; acne; hypokalemia; normal plasma Na$^+$ concentration; amenorrhea; low fasting plasma glucose; physical and mental fatigue; an enlarged clitoris; and metabolic alkalosis. Which of the following endocrine disorders could account for all of these signs and symptoms, together with the laboratory findings?

(A) An adrenocorticotropic hormone (ACTH)–secreting tumor
(B) An 11β-hydroxylase deficiency
(C) A 21-hydroxylase deficiency
(D) An aldosterone-producing adenoma
(E) Primary hypercortisolism

239. Expansion of the antrum causes an increase in all of the following EXCEPT

(A) secretion of gastrin
(B) secretion of pancreatic enzymes
(C) secretion of gastric acid (HCl)
(D) gastric motility
(E) receptive relaxation

240. A 15-year-old patient who was raised as a girl was brought to the physician by her mother because of sexual ambiguity (male pseudohermaphroditism). Bilateral masses were palpable in the inguinal region. Prior to this time the patient presented an external phenotype of a female. Recently the patient exhibited virilization of the external genitalia and developed male axillary and pubic hair together with clitoromegaly. The patient described an increased libido and presented with deepening of the voice and muscle hypertrophy. Facial and body hair were sparse, temporal hair had not receded, acne was absent, and the prostate was not palpable. Laboratory tests revealed a 46,XY karyotype.

With regard to this syndrome, which one of the following conditions would best explain the observations in this patient?

(A) The binding of testosterone and dihydrotestosterone to the receptor is abnormal.
(B) There is a testosterone-secreting tumor.
(C) There is a defect in the conversion of testosterone to dihydrotestosterone.
(D) There was a subnormal secretion of LH during the fetal period of the patient.
(E) There was a subnormal secretion of FSH during the fetal period of the patient.

241. Hypophysectomy results in the functional decline of many endocrine organs. All of the following changes are likely to occur after removal of the pituitary gland EXCEPT

(A) atrophy of the thyroid gland
(B) dwarfism (if performed during early adolescence)
(C) deficiency of aldosterone
(D) cessation of menstrual cycles
(E) impaired testosterone secretion

242. The reflex responsible for withdrawing a limb is characterized by all of the following EXCEPT

(A) local sign
(B) irradiation
(C) unmyelinated afferent fibers
(D) monosynaptic reflex
(E) afterdischarge

243. Hormones with lipolytic activity include all of the following EXCEPT

(A) glucagon
(B) epinephrine
(C) insulin
(D) cortisol
(E) growth hormone (GH)

244. Growth hormone (GH) secretion is increased by all of the following factors EXCEPT

(A) insulin administration
(B) arginine administration
(C) somatostatin administration
(D) onset of sleep
(E) exercise

245. In hyperaldosteronemia, all of the following conditions are likely to be observed EXCEPT

(A) decreased hematocrit
(B) fall in plasma oncotic pressure
(C) increased extracellular fluid (ECF) volume
(D) hyperkalemia
(E) metabolic alkalosis

246. In a patient with intention tremors, which is the most likely site of injury to the central nervous system (CNS)?

(A) Posterior cerebellum
(B) Vestibular apparatus
(C) Cerebral cortex
(D) Reticular formation
(E) Basal ganglia

247. Patients A and B are both 70-kg males. Patient A drinks 2 L of pure water, and patient B drinks 2 L of a 150 mM NaCl solution. As a result of these ingestions, patient B has a

(A) higher free-water clearance
(B) greater change in plasma osmolality
(C) higher urine flow rate
(D) greater change in intracellular fluid (ICF) volume
(E) higher urine osmolality

248. In a patient with rigidity, which is the most likely site of injury to the central nervous system (CNS)?

(A) Posterior cerebellum
(B) Vestibular apparatus
(C) Cerebral cortex
(D) Reticular formation
(E) Basal ganglia

249. In a patient with nystagmus, which is the most likely site of injury to the central nervous system (CNS)?

(A) Posterior cerebellum
(B) Vestibular apparatus
(C) Cerebral cortex
(D) Reticular formation
(E) Basal ganglia

250. The glomerular filtration rate (GFR) can be estimated clinically by which of the following?

(A) Serum inulin concentration
(B) Serum creatinine concentration
(C) Clearance of glucose
(D) Sodium plus potassium excretion
(E) Plasma urea concentration

251. A newborn genotypic male is found to have an adrenogenital (AG) syndrome due to a 17α-hydroxylase defect. In this case of congenital adrenal hyperplasia (CAH), which of the following biochemical reactions in the biosynthesis of gonadal hormones is decelerated?

(A) Pregnenolone → 17α-hydroxypregnenolone
(B) Cholesterol → pregnenolone
(C) Progesterone → corticosterone
(D) Deoxycorticosterone → corticosterone
(E) 17α-Hydroxypregnenolone → 17α-hydroxyprogesterone

252. Which of the following controls body Na^+ content?

(A) Aldosterone
(B) Antidiuretic hormone (ADH)
(C) Atrial natriuretic peptide (ANP)
(D) Renin
(E) Angiotensin I

253. A decrease in cortisol secretion would lead to

(A) increased storage of glycogen in the liver
(B) decreased adrenocorticotropic hormone (ACTH) secretion
(C) decreased adrenomedullary synthesis of epinephrine
(D) increased plasma glucose concentration
(E) increased hepatic protein synthesis

254. Which of the following is a substrate for dipeptidyl carboxypeptidase or kininase II?

(A) Aldosterone
(B) Antidiuretic hormone (ADH)
(C) Atrial natriuretic peptide (ANP)
(D) Renin
(E) Angiotensin I

255. Which of the following is produced by modified smooth muscle cells?

(A) Aldosterone
(B) Antidiuretic hormone (ADH)
(C) Atrial natriuretic peptide (ANP)
(D) Renin
(E) Angiotensin I

Questions 256–260

Questions 256–260 are based on the table. Match each person described below with the set of blood data that best coincides with that person's condition.

	Arterial PO_2 (mm Hg)	Arterial PCO_2 (mm Hg)	O_2 Content (ml/dl)	Arterial pH
(A)	98	40	arterial = 10	7.40
(B)	50	65	arterial = 15	7.32
(C)	50	40	arterial = 16	7.38
(D)	105	35	venous = 18	7.45
(E)	50	32	arterial = 10	7.45

256. A healthy 40-year-old man who has been mountain climbing for two days

257. A 30-year-old anemic woman

258. A 73-year-old man who is hypoventilating

259. A 45-year-old woman who is hyperventilating

260. A 56-year-old man with moderately severe obstructive lung disease

Questions 261–264

Questions 261–264 are based on this figure. Match each site of secretory activity described below with the appropriate lettered region of the nephron.

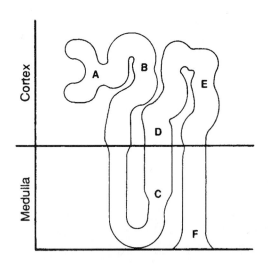

261. Primary site of H^+ secretion

262. Site of K^+ secretion

263. Primary site of NH_4^+ secretion

264. Site of para-aminohippuric acid (PAH) secretion

265. Which of the following substances is the most important for absorption of iron from the intestine?
(A) Intrinsic factor
(B) Ferritin
(C) Bile salts
(D) Vitamin D
(E) Trypsin

266. Untreated type I diabetes mellitus is associated with all of the following biochemical changes EXCEPT

(A) positive nitrogen balance
(B) ketonemia
(C) ketonuria
(D) low plasma C-peptide concentration
(E) glycosuria

267. Which of the following substances is the most important for the absorption of cholesterol from the intestine?

(A) Intrinsic factor
(B) Ferritin
(C) Bile salts
(D) Vitamin D
(E) Trypsin

268. Small solutes are transported across the glomerular capillaries by the process of

(A) simple diffusion
(B) bulk flow
(C) facilitated diffusion
(D) primary active transport
(E) secondary active transport

269. Which of the following conditions would simultaneously increase the aortic systolic pressure and decrease the aortic pulse pressure?

(A) Increased heart rate
(B) Increased arterial compliance
(C) Decreased peripheral resistance
(D) Increased stroke volume
(E) Increased elastic constant

270. Lesions within the basal ganglia produce all of the following signs EXCEPT

(A) hypotonia
(B) hemiballism
(C) tremor
(D) hypokinesia
(E) athetosis

Questions 271–275

The following information was obtained from a healthy 24-year-old man who was studied in a renal laboratory:

Inulin Concentration (mg/ml)	Glucose Concentration	Urine Flow Rate	Hematocrit Ratio
Urine = 150	Urine = 0 mg/ml	1.2 ml/min	0.40
Renal arterial plasma = 1.50	Plasma = 90 mg/dl		
Renal venous plasma = 1.20			

Using this data, match each of the following measurements of renal function with the appropriate lettered value.

(A) 0.20
(B) 108 mg/min
(C) 120 ml/min
(D) 600 ml/min
(E) 1000 ml/min

271. Glomerular filtration rate (GFR)

272. Renal blood flow

273. Filtration fraction

274. Renal plasma flow

275. Filtered load of glucose

Questions 276–278

For each acid-base disturbance in Questions 276–278, select from the table the characteristic set of body fluid changes.

	Plasma pH	Plasma [HCO_3^-] (mEq/L)	Urine pH
(A)	7.27	37	acid
(B)	7.31	16	acid
(C)	7.40	15	alkaline
(D)	7.40	24	acid
(E)	7.55	22	alkaline

276. Hyperventilation

277. Chronic respiratory tract obstruction

278. Diabetic ketoacidosis

ANSWERS AND EXPLANATIONS

1. The answer is E [Chapter 6 I C 3 b]. In the dark, rods and cones are depolarized by the flow of Na^+ into the cell through Na^+ channels that are kept open by cyclic guanosine monophosphate (cGMP). When light strikes the eye, rhodopsin is activated. Rhodopsin activates a G protein called transducin, which in turn activates a phosphodiesterase that hydrolyzes cGMP. When cGMP levels fall, cGMP is removed from its binding site on the Na^+ channels, closing the Na^+ channel and causing the photoreceptor to hyperpolarize.

2. The answer is E [Chapter 25 II C 2 b]. Changes in the glomerular filtration rate (GFR) are a determinant of glomerulotubular balance (GTB), not the other way around. A small increment in efferent arteriolar resistance increases GFR and reduces renal plasma flow (renal blood flow). Prostaglandin E_2 (PGE_2) and a decrease in afferent arteriolar resistance cause both an increase in GFR and renal plasma flow (renal blood flow). However, a high plasma catecholamine (norepinephrine) level increases both afferent and efferent arteriolar resistances. It should be noted that the diameter of the afferent arteriole is larger than that of the efferent arteriole. This fact explains a greater constrictive effect on the efferent arteriole with the same catecholamine concentration. Thus, a high level of catecholamine increases GFR slightly and decreases renal plasma flow (renal blood flow).

3. The answer is D [Chapter 30 II D 1 b]. Renal effects of aldosterone include: (1) increased number of luminal Na^+ and K^+ channels in principal cells of the collecting duct, (2) increased number of luminal H^+ transporters (H^+–ATPase pumps) in the intercalated A-type cells, and (3) increased number of Na^+–K^+–ATPase pumps in the basolateral border of the principal cells. The cellular aldosterone receptors are found in the nucleus, not on the basolateral border of target cells.

4. The answer is D [Chapter 35 I B 1 b (1) (a), 2 a Chapter 32 III D 2, IV B 6, Chapter 36 III C 3]. Extracellular HCO_3^- is not an effective buffer for H_2CO_3. The HCO_3^- buffer system plays no role in the buffering of H_2CO_3, but it is an effec-

tive buffer for noncarbonic acids. HCO_3^- cannot buffer H_2CO_3, because the combination of H^+ with HCO_3^- results in regeneration of H_2CO_3 as:

$$H_2CO_3 + HCO_3^- \leftrightarrows HCO_3^- + H_2CO_3$$

Most buffering of H_2CO_3 occurs within the erythrocytes by hemoglobin. In contrast, the non-HCO_3^- buffer systems (hemoglobin, protein, phosphate) can buffer both noncarbonic acids and H_2CO_3. The HCO_3^-/CO_2 buffer system accounts for 97%–98% of the buffering in the extracellular fluid (ECF), which includes the interstitial fluid, lymph, and cerebrospinal fluid (CSF). A stipulation here is that HCO_3^- is a major buffer for noncarbonic acids.

5. The answer is E [Chapter 53 II B 1 a]. The storage of thyroid hormone is unique in that it is stored as thyroglobulin in the colloid, which constitutes a small fraction of the extracellular fluid (ICF) [namely, transcellular fluid]. Thyroid hormone is stored in large quantities outside the follicular cells.

6. The answer is C [Chapter 49 I E 1 c (3), 3 a, Figure 49-4]. The antipyretic effect of cortisol is due to a decrease in pyrogen [interleukin-1 (IL-1)] from granulocytes. The anti-inflammatory effects of exogenous cortisol result from its ability to decrease capillary membrane permeability and probably also its ability to stabilize lysosomal membranes and decrease the formation of bradykinin. Glucocorticoids inhibit the enzyme phospholipase A_2, which is also known as macrocortin. This decreases the release of arachidonic acid and substances produced from it such as leukotrienes, prostaglandins, thromboxanes, and prostacyclin. Endogenous cortisol does not exert significant anti-inflammatory action.

7. The answer is C [Chapter 51 I K 2 a (1), L 1 a]. Estradiol secreted by the granulosa cells of the follicle causes proliferation of the endometrium to form a new stratum functionale. Injection of estradiol will produce ovarian atrophy through its negative feedback effect on FSH secretion. Menstruation begins with the cessation of estradiol and progesterone secretion by the corpus luteum, which remains viable for 14 days. Luteinizing hormone evokes ovulation and the formation of the corpus luteum and the secretion of estradiol and progesterone in the early luteal phase. The highest plasma levels of FSH are associated with ovulation. The rise of FSH late in the luteal phase initiates the development of follicles and the beginning of the next menstrual cycle; however, this titer of FSH is lower than the midcycle titer of the FSH surge.

8–9. The answers are: 8-C [Chapter 16 VI A 1], **9-B** [Chapter 18 III B 2 a (1) (b); Figure 18-6]. Lung compliance is calculated as the change in volume per unit change in distending pressure. Since alveolar pressure is zero at the beginning and end of inspiration, the transmural (distending) pressure for the lung is zero minus the interpleural pressure. Only the change in interpleural pressure between the beginning and end of inspiration is given. This difference divided into the tidal volume gives the lung compliance during dynamic conditions, or 150 and 60 ml/cm H_2O. Note that compliance is expressed as volume/pressure.

The change in this patient's lung compliance when she alters her respiratory rate is termed frequency-dependent compliance. Frequency-dependent compliance occurs in the presence of high airway resistance, which causes some acini not to fill completely at rapid rates of respiration, as the result of long time constants. Thus, frequency-dependent compliance indicates the presence of high airway resistance, which is synonymous with obstructive lung disease.

10. The answer is A [Chapter 7 II A 2 b, C]. Small motoneurons usually fire before large motoneurons during the performance of a movement. The small motoneurons innervate small, fatigue-resistant muscle fibers that generate long-lasting muscle twitches. Because the duration of the twitch is longer than in other muscle fibers, the frequency of firing required for tetanus is lower. Slow-twitch fibers cannot produce a large amount of force. Because they have a rich capillary supply, slow-twitch fibers do not need to rely on glycolysis as a source of adenosine triphosphate (ATP) and, therefore, are more resistant to fatigue.

11. The answer is D [Chapter 16 III C 1]. The alveolar CO_2 tension is directly proportional to the rate at which CO_2 is produced by metabolism and inversely proportional to alveolar ventilation. The increased minute ventilation would not alter the metabolic rate signifi-

cantly, so any changes in CO_2 tension must be related to alveolar ventilation. Alveolar ventilation is the difference between minute ventilation and dead space ventilation. During control conditions, alveolar ventilation is (O.5 L · 15) − (0.2 L · 15) = 4.5 L/min, which is unchanged by the alteration in respiratory pattern [30 · (0.35 L − 0.2 L)]. An increase in alveolar ventilation would cause a decrease in CO_2 tension, which would lead to respiratory alkalosis (i.e., increased arterial pH).

12. The answer is C [Chapter 29 II B 1, Figures 29-1A and 29-3; Table 29-1; Chapter 25 I A 1]. A decrease in plasma osmolality (osmolarity) leads to a decrease in antidiuretic hormone (ADH) secretion. This results in an increase in free-water clearance and diuresis. These osmoreceptors are found in the vicinity of the supraoptic nucleus of the hypothalamus. ADH augments the water permeability of the cortical collecting duct and the water and urea permeabilities of the medullary collecting duct. It increases renal water reabsorption, resulting in the excretion of a small volume of hypertonic urine. The major stimuli for ADH are an increase in the plasma osmolality and a decrease in the effective circulating blood volume. Aldosterone promotes Na^+ reabsorption, which leads to water retention.

13–15. The answers are: 13-C, 14-A, 15-E [Chapter 16 II C 4 a]. This patient's functional residual capacity (FRC) is 2.7 L. The dilution test measures the FRC, the lung volume at the beginning of the test. Because the volume of gas in the spirometer is kept constant, the degree of dilution produced by the lungs after equilibration must be determined by calculating the ratio of the initial fraction of helium to the fraction of helium following equilibration (F_1/F_2), which equals 0.05 ÷ 0.03, or 1.67. Thus, the volume of the spirometer plus the lung volume is 1.67 times the volume of the spirometer, or 1.67 · 4 (6.7 L). Subtracting the volume of the spirometer leaves the lung volume at the start of the test (i.e., FRC), or 6.7 − 4 (2.7 L).

This patient's residual volume (RV) is 0.7 L. Because FRC is the sum of RV and expiratory reserve volume (ERV), RV is determined as:

$$RV = FRC - ERV, \text{ or } 2.7 - 2.0 = 0.7 \text{ L.}$$

This patient's total lung capacity (TLC) is 5.7 L. TLC is the sum of vital capacity (VC) and RV, or 5 + 0.7 = 5.7 L.

16. The answer is E [Chapter 30 III A-C, Figure 30-2, Tables 30-1, 30-2, and 30-3]. Atrial natriuretic peptide (ANP) is secreted by the atrial myocytes in response to increased blood volume. ANP prevents angiotensin formation by inhibiting renin release. The cardiac hormones inhibit angiotensin II and adrenocorticotropic hormone corticotropin (ACTH)—two stimuli for aldosterone secretion. Angiotensin II is the primary stimulus for aldosterone secretion. Angiotensin II synthesis is regulated by renin release from the juxtaglomerular cells. The principal stimuli for renin secretion are decreased perfusion pressure in the afferent arterioles, decreased [Na$^+$] in the macula densa area of the nephron, and norepinephrine secretion from the sympathetic neurons innervating the juxtaglomerular cells. All actions of renin are mediated through the generation of angiotensin II. Other stimuli for aldosterone include ACTH, a high plasma [K$^+$], and a low plasma [Na$^+$]. The stimulatory effect of ACTH on aldosterone secretion is significant but short-lived and is not a major factor in the control of aldosterone production.

17–18. The answers are: 17-C [Chapter 4 III C 3; IV B 2], **18-D** [Chapter 4 II C 2 b; Table 4-1], The amount of Ca^{2+} released from the sarcoplasmic reticulum (SR) of the smooth and cardiac muscle cells is normally varied to control contractile force. In skeletal muscle, maximal amounts of Ca^{2+} enter the cell with each contraction.

Skeletal and smooth muscles are able to recruit additional fibers when more force is required. The heart must contract in a coordinated fashion so that all of its muscle fibers are recruited at the same time. Smooth, cardiac, and skeletal muscles all are able to influence the force of contraction by varying the initial length (preload) of their sarcomeres.

19. The answer is C [Chapter 6 II C 2]. Sound stimuli striking the tympanic membrane are amplified by the auditory ossicles before reaching the oval window. Amplification is necessary for sounds to pass from an air to a fluid environment.

20. The answer is D [Chapter 12 II B 2 b]. Pco_2 is the most important factor that regulates resistance in the cerebral vessels. Hyperventilation, which reduces the Pco_2, produces a marked vasoconstriction of cerebral vessels that, at times, may lead to hypoxia sufficiently severe to cause dizziness and even fainting.

21. The answer is B [Chapter 31 IV A, B Figure 31-1]. Atrial natriuretic peptide (ANP) has multiple important effects that are involved in the control of renal NaCl and water excretion. They are: (1) increased glomerular filtration rate (GFR), (2) decreased renin secretion, (3) decreased aldosterone secretion, (4) decreased NaCl and water reabsorption by the collecting duct, and (5) decreased antidiuretic hormone (ADH) secretion and action of ADH on the collecting duct.

22. The answer is C [Chapter 26 II B 2, IV A 3, B 2, Table 26-2]. Glomerulotubular balance (GTB) describes a fundamental property of the kidney. In GTB, the tubular reabsorption of filtrate (Na$^+$ and H$_2$O) is adjusted in proportion to the glomerular filtration rate (GFR) such that the fractional tubular reabsorption remains constant despite changes in GFR. Thus, the *absolute* level of tubular reabsorption is directly related to the GFR. When the filtered load of Na$^+$ is increased due to increased GFR (with constant plasma [Na$^+$]), GTB is observed. And when the filtered load of Na$^+$ is increased due to increased plasma [Na$^+$] (with constant GFR), GTB is *not* observed. This mechanism prevents the distal fluid (and solute) delivery from exceeding the reabsorptive capacity of the collecting duct. It is important to appreciate that the GFR, not the filtered load, is the major determinant of GTB. When the filtered load of Na$^+$ is raised by increasing the plasma [Na$^+$] (with constant GFR), the absolute rate of Na$^+$ reabsorption declines. The changes in Na$^+$ excretion do change slightly with changes in GFR, but the excretion rates are markedly attenuated with changes in filtered load due to changes in GFR. GTB serves to regulate the extracellular fluid (ECF) volume and, therefore, blood pressure over time.

23. The answer is B [Chapter 25 II A 3, 5 c]. Oxygen consumption in the kidney changes in response to blood flow, unlike in other organs. Thus, an increase in renal blood flow leads to an increase in renal oxygen utilization. An increase in inulin clearance is indicative of an increase in GFR and an increase in the filtered load of Na$^+$. According to the concept of glomerulotubular balance (GTB), there is a constant fraction, but an increased amount of Na$^+$ reabsorbed. Most of the energy required by the kidney is utilized to reabsorb Na$^+$.

24. The answer is D [Chapter 27 I A 1 B 2 Figure 27-1 A and B]. The transport (tubular) maximum (Tm) is the maximal rate of **active reabsorption** *or* **active secretion** that can occur with saturation of all of the protein-carriers. Below the renal threshold, all of the substance is actively reabsorbed because all the carriers are not saturated. As the plasma concentration increases **beyond** the Tm, a smaller **fraction** (but constant amount) is reabsorbed. Thus, below the saturation of the carrier with substrate (Tm), all of the substance will be transported. It is important to remember that although there is no renal threshold for **secreted** substances, there is a Tm for secreted substances.

25. The answer is E [Chapter 28 I D 2 a (4), II B 2 a]. In the thin ascending limb of the loop of Henle (ALH), the Na^+ concentration is greater than the surrounding interstitium. However, the urea concentration of the tubular fluid is less than that of the interstitial fluid (ISF), and urea passively diffuses into the tubular fluid of the ALH. Overall, the movement of NaCl out of the thin ALH is greater than the movement of urea into the lumen of the ALH. The high Na^+ concentration along the thin ALH is the gradient that drives the **passive** reabsorption of Na^+. In all of the other listed segments of the nephron, the tubular Na^+ concentration is either **equal** to the interstitium (proximal tubule) or **less than** the interstitium (thick segment, medullary collecting duct or distal tubule). It should be pointed out that the osmolality at the bend of the loop of Henle and the interstitium are equal. The tubular fluid NaCl concentration is greater than the interstitium, but the tubular fluid urea concentration is less than the interstitium. The maximal osmolality that the fluid within the medullary collecting duct can attain is equal to that in the surrounding medullary interstitium.

26. The answer is C [Chapter 28 II B 2 d e Figure 28-2]. The ascending limb of the loop of Henle (ALH) has a high passive transport of NaCl because not only is the thin segment permeable to NaCl, but also the thick segment actively reabsorbs NaCl via the $Na^+–2Cl^-–K^+$ cotransporter. The entire ALH is water impermeable, and the thin ALH is also moderately urea permeable. The removal of water from the thin descending limb of the loop of Henle (DLH) and the small addition (secretion) of urea into the thin ALH account for the higher urea concentration in the thin ALH (compared to the thin DLH). In addition, the NaCl concentration is higher in the thin ALH because of water reabsorption by the thin DLH. The osmolality of the tubular fluid in the thin ALH is lower than that in the collecting duct due to the equilibration of the collecting duct fluid with the medullary interstitium in the presence of antidiuretic hormone (ADH). The osmolality of the tubular fluid in the thin (and thick) segments is hyposmotic due to NaCl reabsorption. Lastly, in a state of dehydration (i.e., with a maximally concentrated urine), the tubular fluid in the thin ALH is hyperosmotic to plasma, even though NaCl is being reabsorbed from this segment.

27. The answer is D [Chapter 43 VII C 2, E 4–5]. Ca^{2+} is absorbed from the duodenum by a membrane-bound carrier on the luminal surface of the enterocyte that is formed in response to the presence of vitamin D. Once inside the enterocyte, the Ca^{2+} is extruded from the serosal surface of the cell by an active transport system.

28. The answer is D [Chapter 30 II D 3, Figure 30-1, Chapter 3 II B 2, Figure 37-2]. Aldosterone has three major renal effects: (1) Na^+ reabsorption by the principal cells of the collecting duct; (2) K^+ secretion by the principal cells of the collecting duct; and (3) H^+ secretion by the A-type intercalated cells. In addition, aldosterone has an important secondary effect on water reabsorption that is linked to its positive effect on Na^+ balance. Aldosterone mediates these effects by increased synthesis of Na^+ and K^+ channels, H^+ transporters ($H^+–ATPase$ pumps), and $Na^+–K^+–ATPase$ pumps.

29. The answer is A [Chapter 22 III G 5 H 2]. Aldosterone is the major Na^+-conserving hormone and, therefore, this hormone is the major volume regulator of the extracellular fluid (ECF), inasmuch as Na^+ salts are the major determinants of the ECF volume. If blood pressure is viewed as being equal to the product of cardiac output and total peripheral resistance, then aldosterone indirectly regulates cardiac output (a volume per time) through its effect on Na^+ retention. Angiotensin II plays a role in the regulation of peripheral resistance. Therefore, it is useful to conceptualize:

$$\text{Blood pressure} \propto \text{Cardiac output} \times \text{Total peripheral resistance}$$

It is important to appreciate that antidiuretic hormone (ADH) regulates the osmolality (concentration) of the plasma and, therefore, is the osmoregulator.

30. The answer is D [Chapter 25 II and II A 5 c]. In general, an increase in renal blood flow is a major determinant of the glomerular filtration rate (GFR) except in the setting of a fall in efferent arteriolar resistance. The filtration of plasma by the glomerulus increases the plasma protein concentration, reaching a maximum concentration at the end of the capillary network. This increase in capillary oncotic pressure decreases the net filtration pressure. Vasoconstriction of the afferent arteriole decreases glomerular capillary hydrostatic pressure, and filtration declines because capillary hydrostatic pressure is the primary determinant of GFR. The increase in the hydrostatic pressure within Bowman's space retards glomerular filtration. Vasodilation of the efferent arteriole leads to a fall in glomerular capillary pressure and a resultant reduction in GFR despite an increase in renal blood flow. It is imperative to appreciate that the increase in renal blood flow together with the fall in GFR accounts for the decline in filtration fraction.

31. The answer is E [Chapter 22 III Table 22-5]. A 150 mmol/L NaCl solution is equivalent to a 300 mOsm/kg H_2O solution, which is isosmotic to plasma. Therefore, the entire liter remains in the extracellular fluid (ECF) because there is no osmotic gradient for the diffusion of water.

32. The answer is C [Chapter 22 II A 1, 2 b, B 1 c]. Determining the answer to this question requires an understanding of the dilution principle.

$$V = \frac{A - E}{c}$$

$$= \frac{(1 - 0.2)}{0.08} = \frac{0.8}{0.08} = 10 \text{ L}$$

where V = volume, A = amount, and c = concentration. Application of arithmetic yields the answer, 10 L.

33. The answer is D [Chapter 23 III Table 23-1; III H 2, Figure 27-8 A]. Of the transporters listed, only the H^+–K^+–ATPase pump represents a primary active transport system in which transport is coupled directly to energy derived from metabolic processes. The transport is energized by ATP. Furthermore, the solutes move from an area of lower concentration to an area of higher concentration. The Na^+–glucose and Na^+–amino acid symporters together with the Na^+–Ca^{2+} antiporter are examples of Na^+-coupled transport where one solute (glucose, amino acid, Ca^{2+}) is trans-

ported against its chemical (glucose) or electric (Ca^{2+}) gradient. The energy for the uphill transport is derived from the downhill movement of the other solute (Na^+). The influx of Na^+ via luminal conductive channels is a passive process.

34. The answer is D [Chapter 24 I Figures 24-1 and 24-2; Chapter 27 II Figure 27-1 C]. Clearance, which is inversely related to reabsorption, occurs via filtration, secretion, and excretion. [It should not be equated with excretion ($U_x \cdot \dot{V}$).] To arrange these substances from lowest to highest clearance, it is helpful to arrange them from the highest reabsorption to the lowest reabsorption. Inulin is always the reference point, because it is only filtered—neither reabsorbed nor secreted. Substances with clearances lower than inulin are reabsorbed on a net basis, and substances with clearances above inulin are secreted on a net basis. The substance with the highest reabsorption (lowest clearance) is glucose (100% reabsorption), followed by Na^+ (> 99% reabsorption), urea (40%–50% reabsorption), and inulin (0% reabsorption). The clearance of creatinine is 10%–20% higher than it is for inulin, and the clearance of *para*-aminohippuric acid (PAH) is about five times higher than that for inulin, which means at low plasma concentrations it is almost completely (90%) cleared, making it the substance with the highest clearance.

35. The answer is D [Chapter 32 I A Table 32-1]. Most of the body's daily CO_2 production occurs from chemical reactions of the tricarboxylic acid cycle. From this metabolic activity, humans produce approximately 13,000 mmol of CO_2 daily, or in acid-base terms, approximately 13,000 mEq of H^+ per day. The mammalian body produces large amounts of acids from two major sources. The volatile acid H_2CO_3 is produced from CO_2, the end product of oxidative metabolism. A variety of nonvolatile acids (e.g., H_2SO_4, H_3PO_4) are produced from dietary substances.

36. The answer is E [Chapter 33 I A, C]. The first four choices are associated with the generation of H^+ ions that would tend to acidify the body fluids. An example of an alkalinizing amino acid is an anionic acid such as aspartate and glutamate, not given as a possible answer choice. On the other hand, substances such as acetate, citrate, lactate, and ascorbate are anions that are metabolized to HCO_3^-. Indeed, even the anions of ketoacids, in the presence of insulin, are metabolized to HCO_3^-. The citrate in blood that is anticoagulated with acid-citrate-dextran can be metabolized to HCO_3^-. However, more than 8 U of blood must be given acutely to produce a significant elevation in plasma HCO_3^- concentration.

37. The answer is D [Chapter 35 I B 1 a (2) (a), b (1) (a) Chapter 32 III D 2, IV B 6, Chapter 36 III C 3]. Bicarbonate (HCO_3^-) is an effective buffer for noncarbonic acids, such as sulfuric, phosphoric, hydrochloric, lactic, and keto acids. It is not a buffer for carbonic acid, because this acid is regenerated in the presence of HCO_3^- as:

$$H_2CO_3 + HCO_3^- \rightarrow HCO_3^- + H_2CO_3$$

38–41. The answers are 38-D, 39-C, 40-A, 41-B [Chapter 38 IV B 1, 2, Figures 38-6, 38-7; V A B, Figure 38-8]. In analyzing these four uncompensated acid-base disturbances, it is important to consider the CO_2 tension and [HCO_3^-] rather than the pH, because CO_2 tension and [HCO_3^-] are the key determinants of the cause of, and compensation for, these disturbances.

Point D represents a patient with increased pH ($\downarrow$[H^+]) brought about by respiratory alkalosis. This condition is characterized by a primary decrease in CO_2 tension (hypocapnia) and a variable secondary decrease in plasma [HCO_3^-]. Metabolic acidosis also is characterized by declines in these two variables, but the pH is decreased ($\uparrow$[H^+]) as well. Respiratory alkalosis is defined as alveolar ventilation greater than the existing need of the body to eliminate CO_2. This excess in alveolar ventilation, called hyperventilation, results in a reduced arterial CO_2 tension. Hyperpnea is the general term used to describe any increase in ventilatory effort. With respiratory alkalosis there is a decline in the [total CO_2].

Point C represents a patient with decreased pH ($\uparrow$[H^+]) caused by respiratory acidosis. This clinical disorder is characterized by a primary increase in CO_2 tension (hypercapnia) and a variable secondary increase in plasma [HCO_3^-]. The common denominator in respiratory acidosis is hypoventilation, which is defined as alveolar ventilation insufficient to excrete CO_2 rapidly enough to meet the existing needs of the body. With respiratory acidosis, there is a relatively small increment in the [total CO_2], because the major fraction of the CO_2 content is composed of HCO_3^-.

Point A represents a patient with diabetes mellitus, which is the most common cause of ketoacidosis. This overproduction of ketoacids is caused by a deficiency of insulin, which leads to (1) increased lipolysis and an increased delivery of free fatty acids to the liver and (2) the preferential conversion of free fatty acids to ketoacids rather than to triglycerides. Thus, metabolic acidosis is characterized by a low arterial pH ($\uparrow$[H^+]), a reduced [HCO_3^-], and a compensatory hyperventilation resulting in hypocapnia. The renal compensatory response for respiratory alkalosis also diminishes the plasma [HCO_3^-], but the pH in that disorder is elevated ($\downarrow$[H^+]). Overproduction of ketoacids causes acidosis by two mechanisms: (1) a decrease in plasma [HCO_3^-] with an increase in the anion gap and (2) overloading of the renal capacity to excrete H^+ resulting in a loss of Na^+ and a failure to recover $NaHCO_3$. In metabolic acidosis, there is a decline in the [total CO_2]. Furthermore, ketoacidosis, like lactic acidosis, differs from other forms of metabolic acidosis in that the anion associated with H^+ can be metabolized back to HCO_3^-, as

$$\beta\text{-hydroxybutyrate}^- + O_2 \rightarrow CO_2 + H_2O + HCO_3^-$$

β-hydroxybutyrate represents about 75% of the circulating ketoacids in diabetic ketoacidosis. It can be seen from the above chemical equation that the metabolism of the β-hydroxybutyrate anion results in the regeneration of the HCO_3^- that was neutralized in buffering the H^+. Since the HCO_3^- is replaced by an anion that is metabolized back to HCO_3^-, there is no actual loss of HCO_3^- from the body in ketoacidosis (or lactic acidosis). Insulin administration decreases the accumulation of β-hydroxybutyric acid and allows the metabolism of the acid anions back to HCO_3^-.

Point B represents a patient with metabolic alkalosis. Excessive ingestion of $NaHCO_3$ can result in metabolic alkalosis and an increase of pH ($\downarrow$[H^+]). Metabolic alkalosis is characterized by an increase in the plasma [HCO_3^-] and a compensatory increase in the CO_2 tension produced by a decline in alveolar ventilation. Since elevation of plasma [HCO_3^-] can be due to the renal compensation for chronic respiratory acidosis, the diagnosis of metabolic alkalosis cannot be made without measuring the pH. Metabolic alkalosis is associated with a large increase in the [total CO_2].

42. The answer is B [Chapter 38 IV B 1 a, 2 d, V B 1, Figure 38-8, and Case 1; Chapter 39 IV A, V C, Figure 39-1]. This diabetic patient has metabolic acidosis resulting from ketoacidosis. The ketoacidosis is attributable mainly to the formation of β-hydroxybutyric acid from the partial oxidation of fatty acids. The high concentration of ketoacids in the form of anions is responsible for the increased anion gap; however, it is H^+ retention, not anion accumulation, which is responsible for the acidosis. Osmotic diuresis accounts for this patient's dehydration, which is not only water loss but also increased renal excretion of Na^+, K^+, Cl^-, and glucose. Na^+ and K^+ also are lost when they are excreted in association with the excess quantities of organic anions. In this case, the decline in plasma bicarbonate ($[HCO_3^-]$) is the primary change, and the decreased CO_2 tension (i.e., hyperventilation) is the compensatory response. Complete compensation is evidenced by the normal pH of 7.39 and the near normal ratio of $[HCO_3^-]/S \cdot P_{CO_2}$ (19:1). It is possible to have an acidosis with a normal blood pH, or $[H^+]$, because secondary changes diminish the extent of the acid-base imbalance.

43. The answer is A [Chapter 54 VIII C, Figures 54-7 and 54-9]. The major difference between the actions of vitamin D_3 and PTH is the effect on renal phosphate transport, where vitamin D_3 promotes proximal reabsorption of phosphorus. The other actions of these two calcitropic hormones are similar. The major action of $1,25(OH)_2D_3$ is to stimulate absorption of Ca^{2+} by the intestinal enterocytes of the duodenum against a concentration gradient. Because of the intestinal and renal actions of D_3 on phosphate retention, it is the only hyperphosphatemic hormone. The osteoblasts have receptors for vitamin D_3 and PTH. Lastly, $1,25(OH)_2D_3$ increases the production of intestinal mucosal Ca^{2+} transport proteins called calbindins.

44. The answer is A [Chapter 30 I A 1, Chapter 49 I B 2 a] Aldosterone, the most potent endogenous mineralocorticoid, acts primarily on the renal collecting ducts to promote Na^+ reabsorption and K^+ and H^+ excretion. It has similar effects on sweat, salivary, and intestinal glands. Thus, aldosterone controls the Na^+ content of the body. In turn, the Na^+ content and its accompanying ions determines the volume of the various fluid compartments. Aldosterone also increases Na^+ reabsorption by the connecting segment of the nephron. Aldosterone is synthesized in and secreted from the outermost layer of the adrenal cortex, called the zone glomerulosa.

45. The answer is D [Chapter 45 IV F 7 a–d, Figure 45-3]. A shift from curve A to curve B

indicates that more hormone (increased concentration) is required to produce the same maximal response. This suggests that there are fewer hormone receptors on the target cells than previously. If the number of target cells had increased or decreased, the maximal response would have increased or decreased. A competitive inhibitor (not listed as a choice) could also have produced the observed shift in the dose (concentration)-response curve.

46. The answer is E [Chapter 46 III A 1 b, B 1, 2 b, Table 46-1]. The hypothalamic hormones include the hypophysiotropic hormones (releasing/inhibiting hormones) produced by the tuberal nuclei (e.g., arcuate nucleus), and oxytocin and antidiuretic hormone (ADH) [vasopressin] produced by the supraoptic and paraventricular nuclei. Thus, both parvicellular and magnocellular neurosecretory neurons are sources of hypothalamic hormones.

Because these hormones are produced by neurosecretory neurons (peptidergic neurons), they are all neuropeptides, with the important exception of prolactin-inhibiting factor (PIF), which has been identified as the catecholamine dopamine. The hypophysiotropic hormones are delivered to the adenohypophysis (pars distalis) via the hypophysial portal vessels, and oxytocin and ADH are delivered to the pars nervosa (posterior pituitary) by axoplasmic flow (not portal vessels). The releasing/inhibiting factors pass through fenestrations in the portal system capillaries, connecting the median eminence with the anterior pituitary. These fenestrations overcome the blood–brain barrier, which otherwise would restrict passage of the polypeptides. It is important to appreciate that the pituitary gland lies outside the blood–brain barrier. The anterior pituitary hormones are chemically classified as peptide hormones; however, they are not neuropeptides.

47. The answer is D [Chapter 47 IV A 2 a, Table 47-1]. Of the substances listed, only arginine is a secretogogue for growth hormone (GH). Arginine is also an effective stimulus for insulin secretion, resulting in hypoglycemia, which triggers secretion of GH. The other substances listed are inhibitors of somatotropin secretion.

48. The answer is D [Chapter 48 V A Figure 48-2]. The substrate for dopamine β-hydroxylase is dihydroxyphenylethylamine (dopamine), which is converted to norepinephrine within the cytoplasmic granules of the adrenomedullary chromaffin cell or within the vesicle of the postganglionic sympathetic neuron. The other substrates and their enzymes are: epinephrine or norepinephrine/catechol-O-methyltransferase (COMT) or monoamine oxidase (MAO), tyrosine/tyrosine hydroxylase, phenylalanine/phenylalanine hydroxylase, and dihydroxyphenylalanine (dopa)/dopa decarboxylase.

49. The answer is D [Chapter 49 II C 4 f Figure 49-7]. The 17α-hydroxylase deficiency affects the function of the adrenal cortex and the gonad in the same patient because this enzyme is necessary for both glucocorticoid and sex steroid synthesis. Thus, a male has incomplete differentiation of the external and internal genitalia, leading to sexual ambiguity as evidenced by the female phenotype. This is termed male pseudohermaphroditism because there is a lack of ovarian tissue but an appearance of both testicular and ovarian *function*. Because a female does not exhibit virilization due to elevated androgen secretion, she does not present with female pseudohermaphroditism.

Thus, this boy has deficiencies in adrenal cortisol and testicular androgen (testosterone) production together with elevated mineralocorticoid synthesis [deoxycorticosterone (DOC)]. His plasma aldosterone levels will also be below normal.

50. The answer is B [Chapter 48 V A 2, Chapter 49 I E 8]. Norepinephrine can be converted to epinephrine by methylation with the epinephrine-forming enzyme, phenylethanolamine-N-methyltransferase (PNMT), which is highly localized in the cytosol of the adrenomedullary chromaffin cells. The methyl group donor in this reaction is S-adenosylmethionine. Very high local concentrations of cortisol from the adrenal cortex reach the adrenomedullary chromaffin cells via the adrenal portal system. PNMT is inducible by glucocorticoids. The secretion of adrenomedullary catecholamine is stimulated by acetylcholine (ACh) from the preganglionic nerve endings, which innervates the chromaffin cells. Thus, the adrenal medulla is a functional extension of the nervous system. The synthesis of epinephrine in the adrenal medulla depends on PNMT, cortisol corticotropin (adrenocorticotropic hormone, ACTH), and the corticotropin-releasing hormone.

51. The answer is C [Chapter 50 I D 2 a, II B 4 b (1), Figures 50-2; Case 50, Figures 50-10 and 50-11]. The statements in choices A and B are true but it is not antimüllerian hormone (AMH) that causes the wolffian ducts to differentiate into the male internal genitalia nor that causes the müllerian ducts to develop into the female internal genitalia. Rather, it is testosterone that causes the wolffian ducts to develop and the absence of testosterone that allows the müllerian ducts to develop. The regression of the müllerian ducts is a response to AMH leaving the wolffian ducts intact. The testes develop from the gonadal ridge in response to the Y chromosome-specific testis-determining gene, not AMH. The notion that testosterone (choice E) induces the wolffian ducts to develop into male external genitalia is erroneous because the wolffian ducts develop into the male *internal* genitalia in response to testosterone and not the male *external* structures.

52. The answer is E [Chapter 51 I G 2, Table 51-2]. Human menopausal gonadotropin (hMG) is extracted from the urine of postmenopausal women who have expected elevated levels of urinary FSH and LH, especially elevated FSH. Therefore, the predominant activity of this urinary extract is FSH-like. Therefore, hMG can be used clinically to promote follicular development in women and to stimulate the FSH-dependent stages of spermatid development. Both hMG and HCG (human chorionic gonadotropin) are used to treat women with hypothalamic hypogonadism or women who fail to ovulate with clomiphene citrate treatment. The placental hormone HCG is devoid of FSH activity and resembles LH in its ability to stimulate ovulation in women and testosterone secretion in men.

53. The answer is B [Chapter 48 V B; Chapter 52 I E 1 a, Table 52-6]. Glucagon stimulates insulin secretion and epinephrine inhibits insulin secretion. Epinephrine also increases glucagon secretion. Both hormones activate the phosphorylase enzyme, which depolymerizes glucose and leads to the elevation of blood glucose via glycogenolysis. Both hormones are gluconeogenic, which augments the blood glucose even further. Hypoglycemia is a potent stimulus to both hormones.

54. The answer is E [Chapter 53 VI D 3 e, Table 53-2]. Hypothyroid states are characterized by a decline in T_4 and T_3, which is not the case here. The hallmark of primary hypothyroidism is an elevated thyroid-stimulating hormone (TSH) concentration, generally in conjunction with low T_4 and free T_4 concentrations. Secondary hypothyroidism is consistent with a decline in TSH, but the elevated plasma levels with the low TSH rule out this diagnosis. The administration of exogenous thyroid hormone would lead to TSH suppression by negative feedback; however, there would be a concomitant disuse atrophy of the thyroid gland caused by low pituitary TSH. The last possibility of thyrotoxicosis (Graves' disease) is consistent with neurologic and cardiac findings and, most of all, with the large diffuse hyperthyroid goiter caused by thyroid-stimulating immunoglobulins directed against the TSH receptor. Many of the manifestations of thyrotoxicosis and of sympathetic nervous system activation are similar. Indeed, thyroid hormones increase the number of beta-adrenergic receptors in cardiac and skeletal muscle (vasculature) and adipocytes. It is important to appreciate that sympathetic nervous system activity is not increased in hyperthyroid patients and that alterations in cardiac function are due to increased circulatory demands that result from the hypermetabolism and the need to dissipate the excess heat produced. At rest, peripheral resistance is decreased because of vasodilation, while cardiac output is increased as a result of increases in stroke volume and heart rate. Thyroid hormones in excess have a direct inotropic effect. Widening of the pulse pressure in thyrotoxicosis is due to the increase in systolic pressure and the decrease in diastolic pressure. It may be useful to treat this patient with beta-adrenergic receptor antagonists to block the cardiac manifestations of thyrotoxicosis. Lastly, it should be borne in mind that radiodine (I-131) is the most common therapy for Graves' disease.

55. The answer is D [Chapter 53 VI C 1, D 1 a b, 2 b (1) (6)]. Propylthiouracil is a thionamide (thiocarbamide) used as an antithyroid drug (ATD) because it inhibits organification of iodide and coupling of the iodotyrosyl residues on the thyroglobulin molecule. These drugs reduce plasma thyroid hormone levels to subnormal levels, resulting in the elevated secretion of thyroid-stimulating hormone (TSH) and the formation of a hypothyroid goiter. Therefore, these ATDs sensitize the pituitary thyrotropes to thyroid-releasing hormone (TRH), causing them to secrete more TSH.

56–58. The answers are: 56-A [Chapter 10 II B 2 a; III A], **57-D** [Chapter 10 II B 1 e (2)], **58-**

D [Chapter 10 II B 2 a–b]. Cell A is most likely found in the sinoatrial (SA) node. SA cells are characterized by relatively low membrane potentials, spontaneous depolarization (which indicates pacemaker activity), and a relatively fast rate of depolarization.

Cells A and B could exhibit pacemaker activity, because they are capable of diastolic (spontaneous) depolarization (i.e., a decrease in the diastolic membrane potential). The decrease in membrane potential is caused by the decline in K^+ conductance (G_K). Less K^+ leaves the cell during diastole, while Na^+ continues to leak into the cell. The membrane potential declines until threshold is reached, at which time an all-or-none action potential is generated.

Pacemaker cells, such as A and B, are slow fibers. Slow fibers lack Na^+ channels which, in fast fibers, open once the threshold potential is reached, allowing the rapid influx of Na^+. Slow fibers have "slow channels," which apparently limit the rate of ion entry and prolong phase 0 (i.e., depolarization).

59. The answer is C [Chapter 42 II B]. Receptive relaxation occurs when food enters the stomach. Although a small amount of receptive relaxation occurs as part of the esophageal reflex, the relaxation of the orad stomach necessary to accommodate the food entering it during a meal is brought about by a vagovagal reflex initiated by the presence of food in the stomach. Chewing is entirely dependent on a nonvagal reflex involving stretch receptors and motor efferents in the jaw muscles. Swallowing is coordinated by a swallowing center in the brain stem and does not involve vagal reflexes. Although gastric emptying is modified to some extent by vagovagal reflexes responding to gastric distention and the presence of chyme in the intestine, local reflexes and hormones are primarily responsible for regulating the rate of gastric emptying. Intestinal contractions are controlled almost entirely by local reflexes and the presence of circulating hormones.

60. The answer is C [Chapter 17 III C]. O_2 delivery to the tissues is the product of arterial O_2 content and cardiac output, which normally equals 1 L/min. Of the factors listed, only a 50% reduction in normal hemoglobin concentration would reduce O_2 delivery by half. This would produce a proportional change in O_2 content and an equivalent change in the O_2 delivery. Because of the non-linear relationship between O_2 tension and hemoglobin saturation, changing the arterial O_2 tension, ventilation rate, or inspired O_2 tension would have a relatively small effect on O_2 delivery.

61. The answer is A [Chapter 6 II C 2]. The auditory ossicles amplify the pressure of the sound stimulus so that sound can pass from air to the fluid environment of the inner ear. Without amplification of the stimulus, the sound reaching the inner ear would be too weak for detection because 99.9% of the sound is normally reflected at the air-fluid interface.

62. The answer is D [Chapter 10 IV B 3 b]. The hexaxial reference system consists of reference lines generated from the three standard (bipolar) limb leads and the three augmented limb leads. The three bipolar limb leads are separated by 60°; thus they lie at 0°, 60°, 120°, 180°, and 240°. The augmented limb leads bisect the angles provided by the bipolar leads; therefore, the hexaxial reference system provides reference lines at every 30°. The hexaxial reference system is in the frontal plane, whereas the precordial (V) leads lie in the horizontal plane.

63. The answer is B [Chapter 25 II C 1 b; Figure 25-6; Table 25-2]. The filtration fraction is that fraction of the plasma flowing through the kidneys that is filtered into Bowman's capsule. Normally about one-fifth of the plasma entering the 2 million glomerular capillaries is filtered. The filtration fraction is the ratio of the glomerular filtration rate (GFR) [125 ml/min] to the renal plasma flow (625 ml/min). Both the GFR and renal plasma flow are regulated in parallel at the afferent arteriole (e.g., constriction decreases both) and inversely at the efferent arteriole (e.g., constriction augments GFR and reduces renal plasma flow). As a result, only changes in efferent arteriolar resistance, not those in afferent arteriolar resistance, affect the ratio of the GFR to the renal plasma flow. Since fluid movement across the glomerulus is governed by Starling's forces, it is proportional to the permeability and surface area of the filtering membrane and to the balance between the hydrostatic and oncotic forces. Ureteral obstruction results in an increase in the hydrostatic pressure in Bowman's capsule, reducing the hydrostatic pressure gradient and, therefore,

the GFR and the filtration fraction. An increase in the plasma oncotic pressure contributes to a decrease in GFR as do decreases in the glomerular capillary hydrostatic pressure and the glomerular filtration area.

64. The answer is D [Chapter 10 IV D 1 c]. The T wave in a normal electrocardiogram is an upward deflection representing ventricular repolarization and occurs during the latter half of ventricular systole.

65. The answer is B [Chapter 38 IV B 2 a, V A 1; Chapter 39 V A Figures 38-8 and 39-1]. In respiratory acidosis, there is a primary increase in plasma CO_2 tension (P_{CO_2}). The renal compensation for respiratory acidosis is increased HCO_3^- reabsorption, which increases the plasma $[HCO_3^-]$. With partial compensation, the pH would not return to normal. Only one set of data (B) indicates hypercapnia with a decrease in pH. Note that the pH and the $[HCO_3^-]/S \cdot P_{CO_2}$ ratio are below normal in this patient, which is consistent with acidosis.

66–68. The answers are: 66-D [Chapter 19 I E 2], **67-E** [Chapter 20 C 2], **68-A** [Chapter 13 II A; Chapter 17 II A]. The major drive for respiration comes from the medullary chemoreceptors, which respond to local H^+ concentration, which, in turn, depends on the CO_2 tension in the surrounding tissues. During the period of increased ventilation, the CO_2 tension in the body is reduced, thus eliminating the respiratory drive until CO_2 again reaches a threshold value at the end of apnea. The medullary chemoreceptors do not respond to changes in O_2 tension and, thus, are not the cause of the apnea.

During positive-pressure ventilation, the intrathoracic pressure increases, which reduces the pressure gradient between the peripheral tissues and the right side of the heart. Thus, venous return and cardiac output decline during positive-pressure ventilation, and the tissues remove more O_2 from each unit of blood as the blood flows through systemic capillaries. Consequently, during positive-pressure ventilation, venous blood contains less O_2 than normal and the mixed venous O_2 tension decreases. The mixed venous O_2 tension would not be less than 40 mm Hg because of the hypoxia that would occur from breathing this gas mixture, which contains only 0.9% less O_2

than air; the hyperventilation would more than make up for the slight reduction in O_2 tension. Hyperventilation causes a decrease in CO_2 tension and an increased pH, both of which would reduce the P_{50} of hemoglobin, not increase it.

The arteriovenous O_2 content difference is calculated by dividing the O_2 consumption by the cardiac output: 240 ml/min ÷ 6 L/min = 40 ml O_2/L of blood. Because the measurements in the question are given in ml/dl, the correct answer is 4 ml/dl.

69. The answer is A [Chapter 22 III D 4 a, Chapter 39 IV A 1 b]. Severe diarrhea causes volume depletion and electrolyte loss, which defines a state of dehydration. It is important to remember that volume depletion refers to effective circulating blood volume. Because intestinal secretions are rich in K^+ and HCO_3^-, diarrhea causes K^+ depletion and HCO_3^- loss, which lead to hypokalemia and metabolic acidosis, respectively. Vomiting, excessive sweating, and water deprivation can lead to volume depletion but not acidosis. In fact, vomiting causes loss of high concentrations of gastric H^+ and Cl^-, which leads to metabolic alkalosis and hypochloremia. Daily sweat production can exceed 10 L in subjects exercising in a hot climate. Severe sweating is associated with a significant loss of K^+, which may contribute to heat stroke.

70. The answer is A [Chapter 54 VIII C 1, Table 54-1, Figure 54-9]. Calcitriol promotes renal tubular reabsorption of both Ca^{2+} and HPO_4^{2-}, leading to hypercalcemia and hyperphosphatemia. Calcitonin has the opposite effects, promoting the excretion of both electrolytes and, thus, leading to hypocalcemia and hypophosphatemia. Aldosterone favors increased reabsorption of Na^+ and increased excretion of K^+, leading to hypokalemia and alkalemia; the [Na^+] usually remains within normal limits because of a commensurate increase in water reabsorption. Progesterone has an anti-aldosterone—like effect, in that it promotes Na^+ excretion.

71. The answer is C [Chapter 22 III A 2 a b]. The initial shrinkage of the red blood cell results from a higher osmotic pressure in the solution than within the cell. However, since the red blood cell eventually returns to its initial volume, the solution must be isotonic. The particles producing the higher osmotic pressure in the solution have reflection coefficients of less than 1 and, thus, are able to diffuse across the membrane. Although these particles initially cause water to flow out of the cell, they eventually reach diffusional equilibrium across the cell membrane and, thus, are unable to keep the water from returning to the cell.

72. The answer is E [Chapter 10 IV B 2]. The terms chest leads, V leads, and precordial leads are synonymous. To determine the axis of any lead, a line is drawn from the electrode site to the electrical zero reference point for the system which, theoretically, lies within the heart. Thus, the axis for each V lead runs from the surface of the chest wall to the heart, which is essentially a horizontal direction.

73. The answer is C [Chapter 30 V A]. Spironolactone is a competitive aldosterone antagonist that interferes with the aldosterone-stimulated Na^+ reabsorption in the distal tubular cell and in the collecting duct. Inhibition of Na^+ reabsorption (elevated Na^+ excretion) is associated with a marked decrease in urinary excretion of K^+ and H^+. Spironolactone is effective as a diuretic in normal subjects or in patients on a low-Na^+ diet, but not in adrenalectomized patients.

74. The answer is A [Chapter 7 II A 2 b]. Fatigue-resistant muscle fibers can contract for long periods of time without fatiguing because their rich capillary supply and a high concentration of mitochondria enable them to generate the amount of adenosine triphosphate (ATP) required for their activity. However, these muscles cannot contract as rapidly [and thus have lower myosin—adenosine triphosphatase (ATPase) activity] or produce as much force as the non-fatigue resistant muscles. Fast-twitch fatigable muscle fibers utilize anaerobic metabolic pathways to provide ATP and therefore have much higher concentrations of glycolytic enzymes than fatigue-resistant fibers.

75. The answer is B [Chapter 16 VIII C]. The alveolar ventilation in patient B is greater than in patient A. Alveolar ventilation is the minute ventilation minus the dead space ventilation, or the respiratory rate times the difference between the tidal volume and the dead space.

Thus, patient B has an alveolar ventilation of 10 · (400 − 150) = 2500 ml/min, whereas patient A has an alveolar ventilation of 20 · (200 − 150) = 1000 ml/min. Dead space ventilation in patient A is 3000 ml/min, whereas in patient B it is 1500 ml/min.

76. The answer is D [Chapter 42 II F]. Gastric motility is controlled primarily by enterogastric reflexes that are elicited when chyme enters the small intestine. The reflexes are both neural and hormonal and act to inhibit gastric contractions. They prevent food from entering the intestine too rapidly. Although distention of the antrum will elicit neuronal and hormonal excitatory reflexes, these reflexes are overcome by the inhibitory enterogastric reflexes.

77. The answer is D [Chapter 51 I H 4 d, J 3 h (1) (2)]. During the postovulatory phase of the menstrual cycle, the thickened, secretory endometrium depends on the continued presence of estradiol and progesterone. If fertilization does not occur, the corpus luteum remains functional for 13–14 days and then undergoes regression (luteolysis). After the regressing corpus luteum loses its ability to produce adequate amounts of estradiol and progesterone, the innermost layer (adluminal, or stratum functionale, layer) of the endometrium becomes ischemic, degenerates, becomes necrotic, and is sloughed into the uterine cavity. The loss of proliferated endometrium (stratum functionale) is accompanied by bleeding known as menstruation (menses). The discontinuation of oral contraceptives after 3 weeks also permits menstruation.

78. The answer is B [Chapter 10 IV D 2 c]. A positive QRS complex recorded from a unipolar electrode indicates that the electrical vector is directed toward the electrode. With positive QRS complexes in leads aVr and aVf, the vector must lie in the right axis deviation (RAD) quadrant. A mean electrical axis between 0° and 90° would indicate that the vector lies in the normal quadrant, whereas left ventricular hypertrophy would place the vector in the left axis deviation (LAD) quadrant.

79. The answer is E [Chapter 22 III H Table 22-5]. As a result of the hemorrhage, this patient has undergone the loss of water and electrolytes in isotonic concentration leading to

dehydration [reduced extracellular fluid (ECF) volume]. In this patient, there will be no net water movement across the cell membranes because both NaCl and water are administered as 1 L of isotonic (isosmotic) NaCl. Because the administered NaCl will remain initially in the extracellular space, the only effects will be a 1 L increase in the ECF volume and a dilution of the plasma protein concentration, the latter effect accounting for the decrease in the plasma colloid oncotic pressure. A 0.9% NaCl solution is isotonic because it maintains the normal red blood cell volume. Furthermore, this 0.9% NaCl solution contains dissociated Na^+ and Cl^-, each in a concentration of 150 mEq/L. Because NaCl is an electrolyte, this same solution is equivalent to a concentration of 300 mOsm/L, assuming 100% dissociation of NaCl. Thus, a 150 mmol/L NaCl solution is isotonic and isosmotic to human plasma. Following the infusion of 1 liter of saline the ISF volume increases by 750 ml and the plasma volume increases by 250 ml.

80. The answer is A [Chapter 3 III B 2 b; Table 3-1]. The pacemaker cells of the heart contain muscarinic receptors, which are activated by acetylcholine (ACh). When the ACh receptor on these cells is activated, K^+ conductance is increased, which causes the membrane to hyperpolarize and slows pacemaker activity.

81. The answer is C [Chapter 48 VIII A 3 b c, Chapter 52 D 1 c d, Figure 52-4, Table 52-5]. Epinephrine is a potent hyperglycemic agent for several reasons. It stimulates α-adrenergic receptors on the pancreatic beta cell, inhibiting insulin secretion and, therefore, subsequent facilitated transport of glucose by muscle and adipose tissue. Epinephrine also promotes hepatic and muscle glycogenolysis by activating cyclic adenosine 3′,5′-monophosphate (cAMP)-dependent phosphorylase; glycolysis in muscle leads to an increase in the plasma level of lactate, which provides the liver with an important glyconeogenic substrate. The lipolytic effect of epinephrine mobilizes free fatty acids, which enhances gluconeogenesis. Additionally, catecholamines directly inhibit peripheral glucose uptake, partly due to the suppression of glucose transporters. All of these effects of epinephrine are amplified in the absence of insulin.

82. The answer is D [Chapter 16 V B 1 a]. The interpleural pressure during the expiratory maneuver would be 15 cm H_2O. Before the Valsalva maneuver, the transmural pressure across the lungs (i.e., the transpulmonary pressure) is equal to the alveolar pressure minus the interpleural pressure, or $0 - (-5) = 5$ cm H_2O. Because lung volume remained constant, the transmural pressure must also remain constant during the Valsalva maneuver, so that when the alveolar pressure increases to 20 cm H_2O, the interpleural pressure must equal 15 cm H_2O in order to maintain the difference of 5 cm H_2O between the inside and outside of the lungs.

83–85. The answers are: 83-B [Chapter 11 II A 2], **84-E** [Chapter 11 II A 3 b], **85-D** [Chapter 11 II A 3 c]. The ventricular volume curve is distinctive because of the decline during systole and the rise during diastole, which can be timed from the relationship with the electrocardiogram (EKG) tracing.

Rapid filling begins with the opening of the atrioventricular (AV) valves early in diastole. Diastole normally begins shortly after the end of the T wave and is indicated by the occurrence of the second heart sound (S_2, not shown).

The duration of diastole (interval C) is largely determined by the heart rate; obviously, when the heart rate increases, the duration of the cardiac cycle shortens. The period of systole also shortens with an increase in heart rate, but is not affected as much as diastole. At very high heart rates, the stroke volume is reduced because the abbreviated diastole renders the ventricular filling time inadequate. Thus, it is important to terminate ventricular tachycardia because of the reduced cardiac output that results from the rapid rate.

86. The answer is E [Chapter 7 VI A 2 a, C 1]. The flocculonodular lobe is also called the vestibulocerebellum to indicate its association with the vestibular system. Lesions within the flocculonodular lobe, like those within the vestibular system, result in a loss of balance (i.e., ataxia). The inability to make rapid, alternating movements (dysdiadochokinesia) or to smoothly reach toward a target is a sign of posterior cerebellar disease. Resting tremors or spontaneous movements are signs of basal ganglia disease. A loss of muscle strength is related to lower motor neuron or muscle disease.

87. The answer is D [Chapter 22 III E 1 a b, Tables 22-1 and 22-4, Figures 22-2]. Assuming complete dissociation, this 0.15 mol/L solution of sodium chloride (NaCl) is equivalent to a solution of 300 mOsm/L (0.15 mol/L of Na^+ + 0.15 mol/L of Cl^-). Because this NaCl solution is osmotically balanced with body fluids, there is no shift of water between the major fluid compartments. Thus, the extracellular fluid (ECF) volume increases with no change in the osmolar concentration of the ECF or intracellular fluid (ICF) compartment.

88. The answer is B [Chapter 38 II B 1 b, V B 2, Figure 38-8; Chapter 39 IV B 1, 2, Figure 39-1]. The severe loss of gastric fluid in this patient would produce metabolic alkalosis due to the loss of HCl (a noncarbonic acid). She also would exhibit hypovolemia due to the fluid loss. The development of alkalosis is sensed by the chemoreceptors controlling ventilation, resulting in hypoventilation, and an increase in the arterial CO_2 tension (hypercapnia), which reduces the pH toward normal. The kidneys would be expected to excrete the excess bicarbonate, raising the urinary pH.

89. The answer is A [Chapter 41 III B 2]. The formation of HCl by the parietal cells is a two-step process. First, Cl^- is transported into the parietal cell canaliculi. The negative potential developed by the flow of Cl^- allows K^+ to flow into the canaliculi. The K^+ is then actively transported out of the canaliculi in exchange for H^+. Since both K^+ and H^+ are transported against their concentration gradients, an active transport system (H^+-K^+-ATPase) is required.

90. The answer is A [Chapter 49 II C 4 a–f, Figure 49-7]. A deficiency of 17α-hydroxylase leads to reduction in the 17α-hydroxylation of pregnenolone and progesterone, resulting in hypogonadism and elevated blood gonadotropin levels. This enzyme deficiency also leads to increased production of 11-deoxycorticosterone (11-DOC). This mineralocorticoid causes Na^+ retention, extracellular volume expansion, and hypertension—effects that suppress renin and aldosterone secretion. The 17α-hydroxylase defect also affects the gonads, preventing testicular and adrenal androgen synthesis in males and ovarian estrogen synthesis in females and, thus, resulting in a female phenotype regardless of genotypic sex. These patients require not only cortisol to suppress adrenocorticotropic hormone (ACTH) secretion but also sex steroid treatment consistent with the genotypic sex. The two substrates for 17α-hydroxylase are pregnenolone and progesterone.

91. The answer is C [Chapter 41 III D; V; Chapter 42 VII B 2]. A significant amount of protein digestion occurs in the stomach because of the action of hydrochloric acid (HCl), which begins to break proteins apart, and pepsin, a protease enzyme secreted by gastric chief cells. These protein digestion products then act as secretagogues that stimulate the secretion of pancreatic proteases.

92. The answer is C [Chapter 34 IV C 2 b, V B 2; Chapter 38 III B 2, IV C 1]. From the data given, this patient's arterial CO_2 tension (PCO_2) is determined to be 50 mm Hg (normal = 40 mm Hg). The Henderson equation is used to estimate PCO_2, but $[H^+]$ must be determined first by using the Henderson-Hasselbalch equation. Given a pH of 7.5, $[H^+]$ is calculated as:

$$[H^+] = antilog\ (9 - pH)$$

$$= antilog\ (9 - 7.5)$$

$$= antilog\ 1.5 = 31.6\ nmol/L$$

Substituting to solve for PCO_2,

$$PCO_2 = \frac{[H^+]\ [HCO_3^-]}{24}$$

$$= \frac{(31.6\ nmol/L)\ (38\ mmol/L)}{24}$$

$$= 50\ mm\ Hg$$

This patient's increased bicarbonate concentration ($[HCO_3^-]$) indicates a metabolic alkalosis. The elevated bicarbonate levels suppress respiratory drive, leading to compensatory elevation of CO_2 tension. Note that unit analysis cannot be used in this equation.

93. The answer is D [Chapter 10 IV A 2, B 2, C 2]. The largest deflection in the electrocardiogram (EKG) occurs when the electrical vector is parallel to the lead axis. Lead aVL lies at −30, and therefore should exhibit the largest deflection of any lead.

94–97. The answers are: 94-D, 95-B, 96-D, 97-B [Chapter 22 A 2, B 1 a b, 2, II B 1 c,

Table 22-1], The man's plasma volume is equal to the Evans blue space, which is 3 L. Because his plasma volume represents 60% of his blood volume, the total blood volume is calculated by dividing the Evans blue space by 0.6, or:

$$Blood\ volume\ (L) = \frac{plasma\ volume\ (L)}{(1 - hematocrit)}$$

$$Blood\ volume = \frac{3\ L}{0.6} = 5\ L$$

The interstitial fluid volume cannot be calculated directly by the dilution principle because there is no substance that is confined to the interstitial fluid space. Because the interstitial fluid space constitutes part of the extracellular fluid (ECF) volume, it can be determined by subtracting the plasma volume from the ECF. The ECF volume of this man is equal to the inulin space. Therefore, the interstitial fluid volume equals the inulin space minus the Evans blue space (8 L − 3 L), or 5 L.

The ECF volume is determined directly by the dilution of such substances as inulin, mannitol, sucrose, thiosulfate, radiosodium, and radiochloride. Thus, the volume of the ECF is equal to the inulin space, which is given as 8 L.

The mathematical relationship between lean body mass (LBM) and total body water (TBW) is:

$$TBW\ (L) = 0.7\ LBM\ (kg)$$

Therefore,

$$LBM\ (kg) = \frac{TBW\ (L)}{0.7}$$

Because the total body water is given as the tritiated water space, the calculation is:

$$LBM\ (kg) = \frac{35\ L}{0.7} = 50\ L$$

Because 50 L of water weighs 50 kg, the 50 kg LBM must be subtracted from the 60 kg body weight, leaving 10 kg (i.e., the weight of the body fat).

98. The answer is B [Chapter 29 I A–B] Antidiuretic hormone (ADH), also known as arginine vasopressin, is an octapeptide synthesized mainly in the supraoptic nucleus of the ventral diencephalon. ADH also can be classified as a nonapeptide, if the single cystine moiety is counted as two cysteine residues.

ADH is stored in the pars nervosa, from which it is secreted.

ADH regulates plasma osmolality, which normally is about 300 mOsm/kg. It promotes water reabsorption mainly from the tubular fluid in the renal collecting ducts by increasing the water permeability of these cells. ADH allows humans to elaborate a small volume, hypertonic urine in order to conserve water. Because ADH promotes free-water reabsorption, it determines the plasma [Na^+].

99. The answer is C [Chapter 6 I B (3)]. The axial length of the eye in an individual with normal eyesight (i.e., an emmetrope) is equal to the eye's focal length, which is equal to the reciprocal of its power. Because the power of the eye is 60 diopters (D), the axial length is 0.0167 meters (16.7 mm). The power of a lens required to focus an image at a given distance from the lens can be determined using the lens formula:

$$P = \frac{1}{o} + \frac{1}{i} = \frac{1}{f}, \text{ where}$$

o, i, and f are the object, image, and focal distances respectively (in meters) and P is the power of the lens (in diopters). Because the axial length is 0.0167 meters and the object is placed 0.25 meters from the lens, the total power of the lens must be 64 diopters in order to focus the object. Thus, the converging power of the lens must increase by 4 diopters.

100. The answer is C [Chapter 24 II A 1 a (1), Figure 24-2]. The Na^+-dependent reabsorption of glucose is blocked by phlorizin, a phenolic glycoside. Thus, this competitive inhibitor virtually blocks the secondary active transport of glucose by the proximal tubule, which leads to glycosuria. Therefore, following phlorizin administration, the clearance of glucose becomes equal to the clearance of inulin. Curve C depicts the clearance curve for a filtered substance that is neither reabsorbed nor secreted, such as inulin.

101. The answer is B [Chapter 11 II A 2 b (2)]. Closure of the AV valves isolates the left ventricular chamber, because the aortic valves are closed also as a result of the diastolic aortic pressure. Because both inflow and outflow valves are closed, there is no change in ventricular volume for a time; hence, the interval is called isovolumic (equal or constant volume) contraction.

102. The answer is A [Chapter 16 III C 1–2]. This patient has an alveolar-to-arterial O_2 tension difference of 35 mm Hg. To calculate this, the alveolar O_2 tension (PAO_2) must be determined using the alveolar gas equation. Given an arterial CO_2 tension of 30 mm Hg, the alveolar O_2 tension is determined as:

$$PAO_2 = (760 - 47) \cdot 0.21 - 30$$
$$= 150 - 30 = 120 \text{ mm Hg}$$

Thus, the alveolar-to-arterial O_2 tension difference is 120 − 85, or 35 mm Hg. This patient's low arterial CO_2 tension and high pH indicate that he has respiratory alkalosis; thus, he has been hyperventilating and does not have metabolic alkalosis. Respiratory alkalosis causes a decrease in plasma bicarbonate levels due to the slope of the blood buffer line. Lastly, chronic obstructive pulmonary disease (COPD) leads to hypoxia and CO_2 retention, not hyperventilation.

103. The answer is B [Chapter 24 A b (2); Chapter 27 B 1 a, b (2)]. To measure the reabsorptive capacity it is necessary to subtract the amount excreted ($\dot{E}$) from the amount filtered ($\dot{F}$). Therefore, the filtered load must be determined first from the product of GFR (C_{in}) and the plasma glucose concentration.

The filtered load can be determined by $C_{in} \cdot P = \dot{F}$:

$$C_{in} = \frac{U_{in} \cdot \dot{V}}{P_{in}} = \frac{90 \cdot 2}{1.5}$$
$$= 120 \text{ ml/min}$$

$$F = C_{in} \cdot P_{GI} = 120 \cdot 0.9 = 108 \text{ mg/min}$$

The amount excreted = $U_{GI} \cdot \dot{V}$. Because glucose does not appear in the urine, the excretion of glucose is zero. The amount filtered is completely reabsorbed and, therefore, the amount filtered is equal to the amount reabsorbed, because the plasma glucose concentration is below the renal threshold (180 mg/ml).

104. The answer is B [Chapter 24 A b (2); Chapter 27 B 1 a, b (2)]. To assess the process used by the kidney to transport substance X, it is necessary to calculate the clearance of substance X and compare it with the clearance of inulin (120 ml/min):

$$C_x = \frac{U_x \cdot \dot{V}}{P_x}$$

$$= \frac{100 \cdot 2}{2} = 100 \text{ ml/min}$$

The clearance of substance X (100 ml/min) is less than the clearance of inulin; therefore, on a net basis substance X is reabsorbed. Furthermore, because the clearance of X is less than the clearance of inulin, substance X cannot be used to measure the glomerular filtration rate (GFR).

105. The answer is B [Chapter 27 I B II A, B, Figure 27-1 A]. At plasma glucose concentrations below the renal threshold, the filtered glucose has not exceeded the maximum carrier-mediated transport rate (Tm) for glucose. Therefore, all the glucose that is filtered is reabsorbed until the Tm is reached.

106. The answer is D [Chapter 27 I B II A, B, Figure 27-1 A]. The excretion curve for glucose (curve D) intersects the reabsorption curve for glucose (curve Z) at point D. At this point, the excretion rate of glucose is equal to the reabsorption rate of glucose.

107. The answer is B [Chapter 27 I B II A, B, Figure 27-1 A]. Below the renal threshold for glucose (point C), the carriers are not saturated with glucose, and the transport of glucose is a first-order reaction. Not until the transport maximum for glucose is reached does the transport of glucose become a zero-order reaction (i.e., the transport curve exhibits saturation kinetics, which is characteristic of all carrier-mediated transport curves). Therefore, below the renal threshold, all the filtered glucose is reabsorbed.

108. The answer is A [Chapter 27 I B II A, B, Figure 27-1 A]. Curve X is the filtered load curve for glucose; curve Z depicts the reabsorption of this glucose. However, inulin is a substance that is only filtered and neither reabsorbed nor secreted. Because all the filtered inulin is excreted, the filtered load curve and the excretion curve for inulin are the same curve, curve X.

109. The answer is B [Chapter 23 III C; Chapter 27 III B 1–3 Figure 27-3]. Two-thirds of proximal Na^+ reabsorption is transcellular and active, while one-third of the proximal reab-

sorption is paracellular and passive. In the thin ascending limb of the loop of Henle (ALH), NaCl transport occurs by simple diffusion while the Na^+ transport in the thick ALH is activated via the Na^+–2Cl^-–K^+ symporter, an electroneutral transporter. In the collecting duct, Na^+ is transported through Na^+-conductive channels in the luminal membrane of the **principal** cell. It is important to appreciate that the Na^+ entering the epithelial (luminal) cells is actively transported by the basolateral Na^+–K^+–ATPase pump or can leave the cell via the 3 HCO_3^-–Na^+ cotransporter.

110. The answer is A [Chapter 25 I A]. Starling forces regulate NaCl and water reabsorption across the proximal tubule. Starling forces between the intercellular space and the peritubular capillaries facilitate the movement of the reabsorbed substances into the capillaries. Starling forces that favor reabsortion are the capillary oncotic pressure and the hydrostatic pressure in the intercellular space. The opposing Starling forces are the interstitial oncotic pressure and the capillary hydrostatic pressure. Starling forces do not affect transport by the loop of Henle, distal tubule, and collecting duct because these segments are less permeable to water than the proximal tubule.

111. The answer is A [Chapter 28 I B, D 3, V A 2 b, D 1 Figure 28-2; Chapter 29 III C 1, Figure 29-4]. Antidiuretic hormone (ADH) increases the permeability of the medullary collecting duct to both water and urea. In the presence of ADH, the osmolality of the tubular fluid in the collecting duct increases as water is reabsorbed, and the urea permeability of medullary collecting duct also increases. Because water reabsorption increases the tubular fluid urea concentration in the collecting duct, some urea diffuses into the interstitium. The urine produced when ADH is high can attain an osmolality of 1200 mOsm/kg H_2O and contains high concentrations of urea and other unreabsorbed solutes. Because urea in the tubular fluid equilibrates with urea in the interstitium, its concentration in urine is similar to that in the interstitium. The medullary osmolality would decrease with a decrease in NaCl reabsorption by the ascending limb of the loop of Henle (ALH) or by the suppression of ADH secretion by water ingestion. Finally, an increase in vasa recta flow rate would also dissipate the medullary interstitial gradient.

112. The answer is A [Chapter 22 III H 1, Table 22-4; Chapter 29 II A 1 a (2) (a), Figures

29-1A and 29-3]. The major physiologic stimulus for antidiuretic hormone (ADH) secretion is an increase in plasma osmolality (P_{osm}). This site of stimulation is the hypothalamus where the osmoreceptors (chemoreceptors) are located. Hypernatremia is not a stimulus for aldosterone or renin secretion. The release of ADH would lead to increased free-water reabsorption (a decrease in free-water excretion). Finally, with the hypernatremia there is a reduction in aldosterone secretion, which would lead to increased excretion of Na^+.

113. The answer is E [Chapter 30 III B 3, 5 c, d, Figure 30-4]. A drug that blocks angiotensin-converting enzyme (ACE) would be expected to lead to an increase in angiotensin I, which is proximal to the block, as well as an increase in renin secretion. Now the negative feedback by aldosterone on renin secretion is lost. With the decline in angiotensin II and aldosterone, there is a much reduced Na^+ reabsorption by the proximal tubules and the collecting ducts. The resultant loss of body Na^+ causes contraction of the extracellular fluid (ECF) volume; a fall in blood pressure; and a predicted compensatory increase in sympathetic nervous system activity, which increase norepinephrine secretion.

114. The answer is E [Chapter 54 VII C 6]. Of the actions listed for PTH, the only correct physiologic action is renal gluconeogenesis in the proximal tubule. Otherwise, PTH promotes Ca^{2+} retention via its renal and bone effects. It is important to appreciate that the increase in intestinal Ca^{2+} absorption assigned to PTH is mediated by $1,25(OH)_2D_3$, which is increased via the PTH activation of renal 1α-hydroxylase. Therefore, intestinal Ca^{2+} and phosphate are not major actions of PTH.

115. The answer is B [Chapter 54 VI A 4, Figure 54-4]. Elevated PTH levels lead to activation of renal 1α-hydroxylase activity and the subsequent elevation of the synthesis of $1,25(OH)_2D_3$. Hypophosphatemia is another direct stimulus for 1α-hydroxylase. Further, hypocalcemia indirectly leads to increased $1,25(OH)_2D_3$ synthesis via the resultant increase in PTH secretion. The consequences of decreased phosphate loads are problematic because low phosphate loads raise plasma ionized calcium concentration, increase synthesis of $1,25(OH)_2D_3$ which, in turn, increases intestinal absorption of both Ca^{2+} and phosphate

and bone resorption. The decreased plasma PTH level leads to an increased retention of tubular phosphate. Of these choices, only hepatic (or renal) disease causes a reduction in calcitriol synthesis. In hepatic disease there is a decline in 25-hydroxylase activity with a consequent reduction in $25\ OH\ D_3$ synthesis. This form of vitamin D_3 is the substrate for renal formation of calcitriol. Increased oral phosphate will complex with Ca^{2+} in the gut, decreasing the amount of Ca^{2+} available for absorption, and can complex with Ca^{2+} in the bone, resulting in a decreased filtered load of Ca^{2+}.

116. The answer is C [Chapter 28 IV A 2, B 1 c, Figure 28-3]. The highest tubular fluid urea concentration along the nephron is found in the medullary collecting duct in the presence of antidiuretic hormone (ADH). ADH increases the permeability of the collecting duct to water and urea. The reabsorption of water in the collecting duct leads to the increased concentration of urea and subsequently its reabsorption into the medullary interstitium. Urea can enter the thin ascending limb of the loop of Henle (ALH) and, to a much lesser extent, the thin descending limb of the loop of Henle (DLH).

117. The answer is B. [Chapter 22 III G 2, H 1, Table 22-4]. Antidiuretic hormone regulates Na^+ concentration by its action on free-water reabsorption, and aldosterone regulates plasma volume by its effect on the *amount* of Na^+ reabsorbed. Aldosterone does not determine the Na^+ *concentration*. Changes in Na^+ concentration are almost always due to changes in water balance, which is regulated by ADH. Thus, plasma Na+ concentration is an index of water metabolism and not Na^+ metabolism.

118. The answer is D [Chapter 45 IV F, Table 45-2]. Hormone receptors are proteins whose concentration and activity are regulated. Increased or decreased concentrations of receptors enhance or reduce the biological response, respectively. In hyperthyroidism, thyroid hormone increases β-adrenergic receptors (e.g., in the myocardium) without altering plasma concentration of catecholamines. Resulting biological effects are similar to those resulting from an infusion of epinephrine. Homologous (the same hormone) and heterologous (another hormone) regulation of receptors occurs commonly and is an important mechanism for regulation and integration of endocrine responses. For example, follicle-stimulating hormone (FSH) stimulates the production of luteinizing hormone (LH) receptors in ovarian granulosa cells and testicular Leydig cells. Thus, regulation of receptors is as common and as important as regulation of hormone biosynthesis and metabolism. All hormones are allosteric effectors and require specific allosteric (hormone receptors) for biological activity.

Finally, at the level of the receptor, many peptide hormones produce a maximal biological response when only a fraction of the total cell-surface receptors are occupied. For example, insulin stimulation of glucose transport in adipocytes is maximal when only about 2% of all insulin receptors are occupied.

119. The answer is C [Chapter 47 II A 2 a, 3 b]. Of the tissues listed, only the pars distalis synthesizes hormones (pituitary tropic hormones). The median eminence and the pars nervosa do not synthesize hormones. Rather, they are storage depots and release centers for hypothalamic hormones [hypophysiotropic hormones, oxytocin, and antidiuretic hormone (ADH)]. The pars tuberalis does not produce hormones, and in humans, the pars intermedia is a vestigial structure that is essentially devoid of function in hormone biosynthesis.

120. The answer is D [Chapter 47 IV A 3 d]. Growth hormone (GH) counteracts the action of insulin, thereby decreasing the uptake of glucose by muscle and fat (GLUT-4). For this reason, it is common for acromegalic patients to exhibit insulin resistance (glucose intolerance). All of the other choices result in increases in response to high levels of GH.

121. The answer is A [Chapter 48 II A 2]. The adrenal medulla is a unique autonomic neuroeffector in that it receives only a sympathetic preganglionic innervation. The major secretory product in the adult is epinephrine. Acetylcholine (ACh) precedes adrenomedullary catecholamine secretion by depolarization of the chromaffin cells. Bilateral adrenalectomy results in a precipitous decline in plasma epinephrine with little change in plasma norepinephrine. Hence, the major source of epinephrine in the body is the adrenal medulla, and the major source of norepinephrine is the postganglionic neuron pool of the sympathetic nervous system.

122. The answer is D [Chapter 49 II C 2, Figure 49-7]. The boy is dehydrated, which is consistent with a fall in mineralocorticoid secretion, namely, a 21-hydroxylase deficiency. This deficiency would also cause the accelerated sexual development. Therefore, the diagnosis is a 21-hydroxylase deficiency leading to sexual precocity (pseudosexual precocity) and loss of Na^+, hypotension, increased plasma renin activity, and dehydration [decreased extracellular fluid (ECF) volume]. His plasma K^+ concentration would be elevated, and his acid–base state would be metabolic acidosis, not metabolic alkalosis.

The boy exhibits sexual precocity due to the elevation of plasma 17-ketosteroids [dehydroepiandrosterone (DHEA)], some of which are converted into testosterone. He exhibits advanced linear growth due to the hyperandrogenism. Therefore, in his early life he will be taller than his age-matched cohorts. As an adult he will be shorter than his cohorts due to earlier epiphysial closure. He clearly has congenital adrenal hyperplasia (CAH).

If he had an 11β-hydroxylase deficiency, he would be hypertensive because of the increased Na^+ retention resulting from hypermineralocorticoidism of deoxycorticosterone (DOC). The sexual manifestations would be consistent with this deficiency.

It is important to appreciate that this patient has the same electrolyte and blood pressure changes observed in primary adrenal insufficiency; however, this patient would differ in that his adrenal cortices would be hypertrophic. Bilateral atrophy of the adrenal glands is characteristic of patients with Addison's disease.

123. The answer is A [Chapter 50 IV B 3, Figures 50-7 and 50-8; VI B 2 Table 50-7]. The continued injection of high amounts of testosterone will cause prostatic hypertrophy, but such treatment also increases negative feedback inhibition of Gn RH, LH, and FSH, leading to declines in spermatogenesis, inhibin secretion (Sertoli cell), testosterone secretion (Leydig cell), and testicular size.

124. The answer is D [Chapter 47 II C 1 Figure 46-2]. This woman's inability to lactate and to menstruate following parturition stems from pituitary failure related to the massive bleeding she experienced during delivery. Most likely, this woman has postpartum pituitary necrosis (Sheehan's syndrome), resulting from ischemia of the hypophysial portal system, which supplies 90% of the blood to the anterior pituitary gland. The resultant pituitary failure may be complete (panhypopituitarism) or partial. In this case, the acidophils responsible for production of prolactin, follicle-stimulating hormone (FSH), and luteinizing hormone (LH) were affected, resulting in this patient's inability to lactate and to menstruate. This patient also would exhibit hypoglycemia because of low plasma growth hormone (GH) levels and low plasma adrenocorticotropic hormone (ACTH) levels, which would lead to decreased secretion of cortisol (a potent hyperglycemic hormone) and decreased synthesis of epinephrine (a hyperglycemic hormone that depends on cortisol). The decreased levels of these hyperglycemic hormones would cause insulin sensitivity.

Because aldosterone secretion does not depend mainly on ACTH secretion, this patient should be able to regulate Na$^+$ balance. She also should have normal antidiuretic hormone (ADH) activity, because the supraoptic nuclei and pars nervosa are not perfused by the hypophysial portal system. Thus, this patient should demonstrate normal water balance.

125. The answer is A [Chapter 38 Case 1, Discussion of Question 7]. In type 1 diabetes antidiuretic hormone (ADH) secretion is elevated in response to hyperglycemia; however, the osmotic load in renal tubules provides a larger vector, which leads to diuresis. This osmotic diuresis leads to urinary loss of Na$^+$ and K$^+$. The association of these cations with the high concentration of tubular fluid ketoacid anions contributes further to their loss. Insulin lack also decreases K$^+$ influx into cells and leads to hyperkalemia. The ketoacidosis increases alveolar ventilation, leading to a reduced PCO$_2$. Since the compensatory response is renal, there is an increase in titratable acid and ammonium excretion. The increased loss of H$^+$ in the form of titratable acid leads to the excretion of an acid urine. The increased renal secretion of H$^+$ promotes the renal retention of HCO$_3^-$, which depends on acid secretion.

126. The answer is E [Chapter 52 IX Table 53-2]. From the clinical manifestations, this woman has adult hypothyroidism (myxedema). The increased sensitivity of the pituitary thyrotropes indicates that the plasma thyroid hormone levels are low. The hypersensitivity of the thyrotropes is clearly demonstrated by the release of thyrotropin (TSH) in response to the thyroid-releasing hormone (TRH)-stimulation test. This response rules out any malfunction in the pituitary or thyroid glands.

127. The answer is D [Chapter 29 II A 1 a Table 29-1, Figures 29-1 A and B and 29-3]. Drinking and absorbing 0.5 L of 600 milliosmolar NaCl (hypertonic NaCl) would increase the osmolality of the extracellular fluid (ECF), thus increasing antidiuretic hormone (ADH) secretion. One liter of isotonic saline (A) would not alter osmolality but would expand plasma volume, causing atrial, venous, and arterial baroreceptors to send increased signals to the hypothalamus, and inhibit ADH secretion. Weightlessness (B) shifts blood for the limbs to the abdomen and chest causing the baroreceptors to be stimulated, and again suppressing ADH secretion. In right heart failure (C), the backed-up blood distends the atria and large veins, causing baroreceptors stimulation and inhibition of ADH secretion. Drinking 1 L of tap water (E) would have the opposite effect on ECF osmolality and ADH secretion.

128. The answer is A [Chapter 30 III Table 30-1]. Aldosterone secretion is primarily stimulated by an increase in plasma K$^+$ concentration (hyperkalemia) and the renin–angiotensin II–aldosterone system through a chemoreceptor (macula densa) and a baroreceptor (juxta-glomerular cell). Thus, a decreased NaCl delivery (load) to the macula densa leads to increased renin secretion, with a consequent increase in aldosterone secretion. Hypervolemia produced by the infusion of an isotonic NaCl solution is a negative signal for aldosterone secretion.

129. The answer is B [Chapter 26 I Figure 26-1]. The cardiac effects of increased sympathetic discharge are increased contractility and heart rate. With a fall in the effective circulating volume (ECV), there is an increase in sympathetic neural tone and the secretion of catecholamines (norepinephrine and epinephrine) as evidenced by tachycardia and increased afterload (peripheral resistance). Volume depletion induces a characteristic sequence of compensatory hemodynamic responses. The initial volume deficit results in decreases in the plasma volume and venous return to the heart. Cardiopulmonary receptors in the atria and pulmonary veins sense the decline in the venous return, leading to sympathetically mediated vasoconstriction in the skin and skeletal muscle, resulting in increased peripheral vascular resistance (PVR). The fall in cardiac output lowers the systemic arterial pressure, which is sensed by the carotid sinus and aortic arch baroreceptors. This decline potentiates the increase in sympathetic activity that now involves the splanchnic and renal circulations.

The renal effects of increased sympathetic output include afferent and efferent arteriolar constriction, increased filtration fraction [larger decline in renal blood flow compared to glomerular filtration rate (GFR)], and greater angiotensin II formation due to increased renin secretion. The octapeptide contributes to the vasoconstriction and both direct and indirect (aldosterone) increases in Na$^+$ and water retention. Effective volume depletion and increased solute-free water reabsorption increase antidiuretic hormone (ADH) [reduced solute-free water excretion].

130. The answer is B [Chapter 22 III D 4 b, Figure 22-2A2, F 2, Case 1]. The excessive sweating that occurs in this environment leads to hyperosmotic dehydration. Sweat is a hypotonic fluid, and therefore the body loses proportionately more water than solute. At osmotic equilibrium, both the extracellular fluid (ECF) and intracellular fluid (ICF) lose volume, and the osmolarity of both compartments is elevated.

To determine the answer, it is necessary to look at each variable singly (i.e., to look first at the answers in the downward and vertical direction and then move to the right at the next variable). Thus, the ICF volume decreases, the ICF osmolarity increases, the ECF Na$^+$ concentration is elevated, and the ECF osmolarity (due mainly to Na$^+$) is increased (choice B). The increased ECF osmolarity and the decreased ECF volume stimulate antidiuretic hormone (ADH) secretion and the formation of a small-volume hypertonic urine (increased U_{osm}), together with an increased thirst drive. The decrease in ECF volume also triggers renin release, leading to angiotenin II formation, which, in turn, stimulates aldosterone and ADH secretion along with thirst drive. It is imperative to appreciate that loss of sweat requires water retention (ADH) and Na$^+$ retention (aldosterone). In short, hypovolemia necessitates Na$^+$ to cause volume repletion. Replacement of water without Na$^+$ retention leads to a continued thirst drive due to a hypovolemic stimulus.

131. The answer is D [Chapter 27 I B 1 a]. The filtered load is calculated as the product of the glomerular filtration rate (GFR) and plasma solute (inulin) concentration. However, the GFR is not known, but because inulin is only filtered (not reabsorbed or secreted), the amount excreted and the filtered load are the same. Therefore, it is necessary only to calculate the amount excreted ($\dot{E}$), which is the product of urinary solute (inulin) concentration and urine flow rate ($\dot{V}$).

$$\dot{E} = U_{in} \cdot \dot{V}$$

$$\dot{E} = 480 \cdot 1.5 = 720 \text{ mg/min}$$

Note that the filtered load (GFR $\cdot$ P) is equal to $C_{in} \cdot P_{in}$. The C_{in} is also the GFR ($U_{in} \div P_{in}$) which is 120 ml/min.

132. The answer is B [Chapter 23 III C 5, Figure 23-2B Chapter 27 III C 7 b]. Bulk flow (convection) is the movement "en masse" of a given volume of fluid that occurs when water flows through a channel. All of the other transporters listed exist either in the luminal membrane (Na$^+$–glucose cotransport, Na$^+$–H$^+$ countertransport, and Na$^+$ conductive channels) or in the basolateral membrane (Na$^+$–K$^+$–ATPase pump).

Water can move through a membrane by diffusion (osmosis) or bulk flow. The driving force for bulk flow is a hydrostatic pressure gradient. The existence of bulk flow can generate another transport mechanism for dissolved solutes called solvent drag where the solutes are swept along in the moving stream of solvent. It is important to differentiate diffusion from bulk flow where the driving force for diffusion is a concentration gradient.

133. The answer is A [Chapter 24 II A 1 b (2), 2 a (2)]. A substance that is filtered and reabsorbed (e.g., glucose, urea) has a clearance lower than inulin, which is not reabsorbed at all. Furthermore, reabsorbed substances have lower clearances than substances that are secreted [e.g., creatinine, *para*-aminohippuric acid (PAH)]. Actively reabsorbed substances (e.g., glucose, amino acids) have lower concentrations in the collecting duct, even though water continues to be reabsorbed, tending to concentrate substances.

134. The answer is A [Chapter 48 VII Table 48-1]. The ciliary muscle is innervated by both postganglionic sympathetic and postganglionic parasympathetic fibers. Only β-adrenergic, not α-adrenergic, receptors are found in this smooth muscle. β-Adrenergic stimulation causes relaxation of the ciliary muscle, which, in turn, increases the tension on the lens, causing the lens to become thinner and adapted for far vision. The parasympathetic innervation of the ciliary muscle causes it to contract, which, in turn, decreases the tension on the lens, causing the lens to become thick and adapted for near vision (accommodation). The heart contains only β-adrenergic receptors, whereas vascular smooth muscle, pancreatic beta cells, and intestinal smooth muscle contain both α- and β-adrenergic receptors. Stimulation of either type of receptor in the intestine causes inhibition of peristalsis.

135. The answer is E [Chapter 32 IV B 5 a b e]. Acids that can be converted to carbonic acid are classified as volatile acids. Carbonic acid is called a volatile acid because it can be dehydrated into CO_2 and H_2O and excreted from the body by pulmonary ventilation. In high amounts, many volatile acids are excreted by the kidneys without being converted to CO_2 and H_2O and, thus, are classified as nonvolatile acids. Examples of such acids are citric, isocitric, acetic, lactic acids, and the ketoacids. Acetic acid levels can increase following the ingestion of even small amounts of vinegar. All of these acids can be either eliminated by pulmonary ventilation or excreted by the kidneys. Thus, it is important to remember that nonvolatile (fixed) acids are dissociated at body pH, and the H^+ can be excreted via the urine.

136. The answer is E [Chapter 35 I A 2 b, B 3]. Carbonate is a major buffer system in bone and, therefore, is not an intracellular buffer; bone contains approximately 35,000 mEq of carbonate that contributes to the buffering of acid and base loads. The intracellular fluid (ICF) does not have a high concentration of the bicarbonate (HCO_3^-) buffer system but does contain significant amounts of the non-HCO_3^- buffer systems. Intracellular protein, with its histidine residues, and organic phosphate are the quantitatively significant non-HCO_3^- buffer systems. Thus, the ICF functions to buffer both noncarbonic and carbonic acids well. The red blood cell compartment, by virtue of its hemoglobin content, is regarded in the physiologic context of body buffers as a part of the extracellular buffer system, although it is clearly intracellular. Hemoglobin is quantitatively more important than the erythrocyte HCO_3^- buffer.

137. The answer is D [Chapter 27 III J 1 a b (1) (2) (3) 2 a (1) (a) (b) (i) (ii) (iii) b (1) (2) Table 27-2; Chapter 37 III A B C, IV A B, V B, C VI A–D]. The total amount of H^+ secreted per day by the kidney is the sum of the H^+ secreted that is needed to reabsorb all the filtered HCO_3^- plus the secreted H^+ that combines with nonbicarbonate buffers to be excreted. Since the amount of HCO_3^- reabsorbed depends on H^+ secretion, then the secretion of H^+ is equal to the filtered load of HCO_3^- plus the excretion rate of H^+ (i.e., NAE).

$$\text{Secreted } H^+/\text{day} = \text{Filtered load} + \text{NAE of } HCO_3^-$$

$$= 170 \text{ L/day} \times 24 \text{ mmol/L}$$

$$= 4080 \text{ mmol/day}$$

$$\text{NAE} = \text{TA} + \text{ammonium} - HCO_3^-$$

$$= 26 \text{ mEq/day} + 48 \text{ mEq/day} - 0 \text{ mEq/day}$$

$$= 74 \text{ mEq/day}$$

$$\text{Total amount of } H^+ \text{ secreted} = 4080 \text{ mEq/day} + 74 \text{ mEq/day}$$

$$= 4154 \text{ mEq/day}$$

where NAE = net acid excretion and TA = titratable acid.

138. The answer is C [Chapter 27 III J 1 a b (1) (2) (3) 2 a (1) (a) (b) (i) (ii) (iii) b (1) (2) Table 27-2; Chapter 37 III A B C, IV A B, V B, C VI A–D]. The reabsorption of HCO_3^- can be determined by examining the urinary HCO_3^- concentration, which is zero in this patient. Thus, the reabsorption of HCO_3^- is 100% and can be calculated from the filtered load of HCO_3^-. Therefore, reabsorption rate ($\dot{R}$) is equal to the filtered load minus the amount excreted. Since the amount excreted is zero, the reabsorption of HCO_3^- is equal to the filtered load or

$$\dot{R} = \text{GFR} \times [HCO_3^-]$$

$$= 170 \text{ L/day} \times 24 \text{ mmol/L}$$

$$= 4080 \text{ mmol/day or } 4080 \text{ mEq/day}$$

where GFR = glomerular filtration rate.

139. The answer is C [Chapter 27 III J 1 a b (1) (2) (3) 2 a (1) (a) (b) (i) (ii) (iii) b (1) (2) Table 27-2; Chapter 37 III A B C, IV A B, V B, C VI A–D]. Net acid excretion(NAE) is equal to the sum of the amount of titratable acid (TA) and ammonium (NH_4^+) minus the amount of excreted HCO_3^-. Again, we can quantitatively equate the terms H^+ excretion and the generation of "new" HCO_3^- by the kidney because a HCO_3^- is conserved and added to the blood when a H^+ has combined with a noncarbonate buffer and excreted.

$$NAE = TA + NH_4^+ - HCO_3^-$$

$$= 26 \text{ mEq/day} + 48 \text{ mEq/day} - 0 \text{ mEq/day}$$

$$= 74 \text{ mEq/day}$$

140. The answer is C [Chapter 38 III A Tables 38-3 and 38-4, Figure 38-5 IV A V B 1; Chapter 39 IV A 2]. Metabolic acidosis is an acid-base disturbance characterized by a decreased arterial pH (or increased $[H^+]$), a decreased plasma $[HCO_3^-]$, and a compensatory hyperventilation resulting in a decreased arterial CO_2 tension.

141. The answer is D [Chapter 34 V B 2]. From the data given, this patient's arterial $[H^+]$ is determined to be 32.4 nmol/L. The Henderson equation is used in this case, which is:

$$[H^+] = 24 \frac{P_{CO_2}}{[HCO_3^-]}$$

It is necessary to keep in mind that the units for these factors are: $[H^+]$ (nmol/L), $[HCO_3^-]$ (mmol/L), and P_{CO_2} (mm Hg). Substituting,

$$[H^+] = 24 \frac{30}{22.2}$$

$$= 32.4 \text{ nmol/L}$$

This patient has a partially compensated respiratory alkalosis. Note that her arterial $[H^+]$ and $[HCO_3^-]$ exhibit a parallel decrease.

142–145. The answers are: 142-B, 143-D, 144-B, 145-C [Chapter 38 I B 1 b C 1 a 2 Tables 38-3 and 38-4 III A 1-4 Figure 38-5]. The blood findings indicate that this patient has a respiratory alkalosis, an acid-base disturbance characterized by increased arterial pH (or decreased $[H^+]$), decreased arterial CO_2 tension (hypocapnia), and decreased plasma $[HCO_3^-]$. Note that both $[H^+]$ and $[HCO_3^-]$ are decreased in this patient, which is consistent with the axiom that $[H^+]$ and $[HCO_3^-]$ change in the same direction in respiratory acid-base imbalances. The decline in $[HCO_3^-]$ indicates that renal compensation has begun.

In alkalotic states, the $[HCO_3^-]/S \cdot P_{CO_2}$ ratio exceeds the normal 20:1, owing to either

an increase in $[HCO_3^-]$ (metabolic alkalosis) or a decrease in CO_2 tension (respiratory alkalosis). The normal ratio of 20:1 is derived as:

$$\frac{[HCO_3^-]}{S \cdot P_{CO_2}} = \frac{24 \text{ mmol/L}}{0.03 \cdot 40 \text{ mm Hg}}$$

$$= \frac{24 \text{ mmol/L}}{1.2 \text{ mmol/L}} = \frac{20}{1}$$

In this alkalotic patient, the $[HCO_3^+]/S \cdot P_{CO_2}$ is 30:1. This ratio can be determined by substituting the patient's blood data into the above equation, as:

$$\frac{[HCO_3^-]}{S \cdot P_{CO_2}} = \frac{22.5 \text{ mmol/L}}{0.03 \cdot 25 \text{ mm Hg}}$$

$$= \frac{22.5 \text{ mmol/L}}{0.75 \text{ mmol/L}} = \frac{30}{1}$$

The total CO_2 content for this patient is approximately 23 mmol/L. Total CO_2 equals the sum of all forms of CO_2 in the blood (i.e., HCO_3^-, H_2CO_3, dissolved CO_2, and CO_2 bound to proteins). Dissolved CO_2 content ($[CO_2]$) is calculated as

$$[CO_2] = 0.03 \cdot P_{CO_2}$$

$$= 0.03 \cdot 40 \text{ mm Hg}$$

$$= 1.2 \text{ mmol/L}$$

Since $[H_2CO_3]$ is negligible, the total CO_2 content normally exceeds the $[HCO_3^-]$ by 1.2 mmol/L and therefore equals 25.2 mmol/L when normal plasma $[HCO_3^-]$ and CO_2 tension values exist, as:

$$\text{total } CO_2 \text{ content} = [HCO_3^-] + (S \cdot P_{CO_2})$$

$$= 24 \text{ mmol/L} + 1.2 \text{ mmol/L}$$

$$= 25.2 \text{ mmol/L}$$

Total CO_2 content is decreased in respiratory alkalosis. From this patient's blood data, the CO_2 content is calculated as

$$\text{total } CO_2 \text{ content} = [HCO_3^-] + (S \cdot P_{CO_2})$$

$$= 22.5 \text{ mmol/L} + 0.75 \text{ mmol/L}$$

$$= 23.25 \text{ mmol/L}$$

Respiratory alkalosis decreases the renal reabsorption of HCO_3^-, causing a transient HCO_3^- diuresis and a decline in net acid secretion. Since the major change in respiratory alkalosis is a decrease in arterial CO_2 tension, the compensation will be in the alternate variable (kidney) and in the same direction as the primary event. Thus, there is a decline in plasma $[HCO_3^-]$, which is indicative of a partial renal response (i.e., increased HCO_3^- excretion).

146. The answer is E [Chapter 54 X C 1 b, Table 54-3]. The fall in plasma calcium (hypocalcemia) together with the fall in plasma phosphate (hypophosphatemia) is indicative of dietary vitamin D deficiency. This patient is diagnosed with secondary hyperparathyroidism. Hypocalcemia secondary to vitamin D deficiency or resistance to calcitriol is easily differentiated by the following reasoning. The primary cause of hypocalcemia in vitamin D deficiency is decreased intestinal absorption of Ca^{2+} or low dietary CA^{2+}. In the setting of normal renal function, the hypocalcemia of vitamin D deficiency, unlike that of hypoparathyroidism, is accompanied by hypophosphatemia and increased renal phosphate clearance (hyperphosphaturia). This increase in phosphate clearance is a result of compensatory (secondary) hyperparathyroidism, which is a direct result of the hypocalcemic stimulus to PTH secretion and of stimulation of PTH gene expression and parathyroid cell proliferation by hypocalcemia and low levels of $1,25(OH)_2D_3$. Therefore, measurements of serum phosphate and PTH are very useful in distinguishing these disorders from hypoparathyroidism. This secondary hyperparathyroidism results in increased Ca^{2+} mobilization from the skeleton, increased renal reabsorption of Ca^{2+}, and increased renal 1α-hydroxylation of 25 OH D_3. The hypocalcemia in this patient accounts for the tetany. Vitamin D deficiency can also be caused by malabsorption. Because vitamin D is a fat-soluble vitamin, its absorption is dependent on emulsification by bile acids. Both 25 OH D_3 and $1,25(OH)_2D_3$ are secreted into the bile and undergo enterohepatic circulation; therefore, intestinal disease may also cause vitamin D deficiency due to excessive intestinal losses. Primary hyperthyroidism is related to the absence of normal negative feedback of PTH by serum Ca^{2+}. With virtually all other hypercalcemic conditions, the parathyroid glands are suppressed, and PTH levels are low. The major cause of primary hypoparathyroidism is thyroid surgery. It is characterized by hypocalcemia and hyperphosphatemia due to low plasma PTH concentration. Secondary hypoparathyroidism is caused by vitamin D excess.

147. The answer is B [Chapter 47 IV A 4 a c (1)]. Somatostatin receptors have been demonstrated in more than 90% of growth hormone (GH)–secreting pituitary tumors. Octreotide, an analogue of somatostatin, binds to somatostatin receptors. Therefore, somatostatin (octreotide) receptor scintigraphy (iodide- or indium-labeled) is used to obtain images of GH-secreting tumors. Indium–octreotide imaging is potentially useful for visualization of tumors that escape detection with magnetic resonance imaging (MRI).

148. The answer is D [Chapter 48 VIII Q 3 a b c, Table 48-1]. In the pancreas, epinephrine stimulates glucagon secretion and inhibits insulin secretion, both hyperglycemic effects. Epinephrine also stimulates adrenocorticotropic hormone (ACTH) secretion, which, in turn, leads to secretion of cortisol, which is a major hyperglycemic hormone. Epinephrine is a potent hyperglycemic hormone, due mainly to its effects on the liver and pancreas. In the liver, it promotes glycogenolysis and gluconeogenesis, and the glucose-6-phosphate formed by glycogenolysis is hydrolyzed to glucose. Epinephrine-induced glycogenolysis in muscle leads to formation of lactic acid, which is converted to glucose in the liver, further elevating blood glucose.

149. The answer is D [Chapter 50 I D 2 a (3), Figure 50-2]. Unilateral (right side) orchidectomy (or orchiectomy) at 5 weeks removes the Sertoli cells that secrete antimüllerian hormone (AMH) and the Leydig cells that secrete testosterone. Since AMH acts as a paracrine substance (local hormone) then the müllerian duct will remain on the right side only in males. However, testosterone secreted by the intact left testis will promote bilateral virilization of the male structures because testosterone acts systemically, i.e., it is secreted into the bloodstream and circulates throughout the body as an endocrine and not a paracrine substance. Descent of the left testis between 34 and 35 weeks gestation will still occur because the three necessary factors are present: AMH, intra-abdominal pressure, and androgens.

150. The answer is B [Chapter 51 I G 2, Table 51-2]. It is primary ovarian failure and the reduction in estrogen and progesterone that causes the elevated gonadotropins associated with menopause. The lack of estrogen and progesterone results in a marked reduction in negative feedback at the level of the pituitary and the resultant elevation in gonadotropin secretion.

151. The answer is C [Chapter 52 I C 6, 7; II D 7]. This woman has type 2 diabetes diagnosed one year earlier. Pregnancy represents a stressful condition, which aggravated her preexisting diabetes because of the increased production of diabetogenic hormones such as cortisol and chorionic somatomammotropin (hCS or hCG). Gestational diabetes is a potential problem during pregnancy in patients without previous glucose intolerance. The absence of ketosis and insulin dependence suggests that she is not a type 1 diabetic. Her normal blood pressure and regulated blood glucose (although above normal) rule out a pheochromocytoma that leads to hypertension and blockade of insulin secretion. Elevated secretion of somatostatin, which blocks both glucagon and insulin secretion, would lead to hypoglycemia, which is inconsistent with her data.

152. The answer is C [Chapter 53 VI A 2 b]. The formation of a goiter in the context of an elevated plasma T_4 level presents a paradox. The goiter is caused by elevated thyroid-stimulating hormone (TSH) and, therefore, there must be a reduction in negative feedback to the brain–pituitary functional unit. It is the T_3 formed within the pituitary by the monodeiodination (5'-deiodinase) of T_4 that exerts a negative influence on both thyroid-releasing hormone (TRH) and TSH secretion. Countering this negative feedback of T_3 on the brain–pituitary is the stimulatory effect of TRH on TSH biosynthesis. A reduction in the nuclear content of T_3 in the pituitary diminishes this negative feedback and promotes TSH synthesis and secretion with a subsequent thyroid gland hypertrophy. Therefore, TSH levels are elevated because of the reduced conversion of T_4 to T_3. This also explains the elevation in circulating T_4. The inhibition of the coupling reactions would lead to a decline in plasma T_4 and T_3 with an increase in plasma TSH. The stimulation of iodotyrosine deiodinase activity would provide for increased synthesis of thyroid hormones from this "second iodide" pool, which would not cause an elevation of TSH. Likewise, stimulation of the iodide pump would tend to promote thyroid hormone synthesis, which also would not increase TSH. Lastly, if this unknown drug blocked synthesis of TRH, then there would be decrements in both TRH and TSH secretion and, in turn, a decline in thyroid hormone secretion.

153–158. The answers are: 153-D [Chapter 11 IV A; Figure 11-7B], **154-B** [Chapter 11 IV D; Figure 11-7C], **155-A** [Chapter 11 II A 2 b (1)], **156-D** [Figure 11-7], **157-C** [Figure 11-7], **158-C** [Figure 11-7A]. Loop ACDI shows the effect of an increased afterload. The increased ventricular pressure reflects an increase in arterial resistance, which increases the afterload. The maximal pressure—volume point for loop ACDI lies on the same line as that for the normal pressure—volume loop, which indicates that there is no change in contractility. The stroke volume represents the difference in volume between the vertical lines for any loop. In this case, the increased afterload decreases the stroke volume. The ventricular end-diastolic volume (VEDV) is indicated by point A; all three loops start at the same VEDV. Pre-load is a synonym for VEDV.

An increase in contractility causes the maximal pressure—volume relationship to move to the left and assume a steeper slope. Stroke volume increases and there is a smaller volume of blood that remains in the ventricles at the end of systole. Mitral valve closure occurs at the onset of systole (point A) and represents the beginning of the isovolumic contraction period. During this interval, as the name implies, the ventricular volume remains constant and ventricular pressure rises until it exceeds the pressure in the aorta.

Ventricular filling occurs during diastole (i.e., the interval between points A and H) and is the increase in volume that occurs in preparation for the next contraction. During steady-state conditions, the ventricular filling equals the stroke volume that is ejected during the next systole. Changes in venous return, the duration of diastole, the afterload, and ventricular contractility can all influence ventricular filling and the stroke volume in a complex fashion. The slope of the line from point G to point A has the units of mm Hg/ml, which are compatible with elastance. Compliance is the reciprocal of elastance and has units of ml/mm Hg. The line from point G to point A occurs during diastole; therefore, the slope is a measure of the diastolic elastance of the ventricles.

Points D, E, and F represent the ventricular end-systolic volume (VESV). Stroke volume is represented as the width of each loop (i.e., A-I, A-H, or A-G). The VEDV occurs at point A for all three loops. The diastolic reserve volume is the volume of blood that the ventricle can hold from the end-diastolic point to the maximal volume— this volume is not shown on the graph. The residual volume represents a minimal volume of blood that lies between the trabeculae carneae and the papillary muscles. This volume is a part of the VESV and is never ejected from the ventricles.

159. The answer is D [Chapter 27 III J 2 a (1) (a) (b) (c); Chapter 37 III A 3 a b 4, Figure 37-2 V B 2]. The primary effect of carbonic anhydrase inhibitors such as acetazolamide is to inhibit both H^+ secretion and $NaHCO_3$ reabsorption, making the urine alkaline. NH_4^+ excretion is reduced as a result of the diminished H^+ secretion. Carbonic anhydrase inhibitors restrict H^+ secretion by inhibiting the intracellular hydration of CO_2, a primary source of intracellular H^+. The decline in H^+ secretion inhibits the Na^+-H^+ exchange at the luminal membrane of the proximal tubule. HCO_3^- reabsorption is also inhibited because only a limited amount of HCO_3^- can be reabsorbed by the distal segment. The elevated intraluminal HCO_3^- augments Na^+ and K^+ excretion and results in $NaHCO_3$ diuresis. Carbonic anhydrase inhibitors also block the dehydration of H_2CO_3 formed in the tubular lumen. Chronic doses of such drugs can lead to hyperchloremic acidosis (metabolic acidosis).

160. The answer is A [Chapter 7 III B 1 c (2)]. Reciprocal innervation is a neuronal innervation pattern in which, when one motoneuron is excited, its antagonistic motoneuron is inhibited. Inhibition of flexors during an extension is an example of reciprocal innervation. This pattern of innervation allows movement to occur unimpeded by the activity of antagonistic muscles.

161. The answer is D [Chapter 46 II Figure 46-1]. In humans, there is a diurnal variation in the secretory patterns of adrenocorticotropic hormone (ACTH) and cortisol (hydrocortisone) and in the excretion of 17-hydroxycorticoids. In individuals who sleep regularly from about 11:00 P.M. to 7:30 A.M., the peak of this circadian rhythm occurs between 6 A.M. and 8 A.M., while the nadir is observed between midnight and 2 A.M. Thus, the peak plasma level of glucocorticoid is entrained to the activity cycle with maximal ACTH-cortisol secretion appearing about 1 hour after awakening. Changes in sleep periods or in longitude cause phase shifts in the ACTH-cortisol secretory pattern; however, the rhythm itself persists. There is an abrogation of the pituitary-adrenocortical rhythm in patients with hypercortisolism.

162. The answer is C [Chapter 17 III C, Chapter 13 II A]. This patient's O_2 consumption is

520 ml/min/m². O_2 consumption can be determined using the Fick principle, an important concept that has wide applicability in physiology and medicine. To solve for O_2 consumption ($\dot{V}O_2$), the Fick principle is expressed as:

$$\dot{V}O_2 = \dot{Q} \cdot (CaO_2 - C\bar{v}O_2), \text{ where}$$

$\dot{Q}$ = blood flow and $CaO_2 - C\bar{v}O_2$ = the arteriovenous O_2 difference.

In this problem, the cardiac index equals the blood flow. Because arterial hemoglobin saturation is assumed to be 100%, the arterial O_2 content (CaO_2) equals the O_2 capacity, which equals hemoglobin · 1.34, or 16 ml/dl (160 ml/L). Using these values in the above formula gives:

$$\dot{V}O_2 = 6.5 \cdot (160 - 80)$$

$$= 520 \text{ ml/min}$$

It is important to use similar units for blood flow and O_2 content. In addition, converting O_2 content to ml/L before calculating is recommended.

163. The answer is B [Chapter 51 I H, J, K, Figures 51-4 and 51-6]. The menstrual cycle consists of four phases. These phases (with synonymous terms) are: menses (4–5 days), the preovulatory phase (also called follicular, estrogenic, or proliferative phase; 10–12 days), the ovulatory phase, and the postovulatory phase (also called luteal, progestational, or secretory phase; 14 days).

164. The answer is B [Chapter 34 V B 2]. From the data given, this patient's arterial bicarbonate concentration ($[HCO_3^-]$) is determined to be 14.7 mmol/L (mEq/L). Arterial $[HCO_3^-]$ is easily estimated using the Henderson equation, which is stated as:

$$[HCO_3^-] = 24 \frac{PCO_2}{[H^+]}$$

where $[HCO_3^-]$ is expressed in mmol/L, $[H^+]$ in nmol/L, and PCO_2 in mm Hg. Substituting,

$$[HCO_3^-] = 24 \frac{30}{49}$$

$$= 14.7 \text{ mmol/L}$$

The acid-base disturbance in this case is an almost completely compensated metabolic acidosis (pH 7.31) as pH = 9 – log [H+]

$$= 9 - \log 49$$
$$= 9 - 1.69 = 7.31$$

165. The answer is E [Chapter 30 II A 3; Chapter 39 IV A 1 b]. Although acidosis can result from loss of fluid from both the intestine and the colon, only the colon secretes K^+. Thus, excessive fluid loss from the colon will result in both acidosis and hypokalemia.

166–167. The answers are: 166-B [Figure 11-2A], **167-A** [Chapter 11 II C 3 a (1)]. The systolic gradient that occurs between the ventricular and aortic pressures is diagnostic of aortic valve stenosis. Normally, the aortic valve provides a negligible resistance and the aortic pressure is nearly identical to the ventricular pressure during the phase of rapid ventricular ejection. Pulmonary valve stenosis would produce similar tracings upon measurement of the right ventricular and pulmonary pressures; however, the pressures are proportionately reduced for the right-sided events because of the low resistance of the pulmonary circulation.

Semilunar (e.g., aortic or pulmonary) valve stenosis represents an impediment to the ejection of blood from the ventricle and results in a systolic ejection murmur. An ejection murmur is diamond-shaped (i.e., it is a crescendo—decrescendo sound that has maximal intensity in midsystole when the pressure gradient is largest).

168–170. The answers are: 168-B [Chapter 20 II C 1 d; Table 20-1], **169-E** [Chapter 18 IV A 2 b (3) (b)], **170-A** [Chapter 18 IV A 2 b; Chapter 20 II C 1 d]. A right-to-left anatomic shunt causes mixed venous blood to enter the systemic circulation without being oxygenated, leading to hypoxia and an increased alveolar—arterial O_2 tension difference. Ventilation—perfusion imbalance also leads to hypoxia but is not the cause in this patient. With ventilation—perfusion imbalance, arterial O_2 tension should exceed 500 mm Hg when the patient breathes 100% O_2 at sea level, and the alveolar O_2 tension should be 673 mm Hg (which can be calculated using the alveolar gas equation). A left-to-right anatomic shunt does not cause hypoxia, because oxygenated blood (from the left side of the circulation) enters the right ventricle or the pulmonary artery. Administration of 100% O_2 will completely correct hypoxia resulting from diffusion abnormalities or hypoventilation.

The fraction of the cardiac output that represents shunted blood can be calculated using the shunt equation:

$$\frac{\dot{Q}_S}{\dot{Q}_T} = \frac{(CiO_2 - CaO_2)}{(CiO_2 - C\bar{v}O_2)}, \text{ where}$$

$\dot{Q}_S$ = the shunted flow

$\dot{Q}_T$ = cardiac output

CiO_2 = pulmonary capillary O_2 content

CaO_2 and $C\bar{v}O_2$ = arterial and venous O_2 content, respectively

The calculation usually is sufficiently accurate only if hemoglobin O_2 is used and the dissolved O_2 is disregarded. In the pulmonary capillaries, hemoglobin should be 100% saturated while the patient is breathing 100% O_2 so that:

$$CiO_2 = O_2 \text{ capacity}$$

$$= 18 \text{ g hemoglobin/dl} \cdot 1.34 \text{ ml } O_2/g$$

$$= 24.1 \text{ ml/dl}$$

Arterial O_2 content can be determined as:

$$CaO_2 = CiO_2 \cdot \text{hemoglobin saturation}$$

$$= 24.1 \text{ ml/dl} \cdot 0.85$$

$$= 20.5 \text{ ml/dl}$$

Venous O_2 content can be determined if it is remembered that the normal venous O_2 tension also is 40 mm Hg, which is equivalent to 75% hemoglobin saturation, giving:

$$C\bar{v}O_2 = 24.1 \cdot 0.75$$

$$= 18.1 \text{ ml/dl}$$

Thus,

$$\frac{\dot{Q}_S}{\dot{Q}_T} = \frac{24.1 - 20.5}{24.1 - 18.1}$$

$$= \frac{3.6}{6.0} = 0.6$$

To determine the site of a right-to-left shunt, the O_2 tension must be measured in the left ventricle and atrium rather than the right (i.e., the unsaturated venous blood is used to locate the point where the O_2 tension drops). Thus, if there were an interatrial septal defect with right-to-left flow, the O_2 tension in the left atrium would be lower than the O_2 tension in the pulmonary veins. A ventricular septal defect would show a drop in O_2 tension in the left ventricle compared with that in the left atrium. If the O_2 tension were low and equal in the pulmonary veins, left atrium, and left ventricle, then the shunt would necessarily be within the lungs, which could indicate the presence of an arteriovenous anastomosis.

171. The answer is B [Chapter 48 VIII A 3 a (1), Table 48-1]. Pheochromocytoma is an adrenomedullary tumor characterized by the hypersecretion of catecholamines, usually norepinephrine. Catecholamines block insulin release (hypoinsulinemia) and increase both gluconeogenesis and fatty acid mobilization, which account for glucose intolerance, fasting hyperglycemia, and glycosuria. The breakdown of muscle glycogen leads to elevated plasma pyruvate or lactate levels. The metabolic features of pheochromocytoma resemble hyperthyroidism and include tremor, weight loss, heat intolerance, and increased basal metabolic rate. The cardinal sign is hypertension, which may be persistent or paroxysmal. Patients usually complain of attacks that may be precipitated by emotion or physical exercise, which consist of pounding headaches, sweating, pallor, pain or "tightness" in the chest, apprehension, paresthesia, nausea, and vomiting. In this patient, the attacks were provoked by mechanical pressure that was exerted on the tumor by changes in body position.

172. The answer is B [Chapter 7 III B 1 d (2); Figure 7-4]. Unloading (i.e., the reduction in Ia afferent activity that accompanies muscle shortening) can be prevented if the intrafusal and extrafusal muscle fibers are coactivated so that tension on the intrafusal muscle fibers is maintained during shortening. Therefore, gamma motoneurons, which innervate intrafusal muscle fibers, can prevent unloading. Alpha motoneurons innervate extrafusal muscle fibers; Ib afferent fibers innervate Golgi tendon organs; and the free nerve endings of C fibers contain pain, temperature, and mechanical receptors.

173. The answer is D [Chapter 16 IV B 1 b (1) (c), 2 b (1)]. The man can lie under 68 cm of water. Calculation of this depth requires converting the pressure given in mm Hg to a pressure expressed in cm H_2O: 50 mm Hg · 1.36 cm H_2O (mm Hg) = 68 cm H_2O. This man's alveolar pressure is equal to the atmospheric pressure when he is under water, whereas the pressure outside his chest wall is 68 cm H_2O higher. To expand his lungs, this man must generate a pressure slightly more negative than −68 cm H_2O. Under these conditions, the man is undergoing negative-pressure breathing, which, if prolonged, can lead to pulmonary edema.

174. The answer is B [Chapter 52 I B 2 a]. In a normal subject the elevated insulin could be caused by elevated glucose, which is clearly not the case here. Elevated glucagon (glucagonoma) would lead to elevated insulin; however, there would be an expected hyperglycemia, which is not observed. Further, with glucagon-stimulated insulin secretion there would be an elevated C-peptide concentration because endogenous insulin secretion is accompanied by the secretion of equimolar amounts of C-peptide. This is not consistent with the data. Similarly, an insulinoma would lead to elevated levels of both insulin and C-peptide with a concomitant hypoglycemia, all of which is inconsistent with the data in terms of the plasma C-peptide level. The most consistent abnormality with an insulinoma is the failure of a normal decrease in insulin secretion as the plasma glucose level declines in the postprandial state. A somatostatinoma would reduce plasma insulin, C-peptide, and glucagon with a resultant hypoglycemia. Only the hypoglycemia and reduced plasma C-peptide would be expected, but the expected decline in plasma insulin level was not observed. It now becomes apparent that this patient had an overdose of exogenous insulin that caused the hyperinsulinemia and hypoglycemia without the increase in C-peptide concentration.

175. The answer is C [Chapter 26 III C 1 a b, Figure 26-2]. Tubuloglomerular feedback (TGF) is an autoregulatory mechanism that serves to regulate primarily the glomerular filtration rate (GFR), with changes in renal plasma flow (renal blood flow) as a secondary consequence. An increase in arterial blood pressure raises both the glomerular capillary hydrostatic pressure and RBF. The increase in glomerular capillary pressure raises the GFR, and consequently the distal delivery of NaCl (and NaCl transport) in the region of the macula densa which serves as the receptor for this reflex. The increased NaCl concentration, load, and transport to the macula densa sends a vasoconstrictive signal to the afferent arteriole which increases afferent arteriolar resistance, decreases glomerular capillary pressure and GFR (as well as renal blood flow). This constriction of the afferent arteriole reduces the NaCl concentration (and load) at the macula densa and serves to prevent the distal tubular fluid (and electrolyte) delivery from exceeding the limited reabsorptive capacity of the collecting duct. In summary, there is a direct relationship between distal NaCl load and afferent arteriolar resistance or there is an inverse relationship between distal NaCl load and GFR.

176. The answer is D [Chapter 25 II B 2, Figure 25-5]. The simplest flow (Q) equation that summarizes the relationship between the hydrostatic pressure gradient (ΔP) and resistance (R) is:

$$Q = \frac{\Delta P}{R}$$

The pressure gradient is the hydrostatic pressure difference between the renal artery and renal vein. The resistance to blood flow can be determined by dividing this hydrostatic pressure gradient by the renal blood flow:

$$R = \frac{\Delta P}{Q}$$

177. The answer is C [Chapter 6 II C 2 a (2); Figure 6-11]. The middle ear amplifies the pressure of the sound stimulus so that an adequate signal can reach the inner ear, even though 99.9% of the sound is reflected at the air—fluid interface. Because the middle ear cannot amplify all sounds equally well, some sound frequencies are detected at lower strengths than others. Fortunately, the sounds that are heard at the lowest intensities (e.g., between 500 and 5000 Hz) are the sounds that are used for speech.

178–179. The answers are: 178-E [Chapter 11 II A 3; Figure 11-7], **179-B** [Chapter 11 II A 2 b (2)]. Opening of the mitral valve signals the onset of ventricular filling, which occurs when ventricular pressure and volume are at their lowest point (i.e., point E on the pressure—volume loop).

By definition, isovolumic ("equal volume") contraction must be represented by a vertical line on the pressure—volume loop. Isovolumic contraction is the first period of ventricular systole after the mitral valve closes; at the onset of isovolumic contraction, the ventricular pressure rises to reach the aortic diastolic pressure. Isovolumic contraction ends when the semilunar valve opens and ventricular ejection begins. The onset of ejection is signaled by the point where ventricular volume begins to decrease.

180. The answer is C [Chapter 37 V B 2, VI B Table 37-1]. The kidney excretes H^+ as NH_4^+ and titratable acid. Titratable acid exists mainly in the form of $H_2PO_4^-$. The titratable acid is excreted mainly as NaH_2PO_4, which is also called acid phosphate, monosodium phosphate, or monobasic phosphate. The normal kidney excretes almost twice as much acid combined with NH_3 than it excretes titratable acid. The rate of NH_4^+ excretion increases during metabolic acidosis.

181. The answer is D [Chapter 47 II C 1, Figure 46-2]. This woman's inability to lactate and to menstruate following parturition stems from pituitary failure related to the massive bleeding she experienced during delivery. Most likely, this woman has postpartum pituitary necrosis (Sheehan's syndrome) resulting from ischemia of the hypophysial portal system, which supplies 90% of the blood to the anterior pituitary gland. The resultant pituitary failure may be complete (panhypopituitarism) or partial. In this case, the acidophils responsible for production of prolactin, follicle-stimulating hormone (FSH), and luteinizing hormone (LH) were affected, resulting in this patient's inability to lactate and to menstruate. This patient also would exhibit hypoglycemia because of low plasma growth hormone (GH) levels and low plasma adrenocorticotropic hormone (ACTH) levels, which would lead to decreased secretion of cortisol (a potent hyperglycemic hormone) and decreased synthesis of epinephrine (a hyperglycemic hormone that depends on cortisol). The decreased levels of these hyperglycemic hormones would cause insulin sensitivity. Because aldosterone secretion does not depend mainly on ACTH secretion, this patient should be able to regulate Na^+ balance. She also should have normal antidiuretic hormone (ADH) activity, because the supraoptic nuclei and pars nervosa are not perfused by the hypophysial portal system. Thus, this patient should demonstrate normal water balance.

182. The answer is C [Chapter 18 III A 1 b]. The lung is a passive structure whose transmural pressure varies as a function of volume and phase of respiration. At residual volume (RV), the transpulmonary pressure may be negative at the base of the lung, because interpleural pressure could be positive owing to the hydrostatic effects of lung weight and the decreased retractile force at low lung volume. The transpulmonary pressure always is greater at the apex than at the base when standing because of the hydrostatic effects of gravity. Thus, the airways and alveoli at the apex of the lung always are more distended than those at the base of the lung of a person who is standing.

183–186. The answers are: 183-C, 184-B, 185-D, 186-A [Chapter 16 IV A 1–2; VIII C; Chapter 18 IV A 2; Chapter 39 IV A]. This patient's blood data are almost consistent with a ventilation-perfusion abnormality. Although the CO_2 tension is normal, the O_2 tension is decreased, as are pH and $[HCO_3^-]$. These latter two findings indicate a metabolic acidosis that is most likely due to accumulation of lactic acid caused by the decreased O_2 tension and cardiac output. Ventilation—perfusion abnormalities are the most common cause of clinical hypoxia. A variety of factors affecting the lungs and cardiovascular system may cause these abnormalities.

Given a predicted dead space of 150 ml, this patient's calculated alveolar ventilation is 7.2 L/min. Alveolar ventilation is the volume/min that is effective in gas exchange, which is calculated as follows: (tidal volume − dead space) · respiratory rate. Thus, in this patient, the alveolar ventilation equals (0.6 − 0.15) · 16 = 7.2 L/min.

This patient's O_2 tension value while breathing 40% O_2 (120 mm Hg) indicates an increase in the alveolar-to-arterial O_2 tension difference. Applying the alveolar gas equation, the alveolar O_2 tension is calculated as

$$alveolar\ P_{O_2} = (760 - 47) \cdot 0.40 - \frac{43}{0.8}$$

$$= 230\ mm\ Hg$$

Thus, there is a difference of 110 mm Hg in alveolar-to-arterial O_2 tension in this patient (230 − 120 = 110). Normally, the alveolar-to-arterial O_2 tension is 5–10 mm Hg. The large difference in this patient results from a physiologic shunt secondary to the ventilation-perfusion abnormality. Changes in the hemoglobin concentration do not affect the arterial O_2 tension, which depends solely on the amount of O_2 that is in physical solution in the blood.

This patient's respiratory compliance is 0.03 L/mm Hg. The compliance of the respiratory system is calculated as the change in volume (i.e., tidal volume) divided by the change in distending pressure. Because the respirator is delivering intermittent positive pressure (i.e., 20 mm Hg in order to distend the lungs to accept the delivered volume), the pressure in the lungs at the end of expiration is zero (i.e., atmospheric). Thus, compliance of the respiratory system is 0.6 L/20 mm Hg = 0.03 L/mm Hg. Normal respiratory compliance is about 0.1 L/mm Hg. The decreased compliance ("stiff lungs") in this patient could be a result of the pulmonary edema.

187. The answer is B [Chapter 42 VII C 2 d (3)]. Although fats can be absorbed all along the intestine, from the point at which the bile duct enters the duodenum until the bile salts are absorbed from the terminal ileum, almost all of the digested lipids are absorbed by the time the chyme reaches the midjejunum. Little, if any, lipid absorption occurs in the ileum.

188. The answer is D [Chapter 9 II C; Chapter 13 II A]. The data can be used to calculate the cardiac output using the Fick principle:

$$Q = \frac{\dot{V}_{O_2}}{Ca_{O_2} - C\bar{v}_{O_2}},\ where$$

$$Q = cardiac\ output$$

$$\dot{V}_{O_2} = O_2\ consumption\ (ml/min)$$

$$Ca_{O_2} = arterial\ O_2\ content$$

$$C\bar{v}_{O_2} = mixed\ venous\ O_2\ content$$

Mixed venous blood from the right ventricle or pulmonary artery must be used to calculate the cardiac output. For this calculation, as in all others, the units must be consistent so every volume can be expressed in ml:

Cardiac output (Q) = 210 (ml/min)/(0.18 ml O_2/ml blood) − (0.11 ml O_2/ml blood) = 210/0.07 = 3000 ml/min.

The normal cardiac output is approximately 5 L/min (5000 ml/min). Therefore, choices B ("cardiac output is approximately 1470 ml/min") and E ("cardiac output is extremely high") are incorrect. The amount of O_2 transferred to the tissues is given by the difference between the arterial and venous O_2 content, not the sum. The arterial O_2 content is equal to or only slightly less than the pulmonary venous oxygen content. (Thebesian venous flow into the left ventricle may account for the slightly lower arterial O_2 content.) Stroke volume is equal to the cardiac output divided by the heart rate (3000/75 = 40 ml). In this patient, the stroke volume of 40 ml is less than the normal stroke volume of 70 ml, leading to a lower than normal cardiac output.

189. The answer is D [Chapter 42 VII E 3]. Although intrinsic factor is secreted by parietal cells in the stomach, it is not able to bind vitamin B_{12} in the stomach because the vitamin is bound to another protein, called protein R. When the vitamin reaches the intestine, the R protein is removed, and intrinsic factor is able to bind to the vitamin B_{12}. The B_{12}-intrinsic factor complex is absorbed in the terminal ileum.

190. The answer is C [Chapter 51 II B 4 b (2) Figure 51-11]. The corpus luteum is the initial source of plasma progesterone and 17α-hydroxyprogesterone, which peak at 3–4 weeks postconception. At 6–8 weeks postconception, the progesterone reaches its lowest point, while the 17α-hydroxyprogesterone continues to decline. Since the placenta cannot synthesize 17α-hydroxyprogesterone, the secondary rise in progesterone reflects placental (trophoblast) function, and the 17α-hydroxyprogesterone curve is a correlate of corpus luteal function of pregnancy. The theca interna and adrenal glands do not secrete progesterone. The decidua is not the source of any hormones but is a specialized region of the endometrium that develops into the maternal component of the placenta.

191–192. The answers are: 191-B, 192-C, 193-C [Chapter 16 IV D; VIII B 2 a (2) (b) (ii), C 1; Chapter 38 V A 1; Chapter 39 IV C, V A; Figure 38-1] The increased CO_2 tension (P_{CO_2}) in this patient indicates that alveolar ventilation is inadequate. Minute ventilation may be normal or increased while alveolar ventilation is reduced, because the total dead space increases secondary to ventilation—perfusion abnormalities caused by the pulmonary disease. (It is important to remember that total dead space equals alveolar dead space plus anatomic dead space.) The normal arterial pH in this patient indicates that renal compensation has occurred. Renal compensation may require 1–2 weeks, meaning that the abnormality is chronic, ruling out acute respiratory failure. Anemia and carbon monoxide poisoning are not viable alternatives, since arterial O_2 tension is normal in these two conditions. An anatomic shunt causes hypoxia and typically results in a lowered CO_2 tension as a result of the increased ventilation that results from this type of hypoxia.

Smoking causes inflammation and edema in the airways (bronchitis), which can lead to infection of the airways and consequent mucus production. The resultant airway narrowing increases airway resistance and the work of breathing. If respiratory work increases suffi-

ciently, there will be respiratory muscle fatigue and a decrease in alveolar ventilation, which results in hypercapnia and hypoxia. These latter events cause pulmonary artery vasoconstriction and pulmonary hypertension.

This patient has respiratory acidosis, by definition, because of the hypercapnia. Respiratory acidosis is compensated by renal retention of HCO_3^- (normal = 24 mEq/L). Metabolic or lactic acidosis is not present because of the increased HCO_3^- levels. Respiratory alkalosis is produced by a decrease in CO_2 tension.

194–197. The answers are: 194-D [Chapter 14 III C 2], **195-B** [Chapter 14 III C 1], **196-B** [Chapter 14 III C 1 b (1)], **197-E** [Chapter 14 III C 2]. Stimulation of the right vagus nerve can cause marked cardiac slowing. From the record, it is obvious that the major effect of the intervention at time 1 was a slowing of the heart rate. Although vagal stimulation can cause marked cardiac slowing, the ventricular end-diastolic volume (VEDV) increases so that stroke volume increases sufficiently to compensate for the reduced heart rate. Cardiac output must have remained relatively constant because there is little change in arterial pressure and total peripheral resistance. (Recall that cardiac output equals arterial pressure divided by total peripheral resistance.) Electrical stimulation of the superior cervical ganglion or administration of a cholinergic blocking drug would increase the heart rate. Electrical stimulation of the lumbar sympathetic nerve roots would cause a significant rise in resistance in the lower portion of the body. The administration of a β-adrenergic blocking drug would reduce the heart rate, but it would also reduce cardiac contractility and therefore, cardiac output.

There is obviously a rise in heart rate, arterial pressure, and total resistance at time 2. The only factor that is listed that could cause this sequence of changes is stimulation of the portion of the sympathetic system that controls the heart (i.e., the superior cervical ganglion).

An α-adrenergic drug was most likely administered at time 3. Cholinergic blocking drugs and β-adrenergic agonists are incorrect choices because both drugs would increase, rather than decrease, the heart rate. A β-adrenergic blocking drug would not cause such a rise in arterial pressure, although it would produce a drop in heart rate. An α-adrenergic blocking drug would cause a decrease, rather than an increase, in peripheral resistance.

All adrenergic drugs would increase the heart rate as a direct effect on the sinoatrial (SA) node, isoproterenol having the greatest effect and norepinephrine the least. A drug such as epinephrine, which has both α- and β-adrenergic properties, can increase contractility and peripheral resistance so that a large increase in arterial pressure occurs. The increased arterial pressure then affects the baroreceptors and results in a reflex slowing of cardiac rate. When activated, chemoreceptors lead to a rise in heart rate as well as an increase in contractility. Ventricular extrasystoles have no effect on peripheral resistance. The effect of the drug on ventricular muscle would not alter heart rate.

198. The answer is D [Chapter 17 III A 2 a]. A drop in arterial O_2 tension from 100 mm Hg to 27 mm Hg would decrease the O_2 content of the blood by about 50%. The key to answering this question is to recognize that 27 mm Hg is the normal value for the P_{50}, which is the O_2 tension at a hemoglobin saturation of 50%. Since hemoglobin is nearly 100% saturated at an O_2 tension of 100 mm Hg, then O_2 content must decrease by 50%.

199. The answer is D [Chapter 25 I A 1, Figure 25-1]. The oncotic and hydrostatic pressures within the capillary and within the interstitium contribute to the regulation of fluid exchange between the plasma and the interstitial fluid (or Bowman's capsule). To determine whether there is a net reabsorption or filtration, it is necessary to compare the magnitude and direction of these two different pressures as

Outward Forces (mm Hg)

Capillary hydrostatic pressure	=	47
Bowman's capsule oncotic pressure	=	0
		47

Inward Forces (mm Hg)

Bowman's capsule hydrostatic pressure	=	10
Capillary oncotic pressure	=	28
		38

Because the outwardly directed forces exceed the inwardly directed forces, there will be an effective filtration pressure (EFP) of 9 mm Hg. Note that the oncotic pressure in Bowman's capsule is assigned a value of zero because the fluid in this region is an ultrafiltrate of plasma.

200. The answer is A [Chapter 48 V A 2; Chapter 49 I E 8]. Hydrocortisone (cortisol) directly increases epinephrine-forming enzyme activity. Epinephrine is synthesized in the adrenal medulla and certain brain neurons from norepinephrine by the action of the enzyme phenylethanolamine-N-methyltransferase (PNMT). The adrenal cortex and adrenal medulla are related both anatomically and functionally. Venous blood from the sinusoids of the cortex enters the adrenal portal system and perfuses the adrenal medulla before entering the systemic circulation. Therefore, the chromaffin cells are exposed to a high concentration of cortisol. Adrenocorticotropic hormone (ACTH) indirectly activates the epinephrine-forming enzyme, because it stimulates the secretion of cortisol.

201. The answer is C [Chapter 11 II A 2 b (3) (a)]. Opening of the aortic valve, which indicates the onset of rapid ventricular ejection, occurs when the pressure in the left ventricle exceeds the pressure in the aorta, and blood begins to flow out of the ventricle. Because the rate of ventricular contraction is initially high, the blood leaves the ventricle rapidly during this interval, causing aortic pressure to increase rapidly in association with the pressure in the ventricle.

202. The answer is B [Chapter 12 I C 5 b]. Histamine, released from mast cells in areas of inflammation, results in an increased permeability of microvessels, primarily the postcapillary venules.

203. The answer is D [Chapter 27 I A 1, B 1 a b (2), Figure 27-1A]. Transport maximum (Tm) can only be determined if two conditions are met: (1) the substance must appear in the urine, and (2) the amount reabsorbed (or secreted) must show two values to be the same, indicating that a maximum rate of transport has been attained. In the example, no calculations are necessary because two values for reabsorption rate are the same, namely 400 mg/min. It should be remembered that the reabsorption rate is the difference between the filtered load and the amount excreted.

204. The answer is C [Chapter 26 III C 1 a b, Figure 26-2]. The tubuloglomerular feedback (TGF) mechanism is activated by an increased NaCl concentration (load or delivery) to the macula densa chemoreceptor. This increased distal NaCl load (transport) transmits a vaso-constrictive signal to the afferent arteriole, which leads to a reduction in glomerular filtration rate (GFR).

205. The answer is E [Chapter 25 III C 2, 4]. The clearance of *para*-aminohippuric acid (PAH) [at low plasma concentrations] measures the **effective** renal plasma flow, meaning plasma that flows past those portions of the nephron that can effectively secrete PAH (i.e., some blood perfuses some renal tissues that cannot secrete PAH and, therefore, the clearance of PAH underestimates by 10% the true renal plasma flow). To determine effective renal plasma flow (ER*PF*):

$$ER{\it PF} = C_{PAH} = \frac{U_{PAH} \cdot V}{P_{PAH}}$$

$$= \frac{48 \cdot 2}{0.2}$$

$$= 480 \text{ ml/min}$$

$$ER{\it BF} = C_{PAH} \div (1 - \text{Hematocrit})$$

$$= \frac{480}{0.6} = 800 \text{ ml/min}$$

206. The answer is C [Chapter 7 IV A 2 b]. Elimination of inhibitory control over the neurons within the reticular formation that are responsible for activating the spinal motoneurons during a movement produces spasticity [i.e., continuous contraction of antigravity (or physiologic extensor) muscles]. Loss of inhibition can occur when lesions damage the inhibitory upper motor neurons in the cerebral cortex or their axons within the internal capsule.

207. The answer is D [Chapter 28 II B 2 d e, Figure 28-2]. NaCl transport is an active process via the Na^+–$2Cl^-$–K^+ cotransporter. Twenty-five percent of the Na^+ reabsorption occurs in the thin segment of the loop of Henle, and this transport is passive. About one-half occurs via transcellular transport, and the other one-half takes place via paracellular transport. The fluid entering the descending limb of the loop of Henle (DLH) is isosmotic to plasma, while the fluid leaving the thick segment is hyposmotic to plasma. The thin DLH has a high water permeability and a low solute permeability, while the thick DLH has a high solute (NaCl) permeability and is water impermeable.

208. The answer is A [Chapter 28 V B 1, 3 D 1 E 2 a, Figures 28-6 and 28-7]. The high urine osmolality is indicative of elevated antidiuretic hormone (ADH) secretion as is also the low urine flow (0.6 L/day). Thus, there is increased free-water reabsorption. The calculation of osmolal clearance (C_{osm}) shows:

$$C_{osm} = \frac{U_{osm} \cdot \dot{V}}{P_{osm}} = \frac{1100 \cdot 0.6}{260}$$

$$= 2.5 \text{ L/day}$$

The C_{osm} is the volume of plasma cleared of solutes per time.

To calculate free-water reabsorption ($T^c_{H_2O}$):

$$T^c_{H_2O} = C_{osm} - \dot{V}$$

$$= 2.5 - 0.6$$

$$= 1.9 \text{ L/day (negative free-water clearance)}$$

A large increase in aldosterone secretion would cause expansion of the extracellular fluid (ECF) volume due to distal nephron Na^+ reabsorption and a resultant increase in blood pressure. High aldosterone secretion also promotes the secretion and excretion of K^+. (The plasma K^+ concentration is close to the upper limit of the normal range.) High levels of angiotensin II would also increase proximal Na^+ reabsorption and an expansion of the ECF volume. This would tend to raise blood pressure. More importantly, angiotensin II causes a rise in blood pressure due to vasoconstriction. The absence of ADH or aldosterone would be associated with fluid loss (low ADH) and elevated Na^+ excretion with osmotic diuresis (low aldosterone) with a resultant decline in blood pressure.

209. The answer is A [Chapter 25 I C 4, II C 1 a b (1) 2 a, Table 25-2]. Most of the reabsorption of filtrate occurs in the peritubular capillaries. Stimulation of sympathetic nerves increases the fraction of filtrate reabsorbed here for two reasons. One, vasoconstriction upstream in the afferent and efferent arterioles lowers peritubular capillary hydrostatic pressure, which reduces the magnitude of a force that opposes reabsorption. Two, the increase in filtration fraction when renal plasma flow decreases leads to increases in the protein concentration in the peritubular capillaries (oncotic pressure), a force that promotes reabsorption of filtrate by the peritubular capillaries. Sympathetic stimulation decreases filtration primarily because of a decrease in glomerular capillary hydrostatic pressure. Thus, sympathetic stimulation decreases renal plasma flow and increases filtration fraction because of a smaller decline in the glomerular filtration rate (GFR). In addition, a slower blood flow through the glomerular capillaries promotes the filtration of a greater fraction of the plasma.

210. The answer is B [Chapter 22 III E 1, Figure 22-2]. The infusion of 1 L of isosmotic NaCl would increase the volume of the extracellular fluid (ECF) by 1 L, with 750 ml entering the interstitial fluid (i.e., edema) and 250 ml remaining in the plasma. Sympathetic stimulation causes vasoconstriction of precapillary sphincters, leading to a reduction in capillary hydrostatic pressure and, in turn, a reduction in fluid transfer to the interstitial fluid (ISF). Choices C, D, and E all have increased plasma oncotic pressure, which favors the withdrawal of fluid from the ISF. In addition, it is important to realize that Na^+ and Cl^- are not effective osmoles between the capillaries and the ISF (low reflection coefficient). Therefore, NaCl can leave the plasma readily through the capillaries and move into the ISF.

211. The answer is E [Chapter 22 III E 1 b (1) (2)]. The administration of 1 L of isosmotic NaCl increases the volume of the extracellular fluid (ECF) by 1 L. The distribution of this solution will be: intracellular fluid (ICF) [0 ml], ECF (1000 ml) [interstitial fluid (667 ml and plasma (333 ml)].

212. The answer is A [Chapter 23 III A 2, Figure 23-2, Chapter 1 III 3 A 2]. Facilitated diffusion is a type of passive transport that depends on the binding of a solute with a carrier-protein that enhances its rate of transport. Because it is a passive transport system, it involves the downhill movement of a solute along its concentration (chemical) gradient. Facilitated diffusion requires a carrier-protein, and it exhibits specificity for substrate, competition for similar substrates, and saturability of the carrier protein with the solute. The last

characteristic defines a maximal rate of transport when the carrier is saturated with solute.

213. The answer is D [Chapter 24 I Figure 24-2; Chapter 25 III C 1]. Clearance, which is measured in units of ml/min, is not equivalent to the amount excreted ($U_x \cdot \dot{V}$) but rather the ratio of the excretion rate to the plasma concentration. Inulin clearance does not vary as a function of plasma inulin concentration, because as the plasma concentration increases, so does the excretion rate; inulin is not reabsorbed or secreted and the filtered load is equal to the amount excreted. However, the clearance of *para*-aminohippuric acid (PAH) declines when the transport maximum is exceeded; the clearance of PAH becomes progressively more a function of the glomerular filtration rate (GFR).

214. The answer is C [Chapter 48 VIII A 3 b c; Chapter 52 I D 1 c d, Figure 52-4, Table 52-5]. Epinephrine is a potent hyperglycemic agent for several reasons. It stimulates α-adrenergic receptors on the pancreatic beta cell, inhibiting insulin secretion and, therefore, subsequent facilitated transport of glucose by muscle and adipose tissue. Epinephrine also promotes hepatic and muscle glycogenolysis, leading to an increase in the plasma level of lactate, which provides the liver with an important glyconeogenic substrate. The lipolytic effect of epinephrine mobilizes free fatty acids, which enhances gluconeogenesis. In addition, catecholamines directly inhibit peripheral glucose uptake, partly due to the suppression of glucose transporters that are activated by insulin.

215. The answer is C [Chapter 35 I B 1 a (2)]. More than 90% of the buffer capacity is attributed to the hemoglobin buffer system. Thus, the nonbicarbonate buffer in the erythrocyte is quantitatively greater than the bicarbonate buffer in the red cells. It is important to reiterate that the nonbicarbonate buffer systems can effectively buffer both noncarbonic and carbonic acids and that the bicarbonate buffer system is an effective buffer for noncarbonic acid and plays no role in the buffering of carbonic acid.

216. The answer is B [Chapter 36 II A 1]. About 90% of the CO_2 is carried in plasma as a derivative, namely, HCO_3^-. About 5% of the CO_2 is normally carried as carbamates of hemoglobin and protein, with another 5% of the CO_2 carried in physical solution.

217. The answer is B [Chapter 14 II B 2 b]. Angiotensin II is one of the most powerful vasoconstrictor substances in the body.

218. The answer is A [Chapter 38 III Figure 38-5 IV B 2 b c V A 2, Figure 38-8; Chapter 39 IV D, V B, Figure 39-1]. Respiratory alkalosis is an acid-base disturbance characterized by an increased arterial pH (or decreased [H^+]), a decreased CO_2 tension (hypocapnia), and a variable reduction in arterial [HCO_3^-] due to renal compensation.

219. The answer is D [Chapter 54 X C 2 a (1) (2) (3)]. Low blood Ca^{2+} and high blood phosphate concentrations are consistent with hypoparathyroidism. Lack of PTH decreases bone resorption, decreases renal reabsorption of Ca^{2+}, and increases renal reabsorption of phosphate (causing hypophosphaturia). Because the patient responded to exogenous PTH with an increased phosphate excretion, the renal PTH receptor is functional. Consequently, pseudohypoparathyroidism is excluded. Vitamin D intoxication would cause hypercalcemia, not hypocalcemia. Vitamin D deficiency would cause hypocalcemia and hypophosphatemia. In conclusion, this patient is an example of true (primary) hypoparathyroidism in which PTH secretion rather than PTH responsiveness is defective.

220. The answer is D [Chapter 47 III]. Antidiuretic hormone (ADH) and oxytocin are secreted by the posterior pituitary.

221. The answer is C [Chapter 49 II A 2, Figures 49-6 C and 49-7 (panel 2)]. Patients with secondary adrenal insufficiency exhibit a decline in corticotropin [adrenocorticotropic hormone (ACTH)] and cortisol. The hypofunction of the pituitary leads to the hypocortisolism. Thus, these patients are responsive to exogenous ACTH. It is important to appreciate that aldosterone secretion is normal, because the major regulators of aldosterone secretion are the renin–angiotensin II system and hypokalemia. In short, these patients can maintain Na^+, K^+, and acid–base balance. Thus, concentrations of Na^+, K^+, HCO_3^-, Cl^-, and creatinine are normal. Panhypopituitarism is a cause of secondary adrenal insufficiency.

222. The answer is E [Chapter 50 I D 2 b c, Figures 50-2 and 50-3]. Testosterone causes the growth and development of the male internal genitalia while dihydrotestosterone promotes growth and development of the male external genitalia (and prostate). However, testosterone is the precursor of dihydrotestosterone, which is formed by the action of 5α-reductase on testosterone. Therefore, testosterone is a requirement for the growth and differentiation of both the male internal and external genitalia. The other steroids listed, DHEA and androstenedione, are both 17-ketosteroids, which have very little androgenic activity.

223. The answer is D [Chapter 51 I A 2 c (3) (b), D 4 c (2), H 2 d (3), Figure 51-1, II A 1 c (1)]. The second meiotic division of the oocyte is not completed until just after fertilization. From the third month of embryonic life, the primary oocytes are arrested in the diplotene phase of the early prophase of meiosis. Completion of this first division occurs just prior to ovulation by the extrusion of the first polar body, resulting in the formation of a secondary oocyte with a haploid number of chromosomes (22 autosomes and 1 sex chromosome). The onset of ovulatory menstrual cycles may lag several months behind the first menses, which usually occurs between the ages of 12 and 14 years. The second meiotic division occurs just after conception, yielding a fertilized ovum (zygote) and a second polar body.

224. The answer is A [Chapter 53 IV B 3 c]. Thyroperoxidase (thyroid peroxidase; TPO) catalyzes the oxidation of iodide by H_2O_2, the iodination of tyrosyl residues within thyroglobulin to yield hormonally inactive iodotyrosines, and the coupling of iodotyrosines in thyroglobulin to form the hormonally active iodothyronines T_4 and T_3. The hydrolysis of thyroglobulin to yield free T_4 and T_3 requires a lysosomal protease. The conversion of T_4 to T_3 takes place in the liver, kidney, and pituitary and requires 5'-deiodinase. The uptake of iodide is mediated by an ATP-dependent Na^+-iodide symporter. All of the steps leading to thyroid hormone synthesis are enhanced by thyrotropin (thyroid-stimulating hormone; TSH).

225. The answer is A [Chapter 12 II C 2 b]. An increased blood flow to skeletal muscles (i.e., a functional hyperemia) occurs during exercise in response to metabolic factors. The increased flow results from a local decrease in vascular resistance brought about by an increase in tissue temperature, osmolality, pH and CO_2 tension (PCO_2), and a decrease in the local O_2 tension (PO_2). None of these factors alone appears to be able to duplicate the effects of exercise.

226. The answer is C [Chapter 53 IV B 3 c]. Thyroid peroxidase (TPO) catalyzes all of the biosynthetic reactions of thyroid hormone excluding the active uptake of iodide. Of the choices given, only thyroglobulin is the substrate for TPO, that is, the tyrosyl residues that are linked to thyroglobulin by peptide bonds. The important point is that free tyrosine is not iodinated by TPO. Thus, TPO acts on thyroglobulin-linked tyrosyl residues to produce the iodotyrosyl residues monoiodotyrosine (MIT) and diiodotyrosine (DIT).

227–229. The answers are: 227-B [Chapter 17 III A 2, 3, 4], **228-D** [Chapter 18 II C 1], **229-B** [Chapter 20 II D]. This man's arterial O_2 content is 12 ml/dl. To calculate this, it is important to recognize that the normal P_{50} is 27 mm Hg, meaning that this man's arterial hemoglobin saturation must be 50%. One reason that this man's hemoglobin saturation is low is his exposure to a low barometric pressure at an altitude of 11,500 feet. The barometric pressure at this altitude is about 490 mm Hg, providing an alveolar O_2 tension of about 50 mm Hg. The O_2 capacity is calculated from the hemoglobin concentration as follows: 18 g/dl · 1.34 ml/g = 24.12 ml/dl. Disregarding the small amount of O_2 that is dissolved in plasma, the arterial O_2 content would equal the O_2 capacity · saturation, or 24.12 · 0.5 (12 ml/dl).

This man's pulmonary artery pressure is likely to be higher than normal because of hypoxic pulmonary vasoconstriction (HPV). At high altitudes there would be an increased resistance to flow through the pulmonary vasculature. This increased resistance is the result of smooth muscle contraction in the walls of the pulmonary blood vessels in response to an unknown mediator brought on by hypoxia. The cardiac output in people who live for long periods at high altitudes is in the normal range, although it increases upon initial exposure to such altitudes. Chemoreceptors have no significant effect on the pulmonary circulation.

Venous hemoglobin saturation is decreased at high altitudes, because the hemoglobin starts in the lungs somewhat unsaturated because of the low O_2 tension. Residents at high altitudes have an increased hemoglobin concentration as a compensation for the low O_2 tension in the tissues. If hemoglobin concentration rises sufficiently, the O_2 content may be in the normal range, but the hemoglobin saturation would be reduced secondary to the low O_2 tension. Although cardiac output is normal in people acclimated to high altitude, the venous hemoglobin saturation *is* above normal in people with increased cardiac output. The fact that less O_2 is removed from each unit of blood when O_2 delivery is increased by the higher cardiac output accounts for this phenomenon.

230. The answer is D [Chapter 24 II a (3), Figure 24-2; Chapter 25 I C 4, II C 1 a b]. Because approximately 20% of the renal plasma flow is filtered [filtration fraction (FF) × 100], the maximum clearance that a substance can have is five times that of a marker for glomerular filtration rate (GFR) [inulin, creatinine]. Exceptions are substances that are both synthesized and secreted by the tubular cells.

231. The answer is B [Chapter 24 I A 2, II A 1 b (1)]. The filtered load is equal to the excretion rate ($\dot{F} = \dot{E}$), which indicates that all of the filtered substance appears in the final urine because it is not reabsorbed or secreted. Inulin is the only substance listed to which this applies. Note that only for substances only filtered does the filtered load equal the excretion rate.

$$\text{Filtered load} = P_x \cdot C_x$$

$$= 125 \cdot 1 = 125 \text{ mg/min}$$

$$\text{Excretion} = U_x \cdot \dot{V}$$

$$= 125 \cdot 1 = 125 \text{ mg/min}$$

$$\text{Also, Clearance} = \frac{U_x \dot{V}}{P_x}$$

$$= \frac{125\,(1)}{1} = 125 \text{ mg/min}$$

232. The answer is D [Chapter 23 II A 2, Chapter 25 I C, Figure 25-3]. The concentrations of all non–protein-bound substances in the plasma is the same as the concentrations in the glomerular filtrate in Bowman's space and in the efferent arteriole. However, the concentration of protein or protein-bound substances (Ca^{2+} or HPO_4^{2-}) is not the same. Because the formation of filtrate by bulk flow equals the glomerular filtration rate (GFR) [120 ml/min], the movement of water across the glomerular capillaries significantly increases the concentration of the plasma proteins. As a result, the oncotic pressure in the efferent arteriole is considerably higher than that in Bowman's space. Conversely, the oncotic pressure in Bowman's space is lower than that in the efferent arteriole.

233. The answer is C [Chapter 53 IV B 4 b]. Thyroid hormone biosynthesis occurs in four steps: (1) active uptake of inorganic iodide (I^-), (2) oxidation of inorganic iodide to active iodide (I^+, known as iodinium), (3) formation of iodotyrosines by the iodination of tyrosine residues within the matrix of thyroglobulin, and (4) coupling (condensation) of iodotyrosines to form iodothyronines. All four steps require thyroid-stimulating hormone (TSH); steps 2, 3, and 4 are catalyzed by the membrane-bound enzyme thyroid peroxidase. Diiodotyrosine and monoiodotyrosine have no biologic activity; however, the iodothyronines—T_3 and T_4 (thyroxine)—are biologically active. Therefore, thyroxine synthesis requires TSH, active iodide, thyroglobulin, thyroid peroxidase, and the coupling of two molecules of diodotyrosine.

234. The answer is E [Chapter 6 I C 4]. Rods adapt to a light stimulus more slowly than cones and, therefore, are capable of summating successive light stimuli that, individually, would be too weak to be detected. The ability of rods to detect low levels of light is enhanced because rods can detect scattered light within the eye, they have larger receptor fields than cones (allowing light from a wider area of the eye to stimulate the ganglion cells), and they produce a larger receptor potential than cones do in response to a light stimulus.

235. The answer is C [Chapter 47 IV B 2 b]. Like all anterior pituitary hormones, prolactin is secreted in an episodic pattern. It is synthesized in the lactotropes, which are pituitary acidophil cells located in the pars distalis. Prolactin is unique among the anterior pituitary hormones—it is under tonic hypothalamic in-

hibition via prolactin-inhibiting factor (PIF) [dopamine] produced by tuberoinfundibular neurosecretory neurons of the parvicellular neurosecretory system. The hormone is not colocated or cosecreted with somatotropin (GH). The putative prolactin-releasing factors (PRFs) include thyrotropin-releasing hormone (TRH). The human pars intermedia, a vestigial organ, is not a major source of hormones.

236. The answer is B [Chapter 52 I D 4 a]. Insulin is stimulatory to K^+ uptake by cells, and high concentrations of exogenous insulin cause extracellular hypokalemia. This hypokalemic action of insulin is due to the increased K^+ uptake by muscle and liver. Although the primary stimulus to the alpha cell is hypoglycemia, hypoglycemia-induced catecholamine release undoubtedly plays a role. Hypoglycemia also is a potent stimulus for the release of growth hormone (GH, somatotropin) and adrenocorticotropic hormone (ACTH, corticotropin). Among the stimuli for ACTH release are pain, anxiety, pyrogens, and hypoglycemia.

237. The answer is C [Chapter 47 I B]. The neural lobe of the pituitary gland, or neurohypophysis, is derived from the neural tube (neural ectoderm). The neural crest gives rise to a wide variety of cells, including neurons with perikarya outside the central nervous system (CNS), parafollicular cells of the thyroid gland, fibroblasts, dentin-producing cells, vascular smooth muscle cells, melanocytes, and Schwann cells. Also derived from the neural crest are the cartilage and bone of the skull and the adrenal medulla.

238. The answer is B [Chapter 49 II C 3, Figure 49-7]. This woman presents with the signs of hyperandrogenism and hypermineralocorticoidism. These two findings suggest congenital adrenal hyperplasia (CAH). However, the 21-hydroxylase deficiency does not lead to hypertension because there is a deficiency in both mineralocorticoids (aldosterone) and glucocorticoids (cortisol). Moreover, the 17α-hydroxylase deficiency does not lead to female pseudohermaphroditism due to the hypersecretion of androgens. In fact, a 17α-hydroxylase deficiency causes not only a decline in cortisol secretion but also a decline in gonadal steroid secretion. The 17α-hydroxylase deficiency is associated with elevated deoxycorticosterone (DOC) secretion and hypertension due to excessive Na^+ and water reabsorption.

This leaves the biochemical lesion of 11β-hydroxylase deficiency, which would cause hypertension due to elevated DOC secretion and virilization due to increased DHEA secretion. The elevated DOC causes aldosterone-like effects including hypokalemia, normal plasma Na^+ concentration, depressed plasma renin activity, and metabolic alkalosis. The low cortisol explains the fatigue, hypoglycemia, and elevated corticotropin secretion. The increased ACTH secretion causes the hyperpigmentation and the hypersecretion of mineralocorticoid (DOC) is due to the 11 β-hydroxylase deficiency.

239. The answer is E [Chapter 41 II B 2, F 1 a, 2 a; III A 2 b (2), B 3 a; Chapter 42 III C 2]. Receptive relaxation occurs when the proximal stomach (fundus and corpus) is stretched by the presence of food. Distention of the antrum causes gastrin to be released from G cells. Gastrin enhances gastric acid (HCl) and pancreatic enzyme secretion as well as gastric motility. In addition, expansion of the antrum initiates a vagovagal reflex that enhances antral contractions.

240. The answer is C [Chapter 50 I D 1, 2 a b c, Figures 50-2 and 50-3 III C 1 b c, V Tables 50-4, 50-5 and 50-6 Case 50, Figure 50-11 and Table 50-9]. The cause of this male pseudohermaphroditism is a deficiency in 5α-reductase, which converts testosterone into dihydrotestosterone. Dihydrotestosterone is required for the development of the male external genitalia and the prostate. Its absence explains the external female phenotype. Testosterone is required for the development of the internal genitalia. Thus, this patient would have had normal wolffian duct development with the absence of müllerian duct derivatives. These patients have normal testosterone levels and well developed testes with incomplete spermatogenesis. The plasma level of dihydrotestosterone is low with normal to slightly elevated plasma LH levels. This patient has a blind vaginal pouch. Affected males virilize to a variable degree without gynecomastia. The decreased level of spermatogenesis is expected in that dihydrotestosterone does not play a major role in gametogenesis. In such patients reared as females, gonadectomy before puberty, plastic repair of the genitalia, and

estrogen replacement at an age appropriate for puberty are indicated.

241. The answer is C [Chapter 30 II A 1 b (1)]. Aldosterone secretion is not significantly depressed following hypophysectomy and these patients can regulate Na^+ and K^+ balance. However, hypophysectomy without hormone replacement therapy is incompatible with human life. The pituitary gland is essential for cellular differentiation, somatic growth, adaptation to stress, and reproduction. If the pituitary gland is removed from young, rapidly growing animals, dwarfism occurs as a result of the absence of growth hormone (GH). Atrophy of the gonads, thyroid gland, and adrenal cortex also occurs in the absence of pituitary tropic hormones.

242. The answer is D [Chapter 7 III A 1, 3]. The withdrawal reflex (i.e., the withdrawal of a limb from a painful or irritating stimulus) is produced by a polysynaptic, not a monosynaptic, reflex. The only spinal cord monosynaptic reflex is the stretch reflex. The afferent fibers of the withdrawal reflex include both small myelinated (Aδ) and unmyelinated (C) fibers. In contrast, the afferent fibers used in the stretch reflex are large myelinated fibers. The withdrawal reflex can initiate withdrawal of only the injured area of the body skin (local sign), or it can produce withdrawal of other, non-injured areas of the body (irradiation). Moreover, the reflex contraction of the muscles producing the withdrawal can outlast the stimulus (afterdischarge). The monosynaptic stretch reflex normally involves only the muscle fibers that are stretched. Spread of activity to other muscles or continuation of muscular activity after the stimulus is withdrawn is a pathological sign.

243. The answer is C [Chapter 52 I D 2 a b, Figures 52-3, 52-4, and Table 52-4]. Insulin is a lipogenic as well as antilipolytic hormone. It decreases the activity of the intracellular lipase, triglyceride lipase ("hormone-sensitive lipase"), by inhibiting the formation of cyclic adenosine 3′,5′-monophosphate (cAMP). Insulin activates the extracellular lipase, lipoprotein lipase, which is responsible for the hydrolysis of plasma lipoproteins. The hydrolysis of triglycerides in the adipocyte delivers long-chain fatty acids and glycerol into the circulation. Lipolysis in adipocytes is mediated by triglyceride lipase. Catecholamines play a primary role in lipolysis, whereas glucagon, growth hormone (GH), cortisol, and adrenocorticotropic hormone (ACTH), have lesser lipolytic effects. Cortisol and T_3 modulate the sensitivity of adipocytes to the lipolytic effects of catecholamines.

244. The answer is C [Chapter 47 IV A 2 a, Table 47-1]. Somatostatin is the growth hormone (GH)-inhibiting hormone produced in the arcuate nucleus of the tuberoinfundibular neural tract. Somatostatin is released from the median eminence and enters the hypothalamic-hypophysial portal system that perfuses the adenohypophysis. This neuropeptide also is produced in the duodenum and the pancreatic delta cells. The plasma GH level is elevated in response to any form of stress as well as to exercise and to deep sleep (stages 3 and 4). Both insulin- and arginine-induced hypoglycemia are potent stimuli for GH secretion and can be used as provocative tests of pituitary GH reserve.

245. The answer is D [Chapter 30 II A, B, C, D, E, IV A 2, B 2, Figures 30-1 and 30-2, and Table 30-4]. Aldosterone acts on the connecting tubule and collecting tubules to increase the reabsorption of Na^+ and the secretion of K^+ and H^+. Thus, excess amounts of this hormone lead to hypokalemia (kaliuresis), alkalemia (alkalosis), and hypertension. By promoting Na^+ retention, excess aldosterone secretion leads to an increase in blood volume via an increase in plasma volume. This effect, in turn, brings about a decline in hematocrit and in plasma oncotic pressure.

246. The answer is A [Chapter 7 VI C 3 c]. The posterior cerebellum (cerebrocerebellum) coordinates the motor programs required for the smooth movement of a limb toward its target. This coordination is lacking in individuals with lesions of the cerebrocerebellum, causing the limb to oscillate as it approaches a target. No tremor is present when the limb is resting.

247. The answer is E [Chapter 28 V A, C, D 2, Figures 28-6 and 28-7]. Patient B has a higher urine osmolality because of the ingestion of isosmotic NaCl (300 mOsm/kg H_2O) compared to patient A, who drank pure water. Patient A will develop hyposmotic overhydration, and patient B isosmotic overhydration.

Each patient will have suppression of antidiuretic hormone (ADH) secretion due to expansion of the ECF and because neither has an increased plasma osmolality. Patient B has a lower free-water clearance, because the excess fluid ingestion included NaCl, and more NaCl would appear in the urine. The ingestion of pure water would increase both the extracellular and intracellular fluid (ECF and ICF), whereas the ingestion of isosmotic NaCl would expand only the ECF. Patient A would exhibit a greater change (decline) in plasma osmolality, whereas patient B would have no change in the ECF osmolality. Patient A would also have a higher urine flow rate because of a greater suppression of ADH secretion due to volume expansion and lower plasma osmolality. Finally, the higher urine osmolality of patient B would be consistent with a lower free-water clearance.

248. The answer is E [Chapter 7 V C 4]. Rigidity is a major sign of Parkinson's disease and results from lesions to the dopaminergic neurons within the substantia nigra nucleus of the basal ganglia. Rigidity differs from spasticity in that both the extensor and flexor muscles at a joint are activated.

249. The answer is B [Chapter 7 IV B 3 a]. Nystagmus is the spontaneous release of the vestibulo-ocular reflex, in which the eye moves slowly toward the edge of the socket and then moves quickly back to the center. Damage to the vestibular apparatus, vestibular nerve, or vestibular nucleus can cause nystagmus. Under normal physiologic conditions, the vestibulo-ocular reflex enables the eye to maintain visual fixation while the head is moving.

250. The answer is B [Chapter 24 II B 2]. The glomerular filtration rate (GFR) is the most common clinical indicator of functional renal mass. The GFR, which can be estimated by measuring plasma creatinine concentration, is inversely related to the plasma creatinine concentration.

251. The answer is A [Chapter 49 II C 4]. A deficiency of 17α-hydroxylase leads to reduction in the 17α-hydroxylation of pregnenolone and progesterone, resulting in hypogonadism and elevated blood gonadotropin levels. This enzyme deficiency also leads to increased production of 11-deoxycorticosterone (11-DOC).

This mineralocorticoid causes Na$^+$ retention, extracellular volume expansion, and hypertension—effects that suppress renin and aldosterone secretion. The 17α-hydroxylase defect also affects the gonads, preventing testicular and adrenal androgen synthesis in males and ovarian estrogen synthesis in females and, thus, resulting in a female phenotype regardless of genotypic sex. These patients require not only cortisol to suppress adrenocorticotropic hormone (ACTH) secretion but also sex steroid treatment consistent with the genotypic sex.

252. The answer is A [Chapter 21 I, E, Figure 21-1 Chapter 22 III G 5, H 2, Table 22-4; Chapter 30 II A 4]. Aldosterone, the most potent endogenous mineralocorticoid, acts primarily on the renal collecting ducts to promote Na$^+$ reabsorption and K$^+$ and H$^+$ excretion. It has similar effects on sweat, salivary, and intestinal glands. Thus, aldosterone controls the Na$^+$ content of the body. In turn, the Na$^+$ content determines the volume of the various fluid compartments. Aldosterone also increases Na$^+$ reabsorption by the connecting segment of the nephron. Aldosterone is synthesized in, and secreted from, the outermost layer of the adrenal cortex, called the zone glomerulosa.

253. The answer is C [Chapter 48 V A 2, Chapter 49 I E 8]. Because cortisol activates the epinephrine-forming enzyme phenylethanolamine-N-methyltransferase (PNMT), a decrease in cortisol secretion would lead to decreased adrenomedullary synthesis of epinephrine. Another effect of cortisol is elevation of blood glucose through gluconeogenesis and inhibition of peripheral glucose transport and utilization. The proteolytic effect of cortisol in extrahepatic tissues leads to increased transport of amino acids to the liver, where these substances are used for gluconeogenesis, glycogenesis, and protein synthesis. Therefore, hypocortisolism would result in decrements in plasma glucose concentration, hepatic glycogen, and hepatic protein. A decline in free blood cortisol levels would also lead to an increase in adrenocorticotropic hormone (ACTH; corticotropin) secretion due to the reduced negative feedback effect of cortisol on the hypothalamic–pituitary complex.

254. The answer is E [Chapter 30 II B 5 c (1), Figure 30-4]. Dipeptidyl carboxypeptidase, also known as angiotensin converting enzyme (ACE) or kininase II, is located mainly on the endothelial surface of pulmonary capillaries. ACE catalyzes the conversion of angiotensin I (an inactive decapeptide) to angiotensin II (an active octapeptide). In addition, ACE simultaneously inactivates the nonapeptide, bradykinin. Thus, ACE leads to the increased formation of angiotensin II (a vasoconstrictor) and the decreased formation of bradykinin (a vasodilator). Angiotensin II functions as a vasoconstrictor and aldosterone-stimulating hormone.

255. The answer is D [Chapter 30 III B 1 a]. Renin is a proteolytic enzyme produced by the juxtaglomerular cells of the afferent arteriole. These cells are modified smooth muscle cells that have acquired secretory function and, thus, are described as myoepithelial cells. Juxtaglomerular cells function as low-pressure baroreceptors that are stimulated by a decrease in renal perfusion pressure caused by a decrease in systemic blood volume or pressure.

256. The answer is E [Chapter 20 II D 1 a], **257-A** [Chapter 20 II C 3], **258-B** [Chapter 16 III C 1 b (2)], **259-D** [Chapter 16 VIII C 1 b (1)], **260-C** [Chapter 20 IV C 1]. While mountain climbing, the arterial O$_2$ tension would be reduced, with arterial CO$_2$ tension reduced by reflex hyperventilation. Because this is acute exposure to high altitude, arterial pH would be increased; not enough time has passed for the kidneys to correct the blood pH. Only one set of blood data (E) coincides with these conditions.

Although the arterial O$_2$ tension is normal in anemia, the arterial O$_2$ content is reduced in proportion to the decrease in hemoglobin concentration. Because the chemoreceptors are not stimulated, ventilation does not change and, thus, arterial CO$_2$ tension and pH are normal. Only one set of blood data (A) coincides with these conditions.

Hypoventilation is synonymous with hypercapnia and, thus, with an increase in arterial CO$_2$ tension. Only one set of blood data (B) reflects this change.

During hyperventilation, arterial CO$_2$ tension decreases and arterial O$_2$ tension increases. Only one set of blood data (D) coincides with these conditions.

Patients with chronic obstructive lung disease typically have a reduced arterial O$_2$ tension owing to the ventilation—perfusion abnormality that is present. In early stages of the disease, these patients have a normal-to-low CO_2 tension and an arterial pH in the normal range, because the kidneys can maintain the correct HCO_3^-/H_2CO_3 ratio. Only one set of blood data (C) coincides with these conditions.

261–264. The answers are: 261-B [Chapter 27 III J 1 b (1) Figure 27-2C, Table 27-2; Chapter 37 III A 1, Figure 37-1], **262-E** [Chapter 27 III H 1, Figure 27-6], **263-B** [Chapter 27 III J 2 b (2), Table 27-2 Chapter 33 II A, Figure 33-1; Chapter 37 V A, Figure 37-4], **264-B** [Chapter 27 II C 1 a]. Most H^+ secretion by the nephron occurs in the proximal tubule by Na^+-H^+ exchange. This active H^+ efflux is linked through a countertransport mechanism to Na^+ influx across the luminal membrane. Most of this secreted H^+ is not excreted but is reabsorbed in the form of H_2O. Most important, any secreted H^+ that combines with HCO_3^- in the lumen forms H_2CO_3, which is dehydrated into CO_2 and H_2O, both of which are reabsorbed. Thus, the secreted H^+ that combines with HCO_3^- does not contribute to the urinary excretion of acid.

K^+ secretion occurs mainly in the cortical collecting duct. The excreted K^+ is derived mainly from K^+ secretion in this region of the nephron. Secretion of K^+ involves active pumping across the peritubular membrane followed by passive diffusion across the luminal membrane into the tubular lumen. The cells of the proximal tubule are the major site of ammonium production. Addition of NH_4^+ to the tubular fluid occurs primarily in the proximal tubule. Thus, the accumulation of ammonia in the lumen involves both nonionic diffusion of NH_3 and transport of NH_4^+.

The proximal tubule is the major site for the active secretion of para-aminohippuric acid (PAH) in its anionic form.

265. The answer is B [Chapter 42 VII C 2, E 4–5]. Iron is absorbed from the duodenum and proximal jejunum by a membrane-bound carrier protein on the luminal surface of the enterocyte. Once inside the cell, iron combines with an iron-binding protein to form a complex called ferritin. Before being extruded from the serosal surface of the cell, the iron dissociates from ferritin.

266. The answer is A [Chapter 52 Case 1 discussion of Question 8]. Untreated diabetes mellitus is associated with negative nitrogen balance. The disease reflects a state of severe insulin deficiency combined with a decreased concentration of plasma C-peptide. Since insulin and C-peptide are secreted in equimolar amounts, C-peptide directly reflects pancreatic beta cell secretory activity and, therefore, endogenous insulin secretion. The most characteristic feature of untreated diabetes mellitus is fasting hyperglycemia due, in part, to the lack of insulin and, in larger part, to the unopposed action of the counter regulatory (insulin-antagonizing) hormones [glucagon, cortisol, epinephrine, growth hormone (GH)]. These four hormones cause the liver to change from a glucose-utilizing to a glucose-producing organ, leading to hyperglycemia and glycosuria. The hormones also increase the rate of lipolysis, which leads to a fatty acid-induced decrease in glucose uptake. Cortisol and glucagon promote muscle proteolysis, leading to hyperaminoacidemia, hyperaminoaciduria, elevated blood urea nitrogen (BUN), and negative nitrogen balance. This hormonal imbalance switches liver fatty acid metabolism from oxidation, reesterification, or both to ketogenesis. The sum of these effects is an increase in blood fatty acids, amino acids, and ketones due to the gradual loss of muscle and adipose tissue. The ketosis leads to ketonemia and, eventually, ketonuria.

267. The answer is C [Chapter 42 VII C 2, E 4–5]. Cholesterol must be dissolved in micelles before it can be absorbed. Micelles are small spherical globules formed from bile salts. The polar, water-soluble end of the bile salt faces outward, and the lipid-soluble tail portion of the bile salt faces inward. Cholesterol dissolves in the interior of the micelle, and, when the micelle makes contact with the intestinal membrane, the cholesterol diffuses from the micelle into the enterocyte.

268. The answer is B [Chapter 23 II A]. The transport of solutes and water across the glomerular capillaries occurs by the process of bulk flow (convection). It is important to understand that there is no concentration (chemical) gradient for solutes; therefore, transport by diffusion must be ruled out. The driving force for bulk flow is the hydrostatic (hydraulic) pressure gradient. In the glomerular capillaries, there are no protein-carriers, which also rules out both primary and secondary active transport systems.

269. The answer is A [Chapter 9 IV B 1, C]. An increased heart rate would simultaneously increase the aortic systolic pressure and decrease the aortic pulse pressure, according to the elastic modulus:

$E = V \cdot dP/dV$, where
E = elastic modulus
V = arterial volume
dP = pulse pressure
dV = arterial uptake during diastole

An increase in heart rate increases cardiac output and raises the arterial volume, which is proportional to the mean aortic pressure. If stroke volume remains constant, then the arterial uptake during diastole will also remain essentially unchanged so that the pulse pressure must decrease to maintain the equation valid. An increased arterial compliance decreases the value of the elastic constant (compliance is the reciprocal of elastance), which lowers systolic pressure. Decreased peripheral resistance decreases the systolic pressure and increases the pulse pressure. An increased stroke volume or an increased elastic constant cause an increase in systolic pressure as well as pulse pressure.

270. The answer is A [Chapter 7 V C]. Hypotonia is a sign of cerebellar disease. Lesions within the basal ganglia produce spontaneous, wild, flinging movements (hemiballismus); tremor; slow, twisting movements (athetosis); or lack of spontaneous movements or difficulty initiating movement (hypokinesia).

271–275. The answers are: 271-C, 272-E, 273-A, 274-D, 275-B [Chapter 21 IV A Table 21-2]. The use of inulin clearance (C_{in}) to measure glomerular filtration rate (GFR) is valid because all of the filtered inulin is excreted in the urine without being reabsorbed or secreted by the renal tubules. Thus, GFR is equal to C_{in}:

$$GFR = C_{in} = \frac{U_{in} \cdot \dot{V}}{P_{in}}, \text{ where}$$

U_{in} and P_{in} = urinary and plasma inulin concentrations, respectively, and $\dot{V}$ = the urinary volume/minute. Substituting

$$GFR = C_{in} \frac{150 \text{ mg/ml} \cdot 1.2 \text{ ml/min}}{1.5 \text{ mg/ml}}$$

$$= \frac{180 \text{ mg/min}}{1.5 \text{ mg/ml}}$$

$$= 120 \text{ ml/min}$$

Note that with a unit analysis, both mg/ml terms cancel out. Renal plasma flow (RPF) is calculated from the clearance of para-aminohippuric acid (PAH); however, there are no PAH data provided for this man. Thus, it is necessary to determine RPF from the filtration fraction (FF), defined as the ratio of GFR to renal plasma flow:

$$FF = \frac{GFR}{RPF}$$

The filtration fraction can also be calculated from the arterial and venous inulin concentrations as:

$$\text{fraction of inulin filtered} = \frac{A_{in} - V_{in}}{A_{in}}, \text{ where}$$

A_{in} and V_{in} are the arterial and venous inulin concentrations, respectively. Substituting,

$$FF = \frac{1.50 \text{ mg/ml} - 1.20 \text{ mg/ml}}{1.50 \text{ mg/ml}}$$

$$= \frac{0.3}{1.50} = 0.20$$

With the filtration fraction and GFR determined, the renal plasma flow is easily determined as:

$$RPF = \frac{GFR}{FF} = \frac{120}{0.2} \text{ ml/min} = 600 \text{ ml/min}$$

Because the filtration fraction equals the ratio of the GFR to renal plasma flow, the filtration fraction also can be calculated using the extraction of a substance such as inulin to determine the renal plasma flow. If the urinary concentration of inulin is 150 mg/ml and the urine flow rate is 1.2 ml/min, the urinary excretion rate of inulin is 180 mg/min. If, when the excretion rate was measured, the inulin concentration was 1.50 mg/ml in renal arterial plasma and 1.20 mg/ml in renal venous plasma, each milliliter of plasma traversing the kidneys must have contributed 0.30 mg to the 180 mg that was excreted. Hence, the renal plasma flow must have been 600 ml/min (180 mg/min divided by 0.3 mg/ml). Thus, with the renal plasma flow determined, the filtration fraction can be calculated as:

$$\frac{GFR}{RPF} = \frac{120 \text{ ml/min}}{600 \text{ ml/min}} = 0.2$$

Once renal plasma flow is determined, renal blood flow (RBF) can also be discerned. Renal blood flow is calculated by dividing the renal plasma flow by the term (1 − hematocrit), or

$$RBF = \frac{RPF}{1 - hematocrit} = \frac{600 \text{ ml/min}}{1 - 0.40}$$

$$= \frac{600 \text{ ml/min}}{0.60} = 1000 \text{ ml/min}$$

The quantity (or amount) of the substance filtered per unit time is termed the filtered load, or amount filtered. It is equal to the product of the GFR (or C_{in}) and the plasma concentration of that substance:

$$\text{Filtered load} = GFR \cdot P_G$$

$$= 120 \text{ ml/min} \cdot 0.9 \text{ mg/ml}$$

$$= 108 \text{ mg/min}$$

Note that the ml terms cancel out with a unit analysis and that it is necessary to express the plasma glucose concentration (P_G) in mg/ml and not in the unit of mg/dl given in the original data.

276–278. The answers are: 276-C, [Chapter 38 III A Figure 38-5; IV B 2 b, Figures 38-6 and 38-7; Chapter 39 IV D 2; V B, Figure 39-1] **277-A,** [Chapter 38 III A Figure 38-5; IV B 2 a, Figures 38-6 and 38-7; Chapter 39 IV C 2; V A, Figure 39-1] **278-B** [Chapter 38 III A Figures 38-5; IV B 1 a, Figures 38-6 and 38-7; Chapter 39 IV A 2; V A, Figure 39-1] Hyperventilation is defined as alveolar ventilation in excess of the body's need for CO_2 elimination, which results in decreased arterial CO_2 tension—the underlying factor in respiratory alkalosis. Although CO_2 tension is not given, it can be calculated using the mathematical relationship: $[HCO_3^-]/S \cdot P_{CO_2} = 20/1$. Applying this equation, it is clear that the values in set C indicate a decrease in CO_2 tension:

$$\frac{15}{S \cdot P_{CO_2}} = \frac{20}{1}, \text{ or } S \cdot P_{CO_2} = 0.75 \text{ mmol/L}$$

Because

$$S \cdot P_{CO_2} = 0.75 \text{ mmol/L}$$

and

$$S = 0.03 \text{ mmol/L/mm Hg,}$$

then

$$P_{CO_2} = \frac{0.75 \text{ mmol/L}}{0.03 \text{ mmol/L/mm Hg}} = 25 \text{ mm Hg}$$

A CO_2 tension of 25 mm Hg is significantly lower than normal (40 mm Hg). In acute respiratory alkalosis, there is a decrease in urinary H^+ excretion and an increase in urinary HCO_3^- excretion. In this case, there has been complete renal compensation, as evidenced by the return of the $[HCO_3^-]/S \cdot P_{CO_2}$ ratio to the normal (20:1), i.e., $15 \div 0.75$.

In chronic respiratory tract obstruction (e.g., due to tracheal stenosis, foreign body, or tumor), alveolar ventilation is insufficient to excrete CO_2 at a rate required by the body, which leads to increased arterial CO_2 tension—the underlying factor in respiratory acidosis. The kidney increases H^+ secretion, resulting in the addition of HCO_3^- to the extracellular fluid (ECF). The values in set A coincide with these changes. In this case, there is partial compensation of the respiratory acidosis as evidenced by the increase in $[HCO_3^-]$. In chronic respiratory acidosis, the respiratory centers become less sensitive to hypercapnia and acidosis and rely on the associated hypoxemia as the primary drive to ventilation. Correction of the low O_2 tension by the administration of O_2 will diminish respiratory drive, resulting in hypoventilation, a further increase in CO_2 tension, and possibly CO_2 narcosis. For this reason, O_2 must be given with extreme caution to patients with chronic hypercapnia.

Metabolic acidosis exhibits the characteristics of increased $[H^+]$ (decreased pH), a reduced $[HCO_3^-]$, and a compensatory hyperventilation resulting in hypocapnia. The kidney responds to the increased H^+ load by increasing the secretion and excretion of NH_4^+ and the excretion of titratable acid ($H_2PO_4^-$). The values in set B coincide with these changes.

Index

References in *italics* indicate figures; those followed by "t" denote tables

839